Comprehensive Handbook of Pediatric Audiology

Comprehensive Handbook of Pediatric Audiology

Richard Seewald, PhD and Anne Marie Tharpe, PhD
Editors

PLURAL PUBLISHING
INC.
SAN DIEGO
OXFORD
BRISBANE

PLURAL PUBLISHING
INC.

5521 Ruffin Road
San Diego, CA 92123

e-mail: info@pluralpublishing.com
Web site: http://www.pluralpublishing.com

49 Bath Street
Abingdon, Oxfordshire OX14 1EA
United Kingdom

Typeset in 10/12 Palatino book by Flanagan's Publishing Services, Inc.
Printed in the United States of America by McNaughton & Gunn

Library of Congress Cataloging-in-Publication Data

Comprehensive handbook of pediatric audiology / [edited by] Richard Seewald and Anne Marie Tharpe.
p. ; cm.
Includes bibliographical references and index.
ISBN-13: 978-1-59756-245-4 (alk. paper)
ISBN-10: 1-59756-245-9 (alk. paper)
1. Hearing disorders in children—Handbooks, manuals, etc. I. Seewald, Richard C. II. Tharpe, Anne Marie.
[DNLM: 1. Hearing Disorders. 2. Child. 3. Hearing Tests. 4. Hearing. 5. Infant. WV 271]
RF291.5.C45C66 2010
618.92'09789—dc22

2010032523

Contents

Foreword

It is difficult to pinpoint when the term *pediatric audiology* actually came into common usage. We can only assume that the concept of pediatric audiology began shortly after the development of the discipline of audiology during and following World War II. Certainly, one of the earliest references to pediatric audiology was made by Canfield in his classic book *Audiology, The Science of Hearing* (1949). Long before the 1940s, however, historical writings clearly show that early civilization experienced and appreciated the problems associated with deafness in childhood. Indeed, the plight of the deaf is referenced in the Bible on several occasions as well as by Greek and Latin writers.

During the Renaissance through to the latter part of the 19th century, we read about teachers and priests who were dedicated to serving children with hearing loss. This was a period in deaf education sometimes referred to as "the age of teaching"; it was an era in which the oral method clashed with teachings that emphasized the use of signs and finger spelling. Such well-recognized teachers as Pedro Ponce de León and Juan Pablo Bonet of Spain, Samuel Heinicke of Germany, Abbe Charles Michel de l'Epee of France, and Thomas Braidwood of Scotland were early pioneers of methods and techniques for educating young deaf children. One well-known scholar who brought specific teaching methods and philosophies from Europe to America was Thomas Gallaudet. After studying with de L'Epee in Paris, Gallaudet returned to the United States and established the first school for deaf children in Hartford, Connecticut in 1817. The school was called the American Asylum for the Education and Instruction of the Deaf and Dumb.

During the early 20th century, pediatric audiology was not yet a recognized specialty, but educational and health care professionals throughout the United States and Europe became involved by necessity in the identification, assessment, and management of very young children with hearing loss. Perhaps most notable was the work of Sir Alexander and Lady Irene Ewing who worked tirelessly to serve young children with hearing loss in Great Britain. As early as 1919, Irene Ewing opened a hearing clinic at Manchester University. More than anyone during this period, the Ewings influenced professionals throughout the world on issues pertaining to the identification and management of childhood deafness. They introduced some of the fundamental concepts now associated with pediatric audiology: the benefits of early identification and intervention including hearing aids, the importance of parent-home training for the development of speech and language, and effective approaches for testing young children with hearing loss. From most accounts, this was the beginning of pediatric audiology.

By the late 1950s and early 1960s, a small group of audiologists was beginning to focus their efforts on young children and we began to hear the term *pediatric audiology* on a more frequent basis; soon thereafter training programs started to offer specialty tracks in pediatric audiology. There were few books dedicated to young children with hearing loss. As there was no single text that met the specific needs of pediatric audiologists or university training programs, several resource books were considered essential reading. These books included *Educational Guidance and the Deaf Child* and *New Opportunities for Deaf Children* by the Ewings; *Auditory Disorders in Children* by Myklebust; *Deafness in Childhood* by McConnell and Ward; and *Hearing and Deafness* by Davis and Silverman.

Clinical protocols related to identification, assessment, and hearing aid fitting for very young children also were limited. Evidence-based procedures had not yet been developed and clinicians working with children were forced to rely mostly on intuition and common sense for their clinical decision-making—clinical practice was probably more art than science. As Liden and Harford observed, pediatric audiologists "waved their magic wand and sprinkled whiffle dust to make the child's invisible reactions visible." (p. 6). Importantly, robust clinical tools commonly used today—such as electroacoustic immittance measures, auditory brainstem responses (ABR), and otoacoustic emissions (OAE)—were not yet available to the pediatric audiologist for the identification, assessment, and management of children with hearing loss. Although the profession of audiology recognized the importance of early identification of hearing loss in children, the average age of identification in the United States was

3 to 4 years and there was a significant lag between the age when the child was identified and the age when the child actually received a hearing aid. Hearing aids were large, unattractive, and produced a great deal of distortion. Receiver buttons were used to modify the electroacoustic responses of hearing aids and Y-cords served to provide a child with bilateral amplification. Hearing aid fitting was accomplished using a comparative approach for aided sound field behavioral thresholds. The hearing aid that provided the most threshold improvement with the least amount of irregularity across frequencies was thought to provide the best speech understanding and subsequently was the hearing aid of choice. Because it was difficult to obtain accurate thresholds on young children using behavioral methodology, the fitting strategy was an ongoing process sometimes taking more than a year to finalize.

The contents of this book, *Comprehensive Handbook of Pediatric Audiology*, serves as a stunning reminder of how far we have come since those early years in our efforts to serve young children with hearing loss and their families. Better graduate education, advanced technology, and solid clinical research have brought about significant improvements in early identification of hearing loss, audiologic assessment, and the selection and evaluation of hearing aids. We now have the ability to identify hearing loss in newborns, obtain reliable frequency-specific threshold information on infants and toddlers, and objectively fit young babies with digital hearing aids and other assistive devices. The advent of cochlear implantation has resulted in significant improvements in the speech, language, and listening skills of children with severe-to-profound bilateral sensorineural hearing loss. We also have witnessed improvements in technology and medical care that have brought about changes in the prevalence of causation and severity of hearing loss. *Comprehensive Handbook of Pediatric Audiology* addresses all of the issues impacting today's young children with hearing loss and their families. It is exciting to see in one volume a comprehensive text on contemporary trends in pediatric audiology.

The proceeds of this book will be dedicated to a student scholarship fund at Vanderbilt University named in memory of Dr. Judith S. Gravel, an outstanding alumna of Vanderbilt University and one of the true giants of pediatric audiology. Judy was the consummate scholar and teacher—her contributions to the field of pediatric audiology were impressive, exemplary, and far reaching. Much of her work provided us with the scientific basis for the identification and assessment of children with hearing loss and influenced clinical practice by improving the management protocols for these children. It was Judy Gravel who originally envisioned the need for such a book in pediatric audiology. Her presence can be seen throughout the entirety of this book simply by reviewing the references at the end of each chapter that highlight her diversity of interest areas and contributions to the profession. Although Judy was taken from us at a young age, her life was filled with love, fun, and accomplishments that far exceeded her years. To be sure, we are all so very fortunate that she shared her many gifts with us.

Fred H. Bess, PhD

References

Bender, R. (1961). *The conquest of deafness.* Cleveland, OH: The Press of Western Reserve University.

Canfield, N. (1949). *Audiology: The science of hearing—A developing professional specialty.* Springfield, IL: Charles C. Thompson.

Davis, H., & Silverman, S. R. (1960). *Hearing and deafness.* New York, NY: Holt, Rinehart and Winston.

Ewing, I. R., & Ewing, A. W. G. (1944). The ascertainment of deafness in infancy and early childhood. *Journal of Laryngology and Otology, 59*, 309–333.

Ewing. I. R., & Ewing, A. W. G. (1954). *Speech and the deaf child.* Manchester, UK: Manchester University Press.

Ewing, Sir Alexander. (1957). *Educational guidance and the deaf child.* Manchester, UK: Manchester University Press.

Ewing, Sir Alexander. (1959). *New opportunities for deaf children.* Manchester, UK: Manchester University Press.

Liden, G., & Harford, E. R. (1985). The pediatric audiologist: From magician to clinician. *Ear and Hearing, 6*(1), 6–9.

McConnell, F., & Ward, P. H. (Eds.). (1967). *Deafness in childhood.* Nashville, TN: Vanderbilt University Press.

Myklebust, H. (1954). *Auditory disorders in children: A manual for differential diagnosis.* New York, NY: Grune and Stratton.

Whetnall, E., & Fry, D. B. (1964). *The deaf child.* London, UK: Heinemann.

Acknowledgments

The concept and original outline for this book was developed at a meeting with Dr. Judith Gravel in July 2006. Judy was a big dreamer and saw a great need for a comprehensive text in the area of pediatric audiology. With a twinkle in her eye, she referred to this book as "the mothership." By the end of this meeting, the table of contents included 55 chapters covering every conceivable topic related to the basic sciences, screening, assessment, and management associated with childhood hearing and hearing impairment. It was her vision and passion that led to the development of this book. Two weeks following the July 2006 meeting with Judy, she was diagnosed with cancer. We lost Judy on December 31st, 2009. Throughout her courageous battle with cancer, we asked Judy on numerous occasions if she wanted to continue the work on the book. Our queries were always greeted with silence. When Judy became silent, the answer was always clear. To discontinue work on this project was never an option for Judy. Although we have lost 14 of the original chapters somewhere along the way, we have done all that we could to ensure that this book lives up to Judy's dream. We thank you Judy.

It is possible that our work on this project had more missed deadlines than the book has pages. Throughout this journey we have always had the support, expertise, and patience of the exceptional group at Plural Publishing. Specifically, we would like to thank the late Sadanand Singh, Brad Stach, and Angie Singh for their genuine encouragement and support from the very start. Throughout the process, Casey Stach, Lauren Narasky, Sandy Doyle, and Stephanie Meissner have always been there to support and help us with even the smallest editorial detail. We cannot imagine having a more positive and informed group with whom to work.

This project would not have been completed without the administrative and editorial assistance of Carol Van Evera who spent countless hours interacting with authors, copy editing, formatting chapters, searching for missing references, and keeping us organized throughout the past four years. Her enormous contributions to the project are gratefully acknowledged. We also are appreciative of the "detail" work that Tammy Ezell contributed just when we thought we were about finished. We would like to thank the 68 authors who took time from their research, clinical, and administrative activities to share their knowledge, experiences, and wisdom with the readers of this volume.

Finally, we would like to thank our life partners Carol and Jim for their unqualified support of our work on this project—work that has taken far longer than we first told them it would.

Richard Seewald and Anne Marie Tharpe

Contributors

Oliver F. Adunka, MD
Assistant Professor
Department of Otolaryngology-Head and Neck Surgery
University of North Carolina at Chapel Hill
Chapel Hill, North Carolina, USA
Chapter 8

Prudence Allen, PhD
Director
National Centre for Audiology
Associate Professor
School of Communication Sciences and Disorders
Faculty of Health Sciences
University of Western Ontario
London, Ontario, Canada
Chapter 14

Rachel K. Allen, AuD, CCC-A
Department of Otolaryngology,
Head and Neck Surgery
Indiana University Medical Center
Clarian Health Partners
Riley Hospital for Children
Indianapolis, Indiana, USA
Chapter 36

Marlene Bagatto, AuD
Research Associate
Child Amplification Laboratory
National Centre for Audiology
University of Western Ontario
London, Ontario, Canada
Chapter 25

Anuradha R. Bantwal, MSc
Lecturer (Speech and Hearing)
Department of Audiology
Ali Yavar Jung National Institute for the Hearing Handicapped
Kishenchand Marg, Bandra Reclamation (West)
Mumbai, India
Chapter 21

Kathryn L. Beauchaine, MA
Audiologist
Department of Audiology
Boys Town National Research Hospital
Omaha, Nebraska, USA
Chapter 32

Fred H. Bess, PhD
Professor and Director
National Center for Childhood Deafness and Family Communication
Department of Hearing and Speech Sciences
Vanderbilt University School of Medicine
Vanderbilt Bill Wilkerson Center
Nashville, Tennessee, USA
Chapter 10

Craig A. Buchman, MD
Professor and Chief
Division of Otology/Neurotology and Skull Base Surgery
Director, University of North Carolina Ear and Hearing Center
Medical Director, Carolina Children's Communication Disorders Program
Department of Otolaryngology-Head and Neck Surgery
University of North Carolina at Chapel Hill
Chapel Hill, North Carolina, USA
Chapter 8

Monica L. Burch, AuD, CCC-A
Department of Otolaryngology-Head and Neck Surgery
Indiana University Medical Center
Clarian Health Partners
Riley Hospital for Children
Indianapolis, Indiana, USA
Chapter 36

Neha Chhabria, MA-SLP
Lecturer
Department of Audiology
Ali Yavar Jung National Institute for the Hearing Handicapped
Kishenchand Marg, Bandra Reclamation (West)
Mumbai, India
Chapter 21

Patricia M. Chute, EdD
Dean, School of Health Professions
New York Institute of Technology
Old Westbury, New York, USA
Chapter 41

Kathleen R. Corbin, MA, CCC-A
Department of Otolaryngology-Head and Neck Surgery
Indiana University Medical Center
Clarian Health Partners
Indianapolis, Indiana, USA
Chapter 36

Kathleen A. Daly, PhD, MPH
Professor
Departments of Otolaryngology and Epidemiology
Director of the Otitis Media Research Center
University of Minnesota
Minneapolis, Minnesota, USA
Chapter 9

Adrian Davis, OBE, FFPH, FSS, FRSA, PhD
Director NHS Newborn Hearing and Physical Examination Programme
National Lead for Physiological Measurement and Audiology
Ear Institute
University College London and
Royal Free Hampstead NHS Trust
London, UK
Chapter 5

Katrina A. S. Davis, BA (Hons) Cantab, MB BChir
Specialist Trainee,
South London and Maudsley NHS Foundation Trust
KCL Institute of Psychiatry
Denmark Hill
London, UK
Chapter 5

William W. Dickinson, AuD
Assistant Professor
Department of Hearing and Speech Sciences
Vanderbilt University School of Medicine
Clinical Director of Hearing Technologies
Vanderbilt Bill Wilkerson Center
Nashville, Tennessee, USA
Chapter 34

Allan O. Diefendorf, PhD
Professor
Department of Otolaryngology, Head and Neck Surgery
Indiana University School of Medicine
Director, Audiology and Speech Language Pathology
Indiana University Medical Center and Clarian Health Partners
Riley Hospital for Children
Indianapolis, Indiana, USA
Chapters 23 and 36

Darcia M. Dierking, AuD
Audiologist
Department of Audiology
Boys Town National Research Hospital
Omaha, Nebraska, USA
Chapter 32

Laura Dreisbach, PhD
Associate Professor

School of Speech, Language, and Hearing Sciences
SDSU/UCSD Joint Doctoral Program in Audiology
San Diego State University
San Diego, California, USA
Chapter 19

Andrée Durieux-Smith, PhD
Professor Emeritus
Faculty of Health Sciences
University of Ottawa
Ottawa, Ontario, Canada
Chapter 30

Carolyne Edwards, MClSc, MBA
Director, Auditory Management Services
Faculty, Gestalt Institute of Toronto
Toronto, Ontario, Canada
Chapter 33

Laurie S. Eisenberg, PhD
Scientist III
Division of Communication and Auditory Neuroscience
Children's Auditory Research and Evaluation (CARE) Center
House Ear Institute
Los Angeles, California
Clinical Professor of Otolaryngology
Member, Neuroscience Graduate Program
University of Southern California
Los Angeles, California, USA
Chapter 12

Leisha Eiten, AuD, CCC-A
Clinical Coordinator
Boys Town National Research Hospital
Omaha, Nebraska, USA
Chapter 26

Kris English, PhD
Associate Professor
School of Speech-Language Pathology and Audiology
University of Akron
Akron, Ohio, USA
Chapter 39

Elizabeth Fitzpatrick, PhD
Assistant Professor
Audiology-Speech-Language Pathology Program
Faculty of Health Sciences
University of Ottawa
Ottawa, Ontario, Canada
Chapter 30

Karen A. Gordon, PhD, CCC-A, Reg. CASLPO
Associate Professor
Department of Otolaryngology-Head and Neck Surgery
University of Toronto
Scientist, Research Institute
Director of Research, Archie's Cochlear Implant Laboratory
The Hospital for Sick Children
Toronto, Ontario, Canada
Chapter 27

Christine E. Griffiths, AuD, CCC-A
Department of Otolaryngology-Head and Neck Surgery
Indiana University Medical Center
Indiana University School of Medicine
Indianapolis, Indiana, USA
Chapter 36

James W. Hall III, PhD
Clinical Professor
Department of Speech, Language, and Hearing Sciences
College of Public Health and Health Professions
University of Florida
Gainesville, Florida
Extraordinary Professor
Department of Communication Pathology
University of Pretoria
Pretoria, South Africa
Chapter 21

Melody Harrison, PhD, CCC-SLP
Professor
Division of Speech and Hearing Sciences
University of North Carolina School of Medicine
Chapel Hill, North Carolina, USA
Chapters 31 and 38

Robert V. Harrison, PhD, DSc
Senior Scientist, the Hospital for Sick Children
Neuroscience and Mental Health Program
Professor, Department of Otolaryngology–Head and Neck Surgery
Department of Physiology, University of Toronto
Toronto, Ontario, Canada
Chapter 2

Mark Hill, PhD
Senior Lecturer
School of Medical Sciences
Faculty of Medicine
University of New South Wales
Sydney, Australia
Chapter 1

Bill Hodgetts, PhD
Assistant Professor
Faculty of Rehabilitation Medicine
University of Alberta
Program Director, Bone Conduction Amplification
Institute for Reconstructive Sciences in Medicine (iRSM)
Misericordia Hospital
Edmonton, Alberta, Canada
Chapter 28

Linda J. Hood, PhD
Professor
Department of Hearing and Speech Sciences
Vanderbilt University School of Medicine
Associate Director for Research
National Center for Childhood Deafness
Vanderbilt Bill Wilkerson Center
Nashville, Tennessee
Honorary Professor, School of Health and Rehabilitation Services
University of Queensland, Australia
Chapter 6

Derek Houston, PhD
Associate Professor and Philip F. Holton Scholar
Department of Otolaryngology-Head and Neck Surgery
Indiana University School of Medicine
Indianapolis, Indiana, USA
Chapter 3

Lisa L. Hunter, PhD
Senior Clinical Director
Division of Audiology
Cincinnati Children's Hospital Medical Center
Associate Professor
Department of Otolaryngology
University of Cincinnati
Cincinnati, Ohio, USA
Chapters 9 and 18

Martyn Hyde, PhD
Professor
Department of Otolaryngology-Head and Neck Surgery
University of Toronto
Director, Research and Development
Hearing, Balance and Speech Department
Mount Sinai Hospital, Toronto
Consultant, Infant Hearing Program
Ontario Ministry of Children and Youth Services
Toronto, Ontario, Canada
Chapter 16

Karen C. Johnson, PhD
Advanced Research Associate and Clinical Research Coordinator
House Ear Institute
Los Angeles, California, USA
Chapter 12

Bronya J. B. Keats, PhD
Professor, Division of Biomedical Science and Biochemistry
Research School of Biology

Australian National University
Canberra ACT, Australia
Professor and Head Emeritus
Department of Genetics
Louisiana State University Health Sciences Center
New Orleans, Louisiana, USA
Chapter 6

Jack E. Kile, PhD
Professor Emeritus
University of Wisconsin-Oshkosh
Oshkosh, Wisconsin, USA
Chapter 32

Lori J. Leibold, PhD
Assistant Professor
Department of Allied Health Sciences
University of North Carolina at Chapel Hill
Chapel Hill, North Carolina, USA
Chapter 4

Dawna Lewis, PhD
Staff Scientist
Boys Town National Research Hospital
Omaha, Nebraska, USA
Chapter 26

Robert H. Margolis, PhD
Professor of Audiology
Department of Otolaryngology
University of Minnesota
Minneapolis, Minnesota, USA
Chapter 18

Patti F. Martin, PhD
Director
Audiology and Speech Pathology
Arkansas Children's Hospital
Little Rock, Arkansas, USA
Chapter 24

Amy S. Martinez, MA
Advanced Research Associate, Clinical Research Coordinator
House Ear Institute
Los Angeles, California, USA
Chapter 12

Marilyn Neault, PhD, CCC-A
Children's Hospital Boston at Waltham
Habilitative Audiology Program
Waltham, Massachusetts, USA
Chapter 35

Mary Ellen Nevins, EdD
National Director, Professional Preparation in Cochlear Implants (PPCI)
Independent Contractor to
Children's Hospital of Philadelphia
Philadelphia, Pennsylvania, USA
Chapter 41

Robert J. Nozza, PhD
Pediatric Audiologist
Fernandina Beach, Florida, USA
Chapter 17

James E. Peck, PhD
Emeritus Associate Professor
Division of Communicative Sciences
Department of Otolaryngology and Communicative Sciences
University of Mississippi Medical Center
Jackson, Mississippi, USA
Chapter 15

Harold C. Pillsbury, MD
Professor and Chairman
Department of Otolaryngology-Head and Neck Surgery
University of North Carolina at Chapel Hill
Chapel Hill, North Carolina, USA
Chapter 8

Heather Porter, AuD
Research Associate
Department of Hearing and Speech Sciences
Vanderbilt University School of Medicine
Vanderbilt Bill Wilkerson Center
Nashville, Tennessee, USA
Chapter 10

Aneesha Pretto, MS, CCC-SLP
Research Associate
Division of Speech and Hearing Sciences
University of North Carolina School of Medicine
Chapel Hill, North Carolina, USA
Chapter 38

Beth A. Prieve, PhD
Professor
Department of Communication Sciences and Disorders
Syracuse University
Syracuse, New York, USA
Chapter 19

Vidya Ramkumar, MASLP
Lecturer
Department of Speech, Language and Hearing Sciences
Sri Ramachandra University
Porur, Chennai, India
Chapter 21

Gary Rance, PhD
Associate Professor
Wagstaff Research Fellow in Otolaryngology
Department of Otolaryngology and School of Audiology
University of Melbourne
Melbourne, Victoria, Australia
Chapter 13

Baljit K. Rehal, AuD, CCC-A
Department of Otolaryngology-Head and Neck Surgery
Indiana University Medical Center
Clarian Health Partners
Indianapolis, Indiana, USA
Chapter 36

Amy McConkey Robbins, MS, CCC-SLP
Adjunct Assistant Professor
Department of Hearing and Speech Sciences
Vanderbilt University School of Medicine
Vanderbilt Bill Wilkerson Center
Nashville, Tennessee
Speech-Language Pathologist
Communication Consulting Services
Indianapolis, Indiana, USA
Chapter 40

Jackson Roush, PhD
Professor and Director
Division of Speech and Hearing Sciences
University of North Carolina School of Medicine
Chapel Hill, North Carolina, USA
Chapter 17

Patricia A. Roush, AuD
Director of Pediatric Audiology
University of North Carolina Hospitals
Associate Professor
Department of Otolaryngology-Head and Neck Surgery
University of North Carolina School of Medicine
Chapel Hill, North Carolina, USA
Chapter 37

Hollea M. Ryan, AuD
Research Associate
Department of Hearing and Speech Sciences
Vanderbilt University School of Medicine
Vanderbilt Bill Wilkerson Center
Nashville, Tennessee, USA
Chapter 29

Diane L. Sabo, PhD
Director
Audiology and Speech-Language Pathology
Children's Hospital of Pittsburgh
Associate Professor
Department of Communication Sciences and Disorders
University of Pittsburgh
Pittsburgh, Pennsylvania, USA
Chapter 24

Susan Scollie, PhD
Associate Professor
School of Communication Sciences and Disorders
Principal Investigator

National Centre for Audiology
University of Western Ontario
London, Ontario, Canada
Chapter 25

Richard Seewald, PhD
Distinguished University Professor Emeritus
School of Communication Sciences and Disorders
National Centre for Audiology
Faculty of Health Sciences
University of Western Ontario
London, Ontario, Canada

David R. Stapells, PhD
Hamber Professor of Clinical Audiology
School of Audiology and Speech Sciences
University of British Columbia
Vancouver, British Columbia, Canada
Chapter 20

Arnold Starr, MD
Research Professor, Neurology
School of Medicine
University of California, Irvine
Irvine, California, USA
Chapter 13

Anne Marie Tharpe, PhD
Professor and Chair
Department of Hearing and Speech Sciences
Vanderbilt University School of Medicine
Associate Director
Vanderbilt Bill Wilkerson Center
Nashville, Tennessee, USA
Chapters 11, 29, and 34

Betty R. Vohr, MD
Professor of Pediatrics
Warren Alpert Medical School of Brown University
Medical Director, Rhode Island Hearing Assessment Program
Director, Neonatal Follow-up
Women and Infants Hospital
Providence, Rhode Island, USA
Chapter 7

Amanda S. Weinzierl, AuD, CCC-A
Department of Otolaryngology-Head and Neck Surgery
Indiana University Medical Center
Clarian Health Partners
Riley Hospital for Children
Indianapolis, Indiana, USA
Chapter 36

Lynne A. Werner, PhD
Professor
Department of Speech and Hearing Sciences
University of Washington
Seattle, Washington, USA
Chapter 4

Judith E. Widen, PhD
Associate Professor
Department of Hearing and Speech
University of Kansas Medical Center
Kansas City, Kansas, USA
Chapter 22

Carlton J. Zdanski, MD
Associate Professor
Department of Otolaryngology-Head and Neck Surgery
University of North Carolina at Chapel Hill
Chapel Hill, North Carolina, USA
Chapter 8

Dedication

This book is dedicated to our dear friend and colleague Judith S. Gravel, whose vision for this volume guided our every step. Judy was beautifully unique. She was a scholar, a scientist, a teacher, and a master clinician whose career exemplified the highest standards of professionalism and ethical conduct. Above all, she was a warm and caring person with a remarkable way of bringing out the best in everyone whose life she touched, including children whom she loved the most.

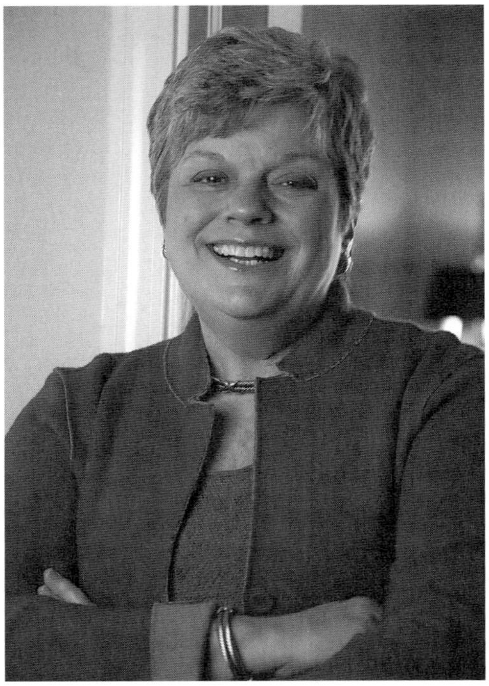

Dr. Judith S. Gravel
December 1948–December 2008

I

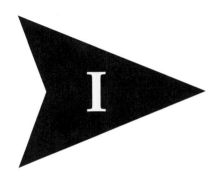

Typical Auditory Development

1

Hearing Development: Embryology of the Ear

Mark Hill

Developmental Origins

Human embryology at the turn of the last century identified selected aspects of ear structural development as part of the overall study of the development of the head and nervous system in studies by Thyng (1914). Studies of animal models played an important role in the early history of auditory embryology. For example, as early as 1911, Jenkinson examined the embryological development of the middle ear in mice. Studies of embryonic human external ears followed in the 1930s (Wood-Jones & Wen, 1934). The chicken model was also used around this time for studying the development of the central auditory pathway (Levi-Montalcini, 1949). In the 1940s and 1950s research focused on the relationship between the developing human auditory system and the general embryonic stages of development (Streeter, 1942, 1948, 1951). It was not until the 1950s that hearing development research took off with many studies on embryologic, anatomic, and neurologic development. Today a search of the Pubmed reference abstract database with "development of hearing" will return almost 6,000 studies. Many of the more recent studies mainly utilize animal models and study the molecular mechanisms of development, which are important in our understanding features of both normal and abnormal embryology. In particular, genetic and teratologic studies have and are identifying a growing number of specific genes and teratogens associated with auditory abnormal embryology.

This chapter introduces the embryology time course of the human ear as divided by the three anatomic divisions (Figure 1–1, external, middle, and inner). The description also will draw on the many animal model studies that have helped us further understand human auditory development. Examples also will be given of embryologic studies currently unravelling the complex signaling pathways involved in development. Many of these pathways involve a regulated sequence of secreted growth factors, transcription factor "switches," gap junctions and adhesive interactions choreographed into a back and forth signaling process between developing ear structures and surrounding tissues. Finally, a brief overview of critical periods of embryologic development in relationship to genetic and environment conditions is given. Note that neurologic and postnatal development is covered elsewhere in this text (see Chapters 2 and 4) and in recent reviews (e.g., Werner, 2007). Human embryology stages and the organ of audition and equilibrium are also described in the online resource UNSW Embryology (http://tiny.cc/Hearing_Development).

General Human Embryology

When staging human prenatal development there is an important consideration and sometimes confusion when reading the literature. Embryologists consider fertilization to initiate development and all following staging commences from this point in time. Clinicians, other than with in vitro fertilization (IVF), cannot easily ascertain the time of fertilization. In this case a far easier and more predictable timing is from when the mother is not pregnant, that is, the last menstrual period (LMP). Therefore, there is often approximately a two-week difference, as fertilization occurs after ovulation

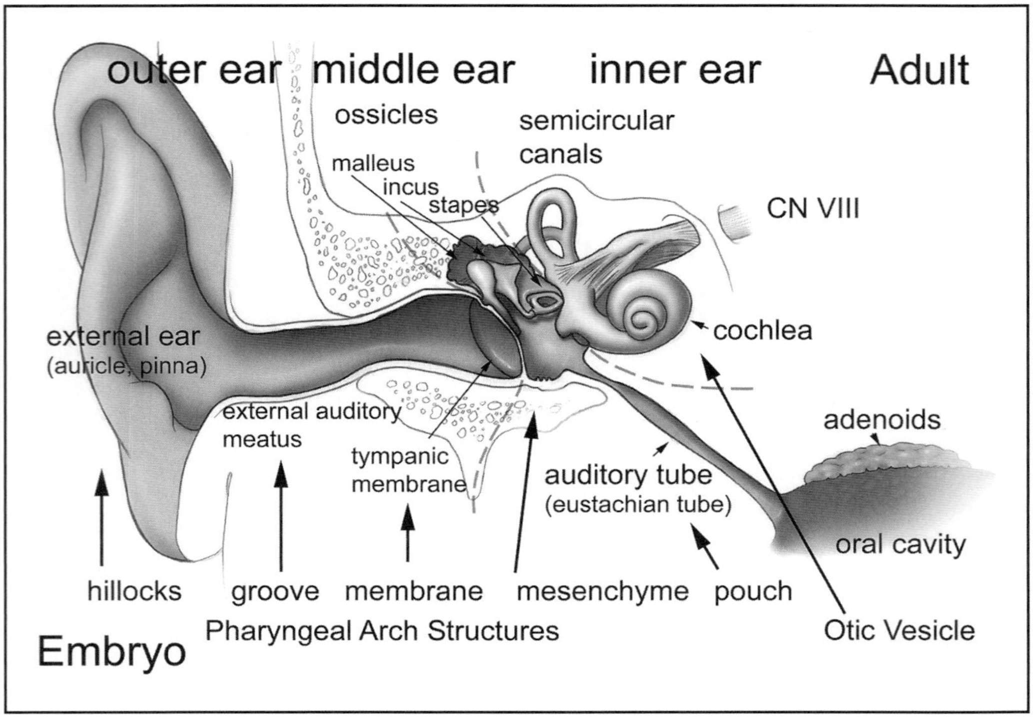

FIGURE 1–1. General anatomy of the adult ear and the equivalent embryonic structures from which each component is derived. The inner ear forms from the surface otic placode forming the otic vesicle (or otocyst), which contributes the membranous labyrinth and cranial ganglia. The middle and external ear form from components from pharyngeal arch one and two. Image based on NIH imagebank and National Institute on Deafness and Other Communication Disorders (NIDCD).

at the midpoint of the menstrual cycle. For example, postfertilization week three is clinically week five LMP. All timings described in this current chapter refer to embryologic dates from fertilization.

In the first three weeks of development, the embryo forms initially as three main layers (trilaminar), or germ layers, from which all tissues of the embryo derive. These three layers are: the ectoderm (forms all neural tissue and the surface epithelium); the mesoderm (forms most connective tissues of the body; muscle, bone, cartilage); the endoderm (forms the lining epithelium of the gastrointestinal, urogenital, and respiratory tract). Each of these layers begins as a simple circular disk of cells stacked like dinner plates. The three layers later will segment themselves into different regions, which contribute to specific tissues. Specialized senses such as hearing and vision will have contributions from all three embryonic germ layers during their complex developmental process.

In the fourth week of development, organogenesis begins throughout the embryo, which converts the trilaminar embryo into anatomically identifiable organs and tissues. In humans the first eight weeks of development are described as the embryonic period when organogenesis occurs, this is followed by the fetal period when continued growth and differentiation of mainly preexisting tissues and organs occurs. Classically, the embryonic period has been divided into 23 Carnegie stages, describing development as a series of observable changes in external appearance and features of the embryo. Stage 1 begins at fertilization, stage 7 at implantation at the end of the first week, and stage 23 the end of the embryonic period in the eighth week. The same classification can be applied to embryos of many different species, allowing direct developmental comparisons although over different time periods for each species stage. This classification has also been useful for studying the embryologic development in human's hearing and balance using a variety of animal models (mainly chicken, mouse, rat, zebrafish), which are referred to within this chapter.

Normal embryonic system development, including hearing, requires a combination of developmental signaling mechanisms. These mechanisms include short and long distance interactions by: secretions (growth factors, hormones, ionic changes), adhesive interactions (cell-cell, cell-extracellular matrix) and a subsequent cascade of transcription factors (DNA binding proteins). These transcription factors activate key genes required at specific developmental stages and eventually the adult pattern of gene expression in that cell or tissue.

Clinically, the embryonic period can also be seen to occupy most of the first trimester and the fetal period occupies the second and third trimester of human development. This division of development is also an important consideration when we look at the critical periods of development that can be impacted by teratogens. This chapter includes a brief coverage of some molecular regulatory mechanisms of normal development, as perturbations of these signaling pathways relate to abnormalities of hearing and balance. The following sections initially cover the early embryonic development of all three anatomic ear divisions, which are followed by later fetal development and detailed development of the cochlear and key auditory components.

Early Inner Ear

The earliest external feature of auditory development is the appearance on the ectoderm of the embryo surface in the head region of otic placodes. These placodes form as a pair of the series of placodal regions that form initially at the edge of the neural plate. The otic placodes are two small circular regions of ectoderm on the lateral surface of the developing head and the first "visible" pair of sensory placodes that eventually will contribute to each sensory system (hearing, vision, smell, and taste). In other species, there can be additional sensory placodes that contribute to sensory systems not present in humans. The otic placode lies closely associated with, but separate from, the neural tube level that corresponds to the hindbrain region of the neural tube. This localization with the neural tube later can be further positioned as adjacent to rhombomere 5 and 6 segmental subdivisions of the hindbrain.

The otic placode is a single layer of ectodermal cells organized in a columnar epithelium, which differs in cell shape from the surrounding cuboidal epithelia that will contribute the epithelia of the skin. In the zebrafish model, a number of specific genes are involved in initial induction of the otic placode including both growth factors (fgf3 and fgf8) and transcription factors (dlx3b, dlx4b, and foxi1) (Solomon, Kwak, & Fritz, 2004).

Proliferation of the otic placode cells leads to an inward folding, or invagination, giving the external appearance of a depression on the lateral sides of the early developing neck region. The epithelium is still a single layer of cells, which continues to invaginate until the edges of the disk of cells come into apposition on the embryo surface. In the mouse model, placodal invagination but not specification requires placodal expression of the transcription factor Sox9 (Barrionuevo et al., 2008).

Further invagination leads to the edges of the placode coming into close appostion and then fusing to form a hollow fluid-filled sac, this structure is then renamed as the otic vesicle or otcyst (Figure 1–2). The otic vesicle is the primordium of all the inner ear structures, including the cochleovestibular neurons of the future cranial nerve eight (CN VIII). The otic vesicle is now lost from the embryo surface and sits embedded within the mesenchyme, embryonic connective tissue, behind the first and second pharyngeal arches. The otic vesicle is surrounded by a number of developmental structures including the 5th rhombomere (medially), the anterior cardinal vein (laterally) and developing cranial ganglia (rostrocaudally). These events of otic placode formation, invagination and otic vesicle formation all occur within the third week of human development.

Otic Vesicle Development

The inner ear membranous labyrinth has two major linked components, the vestibular system (semicircular canals) and the auditory system (cochlea duct). Both are derived from the otic vesicle. This section will detail the early events of otic vesicle differentiation followed by specific notes on the later development of both systems.

By the fourth week the otic vesicle is a spherical epithelial fluid-filled ball at the level of rhombomeres 5 and 6 (Hatch, Noyes, Wang, Wright, & Mansour, 2007). During this week neuroblasts delaminate to form the primordial of the vestibulocochlear (statoacoustic) ganglion, the vesicle elongates, and the walls also change in relative thickness. This initial elongated portion of the otic vesicle will form the endolymphatic sac.

The beginning of otic vesicle differentiation is the localized expression of transforming growth factor-beta2 (Okano et al., 2005). The site (see Figure 1–2) of this expression in the otic wall locates cells that will delaminate and contribute to formation of the statoacoustic ganglion or cranial nerve CN VIII (Andermann, Ungos, & Raible, 2002; Represa, Moro, Gato, Pastor, & Barbosa, 1990). These cells remain adjacent to the otic vesicle residing in the surrounding cellular mesenchyme, a mixture of mesoderm and neural crest cells, the latter contributing to the ganglia (Bruska &

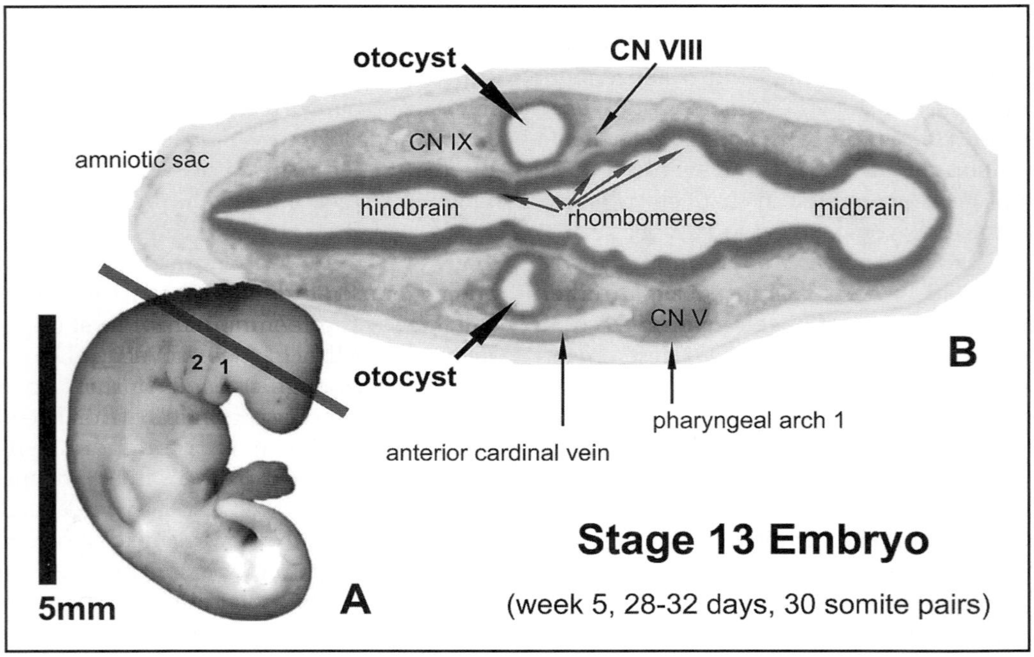

FIGURE 1–2. Stage 13 embryo (week 5) showing otocyst that will form the inner ear. **A.** Ventrolateral view of the whole embryo with 5-mm scale bar. At this stage of development no middle or external ear structures are apparent and will be derived later from pharyngeal arches one and two (*labeled*). **B.** The gray bar through the head indicates the plane of cross-section, which is a cross-section of the head showing the size and position of the otic vesicles. At this stage of development they lie within the head mesenchyme behind pharyngeal arch one and two and in close apposition to the developing hindbrain. Note the close position of the otic vesicle to the rhombomeres, hindbrain folds that represent the initial segmentation of the hindbrain. Also shown are developing cranial ganglia and blood vessel lying adjacent to the otic vesicles. The wall of the otic vesicle at this stage is a simple epithelium.

Wozniak, 2000; Wikstrom & Anniko, 1987). Cells within the ganglia differentiate into both neural and supporting glial cells. The neural cells eventually develop a bipolar morphology, extending central processes toward the neural tube and peripherally into the sensory epithelium of the vestibular apparatus and cochlea. Ganglionic neuron processes extend centrally toward the neural tube region that will form the medial geniculate nuclei. Division of the cochlear ganglion (spiral) from the vestibular ganglion have been identified to occur in human embryos between Carnegie stages 18 and 19 (44 to 46 postovulatory days) (Ulatowska-Blaszyk, & Bruska, 1999). Growth of processes toward the sensory epithelia is potentially driven by chemoattractant and repulsion cues (see review, Fekete & Campero, 2007). The neurotrophin family and their high-affinity Trk receptors control innervation of the cochlea during embryonic development. Mouse models point to a role for both brain-derived neurotrophic factor (Bdnf) and neurtrophin 3 (Nt3) (Schimmang et al., 2003).

The cochlea ganglion neurons differentiate to form two distinct populations on the basis of their location within the ganglia and soma size, central Type I large and peripheral Type II small cells. Note that more Type II ganglion cells have been identified in neonates, within the middle and apical turns, than in adults (Chiong, Burgess, & Nadol, 1993). This suggests an ongoing postnatal differentiation within the ganglion. An earlier study identified the associated glial cells do not myelinate the ganglion fibers, either in the fetus or neonate, and only thin myelination was observed in the elderly (Arnold, 1987). A more recent study identified in the fetal period cochlear, Schwann cell myelination (24 weeks) distally, and a later glial myelination (26 weeks) proximally (Moore & Linthicum, 2001).

In the fourth week the endolymphatic sac extends initially from the otic vesicle as a small diverticulum, with the main otic body forming the primordia of the utricle and the saccule (Figure 1–3). Regional differentiation of the utricle and saccule is regulated by the transcription factors Otx1 (Beisel, Wang-Lundberg, Maklad, & Fritzsch, 2005) and Pax5 (Kwak et al., 2006), both members of the homeobox gene family. The endolymphatic sac's mature function is both secretory and absorptive. The endolymphatic sac begins initially as an extending "single-lumen pouchlike structure," which in humans goes on to develop through fetal into the first postnatal year into a series of tubular structures (Bagger-Sjoback, 1991; Ng, 2000; Ng & Linthicum, 1998). This mature tubular structure is not seen in other species (Ng & Linthicum, 1998).

The adult endolymphatic sac is filled with endolymphatic fluid with a unique composition of high potassium and low sodium ions (Grunder, Muller, & Ruppersberg, 2001). Both the vestibular and cochlear epithelial cells secrete endolymphatic fluid. It is not known in humans at what stage of development this ionic status is achieved. In the rat, adult sodium levels are seen in the first week after birth, while both potassium and chloride levels were below the normal adult levels (Bosher & Warren, 1971). A similar postnatal increase in potassium ion levels occurs in the mouse (Anniko & Nordemar, 1980; Anniko & Wroblewski, 1981), and in chickens this rise occurs before hatching (Masetto, Zucca, Botta, & Valli, 2005).

The otic vesicle in the fifth week (at stage 16) extends a second process at the region where the saccule is forming and at the opposite pole from the developing endolymphatic sac (Yasuda, Yamada, Uwabe, Shiota, & Yasuda, 2007). This otic extension is the initial primordia of the cochlear duct and at this stage is

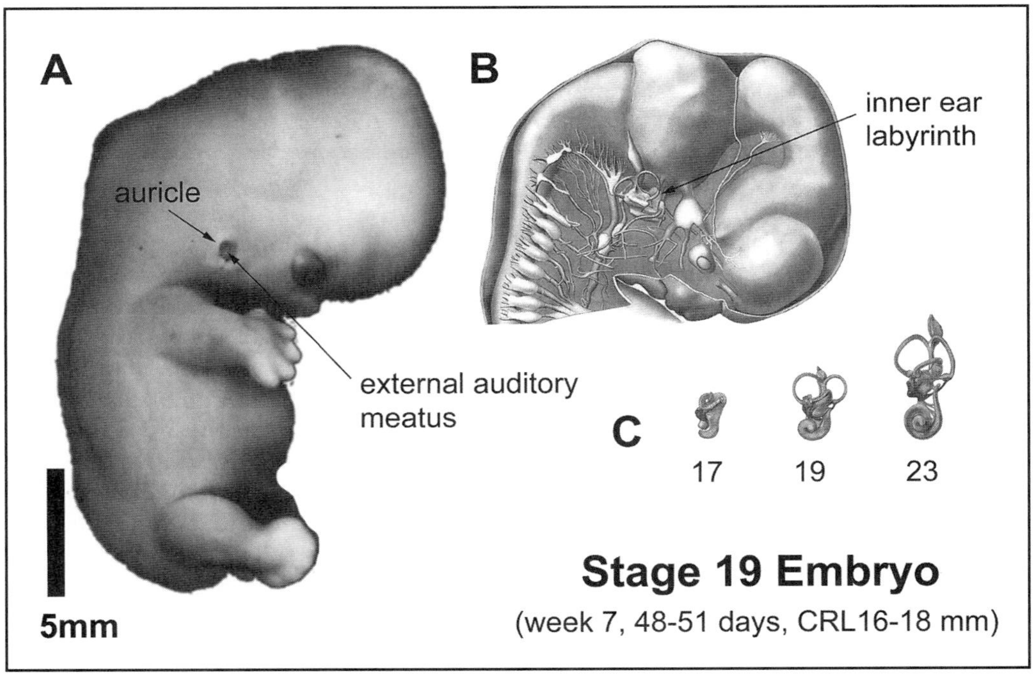

FIGURE 1–3. Stage 19 embryo (week 7) showing the ear development features. **A.** Lateral view of the whole embryo with 5-mm scale bar. Note the pharyngeal arches have differentiated and are no longer visible on the surface. The external ear (auricle) has formed from hillocks on pharyngeal arch one and arch two. Note the relative position of the ear just above the neck and at the level of the lower jaw. The external auditory meatus is enlarged and ends at a meatal plug. **B.** Historic image (Thyng, 1914) cutaway view of same stage embryo showing the position and appearance of the inner ear relative to the developing brain and other cranial ganglia. **C.** The relative size and shape of the inner ear labyrinth at weeks 6, 7, and 8; by the end of the embryonic period (week 8) it approximates the shape of the adult structure.

a simple epithelial fluid-filled sac. Over the next two weeks (week 5 to 7) from stage 16 to 22, the cochlea not only elongates and rotates, it begins to differentiate the organ of Corti, but this will not fully form until well into the fetal period. The cochlear ganglion neurons grow into this developing structure and will contact developing hair cells within the organ of Corti. As in other developing neuronal systems, neuronal development and survival appears to be mediated by target-derived secreted growth factors,in this system both brain-derived neurotrophic factor (BDNF) and neurotrophin 3 (NT-3; Bernd, Zhang, Yao, & Rozenberg, 1994; Camarero et al., 2001; Fekete & Campero, 2007; Fritzsch, Pirvola, & Ylikoski, 1999; Hossain, Brumwell, & Morest, 2002; Wei, Jin, Jarlebark, Scarfone, & Ulfendahl, 2007). Similarly, hair cell survival is also regulated by the growth BDNF and fibroblast growth factor-2 (FGF-2; Cristobal et al., 2002). The other regulatory factor for spiral ganglion neuron development is hormonal and related to fetal thyroid hormone (Parazzini et al., 2002; Rueda, Prieto, Cantos, Sala, & Merchan, 2003). Initial synaptogenesis between developing hair cells and the ganglionic neurons is directly onto neuronal cell bodies (somatic synapses) and only later do a network of dendritic spinous synapses form (Sobkowicz, Slapnick, & August, 2002).

It is during the seventh week of development that the otic vesicle begins formation of the vestibular semicircular canals (see Figure 1–3). Semicircular canal development appears to be initiated by fibroblast growth factor locally up-regulating bone morphogenetic protein 2 (Bmp2) expression (Chang, Brigande, Fekete, & Wu, 2004). A related BMP4 (Omata et al., 2007) and neuronal calcium sensor-1 (Ncs-1; Blasiole et al., 2005) appear to also control early development of the semicircular canals. Three otic vesicle out-pocketings from the utricular region indicate the location of the future semicircular canals. A recent study in human embryos (Yasuda et al., 2007) has established the morphogenesis time course of the three semicircular canals. At stage 17 the anterior and posterior semicircular ducts begin to form. By stage 18 the epithelia at the core of these outpocketings fuse, die by apoptosis, and are replaced by mesenchyme. By stage 19 these canals have the structural "loop" appearance. The lateral semicircular canal appears slightly delayed, but by stage 19 has a similar morphology.

Chondrification of surrounding mesenchyme begins in the first week of fetal development (week 9) forming the otic capsule (Figures 1–4 and 1–5). In the second trimester (week 12 to 16) the cartilage adjacent to the membranous labyrinth breaks down forming the perilymphatic space in which the membranous labyrinth will now float. Ossification of the surrounding capsule, the bony labyrinth, occurs between weeks 16 and 24 of fetal development. The bony labyrinth anatomically is within the petrous portion of the temporal bone and encloses all the inner ear structures. The human bony labyrinth is unique and differs from even those of other primates, in size, shape, and orientation. These differences are thought to derive from the cranial base and the upright bipedal locomotion in humans.

Cochlear Development

The otic vesicle pseudostratified epithelial cells differentiate through regulated signaling into four distinct pathways forming cochlear prosensory cells, vestibular prosensory cells, neurons in the auditory and vestibular ganglia and nonsensory epithelia (Kelley, 2007). Within the cochlea duct a chamber, sensory cells, support cells and specialized extracellular matrices will eventually differentiate from this primordia formed by the otic vesicle. The mesenchyme surrounding the cochlear duct along its length, vacuolates to form a series of fluid-filled spaces. These spaces coalesce either side of the cochlear duct to form two parallel perilymphatic cavities, the scala vestibuli and scala tympani. The remaining mesenchyme will chrondrify and later ossify through the fetal period to form the bony labyrinth in which the membranous labyrinth resides. The adult cochlear size is achieved by 16 to 17 weeks gestation (see Figure 1–4).

The specialized auditory component within the cochlea is referred to as the organ of Corti, named after the Italian anatomist Marquis Alfonso Giacomo Gaspare Corti (1822–1876) who carried out microscopic analysis of human and other species cochleas. The most studied animal model of cochlea development is that of the mouse (then guinea pig and gerbil), with several knockouts mimicking human hearing loss and in contrast to humans, where the onset of hearing occurs postnatally. The molecular differentiation of the individual cells that form the specialized organ of Corti has been recently reviewed (Kelley, 2007).

The first structure to form is Kollicker's organ, or greater epithelial ridge, a transient epithelial structure lying beneath the tectorial membrane from which some of the specialized cells of the organ of Corti are formed. The adjacent lesser epithelial ridge is separated initially by a notch from the greater epithelial ridge and will contribute the outer hair cells. Follow-

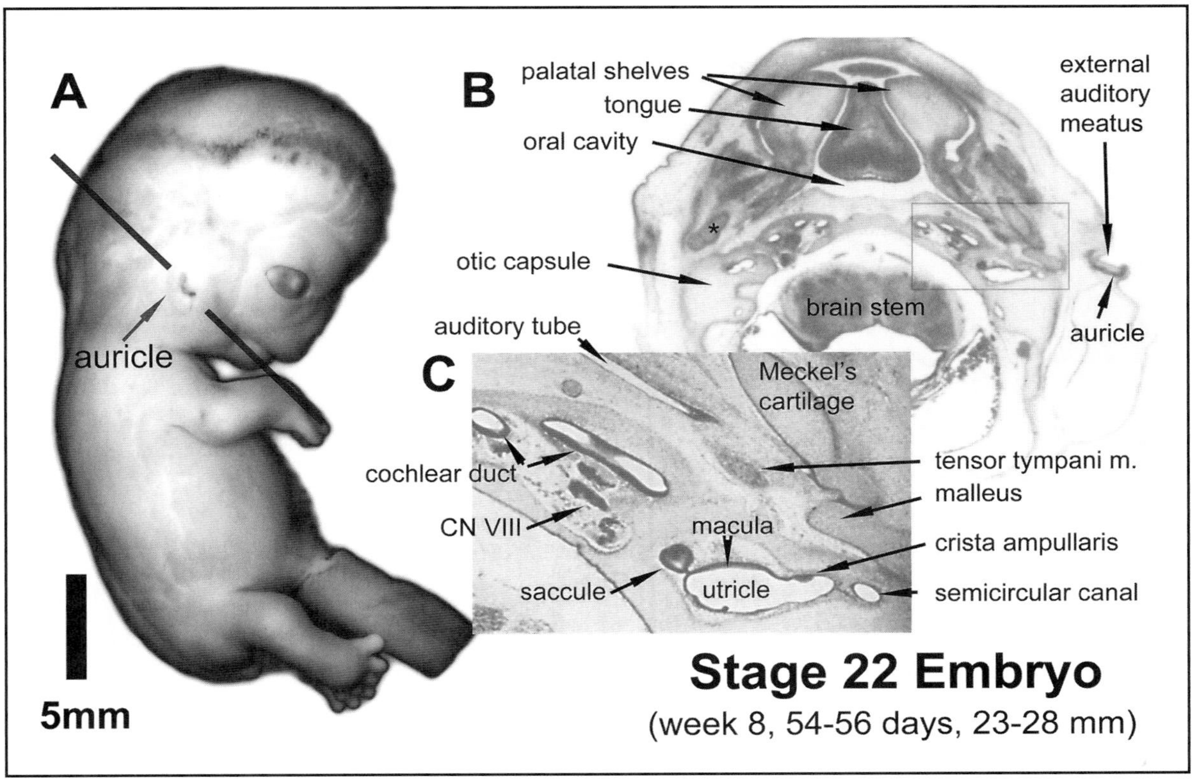

FIGURE 1–4. Stage 22 embryo (week 8) showing the embryo near the end of the embryonic period. **A.** Lateral view of the whole embryo with 5-mm scale bar. Note the well-developed external ear with simplified adult structure and narrower meatal opening. The gray bar through the head indicates the plane of cross-section for (**B**) and (**C**). **B.** Cross-section of the head at the plane of the skull base and oral cavity to the top. The otic capsule is well formed by this stage containing all the membranous labyrinth structures. It is still a cartilaginous structure ventral to the brainstem and lying behind the oral cavity. The tongue occupies the floor of the oral cavity with the unfused palatal shelves lying lateral and the auditory tubes clearly shown on the posterior wall. The external ear is visible on the right hand side of the head with a band of cartilage (dark stain) within the auricle. **C.** The gray box indicates this region: detail of inner and middle ear development. The middle ear cavity has not yet formed and the ossicles (malleus shown) are embedded in mesenchyme that is being lost. The tensor tympani muscle is differentiating in the adjacent mesenchyme. The inner ear membranous labyrinth has formed its adult external structure. The section through the turns of the cochlear duct shows the internal cochlea structure is still underdeveloped; in contrast, the balance region is more developed.

ing generation of the hair and pillar cells, Kollicker's organ will then regress and generate the inner sulcus.

A study has been made of early human organ of Corti development (Pujol & Lavigne-Rebillard, 1985), and a recent detailed histological study has been made of the human timeline of development of both the temporal bone and the organ of Corti (Bibas et al., 2008) (Table 1–1 and Figure 1–3). The recent morphologic developmental timeline suggests that auditory function begins after the week 20 (LMP) time point, later than the week 14 suggested by other studies. Note that not only the cochlea, but also the cochlea nerve and central pathways need to develop for a functioning central neural pathway to occur (Sanchez Del Rey, Sanchez Fernandez, Martinez Ibarguen, & Santaolalla Montoya, 1995).

Audition through the fetal period is by bone conduction, not mediated by the middle ear. Bone conduction occurs from the developing skull and its contents, including the brain and fluids, low frequency vibrat-

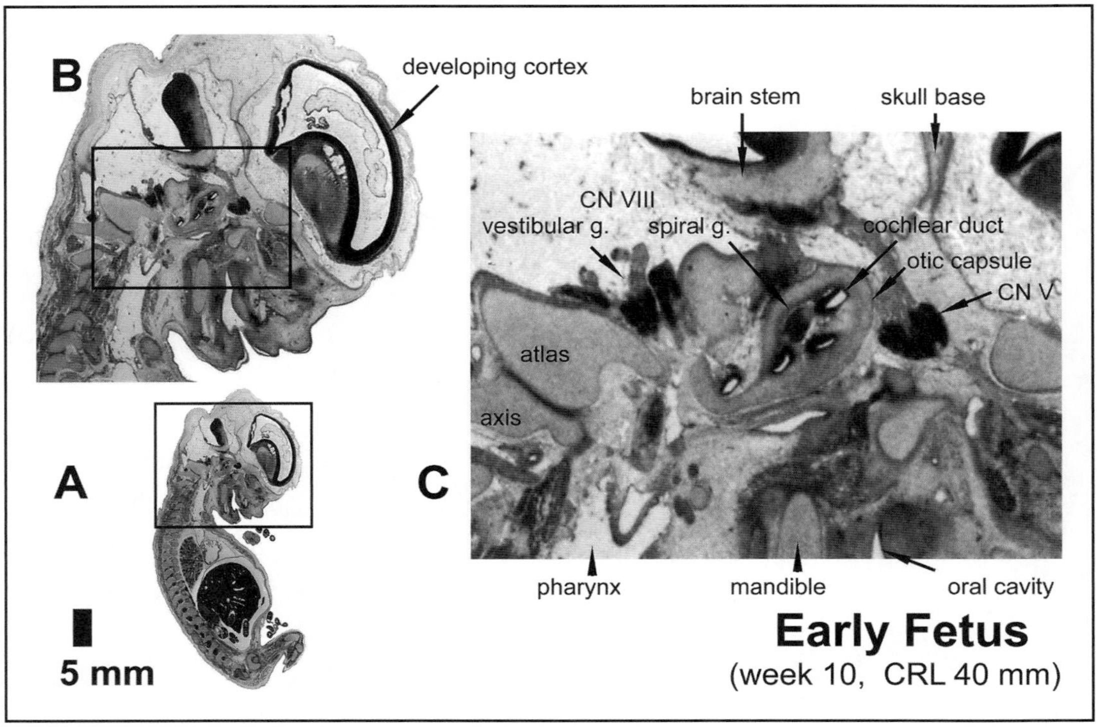

FIGURE 1–5. Fetal development (week 10) showing the early fetal cochlea. **A.** Sagittal section through the whole fetus with 5-mm scale bar. **B.** The gray box indicates this region; enlarged view of head showing the anatomic position and size of the cochlea relative to the developing brain, mouth and vertebral column. Note the large trigeminal ganglia (CN V) and relatively underdeveloped cortex above the basal ganglia. **C.** The gray box indicates this region; enlarged view of cochlea showing sections through turns of the cochlear duct in the otic capsule. The cranial ganglia CN VIII (vestibulocochlear nerve, auditory-vestibular nerve or statoacoustic nerve) has clearly separated vestibular and cochlear divisions. Note the position of the oral cavity, mandible, and pharynx lying directly beneath the otic capsule.

ing from sound-induced fluid vibrations of amniotic fluid (Sohmer, Perez, Sichel, Priner, & Freeman, 2001).

A key regulator in hair cell production is Math1, the homolog of the *Drosophila* proneural gene atonal, which regulates the total number of hair cells produced. This gene is in turn negatively regulated by the Hes (hairy and enhancer of split) family of factors, which has been shown to be a general negative regulator of neurogenesis (Zheng, Shou, Guillemot, Kageyama, & Gao, 2000).

Another gene involved in early hair cell proliferation, but not differentiation, is the expression of the retinoblastoma protein pRb (Sage et al., 2006). Later differentiation of hair and support pillar cells appears to rely initially on a lateral inhibition process mediated through the Notch signaling pathway (Daudet, Ariza-McNaughton, & Lewis, 2007). Outer hair cell differentiation also requires further signaling by the Pou4f3 (Brn3.1, Brn3c) transcription factor activation of growth factor-independent 1 (Gfi 1; Hertzano et al., 2004). Mouse Pou4f3 knockout, a model for human autosomal dominant nonsyndromic progressive hearing loss, shows a specific developmental degeneration of outer hair cells (Hertzano et al., 2004).

Later hair cell neural transmission occurs through voltage-gated calcium channels opening when mechanical stimulation depolarizes the hair cell membrane, and the resulting calcium influx triggers neurotransmitter release. In animal models, these channels are expressed very early in hair cell development and may have additional developmental functions within these cells (Hafidi & Dulon, 2004; Waka, Knipper, & Engel,

Table 1–1. Late Embryonic and Fetal Development of Both the Cochlea and Organ of Corti

LMP Week	*Postovulatory Week*	*Event*
10	8	tectorial membrane primordium found throughout cochlea turns
14	12	hair cells at the basal turn
		oval space located between inner and outer hair cells in the basal turn
14–15	12–13	Hensen's cells present
17	15	pillar cells present
		spiral limbus increases in size
		Kollicker's organ
20	18	tunnel of Corti opens
21–25	19–23	tunnel of Corti continues to open upward from the base
25	23	cochlea is adult size
26	24	inner sulcus a single layer of flattened cells
		supporting cells become columnar

Note: Data from A. G. Bibas et al. (2008), based on the study of 81 human fetal temporal bones.

2003). Finally, fetal thyroid hormone contributes a hormonal role in the differentiation of hair cells and their subsequent innervation by spiral ganglion neurons (Rueda et al., 2003).

The stria vascularis within the cochlea produces by ionic regulation endocochlear potential and contacts both perilymph and endolymph fluids (Johnson & Spoendlin, 1966; Nin et al., 2008). In humans, the earliest strial cell differentiation occurs during week 9 (11 weeks LMP) as a ridge of epithelial cells on the lateral wall of the cochlear duct (Bibas, Liang, Michaels, & Wright, 2000). By week 12 (14 weeks LMP) the three major strial cell types are present: marginal, intermediate and basal cells (Lavigne-Rebillard & Bagger-Sjoback, 1992). The intermediate cells of the stria vascularis are neural crest-derived melanocytes, which are capable of continuous replication (Conlee, Gerity, & Bennett, 1994). By week 19 (21 weeks LMP) the stria vascularis appears adult in structure, but is not mature until the third trimester (Lavigne-Rebillard & Bagger-Sjoback, 1992). Atrophy occurs postnatally in the elderly of both the stria vascularis and spiral ganglion (Suzuki et al., 2006).

Vestibular Development

The short tube of the ductus reuniens connects the cochlear duct to the vestibular components of the membranous labyrinth (see Figure 1–4). The saccule and utricle are the two dilatations of the membranous labyrinth in the vestibule. The utricle is a connecting chamber that communicates with the semicircular canals. The saccule communicates with the utricle and the two combine to form the endolymphatic duct, a sac that ends blindly in the temporal bone.

In the utricle and saccule are the maculae utriculi and maculae sacculi, respectively. These lie perpendicular to one another, and each consists of supporting (sustentacular) cells and hair cells. The hair cells have long cilia that are embedded in an otolithic membrane. The otolithic membrane contains otoliths, which are small crystalline bodies of calcium carbonate. Position changes of the head stimulate the otolithic membrane and this stimulation is picked up by nerve endings between the hair cells. The maculae are concerned with the detection of linear movement of the head. The semicircular canals achieve adult size by 17 to 19 weeks gestation, with the lateral canal being the most slowly growing.

Early Middle Ear

Middle ear development begins closely associated with head formation and involves both the foregut tube (pharynx) and the pharyngeal arches. Pharyngeal arches form the main anatomic structures of the head and neck, including all components of the middle and outer ear.

Pharyngeal arches (branchial arches) are named by their location and shape, wrapping externally around the ventral surface of the pharynx and forming an "arch" shape. In humans, a series of five pharyngeal arches (1, 2, 3, 4, 6) form in sequence rostrocaudally (head to tail); arch 5 apparently does not form and arches 4 and 6 soon fuse together. This leaves a series of 4 externally visible arches in the head region, with arch 2 eventually growing over the inferior arches so that they are lost from the embryo surface.

Pharyngeal arches 1 and 2 are the main contributors to the middle and outer ear. Each of the arches has a similar overall structure with contributions from all 3 germ cell layers, but each arch will form different anatomical components of the head and neck. Each arch is covered with ectoderm (embryo surface) and lined with endoderm (pharynx) and separated from each other by a membrane formed by these two layers. The arches are composed of unsegmented head mesoderm, which is invaded by neural crest cells to form initially mesenchyme, a term used to describe an embryonic undifferentiated connective tissue. The mesenchyme differentiates to form the same series of components within each arch: a band of cartilage, an artery, and a vein. During later development these pharyngeal arch structures are extensively remodeled.

Middle Ear Auditory Ossicles

The three middle ear bones or auditory ossicles (malleus, incus, stapes) are formed from the cartilage template found within pharyngeal arch 1 and 2. These bones are commonly named the hammer (malleus), anvil (incus) and stirrup (stapes), and the cartilage bands are historically named after two German anatomists and are called Meckel's cartilage (first pharyngeal arch; named after Johann Friedrich Meckel, 1781–1833) and Reichert's cartilage (second pharyngeal arch; named after Karl Bogislaus Reichert, 1811–1883). There are several theories as to how each arch cartilage contributes individual components of the middle ear ossicles (Whyte et al., 2008; Whyte Orozco et al., 2003). Meckel's cartilage first appears histologically at stage 16 (Orliaguet, Darcha, Dechelotte, & Vanneuville, 1994) and Reichert's cartilage slightly later.

The early stages of auditory ossicle development all occur within the solid mesenchyme of the pharyngeal arches until the eighth month of development, then within a fluid-filled space for the final month, and finally only postnatally in the neonate in the air-filled tympanic cavity. This transition in auditory ossicle environment means that the middle ear does not function correctly until after birth, and any prenatal conduction to the cochlea must be mediated through bone conduction. During development of the tympanic cavity, the auditory ossicles are held in their correct anatomic positions by supporting ligaments. Arch cartilages ossify by the process of endochondral ossification, where a preexisting cartilage template is first formed and later replaced by bone. Endochondral ossification is the main process of bone formation throughout the entire skeleton, except for the cranial vault and the clavicle that ossify by a process of intramembranous ossification.

Initially, the malleus and incus form as a single structure, and it is only later that they separate to form two separate bones. Ossification continues through the entire fetal period, and the newly formed bones also have a transient bone marrow cavity (Yokoyama, Iino, Kakizaki, & Murakami, 1999). The marrow cavity is still present at birth, in both the malleus and the incus, and with continued ossification is lost during the first two years after birth. Postnatally, first the malleus and then the incus lose their marrow spaces (Yokoyama et al., 1999).

Middle Ear Muscles

The middle ear also contains the two smallest muscles of the body, the stapedius and tensor tympani muscles, which both differentiate from arch mesenchyme (see Figure 1–5). These muscles form and differentiate in a similar fashion to other developing skeletal muscle. Initially myoblasts proliferate under the influence of growth factors in the region of where the muscle will form. Myoblasts are the embryonic undifferentiated single cells of all skeletal muscles. The myoblasts' numbers reach a critical concentration, often depleting locally secreted growth factors, migrate, align, and commence to fuse plasma membranes. These fusion events form multinucleated myotubes, into which additional myoblasts continue to fuse at each end. The mechanisms regulating myoblast fusion are still being investigated (suggested signaling mechanisms include: adhesion, immunoglobulin superfamily proteins, metalloproteases, potassium ion channels, and calcium). These myotubes that form are the second main stage of muscle cellular differentiation.

Depending on the size and structure of the muscle, a later second round of myoblast fusion events may occur around these early forming primary myotubes. The myotubes begin to upregulate and express the contractile proteins involved in forming the molecular contractile apparatus within muscle. Striated muscle contractile apparatus is called the sarcomere, which is the basic unit of contraction. The two major proteins are actin and myosin, which interact to shorten the single sarcomere, and the serial organization of thousands of sarcomeres within the muscle fiber leads to overall anatomical contraction. Sarcomeres initially form at the edge of developing myotubes and in many cases require innervation to complete their organization to form the mature muscle fiber. Innervation of muscle is therefore the final key to skeletal muscle differentiation, and functioning, denervated muscle will atrophy.

The type (isoform) of myosin and actin expressed by individual muscle fibers determines the contractile properties of the muscle fiber: slow (type 1) or fast (type 2A, 2X, 2B) twitch; oxidative (1, 2A), glycolytic (2B), or a mixture of both (2X) metabolisms. The adult muscle fiber isoform will then be regulated by the activity type of the innervating neuron. There is also some evidence to suggest a role for some hormonal regulation of muscle differentiation pattern. A single neuron will innervate a group of fibers all with the same contractile properties. The neuron together with the group of individual muscle fibers it innervates is called a motor unit.

Little is known about either the developmental or adult muscle fiber types present in the human tensor tympani and stapedius muscles. In other skeletal muscles, the initial myotubes form as primary embryonic slow fibers being surrounded later by secondary fast fibers. Both primary and secondary fibers are then converted into their final adult fiber type by the innervating neuron. There is some fiber type analysis from animal model studies including: avian (Counter, Hellstrand, & Borg, 1987), rabbit (Vita, Muglia, Germana, Pennica, & Carfi, 1983), and cat (Lyon & Malmgren, 1982, 1988). The adult tensor tympani is classified as a mixed muscle containing slow (type 1) and fast (type 2A, and probably 2X) muscle fibers. The adult mammalian stapedius muscle contains mainly (77%) fast oxidative glycolytic type muscle fibers and the avian muscle only contains fast fibers (Counter et al., 1987).

Both muscles carry out their contractile function postnatally. The tensor tympani's contraction pulls the malleus and tenses the tympanic membrane dampening auditory ossicle movement. The tensor tympani muscle cells arise from beside the auditory tube, the cartilaginous portion, and the muscle inserts into the malleus at the manubrium near the root. The tensor tympani will be innervated by cranial nerve five (CN V, trigeminial nerve). The second muscle, the stapedius muscle, will contract to pull the stapes and dampens auditory ossicle movement. This muscle is innervated by cranial nerve seven (CN VII, facial nerve). The main cranial nerve associated with hearing and balance is cranial nerve eight (CN VIII, vestibulocochlear nerve) or auditory-vestibular nerve or statoacoustic nerve. A brief summary of cranial nerve development is described later in this chapter and elsewhere (see Chapter 2).

Middle Ear Auditory Tube and Tympanic Cavity

The auditory tube, eustachian tube (named after Bartolomeo Eustachi, 1500–1574), otopharyngeal or pharyngotympanic tube develops from the first pharyngeal pouch and is lined with endoderm. This narrow cavity links the pharynx to the middle ear and is continuous with the tympanic cavity (see Figure 1–5). The auditory tube has two main functions: ventilation, to allow the equalization of pressure in the middle ear, and clearance, to allow the middle ear fluid continuously produced by the epithelial lining to drain from the middle ear.

In normal human development, the auditory tube has an almost straight posterolateral to anteromedial pathway. The main growth of the auditory tube occurs in extension and lumen of the cartilaginous portion in the fetal period between weeks 16 to 28 (Swarts, Rood, & Doyle, 1986).

At birth, and in the young child, the tube is both shorter (8–9 mm) compared to the adult length (17–18 mm), runs almost horizontal and is narrower in diameter. Head growth in the child to adult size results in a longer wider tube that runs at approximately 45 degrees to the horizontal. The auditory tube is also normally closed and is opened by muscles—in the infant this is only a single muscle, the tensor palati muscle. In the adult the auditory tube is now opened by two separate muscles, the tensor palati and levator palati muscles.

The above developmental factors combine to contribute to the increased frequency of middle ear infections arising in the young child. The short length leads to easier transmission of infection from oral cavity to middle ear. The opening beside the adenoids and narrow lumen leads to easy blockage during infection and inflammation. Finally, the almost horizontal pathway leads to poor middle ear drainage.

The middle ear cavity or tympanic cavity is formed by an expansion of the pharynx. The initial early cavity lining is formed by the pharyngeal endoderm epithelium. The epithelium will then continue to expand, to eventually line the entire mastoid antrum.

The adult middle ear, like the inner ear, eventually will lie within the petrous portion of temporal bone. Initially, both the middle and inner ear form within mesenchyme, embryonic connective tissue, forming the otic capsule, and this will also form the base of the skull. The mesenchyme differentiates first to form cartilage, forming a structure known as the chondrocranium. This initial cartilage is gradually replaced by bone forming at a number of sites within the cartilage, ossification centers. The initial bone that is formed also contains marrow spaces that disappear with ongoing ossification (Yokoyama et al., 1999). Between the weeks 16 to 24, centers of ossification appear in the remaining cartilage of the otic capsule, and these continue to ossify to eventually form mastoid process of temporal bone (Nemzek et al., 1996).

Early External Ear Development

The outer ear consists of the auricle (pinna), the external auditory meatus (ear canal) and the outer layer of the tympanic membrane. The first and second pharyngeal arches contribute the auricle, each contributing three auricular hillocks. Each of the auricular hillocks (small hills) is a mesenchymal swelling covered in ectoderm observable on the embryo surface and will contribute an individual anatomic component of the external ear (Figure 1–6). These hillocks are initially located low on the developing head, at the level of the neck, and both change their relative position with head growth and are extensively remodeled during late embryonic period (weeks 5 to 8). By the end of week 8 the basic structure of the external auricle has been formed, but it still lies well below its final anatomic position. Some abnormalities of external ear structure and position are both indicators of developmental problems requiring further investigation; this is discussed later in the chapter. These abnormalities can relate not only to the development of hearing, but other internal systems that develop over a similar time course.

The external auditory meatus develops from the first pharyngeal cleft, which lies externally between the first two arches. It is the only cleft that will form a structure in the developing embryo. The embryonic canal is blocked by a temporary meatal plug, which forms at the end of the embryonic period and remains for a variable period through fetal development. The epithelial lining is derived from the ectoderm germ layer and also contributes the outer layer of the tympanic membrane. Failure of the meatal plug to degenerate can lead to deafness. A detailed time course of human meatal development has been previously described and published by Nishimura and Kumoi (1992).

Later in the fetal period, toward the end of the second trimester, within the epithelium two types of associated glands differentiate, sebaceous and modified apocrine glands, which in the postnatal period begin to secrete cerumen, or earwax (Wright, 1997). The cerumen is composed of exfoliated epithelial keratin and gland secretions also containing antimicrobial peptides (Supp, Karpinski, & Boyce, 2004). These glandular secretions are altered postnatally and mature at puberty (Wright, 1997).

After the embryonic period, both the auricle and external canal continue to grow through the fetal period and into the postnatal period, reaching their young adult size at about 9 years of age (Wright, 1997). The external ear then continues to grow in size slowly through the entire adult life.

The tympanic membrane or eardrum has contributions from all three germ layers. The external auditory meatus is lined with surface ectoderm, which is continuous with the outer tympanic membrane. The tympanic cavity forms from the pharynx and is lined with endoderm, which is continuous with the inner tympanic membrane. Lying between the two layers is a thin layer of mesenchymal connective tissue, the fibrous stratum.

Cranial Nerve Development

There are twelve pairs of cranial nerves numbered in rostrocaudal (head to tail) sequence and developing initially beside the neural tube at the level of the hindbrain. The cranial nerves are traditionally numbered by Roman numerals as well as having names based on their adult function. As discussed previously, the

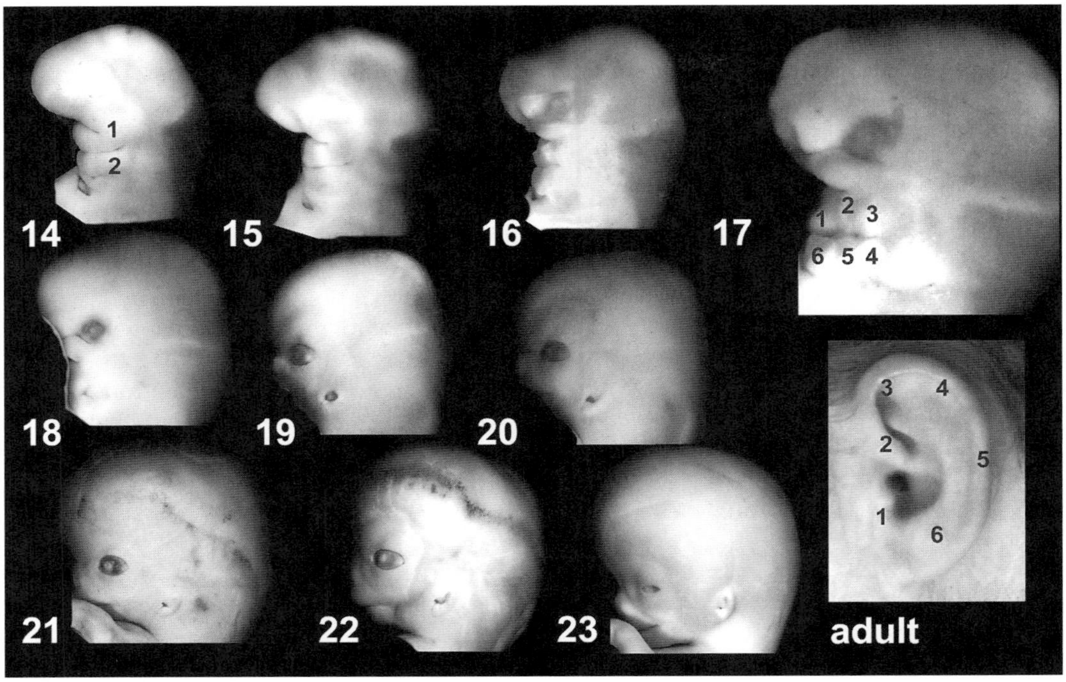

FIGURE 1–6. Embryonic development of the external ear from stage 14 (week 5) to stage 23 (week 8) compared to the adult ear. Lateral view of the heads are shown not to scale and there is a 5–fold increase in size between stages 14 and 23. Week 5 (stage 14 to 15) pharyngeal arches one and two are visible separated by the first pharyngeal groove, which will form the external auditory meatus. Week 6 (stage 16 and 17) separate hillocks appear on the surfaces of pharyngeal arches one and two, which will contribute the structure of the external ear. Stage 17 is enlarged to show the numbered hillocks, and equivalent regions are shown in the adult ear. Importantly, note the changing relative position of the external ear with head growth and development from below the lower jaw to between the level of the nose and eye by the end of the embryonic period. Embryo images are modified from the Kyoto collection, courtesy of Professor Kohei Shiota.

middle ear muscles are supplied by motor divisions of different cranial nerves. The tensor tympani will be innervated by the mandibular division of the trigeminial nerve (CN V). The stapedius muscle is innervated by the tympanic branch of the facial nerve (CN VII), while the cochlea and vestibular apparatus are supplied by statoacoustic or vestibulocochlear ganglion (CN VIII).

Abnormalities

Human pregnancy and development are generally robust processes, and in dealing with abnormalities this can sometimes be forgotten. All abnormalities of human development can be grouped into three main categories: genetic, environmental, and unknown (or undetermined). The complex origins of all components of hearing and the long time course of development exposes this system to a large number of different environmental effects. To further complicate diagnosis and prognosis, all the environmental factors below have different combinatorial effects, and exposure at different times of the pregnancy can also lead to entirely different developmental outcomes. The sensory systems too have the combined effects of abnormalities in both or either the sensory components or structures (conductive) and the sensorineural neural pathway. This also may mean that an abnormality will occur in combinations of outer, middle, and inner ear structures. Two notable recent changes in our general understanding of human abnormalities include increasing fetal alcohol syndrome and the fetal origins hypothesis that states that prenatal developmental effects impact postnatally on lifelong health outcomes.

The external ear (auricle) is also an excellent indicator or marker for other not as easily detectible internal developmental abnormalities. The commonly detected abnormalities include sinuses, tags, and position on the head. In many cases this is related to the development of the external ear and head overlapping with these internal systems—for example, the correlation of ear abnormalities with kidney developmental abnormalities. Another currently relevant correlation is a low or uneven ear/head position with the growing occurrence of fetal alcohol syndrome.

This chapter includes a brief overview and a few sample disorders of some hearing abnormalities, due to the large number of different genetic associations. More details are shown online at UNSW Embryology, hearing and balance abnormalities notes (http://embryology.med.unsw.edu.au/Notes/ear2.htm).

Genetic

In human development, the majority of major genetic abnormalities are thought to be lost in the first two weeks of development as the zypote, then morula and blastocyst fails to develop correctly and complete implantation. Genetic abnormalities can be further grouped into chromosomal aneuploidies (abnormal chromosome numbers, e.g., Down syndrome, trisomy 13), translocation of chromosomal segments, and, finally, single gene mutations. The single gene mutations can be of four main types; autosomal (nonsex chromosome) and X-linked and in both cases can be a dominant (expressed) or a recessive (carrier) trait. These genetic mutations are now often well documented in terms of systematic effects. Single gene mutations are also defined by the gene location using the following combination of: chromosome number (1 to 22, X or Y), letter (p or q, referring to the short or long "arm" of each chromosome) and number (variable referring to position with reference to banding pattern on folded chromosome). The gene location as yet may not be exactly located or may span two reference locations.

The database Online Mendelian Inheritance in Man (OMIM; http://www.ncbi.nlm.nih.gov/sites/entrez?db=omim) is a readily available and searchable compendium of these human genes and genetic phenotypes and contain both reference links for this next section of notes and detailed clinical synopses. A search of OMIM with the term "hearing," results in more than 900 different entries, and nearly 400 entries have a clinical synopsis. Many of these genetic disorders that affect hearing are also part of multisystem genetic syndromes.

Environmental

The many different environmental effects, described as "teratogens," have been more typically described as "maternal effects." This term, however, is both outdated and stigmatizing to parents. Some environmental effects can be directly due to maternal behavior/lifestyle (e.g., diet, drugs, smoking, alcohol) or a preexisting maternal condition (e.g., diabetes), often before pregnancy has been detected. However there are many other developmental environmental effects that are not directly controlled by the mother. These include: infections (bacterial, viral, parasites), hyperthermia, environmental contaminants (heavy metals, polychlorinated biphenyls), and radiation.

External Ear

Low or uneven set ears indicates a developmental abnormality of head growth and development and can be unique to the ear or relate to other conditions. Some of these external abnormalities are indicative of middle ear bone abnormalities: thickened lobes (abnormal incus and stapes), smaller "cup" ears with absent cartilage (Mennonite genetic kindred absence of incus and stapes), or absent superior crus (congenital ossicle fixation). Other nonhearing-associated abnormalities include Klippel-Feil syndrome, cardiac, and urogenital (kidney and gonad) abnormalities.

Anotia or absence of the ear is due to the pharyngeal arch hillocks failing to form and impacts also on the external auditory meatus and middle ear bones and is sometimes grouped with microtia. Known genetic associations include: mandibulofacial dysostosis, Treacher Collins syndrome (5q32-q33.1), hemifacial microsomia (14q32), and congenital aural atresia (18q22.3-q23).

Microtia or small ear has a cup ear or overfolded auricle and may have absence of the external auditory meatus. Genetically, there are nearly 40 different associations including syndromes, hearing and vision abnormalities, neurologic abnormalities, clefting of the palate and face, and other musculoskeletal abnormalities. Environmentally, maternal drugs including thalidomide and retinoic acid have also caused microtia. This condition is repaired surgically using cartilage derived from the rib to reconstruct the external ear. Auriculocondylar syndrome (question mark ear) also can be repaired by this cartilage transfer operation; it is a rare syndrome with variable hearing loss and facial effects.

Auricular fistulas (an abnormal connection or passageway) and sinuses (cavities) can usually be harmless. Preauricular sinus occurs in 0.25% births, is bilateral (hereditary) in 25 to 50% of cases, and unilateral (mainly the left). They are developmental and generally occur on the surface in the anterior margin of the ascending limb of the helix, and the duct runs inward to the perichondrium of the auricular cartilage and in some cases extends into the parotid gland. Some genetic associations vary from prevalent to rare syndromes and include: hemifacial microsomia (914q32), Townes and Brocks syndrome (16q12.1), branchiooculofacial syndrome (96p24), and velocardiofacial syndrome (22q11.2). Sinuses postnatally are also a common site of infections.

Auricular appendages (tags) bilateral or unilateral (one or both ears) are quite common and often not associated with other developmental conditions other than those shown above. Stenosis (narrowing) of the external auditory meatus is uncommon and postnatally can be due to chronic otitis externa or acquired atresia. The condition can be treated surgically by meatoplasty (reconstructive surgery of the canal) alone, though acquired atresia requires removal of the soft tissue plug and a split skin graft.

The external ear can also be diagnostic for fetal alcohol syndrome (FAS), the most serious of the fetal alcohol spectrum disorders (FASD). FASD is an umbrella term used to describe the range of effects that can occur in an individual whose mother drank alcohol during pregnancy, and is not intended as a clinical diagnosis. The effects may include physical, mental, behavioral, and/or learning disabilities with possible lifelong implications. There is also evidence that FAS is directly associated with: delayed auditory function, sensorineural hearing loss, and intermittent conductive hearing loss due to recurrent serous otitis media (Church & Abel, 1998). Fetal alcohol effect (FAE) is the less obvious form and has the neurological effects without the external physiologic features and presents as learning difficulties or delayed milestones. The FAS infant will have lower or uneven external ear position. The auricle also may feature a curve at the top part of the ear, which is underdeveloped and folded over parallel to the curve beneath. This appearance is often described as a "railroad track" ear.

Middle Ear

There are many middle ear abnormalities, which mainly effect the middle ear ossicle formation and can also incorporate effects on the facial nerve. The majority (90%) of Trisomy 21 (Down syndrome) infants have a hearing loss due to conduction abnormalities.

Absence of middle ear ossicles can be associated with a range of conditions and syndromes, including dwarfism and achondrogenesis. The most common bones to be absent are the incus and stapes. Fixation of the stapes by fibrous tissue can occur in association with cochlear abnormalities of oval window absence and in several syndromes including: X-linked deafness 2 DFNX2 (Xq21.1), branchiootorenal syndrome (8q13.3; Senel et al., 2009), and Beckwith-Wiedemann syndrome (11p15.5, 11p15.5, 11p15.5, 5q35; Paulsen, 1973).

Persistent stapedial artery occurs in the fetus, as the stapedial artery initially lies between the foramen of the stapes and is lost before birth. If this regression fails it can lead to a persistent stapedial artery that will affect conduction through the middle ear ossicle chain. This condition can be seen in hemifacial microsomia (14q32), a reasonably common sporadic and rare familial autosomal dominant abnormality of the first and second pharyngeal arch derivatives (Carvalho, Song, Vargervik, & Lalwani, 1999).

The middle ear cavity itself can either be delayed in formation or size, leading to variable conduction effects. This can be seen with oligohydramnios caused by renal agenesis, such as in branchiootorenal syndrome (8q13.3).

Inner Ear

Inner ear cochlear and semicircular canal abnormalities are generally due to many different genetic effects and are both conducting and sensorineural related. In addition to specific gene mutations, the trisomies (chromosomal aneuploidy) have inner ear abnormalities. Infants with Trisomy 21 (Down syndrome) can have a range of conduction defects and reported more recently inner ear defects (Blaser et al., 2006). Infants with Trisomy 13 (Patau syndrome) can have both an underdeveloped cochlear duct and saccule. Infants with Trisomy 18 (Edwards syndrome) lack spiral ganglia and have other middle ear abnormalities.

Michel aplasia is an extremely rare abnormality showing complete absence of the inner ear labyrinth and can also be seen in the condition labyrinthine aplasia, microtia, and microdontia (LAMM) caused by mutations in the fibroblast growth factor 3 gene (11q13).

Pendred syndrome (7q31) is one of the most common (1 to 10% of hereditary deafness) inner ear deafness syndromes, autosomally recessive with abnormalities of the cochlea, enlarged vestibular aqueduct, sensorineural hearing loss, and diffuse thyroid enlargement (goiter; Phelps et al., 1998). The condition is caused by a mutation in the gene encoding an anion transporter (SLC26A4) protein called pendrin (Everett et al., 1997). More recently, a growing number of human genetic studies and animal model studies have identified gene mutations (OMIM 67 entries) that can impact general cochlear and specifically hair cell development.

Several examples of prenatal infections that impact inner ear development are also mentioned. Rubella is the most well-known viral infection with severe impact on hearing through effects on cochlear duct and saccular development (Vermeif-Keers, 1975). In some countries with poor vaccination records gestational rubella can be responsible for a significant proportion of reported deafness (Bento, Castilho, Sakae, Andrade, & Zugaib, 2005; Niedzielska, Katska, & Szymula, 2000). Other viral infections have also been shown to impact hearing: cytomegalovirus inner ear vascular effects and herpes simplex 2 viremia can cause both hemorrhagic and necrotic lesions. Toxoplasmosis infection caused by the protist *Toxoplasma gondii* being present in uncooked meat and contact with cat feces, is rarely serious postnatally in children or adults. In contrast, a maternally derived infection of the fetus can lead to spontaneous abortion and a range of developmental effects including deafness (Brown, Chau, Atashband, Westerberg, & Kozak, 2009).

This chapter has provided a brief introduction to the normal and abnormal development of hearing and the related genetic and environmental effects. Other chapters in this textbook will expand on the clinical aspects of these topics and additional disorders, as well as cover issues relating to neonatal hearing testing and diagnosis.

Acknowledgments. The author wishes to thank Judith Gravel, Richard Seewald, and Anne Marie Tharpe for the invitation to contribute this chapter. I also thank my wife Leighana for her understanding and support during preparation of this chapter. I apologize to any of my colleagues whose work was not cited in this review because of length constraints.

References

Andermann, P., Ungos, J., & Raible, D. W. (2002). Neurogenin1 defines zebrafish cranial sensory ganglia precursors. *Developmental Biology, 251*(1), 45–58.

Anniko, M., & Nordemar, H. (1980). Embryogenesis of the inner ear. IV. Post-natal maturation of the secretory epithelia of the inner ear in correlation with the elemental composition in the endolymphatic space. *Archives of Otolaryngology-Head and Neck Surgery, 229*(3–4), 281–288.

Anniko, M., & Wroblewski, R. (1981). Elemental composition of the developing inner ear. *Annals of Otology, Rhinology and Laryngology, 90*(1 Pt. 1), 25–32.

Arnold, W. (1987). Myelination of the human spiral ganglion. *Acta Otolaryngologica, Suppl., 436*, 76–84.

Bagger-Sjoback, D. (1991). Embryology of the human endolymphatic duct and sac. *Journal of Oto-Rhino-Laryngology and Its Related Specialties, 53*(2), 61–67.

Barrionuevo, F., Naumann, A., Bagheri-Fam, S., Speth, V., Taketo, M. M., Scherer, G., . . . Neubüser, A. (2008). Sox9 is required for invagination of the otic placode in mice. *Developmental Biology, 317*(1), 213–224.

Beisel, K. W., Wang-Lundberg, Y., Maklad, A., & Fritzsch, B. (2005). Development and evolution of the vestibular sensory apparatus of the mammalian ear. *Journal of Vestibular Research, 15*(5–6), 225–241.

Bento, R. F., Castilho, A. M., Sakae, F. A., Andrade, J. Q., & Zugaib, M. (2005). Auditory brainstem response and otoacoustic emission assessment of hearing-impaired children of mothers who contracted rubella during pregnancy. *Acta Otolaryngologica, 125*(5), 492–494.

Bernd, P., Zhang, D., Yao, L., & Rozenberg, I. (1994). The potential role of nerve growth factor, brain-derived neurotrophic factor and neurotrophin-3 in avian cochlear and vestibular ganglia development. *International Journal of Developmental Neuroscience, 12*(8), 709–723.

Bibas, A., Liang, J., Michaels, L., & Wright, A. (2000). The development of the stria vascularis in the human foetus. *Clinical Otolaryngology and Allied Sciences, 25*(2), 126–129.

Bibas, A. G., Xenellis, J., Michaels, L., Anagnostopoulou, S., Ferekidis, E., & Wright, A. (2008). Temporal bone study of development of the organ of Corti: Correlation between auditory function and anatomical structure. *Journal of Laryngology and Otology, 122*(4), 336–342.

Blaser, S., Propst, E. J., Martin, D., Feigenbaum, A., James, A. L., Shannon, P., . . . Papsin, B. C. (2006). Inner ear dysplasia is common in children with Down syndrome (trisomy 21). *Laryngoscope, 116*(12), 2113–2119.

Blasiole, B., Kabbani, N., Boehmler, W., Thisse, B., Thisse, C., Canfield, V., . . . Levenson, R. (2005). Neuronal calcium sensor-1 gene ncs-1a is essential for semicircular canal formation in zebrafish inner ear. *Journal of Neurobiology, 64*(3), 285–297.

Bosher, S. K., & Warren, R. L. (1971). A study of the electrochemistry and osmotic relationships of the cochlear fluids in the neonatal rat at the time of the development of the endocochlear potential. *Journal of Physiology, 212*(3), 739–761.

Brown, E. D., Chau, J. K., Atashband, S., Westerberg, B. D., & Kozak, F. K. (2009). A systematic review of neonatal toxoplasmosis exposure and sensorineural hearing loss. *International Journal of Pediatric Otorhinolaryngology, 73*(5), 707–711.

Bruska, M., & Wozniak, W. (2000). The origin of cells of the cochlear ganglion in early human embryos. *Folia Morphol (Warsz), 59*(4), 233–238.

Camarero, G., Avendano, C., Fernandez-Moreno, C., Villar, A., Contreras, J., de Pablo, F., . . . Varela-Nieto, I. (2001). Delayed inner ear maturation and neuronal loss in postnatal Igf-1-deficient mice. *Journal of Neuroscience*, *21*(19), 7630–7641.

Carvalho, G. J., Song, C. S., Vargervik, K., & Lalwani, A. K. (1999). Auditory and facial nerve dysfunction in patients with hemifacial microsomia. *Archives of Otolaryngology-Head and Neck Surgery*, *125*(2), 209–212.

Chang, W., Brigande, J. V., Fekete, D. M., & Wu, D. K. (2004). The development of semicircular canals in the inner ear: Role of FGFs in sensory cristae. *Development*, *131*(17), 4201–4211.

Chiong, C. M., Burgess, B. J., & Nadol, J. B., Jr. (1993). Postnatal maturation of human spiral ganglion cells: Light and electron microscopic observations. *Hearing Research*, *67*(1–2), 211–219.

Church, M. W., & Abel, E. L. (1998). Fetal alcohol syndrome. Hearing, speech, language, and vestibular disorders. *Obstetrics and Gynecology Clinics of North America*, *25*(1), 85–97.

Conlee, J. W., Gerity, L. C., & Bennett, M. L. (1994). Ongoing proliferation of melanocytes in the stria vascularis of adult guinea pigs. *Hearing Research*, *79*(1–2), 115–122.

Counter, S. A., Hellstrand, E., & Borg, E. (1987). A histochemical characterization of muscle fiber types in the avian M. stapedius. *Comparative Biochemistry and Physiology A*, *86*(1), 185–187.

Cristobal, R., Popper, P., Lopez, I., Micevych, P., De Vellis, J., & Honrubia, V. (2002). In vivo and in vitro localization of brain-derived neurotrophic factor, fibroblast growth factor-2 and their receptors in the bullfrog vestibular end organs. *Brain Research Molecular Brain Research*, *102*(1–2), 83–99.

Daudet, N., Ariza-McNaughton, L., & Lewis, J. (2007). Notch signalling is needed to maintain, but not to initiate, the formation of prosensory patches in the chick inner ear. *Development*, *134*(12), 2369–2378.

Everett, L. A., Glaser, B., Beck, J. C., Idol, J. R., Buchs, A., Heyman, M., . . . Green, E. D. (1997). Pendred syndrome is caused by mutations in a putative sulphate transporter gene (PDS). *Nature Genetics*, *17*(4), 411–422.

Fekete, D. M., & Campero, A. M. (2007). Axon guidance in the inner ear. *International Journal of Developmental Biology*, *51*(6–7), 549–556.

Fritzsch, B., Pirvola, U., & Ylikoski, J. (1999). Making and breaking the innervation of the ear: Neurotrophic support during ear development and its clinical implications. *Cell Tissue Research*, *295*(3), 369–382.

Grunder, S., Muller, A., & Ruppersberg, J. P. (2001). Developmental and cellular expression pattern of epithelial sodium channel alpha, beta and gamma subunits in the inner ear of the rat. *European Journal of Neuroscience*, *13*(4), 641–648.

Hafidi, A., & Dulon, D. (2004) Developmental expression of Ca(v)1.3 (alpha1d) calcium channels in the mouse inner ear. *Brain Research Developmental Brain Research*, *150*(2), 167–175.

Hatch, E. P., Noyes, C. A., Wang, X., Wright, T. J., & Mansour, S. L. (2007). Fgf3 is required for dorsal patterning and morphogenesis of the inner ear epithelium. *Development*, *134*(20), 3615–3625.

Hertzano, R., Montcouquiol, M., Rashi-Elkeles, S., Elkon, R., Yucel, R., Frankel, W. N., . . . Avraham, K. B. (2004). Transcription profiling of inner ears from Pou4f3(ddl/ddl) identifies Gfi1 as a target of the Pou4f3 deafness gene. *Human Molecular Genetics*, *13*(18), 2143–2153.

Hossain, W. A., Brumwell, C. L., & Morest, D. K. (2002). Sequential interactions of fibroblast growth factor-2, brain-derived neurotrophic factor, neurotrophin-3, and their receptors define critical periods in the development of cochlear ganglion cells. *Experimental Neurology*, *175*(1), 138–151.

Jenkinson, J. W. (1911). The development of the ear-bones in the mouse. *Journal of Anatomy and Physiology*, *45*(Pt. 4), 305–318.

Johnson, R. L., & Spoendlin, H. H. (1966). Structural evidence of secretion in the stria vascularis. *Annals of Otology, Rhinology and Laryngology*, *75*(1), 127–138.

Kelley, M. W. (2007). Cellular commitment and differentiation in the organ of Corti. *International Journal of Developmental Biology*, *51*(6–7), 571–583.

Kwak, S. J., Vemaraju, S., Moorman, S. J., Zeddies, D., Popper, A. N., & Riley, B. B. (2006). Zebrafish pax5 regulates development of the utricular macula and vestibular function. *Developmental Dynamics*, *235*(11), 3026–3038.

Lavigne-Rebillard, M., & Bagger-Sjoback, D. (1992). Development of the human stria vascularis. *Hearing Research*, *64*(1), 39–51.

Levi-Montalcini, R. (1949). The development to the acoustico-vestibular centers in the chick embryo in the absence of the afferent root fibers and of descending fiber tracts. *Journal of Comprehensive Neurology*, *91*(2), 209–241.

Lyon, M. J., & Malmgren, L. T. (1982). A histochemical characterization of muscle fiber types in the middle ear muscles of the cat. 1. The stapedius muscle. *Acta Otolaryngologica*, *94*(1–2), 99–109.

Lyon, M. J., & Malmgren, L. T. (1988). Muscle fiber types in the cat middle ear muscles. II. Tensor tympani. *Archives of Otolaryngology-Head and Neck Surgery*, *114*(4), 404–409.

Masetto, S., Zucca, G., Botta, L., & Valli, P. (2005). Endolymphatic potassium of the chicken vestibule during embryonic development. *International Journal of Developmental Neuroscience*, *23*(5), 439–448.

Moore, J. K., & Linthicum, F. H., Jr. (2001). Myelination of the human auditory nerve: different time courses for Schwann cell and glial myelin. *Annals of Otology, Rhinology and Laryngology*, *110*(7 Pt. 1), 655–661.

Nemzek, W. R., Brodie, H. A., Chong, B. W., Babcook, C. J., Hecht, S. T., Salamat, S., . . . Seibert, J. A. (1996). Imaging findings of the developing temporal bone in fetal specimens. *AJNR American Journal of Neuroradiology*, *17*(8), 1467–1477.

Ng, M. (2000). Postnasal maturation of the human endolymphatic sac. *Laryngoscope*, *110*(9), 1452–1456.

Ng, M., & Linthicum, F. H. (1998). Morphology of the developing human endolymphatic sac. *Laryngoscope, 108*(2), 190–194.

Niedzielska, G., Katska, E., & Szymula, D. (2000). Hearing defects in children born of mothers suffering from rubella in the first trimester of pregnancy. *International Journal of Pediatric Otorhinolaryngology, 54*(1), 1–5.

Nin, F., Hibino, H., Doi, K., Suzuki, T., Hisa, Y., & Kurachi, Y. (2008). The endocochlear potential depends on two K+ diffusion potentials and an electrical barrier in the stria vascularis of the inner ear. *Proceedings of the National Academy of Sciences, USA, 105*(5), 1751–1756.

Nishimura, Y., & Kumoi, T. (1992). The embryologic development of the human external auditory meatus. Preliminary report. *Acta Otolaryngologica, 112*(3), 496–503.

Okano, J., Takigawa, T., Seki, K., Suzuki, S., Shiota, K., & Ishibashi, M. (2005). Transforming growth factor beta 2 promotes the formation of the mouse cochleovestibular ganglion in organ culture. *International Journal of Developmental Biology, 49*(1), 23–31.

Omata, Y., Nojima, Y., Nakayama, S., Okamoto, H., Nakamura, H., & Funahashi, J. (2007). Role of Bone morphogenetic protein 4 in zebrafish semicircular canal development. *Developmental Growth and Differentiation, 49*(9), 711–719.

Orliaguet, T., Darcha, C., Dechelotte, P., & Vanneuville, G. (1994). Meckel's cartilage in the human embryo and fetus. *Anatomical Record, 238*(4), 491–497.

Parazzini, M., Ravazzani, P., Medaglini, S., Weber, G., Fornara, C., Tognola, G., . . . Grandori, F. (2002). Click-evoked otoacoustic emissions recorded from untreated congenital hypothyroid newborns. *Hearing Research, 166*(1–2), 136–142.

Paulsen, K. (1973). Otological features in exomphalos-macroglossia-gigantism syndrome (Wiedemann's syndrome). *Z Laryngology Rhinology and Otology, 52*(11), 793–798.

Phelps, P. D., Coffey, R. A., Trembath, R. C., Luxon, L. M., Grossman, A. B., Britton, K. E., . . . Reardon, W. (1998). Radiological malformations of the ear in Pendred syndrome. *Clinical Radiology, 53*(4), 268–273.

Pujol, R., & Lavigne-Rebillard, M. (1985). Early stages of innervation and sensory cell differentiation in the human fetal organ of Corti. *Acta Otolaryngologica, Suppl., 423*, 43–50.

Represa, J. J., Moro, J. A., Gato, A., Pastor, F., & Barbosa, E. (1990). Patterns of epithelial cell death during early development of the human inner ear. *Annals of Otology, Rhinology and Laryngology, 99*(6 Pt. 1), 482–488.

Rueda, J., Prieto, J. J., Cantos, R., Sala, M. L., & Merchan, J. A. (2003). Hypothyroidism prevents developmental neuronal loss during auditory organ development. *Neuroscience Research, 45*(4), 401–408.

Sage, C., Huang, M., Vollrath, M. A., Brown, M. C., Hinds, P. W., Corey, D. P., . . . Chen, Z. Y. (2006). Essential role of retinoblastoma protein in mammalian hair cell development and hearing. *Proceedings of the National Academy of Sciences, USA, 103*(19), 7345–7350.

Sanchez Del Rey, A., Sanchez Fernandez, J. M., Martinez Ibarguen, A., & Santaolalla Montoya, F. (1995). Morphologic and morphometric study of human spiral ganglion development. *Acta Otolaryngologica, 115*(2), 211–217.

Schimmang, T., Tan, J., Muller, M., Zimmermann, U., Rohbock, K., Kopschall, I., . . . Knipper, M. (2003). Lack of Bdnf and TrkB signalling in the postnatal cochlea leads to a spatial reshaping of innervation along the tonotopic axis and hearing loss. *Development, 130*(19), 4741–4750.

Senel, E., Kocak, H., Akbiyik, F., Saylam, G., Gulleroglu, B. N., & Senel, S. (2009). From a branchial fistula to a branchiootorenal syndrome: A case report and review of the literature. *Journal of Pediatric Surgery, 44*(3), 623–625.

Sobkowicz, H. M., Slapnick, S. M., & August, B. K. (2002). Differentiation of spinous synapses in the mouse organ of corti. *Synapse, 45*(1), 10–24.

Sohmer, H., Perez, R., Sichel, J. Y., Priner, R., & Freeman, S. (2001). The pathway enabling external sounds to reach and excite the fetal inner ear. *Audiology and Neuro-Otology, 6*(3), 109–116.

Solomon, K. S., Kwak, S. J., & Fritz, A. (2004). Genetic interactions underlying otic placode induction and formation. *Developmental Dynamics, 230*(3), 419–433.

Streeter, G. L. (1942) Developmental horizons in human embryos: Description of age group XI, 13 to 20 somites and age group XII, 21 to 29 somites. *Contributions to Embryology, 30*, 211–245.

Streeter, G. L. (1948) Developmental horizons in human embryos: Description of age groups XV, XVI, XVII and XVIII, being the third issue of a survey of the Carnegie Collection. *Contributions to Embryology, 32*, 133–203.

Streeter, G. L. (1951) Developmental horizons in human embryos: Description of age groups XIX, XX, XXI, XXII and XXIII, being the fifth issue of a survey of the Carnegie Collection. *Contributions to Embryology, 34*, 165–196.

Supp, D. M., Karpinski, A. C., & Boyce, S. T. (2004). Expression of human beta-defensins HBD-1, HBD-2, and HBD-3 in cultured keratinocytes and skin substitutes. *Burns, 30*(7), 643–648.

Suzuki, T., Nomoto, Y., Nakagawa, T., Kuwahata, N., Ogawa, H., Suzuki, Y., . . . Omori, K. (2006). Age-dependent degeneration of the stria vascularis in human cochleae. *Laryngoscope, 116*(10), 1846–1850.

Swarts, J. D., Rood, S. R., & Doyle, W. J. (1986). Fetal development of the auditory tube and paratubal musculature. *Cleft Palate Journal, 23*(4), 289–311.

Thyng, F. W. (1914). The anatomy of a 17.8mm human embryo. *American Journal of Anatomy, 14*, 31–113.

Ulatowska-Blaszyk, K., & Bruska, M. (1999). The cochlear ganglion in human embryos of developmental stages 18 and 19. *Folia Morphol (Warsz), 58*(1), 29–35.

Vermeif-Keers, C. (1975). Primary congenital aphakia and the rubella syndrome. *Teratology, 11*(3), 257–265.

Vita, G., Muglia, U., Germana, G., Pennica, F., & Carfi, F. (1983). Histochemical characteristics of rabbit stapedius muscle. *Experimental Neurology, 81*(2), 511–516.

Waka, N., Knipper, M., & Engel, J. (2003). Localization of the calcium channel subunits Cav1.2 (alpha1C) and Cav2.3 (alpha1E) in the mouse organ of Corti. *Histology and Histopathology, 18*(4), 1115–1123.

Wei, D., Jin, Z., Jarlebark, L., Scarfone, E., & Ulfendahl, M. (2007). Survival, synaptogenesis, and regeneration of adult mouse spiral ganglion neurons in vitro. *Developmental Neurobiology*, *67*(1), 108–122.

Werner, L. A. (2007). Issues in human auditory development. *Journal of Communication Disorders*, *40*(4), 275–283.

Whyte, J., Cisneros, A., Yus, C., Obon, J., Whyte, A., Serrano, P., . . . Vera, A. (2008). Development of the dynamic structure (force lines) of the middle ear ossicles in human foetuses. *Histology and Histopathology*, *23*(9), 1049–1060.

Whyte Orozco, J., Cisneros Gimeno, A. I., Urieta Carpi, J. J., Yus Gotor, C., Ganet Sole, J., Torres del Puerto, A., . . . Sarrat Torreguitart, R. (2003). [Ontogenic peculiarities of the human tympanic ossicular chain]. *Acta Otorrinolaringol Esp.*, *54*(1), 1–10.

Wikstrom, S. O., & Anniko, M. (1987). Early development of the stato-acoustic and facial ganglia. *Acta Otolaryngologica*, *104*(1–2), 166–174.

Wood-Jones, F., & Wen, I. C. (1934). The development of the external ear. *Journal of Anatomy*, *68*(Pt. 4), 525–533.

Wright, C. G. (1997). Development of the human external ear. *Journal of the American Academy of Audiology*, *8*(6), 379–382.

Yasuda, M., Yamada, S., Uwabe, C., Shiota, K., & Yasuda, Y. (2007). Three-dimensional analysis of inner ear development in human embryos. *Anatomical Science International*, *82*(3), 156–163.

Yokoyama, T., Iino, Y., Kakizaki, K., & Murakami, Y. (1999). Human temporal bone study on the postnatal ossification process of auditory ossicles. *Laryngoscope*, *109*(6), 927–930.

Zheng, J. L., Shou, J., Guillemot, F., Kageyama, R., & Gao, W. Q. (2000). Hes1 is a negative regulator of inner ear hair cell differentiation. *Development*, *127*(21), 4551–4560.

2

Development of the Auditory System From Periphery to Cortex

Robert V. Harrison

Introduction

At birth, the human cochlea is almost fully developed; however, the central auditory pathways are definitely not "ready to go" from day one. The system takes over a decade for its maturation and, even beyond then, "plasticity" in some auditory brain areas continues throughout life. In pediatric audiology, the important questions are not only about how hearing loss affects an infant's immediate communication skills, but also about the long-term impact of early impairment on the development of the auditory brain. Importantly, before we can optimize interventions for hearing loss in children, we must fully appreciate the developmental processes that the treatment or therapy will impact, and how we can take advantage of this development. One obvious example of how we already capitalize on auditory development is the cochlear implantation of congenitally deaf infants. Our knowledge of age-related plasticity has prompted us to pursue early detection of hearing loss through newborn hearing screening, and to provide an implant as early as possible. We now appreciate that the auditory system specifically develops to take advantage of the very limited sound information provided by an implant device, such that eventually communication ability in such children approaches normal.

This chapter provides an outline of important stages in the normal development of the auditory system, as well as describe how hearing loss can influence such development. The coverage will deal with fundamental physiologic concepts rather than specific clinical issues, which are comprehensively covered in other sections of this handbook. The chapter describes some basic aspects of developmental plasticity in the auditory system and discusses associated concepts, such as age-related plasticity and whether there are sensitive periods during development. This provides a useful background to later chapters in this handbook dealing with hearing loss and child development, and the early identification of hearing loss in childhood.

The Beginning and the End of Hearing Development

Perhaps the first task in considering the development of the auditory system is to define a starting point and to ask when we first hear. This question is more philosophical than biological, not least because it depends on what we mean by "hear." Does hearing start when cochlear hair cells can first be activated by acoustic signals? If we can detect that neurons in the auditory brainstem are excited by acoustic stimuli (e.g., with auditory brain stem response [ABR] tests) or if we can record middle latency responses from auditory cortex, does that imply "hearing" or do we require behavioral evidence? Even if there is a behavioral response such as a head orientation or an eye blink (startle) reflex, is this "hearing" or do we need proof of conscious perception of sound? Determination of when we first hear sound is not so simple, and when a question is posed such as, "Can my baby hear in utero?" the answer is not so easy.

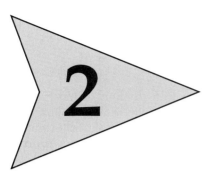

At the other end of the developmental time continuum, we can also ask when the development of the auditory system is complete. If we consider simple patterns of neural activity in primary auditory cortex we might say at age 1 to 2 years in humans. If we consider more complex processing in core auditory areas, we can consider late puberty to be a significant end point. However, as we must all recognize, higher levels of cortex, including auditory memory, speech/language regions and speech motor areas are always developing, always "plastic." If we consider that brain neuroplasticity is the norm, then the development of the auditory system never really ends. In between these not so easily defined endpoints, we do have a mainline auditory system development, which has been studied anatomically and physiologically in various animal models, and which in humans can be monitored by various test methods.

In the context of pediatric audiology, we obviously need to understand the system development and, most importantly, appreciate the concept of age-related plasticity in the auditory system. In other words, how does the plasticity (the ability of neural networks to remodel) of the developing auditory system reduce over time. Furthermore, we need to recognize that there might be sensitive (or critical) periods during development such that intervention strategies can be planned for maximal benefit. In this chapter we first consider some important developmental epochs at the level of the inner ear, including when cochlear hair cells connect up with the brain, when other components of the organ of Corti (e.g., tectorial membrane) are ready to optimally activate hair cells and thus when environmental acoustic stimuli can effectively activate the cochlea. This is followed by a brief description of central auditory pathway development up to core auditory cortex based on both animal models and human data. Some of the work reviewed relates to normal auditory system maturation, and other studies show us the effects of hearing impairment on system development. A particular emphasis is on research that indicates how acoustically driven activity of the auditory system acts to guide its development. In the final section, clinical issues that relate to developmental plasticity are discussed.

The Early Growth of the Auditory Periphery

The sequence of embryologic development of the inner ear has been extensively studied in various animal models and is well described in Chapter 1 of this volume. In the human, when cochlear hair cells start to differentiate within the otocyst (about 2 months after conception), there is evidence of the formation of presynaptic structures (Pujol, 1986). Within a few weeks the hair cells have formed synaptic connections with cochlear afferent neurons; however, hair cell function in terms of the transduction of mechanical stimuli lags behind. At this time the stereocilia are still not fully developed, and the final maturation of the tectorial membrane is incomplete (Lim & Anniko, 1986). Figures 2–1, 2–2, and 2–3 illustrate some salient features of tectorial membrane development. Note in particular that both inner hair cells (IHCs) and outer hair cells (OHCs) are well differentiated and innervated long before the tectorial membrane has grown into position. Before this time, hair cells may transduce some mechanical signals, but the role of OHCs as a biomechanical amplifier, and the normal mode of stimulation of the IHCs (fluid streaming in the subtectorial space) is not possible. As a result low threshold signal detection and cochlear frequency selectivity is not evident until late stages of gestation.

When an animal is born, the state of these important developmental stages differs considerably between species. Many altricious mammals are born in an immature state (e.g., mice and rats) and have a postnatal onset of hearing. On the other hand the human is a relatively precocious species and has a well-developed cochlea at birth similar to, for example, the chinchilla (which makes the latter an appropriate animal model for studies related to human auditory development). To illustrate such species differences Figure 2–2 shows the sensory epithelium of the mouse cochlea at birth compared with that of the chinchilla.

In the mouse (left-hand panel) note the excessive tissue on the surfaces of cells surrounding the hair cells. This is evidence of the subtectorial meshwork, which after birth is still active in secreting and forming the tectorial membrane. At this stage the normal deflection of outer hair cell stereocilia by tectorial membrane or by fluid motion beneath it (to activate inner hair cells) is clearly not optimal. Contrast this to the sensory epithelium of the newborn chinchilla (right panel) where the subtectorial space (surface of the reticular lamina) is clear (Harrison, Cullen, Takeno, & Mount, 1996). Figure 2–3 summarizes the sequence of anatomical and functional development as the cochlea develops with specific reference to the human inner ear (Pujol, 1986; Romand, 1983).

Connecting the Cochlea to the Brain

Not only does the human cochlea function well before birth, but cochlear afferent connections from hair cells to the cochlear nucleus of the brainstem are also well established. Essentially the auditory nuclei of the

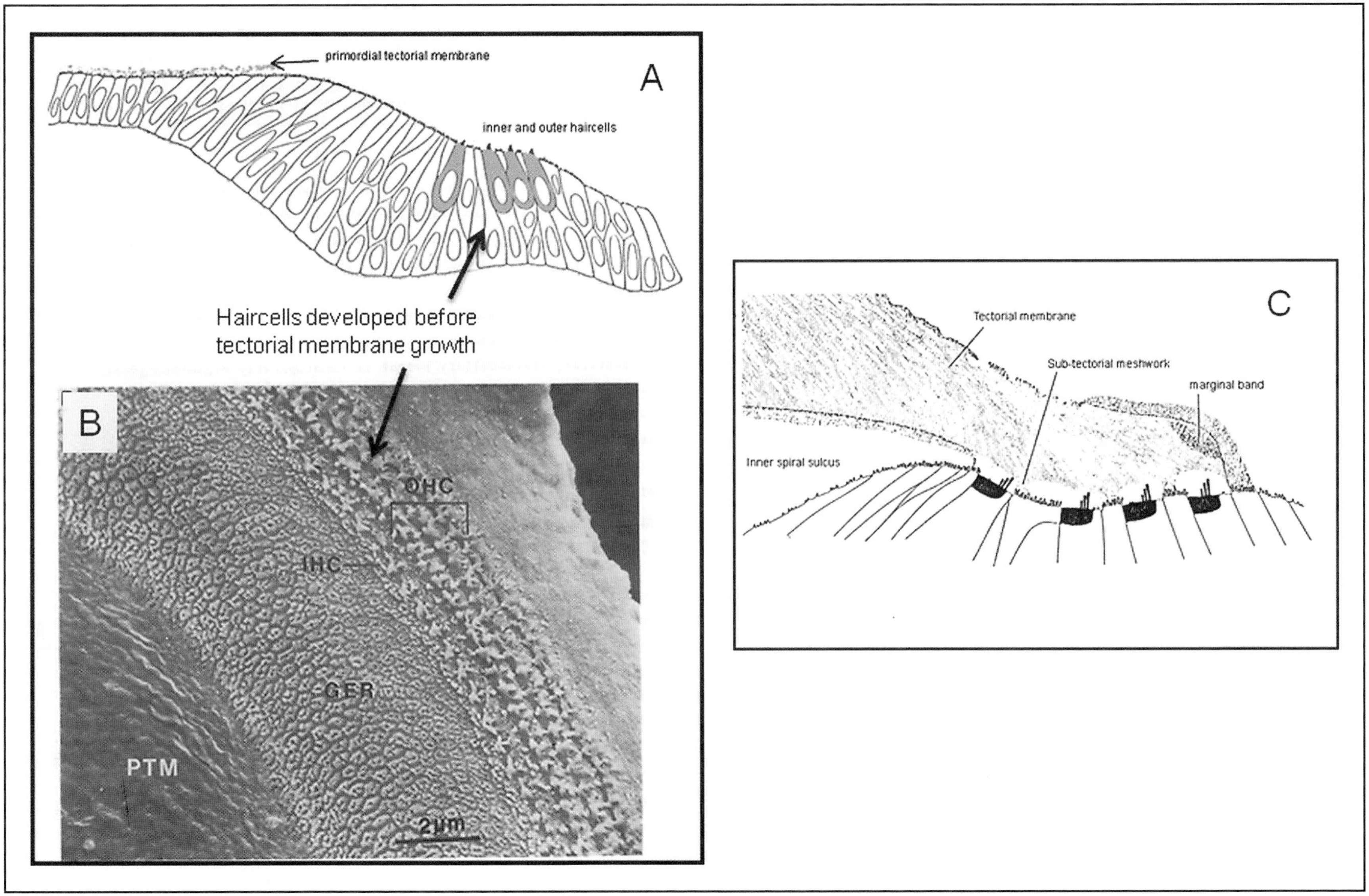

FIGURE 2–1. Some aspects of early tectorial membrane growth. **A.** Cross-sectional view at initial stage of membrane production. **B.** SEM view of immature sensory surface. **C.** Intermediate stage of membrane maturation. Adapted from data of Lim and Anniko (1986).

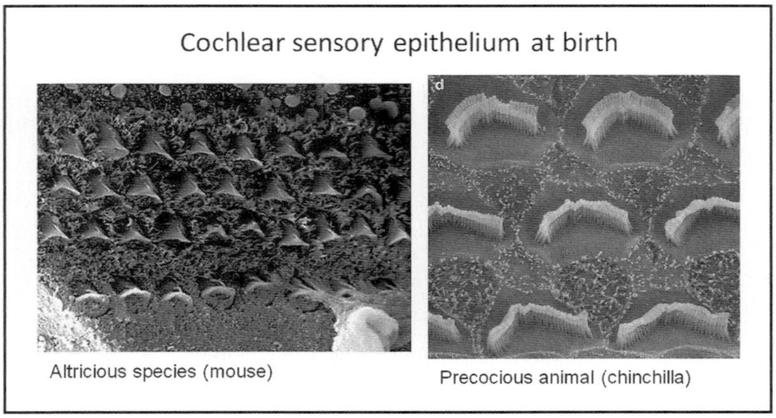

FIGURE 2–2. Scanning electron micrographs of the cochlear sensory epithelium, at birth, in an altricious species (mouse; *left panel*) compared with a precocious animal (chinchilla; *right panel*).

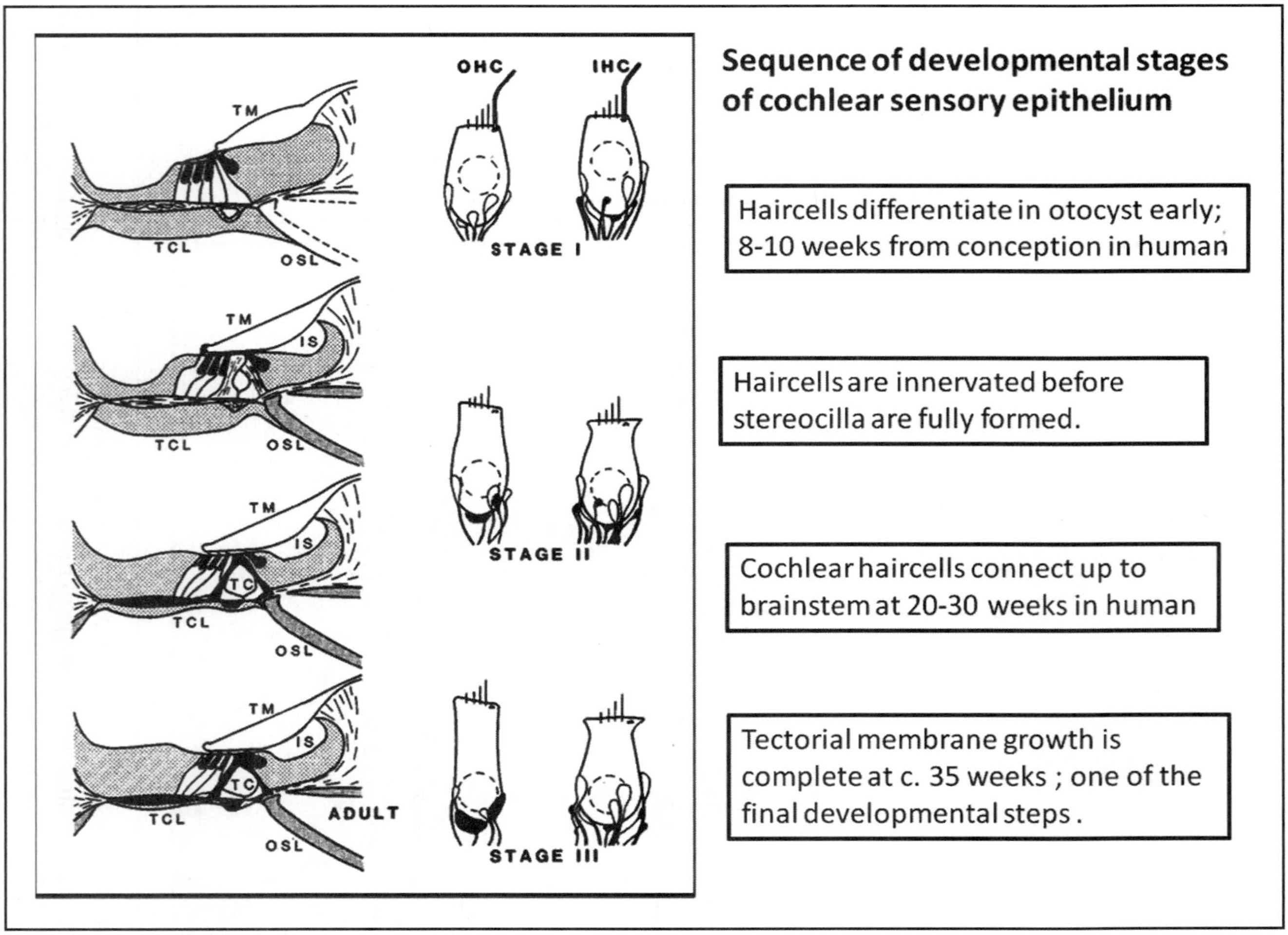

Sequence of developmental stages of cochlear sensory epithelium
Haircells differentiate in otocyst early; 8-10 weeks from conception in human
Haircells are innervated before stereocilla are fully formed.
Cochlear haircells connect up to brainstem at 20-30 weeks in human
Tectorial membrane growth is complete at c. 35 weeks ; one of the final developmental steps .
OHC
IHC
TM
TCL
OSL
IS
TC
STAGE I
STAGE II
STAGE III
ADULT

FIGURE 2–3. Timeline of some key anatomic changes to the organ of Corti during development. Cochlear afferents are unshaded; efferents are shaded. OHC, outer hair cell; IHC, inner hair cell; OSL, osseous spiral lamina; TC, tunnel of Corti; TCL, tympanic covering layer; TM, tectorial membrane. Based on data of Romand (1983) and Pujol (1986). Adapted with permission from R. Romand, (1983). *Development of the Auditory and Vestibular Systems* (Figure 3–3). New York, NY: Academic Press. Copyright Academic Press 1983.

brainstem and midbrain arise at about the same time as the inner ear formation. Immature neurons derived from the otocyst produce centrally directed processes, which grow toward, and split to send branches to the three brainstem areas that are to become anteroventral-cochlear nucleus (AVCN), posteroventral-cochlear nucleus (PVCN), and dorsal cochlear nucleus (DCN). These neurons connect hair cells along the cochlear length with target cells in the cochlear nucleus in a topographic fashion, resulting in the systematic tonotopic mapping seen in the mature subject. Strictly speaking, the neural projections should be described as cochleotopic rather than tonotopic, but most often (but not always) the terms can be interchanged. This ordered "wiring pattern" occurs before the system has auditory input, that is, before there is acoustically activated neural activity. However, there may be a role for spontaneous (intrinsically arising) neural activity in these early developmental stages. When the neural connections have been established, the maintenance and survival of target cells in cochlear nucleus does depend on activity in cochlear nerve whether intrinsic (spontaneous activity) or extrinsic (stimulus driven). For a more comprehensive review, see Rubel, Parks, and Zirpel (2004).

When Do We First "Hear"?

In humans, anatomic connections of cochlea to brain occur between 20 to 30 weeks of gestation (i.e., 10–20 weeks before birth; see Figure 2–3), and toward the end of that period there is some evidence of auditory function. For example, ABR waveforms can be measured in 15-week premature neonates (Graziani, Weitzman, & Velasco, 1968), and sound-evoked blink startle reflex (ultrasound imaging in utero) shows responses at 24 to 25 weeks gestational age (Birnholz & Benacerraf, 1983). As mentioned earlier, tectorial membrane maturation is required for low threshold cochlear activation and for cochlear frequency selectivity; these do not develop until 30 to 35 weeks of gestation. The sensory epithelium of mid-frequency regions of the cochlea are the first to develop and connect with the brainstem. The development of more apical and basal areas follows later such that even 6 months after birth, high and low frequency thresholds continue to improve (e.g., Olsho, 1986; Trehub, Schneider, & Endman, 1980). It is clear that mid-frequency regions of the cochlea and neural connections through much of the auditory pathway can be activated during the third trimester; however, does this mean that the unborn baby can "hear" in the normal perceptual sense, and if so, what can he or she possibly hear? Clearly environmental sounds will be much attenuated by the completely fluid-filled system. Normal middle-ear impedance matching mechanism will not work, and the cochlea will be essentially stimulated by something similar to a bone conduction pathway. On the other hand, maternal sounds (e.g., mother's voice and heart beat) will be somewhat effective as stimuli, as will acoustic signals directly applied to the body in the mode of a bone conduction hearing aid.

Central Auditory Pathway Development

At the same time that the cochlea is linking to the brainstem, more central nuclei in the superior olivary complex, auditory midbrain and thalamus are forming and connecting. In these locations, neuron formation and migration, axon outgrowth and synaptic connections to other target cells are also made before there is any acoustic driven activity, but there may be an important role for spontaneous activity in the system, especially for the consolidation of synapses. There does not appear to be any particular sequence of connectivity (e.g., from the peripheral to central), but rather there is overlapping development of connections, and both the ascending and descending neural pathways appear to be formed at the same time (Rubel et al., 2004). As is the case in the cochlear nucleus, more central connections are topographically organized so as to result in relatively good cochleotopic/tonotopic mapping throughout, and this initial order does not depend on stimulus driven neural activity (which is not yet present). Again it is likely that intrinsically arising (spontaneous) neural activity has a significant role (Lippe, 1994). Later on it is clear that acoustically driven neural signals will act to consolidate synaptic connections and refine cochleotopic projections. There is good evidence (some of which is reviewed below) that abnormal patterns of activity at the cochlear nerve level during an early postnatal period can have significant influence on tonotopic organization in central auditory areas.

Developmental Plasticity of the Binaural System

The earliest studies of plasticity in auditory system development were anatomic studies by Levi-Montalcini (1949) who demonstrated that unilateral otocyst removal (in chick embryo) resulted in very abnormal central auditory neuron projections. Many other more recent studies in mammals have similarly shown that unilateral cochlear ablation results in the development of unusual innervations patterns in the brainstem (e.g., Hashisaki & Rubel, 1989; Kitzes, 1984; Moore & Kitzes, 1985; Parks & Jackson, 1986). Example findings are illustrated in Figure 2–4. The left-hand panel shows some effects of neonatal cochlear ablation (in gerbil) on brainstem "wiring." During normal development, target neurons of the medial and lateral nuclei of the superior olive and the medial nucleus of the trapezoid body receive input from both cochleas, but after cochlear ablation these nuclei each receive two inputs originating from the same, unablated side (Kitzes, 1986). In the right-hand panel, we note that unilateral otocyst removal results in aberrant neural projections to central auditory nuclei (Parks & Jackson, 1986). The abnormal neural connections that result from neonatal cochlear ablation significantly change the response properties of neurons in the brainstem and midbrain, and needless to say these nuclei can no longer serve to compare input from two ears.

It might be supposed that there are few clinical situations in pediatric audiology where the extreme condition of complete unilateral profound hearing loss exists; however, consider an infant with a cochlear implant. In this case, from an early age (of cochlear implantation) there is effectively a unilateral auditory input stimulating the development of the auditory brain. There are some parallels between an infant with a cochlear implant and an animal model in which one cochlea operates whilst the other does not. Is it possible that some of the abnormal neural connections seen in animal models of unilateral cochlear ablation will arise in the unilaterally implanted infant? We do have to consider, as previously noted above, the issue of precocious (well-developed at birth) versus altricious species. For any infant given a cochlear implant, the new electrically generated activity patterns will be imposed on an already well-formed central auditory system and thus, might not produce the radically abnormal innervation patterns found in the animal models. On the other hand, if there has been no extrinsic input to an infant because of profound deafness, the system may still be awaiting consolidation by stimulus driven activity. If this comes from one side only final innervations patterns could be significantly abnormal.

Perhaps more clinically relevant are studies in which the balance of input to the two ears has been less extensively altered, for example by unilateral plugging (unilateral conductive hearing loss). Experimental manipulations like this have been shown, in some animal models, to result in significant impairment in bilateral function. For example, experiments in the barn owl (Knudsen, 1984; Knudsen, Esterly, & Knudsen, 1984) and in the ferret (Moore, Hutchings, King, & Kowalchuk, 1989; Moore, King, McAlpine, Martin, & Hutchings, 1993; Moore et al., 1999) show that early disruption by bilateral input can result in significant impairment of sound localization ability. In humans, the most common condition in which there is an unbalanced auditory input during early life is that resulting from chronic or recurring otitis media in infants. There is some evidence that such a condition can result in impaired auditory function (e.g., Hogan & Moore, 2003) and perhaps delays in language development. Another condition in which unbalanced auditory input could occur is when an infant is provided with unilateral hearing aid amplification. Of course, our standard practice for infant aiding is bilateral amplification because of the improved threshold sensitivity, signal detection in noise and sound localization. We could add a possible further benefit of providing a balanced binaural input during early system maturation. In summary, we can think of the auditory system as being a fully integrated binaural system that requires, during development (and perhaps later), a balanced input from both sides. Experimental or clinical situations when balanced input is not the case potentially will result in some degree of abnormal function. For readers interested in a more comprehensive review of the plasticity of binaural hearing, see Moore and King (2004).

Intrinsic Versus Extrinsic Influences During Development

Another concept to keep in mind when considering auditory system development is the issue of extrinsic versus intrinsic influences. Extrinsic means acoustically-driven neural activity from the periphery as opposed to intrinsically arising signals such as spontaneous discharge, activity from descending auditory pathways or, at the highest levels, corticocortical connections. Mention has already been made of the possible role of spontaneous neural activity in the formation and /or consolidation of synaptic connections in the auditory brainstem. In studies of the auditory brainstem there is some evidence that spontaneous discharge in cochlear afferent neurons (preceding any acoustically driven neural activity) appears to have a role in establishing central connections (e.g., Lippe, 1994). Similarly, in the visual system, retinal level spontaneous activity appears to have a role in central visual system development (e.g., Cang et al., 2005; Meister, Wong, Baylor, & Schatz,

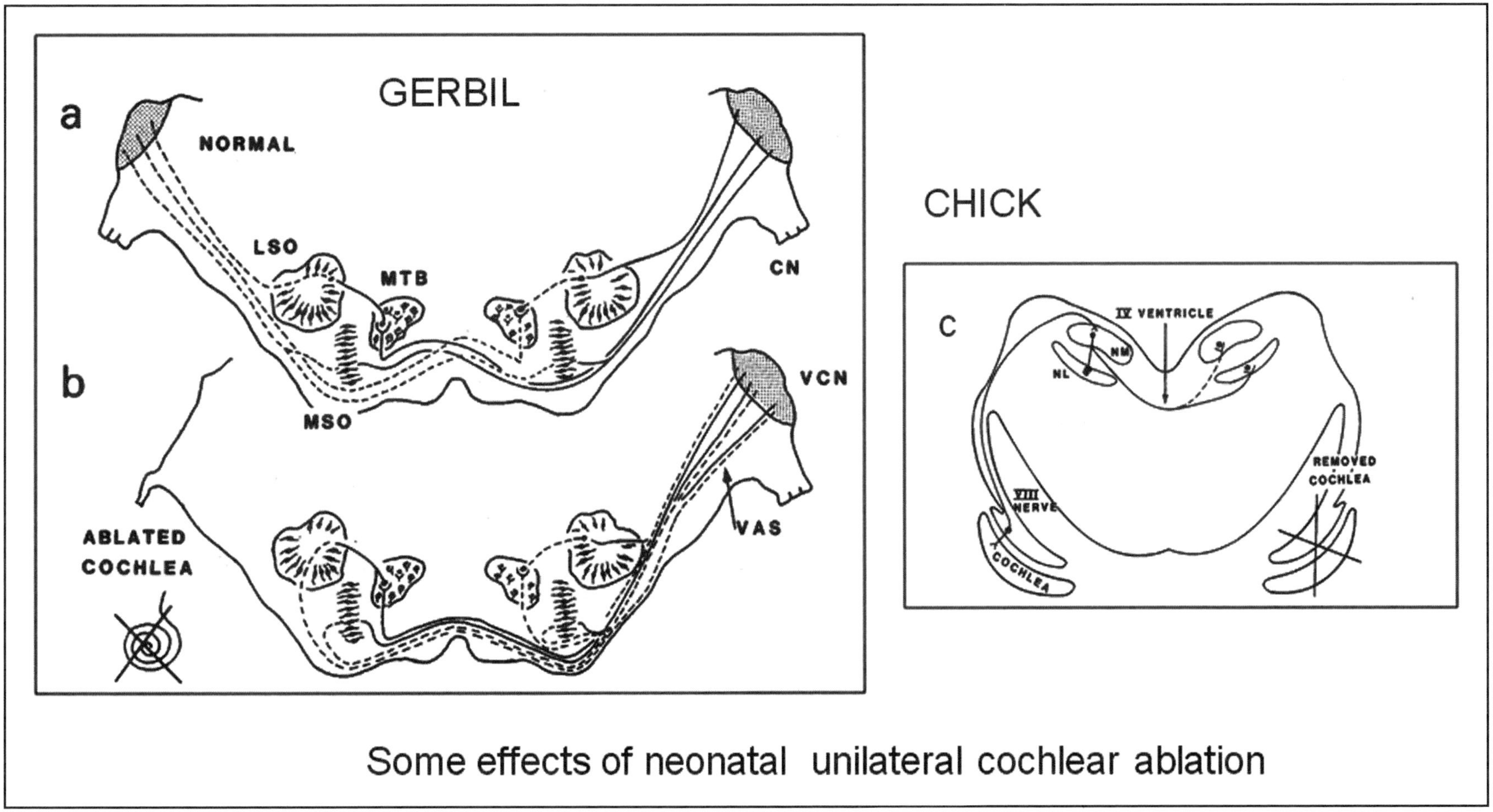

FIGURE 2–4. The effects of unilateral cochlear ablation on the development of neural pathways in the auditory brainstem. Left panel shows abnormal innervations in the superior olive of the gerbil. Adapted with permission from Kitzes (1986). The role of binaural innervations. In: Ruben, Van der Water, and Rubel (Eds.), *The Biology of Change in Otolaryngology* (p. 188). The Netherlands: Elsevier Press. Copyright Elsevier 1986. On the right, aberrant neural pathways after unilateral otocyst removal in the chick. CN, cochlear nerve; LSO, lateral superior olive; MSO, medial superior olive; MTB medial nucleus of trapezoid body; NL, nucleus laminaris; NM, nucleus magnocellularis; VAS ventral acoustic stria; VCN, ventral cochlear nucleus. Adapted with permission from Parks, and Jackson (1986). Early destruction of the inner ear induces formation. In: Ruben, Van der Water, Rubel, (Eds.), *The Biology of Change in Otolaryngology* (p. 226). The Netherlands: Elsevier Press. Copyright Elsevier 1986.

1991). At the level of cortex, other types of intrinsic signals have to be considered, not least activity from other sensory systems, and reciprocal connections with other brain systems. A detailed coverage is not possible here, but for useful discussion see reviews by Pallas (2001) and Newton and Sur (2005).

The Development of Auditory Connections at the Level of Cortex

The number of potential neural linkages and the corresponding complexity of auditory processing increase with ascending level in the auditory system. Up to the thalamic level the system is largely activated by auditory signals originating from the periphery. At the cortical level many more pathways of connectivity develop including projections to multimodal sensory cortex, speech areas, and to nonsensory regions such as memory, motor, and arousal systems; most of these connection pathways are reciprocal. Furthermore, it appears that system plasticity is greater at the cortical level (or at least maintained for longer) than in more peripheral auditory areas. We can gain an impression about the remarkable degree of this cortical plasticity, especially during early development, from experiments in which the sensory inputs to the cortex are rewired, as well as in demonstrations of crossmodal plasticity. In one type of sensory re-routing experiment, visual neurons from the retina have been directed to the early developing medial geniculate nucleus of the (auditory) thalamus (Roe, Pallas, Kwon, & Sur, 1992; Sharma, Angelucci, & Sur, 2000). As a result, cells in the auditory cortex are driven by visual input and develop visual response characteristics normally associated with primary visual cortex (e.g., retinotopic organization and visual contour orientation selectivity).

Such studies reveal how sensory areas that we normally assume to be "devoted" to one sense, can in fact take on a role for neural processing of a different sensory modality. We could say that the auditory cortex is not reserved for hearing. In experimental or natural circumstances when one modality of sensory input is absent, the cortical area normally associated with processing that sensory information becomes used to process some other sensory modality. For example, in congenitally blind humans the visual areas are driven by somatosensory input (Sadato et al., 1996) and also involved in auditory tasks (Kujala et al., 1997). Similarly, visual processing occurs in "auditory" cortical regions of congenitally deaf subjects (Neville, Schmidt, & Kutas, 1983). This extremely plastic reorganization ability in the cortex has some clinical implications. For example, if the auditory cortex of a congenitally deaf adult has been taken over for other functions, will there be adequate cortical space for processing if the subject is provided with a cochlear implant?

Evoked Potential Measures of Human Auditory System Development

Much has been learned about the maturational changes in the human auditory system by systematic studies of auditory evoked potential as a function of age. Some of the classic work in this regard has been documented by Eggermont and colleagues in normal infants and children (Eggermont, 1985, 1988; Eggermont & Salamy, 1988; Ponton, Eggermont, Kwong, & Don, 2000; see also review: Ponton & Eggermont, 2007). Complementary to such monitoring in normal hearing are studies of auditory evoked potentials elicited by electrical stimulation subjects with cochlear implants (e.g., Gordon, Papsin, & Harrison, 2003; Ponton, Don, Eggermont, Waring, & Masuda, 1996; Ponton & Eggermont, 2001; see also Chapter 27 in this volume on cochlear implants for children).

It is clear from these studies that, at birth, ABR and middle latency responses (MLR) from the thalamocortex can be detected, but all differ in amplitude and are longer in latency compared with the adult subject. During maturation, waveform peak latencies become reduced, with the earliest ABR waveform component from cochlear nerve having normal values within a few weeks of birth. Later components such as wave P5, originating from the auditory midbrain, continue to reduce in latency for many months after birth. These ABR changes during development are illustrated in the left panel of Figure 2–5.

On a longer time scale, auditory evoked cortical potentials continue to show modification for many years, in terms of increasing detectability, changes in amplitude and reduction in latency, being finally "mature" (adultlike in waveform morphology) in adolescent children. This is illustrated in Figure 2–5 (right-hand panel; Ponton & Eggermont, 2001). Note in particular the change, with increasing age, of the waveform shape from being one dominant positive peak in the two earliest age groups (5–7y, 8–9y), and thereafter the emergence of a second positive peak to the waveform. These very distinct changes clearly indicate that cortical maturational processes continue through adolescence. These cortical potential waveform changes approximate in time with neurofilament maturation in

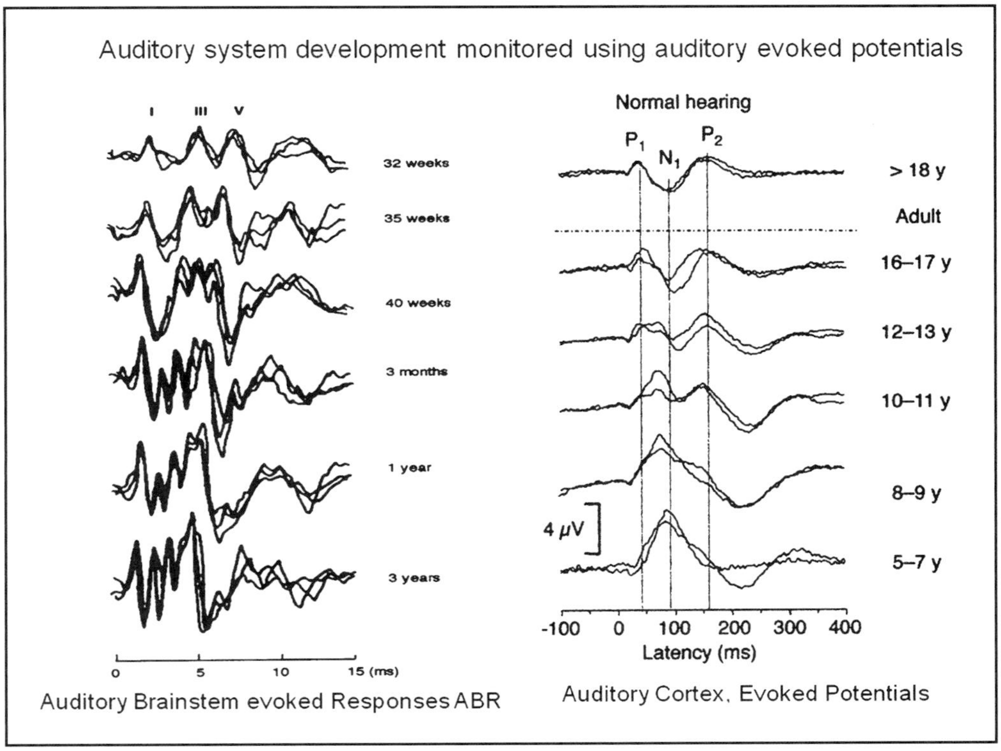

FIGURE 2–5. Auditory system maturation as revealed by auditory evoked potential recordings. *Left panel*, ABR waveforms in normal hearing infants of various ages. *Right panel*, evoked potential from auditory cortex in normal hearing children and adults of various ages. Adapted with permission from C. W Ponton & J. J. Eggermont, (2007). Electrophysiological measures of human auditory system maturation: Relationship with neuroanatomy and behavior. In R. F. Burkard, M. Don, & J. J. Eggermont (Eds.), *Auditory Evoked Potentials. Basic Principles and Clinical Application* (pp. 386, 392). Lippincott Williams and Wilkins. Copyright Lippincott Williams and Wilkins 2007.

deeper cortical layers as shown in human tissue studies by Moore (2002), and may be correlated in some way. Figure 2–6 illustrates the findings of the anatomical study by Moore (left panel). Note in particular the dense labeling in all cortical layers of the 11y specimen compared with those from younger subjects. Thus, we have both functional and anatomical evidence of the relatively lengthy time course of human auditory cortex development.

Another perspective on the developmental progression within the auditory system is to consider when different types of auditory evoked potentials are fully mature (i.e., have adultlike characteristics). As a rule of thumb, cochlear action potentials are mature within weeks of birth, and the ABR is adultlike within 3 to 5 years. Potentials from the thalamocortical input pathways (middle latency response) and the later auditory evoked cortical potentials are mature by about 14 years of age. Later auditory potentials originating in cortical areas beyond primary auditory cortex (e.g., P 300) can take up to 20 years to show full maturity.

These auditory evoked response studies have provided a general picture of the developmental changes in the auditory pathways. Latency and amplitude characteristics of waveform peaks reflect the number and synchronicity of underlying neurons activated by acoustic stimuli, and in general it can be concluded that throughout the system, with age, there is a decrease in neural transmission time, perhaps related to increased myelination of neurons or to increased efficacy of synaptic transmission. Increases in peak amplitudes in waveforms indicate increases in either number of neurons contributing, or more synchronized responses, or perhaps structural/orientation changes to auditory array pathways that create more effective dipole sources for scalp recorded signals. More detailed information

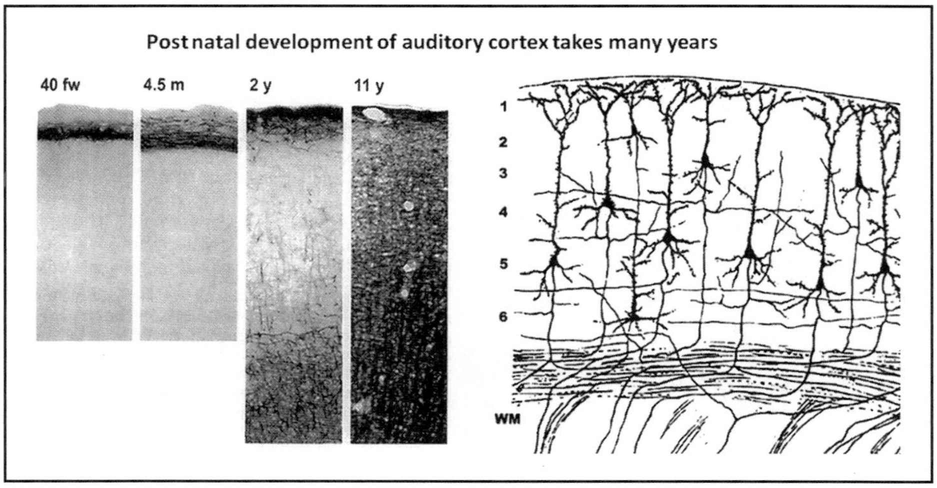

FIGURE 2–6. Long-term postnatal maturation of human auditory cortex. Left panel shows immunolabeled neurofilaments in section of cortical tissue from subjects at 40 fetal weeks (fw), 4.5 months (m), 2 years (y), and 11 years of age (Moore, 2002). For reference, the right panel shows the laminar organization of cortex from the classical work of Ramon and Cajal. Reprinted with permission from Moore, J. K. (2002). Maturation of human auditory cortex: Implications for speech perception. *Annals of Otology, Rhinoloy, Laryngoloy Supplementum, 189*, 7–10. Copyright Annals Publishing Company 2002.

about system development is difficult to judge from such "standard" electrophysiologic studies, not least because scalp recorded signals can have complex waveforms that reflect not only the number and synchronicity of neurons firing, but also on the (multiple) source distribution of contributing current sources. However, there have been many methodological refinements such as multichannel EEG recordings allowing dipole source analysis, and new technologies such as magnetoencephalography (MEG) and functional magnetic resonance imaging (fMRI). Systematic investigations using such tools undoubtedly will provide us with much more detail about human auditory system development.

Development, Maintenance, and Plasticity of Tonotopic Projections

Patterns of neural activity generated at the cochlear level are influential in the development, maintenance, and plasticity of the central auditory brain. When abnormal cochlear activity patterns exist from an early age, tonotopic (cochleotopic) map reorganization occurs in core auditory cortex. In addition, there is significant reorganization to frequency maps at subcortical levels, for example in the auditory thalamus and midbrain. In contrast when cochlear activity pattern changes are induced in an adult model (e.g., by partial cochlear deafferentation) there is reorganization of frequency maps in cortex, but little evidence of midbrain tonotopic map change suggesting an age-related plasticity at subcortical levels in the auditory system.

What Do We Mean by the Term "Plasticity"?

The term "plasticity" has been used by various authors to describe different aspects to brain function, and we should be careful to avoid making inappropriate comparisons of different types of "plasticity." Let us consider some of the different types of plasticity that have been reported. One obvious classification relates to the research methods used to demonstrate plastic change. Plasticity has been demonstrated in anatomical studies (e.g., abnormal neural structures, new or altered axonal pathways). Numerous types of functional studies have revealed plasticity including fMRI measures, evoked potential recordings and physiological experiments at cellular, membrane or ion channel levels. We also have a wide range of behavioral studies from standard audiologic tests through to detailed psychophysical studies that demonstrate plastic change.

Another important dimension of "plasticity" is its time course. Auditory system plasticity has been described over time spans from minutes and hours, through months and years. An example of rapid plasticity is the observation of auditory neuron receptive field alteration (both excitatory and inhibitory frequency tuning curves), which can occur within tens of minutes after induction of cochlear lesions, or partial deafferentation (e.g., Boettcher & Salvi, 1993; Wang, Salvi, & Powers, 1996). It is reasonable to suppose that short-term plastic change reflects relatively small-scale neural alterations, with subtle synaptic modifications to existing neural networks. More extensive auditory system reorganization appears to occur over a longer time course. This is clear from numerous electrophysiologic studies showing a modification of central tonotopic mapping as a result of cochlear lesions or partial deafferentation. In these studies the time course of plastic change appears to be completed over many weeks or months. In such cases very extensive reorganization is often observed, which suggests that long-term processes such as new axonal growth and synaptogenesis have occurred in addition to a consolidation of synaptic changes. To use a computer analogy, short-term plasticity might be considered to be software changes, whereas long-term changes might also include hardwiring modifications.

Most importantly, we should be careful to distinguish the neural plasticity during early development, as opposed to that occurring in the mature subject. It is age related or developmental plasticity that relates most directly to this pediatric audiology text. As mentioned below in relation to tonotopic map reorganization after cochlear lesions, more extensive and also subcortical changes are found when the system input is altered during early development compared to in the adult. In considering animal studies of developmental plasticity, it is important to note, as already emphasized, whether the species is altricious or precocious. The human (peripheral) auditory system is well developed at birth and an animal model of choice would be a precocious species such as chinchilla.

Reorganization of Tonotopic Maps After Cochlear Lesions

Cochleotopic projections can be considered as a mainline organizational feature of the auditory system. Just as the sensory epithelium of the skin surface or the retina has orderly central projections, so too in the auditory system, the topographical order of afferent neurons is well maintained from the sensory epithelium of the cochlea up to cortex (e.g., Merzenich & Brugge, 1973; Reale & Imig, 1980). Strictly speaking, we should refer to this projection system as cochleotopic, in analogy with the similarly organized retinotopic visual system and the somatotopic pathways of the somatosensory system. The interchangeability of the terms "cochleotopic" and "tonotopic" is possible because of the place coding of sound frequency along the cochlear length. However, some caution is advised on the interchangeability of these terms when considering systems having pathologic cochleas; under such conditions, considerable distortion of the normal place coding of sound frequency is possible. The term tonotopic becomes somewhat inappropriate when considering a cochlea electrically stimulated with an electrode array!

The tonotopic map in primary auditory cortex of a normal cat, as determined by recording from cortical neurons at several sites, is shown in Figure 2–7 (Harrison, Nagasawa, Smith, Stanton, & Mount, 1991). Each data point indicates the microelectrode recording site, and the sound frequency to which neuron(s) respond best (characteristic frequency, CF) is indicated in kHz. The isofrequency contours that are drawn through the cortical map are plotted at octave intervals. The right panel simply illustrates the necessary "point-to-point" neural projection system from the cochlear sensory epithelium to achieve the orderly tonotopic mapping at the level of cortex.

Figure 2–8 shows the cortical tonotopic map treated at birth with amikacin, an aminoglycoside antibiotic, which is ototoxic in high concentration. Such treatment results in (bilateral) cochlear hair cell degeneration, particularly in basal (high frequency) regions. In this case, histological examination of the cochlea showed that the basal region of the cochlea was totally damaged (both inner and outer hair cells destroyed), but in more apical areas, above the 6- to 8-kHz region, a normal sensory epithelium was present. This is consistent with the cat's ABR audiogram, which indicates a high frequency hearing loss to sound frequencies above 6 to 8 kHz, but normal response thresholds to lower stimulus frequencies.

The cortical tonotopic map for this subject map is characterized by a normal representation of low frequencies, up to 6 kHz, consistent with a histologically normal apical cochlear region and corresponding normal ABR thresholds. However, the cortical region that has been deprived of normal input by the partial cochlear deafferentation now contains neurons that are all tuned to 6 to 8 kHz (shown as the cross-hatched area).

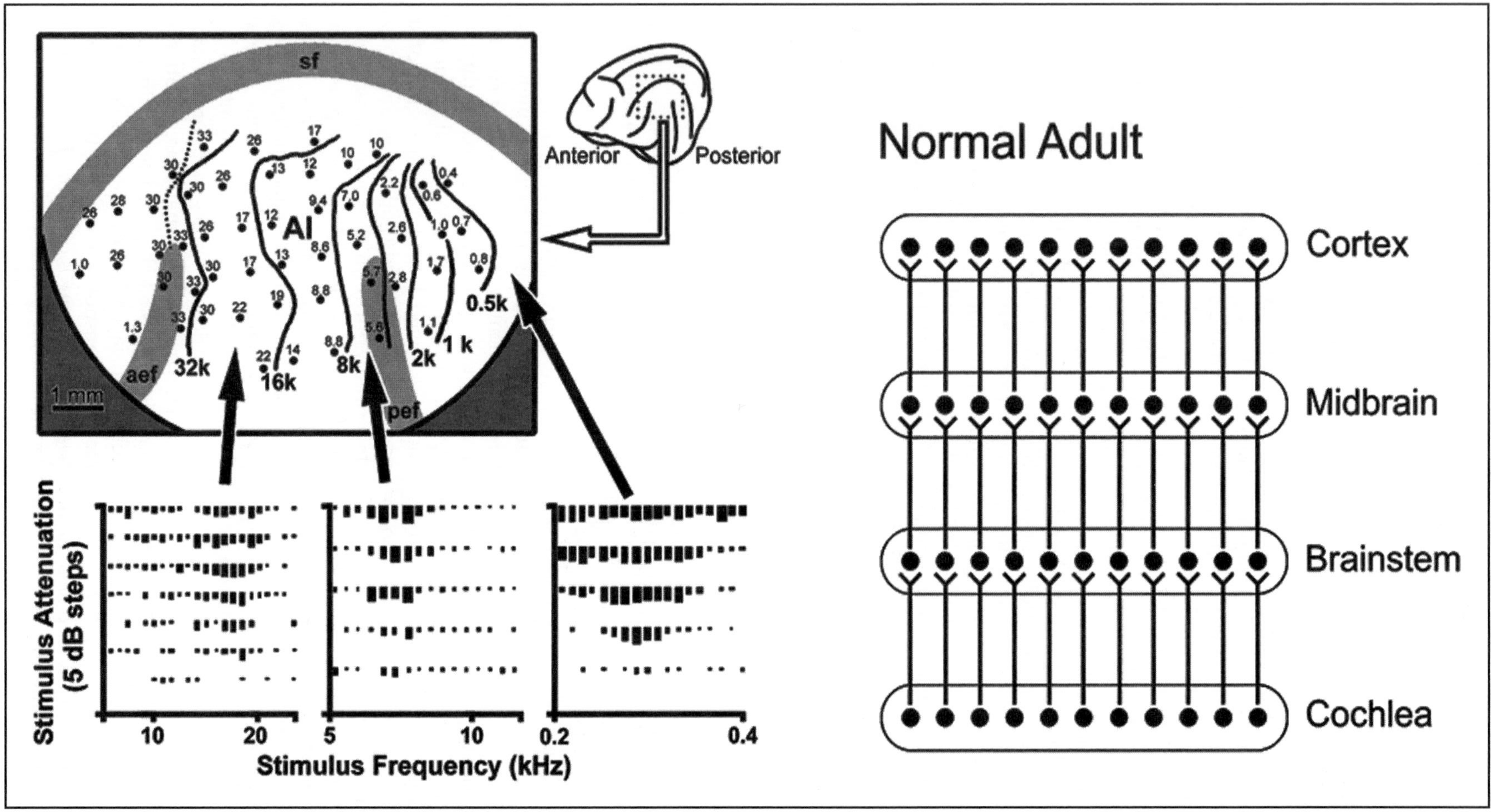

FIGURE 2–7. Cochleotopic or tonotopic map in normal cat auditory cortex as determined by single unit mapping (Harrison et al., 1991). At each indicated electrode position, the frequency tuning of neural units is determined from receptive field raster plots as indicated (*lower panels; three example neurons*). The stimulus frequency that evokes a response at minimum threshold (characteristic frequency; CF) is indicated on the tonotopic map in kHz. Isofrequency contours shown are at octave intervals. sf: sylvian fissure; aef: anterior ectosylvian fissue; pef: posterior ectosylvian fissure. The neural projection system from cochlea to cortex is shown schematically in the right panel.

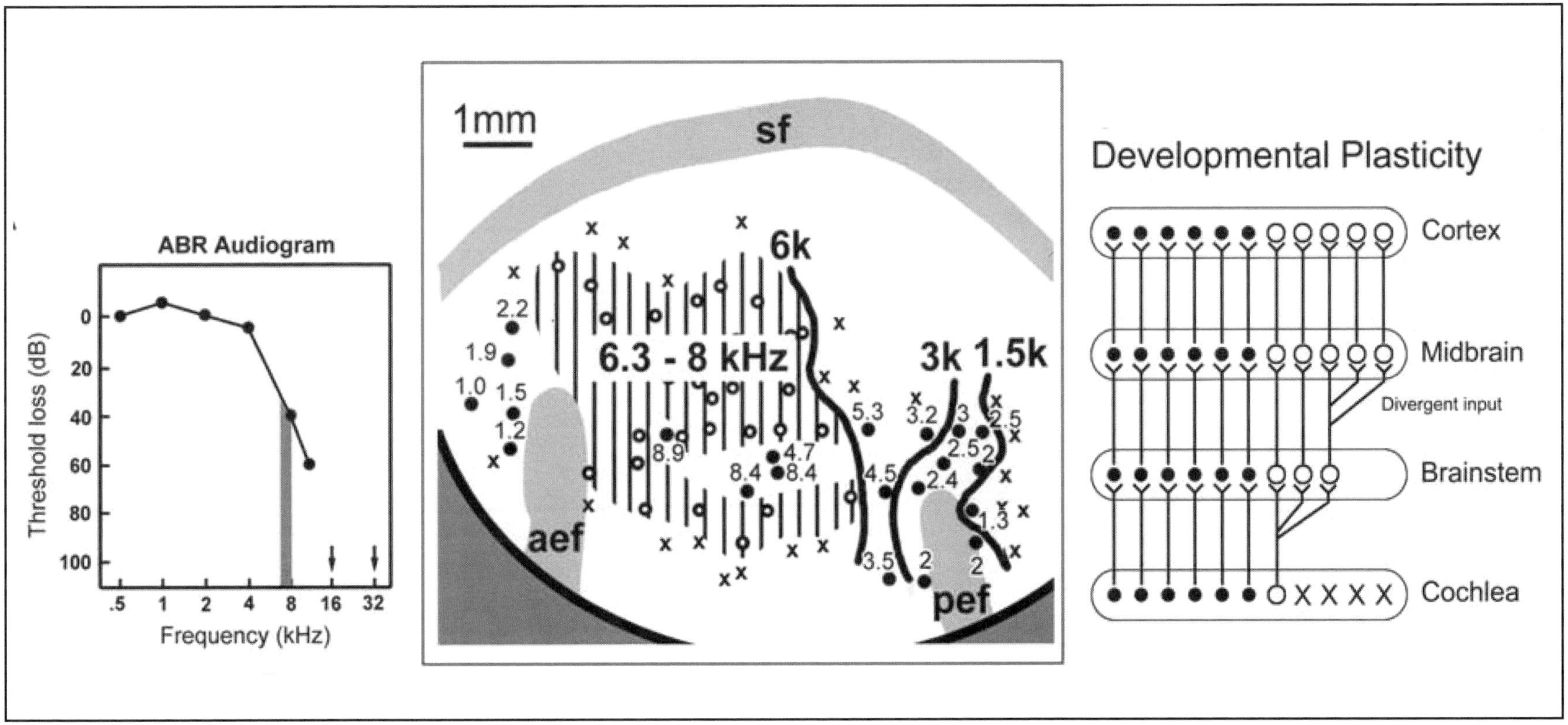

FIGURE 2–8. Abnormal tonotopic maps that developed in a cat after a basal cochlear lesion (amikacin treatment). The effect of the cochlear damage is reflected in the ABR derived audiograms (*left panel*) panels. Tonotopic maps plotted from neuron (characteristic frequency CF) data; isofrequency contours are at octave intervals. Cross-hatching indicates regions in which all neurons have similar tuning properties. Based on data from Harrison et al., 1991. sf: sylvian fissure; aef: anterior ectosylvian fissue; pef: posterior ectosylvian fissure. The right panel shows, schematically, the possible neural projections from cochlear to the cortex to produce the overrepresentation of the 6.3- to 8-kHz region.

This suggests that the boundary region of the cochlear lesion in the 6- to 8-kHz region of the cochlea is abnormally overrepresented in terms of cortical space.

Figure 2–9 shows results from a subject in which an amikacin-induced cochlear lesion was more extensive, with a severe basal lesion and also scattered hair cell loss up to apical, low frequency regions. This is reflected in the ABR audiogram that shows a gradually increasing hearing loss across all frequencies measured. This subject also developed a cortical tonotopic map in which there was a very large isofrequency area (shown cross-hatched) where all neurons have common 6.6-kHz frequency tuning. In addition, the low frequency region of the tonotopic map is severely distorted compared to normal (compare the irregular, closely-space isofrequency contours with those in the normal cat of Figure 2–7). It is reasonable to suppose that abnormal neural activity patterns from partially damaged apical cochlear areas have shaped the cortical map development.

The experimental results described above were from studies in which the cochlear lesions were induced in neonates (Harrison et al., 1991). Qualitatively similar results are found at the cortical level if the lesions are made in the adult animal (Kakigi, Hirakawa, Harel, Mount, & Harrison, 2000; Rajan, Irvine, Wise, & Heil, 1993; Robertson & Irvine, 1989; Schwaber, Garraghty, & Kaas, 1993). However, the spatial extent of such cortical map reorganization is usually much less extensive after cochlear damage in the mature subject compared with that resulting from neonatal lesions.

Tonotopic Map Reorganization After Chronic Local Excitation of the Neonatal Cochlea

The studies outlined above have shown that drastic reductions in neural activity patterns from cochlear lesions can modify the development of central tonotopic projections. What happens if we locally increase cochlear excitation? In one such experiment (Stanton & Harrison, 1996) kittens were reared for many weeks postnatally in an environment where an 8-kHz acoustic signal was constantly present, at a level of 55 to 60 dB SPL (at level ear canal). Being suprathreshold, the stimulus activated cochlear neurons across a 7- to 12-kHz range. The tonal stimulus was frequency modulated (±1 kHz; once per sec) so as to avoid adaptation effects and possible cochlear hair cell trauma. Some months after this initial rearing period, cortical tonotopic maps were assessed as illustrated in Figure 2–10.

Compared to normal age matched control (left panel), a kitten reared in the tonal environment (right panel) showed a significant increase in the cortical space devoted to the frequency region extending from 8 kHz to 12 kHz. Compare the cross-hatched 8- to 16-kHz cortical frequency region in the experimental animal versus the control. It is supposed that the chronic increase in firing rate of neurons in the mid-frequency area of the cochlear level during an early postnatal period caused the overrepresentation of those sound frequencies in auditory cortex. Note also that for the kitten, this environmental tonal stimulus was passive and had no behavioral significance for the kitten. In the mature animal, such stimulus driven cortical reorganization appears only possible when the acoustic stimulus has behavioral significance (e.g., an attention or conditioning task) or in experimental conditions involving forebrain (nucleus basalis) activation (Kilgard & Merzenich, 1998; Weinberger & Bakin, 1998). We could suppose that during an early developmental period when the whole auditory brain is plastic, any stimulus driven activity has the potential to "remodel" the system. After this (critical?) period the cortex remains plastic but only when the acoustic stimulus has some important significance to the subject.

Tonotopic Map Reorganization at Subcortical Levels

Although many experiments show sensory map reorganization at the cortical level, it does not necessarily follow that the neural alterations are intrinsically cortical. Mapping changes can reflect (wholly or in part) rewiring at lower levels in the system. In the case of developmental plasticity of tonotopic maps in auditory cortex this is absolutely the case. In cats with tonotopic map reorganizations shown, for example, in Figures 2–8 and 2–9, neural tracer studies labeling input pathways show that the auditory thalamus has similarly reorganized tonotopic maps (Stanton & Harrison, 2000).

More direct evidence of subcortical frequency map reorganization after cochlear lesions in a developmental model can be observed at the level of the inferior colliculus (IC; Harrison, Ibrahim, & Mount, 1998). The left-hand panel of Figure 2–11 shows, for a normal control animal (chinchilla), the characteristic frequency based tonotopic map within the central nucleus of IC. The upper plot shows the tonotopic progression of neuron CF, as the electrode penetrates IC in a dorsoventral direction (shown in the lower diagrams).

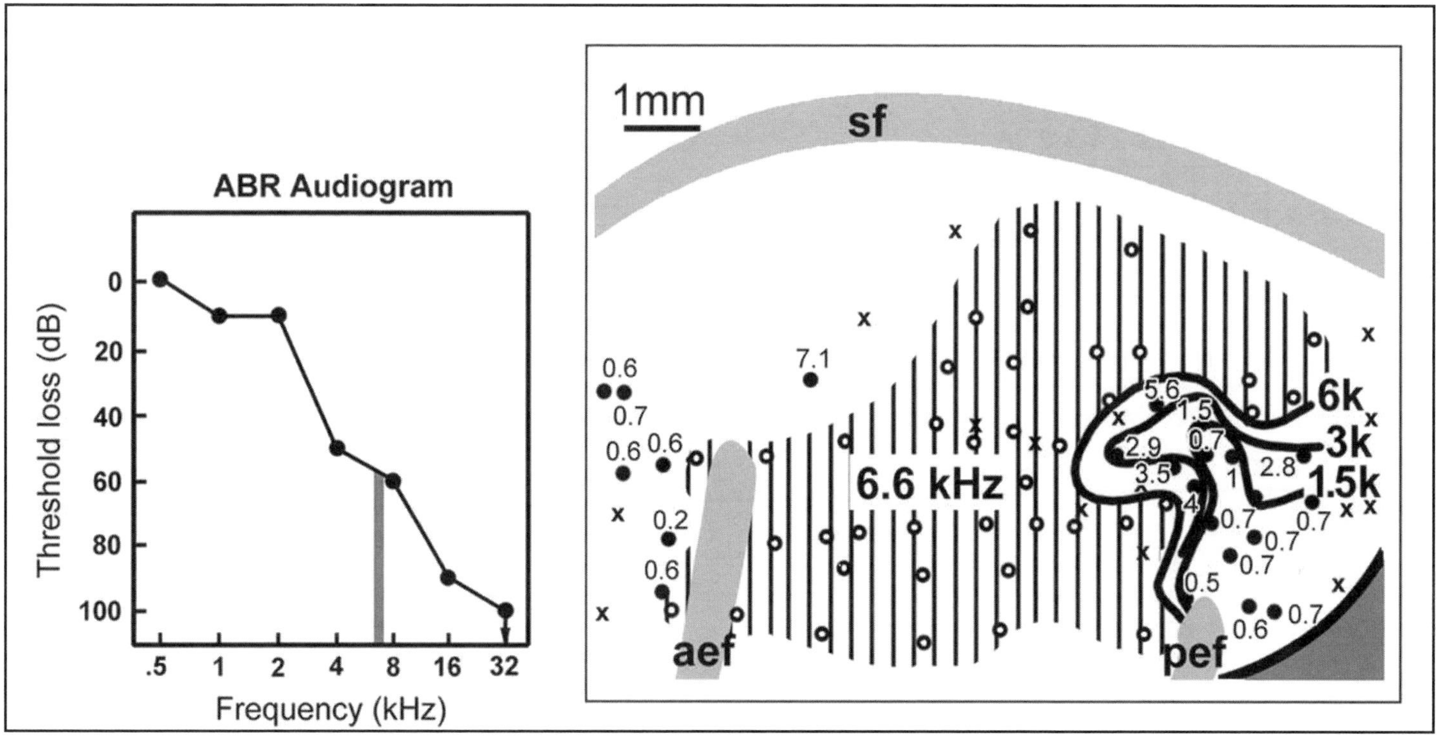

FIGURE 2–9. The cortical frequency map in a kitten reared with a high frequency cochlear hearing loss from birth (as indicated by the ABR audiogram in the left panel). Cross-hatch area show a monotonic area in which all neurons are tuned to c. 6.6 kHz. Based on data from Harrison et al., 1991. sf: sylvian fissure; aef: anterior ectosylvian fissure; pef: posterior ectosylvian fissure.

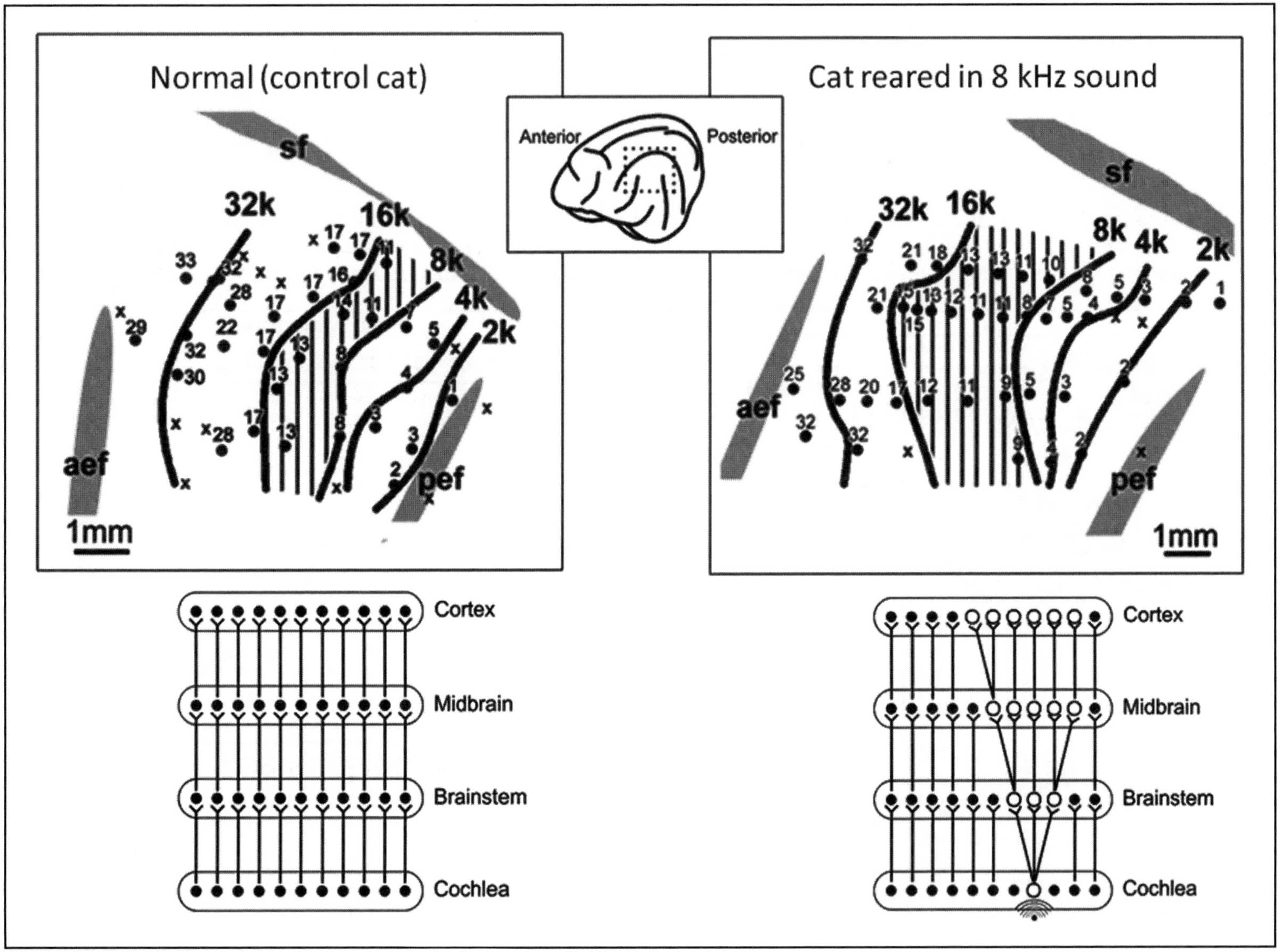

FIGURE 2–10. Tonotopic map in cat auditory cortex resulting from chronic local cochlear activation in the neonate. Isofrequency contours are drawn at octave intervals. The right-hand map is from a cat that spent about a month postnatally in an acoustic environment with a constant 8 kHz signal. The left-hand frequency map is from a normal control subject. In both examples, the 8- to16-kHz octave interval is cross-hatched to emphasize the main difference between the experimental and control subject. Based on data from Stanton and Harrison (1996). The lower diagrams schematically depict the possible wiring patterns of neural projections from the cochlea to cortex. sf: sylvian fissure; aef: anterior ectosylvian fissue; pef: posterior ectosylvian fissure.

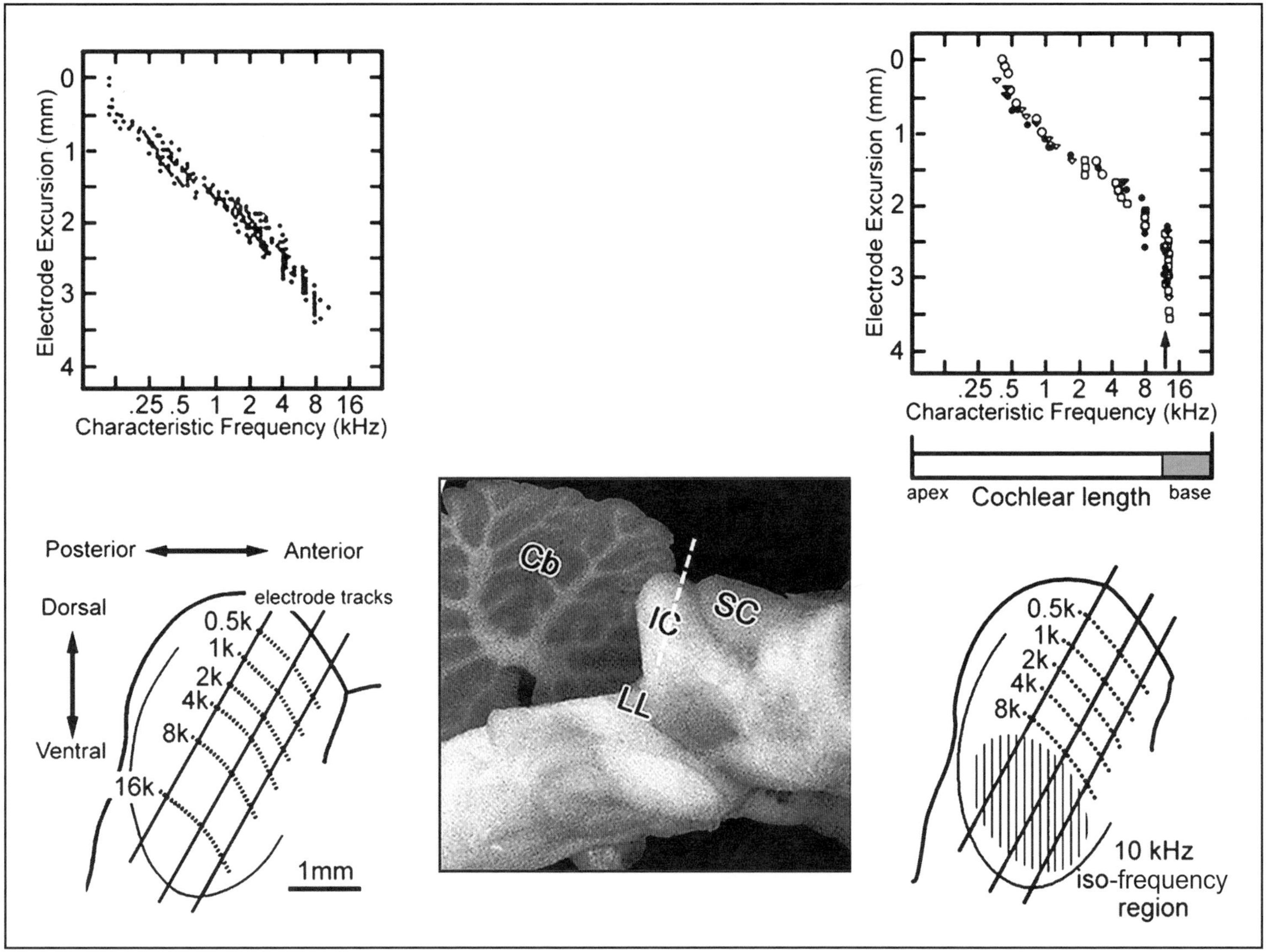

FIGURE 2–11. Tonotopic maps in the inferior colliculus (IC; central nucleus) of the chinchilla. All maps were derived from single neuron recordings in electrode tracks along the dorsoventral axis of IC as shown. The upper graphs plot neuron CF as a function of electrode excursion. The lower diagrams represent the tonotopic maps, with isofrequency contours indicated at octave intervals. Results from a normal animal is shown on the left compared with a subject in which a basal cochlear lesion was made within days of birth (IC tonotopic map derived 4 months later). In the map (*lower right-hand plot*) the cross-hatched area shows the ventral region of IC in which all neurons had a common CF. Based on data from Harrison, Ibrahim, and Mount (1998). Cb: cerebellum; CF: characteristic frequency; IC: inferior colliculus; LL: lateral lemniscus; SC: superior colliculus.

The right-hand panels show IC tonotopic organization after a basal cochlear lesion made (by amikacin drug treatment) in a neonate. The cochlear lesion location is indicated on the bar plot. The graph of unit CF versus position within the dorsoventral IC axis clearly indicates that a large region of IC contains neurons tuned to about 10 kHz (arrow symbol). This region of over-representation of one frequency is analogous to the large monotonic regions found in cortical maps after neonatal cochlear lesions. These results are consistent with the schematic model of connections shown in the right panel of Figure 2–8.

Collectively, these data demonstrate that when cochlear lesions exist during an early developmental period, tonotopic map reorganization occurs not only in auditory cortex but also at subcortical levels. The studies discussed here demonstrate this at thalamic and midbrain levels, and it is likely that similar reorganization also exists at the brainstem level. Can such subcortical reorganization occur in the mature animal after cochlear lesions? Some data suggest that at the level of IC, it does not. In Figure 2–12, the left-hand panel illustrates the tonotopic map change in IC after a neonatal cochlear lesion, compared with a subject in which a similar lesion was made in a mature animal (right-hand panel; based on data from Harrison, 2001). Note that there is no isofrequency region in IC, the de-afferented ventral area of IC being "silent" (no neurons respond to sound stimulation). At the level of the cochlear nucleus, there is also little evidence of tonotopic map reorganization resulting from cochlear lesions made in the mature subject (Kaltenbach, Meleca, & Falzarano, 1996; Rajan & Irvine, 1998). It appears that despite considerable plasticity at all levels of the auditory pathways during early development, plasticity is much reduced in the peripheral pathways as a subject matures.

Mechanisms of (Auditory) Brain Plasticity

Neural plasticity is the result of numerous mechanisms, some of which we understand in detail, some vaguely, and many of which are likely unknown. The development of a functional neural system depends first on the growth of neuronal processes toward target cells and the establishment of synaptic linkages. These initial stages will provide a coarsely connected system, which can be followed by anatomic refinements such as by "pruning" of unwanted or underutilized synaptic connections. For any individual synapse there are many known mechanisms that can adjust its efficacy or "strength." A detailed review of synaptic strengthening mechanisms is beyond the scope of this text, but a few key principles should be mentioned. Two terms that are often cited in this regard are: long-term potentiation (LTP) and Hebbian synaptic strengthening. The former refers to mechanisms in which synaptic transmission is improved after repeated stimulation. A number of pre- and postsynaptic factors have been identified that can achieve this result, including the well known changes to the effectiveness of NMDA postsynaptic receptors (see review by Rauschecker, 1991). Hebbian processes, originally postulated by Donald Hebb (1949), are those where synapses between cells are strengthened when pre- and postsynaptic cells are simultaneously active. The catch phrase here is, "cells that fire together, wire together." Besides synapses, other neuronal structures can modify to improve signal transmission, for example increased myelination of axons as well as other types of neuron-glia cell interactions. All of these known processes are likely in operation during the development of auditory pathways, particularly at early stages when the system is most plastic. In addition to synaptic strengthening there are also mechanisms that will consolidate and maintain any "programmed" neural network.

As mentioned previously, during early development and in later maturation there are both intrinsic and extrinsic factors that play a role in guiding or driving the process. In this chapter we have concentrated on the main extrinsic factor, that is, acoustically driven activity, and have seen that during early development this input certainly does drive the organization of the central auditory brain. To complete this chapter, let us take from this review of auditory system development (from cochlea to cortex) some important concepts that are relevant to clinical issues in pediatric audiology.

Auditory System Plasticity: Some Clinical Implications

What do our new insights about neural plasticity mean in practical terms for healthcare professionals dealing with hearing and deafness? In some areas, the new knowledge may have little immediate impact on healthcare practice, other than offering some further explanations of cause of certain symptoms (e.g., understanding the genesis of some types of tinnitus, or loudness perception disorders). In other areas new scientific information particularly about age-related plasticity of the auditory system has already changed hearing-health care and patient management.

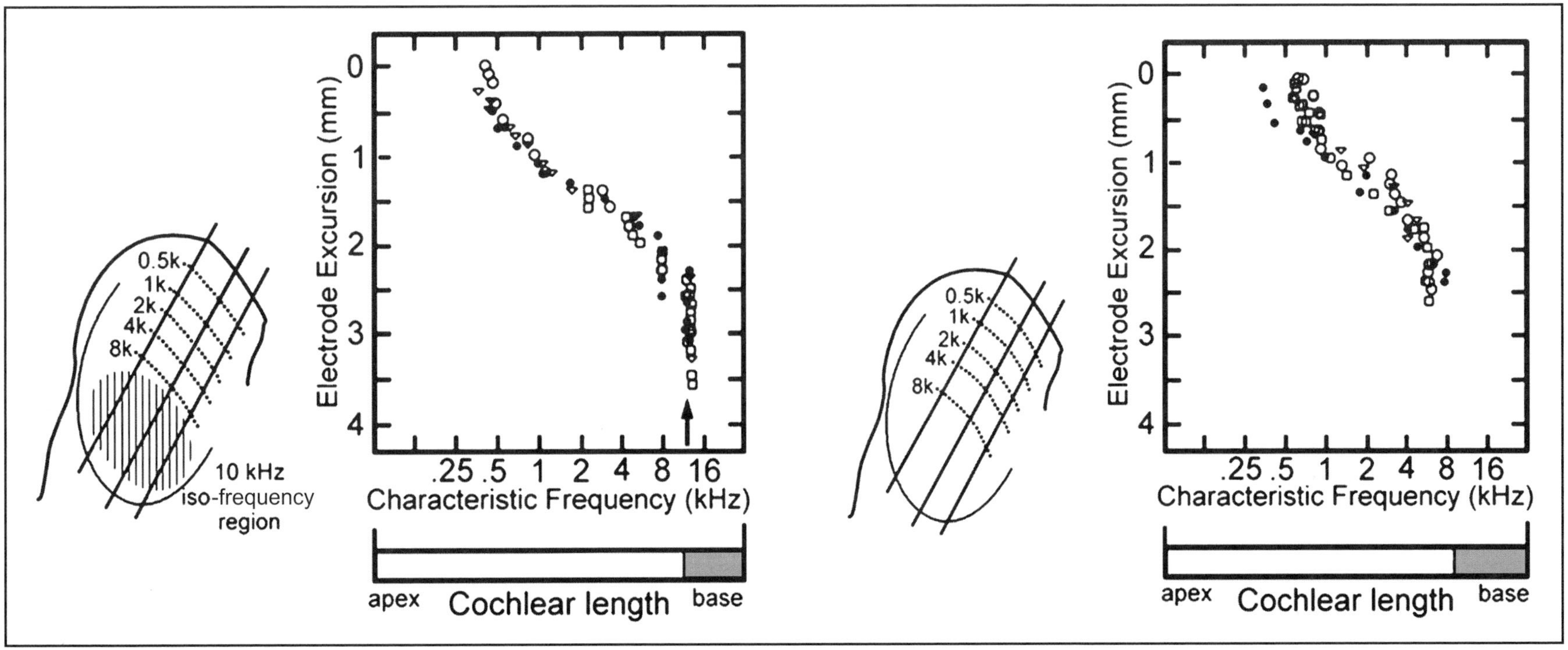

FIGURE 2–12. Tonotopic maps in the central nucleus of the inferior colliculus (chinchilla) after a basal cochlear lesion induced in a neonatal animal (*left panels*) compared with an equivalent lesion in the adult subject. Based on data from Harrison (2001).

Possible Consequences of Abnormal Auditory System Development

Experimental animal studies (e.g., illustrated in Figures 2–8, 2–9, and 2–11) clearly indicate that early sensorineural hearing loss will result in some organizational change at the cortical level. A common feature of reorganization is the isofrequency region where certain sound frequencies (or, strictly speaking, cochlear positions) are over-represented. It is still unclear whether such changes have any functional significance. In other words, we do not know whether reorganization improves auditory processing within the range of the residual hearing. On the negative side, one might speculate that such isofrequency areas will contribute to perceptual problems such as loudness recruitment, and perhaps the generation of certain types of tinnitus. In the experimental animals depicted in Figures 2–8 and 2–9 with large monotonic regions of auditory cortex, certain acoustic stimulus frequencies will activate very extensive areas of auditory cortex. Given that perceptual loudness is related to the number of neurons active, it is difficult to imagine that this degree of cortical activation will not result in a perceived abnormal increase in loudness (loudness recruitment).

In regard to tinnitus, a few speculative comments are worth making. First, certain types of tinnitus could arise from groups of auditory neurons that develop self-perpetuating activity. The brain is full of network connections that might allow this, for example local and reciprocal intracortical connections, or thalamocortical feedback loops. With our understanding that synaptic efficacy can be considerably increased by LTP and Hebbian mechanisms, it is easy to conceive of local circuits being reinforced to the point of "ringing" (i.e., having a positive feedback mode). For this and other reasons, the need for extensive and continuous inhibitory control within the brain is obvious. When there are extensive isofrequency areas in auditory cortex, with the potential for massive synchronous activity, it is possible that such inhibitory mechanism cannot sufficiently suppress positive feedback processes that could lead to self-generated percepts of sound (i.e., tinnitus). An even simpler mechanism for tinnitus production is plausible. Suppose that the synchronous firing of these extensive isofrequency neural population results in them all being connected up together. This is quite feasible; remember Hebb's rule, "cells that fire together, wire together." If we assume that conscious perception has some basis in cortical neuronal activity, then perhaps even very low levels of activity in a vast, linked network of cells could give rise to a chronic sound sensation. See also discussions by Eggermont (2007, 2008).

In light of experimental data on plasticity, one final comment about tinnitus is relevant. There is much discussion about the different types and origins of tinnitus. One distinction, often made, is between "central" and "peripheral" tinnitus. The studies on central auditory plasticity draw attention to the fact that a cochlear lesion can cause central reorganization. It is very plausible that some traumatic event at the cochlear level, causing either less afferent input (after hair cell loss) or more afferent input (injury discharges from damaged or degenerating neurons) could promote central neural connection patterns, which result in cortical over-representation (as in many of the examples shown in this chapter). Although activity in central neurons is presumably the immediate generator of a tinnitus sensation, the intimate link to a causal peripheral lesion somewhat blurs any notion about the real origin of the tinnitus.

Early Hearing Loss Detection and Intervention

The take home message from numerous clinical observations and experimental studies, some described in this text, is that early auditory system development is, in large part, dependent on the pattern of neural activity from the periphery. This means that hearing loss, especially during early development, will significantly impact central auditory brain development. For normal central development it is clear that there needs to be normal (or near normal?) cochlear function during the time window when the system is most plastic and thus influenced by extrinsic signals. Perhaps there is a critical period during which cochlear function needs to be particularly intact. The concepts and concerns raised by developmental neural plasticity experiments (in all sensory systems) have heightened an appreciation about age-related plasticity, and have been responsible for major initiatives for early detection and intervention in sensorineural hearing loss. This has, importantly, led to the implementation of universal infant hearing screening programs in many health care jurisdictions.

Most of the animal studies of plasticity that clearly show central structural and functional alterations, involve extreme experimental manipulations, such as total cochlear ablation or partial deafferentation. However, it is logical to suppose that more subtle types of cochlear dysfunction will alter peripheral stimulation patterns and thus influence auditory system development. Thus, a mild sensorineural hearing loss, or a chronic conductive hearing loss (e.g., from repeated episodes of otitis media), particularly in the very young may well alter normal central pathway development.

Similarly, an asymmetric hearing loss, which might not be considered clinically significant, may also have an impact on binaural auditory system development.

One of the difficulties with testing or "proving" such hypotheses is that any abnormal auditory development will not be immediately apparent, but show up much later in time. For example, neonatal hearing disorders that might lead to problems in language development will only become evident 4 or 5 years later when such development can be assessed. Also a problem in this area is the gathering of solid experimental proof, for example the "gold standard" prospective, randomized controlled study. Rather than dismissing (or ignoring) a potential hearing development problem for lack of real evidence, a good practical strategy is to assume the worst, and make every possible effort to normalize hearing during early postnatal years. Pediatric audiologists and other clinicians already take this approach, for example by making the early detection of hearing problems a priority though neonatal or infant hearing screening programs. Equally important is the timely diagnostic follow up from such screening and the early intervention with hearing aids, cochlear implants, and auditory habilitation training. There are still many unanswered questions about age-related plasticity, most importantly being if there are developmental time windows within which interventions will be most effective. In other words, are there critical periods not to be missed? Importantly, are there stages in development when the door has effectively closed for an intervention (prosthesis or training program)?

When cochlear implants for children became widely available, an important question asked was whether (for congenitally deaf infants) there was a critical or sensitive period after which implantation was of limited benefit. The consensus from many studies was that there was always some benefit, no matter what the duration of deafness, but that children implanted before the age of about six years progressed significantly better in speech understanding tests. The results of one such study (from the present author) is shown in Figure 2–13. Children with severe to profound hearing loss from birth (n = 82) were tested with a battery of speech perception tests before and at regular intervals after receiving a cochlear implant. The children were grouped into subsets by age. In the figure, these age groups are coded with symbols shown in the key to the right of the data. Filled symbols (and dashed

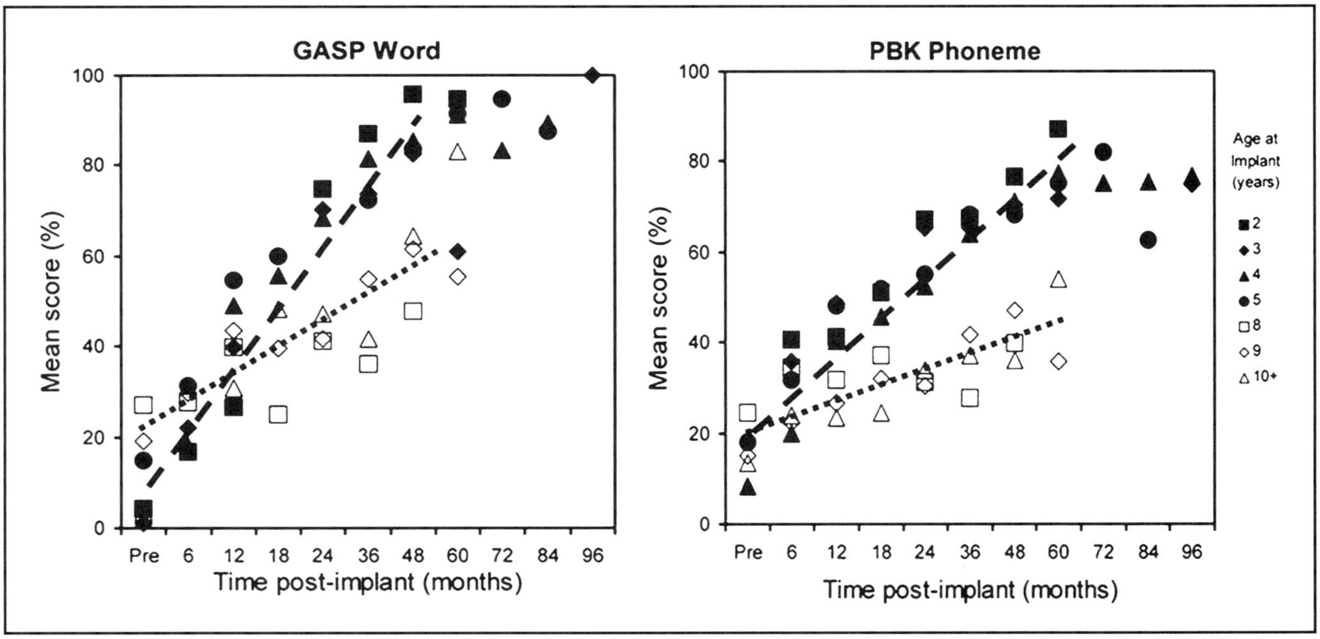

FIGURE 2–13. Development of speech perception in congenitally deaf children (n = 82) with cochlear implantation provided at different ages. Scores in GASP word test (*left panel*) and in the PBK phoneme test (*right panel*), preimplant (Pre) and at intervals up to 96 months postimplantation. Mean values are shown for each age-at-implant group, as indicated by the symbols (*key on far right*). Filled symbols (*dashed line*) represent scores for children who were implanted before 6 years of age; open symbols (*dotted line*) are results from later implanted children (Harrison, Gordon, & Mount, 2005).

line) represent children implanted before 6 years of age, and open symbols (and dotted line) show data from children implanted after 6 years. Note there is a categorical difference in the performance on these typical example tasks (GASP word and PBK phoneme tests) between children implanted before versus after age 6 years (Harrison, Gordon, & Mount, 2005).

Cochlear Implants in Children; Stimulating Central Auditory Development

The central auditory system development is significantly guided by cochlear activity patterns. It follows that a cochlear implant, or other hearing prosthesis provided to a young infant, will have a dual purpose. Not only does the device provide "hearing," but the augmented stimulation of the cochlear nerve will also have an influence on central auditory system development. Many questions arise from this notion. First, is a stimulation paradigm designed to provide good auditory input for hearing, the most optimal for influencing developmental change? Perhaps we should design devices that are constantly active, even when not being used for "hearing," so that they constantly provide stimulation to the developing auditory brain. Another issue relating to cochlear implants is that for the early implanted (congenitally deaf) infant it is likely that the pattern of stimulation from a specific cochlear implant device drives the development of an atypical central auditory system. If so, what does this mean for changing devices or even speech coding paradigms later in life, especially if a critical period of early development is over and the system is less plastic?

A related issue concerns bilateral cochlear implantation. It safely can be argued that to most closely emulate natural auditory system development, we would like a balanced binaural activation implemented as early as possible. Hence, for the congenitally deaf infant, simultaneous binaural cochlear implantation could be recommended. However, what about the provision of a second implant in children already implanted in one ear? If we suppose that activity patterns from one cochlear implant have driven auditory system development in a particular way, can new contralateral activity integrate with the previously established monaural pathway? Is there an overall age-related plasticity during which conversion from monaural to binaural input is useful? Is there a delay between implantation beyond which the benefits of binaural hearing are not realized? These are important questions that presently need addressing.

Conclusions

We now clearly understand that throughout life, the brain, including the auditory areas, maintains some plasticity and can be rewired, reprogrammed and taught new tricks of all kinds. In the adult, plasticity appears to be predominantly at the cortical level, and reprogramming is mainly achieved through active attention to tasks and (sometimes difficult) learning procedures. On the other hand, the developing brain is enormously plastic especially in neonates and young infants. At this stage the developing central auditory system can be significantly influenced by patterns of auditory activity from the periphery. During early development, plasticity is not confined to auditory cortex, and all levels of the pathway (from the brainstem and up) can be (re)organized by auditory input. In pediatric audiology, we must be aware of this plasticity during early years and work to take advantage of this sensitive period in early development. Interventions are more effective at age six months than at six years. We should also bear in mind that early interventions (e.g., provision of hearing aids, cochlear implant and auditory training therapies) will be influential not just in helping a child to hear better in the short term, but also in guiding the long term development of the auditory system.

This chapter has provided only some key studies related to auditory development. Some of the references given are chapters in multiauthor texts dealing broadly with hearing development and plasticity, and generally those volumes provide more comprehensive coverage for those with further interest.

Acknowledgments. The research reported here was funded by the Canadian Institutes of Health Research (CIHR), and the Masonic Foundation of Ontario.

References

Birnholz, J. C., & Benacerraf, B. R. (1983). The development of human fetal hearing. *Science*, *222*, 516–518.

Boettcher, F. A., & Salvi, R. J. (1993). Functional changes in the ventral cochlear nucleus following acute acoustic overstimulation. *Journal of the Acoustical Society of America*, *94*, 2123–2134.

Cang, J., Rentería, R. C., Kaneko, M., Liu X., Copenhagen, D. R., & Stryker, M. P. (2005). Development of precise maps in visual cortex requires patterned spontaneous activity in the retina. *Neuron*, *48*, 797–809.

Eggermont, J. J. (1985). Evoked potentials as indicators of auditory maturation. *Acta Otolaryngologica Suppl (Stockh.), 421*, 41–47.

Eggermont, J. J. (1988). On the rate of maturation of sensory evoked potentials. *Electroencephalography and Clinical Neurophysiology, 70*, 293–305.

Eggermont, J. J. (2007). Pathophysiology of tinnitus. *Progress in Brain Research, 166*, 19–35.

Eggermont, J. J. (2008). Role of auditory cortex in noise- and drug-induced tinnitus. *American Journal of Audiology, 17*, 162–169.

Eggermont, J. J., & Salamy, A. (1988). A maturational time course for the ABR in preterm and full term infants. *Hearing Research, 33*, 37–47.

Gordon, K. A., Papsin, B. C., & Harrison, R. V. (2003). Activity-dependent developmental plasticity of the auditory brainstem in children who use cochlear implants. *Ear and Hearing, 24*, 485–500.

Graziani, L. J, Weitzman, E. D., & Velasco, M. S. (1968). Neurologic maturation and auditory evoked responses in low birth weight infants. *Pediatrics, 41*, 483–494.

Harrison, R. V. (2001). Age related tonotopic map plasticity in the central auditory pathways. *Scandinavian Audiology, 30*(Suppl. 53), 8–14.

Harrison, R. V., Cullen, J. R., Takeno, S., & Mount, R. J. (1996). The neonatal chinchilla cochlea: Morphological and functional study. *Scanning Microscopy, 10*, 889–894.

Harrison, R. V., Gordon, K. A., & Mount, R. J. (2005). Is there a critical period for cochlear implantation in congenitally deaf children? Analyses of hearing and speech perception performance after implantation. *Developmental Psychobiology, 46*, 252–261.

Harrison, R. V., Ibrahim, D., & Mount, R. J. (1998). Plasticity of tonotopic maps in auditory midbrain following partial cochlear damage in the developing chinchilla. *Experimental Brain Research, 123*, 449–460.

Harrison, R. V., Nagasawa, A., Smith, D. W., Stanton, S., & Mount, R. J. (1991). Reorganization of auditory cortex after neonatal high frequency cochlear hearing loss. *Hearing Research, 54*, 11–19.

Hashisaki, G. T., & Rubel, E. W (1989). Effects of unilateral cochlea removal on anteroventral cochlear nucleus neurons in developing gerbils. *Journal of Comprehensive Neurology, 283*, 465–473.

Hebb, D. O. (1949). *The organization of behavior*. New York, NY: Wiley.

Hogan, S. C., & Moore, D. R. (2003). Impaired binaural hearing in children produced by a threshold level of middle ear disease. *Journal of the Association for Research in Otolaryngology, 4*, 123–129.

Kakigi, A., Hirakawa, H., Harel, N., Mount, R. J., & Harrison, R. V. (2000). Tonotopic mapping in auditory cortex of the adult chinchilla with amikacin-induced cochlear lesions. *Audiology, 39*, 53–160.

Kaltenbach, J. A., Meleca, R. J., & Falzarano, P. R. (1996). Alterations in the tonotopic map of cochlear nucleus following cochlear damage. In R. J. Salvi, D. Henderson, F. Fiorino, & V. Colletti (Eds.), Auditory *system plasticity and regeneration* (pp. 317–332). New York, NY: Thieme Medical.

Kilgard, M. P., & Merzenich, M. M. (1998). Cortical map reorganization enabled by nucleus basalis activity. *Science, 279*, 1714–1718.

Kitzes, L. M. (1984). Some physiological consequences of neonatal cochlear destruction in the inferior colliculus of the gerbil, Meriones unguiculatus. *Brain Research, 306*, 171–178.

Kitzes, L. M. (1986). The role of binaural innervation in the development of the auditory brainstem. In R. J. Ruben, T. R. Van De Water & E. W. Rubel (Eds.), *The biology of change in otolaryngology* (pp. 185–199). The Netherlands: Elsevier Science.

Knudsen, E. I. (1984). The role of auditory experience in the development and maintenance of sound localization. *Trends in Neuroscience, 7*, 326–330.

Knudsen, E. I., Esterly, S. D., & Knudsen, P. F. (1984). Monaural occlusion alters sounds localization during a sensitive period in the barn owl. *Journal of Neuroscience, 4*, 1001–1011.

Kujala, T., Alho, K., Huotilainen, M., Ilmoniemi, R. J., Lehtokoski, A., Leinonen, A., . . . Näätänen, R. (1997). Electrophysiological evidence for cross-modal plasticity in humans with early- and late-onset blindness. *Psychophysiology, 34*, 213–216.

Levi-Montalcini, R. (1949). Development of the acoustico-vestibular centers in the chick embryo in the absence of the afferent root fibres and of descending fiber tracts. *Journal of Comparative Neurology, 91*, 209–242.

Lim, D. J., & Anniko, M. (1986). Correlative development of sensory cells and overlying membrane of the inner ear: Micromechanical aspects. In R. J. Ruben, T. R. Van De Water, & E. W. Rubel (Eds.), *The biology of change in otolaryngology* (pp. 55–69). The Netherlands: Elsevier Science.

Lippe, W. R. (1994). Rhythmic spontaneous activity in the developing avian auditory system. *Journal of Neuroscience, 14*, 1486–1495.

Meister, M., Wong, R. O., Baylor, D. A., & Schatz, C. J. (1991). Synchronous bursts of action potentials in ganglion cells of the developing mammalian retina. *Science, 252*, 939–943.

Merzenich, M. M., & Brugge, J. F. (1973). Representations of the cochlear partition on the superior temporal plane of the macaque monkey. *Brain Research, 50*, 275–296.

Moore, J. K. (2002). Maturation of human auditory cortex: Implications for speech perception. *Annals of Otology, Rhinology and Laryngology Supplementum, 189*, 7–10.

Moore, D. R., Hine, J. E., Jiang, Z. D., Matsuda, H., Parsons, C. H., & King, A. J. (1999). Conductive hearing loss produces a reversible binaural hearing impairment. *Journal of Neuroscience, 19*, 8704–8711.

Moore, D. R., Hutchings, M. E., King, A. J., & Kowalchuk, N. E. (1989). Auditory brain stem of the ferret: Some effects of rearing with a unilateral ear plug on the cochlea, cochlear nucleus, and projections to the inferior colliculus. *Journal of Neuroscience, 9*, 1213–1222.

Moore, D. R., & King, A. J. (2004). Plasticity of binaural systems. In R. R. Fay & A. N. Popper (Eds.), *Plasticity of the auditory system* (pp. 96–172). New York, NY: Springer Science.

Moore, D. R., King, A. J., McAlpine, D., Martin, R. L., & Hutchings, M. E. (1993). Functional consequences of neonatal unilateral cochlear removal. *Progress in Brain Research, 97,* 127–133.

Moore, D. R., & Kitzes, L. M. (1985). Projections from the cochlear nucleus to the inferior colliculus in normal and neonatally cochlea-ablated gerbils, *Journal of Comparative Neurology, 240,* 180–195.

Neville, H. J., Schmidt, A., & Kutas, M. (1983). Altered visual-evoked potentials in congenitally deaf adults. *Brain Research, 266,* 127–132.

Newton, J. R., & Sur, M. (2005). Rewiring cortex: Functional plasticity of the auditory cortex during development. In J. Syka, & M. M. Merzenich (Eds), *Plasticity and signal representation in the auditory system* (pp. 127–137). New York, NY: Springer Science.

Olsho, L. W. (1986). Early development of human frequency resolution. In R. J. Ruben, T. R. Van De Water, & E. W. Rubel (Eds.), *The biology of change in otolaryngology* (pp. 71–90). The Netherlands: Elsevier Science.

Pallas, S. L. (2001). Intrinsic and extrinsic factors that shape neocortical specification. *Trends in Neuroscience, 24,* 417–432.

Parks, T. N., & Jackson, H. (1986). Early destruction of the ear induces formation of a new functional brainstem auditory pathway. In R. J. Ruben, T. R. Van De Water, & E. W. Rubel (Eds.), *The biology of change in otolaryngology* (pp. 225–234). The Netherlands: Elsevier Science.

Ponton, C. W., Don, M., Eggermont, J. J., Waring, M. D., & Masuda, A. (1996). Maturation of human cortical auditory function, difference between normal hearing and cochlear implanted children. *Ear and Hearing, 17,* 430–437.

Ponton, C. W., & Eggermont, J. J. (2001). Of kittens and kids: Altered cortical maturation following profound deafness and cochlear implant use. *Audiology and Neurootology, 6,* 363–380.

Ponton, C. W., & Eggermont, J. J. (2007). Electrophysiological measures of human auditory system maturation: Relationship with neuroanatomy and behavior. In R. F., Burkard, M. Don, & J. J. Eggermont (Eds.), *Auditory evoked potentials. Basic principles and clinical application* (pp. 385–402). Baltimore, MD: Lippincott Williams & Wilkins.

Ponton, C. W., Eggermont, J. J., Kwong, B, & Don, M. (2000). Maturation of human central auditory system activity: Evidence from multichannel evoked potentials. *Clinical Neurophysiology, 111,* 220–236.

Pujol, R. (1986). Synaptic plasticity in the developing cochlea. In R. J. Ruben, T. R. Van De Water, & E. W. Rubel (Eds.), *The biology of change in otolaryngology* (pp. 47–54). The Netherlands: Elsevier Science.

Rajan, R., & Irvine, D. R. F. (1998). Absence of plasticity of the frequency map in dorsal cochlear nucleus of adult cats after unilateral partial cochlear lesions. *Journal of Comparative Neurology, 399,* 35–46.

Rajan, R., Irvine, D. R. F., Wise, L. Z., & Heil, P. (1993). Effect of unilateral partial cochlear lesions in adult cats on the representation of lesioned and unlesioned cochleas in primary auditory cortex. *Journal of Comparative Neurology, 338,* 17–49.

Rauschecker, J. P. (1991). Mechanisms of visual plasticity: Hebb synapses, NMDA receptors and beyond. *Physiological Reviews, 71,* 587–615.

Reale, R., & Imig, T. (1980). Tonotopic organization in auditory cortex of the cat. *Journal of Comparative Neurology, 338,* 265–291.

Robertson, D., & Irvine, D. R. F. (1989). Plasticity of frequency organization in auditory cortex of guinea pigs with partial unilateral deafness. *Journal of Comparative Neurology, 282,* 456–471.

Roe, A. W., Pallas, S. L., Kwon, Y. H., & Sur, M. (1992). Visual projections routed to the auditory pathway in ferrets: Receptive fields of visual neurons in primary auditory cortex. *Journal of Neuroscience, 12,* 3651–3664.

Romand, R. (1983). Development of the cochlea. In R. Romand (Ed.), *Development of the auditory and vestibular systems* (pp. 47–88). New York, NY: Academic Press.

Rubel, E. W., Parks, T. N., & Zirpel, L. (2004). Assembling, connecting and maintaining the cochlear nucleus. In R. R. Fay, & A. N. Popper (Eds.), *Plasticity of the auditory system* (pp. 8–48). Baltimore, MD: Springer Science.

Sadato, N., Pascual-Leone, A., Grafman, J., Ibañez, V., Deiber, M. P., Dold, G., & Hallett, M. (1996). Activation of the primary visual cortex by Braille reading in blind subjects. *Nature, 380,* 526–528.

Schwaber, M. K., Garraghty, P. E., & Kaas, J. H. (1993). Neuroplasticity of the adult primate auditory cortex following cochlear hearing loss. *American Journal of Otolaryngology, 14,* 252–258.

Sharma, J., Angelucci, A., & Sur, M. (2000). Induction of visual orientation modules in auditory cortex. *Nature, 404,* 841–847.

Stanton, S. G., & Harrison, R. V. (1996). Neonatal auditory augmentation modifies cochleotopic mapping in primary auditory cortex of the cat. *Auditory Neuroscience, 2,* 97–107.

Stanton, S. G., & Harrison, R. V. (2000). Projections from the medial geniculate body to primary auditory cortex in neonatally deafened cats. *Journal of Comparative Neurology, 426,* 117–129.

Trehub, S. E., Schneider, B. A., & Endman, M. (1980). Developmental changes in infants' sensitivity to octave-band noises. *Journal of Experimental Child Psychology, 29,* 283–293.

Wang, J., Salvi, R. J., & Powers, N. (1996). Plasticity of response properties of inferior colliculus neurons following acute cochlear damage. *Journal of Neurophysiology, 75,* 171–183.

Weinberger, N. M., & Bakin, J. S. (1998). Learning-induced physiological memory in adult primary auditory cortex: Receptive fields plasticity, model, and mechanisms. *Audiology and Neuro-Otology, 3,* 145–167.

3

Infant Speech Perception

Derek Houston

Introduction

Speech perception can be described as a mode of hearing specialized for speech. When people engage in conversation, they do not hear simply the information conveyed in a waveform or a spectrogram. Instead, they perceive linguistic and indexical information that conveys words and sentences as well as identifying qualitative characteristics of the talkers. People are able to extract linguistic and indexical information from speech because of the specialized way the human hearing instrument is tuned. Accordingly, the study of infant speech perception is concerned with the tuning of that instrument during early development.

A complete understanding of how speech perception develops would require descriptions of the initial and end states of infants' speech perception and an explanation of how the change of state happens. The field of infant speech perception is not yet able to describe with certainty exactly what information infants perceive from speech at any stage of development or what drives speech perception to change with development and language experience. Nevertheless, developmental scientists have made a great deal of progress over the last 40 years toward these goals.

Early work in infant speech perception was strongly influenced by Noam Chomsky's theories, which were revolutionizing the field of linguistics at the time. Chomsky (1968, 1975) posited that language was not learnable from the input alone and required a specialized universal language acquisition device that was innately endowed to humans. Because of this prevailing view, most work focused on identifying speech perception skills that were thought to be innate and universal. Gradually, however, infant speech perception scientists have focused increasingly more on what infants are able to learn from the input, and mounting evidence suggests that general learning mechanisms may play a larger role in language acquisition than previously thought (Behme & Deacon, 2008).

This chapter reviews what is known about normal-hearing infants' initial preferences and sensitivities to both suprasegmental properties of speech (e.g., stress, intonation, rhythm) and fine-grained information contained in phonemes. We then discuss learning mechanisms that have been found to play a role in tuning infants' speech perception skills. Finally, we describe the speech perception skills that infants acquire as a result of these learning mechanisms, which put them in a position to build a vocabulary and acquire language.

Birth to Six Months: Initial Preferences and Sensitivities

The aim of this section is to describe infants' speech perception skills during the early postnatal period. This period may not reflect infants' initial state, however, because fetuses are able to hear and learn in utero. Fetuses demonstrate consistent responses to auditory stimulation by 25 to 29 weeks gestational age (Birnholz & Benacerraf, 1983), which means that full-term newborns have more than two months of auditory experience. In utero experience may shape the initial postnatal state, and we consider its role in the initial postnatal state of speech perception.

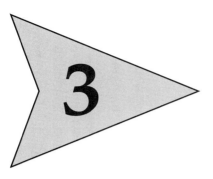

The fetal hearing experience may affect some aspects of speech perception more than others. Studies of the in utero acoustic environment suggest that frequencies above 1000 Hz are attenuated 20 to 30 dB in transmission to fetuses (e.g., Lecanuet et al., 1998), suggesting that they have, at best, limited access to acoustic information important for discriminating segmental information, especially consonants. However, the sound that does reach fetuses provides sufficient information for perception of suprasegmental aspects of speech.

Perception of Suprasegmental Information

Suprasegmental information, such as intonation and rhythm, transmits very well to fetuses. Several research teams have investigated how prenatal experience with suprasegmental information affects infants' early speech perception. One issue of interest is whether or not fetuses encode suprasegmental information into memory. If so, their in utero experience with speech may affect their initial postnatal speech processing and preferences.

Evidence of Early Encoding

There is evidence that fetuses not only have access to auditory information, they also encode speech information into memory—especially suprasegmental information. Both newborns and fetuses demonstrate the ability to discriminate their native language from a foreign language (Kisilevsky et al., 2009; Mehler et al., 1988; Moon, Cooper, & Fifer, 1993; Nazzi, Bertoncini, & Mehler, 1998) and their mother's voice from another woman's voice (DeCasper & Fifer, 1980; Kisilevsky et al., 2003). Because most fine-grained segmental information is filtered out before it reaches the fetus, these findings suggest that fetuses encode some suprasegmental characteristics of speech.

To explore the possibility that suprasegmental properties encoded during the last trimester persist in memory, DeCasper and colleagues investigated newborns' and fetuses' memory of their mothers' speech. They instructed women to read a nursery rhyme three times a day, starting six weeks before their due date. Newborns showed a preference for the familiar nursery rhyme over a novel nursery rhyme (DeCasper & Spence, 1986). A follow-up investigation found that fetuses who were tested two weeks before birth showed differential heart rate responses for the familiar compared to a novel rhyme (DeCasper, LeCanuet, Busnel, Granier-Deferre, & Maugeais, 1994). Thus, four weeks of exposure for a few minutes a day is *sufficient* for fetuses to encode some properties of a nursery rhyme. However, it is unknown at this time how much exposure is *necessary* for fetuses to encode suprasegmental properties of their language, their mother's voice, or a nursery rhyme. Moreover, we do not know how long suprasegmental information like this persists in memory.

Sensitivity to Rhythm and Intonation

The above findings suggest that infants are highly attuned to what they hear in utero. But what aspects of speech are they encoding? One possibility is that infants' ability to discriminate what they hear in utero from novel stimuli may reflect simple pattern-matching skills. However, their discrimination abilities may instead reflect a more general attunement to suprasegmental properties of speech. Nazzi, Bertoncini, and Mehler (1998) investigated this possibility by testing newborn infants' discrimination of languages they were not exposed to in utero. Specifically, they investigated the role of rhythm—the timing of syllables in a language—in infants' language discrimination. French newborns demonstrated discrimination of unfamiliar languages that were rhythmically dissimilar (English and Japanese) but not languages that were rhythmically similar (English and Dutch), suggesting they had a general sensitivity to rhythmic information in speech.

As discussed later in the chapter, infants' sensitivity to the rhythmic properties of speech appears to play an important role in their later speech segmentation skills, that is, their ability to locate word boundaries in the context of fluent speech. It is therefore tempting to assume that infants' ability to discriminate languages that are rhythmically different means that they are especially sensitive to rhythmic properties of speech. However, the rhythm of speech correlates strongly with its intonation, and it is not clear if infants rely mainly on rhythm or intonation to discriminate languages (Ramus, 2002). Whatever the case, infants' sensitivity to suprasegmental properties of speech seems to be general rather than limited to only the speech they were exposed to in utero. In the next section, we discuss the role that infant sensitivity to suprasegmental properties might play in their processing of speech.

Effects of Rhythm and Intonation on Early Speech Processing: Preference for Infant-Directed Speech

Not only are infants able to discriminate suprasegmental properties, several investigations suggest that these properties play a role in infants' attention to speech and what information they extract. With respect to attention, adults speak differently to infants than they do to other adults or even older children, especially when they want to engage infants' attention. *Infant-directed speech* (IDS) and *adult-directed speech* (ADS) differ in their rhythmic and intonational properties. IDS is characterized as being slower (longer durations of syllables and pauses), higher pitched, and having greater pitch excursions than ADS. Infants demonstrate greater attention to IDS than to ADS, at least during the first six months of life (Cooper & Aslin, 1990; Fernald, 1985; Fernald & Kuhl, 1987; Werker & McLeod, 1989).

The advantage of IDS over ADS in capturing infants' attention does not appear to depend much, if at all, on infants' experience with IDS. Cooper and Aslin (1990) assessed attention to IDS and ADS in 2-day-olds and 1-month-olds and found that both groups of infants demonstrated longer looking times when presented with IDS than when presented with ADS. Given our previous discussion of fetal sensitivities to speech, we might speculate that in utero experience plays a role in infants' attention to IDS. However, fetuses are exposed to ADS more than to IDS (unless the pregnant mother speaks more to infants than to adults and older children); thus, it seems very unlikely that newborns' increased attention to IDS could be due to their exposure to speech (which is mainly ADS) during the fetal period.

If infants' attention to IDS is not due to experience, then it is likely something about the acoustic properties of IDS that draws infants' attention to it. To investigate the relative contributions of the pitch (as measured by F0), intensity, and duration characteristics of IDS on capturing infants' attention, Fernald and Kuhl (1987) presented infants with one of three types of IDS and ADS computer-synthesized speech. Each type of synthesized speech preserved one characteristic that differentiated IDS and ADS and equalized the other two characteristics; all speech types were devoid of any lexical information. The investigators found that 4-month-olds showed greater attention to the IDS only when the pitch was preserved, suggesting that the pitch characteristics of IDS is what captures infants' attention (Fernald & Kuhl, 1987). Follow-up studies suggested that the aspect of pitch most important for infants' preference for IDS is intonation rather than the mean pitch height (Fernald, 1993). More recently, however, Singh, Morgan, and Best (2002) found that 6-month-olds preferred speech that conveyed positive affect to speech that conveyed neutral affect, regardless of whether it was IDS or ADS. Moreover, infants showed no preference for IDS over ADS when they controlled for affect. In fact, infants preferred ADS to IDS when presented with positive-affect ADS and neutral-affect IDS. Also, infants respond more positively to IDS that expresses approval than IDS that expresses disapproval (Fernald, 1993). These findings suggest that infants' prefer IDS because it generally conveys a positive affect, which is carried primarily through intonation (Fernald, 1989).

Taken together, research on young infants' sensitivity to suprasegmental information suggests that they are attuned to the rhythmic and intonational properties of speech at birth and even before. They prefer intonation that conveys emotional information. There is no strong evidence that infants have a similar kind of preference for a particular type of rhythm, but they are able to discriminate rhythmic differences at very young ages. It is not clear what drives infants to attend to rhythmic properties. It is possible that because intonation and rhythm are highly correlated, attention to intonation may contribute to sensitivity to rhythm. Infants' attention to rhythmic properties plays an important role in the development of more advanced speech perception skills, as we discuss later in this chapter. For now, however, we continue to focus on speech perception skills during early infancy. We now turn to their perceptual sensitivities to segmental information in speech.

Perception of Segmental Information

Segmental information refers to the acoustic properties of speech that differentiate phonemes. Given that much of the high-frequency acoustic information that distinguishes phonemes is not available to fetuses because of in utero filtering, we might expect young infants to be poor at discriminating phonemes. But despite the lack of experience with high-frequency segmental information in utero, newborns and young infants demonstrate sensitivities to fine-grained changes in segmental information.

Categorical Perception

The earliest infant speech perception research was motivated by findings that adults perceived some acoustic-phonetic dimensions categorically rather than continuously (Liberman, Harris, Hofman, & Griffith, 1957). For example, *voice onset time* (VOT) is the time between the release of an articulation for a stop consonant (e.g., [p, b, t, d, k, g]) and the onset of voicing. Although VOT varies along a continuum, adults perceive VOT categorically (Liberman, Harris, Kinney, & Lane, 1961). In English, stop consonants with relatively short VOTs (0–20 msec) are perceived as *voiced* (e.g., [b, d, g]) and those with relatively long VOTs

(>30 msec) are perceived as *voiceless* (e.g., [p, t, k]). They are considered to be perceived categorically because listeners are very poor at discriminating within-category changes in VOT (e.g., 0 and 20 msec VOTs or 40 and 60 msec VOTs) but can readily discriminate changes in VOT that cross VOT categories (e.g., 20 and 40 msec VOTs) even when the objective differences in VOT are identical. At issue in the late 1960s was whether or not categorical perception was due to innate auditory sensitivities or due to experience—learning the phonology of the ambient language.

To test whether or not infants were innately endowed with speech discrimination abilities that were attuned to language, Peter Eimas and his colleagues tested 1- and 4-month-old infants' ability to discriminate synthesized versions of [ba]-[pa] that varied along the VOT continuum. To test young infants, Eimas, Siqueland, Jusczyk, and Vigorito (1971) used the high amplitude sucking (HAS) paradigm. In the HAS infants suck on a non-nutritive pacifier that is connected to a computer that registers each suck. During the habituation phase, infants are presented with one stimulus each time they suck until their sucking rate decreases to a habituation criterion. They are then presented with a novel stimulus (experimental group) or the same stimulus (control group) and their sucking times are analyzed to determine if the presentation of the novel stimulus elicits an increase in sucking rate, suggesting infants can discriminate the two stimuli. Eimas and colleagues found that 1- and 4-month-old infants showed discrimination of the same VOTs as adults, suggesting that they also perceived VOT categorically. Numerous follow-up studies have shown that infants categorically discriminate voicing, place-of-articulation, and manner-of-articulation (e.g., Eimas, 1974, 1975; Eimas & Miller, 1980a, 1980b; Eimas et al., 1971), suggesting that infants are born with a perceptual system that is tuned to detect acoustic-phonetic properties important for identifying phonemes in many of the world's languages.

Some more recent work suggests that infants' discrimination of consonants is not as fixed or as strictly categorical as previously thought. Maye, Werker, and Gerken (2002) tested the effects of input on infants' discrimination of VOT contrasts. They familiarized infants with repetitions of eight unaspirated alveolar stops that varied in VOT from [da] to [ta]. One group of infants was presented with relatively more tokens from the middle of the VOT range (unimodal distribution), while the other group was presented with relatively more tokens from the two endpoints of the VOT range (bimodal distribution). They then tested infants' discrimination of [da] and [ta] and found that only the group familiarized with the bimodal distribution demonstrated discrimination.

Whereas Maye et al. (2002) found that infants can fail to discriminate across category boundaries under some stimulus conditions, McMurray and Aslin (2005) found that infants can discriminate VOTs within category boundaries under some testing conditions. They used a head-turn preference procedure (described in more detail later) to assess 8-month-olds' discrimination of prototypical and nonprototypical tokens of [ba] and [pa]. Unlike previous studies that used a habituation/dishabituation procedure, McMurray and Aslin (2005) found that infants could discriminate tokens that fell within phoneme categories. Taken together, these findings suggest that while infants may have some initial auditory sensitivities to particular acoustic-phonetic cues, these sensitivities are not rigid and can be influenced by linguistic input.

Although the above work suggests that many consonant contrasts may be perceived categorically, investigations on the perception of vowels suggest that they are perceived more continuously. Unlike consonants, adults discriminate steady-state vowels in a continuous rather than a categorical manner (Fry, Abramson, Eimas, & Liberman, 1962; Pisoni, 1973; Stevens, Liberman, Studdert-Kennedy, & Ohman, 1969). Swoboda, Morse, and Leavitt (1976) discovered that 2-month-olds not only discriminated [i] and [ê] but also discriminated vowel sounds that fell within the same vowel category but differed with respect to formant frequencies, suggesting that, like adults, young infants also perceive vowels in a continuous manner.

Sensitivity to Phoneme Inventory

The above findings suggest that, like their ability to discriminate surprasegmental properties of speech, young infants are able to discriminate segmental properties after little to no experience with language. The above findings tell us very little, however, about infants' ability to encode phonemes into long-term memory. Evidence that they can encode suprasegmental information into long-term memory comes from studies reviewed in the previous section in which infants respond differently to the familiar rhythmic and intonational characteristics of their mothers' speech than to the speech of another woman and to a familiar nursery rhyme than to an unfamiliar one. Responding to familiarity requires not only the ability to discriminate familiar and unfamiliar stimuli, but also the ability to associate a familiar sample of speech to representations of that speech stored in long-term memory. In contrast, a finding of discrimination where one stimulus is presented until habituation is reached and then a novel stimulus is presented requires infants to store speech information into memory for only a very brief period of time.

If infants are able to encode segmental information of the ambient language into their long-term memory as they do suprasegmental information, they should show similar attentional preferences for native segmental information as they do for native suprasegmental information. Jusczyk, Friederici, Wessels, Svenkerud, and Jusczyk (1993) tested this possibility by assessing 6- and 9-month-old English-learning infants' preferences for English words versus foreign words that differed from English words in phoneme inventories, rhythmic properties, or both. Infants demonstrated longer looking times for their native rhythm versus a foreign rhythm (low-pass filtered Norwegian) but not for their native phoneme inventory versus a language with a similar rhythm but dissimilar phoneme inventory (Dutch). Nine-month-olds, in contrast, showed preferences based on both rhythm and phoneme inventories, suggesting that familiarity with native segmental characteristics emerges later than familiarity with native suprasegmental characteristics.

Effects of Language Experience on Speech Discrimination

Many phonemes are common across most languages, and early work on speech discrimination in infants focused on their ability to discriminate those common phonemes. However, some phonemes are particular to one or just a few of the world's languages. For example, in Hindi there are two types of "d" sounds. One is similar to the English "d" ([d]—produced by the tongue releasing down from the teeth); the other—a *retroflex* "d" [ɖ]—is produced by pulling the tongue back from the teeth. Non-Hindi speakers have difficulty hearing the difference between these two "d" sounds. Werker and Tees (1984) wanted to know if infants could discriminate phonemic contrasts that occurred in some languages but which were difficult for adults who did not speak those languages to discriminate. They tested three age groups (6–8 months, 8–10 months, and 10–12 months) from three language backgrounds (English, Hindi, and Nthlakapmx) on several consonant contrasts. Werker and Tees (1984) found that younger infants were able to discriminate all of the contrasts but 10- to 12-month-olds could discriminate only those that were linguistically relevant in their native language, suggesting that consonant discrimination is affected by language input.

The effect of language input on speech discrimination has been investigated with vowels as well. Kuhl, Williams, Lacerda, Stevens, and Lindblom (1992) tested English-learning and Swedish-learning infants' discrimination of variants of the English vowel [i] and the Swedish vowel [y]. The two groups of infants showed different patterns of results, suggesting that language background affected their discrimination of the vowels. Specifically, when infants were presented with variants of [i], English-learning infants were less likely to discriminate two variants that were acoustically similar to the prototypical English [i] than two variants that were less similar to the prototype, even though the variants in each pair were equally similar to each other. Swedish-learning infants, by contrast, were just as likely to discriminate both pairs of the English [i] variants. When infants were presented with variants of the Swedish vowel [y], the group differences were reversed: only the Swedish-learning infants' discrimination was affected by similarity to the prototype. Kuhl (1991, 1993) described these findings as representing a "perceptual magnet effect" in which the distribution of vowel variants in the ambient language shapes infants' perceptual systems such that they perceive variants within a vowel category to be more like the prototype of that category. Polka and Bohn (1996), however, found no evidence of a perceptual magnet effect when they tested English-learning and German-learning infants' discrimination of the German and English contrasts. Instead, these findings and others suggest that vowels on the periphery of the F1/F2 acoustic space serve as universal perceptual attractors (Polka & Bohn, 2003).

These and similar findings (Best, McRoberts, & Sithole, 1988; Trehub, 1976; Tsushima et al., 1994; Werker & Lalonde, 1988) led to a *universalist* view of infant speech discrimination—that infants are born able to discriminate any phonemic contrast that could potentially be relevant to any of the world's languages; and then, with experience, infants lose the ability to discriminate contrasts that are not relevant for their language (e.g., Eimas, Miller, & Jusczyk, 1987; Werker & Pegg, 1992). Since then, however, the picture of infants' speech discrimination abilities has become more complex. For example, while some non-native phoneme contrasts may fall into the same phonemic category in English (e.g., the Hindi [ɖ]), many speech sounds (e.g., African clicks) do not fall into any phonemic category of English speakers. Best, McRoberts, Lafleur, and Silver-Isenstadt (1995) found that such contrasts remain easy to discriminate for English-speaking adults and older infants. These findings provide evidence against a strong universalist view that infants lose the ability to discriminate all sounds that are not linguistically relevant.

One limitation of a universalist view of speech discrimination is that it does not take into consideration subphonemic information that, while not relevant for distinguishing words, is relevant for other aspects of speech perception and language acquisition. Allophones (context-dependent variants of phonemes) specify details for how words are produced in the native language and can play a role in speech segmentation. For example, initial stops are aspirated in English but not in French—"port" is pronounced [p^hort] in English, but in French "porte" (door) is pronounced [port]. Stops are unaspirated in other positions in English (e.g., "sport"). To sound like a native English speaker, English-learning infants must encode allophonic information even though it does not differentiate words. Hohne and Jusczyk (1994) tested infants' discrimination of words and word pairs such as "nitrates" and "night rates." The same strings of phonemes comprise these sequences but differ with respect to some of the allophonic information: the "t" in "nitrates" is aspirated, released, and retroflexed; the "t" in "night rates" is unaspirated, unreleased, and not retroflexed. Also, the "r" is devoiced in "nitrates" but not in "night rates." Two-month-olds demonstrated discrimination of these allophones (Hohne & Jusczyk, 1994). Subsequent investigations of infants' use of allophonic information (discussed below) suggest that infants do not lose their ability to discriminate this fine-grained information.

Another challenge to a universalist view of speech discrimination is that some contrasts, rather than being discriminable universally during early infancy, require language experience before they can be discriminated. Lacerda (1993) found that Swedish-learning 6- to 12-month-olds could discriminate between [a] and [ʌ] but not between [a] and [ɑ], both of which are linguistically relevant in Swedish. Similarly, Lasky, Syrdal-Lasky, and Klein (1975) tested Spanish-learning 4.5- to 6-month-olds on three different VOT contrasts. They found that the Spanish-learning infants were able to discriminate a pair of speech sounds that was irrelevant for Spanish but relevant for English, but did not discriminate a contrast that is distinctive in Spanish. Recent investigations have demonstrated that discrimination of some contrasts improves with language experience from infancy through adulthood (Polka, Colantonio, & Sundara, 2001; Sundara, Polka, & Genesee, 2006; Tsao, Lui, & Kuhl, 2006). For example, English-learning infants and children improve in their ability to discriminate the [d]-[ð] contrast, whereas French-learning infants and children do not (Polka et al., 2001; Sundara et al., 2006). Taken together, the findings point to an early perceptual system that is able to discriminate most contrasts of the world's languages, and then through experience with language input, infants become more sensitive to sounds that are relevant for their language and less sensitive to contrasts that are not linguistically relevant.

Six Months to One Year: Demonstrations of Learning

Given that infants seem to learn something about the organization of sounds in their language by the second half of the first year of life, it is worth considering what kinds of learning mechanisms are required to allow this auditory-perceptual learning to occur. This section will describe some of the specific learning abilities of infants that may interact with their innate auditory and perceptual abilities to transition them from a universal perceiver to having a perceptual system tuned to the native language.

Mechanisms of Learning in Infants

Several learning mechanisms contribute to the development of language-specific speech perception skills. These learning mechanisms include (but are not limited to) recognition memory, associative learning, and statistical learning. Each of these learning mechanisms has been studied extensively by developmental scientists, and a full review of them is beyond the scope of this chapter. Instead, we will briefly describe what these mechanisms are and some evidence that infants possess these learning mechanisms.

Recognition Memory

Recognition is a very basic form of learning. In order to recognize something, it must be encoded into memory. Visual recognition memory has been investigated much more than auditory recognition memory. One way developmental scientists have investigated visual recognition memory is by using habituation/dishabituation paradigms (Colombo, Shaddy, Richman, Maikranz, & Blaga, 2004; Fagan & McGrath, 1981; Rose & Feldman, 1997; Rose, Feldman, & Jankowski, 2001). Infants are presented with an object or photograph of a face repeatedly until they habituate to it (i.e., decrease their looking time). Then they are presented with both a novel and the habituated object. Longer looking to the novel than to the habituated object indicates recognition of the object the child has already seen. Recognition memory improves significantly during the first year of life (Rose et al., 2001) and correlates with later cognitive and language outcomes (Rose, Feldman, & Wallace, 1992; Rose, Feldman, Wallace, & McCarton, 1991), suggesting that it is an important cognitive skill for cognitive and language development.

Some examples of infants' recognition memory for speech have already been reviewed above. Preferences for native language and mother's voice suggest recognition. Work with older infants suggests that infants' representations of speech sounds become more generalizable with experience and development. For example, Houston and Jusczyk (2000) tested infants' ability to recognize familiarized words when presented with a different voice. They found that 10.5-month-olds but not 7.5-month-olds were able to recognize words across talkers of the opposite sex, suggesting that 7.5-month-olds encode talker-specific information in memory and that this affects how they recognize words (see also Houston, 1999; Houston & Jusczyk, 2003). These findings illustrate how the development of recognition memory skills is important for correctly identifying words as novel and old, which is an important skill for learning the meaning of words across different contexts. Later, we discuss some additional examples of how the development of recognition memory skills affects speech perception in infants.

Associative Learning

Associative learning is highly relevant to language acquisition; word learning is a sophisticated type of associative learning. But well before infants utter their first words, their associative learning skills develop in nonlinguistic domains. In the visual domain, early associative learning plays an important role in forming categories of objects. Younger and Cohen (1986) investigated 4-, 7-, and 10-month-olds' use of correlated attributes (e.g., long neck associated with large ears and short neck associated with small ears) to form categories of novel animal drawings. They found that normal hearing 7-month-olds but not 4-month-olds could learn correlations among attributes when all attributes were perfectly correlated and that normal hearing 10-month-olds but not 7-month-olds could learn correlations among attributes when some of the attributes were correlated and others were not. Similar studies have found that older infants can learn correlations among objects' parts and their motion trajectories (Rakison & Poulin-Dubois, 2002).

In the auditory domain, young infants can learn simple associations, such as the relationship between vocal affect and facial expressions (Kahana-Kalman & Walker-Andrews, 2001; Walker, 1982; Walker-Andrews, 1986). Older infants learn to associate complex strings of speech sounds (i.e., words) with objects, actions, attributes, and experiences. The development of associative learning skills plays important roles in various aspects of language acquisition, some of which will be discussed later.

Statistical Learning

Statistical learning is related to associative learning. But rather than learning that x is associated with y, statistical learning involves learning the probability of y given x. In the visual domain, infants' statistical learning skills have been investigated by assessing their ability to learn visual sequences. Young infants (3- to 4-month-olds) can learn simple two- and three-location spatiotemporal patterns (Clohessy, Posner, & Rothbart, 2001; Haith, Hazan, & Goodman, 1988; Wentworth, Haith, & Hood, 2002), whereas older infants are able to learn more complex spatiotemporal sequences (Clohessy et al., 2001; Kirkham, Slemmer, Richardson, & Johnson, 2007).

In a seminal study on auditory statistical learning, Saffran, Aslin and Newport (1996) tested 8-month-olds' ability to detect syllable sequences within a two-minute continuous stream of synthetic CV syllables. The speech stream consisted of four three-syllable sequences with no pauses between sequences. Thus, the only way infants could learn the sequences was by encoding the transitional probabilities of the syllables. For example, if one of the four sequences was /da/ro/pi/ then the probability of /ro/ following /da/ and of /pi/ following /ro/ would both be 1.0. However, /pi/ would be followed by one of three syllables. Saffran et al. found that 8-month-olds showed a novelty preference for sequences that had lower transitional probabilities in the speech stream (e.g., /pi/go/) compared with sequences that had high transitional probabilities (e.g., /da/ro/). These findings and others suggest that infants are sensitive to the statistical properties of speech sounds in their language.

Motivation for Social Interaction and Exploration

Although children readily learn language, it does require some effort. Innate speech perception capacities and learning mechanisms do not by themselves explain language acquisition. Infants' motivations and intentions play an important role in language development (Bloom & Tinker, 2001). Infants are dependent on their caregivers for physical and emotional needs and are thus motivated to communicate with their caregivers (Locke, 1993). What infants attend to in speech depends on their needs, which change with development. At the beginning of life, infants may seek only social-emotional information from speech and may attend mainly to prosodic information. As infants become more sophisticated, they attend to other aspects of speech that are more relevant to language acquisition. Moreover, motivation to attend to one type of information (e.g., prosody for affect) may set the groundwork for acquiring knowledge useful for obtaining other types of information (e.g., word boundaries) that are useful for obtaining later goals (e.g., understanding what the caregiver is trying to communicate).

Infants' speech perception changes through the interaction of cognitive, social, and linguistic factors. With development, infants are motivated for increasingly more sophisticated communication. Attention to speech and increasingly sophisticated learning mechanisms result in infants forming mental representations that shape how speech is perceived. And because the input to the learning mechanisms differs across languages, infants form language-specific representations that result in language-specific perception of speech.

Organizing the Suprasegmentals

We learned earlier that newborns are able to discriminate the rhythmic properties of languages when languages fall into different rhythmic classes. That initial sensitivity to rhythmic information forms the basis for the ability to detect rhythmic information that relates to linguistic units in speech, such as clauses, phrases, and words. Being able to detect these linguistic structures may play a role in infants' ability to develop a vocabulary and acquire a grammar.

Utterance-Level Prosody

Utterances tend to contain one or more clauses, and clauses contain one or more phrases. An implicit understanding of clausal and phrasal organization in speech is important for language comprehension and production. Clauses and phrases influence the prosody of speech. For example, pauses tend to occur more often at clause and phrase boundaries than within clauses or phrases. It is possible that perceiving grammatical units within utterances (e.g., clauses) may be a first step in acquiring a grammar.

Hirsh-Pasek et al. (1987) investigated infants' sensitivity to prosodic markings of clause boundaries in fluent speech. They presented 6- and 9-month-olds with passages of natural infant-directed speech in which 1-second pauses were inserted either between or within clauses. Both groups of infants looked longer when pauses were between clauses than when they were within clauses, suggesting that by 6 months of age, English-learning infants have become familiarized with the prosodic cohesiveness of clauses in English.

Infants' sensitivity to the prosody of syntactic structures appears to also play a role in recognizing familiar sequences of words in the context of fluent speech. Nazzi, Kemler Nelson, Jusczyk, and Jusczyk (2000) investigated this in English-learning infants. Six-month-olds were familiarized with sequences of words (e.g., rabbits eat leafy vegetables) and then presented with passages in which the sequence of words occurred either within a clause (e.g., . . . rabbits eat leafy vegetables . . . .) or between clauses (e.g., . . . rabbits eat. Leafy vegetables . . .). Infants demonstrated recognition of the words only when they occurred within clauses (see also Soderstrom, Seidl, Kemler Nelson, & Jusczyk, 2003). Six- and 9-month-old English-learning infants show similar encoding effects for the prosodic structure of phrases (Soderstrom, Kemler Nelson, & Jusczyk, 2005).

There are several possible prosodic cues that can play a role in infants' perception of prosodic structure cohesiveness (e.g., pauses, lengthening of vowels before clause boundaries, intonation). English-learning infants appear to use multiple cues fairly equally at 4 months of age (Seidl & Cristiá, 2008) but then rely mainly on pitch cues by 6 months of age (Seidl, 2007). The cues that infants rely on also seem to be language dependent (Johnson & Seidl, 2008). Taken together, the studies of infants' sensitivity to prosodic structure suggest that infants may begin parsing speech into prosodic units at a very young age using multiple cues and then eventually learn to rely on particular cues. Statistical and associative learning are involved such that infants learn via statistical learning which prosodic boundaries cues co-occur most often with other prosodic boundary cues and then associate those cues with clausal and phrasal boundaries.

Language discrimination studies provide additional evidence of infants' developing sensitivity to prosodic information. Recall that newborns are able to discriminate languages that differ rhythmically (Nazzi et al., 1998). Nazzi, Jusczyk, and Johnson (2000) found that by 5 months of age, English-learning infants can discriminate their native language (e.g., American English) from languages (e.g., Dutch) and dialects (e.g., British English) within their same rhythmic class but cannot discriminate two foreign languages (e.g., Dutch and German) from the same rhythmic class. The investigators concluded that because 5-month-olds do not show language discrimination based on segmental information in previous work (Jusczyk, Friederici, et al., 1993), their discrimination was most likely due to an increased sensitivity to prosodic information that allowed the infants to detect subtle differences in rhythmic properties between the languages and dialects.

The above findings suggest that infants develop increasing familiarity with the prosodic properties of speech, including prosodic cues to linguistic units. This development suggests that there are learning mechanisms that transform infants from having a universal sensitivity to prosodic information to having a perceptual system tuned to the prosodic properties of the ambient language. First, recognition memory is required to identify units of speech as having rhythmic structure consistent with being clauses or phrases. Second, statistical learning is required to learn that certain rhythmic units (e.g., clauses) tend to co-occur with pauses while other rhythmic units (e.g., a sequence of words across a clause boundary) are not associated with a pause.

Word-Level Prosody

The research reviewed so far has informed us about infants' sensitivity to the organization of large prosodic units and intonational patterns, which may be an important first step in children's acquisition of syntax. But we have said very little so far about infants' sensitivity to smaller rhythmic units. Young infants are able to discriminate isolated words that differ in stress pattern (Jusczyk & Thompson, 1977) just as they are able to discriminate isolated words and syllables that differ by one phoneme (reviewed above). But to what extent are they sensitive to the rhythmic properties of words in the real world? In other words, do infants encode the rhythmic properties of words in the ambient language and build up implicit knowledge—via statistical learning—of the frequencies of different rhythmic patterns of words? Before we review the research that has addressed this question, we should first consider why sensitivity to the rhythmic properties of words might be important for speech comprehension. One important role for the rhythmic properties of words in speech comprehension is the role it plays in the process of segmenting words from the context of fluent speech (i.e., speech segmentation).

Speech segmentation is a major topic in speech science because natural speech does not contain obvious acoustic cues to word boundaries (Cole & Jakimik, 1980). We perceive word boundaries because we are able to segment continuous speech into words (listening to someone speak an unfamiliar language is an easy way to appreciate this fact). Although fluent speech does not reliably contain obvious word boundaries, people are, of course, able to segment fluent speech once they know a language. Knowing the words of a language is probably the most important factor for segmenting speech—recognizing a word informs the listener where the onset of the following word is. But there are also acoustic cues that become useful for segmentation as listeners gain implicit knowledge of the language, including the rhythmic properties of words.

One model of speech segmentation that emphasizes the importance of word rhythm is Anne Cutler's metrical segmentation strategy (MSS) model. The MSS asserts that in some languages, including English, listeners are attuned to strong[1] syllables as the primary acoustic cue for speech segmentation. In languages like English strong syllables can serve as cues for segmentation because of their distribution in the language. Cutler and Carter (1987) conducted a corpus investigation of English and found that approximately 90% of content words in English begin with a strong syllable. Thus, if listeners assumed that every strong syllable they heard marked the onset of a word, they would be correct most of the time. Cutler and colleagues tested this idea experimentally in a number of studies with adults and found that English speakers do indeed tend to perceive strong syllables as word onsets (Cutler & Butterfield, 1992; Cutler & Norris, 1988; McQueen, Norris, & Cutler, 1994).

As important a role that word rhythm may play in adults' ability to segment speech, it may play an even greater role in the development of speech segmentation during infancy. Unlike adults, infants do not have a developed lexicon to help them identify words in fluent speech. And while infants may learn some words from hearing them often in isolation (e.g., "hi," "daddy"), the vast majority of words are not uttered in isolation,

[1]The term "strong syllable" is nearly synonymous with the term "stressed syllable." A strong syllable is any syllable that has a fully realized (i.e., nonreduced) vowel. A stressed syllable is a syllable that is more perceptually salient than its neighboring syllables. To illustrate, take the spondee "mailman." Both syllables are strong because their vowels are fully realized. However, neither syllable has lexical stress because they have similar perceptual salience.

even to infants. An analysis of speech to an infant over a three-week period found that 90 to 95% of utterances contained more than one word (van de Weijer, 1998). Even when caregivers are instructed to teach words, they present the novel words in isolation only 20% of the time (Woodward & Aslin, 1990). Thus, being able to segment words from the context of fluent speech is an important skill for language acquisition.

Understanding the role word rhythm might play in infant speech segmentation returns us to the question of infants' sensitivity to the rhythmic properties of words. To address this question, Jusczyk, Cutler, and Redanz (1993) presented 6- and 9-month-old English-learning infants with lists of strong/weak words and lists of weak/strong words. They found that 9-month-olds oriented longer to the words that follow the predominant stress pattern of English (strong/weak), but 6-month-olds did not. Similarly, Echols, Crowhurst, and Childers (1997) presented infants with trisyllabic weak/strong/weak sequences that contained a pause either before or after the strong syllable. They found that 9-month-old English-learning infants preferred sequences with the pause before the strong syllable, which preserved the strong/weak structure. These findings suggest that over the course of at least six months of exposure to English, infants build up the implicit knowledge that strong/weak words are more common than weak/strong words. In other words, their statistical learning skills enable them to acquire sensitivity to the predominant stress pattern of words in their language.

Findings that English-learning infants become sensitive to the predominant stress pattern of words in their language led Peter Jusczyk and his colleagues to investigate the role of lexical stress in the development of speech segmentation skills. They did this by using a variant of the headturn preference procedure (HPP) to directly assess infants' ability to detect different types of familiarized words in the context of fluent speech. In the HPP infants are first familiarized with two words—one word per trial repeated up to 20 times. Then during a test phase, they are presented with four passages—two of which contain the familiarized words. Their attention to each passage is measured by the amount of time they orient to a light that is located in front of the loudspeaker presenting the passages and which blinks during the presentation of each passage. Seminal work using this methodology suggests that infants orient longer to the presentation of passages containing the familiarized words than to other passages when they are able to segment and recognize the familiarized words from the context of fluent speech (Jusczyk & Aslin, 1995). An alternative version of the HPP involves presenting two of the four passages during the familiarization period and then presenting the two familiarized words and two unfamiliar words during the test phase. These two variants of the HPP have been found to produce identical results (Jusczyk & Aslin, 1995; Jusczyk, Houston, & Newsome, 1999).

Using the HPP, Jusczyk, Houston, and Newsome (1999) assessed 7.5- and 10.5-month-old English-learning infants' ability to segment strong/weak and weak/strong words from fluent speech. They found that 7.5-month-olds were able to segment strong/weak but not weak/strong words from fluent speech. Instead, infants showed evidence of segmenting only the strong syllable of weak/strong words. When 7.5-month-olds were familiarized with just the strong syllable of weak/strong words (e.g., tar from guitar) they oriented longer to passages containing the corresponding weak/strong whole words (e.g., guitar). However, when they were familiarized with the whole words (e.g., guitar), they did not orient longer to the passages containing the familiarized words.[2] In other words, *tar* matched better to what 7.5-month-olds heard in passages containing *guitar* than did *guitar*. By 10.5 months of age, however, English-learning infants show the opposite pattern of results.

Jusczyk, Houston, and Newsome (1999) interpreted the findings with the strong/weak and weak/strong words as follows: English-learning infants begin segmenting words from fluent speech using a type of metrical segmentation strategy: They assume that strong syllables mark word onsets; when a strong syllable is followed by the same weak syllable consistently—as is the case when a strong/weak word occurs often in a passage—then infants will treat the strong/weak word as a cohesive unit. To test this interpretation, they created new passages for the weak/strong words in which each weak/strong word was consistently followed by the same function word (e.g., guitar is). Infants were presented with two of the passages and then tested on either the strong syllables of the target words or with strong/weak nonwords formed from the strong syllable of the weak/strong words and the following function word (e.g., tar-is). Unlike the previous experiment with weak/strong words, 7.5-month-olds did not demonstrate segmentation of the strong syllable from the weak/strong words in the passages. Instead, they demonstrated recognition of

[2]For both conditions, identical results were found when infants were tested with the passages-first variant of the HPP.

the strong/weak pseudowords (e.g., taris). These findings suggest that 7.5-month-old English-learning infants use a strong version of the MSS to segment words from fluent speech such that they segment strong/weak units even when they cross word boundaries.

Using a strong version of the MSS allows English-learning infants to segment most words from fluent speech correctly. However, as seen in the findings of Jusczyk et al. (1999), a strong version of MSS results in mis-segmenting words that do not follow the predominant stress pattern of English. Thus, if infants use a strong version of the MSS, they must eventually adopt a less strong version and incorporate other information in their segmentation strategy. To investigate the use of this strong version of the MSS in older infants, Jusczyk et al. (1999) also tested 10.5-month-olds with the passages in which the weak/strong target words were always followed by the same function word. Unlike 7.5-month-olds, 10.5-month-olds did not demonstrate recognition when presented with the pseudowords (e.g., taris). However, they did demonstrate recognition when presented with the weak/strong words (e.g., guitar) during testing, suggesting that 10.5-month-old English-learning infants correctly segment weak/strong words from fluent speech even when they are consistently followed by the same function word.

Taken together, the above findings and others (Houston, Jusczyk, Kuijpers, Coolen, & Cutler, 2000; Houston, Santelmann, & Jusczyk, 2004; Johnson & Jusczyk, 2001) suggest that infants use statistical learning to infer the rhythmic structure of words in their language, and then that learning influences their processing of fluent speech. The initial segmentation strategy that develops from acquiring knowledge about the rhythmic properties of words does not always result in correct segmentation, so infants must acquire knowledge about other segmentation cues. We discuss what some of those other cues are next.

Meaningful Segmental Information

We learned earlier that young infants demonstrate discrimination of phonetic segments even when the differences between those segments do not differentiate words in their language. We also learned that toward the end of the first year of life, infants lose the ability to discriminate some non-native contrasts. On the surface, it appears that infants become less sensitive to segmental information. However, investigations of infants' sensitivity to segmental properties in their language suggest that infants learn much about how phonetic segments are distributed and organized in the ambient language during the first year of life. This statistical learning about the distributional properties of segmental information, in turn, shapes more advanced speech perception processes, such as infants' perception of word boundaries in fluent speech (i.e., speech segmentation). The following sections review investigations of older infants' sensitivity to several types of segmental information and what role these acquired sensitivities play in segmenting words from fluent speech.

Phonotactic Probabilities

The term "phonotactics" refers to the ordering of segments in languages. Languages differ greatly with respect to what clusters of phonemes are permissible in various positions within and between words and syllables. In English syllables, for example, each consonant before a vowel must be more sonorous than the previous segment and less sonorous than the subsequent segment ([s] is an exception). Thus the word "plan" is possible but the word "lpan" is not in English. Moreover, the word "pkan" is not possible because [p] and [k] have equal sonority. In other languages, such as Polish, syllable-initial consonant clusters can contain two voiceless stops in a row. In addition to phonotactic rules, there are phonotactic probabilities. Phonotactic probabilities refer to the occurrence of segment pairs within and between words and syllables. For example, the pair [s]-[d] occurs more often between words than within words in English whereas the pair [s]-[t] occurs more often within words than between words. Sensitivity to these kinds of phonotactic probabilities can provide information about likely word boundaries in fluent speech.

Infants appear to become sensitive to phonotactic rules and probabilities at around the same time they show sensitivity to the predominant stress pattern of words in their language. Jusczyk, Friederici, Wessels, Svenkerud, and Jusczyk (1993) tested English-learning and Dutch-learning infants with lists of words that were either phonotactically legal in English and not in Dutch or vice versa. Dutch- and English-learning 9-month-olds both oriented longer to lists of words that were legal in their native language. Six-month-olds showed no preferences. Similarly, Friederici and Wessels (1993) found that Dutch-learning 9-month-olds but not 6-month-olds attended longer to non-words with phonotactically permissible word onsets and offsets than to nonwords with phonotactically impermissible onsets and offsets, even though the impermissible onsets were permissible as offsets and vice versa. Jusczyk, Luce, and Charles-Luce (1994) found that 9-month-old English-learning infants attended longer to lists of words with higher phonotactic probabilities than to lists of words with relatively lower phonotactic probabilities even though none of the words had any sequences that were phonotactically impermissible.

Like sensitivity to lexical stress, sensitivity to phonotactic probabilities appears to play a role in infants' segmentation abilities. Mattys and Jusczyk (2001) used the HPP to investigate 9-month-old English-learning infants' segmentation of words from fluent speech that had either easy or difficult phonotactic boundary information. Similar to Jusczyk, Houston, and Newsome (1999), infants were familiarized with two passages, each containing several instances of a target word. In this experiment, however, they manipulated the words that surrounded the target words such that they provided either good or poor phonotactic boundary information. Infants were able to segment the words from fluent speech only when the phonotactic boundary information for the target words was good at either the onset, offset or both. These findings suggest that by 9 months of age, English-learning infants acquire knowledge about the frequency of occurrence of phoneme sequences within words and can use this information to segment words from fluent speech.

Subphonemic Cues

So far, we have reviewed speech cues infants use for segmenting words from fluent speech that are at the clause, phrase, syllable, and phoneme levels of acoustic-phonetic information. As discussed earlier, infants appear to be sensitive not only to these levels of acoustic-phonetic information; they are also sensitive to subphonemic information in speech (Hohne & Jusczyk, 1994; McMurray & Aslin, 2005). It is possible that subphonemic information may play a role in infant speech segmentation. Using the HPP, Jusczyk, Hohne, and Bauman (1999) investigated English-learning infants' sensitivity to allophonic information as a cue to word segmentation. Infants were familiarized with two-syllable items (e.g., nitrates) and tested for recognition of those sequences in fluent speech. Jusczyk et al. found that 10.5-month-olds but not 9-month-olds listened longer to the passages containing the exact match (e.g., nitrates) than to passages containing an allophonic variant (night rates) of the familiarized items, suggesting that only the older infants relied on allophonic information to segment words from fluent speech.

Subsequent investigations have provided additional evidence that infants are sensitive to subphonemic cues to word segmentation. By 8 months of age, English-learning infants' segmentation of three-word sequences is affected by whether they are produced as single words (e.g., catalog) versus three-word phrases (e.g., cat a log; Johnson, 2003; Johnson & Jusczyk, 2001). By 12 months of age, English-learning infants demonstrate sensitivity to subtle acoustic-phonetic word boundary information (e.g., [toga][lore] versus [toe][galore]) when segmenting strong/weak sequences (e.g., toga) from fluent speech (Johnson, 2008). Taken together, these studies suggest that a variety of subphonemic cues play a role in infants' speech segmentation, especially by the end of their first year of life.

Infants' sensitivity to segmental information as cues to word segmentation is acquired as a result of their experience to language and their developing learning mechanisms. Most of the segmental cues to segmentation discussed in this section are not universal across languages. So for these cues to be useful for segmentation, statistical and associative learning is necessary in order to learn which phoneme sequences and subphonemic variants are associated with word boundaries and which are not. However, in order to learn which segmental cues are associated with word boundaries, infants must be able to segment at least some words from fluent speech. As a solution to this apparent chicken-and-egg problem, Jusczyk (1997, 2002) posited that English-learning infants use a divide-and-conquer strategy: they first segment strong/weak units from fluent speech and then analyze the strong/weak units to discover other segmentation cues. This is a plausible strategy for English-learning infants to use because of the rhythmic properties of English words. Recent evidence suggests that in languages with different rhythmic properties, infants adopt other segmentation strategies (Nazzi, Iakimova, Bertoncini, Frédonie, & Alcantara, 2006).

Nonphonetically Based Segmentation Cues

Most work on infant speech segmentation has focused on the role that acoustic-phonetic properties play. However, there are other types of information infants can exploit to segment words from fluent speech. Earlier we reviewed work by Saffran et al. (1996), which found that statistical learning skills enable 8-month-olds to compute transitional probabilities of syllables. For example, if an infant notices that occurrences of the syllable [ma] are usually followed by the syllable [mi] and that what precedes [ma] and what follows [mi] is highly variable, this statistical information may contribute to helping the infant segment [ma]-[mi] as a cohesive unit from fluent speech. And then if an infant is able to recognize a familiar word like "mommy" in an utterance, then that word can serve as a wedge to help segment the surrounding words. A recent investigation found just that. Bortfeld, Morgan, Golinkoff, and Rathbun (2005) tested 6-month-olds' segmentation of words from fluent speech that were preceded by words they already knew (e.g., "mommy"). In contrast to earlier studies showing that 6-month-olds could not segment words from fluent speech (Jusczyk & Aslin, 1995), Bortfeld et al. (2005) found that 6-month-olds could segment words from fluent speech, but only when preceded by a word they already knew. These findings suggest that word recognition plays an important role in segmenting novel words from fluent speech.

Some Afterthoughts

The field of infant speech perception has grown immensely over the last 40 years, and this review of the work is, as a consequence, very incomplete. Many of the most important studies in the field were left out. More thorough reviews of the field can be found elsewhere (Jusczyk, 1997; Saffran, Werker, & Werner, 2006). The purpose of this chapter is to provide some understanding of how our hearing instrument becomes tuned to process speech. We first reviewed some of what is known about infants' early speech perception abilities and then described some of the developments in speech perception during the second half of the first year of life that put infants in a position to segment words from fluent speech. Finally, I described some general learning mechanisms that play a role in the development of speech perception skills.

Gaining a better understanding of how cognitive mechanisms affect speech perception development in typically developing normal-hearing infants contributes to our general understanding of language development. This knowledge also may have clinical implications for infants and children with congenital hearing loss. With impoverished auditory input, general cognitive skills may be particularly important for hearing-impaired infants' ability to achieve successful language outcomes. Future work exploring the links between specific cognitive and speech perception skills in both normal-hearing and hearing-impaired infants could provide valuable information to clinicians, especially if methods of improving cognitive skills in infants can be developed. Moreover, comparing normal-hearing and hearing-impaired infants' speech perception skills can provide insight into the effects of early auditory experience on the development of early speech perception and language skills (Horn, Houston, & Miyamoto, 2007; Houston, Pisoni, Kirk, Ying, & Miyamoto, 2003; Houston, Ying, Pisoni, & Kirk, 2003).

Acknowledgments. Preparation of this chapter was facilitated by a Research Grant from NIDCD (DC006235) and support from the Philip F. Holton Fund. The author would like to thank Carissa Shafto for helpful comments on a previous version of this chapter.

References

Behme, C., & Deacon, S. H. (2008). Language learning in infancy: Does the empirical evidence support a domain specific language acquisition device? *Philosophical Psychology*, *21*(5), 641–671.

Best, C. T., McRoberts, G. W., Lafleur, R., & Silver-Isenstadt, J. (1995). Divergent developmental patterns for infants' perception of two nonnative consonant contrasts. *Infant Behavior and Development*, *18*, 339–350.

Best, C. T., McRoberts, G. W., & Sithole, N. M. (1988). Examination of the perceptual re-organization for speech contrasts: Zulu click discrimination by English-speaking adults and infants. *Journal of Experimental Psychology: Human Perception and Performance*, *14*, 345–360.

Birnholz, J. C., & Benacerraf, B. B. (1983). The development of human fetal hearing. *Science*, *222*, 516–518.

Bloom, L., & Tinker, E. (2001). The intentionality model and language acquisition: Engagement, effort, and the essential tension in development. *Monographs of the Society for Research in Child Development*, *66*(4), 1–91.

Bortfeld, H., Morgan, J. L., Golinkoff, R. M., & Rathbun, K. (2005). Mommy and me: Familiar names help launch babies into speech-stream segmentation. *Psychological Science*, *15*(4), 298–304.

Chomsky, N. (1968). *Language and mind*. New York, NY: Harcourt Brace.

Chomsky, N. (1975). *Reflections on language*. New York, NY: Pantheon Books.

Clohessy, A. B., Posner, M. I., & Rothbart, M. K. (2001). Development of the functional visual field. *Acta Psychologica*, *106*(1–2), 51–68.

Cole, R. A., & Jakimik, J. (1980). A model of speech perception. In R. A. Cole (Ed.), *Perception and production of fluent speech* (pp. 133–163). Hillsdale, NJ: Erlbaum.

Colombo, J., Shaddy, D. J., Richman, W. A., Maikranz, J. M., & Blaga, O. M. (2004). The developmental course of habituation in infancy and preschool outcome. *Infancy*, *5*(1), 1–38.

Cooper, R. P., & Aslin, R. N. (1990). Preference for infant-directed speech in the first month after birth. *Child Development*, *61*, 1584–1595.

Cutler, A., & Butterfield, S. (1992). Rhythmic cues to speech segmentation: Evidence from juncture misperception. *Journal of Memory and Language*, *31*(2), 218–236.

Cutler, A., & Carter, D. M. (1987). The predominance of strong initial syllables in the English vocabulary. *Computer Speech and Language*, *2*, 133–142.

Cutler, A., & Norris, D. (1988). The role of strong syllables in segmentation for lexical access. *Journal of Experimental Psychology: Human Perception and Performance*, *14*(1), 113–121.

DeCasper, A. J., & Fifer, W. P. (1980). Of human bonding: Newborns prefer their mothers' voices. *Science*, *208*, 1174–1176.

DeCasper, A. J., Lecanuet, J. P., Busnel, M. C., Granier-Deferre, C., & Maugeais, R. (1994). Fetal reactions to recurrent maternal speech. *Infant Behavior and Development*, *17*, 159–164.

DeCasper, A. J., & Spence, M. J. (1986). Prenatal maternal speech influences newborns' perception of speech sounds. *Infant Behavior and Development*, *9*, 133–150.

Echols, C. H., Crowhurst, M. J., & Childers, J. (1997). Perception of rhythmic units in speech by infants and adults. *Journal of Memory and Language*, *36*, 202–225.

Eimas, P. D. (1974). Auditory and linguistic processing of cues for place of articulation by infants. *Attention, Perception, & Psychophysics*, *16*, 513–521.

Eimas, P. D. (1975). Auditory and phonetic coding of the cues for speech: Discrimination of the [r-l] distinction by young infants. *Perception, and Psychophysics*, *18*, 341–347.

Eimas, P. D., & Miller, J. L. (1980a). Contextual effects in infant speech perception. *Science*, *209*, 1140–1141.

Eimas, P. D., & Miller, J. L. (1980b). Discrimination of the information for manner of articulation. *Infant Behavior and Development*, *3*, 367–375.

Eimas, P. D., Miller, J. L., & Jusczyk, P. W. (1987). On infant speech perception and the acquisition of language. In H. Stevan (Ed.), *Categorical perception: The groundwork of cognition* (pp. 161–195). New York, NY: Cambridge University Press.

Eimas, P. D., Siqueland, E. R., Jusczyk, P., & Vigorito, J. (1971). Speech perception in infants. *Science*, *171*(968), 303–306.

Fagan, J. F., & McGrath, S. K. (1981). Infant recognition memory and later intelligence. *Intelligence*, *5*, 121–130.

Fernald, A. (1985). Four-month-old infants prefer to listen to motherese. *Infant Behavior and Development*, *8*, 181–195.

Fernald, A. (1989). Intonation and communicative intent in mothers' speech to infants: Is the melody the message. *Child Development*, *60*, 1497–1510.

Fernald, A. (1993). Approval and disapproval: Infant responsiveness to vocal affect in familiar and unfamiliar languages. *Child Development*, *64*(3), 657–674.

Fernald, A., & Kuhl, P. K. (1987). Acoustic determinants of infant preference for Motherese speech. *Infant Behavior and Development*, *10*, 279–293.

Friederici, A. D., & Wessels, J. M. I. (1993). Phonotactic knowledge and its use in infant speech perception. *Perception and Psychophysics*, *54*, 287–295.

Fry, D. B., Abramson, A. S., Eimas, P. D., & Liberman, A. M. (1962). The identification and discrimination of synthetic vowels. *Language and Speech*, *5*, 171–189.

Haith, M. M., Hazan, C., & Goodman, G. S. (1988). Expectation and anticipation of dynamic visual events by 3.5-month-old babies. *Child Development*, *59*, 467–479.

Hirsh-Pasek, K., Kemler Nelson, D. G., Jusczyk, P. W., Cassidy, K. W., Druss, B., & Kennedy, L. (1987). Clauses are perceptual units for young infants. *Cognition*, *26*(3), 269–286.

Hohne, E. A., & Jusczyk, P. W. (1994). Two-month-old infants' sensitivity to allophonic differences. *Perception and Psychophysics*, *56*(6), 613–623.

Horn, D. L., Houston, D. M., & Miyamoto, R. T. (2007). Speech discrimination skills in deaf infants before and after cochlear implantation. *Audiological Medicine*, *5*, 232–241.

Houston, D. M. (1999). *The role of talker variability in infant word representations.* Doctoral dissertation. Johns Hopkins University, Baltimore, MD.

Houston, D. M., & Jusczyk, P. W. (2000). The role of talker-specific information in word segmentation by infants. *Journal of Experimental Psychology: Human Perception and Performance*, *26*(5), 1570–1582.

Houston, D. M., & Jusczyk, P. W. (2003). Infants' long-term memory for the sound patterns of words and voices. *Journal of Experimental Psychology: Human Perception and Performance*, *29*(6), 1143–1154.

Houston, D. M., Jusczyk, P. W., Kuijpers, C., Coolen, R., & Cutler, A. (2000). Cross-language word segmentation by 9-month-olds. *Psychonomic Bulletin & Review*, *7*, 504–509.

Houston, D. M., Pisoni, D. B., Kirk, K. I., Ying, E., & Miyamoto, R. T. (2003). Speech perception skills of deaf infants following cochlear implantation: A first report. *International Journal of Pediatric Otorhinolaryngology*, *67*, 479–495.

Houston, D. M., Santelmann, L., & Jusczyk, P. W. (2004). English-Learning infants' segmentation of trisyllabic words from fluent speech. *Language and Cognitive Processes*, *19*(1), 97–136.

Houston, D. M., Ying, E., Pisoni, D. B., & Kirk, K. I. (2003). Development of pre word-learning skills in infants with cochlear implants. *Volta Review*, *103 (Monograph* 4), 303–326.

Johnson, E. K. (2003). *Word segmentation during infancy: The role of subphonemic cues to word boundaries.* Doctoral dissertation, Johns Hopkins University, Baltimore, MD.

Johnson, E. K. (2008). Infants' use of prosodically conditioned acoustic-phonetic cues to extract words from speech. *Journal of Acoustical Society of America*, *123*(6), EL144-148.

Johnson, E. K., & Jusczyk, P. W. (2001). Word segmentation by 8-month-olds: When speech cues count more than statistics. *Journal of Memory and Language*, *44*, 548–567.

Johnson, E. K., & Seidl, A. (2008). Clause segmentation by 6-month-old infants: A crosslinguistic perspective. *Infancy*, *13*(5), 440–455.

Jusczyk, P. W. (1997). *The discovery of spoken language.* Cambridge, MA: MIT Press.

Jusczyk, P. W. (2002). How infants adapt speech-processing capacities to native-language structure. *Current Directions in Psychological Science*, *11*(1), 18.

Jusczyk, P. W., & Aslin, R. N. (1995). Infants' detection of the sound patterns of words in fluent speech. *Cognitive Psychology*, *29*(1), 1–23.

Jusczyk, P. W., Cutler, A., & Redanz, N. J. (1993). Infants' preference for the predominant stress patterns of english words. *Child Development*, *64*(3), 675–687.

Jusczyk, P. W., Friederici, A. D., Wessels, J., Svenkerud, V. Y., & Jusczyk, A. M. (1993). Infants' sensitivity to the sound patterns of native language words. *Journal of Memory and Language*, *32*, 402–420.

Jusczyk, P. W., Hohne, E. A., & Bauman, A. (1999). Infants' sensitivity to allophonic cues for word segmentation. *Perception and Psychophysics*, *61*, 1465–1476.

Jusczyk, P. W., Houston, D. M., & Newsome, M. (1999). The beginnings of word segmentation in english-learning infants. *Cognitive Psychology*, *39*, 159–207.

Jusczyk, P. W., Luce, P. A., & Charles-Luce, J. (1994). Infants' sensitivity to phonotactic patterns in the native language. *Journal of Memory and Language*, *33*(5), 630–645.

Jusczyk, P. W., & Thompson, E. (1977). Perception of a phonetic contrast in multisyllabic utterances by 2- month-old infants. *Perception and Psychophysics*, *23*(2), 105–109.

Kahana-Kalman, R., & Walker-Andrews, A. S. (2001). The role of person familiarity in young infants' perception of emotional expressions. *Child Development*, *72*(2), 352–369.

Kirkham, N. Z., Slemmer, J. A., Richardson, D. C., & Johnson, S. P. (2007). Location, location, location: Development of spatiotemporal sequence learning in infancy. *Child Development*, *78*(5), 1559–1571.

Kisilevsky, B. S., Hains, S. M., Brown, C. A., Lee, C. T., Cowperthwaite, B., Stutzman, S. S., . . . Wang, Z. (2009). Fetal sensitivity to properties of maternal speech and language. *Infant Behavior and Development*, *32*(1), 59–71.

Kisilevsky, B. S., Hains, S. M., Lee, K., Xie, X., Huang, H., Ye, H. H., . . . Wang, Z. (2003). Effects of experience on fetal voice recognition. *Psychological Science*, *14*(3), 220–224.

Kuhl, P. K. (1991). Human adults and human infants show a "perceptual magnet effect" for the prototypes of speech categories, monkeys do not. *Perception and Psychophysics*, *50*, 93–107.

Kuhl, P. K. (1993). Innate predispositions and the effects of experience in speech perception: The native language magnet theory. In B. de Boysson-Bardies, S. de Schonen, P. Jusczyk, P. McNeilage, & J. Morton (Eds.), *Developmental neurocognition: Speech and face processing in the first year of life* (pp. 259–274). Dordrecht, The Netherlands: Kluwer.

Kuhl, P. K., Williams, K. A., Lacerda, F., Stevens, K. N., & Lindblom, B. (1992). Linguistic experiences alter phonetic perception in infants by 6 months of age. *Science*, *255*, 606–608.

Lacerda, F. (1993). Sonority contrasts dominate young infants' vowel perception. In *PERILUS XVII* (pp. 55–63). Stockholm University, Sweden.

Lasky, R. E., Syrdal-Lasky, A., & Klein, R. E. (1975). VOT discrimination by four to six and a half month old infants from Spanish environments. *Journal of Experimental Child Psychology*, *20*, 215–225.

Lecanuet, J. P., Gautheron, B., Locatelli, A., Schaal, B., Jacquet, A. Y., & Busnel, M. C. (1998). What sounds reach fetuses: Biological and nonbiological modeling of the transmission of pure tones. *Developmental Psychobiology*, *33*(3), 203–219.

Liberman, A. M., Harris, K. S., Hoffman, H. S., & Griffith, B. C. (1957). The discrimination of speech sounds within and across phoneme boundaries. *Journal of Experimental Psychology*, *54*, 358–368.

Liberman, A. M., Harris, K. S., Kinney, J. A., & Lane, H. L. (1961). The discrimination of relative-onset time of the components of certain speech and non-speech patterns. *Journal of Experimental Psychology*, *61*, 379–388.

Locke, J. L. (1993). *The child's path to spoken language*. Cambridge, MA: Harvard University Press.

Mattys, S. L., & Jusczyk, P. W. (2001). Phonotactic cues for segmentation of fluent speech by infants. *Cognition*, *78*(2), 91–121.

Maye, J., Werker, J. F., & Gerken, L. (2002). Infant sensitivity to distributional information can affect phonetic discrimination. *Cognition*, *82*, B101–B111.

McMurray, B., & Aslin, R. N. (2005). Infants are sensitive to within-category variation in speech perception. *Cognition*, *95*(2), B15–B26.

McQueen, J. M., Norris, D., & Cutler, A. (1994). Competition in spoken word recognition: Spotting words in other words. *Journal of Experimental Psychology: Learning, Memory, and Cognition*, *20*(3), 621–638.

Mehler, J., Jusczyk, P., Lambertz, G., Halsted, N., Bertoncini, J., & Amiel-Tison, C. (1988). A precursor of language acquisition in young infants. *Cognition*, *29*(2), 143–178.

Moon, C., Cooper, R. P., & Fifer, W. P. (1993). Two-day old infants prefer their native language. *Infant Behavior and Development*, *16*, 495–500.

Nazzi, T., Bertoncini, J., & Mehler, J. (1998). Language discrimination by newborns: Toward an understanding of the role of rhythm. *Journal of Experimental Psychology: Human Perception and Performance*, *24*(3), 756–766.

Nazzi, T., Iakimova, Bertoncini, J., Frédonie, & Alcantara, C. (2006). Early segmentation of fluent speech by infants acquiring French: Emerging evidence for crosslinguistic differences. *Journal of Memory and Language*, *54*, 283–299.

Nazzi, T., Jusczyk, P. W., & Johnson, E. K. (2000). Language discrimination by English-learning 5-month-olds: Effects of rhythm and familiarity. *Journal of Memory and Language*, *43*(1), 1–19.

Nazzi, T., Kemler Nelson, D. G. K., Jusczyk, P. W., & Jusczyk, A. M. (2000). Six-month-olds detection of clauses embedded in continuous speech: Effects of prosodic well-formedness. *Infancy*, *1*(1), 123–147.

Pisoni, D. B. (1973). Auditory and phonetic memory codes in the discrimination of consonants and vowels. *Perception and Psychophysics*, *13*, 253–260.

Polka, L., & Bohn, O. S. (1996). A cross-language comparison of vowel perception in English-learning and German learning infants. *Journal of the Acoustical Society of America*, *100*(1), 577–592.

Polka, L., & Bohn, O. S. (2003). Asymmetries in vowel perception. *Speech Communication*, *41*(1), 221–231.

Polka, L., Colantonio, C., & Sundara, M. (2001). A cross-language comparison of /d/ - /ð/ perception: Evidence for a new developmental pattern. *Journal of the Acoustical Society of America*, *109*(5), 2190–2201.

Rakison, D. H., & Poulin-Dubois, D. (2002). You go this way and I'll go that way: Developmental changes in infants' detection of correlations among static and dynamic features in motion events. *Child Development*, *73*(3), 682–699.

Ramus, F. (2002). Language discrimination by newborns: Teasing apart phonotactic, rhythmic, and intonational cues. *Annual Review of Language Acquisition*, *2*, 85–115.

Rose, S. A., & Feldman, J. F. (1997). Memory and speed: Their role in the relation of infant information processing to later IQ. *Child Development*, *68*(4), 630–641.

Rose, S. A., Feldman, J. F., & Jankowski, J. J. (2001). Visual short-term memory in the first year of life: Capacity and recency effects. *Developmental Psychology*, *37*(4), 539–549.

Rose, S. A., Feldman, J. F., & Wallace, I. F. (1992). Infant information processing in relation to six-year cognitive outcomes. *Child Development*, *63*, 1126–1141.

Rose, S. A., Feldman, J. F., Wallace, I. F., & McCarton, C. (1991). Information processing at 1 year: Relation to birth status and developmental outcome during the first 5 years. *Developmental Psychology*, *27*(5), 723–737.

Saffran, J. R., Aslin, R. N., & Newport, E. L. (1996). Statistical learning by 8-month-old infants. *Science*, *274*, 1926–1928.

Saffran, J. R., Werker, J., & Werner, L. (2006). The infant's auditory world: Hearing, speech and the beginnings of language. In R. Siegler & D. Kuhn (Eds.), *Handbook of child development*. (pp. 58–108). New York, NY: Wiley.

Seidl, A. (2007). Infants' use and weighting of prosodic cues in clause segmentation. *Journal of Memory and Language*, *57*(1), 24–48.

Seidl, A., & Cristià, A. (2008). Developmental changes in the weighting of prosodic cues. *Developmental Science*, *11*(4), 596–606.

Singh, L., Morgan, J. L., & Best, C. T. (2002). Infants listening preferences: Baby talk or happy talk? *Infancy*, *3*(3), 365–394.

Soderstrom, M., Nelson, D. G. K., & Jusczyk, P. W. (2005). Six-month-olds recognize clauses embedded in different passages of fluent speech. *Infant Behavior and Development*, *28*(1), 87–94.

Soderstrom, M., Seidl, A., Kemler Nelson, D. G., & Jusczyk, P. W. (2003). The prosodic bootstrapping of phrases: Evidence from prelinguistic infants. *Journal of Memory and Language*, *49*(2), 249–267.

Stevens, K. N., Liberman, A. M., Studdert-Kennedy, M. G., & Ohman, S. E. G. (1969). Cross-language study of vowel perception. *Language and Speech*, *12*, 1–23.

Sundara, M., Polka, L., & Genesee, F. (2006). Language-experience facilitates discrimination of /d-th/ in monolingual and bilingual acquisition of English. *Cognition*, *100*(2), 369–388.

Swoboda, P., Morse, P. A., & Leavitt, L. A. (1976). Continuous vowel discrimination in normal and at-risk infants. *Child Development*, *47*, 459–465.

Trehub, S. E. (1976). The discrimination of foreign speech contrasts by infants and adults. *Child Development*, *47*, 466–472.

Tsao, F. M., Liu, H. M., & Kuhl, P. K. (2006). Perception of native and non-native affricate-fricative contrasts: Cross-language tests on adults and infants. *Journal of the Acoustical Society of America*, *120*(4), 2285–2294.

Tsushima, T., Takizawa, O., Sasaki, M., Siraki, S., Nishi, K., Kohno, M., . . . Best, C. (1994). Discrimination of English /r-l/ and /w-y/ by Japanese infants at 6–12 months: Language specific developmental changes in speech perception abilities. In *International conference on spoken language processing*. Yokohama, Japan: The Acoustical Society of Japan.

van de Weijer, J. (1998). *Language input for word discovery*. Nijmegen, The Netherlands: Kluwer.

Walker, A. S. (1982). Intermodal perception of expressive behaviors by human infants. *Journal of Experimental Child Psychology*, *33*(3), 514–535.

Walker-Andrews, A. S. (1986). Intermodal perception of expressive behaviors: Relation of eye and voice. *Developmental Psychology*, *22*(3), 373–377.

Wentworth, N., Haith, M. M., & Hood, R. (2002). Spatiotemporal regularity and interevent contingencies as information for infants' visual expectations. *Infancy*, *3*(3), 303–321.

Werker, J. F., & Lalonde, C. E. (1988). Cross-Language speech perception: Initial capabilities and developmental change. *Developmental Psychology*, *24*, 672–683.

Werker, J. F., & McLeod, P. J. (1989). Infant preference for both male and female infant-directed talk: A developmental study of attentional and affective responsiveness. *Canadian Journal of Psychology*, *43*, 230–246.

Werker, J. F., & Pegg, J. E. (1992). Infant speech perception and phonological acquisition. In C. A. Ferguson, L. Menn, & C. Stoel-Gammon (Eds.), *Phonological development: Models, research, implications* (pp. 285–311). Timonium, MD: York Press.

Werker, J. F., & Tees, R. C. (1984). Cross-Language speech perception: Evidence for perceptual reorganization during the first year of life. *Infant Behavior and Development*, *7*, 49–63.

Woodward, J. Z., & Aslin, R. N. (1990). *Segmentation cues in maternal speech to infants*. Paper presented at the 7th biennial meeting of the international conference on infant studies. Montreal, Quebec, Canada.

Younger, B. A., & Cohen, L. B. (1986). Developmental change in infants' perception of correlations among attributes. *Child Development*, *57*(3), 803–815.

4

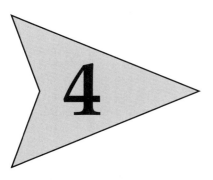

Auditory Development in Normal-Hearing Children

Lynne A. Werner and Lori J. Leibold

Why Study Auditory Development?

One of the first things that students learn when they begin to study pediatric audiology is that infants come into the world ready to learn about sound. Students are often surprised to learn that hearing, although functional, is still immature in infancy and that it continues to develop into adolescence. This may seem particularly perplexing once it is realized that the cochlea of a newborn infant responds much like that of an adult. If the inner ear is mature, why does hearing continue to develop?

Because most people with hearing loss have otherwise normally-functioning brains connected to their disordered ears, it is easy to forget that without that mature brain function, hearing could be difficult or even impossible. In fact, it appears that much of what develops about hearing during infancy and childhood resides not in the peripheral auditory system, but in the nervous system. Infants and children learn about sound, what is important in sound and what is less important, as well as what sounds mean. What infants and children learn about sound eventually makes them rapid and efficient processors of sound, but it takes a long time to learn all the details of complex sounds such as speech.

Obviously, experience with sound is critical to auditory development. Infants and children with hearing loss must pass through the same stages of auditory development as infants and children with normal hearing, but their ability to learn about sound is likely to be limited by their hearing impairment. Very little is known about auditory development in children with hearing loss. However, by carefully documenting how hearing develops in normal-hearing children, we can develop hypotheses about what specific types of auditory experience are important to development. Moreover, understanding the typical developmental time course allows us to predict how a hearing loss, amplification, or electric stimulation would change auditory development.

The studies reviewed in this chapter used behavioral responses to assess a broad range of auditory abilities, from detecting tones in quiet to detecting speech in a background of competing speech. In the study of auditory development, as in audiology, behavior is considered the "gold standard" of hearing. The studies of infants generally use a conditioned-response procedure to assess hearing; infants are rewarded by interesting sounds or interesting sights for responding to the test sounds. Visual reinforcement audiometry (VRA) is a clinical example of this type of procedure. The studies of children generally use the same sort of procedure to test children as one would use to test adults; children are asked to push a button to indicate when they hear the test sound. A detailed account of these methods and their limitations can be found in Werner and Rubel (1992) and in Werner and Marean (1995).

Development of Sound Detection: Absolute Sensitivity

Age-Related Changes

Absolute auditory sensitivity refers to the ability to detect a sound in quiet. In the audiology clinic, the typical measure of absolute sensitivity is the pure-tone audiogram. Several laboratories studying auditory development have consistently and reliably observed systematic age-related changes in absolute sensitivity (e.g., Olsho, Koch, Carter, Halpin, & Spetner, 1988; Tharpe & Ashmead, 2001; Trehub, Schneider, & Endman, 1980; reviewed by Werner, 2007). Although the most substantial of these changes occur during infancy (e.g., Tharpe & Ashmead, 2001), progressive improvements in sound detection have been observed until approximately 10 years of age (e.g., Trehub, Schneider, Morrongiello, & Thorpe, 1988).

Figure 4–1 shows the estimated audibility curve, the function that relates absolute sensitivity to acoustic frequency, at 1 month, 3 months, 6 months, 4 years, 10 years, and for adults, using data published by Werner and Marean (1996). The sounds used in the studies summarized in Figure 4–1 were pure tones or noise bands. It is clear from Figure 4–1 that developmental improvements in absolute sensitivity are not uniform across frequency. The most rapid changes in absolute thresholds occur in early infancy at high frequencies. In contrast, low-frequency thresholds mature more gradually. Whereas the average threshold in quiet at 4000 Hz improves by about 20 dB between 1 and 3 months of age, the average threshold at 500 Hz improves by only 10 dB across the same age span (e.g., Olsho, Koch, Carter, Halpin, et al., 1988). Note that, although absolute sensitivity does not reach adult levels until about 10 years of age at all frequencies, absolute auditory thresholds are within 10 to 15 dB of adults' thresholds by about 6 months of age (e.g., Trehub et al., 1988). Thus, 6-month-old infants generally can respond within audiometrically normal limits by the time that VRA becomes clinically feasible (reviewed by Gravel & Hood, 1998). It should be noted that infants' absolute threshold is even closer to adults' for a broadband noise (Werner & Boike, 2001).

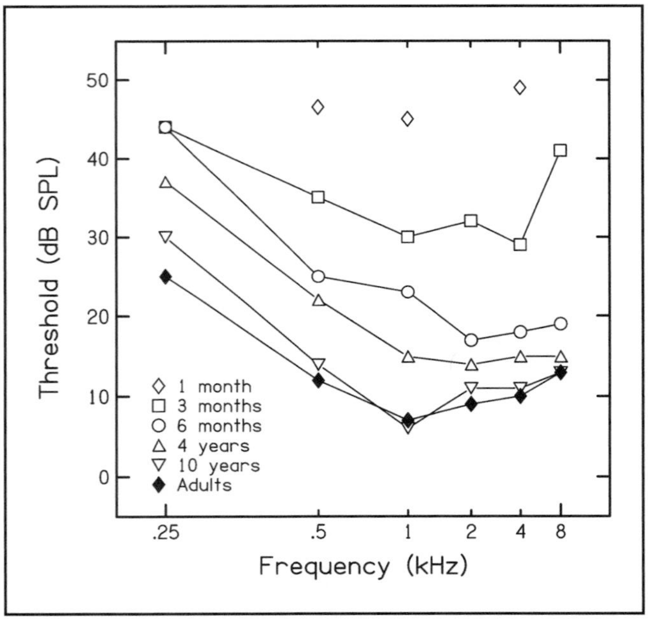

FIGURE 4–1. A summary of the audibility curve at different ages. Notice that absolute thresholds are rather high in the first months after birth. High-frequency thresholds improve the most in the first six postnatal months, so that high-frequency thresholds reach adult values before low-frequency thresholds. Low-frequency thresholds continue to improve into childhood.

Sources of Age-Related Change

The development of the conductive apparatus appears to be an important contributor to age-related changes in the shape of the audibility curve (e.g., Keefe, Bulen, Arehart, & Burns, 1993; Keefe, Burns, Bulen, & Campbell, 1994). Anatomic changes in the ear canal and middle ear system have been documented during infancy and childhood, including a lengthening of the ear canal (e.g., Keefe et al., 1993), an increase in the volume of the middle ear cavities (e.g., Eby & Nadol, 1986), and changes in the density and orientation of surrounding tissues (e.g., Ikui, Sando, & Fujita, 1997; Ruah, Schachern, Zelterman, Paparella, & Yoon, 1991). As a consequence of these anatomic changes, the conduction of sound energy through the conductive apparatus becomes progressively more efficient with increasing age during infancy (Keefe et al., 1993, 1994; reviewed by Keefe & Levi, 1996), and is not adultlike until 11 years of age (Okabe, Sachiko, Hareo, Tanetoshi, & Hiroaki, 1988). Consistent with developmental changes in absolute sensitivity (e.g., Olsho, Koch, Carter, Halpin, et al., 1988; Tharpe & Ashmead, 2001; Trehub et al., 1980), however, the largest improvements in conductive efficiency occur during the first six months of life (Keefe et al., 1993, 1994). For example, the amount of sound energy transmitted through the middle ear is approximately 20 dB less for a one-month-old infant than for an adult at high frequencies, but improves to within 10 dB compared to an adult by six months of age (Keefe et al., 1994). Of particular relevance to pediatric audiologists is the fact that improvements in middle ear efficiency directly influence behavioral thresholds. For example, Werner and Holmer (2002) demonstrated that improvements in middle ear conductance between 3 months of age and adulthood can account for approximately 8 dB of the improvement in behavioral threshold estimates.

Converging evidence indicates that neither the rapid improvements in absolute auditory sensitivity occurring in early infancy nor the later progressive improvements occurring into childhood can be accounted for by maturation of the inner ear. The inner ear starts to function in utero by at least 22 weeks gestational age (e.g., Birnholz & Benacerraf, 1983; Pujol, Lavigne-Rebillard, & Uziel, 1991). In addition, anatomic, histologic, and physiologic data indicate mature cochlear function at term birth (e.g., Bargones & Burns, 1988; Lavigne-Rebillard & Pujol, 1987, 1988).

One physiologic method that has often been used to study cochlear function during infancy is the measurement of otoacoustic emissions (OAEs), sounds that are generated by the cochlea in response to stimulation. OAEs can be measured in the ear canal and provide a noninvasive indicator of normal cochlear function. Abdala, Oba, and Ramanathan (2008) reported that OAE amplitude increased with age at some frequencies in preterm infants, and that the amplitude of OAEs was higher in term infants than in adults, particularly at certain frequencies. The amplitude of OAEs, however, did not change between birth and 6 months postnatal age in full-term infants, an age range over which absolute thresholds change considerably. It appears that most of the reported age-related differences in OAE level reflect infants' immature conductive transmission (Abdala & Keefe, 2006; Keefe & Abdala, 2007).

Inefficient neural transmission through the auditory pathways in the brainstem also appears to play a role in the development of absolute sensitivity during early infancy (e.g., Gorga, Kaminski, Beauchaine, Jesteadt, & Neely, 1989; Ponton, Moore, & Eggermont, 1996; Werner, Folsom, & Mancl, 1994). Moreover, this inefficient neural transmission is related to absolute sensitivity prior to 6 months of age. Werner et al. (1994) demonstrated that auditory brainstem response (ABR) Wave I-V interwave latency predicts high-frequency behavioral thresholds for 3-month-olds, but not for 6-month-olds. One explanation for this result is that improvements in synaptic efficiency in the auditory brainstem occur between 3 and 6 months of age.

Conductive and brainstem immaturities do not account for all of the behavioral threshold immaturities that have been observed. In fact, by 7 months of age only a relatively small effect of conductive immaturity appears to remain (e.g., Keefe et al., 1994).

It has been suggested that infants and young children perform more poorly than adults on behavioral measures because they are inattentive or "off-task" on a certain proportion of trials. Models of inattention, however, account for only a small portion (2–3 dB) of the observed threshold immaturity (e.g., Viemeister & Schlauch, 1992; Wightman & Allen, 1992). Rather, it appears that some of the developmental changes in absolute sensitivity are the result of immature processing efficiency. Processing efficiency is a central phenomenon that is influenced by attention, motivation, memory, and selective attention (e.g., Bargones & Werner, 1994; Bargones, Werner, & Marean, 1995; Werner & Boike, 2001). For example, it has been suggested that infants and young children listen less selectively than adults. Whereas adults listen selectively for an expected signal in a detection task (e.g., Dai, Scharf, & Buus, 1991), infants monitor a broad range of frequencies during detection (Bargones & Werner, 1994). This inability to direct attention to the appropriate frequency appears to account for a substantial part of early behavioral threshold immaturity (e.g., Werner & Boike, 2001). It also explains why infants' absolute thresholds are more like adults' for broadband than for narrowband sounds (e.g., Werner & Boike, 2001).

Development of the Basic Representations of Sound

Acousticians describe sound in two ways—in the time domain and in the frequency domain. The time domain representation of sound is pressure as a function of time and is often referred to as the time waveform. The frequency domain representation of sound has two components: the amplitude of sound as a function of frequency, called the amplitude spectrum, and the phase of sound as a function of frequency, called the phase spectrum. These representations of sound are illustrated in Figure 4–2. The peripheral auditory system also represents sound in the time domain (the "temporal" representation) and in the frequency domain (the "spectral" representation), although neither representation is complete and distortion-free. These neural representations of sound are also shown in Figure 4–2. It is useful to think about hearing and hearing development in terms of the auditory system's representation of the time waveform and the amplitude spectrum.

Development of the Spectral Representation of Sound

A simple way to test a listener's representation of the amplitude spectrum is to measure a threshold for a tone or a narrow band of noise in broadband noise.

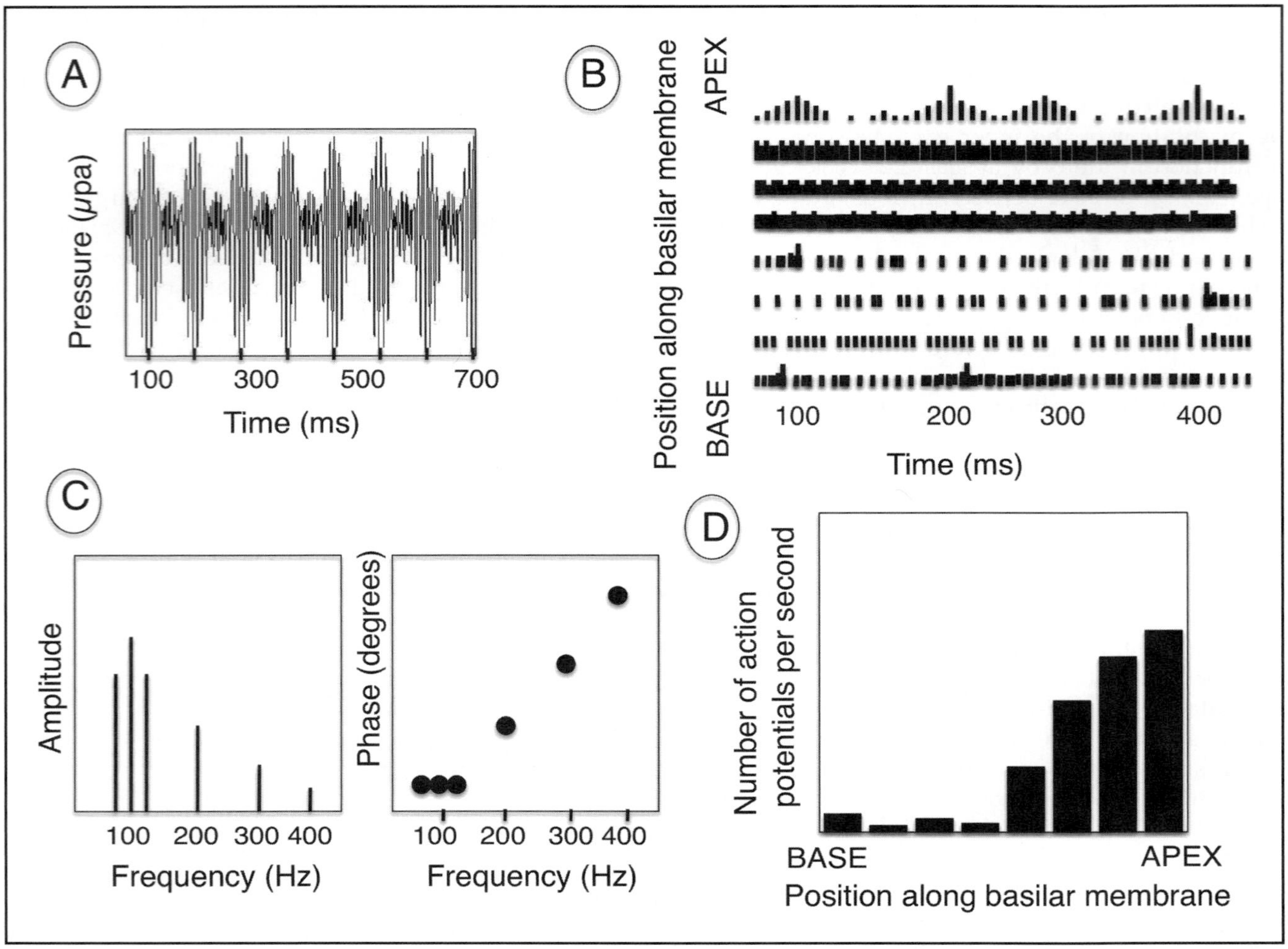

FIGURE 4–2. A comparison of acoustic and neural representations of sound. Sounds can be described in terms of their waveform, pressure as a function of time **(A)**. An equivalent representation is the frequency domain representation **(C)**. The sound is described in terms of its amplitude spectrum—amplitude as a function of frequency—and its phase spectrum—starting phase as a function of frequency. The auditory nerve carries two similar representations of sound. Neurons from each position along the basilar membrane respond in synchrony with the waveform of sound in each frequency band **(B)**. Each bar represents the number of action potentials produced in a group of neurons at a particular position along the basilar membrane at each point in time. A taller bar indicates a larger number of action potentials. The neurons near the apex of the basilar membrane respond more when the amplitude of the waveform is high and less when the amplitude of the waveform is low. The other neural representation of sound is similar to the amplitude spectrum **(D)**. Neurons from each position along the basilar membrane respond to a limited range of frequencies. Neurons respond more when the amplitude of sound within their frequency range is high and less when the amplitude of sound in their frequency range is low. Notice that there is some spontaneous activity in the basal (high-frequency) neurons even though there is no high-frequency energy in the sound **(B and D)**. The phase spectrum of sound is not represented directly in the auditory nerve.

Schneider, Trehub, Morongiello, and Thorpe (1989) measured thresholds for a noise band masked by a broadband noise in listeners ranging from 6 months, through childhood, to adulthood. A summary of their results is shown in Figure 4–3. At 6 months, the masked threshold is about 15 dB higher than in adulthood. This difference grows progressively smaller as children grow older. Schneider et al. report that by 8 years,

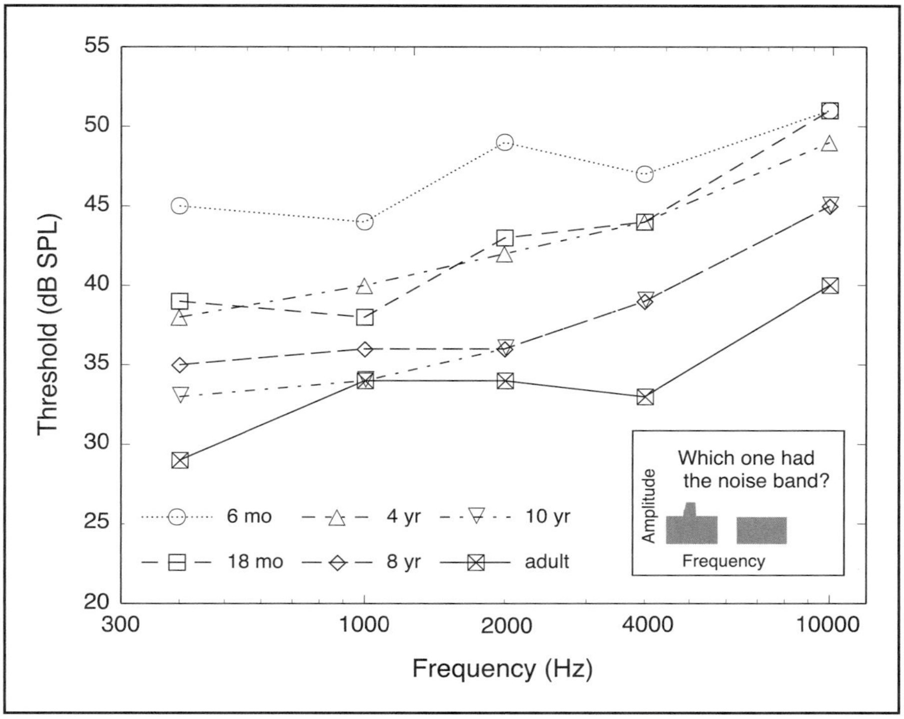

FIGURE 4–3. Threshold for an octave band of noise masked by a broadband noise, as a function of the center frequency of the noise band, for listeners of various ages, as reported by Schneider et al. (1989). Notice that masked threshold improves progressively with age up to about 10 years of age in this study. The masked threshold matures at about the same rate at all frequencies.

the masked threshold is only a little worse than that seen in adults. By some other reports, 6-year-olds are adultlike in threshold for a tone in noise (e.g., Hall & Grose, 1991).

Age-Related Changes

The amplitude spectrum plots amplitude, or intensity, as a function of frequency. Thus, to represent the amplitude spectrum, the auditory system must represent both the frequency and the intensity of sound. Consequently, maturation of the representation of frequency or intensity could be responsible for maturation of the spectral representation of sound. The precision of the representation of frequency, also known as frequency resolution, has been studied in infants and children using several different masking procedures (Hall & Grose, 1991; Olsho, 1985; Schneider, Morrongiello, & Trehub, 1990; Spetner & Olsho, 1990). Spetner and Olsho (1990), for example, tested frequency resolution in 3- and 6-month-old infants at 500, 1000, and 4000 Hz. They found that 6-month-olds were like adults in frequency resolution at all frequencies. Three-month-olds also had mature frequency resolution at 500 and 1000 Hz, but had poorer frequency resolution than adults and older infants at 4000 Hz. Mature frequency resolution has also been reported in preschool children (e.g., Hall & Grose, 1991).

Maturation of the representation of intensity has been studied in two ways. One is intensity discrimination, in which the listener is asked to detect an intensity change in a sound or to choose the more intense of two sounds. The result is expressed as the change in intensity, expressed in dB, that a listener can just discriminate, the intensity difference limen (DL). Several studies have examined the development of intensity discrimination in infants and children; the results of these studies are summarized in Figure 4–4. The performance of 6-month-olds in these studies can be quite variable; in some studies infants could only discriminate a 12 dB change in intensity, while in others they could discriminate a 4 dB change in intensity. Infants

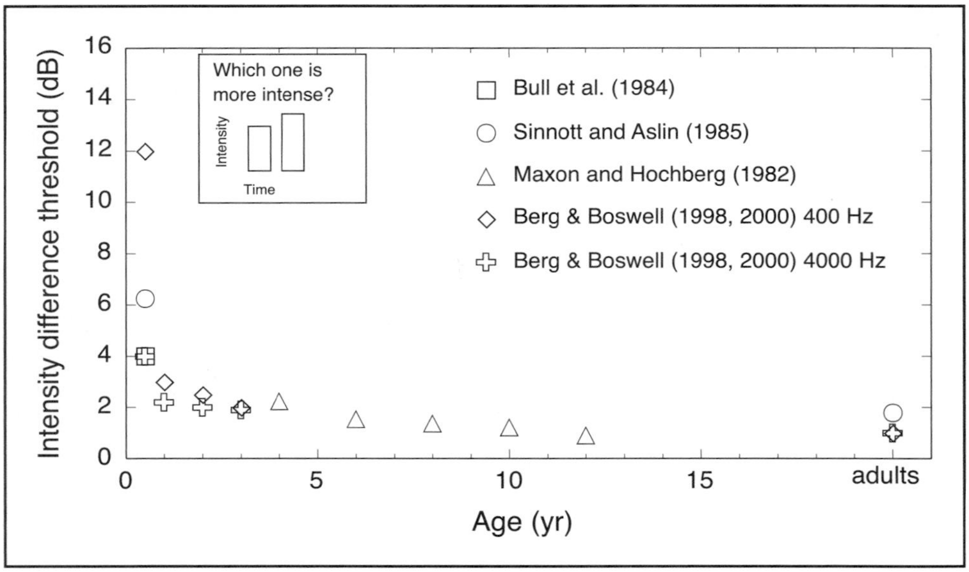

FIGURE 4–4. A summary of the development of intensity discrimination. The listener's task is to respond to the more intense sound. The difference in intensity that a listener can just discriminate gets smaller as the listener gets older, up to about 5 years of age, although even preschool children can discriminate fairly small changes in intensity.

discriminate the smallest intensity changes for broadband sounds and at high frequencies (Berg & Boswell, 1998; Bull, Eilers, & Oller, 1984). At 12 months and beyond, however, intensity discrimination is consistently fairly good, and the intensity DL decreases from about 3 dB at 12 months to 1 to 2 dB at 6 years.

Another way to assess the representation of intensity in the auditory system is to ask the listener to report the loudness of a sound. It is not easy to get an infant to report how loud a sound is, but Leibold and Werner (2002) used the time it took infants to respond to a sound as an indication of loudness. Loudness had been shown in several studies to be related to reaction time in adults; adults respond faster when a sound is louder (e.g., Humes & Ahlstrom, 1984). Leibold and Werner found that infants also responded faster to more intense sounds, but infants' reaction time changed much more for a given change in intensity than adults' did. Thus, it is possible that loudness increases more with an increase in intensity for infants than for adults. By the time a child is 5 years old, it is possible to get them to draw a line or provide a numerical estimate to express how loud something sounds to them. A 5-year-old's performance on these tests is comparable to that of an adult (e.g., Collins & Gescheider, 1989).

Thus, it appears that frequency resolution is immature at birth, at least at high frequencies, but matures during early infancy. The representation of intensity may still be rather immature in infants, but it matures quickly throughout the preschool period. The spectral representation of sound, then, is fairly precise in later infancy and probably adultlike by the time children begin kindergarten.

Sources of Age-Related Change

Postnatal maturation of the cochlea is probably not involved in the early development of the representation of the amplitude spectrum. As noted above, OAEs provide a noninvasive method for studying cochlear function, even in infants. OAEs for newborns increase in amplitude as the intensity of sound is increased in a similar way as OAEs for adults (Abdala, 2000). An OAE at a specific frequency can be "suppressed," or masked, by sounds over about the same range of frequencies in newborns' and adults' ears (Abdala, Keefe, & Oba, 2007). Although some subtle differences between infant and adult cochlear responses have been reported (e.g., Dhar & Abdala, 2007; Moleti et al., 2008), at least some of these differences are actually due to middle ear immaturity (Abdala et al., 2007; Keefe & Abdala, 2007). In general then, these results suggest that both frequency and intensity are represented in a mature way by the newborn's cochlea.

Immature frequency resolution before 6 months of age is apparently due to neural immaturity; frequency resolution measured in the cochlea is mature in newborns (e.g., Abdala & Sininger, 1996), but frequency resolution in the brainstem is immature in young infants as indicated by ABR (Abdala & Folsom, 1995; Folsom & Wynne, 1987). However, ABR results also indicate that frequency resolution is adultlike by 6 months of age (Abdala & Folsom, 1995; Folsom & Wynne, 1987). During the months after birth, it is likely that the connections between neurons in the auditory system are refined with exposure to sound (e.g., Sanes & Constantine-Paton, 1985). The refinement is reflected in maturation of frequency resolution.

There is little evidence, however, that primary neural maturation contributes to age-related improvements in intensity resolution. The ABR increases in amplitude and decreases in latency as the intensity of the evoking sound is increased. If auditory neurons were not representing intensity accurately, we would expect to find that greater increases in intensity might be required to produce a certain amplitude or latency change for infants than for adults. Although ABR amplitude and latencies change as infants grow older, the effect of changing sound intensity is the same for infants as it is for adults (Gorga et al., 1989).

A small contributor to infants' immature tone-in-noise detection thresholds is their inability to stay on task during testing, as noted previously. A more important contributor is the way that infants listen to complex sounds. To detect a tone in noise at a low intensity, a listener must focus on the frequencies close to that of the tone. Adult listeners do this so well that they do not even hear tones that are presented at frequencies far from that of a target tone (e.g., Schlauch & Hafter, 1991). However, infants appear to listen broadly over a wide frequency range even when it would be beneficial to listen selectively (e.g., Bargones & Werner, 1994). It is not clear when children are able to listen as selectively as adults do (Leibold & Neff, 2007). Listening broadly over frequency is likely to be informative when infants and children are just learning about sounds in their environment. However, the disadvantage of broad listening is that competing sounds and noise are more detrimental to hearing for young listeners.

Development of the Temporal Representation of Sound

The auditory system's representation of the time waveform, or temporal characteristics, of sound provides information that the spectral representation cannot. For example, listeners can discriminate smaller changes in the frequency of a sound using its temporal representation (Moore, 1973). Furthermore, some slow changes in a sound over time, such as those that indicate prosody and intonation of speech, are carried by the temporal representation of sound (Rosen, 1989).

Pitch Perception

Age-Related Changes. Pitch is the perceptual dimension along which sounds are arranged from "high" to "low." In general, pitch varies with the frequency of a sound. Olsho, Koch, and Halpin (1987) reported that 3-month-old infants were poorer than adults at discriminating changes in the frequency of pure tones, particularly high-frequency (4000 Hz) tones. In contrast, 6- and 12-month-old infants could discriminate changes in the frequency of a pure tone as well as adults at 4000 Hz, but they were poorer than adults at discriminating changes in frequency and not much better than 3-month-olds, at lower frequencies. Studies of preschool and school-age children indicated that low-frequency pure-tone discrimination continues to improve into the school years, but that high-frequency discrimination is quite good, even in 3-year-olds, as would be predicted from the infant studies (Hill, Hogben, & Bishop, 2005; Maxon & Hochberg, 1982). These age-related changes in pure-tone frequency discrimination are summarized in Figure 4–5.

Real-world sounds are never pure tones. Complex sounds that have distinct pitch consist of a fundamental frequency plus a set of harmonic frequencies. The pitch of such sounds corresponds to the pitch associated with the fundamental frequency, but if the fundamental frequency is filtered out, the remaining harmonics are still perceived as having the pitch of the fundamental. Thus, it is clear that complex pitch involves integrating information across frequency. Moreover, the perception of complex pitch depends on the temporal representation of sound. The development of complex pitch perception has not been well studied. Clarkson and her colleagues (Clarkson & Clifton, 1985, 1995; Clarkson, Martin, & Miciek, 1996; Clarkson & Rogers, 1995; Montgomery & Clarkson, 1997) have demonstrated that 7-month-old infants hear complex pitch much like adults (Figure 4–6), although there are circumstances in which infants of this age do not hear less salient pitches. Although neonates have been shown to discriminate large changes in the pitch of complex tones (Jeffrey & Cohen, 1971), there is no evidence that infants are extracting complex pitch from such sounds. By one report, 4-month-olds hear complex pitch poorly and 2-month-olds not at all

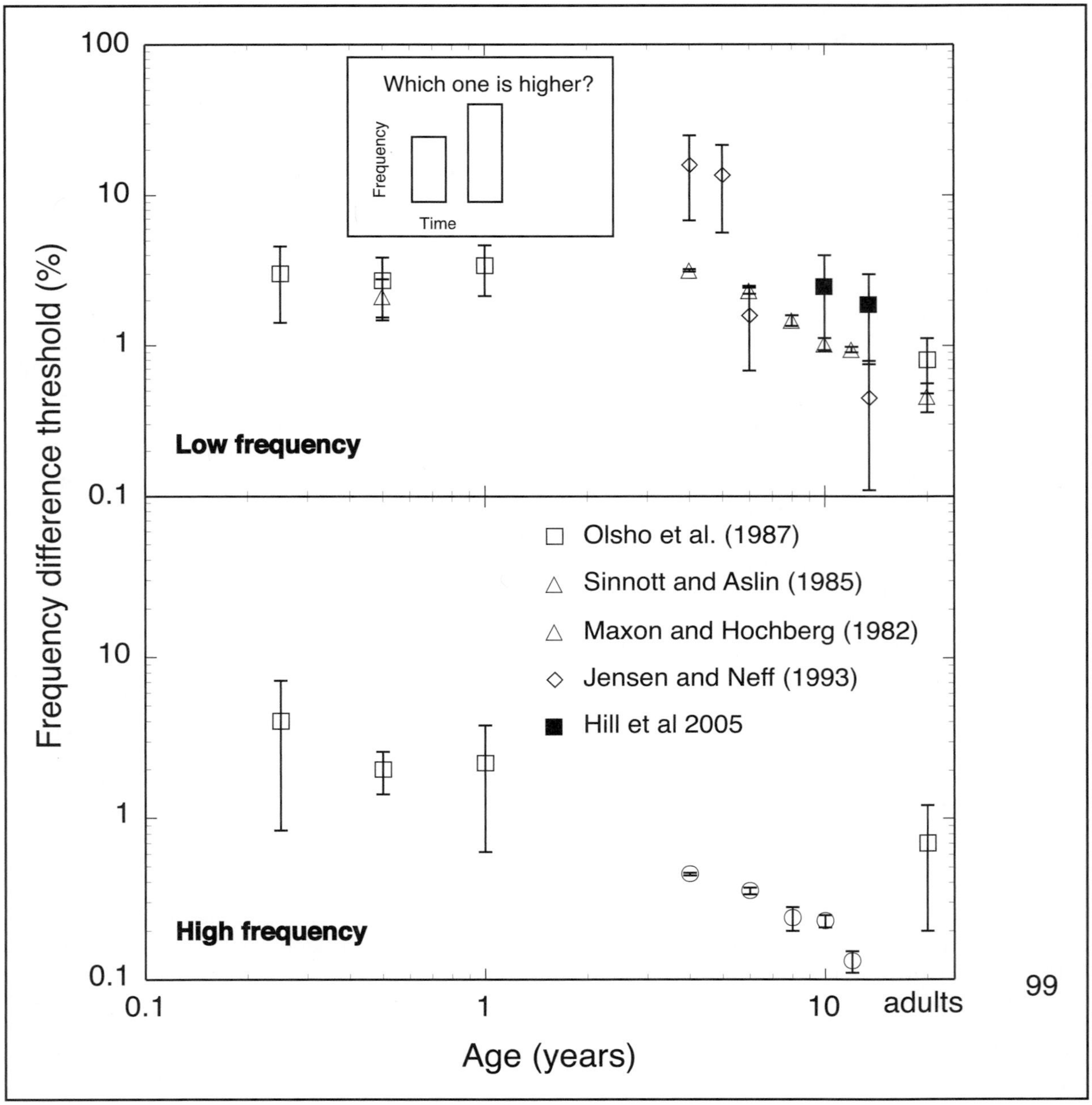

FIGURE 4–5. A summary of the development of frequency discrimination. The listener's task is to respond to the higher frequency tone. The difference in frequency that a listener can just discriminate gets smaller as the listener gets older, and for low-frequency tones this improvement continues into the school years. For high-frequency tones, 6- and 12-month-old infants are not very different from adults; notice that the error bars around the data points for these infants and all of the child groups overlap with the error bars around the adult data point. High-frequency pure-tone discrimination appears to mature earlier than low-frequency.

(Clarkson, Montgomery, Miciek, & Larson, 1998). It is not clear when children are able to hear complex pitch in all of the conditions in which adults hear it, although 5-year-old children have been shown to hear some subtle pitches like adults (Edwards, Giaschi, Low, & Edgell, 2005; Koelsch et al., 2003).

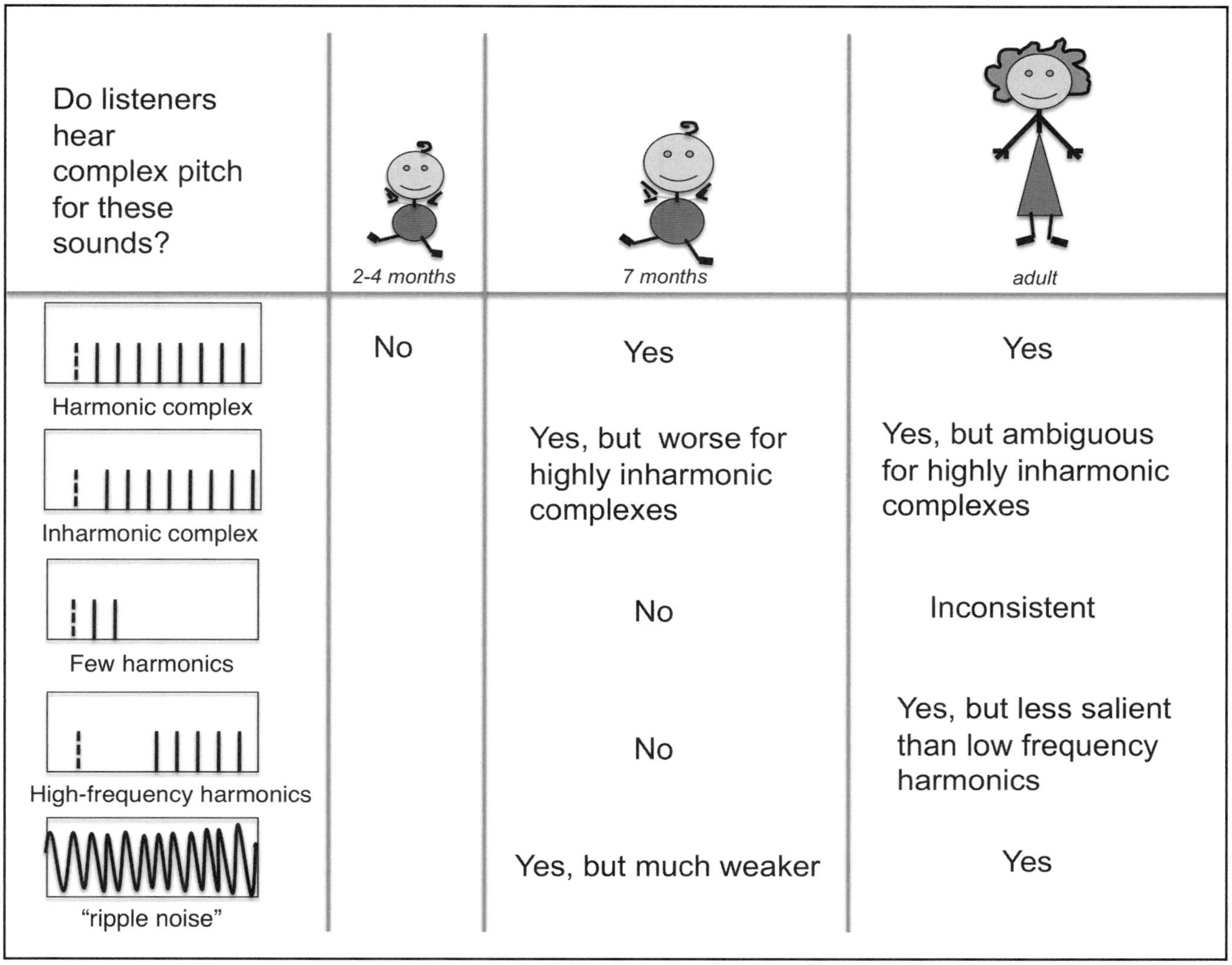

FIGURE 4–6. A summary of the development of complex pitch perception. Adults hear complex pitch in all of the sounds whose amplitude spectra are shown in the left hand column. In each amplitude spectrum, the fundamental frequency of the complex is shown as a dashed line, but is not physically present in the sound. Two-month-old infants do not appear to hear complex pitch, and 4-month-olds hear it poorly. Seven-month-olds and adults hear complex pitch in many of the same sounds, but when the pitch is weak for adults, the pitch is much weaker or absent for 7-month-olds.

Sources of Age-Related Change. Although pitch perception clearly involves the neural representation of the time waveform of sound, the so-called temporal representation, the neural representation of the amplitude spectrum must also be involved. For example, people can discriminate changes in the frequency of pure tones at high frequencies, and the auditory system does not represent high-frequency information temporally (Pickles, 2008). Thus, that 3-month-old infants have particular difficulty discriminating between high-frequency tones is consistent with their immature high-frequency resolution, as described in the previous section of this chapter (Spetner & Olsho, 1990). Similarly, that 6-month-old infants can discriminate high-frequency tones as well as adults is consistent with their mature high-frequency resolution. Because low-frequency pure tone discrimination is likely based on the temporal representation of sound, that even 12-month-old infants are immature at low-frequency pure tone discrimination may mean that infants do not have precise temporal information. However, some evoked potential findings suggest that at least at low levels in the auditory system, the temporal representation of frequency is much like that in adults even in 1-month-old infants (Levi, Folsom, & Dobie, 1995).

The neural representation of both spectral and temporal information is involved in the perception of simple (pure tone) and complex pitch. As described, both the temporal and spectral representations of sound sent to the brain from the ear are mature by one month of age. Thus, it is somewhat surprising that infants younger than 7 months of age do not seem to perceive complex pitch like adults. There are several indications, however, that central processing of the neural representation of sound does not mature until later in childhood. First, recent evidence indicates that although the cortical evoked response to changes in complex pitch are seen even in 2-month-olds, the organization of the response—which parts of the brain respond and when—changes systematically during early infancy (He, Hotson, & Trainor, 2007). He and Trainor (2009), moreover, found that the cortical evoked response to changes in complex pitch occurred in 4-month-olds, but not 2-month-olds, when the fundamental was missing from the complex. Second, training seems to improve performance in both pure-tone frequency discrimination, especially at low frequencies (Olsho, Koch, & Carter, 1988) and discrimination of subtle complex pitch changes (Edwards et al., 2005). Thus, it may be that infants and children have the neural representations they need to perceive pitch, but it takes time for them to learn to use those representations effectively.

Temporal Resolution

Age-Related Changes in Temporal Resolution. The ability to hear changes in a sound over time is called temporal resolution. Information about such changes is carried in the auditory system's temporal representation of sound. Temporal resolution has been measured in a variety of ways, and some of these measures have been applied to infants and children. In gap detection, for example, a listener is asked to detect a short interruption in an ongoing sound. Adults can detect gaps as short as 3 ms in some conditions (e.g., Eddins, Hall, & Grose, 1992). Infants, even 12-month-olds, in contrast, do not detect gaps shorter than about 30 ms (Trehub, Schneider, & Henderson, 1995; Werner, Marean, Halpin, Spetner, & Gillenwater, 1992). By preschool, the gap detection threshold in a 2000-Hz noise band has improved to about 12 ms, and by 6 years of age, gap detection appears to be mature (Wightman, Allen, Dolan, Kistler, & Jamieson, 1989). These age-related changes in gap detection are illustrated in Figure 4–7.

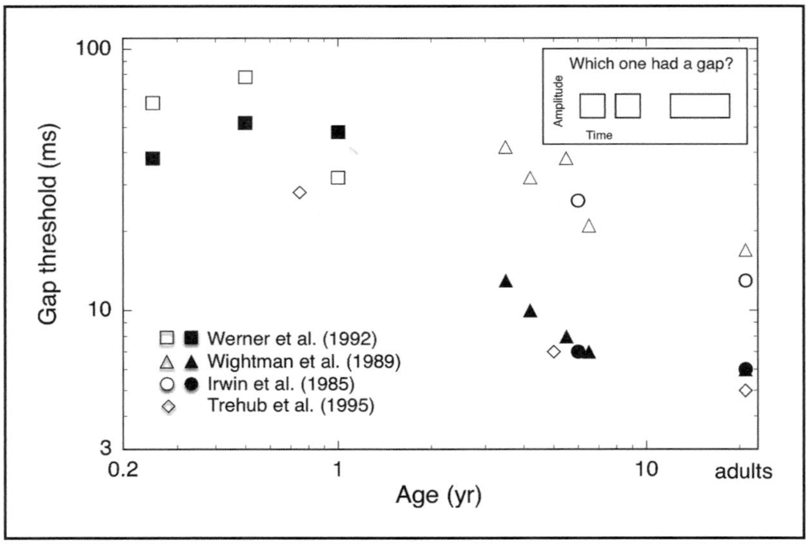

FIGURE 4–7. A summary of the development of gap detection. The listener's task is to respond when a very short interruption in an ongoing sound occurs. The unfilled symbols are gap thresholds for low-frequency sounds, and the filled symbols are gap thresholds for high-frequency sounds. Gap thresholds for both low and high frequency sounds improve with age, but high-frequency gap thresholds approach adult values at younger ages than low-frequency gap thresholds.

An issue with gap detection is that it depends not only on the auditory system's ability to follow a rapid change in sound, but also on the ability to represent a change in intensity. As noted above, the ability to represent a change in intensity may be immature in infants, so it is difficult to interpret the finding of poor gap detection performance. Another measure of temporal resolution is the temporal modulation transfer function (TMTF), which shows the amount of amplitude modulation required to detect modulation at different modulation rates (Viemeister, 1979). When the modulation rate is slow, the auditory system should have no trouble following the modulation, so the amount of modulation needed to hear the change will only depend on the system's ability to represent a change in intensity. However, as the modulation rate increases, the auditory system's ability to follow rapid changes begins to deteriorate. This will be reflected in an increase in the amount of modulation required for modulation detection (Figure 4–8). Thus, the modulation rate at which the amount of modulation required to detect modulation starts to increase is a measure of temporal resolution, independent of intensity resolution. The TMTF of 4-year-old children has been shown to parallel that of adults (see Figure 4–8), indicating mature temporal resolution (Hall & Grose, 1994). Recall that gap detection is immature at this age, however. There are few published data on infants' TMTF, although the data that are available suggest no obvious immaturity in this measure (Werner, 1996).

Sources of Age-Related Change. Electrophysiologic data on temporal resolution are consistent with the idea that temporal resolution is an early-maturing ability. For example, auditory brainstem responses to the sound at the end of a gap in a sound are similar to those of adults at 3 months of age (Werner, Folsom, Mancl, & Syapin, 2001). Furthermore, an evoked potential evoked by amplitude-modulated tones is very similar in 1-month-olds and adults (Levi et al., 1995). Cortical potentials evoked by gaps in sound appear to be adultlike by 6 months of age, and although younger

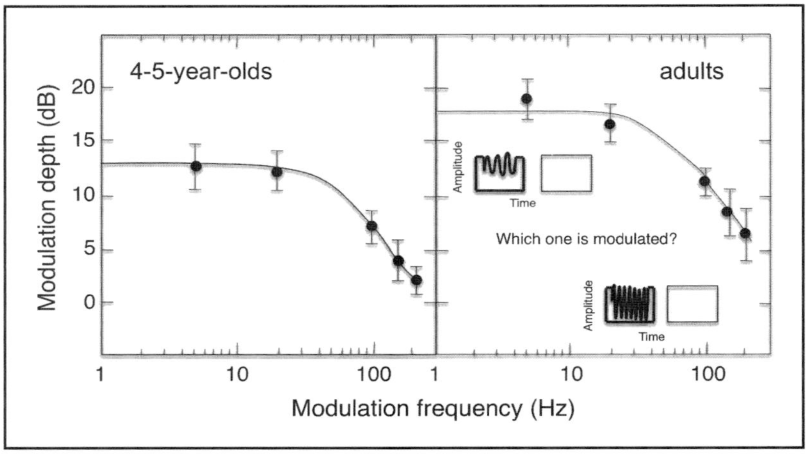

FIGURE 4–8. Temporal modulation transfer functions for 4 to 5-year-old children (*left panel*) and for adults (*right panel*), as reported by Hall and Grose (1994). The listener's task is to respond when the amplitude of a sound changes over time; that is, when the sound is amplitude modulated. In some conditions, the sound's amplitude changes slowly (*see inset at top left of right panel*); in other cases, the sound's amplitude changes rapidly (*see inset at bottom right of right panel*). How rapidly the sound is changing is the "modulation frequency" on the *x*-axis. The more rapid the modulation, the bigger, or "deeper," the modulation has to be for the listener to detect it. Notice that in the inset with the slowly changing sound, the modulation is not as deep as in the inset with the rapidly changing sound. The modulation depth, on the *y*-axis, can be thought of as how far down the amplitude has to go for the listener to detect the change. A value of 0 would mean that the amplitude has to go all the way off, whereas a value of 15 would mean that the amplitude only has to go down some of the way. Each data point plots the depth of modulation required to just detect modulation at a certain modulation frequency; the curves were fit to the data points. This shows that 4 to 5-year-olds generally need deeper modulation than adults do to detect modulation. Children's modulation threshold gets worse as the modulation frequency increases, however, just as adults' does. The curves are offset along the *y*-axis, but they are parallel to each other. This suggests that children's temporal resolution is similar to adults'.

infants demonstrate a cortical response to gaps in sound, the morphology of the response is quite different from that seen in older infants (Trainor et al., 2003). Thus, it is possible that cortical development leads to early changes in temporal resolution, although there is no evidence that behavioral measures of temporal resolution change early in infancy. In sum, the available physiological evidence suggests that changes in a sound over time are accurately represented in the auditory system of infants and children.

If an infant's auditory system can represent temporal modulation in sound, why is an infant's gap detection performance so poor? One possibility is that immature gap detection reflects immature intensity resolution rather than immature temporal resolution. As noted above, infants are not as good as adults at discriminating a change in intensity, and loudness growth may be immature in infants. Although there are few electrophysiologic findings consistent with primary immaturity of the representation of intensity in the infant auditory system, this possibility cannot be dismissed.

Another possible explanation is immature selective attention. A listener will detect a gap in a sound most effectively if attention is focused on the point in time—a very precise point in time—at which a gap might occur. If infants cannot direct attention to a precise point in time, then their gap detection performance would be poor compared to temporally selective adults. This could also explain why infants are particularly poor at detecting very short duration sounds. Werner, Parrish, and Holmer (2009) have recently examined infants' ability to focus on a particular point in time by comparing infants' detection of a tone that occurs at an expected time, compared to tones that occur at unexpected times. Interestingly, Werner et al. (2009) found that, like adults, infants detected tones at expected times better than they detected tones at unexpected times, indicating that they were listening selectively at the expected time. This finding argues against the idea that immature gap detection results from a failure to listen selectively in time, although it is not possible to determine whether infants' temporal attention is as precise as adults' from the results of Werner et al. (2009).

Spatial Hearing

From a developmental perspective, one of the more interesting aspects of hearing is spatial hearing. People are able to localize sound sources in space by using differences in the intensity and timing of sounds at the two ears and by reference to the shape of a sound's amplitude spectrum after it has passed through the external ear. All three of these acoustic cues to a sound source's location depend on the size of the head and the pinnas. Thus, as a child's head and ears grow, the acoustic cues associated with a particular location in space will change. Moreover, a small head and ears will provide a smaller cue than a large head and ears. Thus, infants and children are not only at an acoustic disadvantage when it comes to spatial hearing, but their brains must deal with a continually changing set of acoustic cues.

Age-Related Changes

Given the age-related differences in the acoustics that result from the growth of the head and ears, it will come as no surprise that infants and young children are not as good as adults at identifying the spatial location of a sound. For example, an adult will be able to tell that a sound source has moved by as little as 1° to the left or right (Blauert, 1983). Newborn infants can tell that a sound comes from the left or right (Field, Muir, Pilon, Sinclair, & Dodwell, 1980), but a sound source must move by as much as 27° before a 1-month-old can tell that the sound has moved (Morrongiello, Fenwick, & Chance, 1990). An 18-month-old can tell when a sound has moved left or right by 5°, and a 5-year-old can localize many sounds in the left-right dimension as well as adults (Litovsky & Ashmead, 1997). These age-related changes in the accuracy of sound localization are summarized in Figure 4–9. The ability to localize a sound in elevation—up or down—follows a similar developmental course (Morrongiello & Rocca, 1987).

In most studies of the development of sound localization, however, testing is conducted in a space in which reverberation is minimized. This is important, because in many situations, the sound reaches the ears directly from the source, followed reverberations of the sound ("echoes") from walls and obstacles at other locations. To solve this problem, the auditory system bases its estimate of a sound's location primarily on the first sound that arrives at the ears. This is known as the precedence effect. Newborn infants do not demonstrate the precedence effect; they seem to hear both the direct sound and its echoes. By the time infants are 4 or 5 months old, however, they respond as if the first sound they hear gives the location of a sound source (see Figure 4–9; Clifton, Morrongiello, & Dowd, 1984). At the same time, infants and even

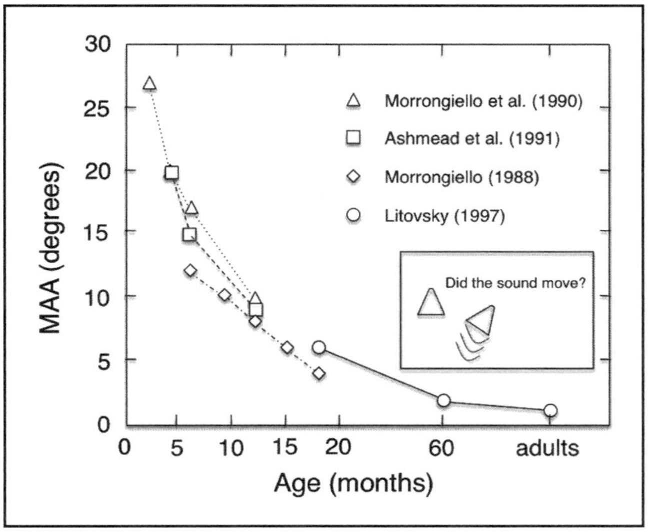

FIGURE 4–9. A summary of the development of the precision of sound localization in the left-right dimension. The listener's task is to respond when the location from which the sound is coming changes. The minimum audible angle is the change in position, expressed in degrees of arc, which the listener can just detect. The MAA improves dramatically throughout infancy and reaches adult values around 5 years of age.

5-year-old children do not localize sound sources as accurately when there is reverberation, suggesting that the precedence effect is still immature at school age (Litovsky, 1997).

Sources of Age-Related Change

There are several possible explanations for infants' and young children's poor sound localization. These are illustrated in Figure 4–9.

As noted above, infants and young children may have difficulty localizing sounds because their small head and ears provide them with less acoustic information about a sound source's location. The data indicate that while the acoustics limit a young child's sound localization, they are not the only limitation. Clifton, Gwiazda, Bauer, Clarkson, and Held (1988) measured the distance between the ears in infants of different ages and calculated what the maximum acoustic differences between the ears would be at each age. What they found was that although the acoustic differences were smaller in younger infants, the differences were not small enough to account for the imprecise sound localization seen in infants.

To use the acoustic information about a sound's location, the ears must accurately represent the frequency, intensity, and timing of the sound, and the brain must be able to calculate the differences between the ears and to extract the shape of a sound's amplitude spectrum. As described above, the representation of sound reaching the brain from the ear is mature rather early in life. Ashmead, Davis, Whalen, and Odom (1991) found, however, that infants were less accurate than adults at estimating differences in the arrival times of sounds at the two ears. This would suggest that the auditory system's ability to calculate differences between the ears is not yet mature in infancy. However, Ashmead et al. (1991) also showed that infant's poor arrival-time calculations were not poor enough to account for their imprecise sound localization.

Finally, to be able to figure out where a sound is coming from, the brain must "translate" an acoustic pattern into a particular spatial location. Although the development of this map of auditory space has not been studied in humans, it is known to depend on experience with sound in other species (Gray, 1992; Knudsen, 1985). Furthermore, people who are deprived of input to one ear for a time during development and then later have hearing in that ear restored, have a normal ability to discriminate the acoustic cues that specify a sound's location, but are unable to say where a sound is coming from (Wilmington, Gray, & Jahrsdorfer, 1994). Thus, the development of sound localization may also depend on the formation of a map of auditory space.

Hearing in Complex Sound Environments

Natural environments contain multiple sources of competing sounds. Each source produces acoustic waveforms that vary in frequency and amplitude across time. In order to make sense of the overlapping mixture of sounds that reach the ears, listeners must determine which components were produced by the same source. This process is often referred to as sound source segregation (Bregman, 1990).

The developing child must learn speech and language in complex sound environments. For example, children are expected to follow directions spoken by their teacher in the classroom, despite hearing the voices of classmates and rumblings of cars driving on a nearby road (Figure 4–10). We do not yet know how children develop the ability to separate and select the most

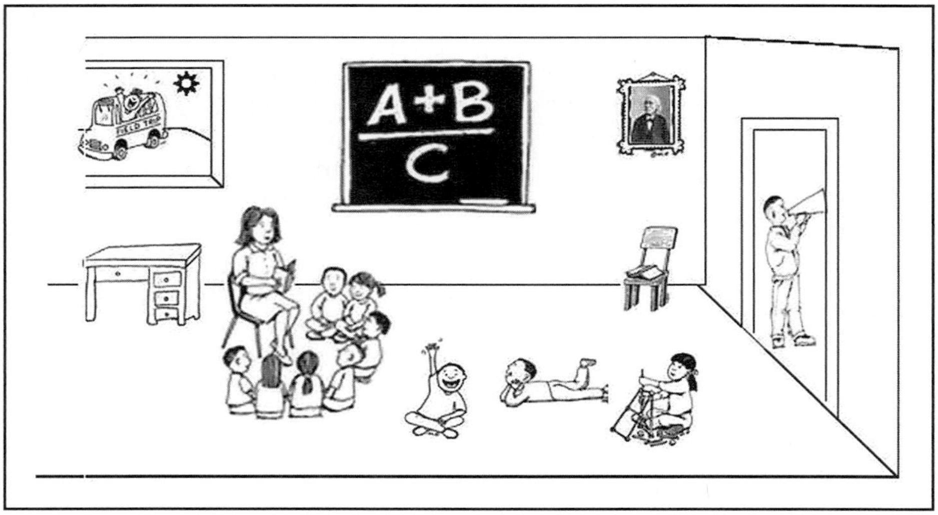

FIGURE 4–10. An illustration of the problem of sound source segregation in the classroom. Children are asked to listen to one sound source—the teacher—in the presence of many other sound sources—other children's voices inside and outside the classroom, a school bus engine, clanking toys. The characteristics of sound that a listener might use to separate the sounds include differences in the fundamental frequency of the teacher and child voices, differences in the spatial location of the teacher and other sound sources, and differences in the pattern of sound over time.

important sounds while ignoring sounds that are unrelated. Emerging data suggest, however, that the complex sound environments typical of everyday life pose considerable difficulty for infants and young children.

Research conducted over the past 30 years has consistently shown that preschoolers and school-aged children require a higher signal-to-noise ratio (SNR) compared to adults to achieve similar levels of performance on speech recognition tests in the presence of noise or speech maskers (e.g., Elliott et al., 1979; Nittrouer & Boothroyd, 1990; Wightman & Kistler, 2005). Similar to the studies of preschoolers and older children, Newman and Jusczyk (1996) found that infants could recognize their name embedded in a background of competing speech, but needed a higher SNR to do so, relative to adults.

The increased susceptibility to interference from competing sounds observed during infancy and childhood appears to be different from the masking described in previous sections of this chapter (reviewed by Werner & Leibold, 2004). For example, Hall, Grose, Buss, and Dev (2002) demonstrated that child-adult differences in spondee word recognition were more pronounced for a 2-talker competing sound than for a speech-shaped noise. These two distracting noises overlapped with the target words to the same extent in frequency and in time, and yet children had relatively greater difficulty hearing the target words when the distracter was speech. The pronounced developmental effects observed with increasing acoustic complexity may reflect immaturity in how children perceptually segregate the target sound from the competing background sounds.

Age-Related Change

Sound source segregation is often examined in adults by assessing auditory stream segregation (Bregman, 1990). Auditory streams can be thought of as sounds coming from different sources. People divide incoming sound complexes into separate auditory streams on the basis of acoustic similarities between frequency components. For example, components that come on and go off together will be heard as coming from the same source, but components with very different frequencies will be heard as coming from different sources (reviewed by Darwin & Carlyon, 1995; Yost, 1997). In a typical auditory streaming task, several components are presented, and one or more acoustic cues are manipulated. Listeners are asked to report whether they heard a single auditory stream or two distinct streams.

Studies of auditory streaming in infants indicate that auditory streaming processes are functional at birth (Demany, 1982; Fassbender, 1993; McAdams & Bertoncini, 1997; Winkler et al., 2003). Moreover, infants appear to be able to use several of the same acoustic cues used by adults to separate streams, including frequency proximity (Demany, 1982; Fassbender, 1993), intensity similarity (Fassbender, 1993), spectral similarity (Fassbender, 1993); timbre (McAdams & Bertoncini, 1997), and spatial location (McAdams & Bertoncini, 1997). However, larger acoustic differences in these potential cues were used for testing infants than for testing adults. In addition, only indirect measures of auditory streaming were used in the infant studies, because infants cannot be asked to say "one stream" or "two streams." Thus, it is as yet undetermined whether auditory streaming processes are fully adultlike during infancy or are functional, but immature.

Few studies have examined the auditory streaming abilities of preschoolers and school-aged children. In a recent study, however, Sussman, Wong, Horvath, Winkler, and Wang (2007) compared auditory streaming in children (5–11 years) and adults as a function of frequency proximity. Listeners heard a sequence of pure tones that differed in frequency. The frequency separation of the alternating pure tones was varied, and listeners were asked if they heard one or two auditory streams. A larger frequency separation was needed for children compared to adults before they would indicate that two streams were presented. Sussman et al. (2007) suggested that auditory stream segregation is functional early in life, but matures with increasing age and experience throughout childhood.

Another promising approach to the study of sound source segregation during infancy and childhood is to examine whether acoustic cues shown to promote sound source segregation in adults provide infants and children with a release from "informational masking" (e.g., Kidd, Mason, Deliwala, Woods, & Colburn, 1994; Neff & Green, 1987; Watson, Wroton, Kelly, & Benbassat, 1975). Informational masking generally refers to masking that occurs even though the spectral and temporal representations of the sound provide enough detail to allow the listener to separate the target sound from the competing sound. For example, in an early study of informational masking, Neff and Green (1987) asked listeners to detect a 1000-Hz pure tone presented simultaneously with a multitonal masker. The individual frequency components of the multitonal masker were varied randomly on each presentation. For many adults, the introduction of variation in the masker had a large and detrimental effect on detection of the 1000-Hz tone even though the masker components were very different in frequency from the 1000-Hz tone.

Interestingly, manipulations of the acoustic properties of sound that promote sound source segregation, including spatial separation, asynchronous temporal onsets and dissimilar temporal modulations, reduce informational masking for most adults who are susceptible to the effect (e.g., Arbogast, Mason, & Kidd, 2002; Durlach et al., 2003; Kidd et al., 1994; Neff, 1995; Oh & Lutfi, 1998). This suggests that informational masking could result from poor sound source segregation.

Researchers interested in auditory development have started to examine whether the acoustic cues that reduce informational masking in adults provide infants and children with a release from informational masking (e.g., Hall, Buss, & Grose, 2005; Leibold & Werner, 2006; Wightman, Callahan, Lutfi, Kistler, & Oh, 2003; Wightman & Kistler, 2005). The results of these initial studies indicate that children benefit from some, but not all, of the cues that improve adults' performance. Whereas the introduction of temporal asynchrony between a pure-tone signal and a multitonal masker improves thresholds for children and adults by a similar amount (Hall et al., 2005; Leibold & Neff, 2007), presenting the signal and masker to opposite headphones results in a large masking release for adults but does not benefit children (Hall et al., 2005; Wightman et al., 2003). For example, Wightman et al. (2003) measured detection thresholds for a 1000-Hz tone in the presence of a random-frequency, multitonal masker. Informational masking was observed for children and adults. However, masking was substantially reduced or eliminated in adults when signal and masker were presented to opposite ears. In contrast, improvement was significantly less for children in that condition.

Sources of Age-Related Change

The basic representation of sound provided to the brain of a typically-developing 6-month-old appears to be adequate to support sound source segregation. Nonetheless, it is clear that the ability to separate target sounds embedded in competing background sounds is not mature until well into childhood. The sources of children's prolonged difficulties in complex sound environments are not well understood, but appear to reflect maturation of higher-level neural structures and nonsensory or "central" auditory processes, such as sound source segregation. Understanding how infants and children perform sound source segregation is critical to understanding how children acquire speech and language in complex natural environments.

An important unresolved question for researchers and audiologists is to understand the influence of listening experience on the development of hearing in complex sound environments. Children become more efficient and flexible listeners as they learn about the important features of sound across different talkers and listening environments, but it is unclear how and when this process unfolds. Moreover, this development might well be prolonged or altered by hearing loss if access to sound is delayed or compromised.

Summary, Conclusions, and Principles of Development

Human auditory development begins before birth and continues into adolescence. The basic auditory capacities, the spectral and temporal representations of sound, are not completely mature at birth, but are apparently adultlike by about 6 months of age. However, the ability to use the information that the ear provides the brain develops over a much longer time course. Infants and children progressively learn to separate a target sound from irrelevant sounds. As children grow older, they become sensitive to aspects of sounds that they previously appeared not to notice. Finally, children are able to choose the most informative aspects of sound to be efficient information processors. In addition, the abilities to break a sound down into separate sources and to match a pattern of sound to a particular location in space take time to develop. Although these abilities are present in rudimentary form in early infancy, they do not function effectively in the most complex listening conditions until adolescence.

References

Abdala, C. (2000). Distortion product otoacoustic emission (2f1-f2) amplitude growth in human adults and neonates. *Journal of the Acoustical Society of America, 107*, 446–456.

Abdala, C., & Folsom, R. C. (1995). The development of frequency resolution in humans as revealed by the auditory brain-stem response recorded with notched-noise masking. *Journal of the Acoustical Society of America, 98*, 921–930.

Abdala, C., & Keefe, D. H. (2006). Effects of middle-ear immaturity on distortion product otoacoustic emission suppression tuning in infant ears. *Journal of the Acoustical Society of America, 120*, 3832–3842.

Abdala, C., Keefe, D. H., & Oba, S. I. (2007). Distortion product otoacoustic emission suppression tuning and acoustic admittance in human infants: Birth through 6 months. *Journal of the Acoustical Society of America, 121*, 3617–3627.

Abdala, C., Oba, S., & Ramanathan, R. (2008). Changes in the DP-gram during the preterm and early postnatal period. *Ear and Hearing, 29*, 512–523.

Abdala, C., & Sininger, Y. S. (1996). The development of cochlear frequency resolution in the human auditory system. *Ear and Hearing, 17*, 374–385.

Arbogast, T. L., Mason, C. R., & Kidd, G. (2002). The effect of spatial separation on informational and energetic masking of speech. *Journal of the Acoustical Society of America, 112*, 2086–2098.

Ashmead, D. H., Davis, D., Whalen, T., & Odom, R. (1991). Sound localization and sensitivity to interaural time differences in human infants. *Child Development, 62*, 1211–1226.

Bargones, J. Y., & Burns, E. M. (1988). Suppression tuning curves for spontaneous otoacoustic emissions in infants and adults. *Journal of the Acoustical Society of America, 98*, 99–111.

Bargones, J. Y., & Werner, L. A. (1994). Adults listen selectively; Infants do not. *Psychological Science, 5*, 170–174.

Bargones, J. Y., Werner, L. A., & Marean, G. C. (1995). Infant psychometric functions for detection: Mechanisms of immature sensitivity. *Journal of the Acoustical Society of America, 98*, 99–111.

Berg, K. M., & Boswell, A. E. (1998). Infants' detection of increments in low- and high-frequency noise. *Perception and Psychophysics, 60*, 1044–1051.

Berg, K. M., & Boswell, A. E. (2000). Noise increment detection in children 1 to 3 years of age. *Perception and Psychophysics, 62*(4), 868–873.

Birnholz, J. C., & Benacerraf, B. R. (1983). The development of fetal hearing. *Science, 222*, 516–518.

Blauert, J. (1983). *Spatial hearing: The psychophysics of human sound localization* (J. S. Allen, Trans.). Cambridge, MA: MIT Press.

Bregman, A. S. (1990). *Auditory scene analysis: The perceptual organization of sound*. Cambridge, MA: MIT Press.

Bull, D., Eilers, R. E., & Oller, D. K. (1984). Infants' discrimination of intensity variation in multitsyllabic stimuli. *Journal of the Acoustical Society of America, 76*, 13–17.

Clarkson, M. G., & Clifton, R. K. (1985). Infant pitch perception: Evidence for responding to pitch categories and the missing fundamental. *Journal of the Acoustical Society of America, 77*, 1521–1528.

Clarkson, M. G., & Clifton, R. K. (1995). Infants' pitch perception: Inharmonic tonal complexes. *Journal of the Acoustical Society of America, 98*(3), 1372–1379.

Clarkson, M. G., Martin, R., & Miciek, S. (1996). Infants' perception of pitch: Number of harmonics. *Infant Behavior and Development, 19*, 191–197.

Clarkson, M. G., Montgomery, C. R., Miciek, S. G., & Larson, M. E. (1998). Perception of the pitch of the missing fundamental by 4-month-old infants. *Infant Behavior and Development, 21*, 343.

Clarkson, M. G., & Rogers, E. C. (1995). Infants require low-frequency energy to hear the pitch of the missing fundamental. *Journal of the Acoustical Society of America, 98*(1), 148–154.

Clifton, R. K., Gwiazda, J., Bauer, J., Clarkson, M., & Held, R. (1988). Growth in head size during infancy: Implications for sound localization. *Developmental Psychology, 24*, 477–483.

Clifton, R. K., Morrongiello, B. A., & Dowd, J. M. (1984). A developmental look at an auditory illusion: The precedence effect. *Developmental Psychobiology, 17*(5), 519–536.

Collins, A. A., & Gescheider, G. A. (1989). The measurement of loudness in individual children and adults by absolute magnitude estimation and cross-modality matching. *Journal of the Acoustical Society of America, 85*, 2012–2021.

Dai, H., Scharf, B., & Buus, S. (1991). Effective attenuation of signals in noise under focused attention. *Journal of the Acoustical Society of America, 89*(6), 2837–2842.

Darwin, C. J., & Carlyon, R. P. (1995). Auditory grouping. In B. C. J. Moore (Ed.), *Hearing* (pp. 387–424). New York, NY: Academic Press.

Demany, L. (1982). Auditory stream segregation in infancy. *Infant Behavior and Development, 5*, 261–276.

Dhar, S., & Abdala, C. (2007). A comparative study of distortion-product-otoacoustic-emission fine structure in human newborns and adults with normal hearing. *Journal of the Acoustical Society of America, 122*, 2191–2202.

Durlach, N. I., Mason, C. R., Shinn-Cunningham, B. G., Arbogast, T. L., Colburn, H. S., & Kidd, G. (2003). Informational masking: Counteracting the effects of stimulus uncertainty by decreasing target-masker similarity. *Journal of the Acoustical Society of America, 114*, 368–379.

Eby, T. L., & Nadol, J. B., Jr. (1986). Postnatal growth of the human temporal bone. Implications for cochlear implants in children. *Annals of Otology, Rhinology, and Laryngology, 85*, 356–364.

Eddins, D. A., Hall, J. W., & Grose, J. H. (1992). The detection of temporal gaps as a function of frequency region and absolute noise bandwidth. *Journal of the Acoustical Society of America, 91*, 1069–1077.

Edwards, V. T., Giaschi, D. E., Low, P., & Edgell, D. (2005). Sensory and nonsensory influences on children's performance of dichotic pitch perception tasks. *Journal of the Acoustical Society of America, 117*, 3157–3164.

Elliott, L. L., Connors, S., Kille, E., Levin, S., Ball, K., & Katz, D. (1979). Children's understanding of monosyllabic nouns in quiet and noise. *Journal of the Acoustical Society of America, 66*, 12–21.

Fassbender, C. (1993). *Auditory grouping and segregation processes in infancy*. Norderstedt, Germany: Kaste Verlag.

Field, T. J., Muir, D., Pilon, R., Sinclair, M., & Dodwell, P. (1980). Infants' orientation to lateral sounds from birth to three months. *Child Development, 51*, 295–298.

Folsom, R. C., & Wynne, M. K. (1987). Auditory brain stem responses from human adults and infants: Wave V tuning curves. *Journal of the Acoustical Society of America, 81*, 412–417.

Gorga, M. P., Kaminski, J. R., Beauchaine, K. L., Jesteadt, W., & Neely, S. T. (1989). Auditory brainstem responses from children three months to three years of age: Normal patterns of response II. *Journal of Speech and Hearing Research, 32*, 281–288.

Gravel, J. S., & Hood, L. J. (1998). Pediatric audiological assessment. In F. Musiek & W. Rintelmann (Eds.), *Contemporary perspectives in hearing assessment* (pp. 305–326). Needham Heights, MA: Allyn and Bacon.

Gray, L. (1992). Interactions between sensory and nonsensory factors in the responses of newborn birds to sound. In L. A. Werner & E. W. Rubel (Eds.), *Developmental psychoacoustics* (pp. 89–112). Washington, DC: American Psychological Association.

Hall, J. W., Buss, E., & Grose, J. H. (2005). Informational masking release in children and adults. *Journal of the Acoustical Society of America, 118*, 1605–1613.

Hall, J. W., & Grose, J. H. (1991). Notched-noise measures of frequency selectivity in adults and children using fixed-masker-level and fixed-signal-level presentation. *Journal of Speech and Hearing Research, 34*, 651–660.

Hall, J. W., & Grose, J. H. (1994). Development of temporal resolution in children as measured by the temporal-modulation transfer-function. *Journal of the Acoustical Society of America, 96*, 150–154.

Hall, J. W., Grose, J. H., Buss, E., & Dev, M. B. (2002). Spondee recognition in a two-talker masker and a speech-shaped noise masker in adults and children. *Ear and Hearing, 23*, 159–165.

He, C., Hotson, L., & Trainor, L. J. (2007). Mismatch responses to pitch changes in early infancy. *Journal of Cognitive Neuroscience, 19*, 878–892.

He, C., & Trainor, L. J. (2009). Finding the pitch of the missing fundamental in infants. *Journal of Neuroscience, 29*, 7718–7722.

Hill, P. R., Hogben, J. H., & Bishop, D. M. V. (2005). Auditory frequency discrimination in children with specific language impairment: A longitudinal study. *Journal of Speech Language and Hearing Research, 48*, 1136–1146.

Humes, L. E., & Ahlstrom, J. B. (1984). Relation between reaction time and loudness. *Journal of Speech and Hearing Research, 27*, 306–310.

Ikui, A., Sando, I., & Fujita, S. (1997). Postnatal change in angle between the tympanic annulus and surrounding structures: Computer-aided three-dimensional reconstruction study. *Annals of Otology, Rhinology, and Laryngology, 106*, 33–36.

Irwin, R. J., Ball, A. K. R., Kay, N., Stillman, J. A., & Rosser, J. (1985). The development of auditory temporal acuity in children. *Child Development, 56*, 614–620.

Jeffrey, W. E., & Cohen, L. B. (1971). Habituation in the human infant. In H. Reese (Ed.), *Advances in infancy research* (Vol. 6, pp. 63–99). New York, NY: Academic Press.

Jensen, J. K., & Neff, D. L. (1993). Development of basic auditory discrimination in preschool children. *Psychological Science*, 4(2), 104–107.

Keefe, D. H., & Abdala, C. (2007). Theory of forward and reverse middle-ear transmission applied to otoacoustic emissions in infant and adult ears. *Journal of the Acoustical Society of America, 121*, 978–993.

Keefe, D. H., Bulen, J. C., Arehart, K. H., & Burns, E. M. (1993). Ear-canal impedance and reflection coefficient in human infants and adults. *Journal of the Acoustical Society of America, 94*, 2617–2638.

Keefe, D. H., Burns, E. M., Bulen, J. C., & Campbell, S. L. (1994). Pressure transfer function from the diffuse field to the human infant ear canal. *Journal of the Acoustical Society of America, 95*, 355–371.

Keefe, D. H., & Levi, E. (1996). Maturation of the middle and external ears: Acoustic power-based responses and reflectance tympanometry. *Ear and Hearing, 17*, 361–373.

Kidd, G., Mason, C. R., Deliwala, P. S., Woods, W. S., & Colburn, H. S. (1994). Reducing informational masking by sound segregation. *Journal of the Acoustical Society of America, 95*, 3475–3480.

Knudsen, E. I. (1985). Experience alters the spatial tuning of auditory units in the optic tectum during a sensitive period in the barn owl. *Journal of Neuroscience, 5*, 3094–3109.

Koelsch, S., Grossmann, T., Gunter, T. C., Hahne, A., Schroger, E., & Friederici, A. D. (2003). Children processing music: Electric brain responses reveal musical competence and gender differences. *Journal of Cognitive Neuroscience, 15*, 683–693.

Lavigne-Rebillard, M., & Pujol, R. (1987). Surface aspects of the developing human organ of corti. *Acta Otolaryngologica, 436*, 43–50.

Lavigne-Rebillard, M., & Pujol, R. (1988). Hair cell innervation in the fetal human cochlea. *Acta Otolaryngologica (Stockh.), 105*, 398–402.

Leibold, L., & Neff, D. L. (2007). Effects of masker-spectral variability and masker fringes in children and adults. *Journal of the Acoustical Society of America, 121*, 3666–3676.

Leibold, L., & Werner, W. A. (2002). Relationship between intensity and reaction time in normal hearing infants and adults. *Ear and Hearing, 23*, 92–97.

Leibold, L. J., & Werner, L. A. (2006). Effect of masker-frequency variability on the detection performance of infants and adults. *Journal of the Acoustical Society of America, 119*, 3960–3970.

Levi, E. C., Folsom, R. C., & Dobie, R. A. (1995). Coherence analysis of envelope-following responses (EFRs) and frequency-following responses (FFRs) in infants and adults. *Hearing Research, 89*, 21–27.

Litovsky, R. Y. (1997). Developmental changes in the precedence effect: Estimates of minimum audible angle. *Journal of the Acoustical Society of America, 102*(3), 1739–1745.

Litovsky, R. Y., & Ashmead, D. H. (1997). Development of binaural and spatial hearing in infants and children. In R. H. Gilkey & T. R. Anderson (Eds.), *Binaural and spatial hearing in real and virtual environments* (pp. 571–592). Manwah, NJ: Lawrence Erlbaum Associates.

Maxon, A. B., & Hochberg, I. (1982). Development of psychoacoustic behavior: Sensitivity and discrimination. *Ear and Hearing, 3*(6), 301–308.

McAdams, S., & Bertoncini, J. (1997). Organization and discrimination of repeating sound sequences by newborn infants. *Journal of the Acoustical Society of America, 102*, 2945–2953.

Moleti, A., Sisto, R., Paglialonga, A., Sibella, F., Anteunis, L., Parazzini, M., & Tognola, G. (2008). Transient evoked otoacoustic emission latency and estimates of cochlear tuning in preterm neonates. *Journal of the Acoustical Society of America, 124*, 2984–2994.

Montgomery, C. R., & Clarkson, M. G. (1997). Infants' pitch perception: Masking by low- and high-frequency noises. *Journal of the Acoustical Society of America, 102*, 3665–3672.

Moore, B. C. J. (1973). Frequency difference limens for short-duration tones. *Journal of the Acoustical Society of America, 54*, 610–619.

Morrongiello, B. A. (1988). Infants' localization of sounds along two spatial dimensions: Horizontal and vertical axes. *Infant Behavior and Development, 11*, 127–143.

Morrongiello, B. A., Fenwick, K., & Chance, G. (1990). Sound localization acuity in very young infants: An observer-based testing procedure. *Developmental Psychology, 26*, 75–84.

Morrongiello, B. A., & Rocca, P. T. (1987). Infants' localization of sounds in the median sagittal plane: Effects of signal frequency. *Journal of the Acoustical Society of America, 82*, 900–905.

Neff, D. L. (1995). Signal properties that reduce masking by simultaneous, random-frequency maskers. *Journal of the Acoustical Society of America, 98*, 1909–1920.

Neff, D. L., & Green, D. M. (1987). Masking produced by spectral uncertainty with multicomponent maskers. *Perception and Psychophysics, 41*(5), 409–415.

Newman, R. S., & Jusczyk, P. W. (1996). The cocktail party effect in infants. *Perception and Psychophysics, 58*(8), 1145–1156.

Nittrouer, S., & Boothroyd, A. (1990). Context effects in phoneme and word recognition by young children and older adults. *Journal of the Acoustical Society of America, 87*, 2705–2715.

Oh, E. L., & Lutfi, R. A. (1998). Nonmonotonicity of informational masking. *Journal of the Acoustical Society of America, 104*, 3489–3499.

Okabe, K., Sachiko, T., Hareo, H., Tanetoshi, M., & Hiroaki, F. (1988) Acoustic impedance measurement on normal ears of children. *Journal of the Acoustical Society of Japan, 9*, 287–294.

Olsho, L. W. (1985). Infant auditory perception: Tonal masking. *Infant Behavior and Development, 8*, 371–384.

Olsho, L. W., Koch, E. G., & Carter, E. A. (1988). Nonsensory factors in infant frequency discrimination. *Infant Behavior and Development, 11*, 205–222.

Olsho, L. W., Koch, E. G., Carter, E. A., Halpin, C. F., & Spetner, N. B. (1988). Pure-tone sensitivity of human infants. *Journal of the Acoustical Society of America, 84*, 1316–1324.

Olsho, L. W., Koch, E. G., & Halpin, C. F. (1987). Level and age effects in infant frequency discrimination. *Journal of the Acoustical Society of America, 82*, 454–464.

Pickles, J. O. (2008). *An introduction to the physiology of hearing* (3rd ed.). Bingley, UK: Emerald Press.

Ponton, C. W., Moore, J. K., & Eggermont, J. J. (1996). Auditory brain stem response generation by parallel pathways: Differential maturation of axonal conduction time and synaptic transmission. *Ear and Hearing, 17*, 402–410.

Pujol, R., Lavigne-Rebillard, M., & Uziel, A. (1991). Development of the human cochlea. *Acta Otolaryngologica (Suppl.), 482*, 7–12.

Rosen, S. (1989). Temporal information in speech and its relevance for cochlear implants. In B. Fraypse & N. Cothard (Eds.), *Cochlear implants: Acquisitions and controversies* (pp. 3–26). Toulouse, France: Impasse La Caussade.

Ruah, C. B., Schachern, P. A., Zelterman, D., Paparella, M. M., & Yoon T. H. (1991). Age-related morphological changes in the human tympanic membrane. A light and electron microscopy study. *Archives of Otolaryngology-Head Neck Surgery, 117*, 627–634.

Sanes, D. H., & Constantine-Paton, M. (1985). The sharpening of frequency tuning curves requires patterned activity during development in the mouse, Mus musculus. *Journal of Neuroscience, 5*, 1152–1166.

Schlauch, R. S., & Hafter, E. R. (1991). Listening bandwidths and frequency uncertainty in pure-tone signal detection. *Journal of the Acoustical Society of America, 90*, 1332–1339.

Schneider, B. A., Morrongiello, B. A., & Trehub, S. E. (1990). The size of the critical band in infants, children, and adults. *Journal of Experimental Psychology: Human Perception and Performance, 16*, 642–652.

Schneider, B. A., Trehub, S. E., Morrongiello, B. A., & Thorpe, L. A. (1989). Developmental changes in masked thresholds. *Journal of the Acoustical Society of America, 86*, 1733–1742.

Sinnott, J. M., & Aslin, R. N. (1985). Frequency and intensity discrimination in human infants and adults. *Journal of the Acoustical Society of America, 78*, 1986–1992.

Spetner, N. B., & Olsho, L. W. (1990). Auditory frequency resolution in human infancy. *Child Development, 61*, 632–652.

Sussman, E., Wong, R., Horvath, J., Winkler, I., & Wang, W. (2007). The development of the perceptual organization of sound by frequency separation in 5- to 11-year-old children. *Hearing Research, 225*, 117–127.

Tharpe, A. M., & Ashmead, D. H. (2001). A longitudinal investigation of infant auditory sensitivity. *American Journal of Audiology, 10*, 104–112.

Trainor, L., McFadden, M., Hodgson, L., Darragh, L., Barlow, J., Matsos, L., & Sonnadara, R. (2003). Changes in auditory cortex and the development of mismatch negativity between 2 and 6 months of age. *International Journal of Psychophysiology, 51*, 5–15.

Trehub, S. E., Schneider, B. A., & Endman, M. (1980). Developmental changes in infants' sensitivity to octave-band noises. *Journal of Experimental Child Psychology, 29*, 282–293.

Trehub, S. E., Schneider, B. A., & Henderson, J. (1995). Gap detection in infants, children and adults. *Journal of the Acoustical Society of America, 98*, 2532–2541.

Trehub, S. E., Schneider, B. A., Morrongiello, B. A., & Thorpe, L. A. (1988). Auditory sensitivity in school-age children. *Journal of Experimental Child Psychology, 46*, 273–285.

Viemeister, N. F. (1979). Temporal modulation transfer functions based upon modulation thresholds. *Journal of the Acoustical Society of America, 66*, 1364–1380.

Viemeister, N. F., & Schlauch, R. S. (1992). Issues in infant psychoacoustics. In L. A. Werner & E. W. Rubel (Eds.), *Developmental psychoacoustics* (pp. 191–210). Washington, DC: American Psychological Association.

Watson, C. S., Wroton, H. W., Kelly, W. J., & Benbassat, C. A. (1975). Factors in the discrimination of tonal patterns. I. Component frequency, temporal position, and silent intervals. *Journal of the Acoustical Society of America, 57*, 1175–1185.

Werner, L. A. (1996). The development of auditory behavior (or what the anatomists and physiologists have to explain). *Ear and Hearing, 17*, 438–446.

Werner, L. A. (2007). Issues in human auditory development. *Journal of Communication Disorders, 40*, 275–283.

Werner, L. A., & Boike, K. (2001). Infants' sensitivity to broadband noise. *Journal of the Acoustical Society of America, 109*, 2101–2111.

Werner, L. A., Folsom, R. C., & Mancl, L. R. (1994). The relationship between auditory brainstem response latencies and behavioral thresholds in normal hearing infants and adults. *Hearing Research, 77*, 88–98.

Werner, L. A., Folsom, R. C., Mancl, L. R., & Syapin, C. (2001). Human auditory brainstem response to temporal gaps in noise. *Journal of Speech, Language, and Hearing Research, 44*, 737–750.

Werner, L. A., & Holmer, N. M. (2002). *Infant hearing thresholds measured in the ear canal*. Paper presented at The American Auditory Society conference, Scottsdale, AZ.

Werner, L. A., & Leibold, L. J. (2004). Ecological developmental psychoacoustics. In J. Neuhoff (Ed.), *Ecological psychoacoustics* (pp. 192–219). San Diego, CA: Elsevier.

Werner, L. A., & Marean, G. C. (1995). *Human auditory development*. Boulder, CO: Westview Press.

Werner, L. A., & Marean, G. C. (1996). Methods for estimating infant thresholds. *Journal of the Acoustical Society of America, 90*, 1867–1875.

Werner, L. A., Marean, G. C., Halpin, C. F., Spetner, N. B., & Gillenwater, J. M. (1992). Infant auditory temporal acuity: Gap detection. *Child Development, 63*, 260–272.

Werner, L. A., Parrish, H. K., & Holmer, N. M. (2009). Effects of temporal uncertainty and temporal expectancy on infants' auditory sensitivity. *Journal of the Acoustical Society of America, 125*, 1040–1049.

Werner, L. A., & Rubel, E. W. (Eds.). (1992). *Developmental psychoacoustics*. Washington, DC: American Psychological Association.

Wightman, F., & Allen, P. (1992). Individual differences in auditory capability among preschool children. In L. A. Werner & E. W. Rubel (Eds.), *Developmental psychoacoustics* (pp. 113–133). Washington, DC: American Psychological Association.

Wightman, F. L., Allen, P., Dolan, T., Kistler, D., & Jamieson, D. (1989). Temporal resolution in children. *Child Development, 60*, 611–624.

Wightman, F. L., Callahan, M. R., Lutfi, R. A., Kistler, D. J., & Oh, E. (2003). Children's detection of pure-tone signals: Informational masking with contralateral maskers. *Journal of the Acoustical Society of America, 113*, 3297–3305.

Wightman, F. L., & Kistler, D. J. (2005). Informational masking of speech in children: Effects of ipsilateral and contralateral distracters. *Journal of the Acoustical Society of America, 118*, 3164–3176.

Wilmington, D., Gray, L., & Jahrsdorfer, R. (1994). Binaural processing after corrected congenital unilateral conductive hearing loss. *Hearing Research, 74*, 99–114.

Winkler, I., Kushnerenko, E., Horvath, J., Ceponiene, R., Fellman, V., Huotilainen, M., . . . Sussman, E. (2003). Newborn infants can organize the auditory world. *Proceedings of the National Academy of Sciences of the United States of America, 100*, 11812–11815.

Yost, W. A. (1997). The cocktail party problem: Forty years later. In R. A. Gilkey & T. R. Anderson (Eds.), *Binaural and spatial hearing in real and virtual environments* (pp. 329–347). Hillsdale NJ: Erlbaum.

II

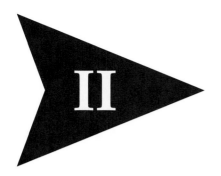

Etiology and Medical Considerations

5

Descriptive Epidemiology of Childhood Hearing Impairment

Adrian Davis and Katrina A. S. Davis

Introduction

The impact of hearing impairment on a newborn or developing child is vast. Not only does hearing impairment impact on method and quality of communication, but research also indicates potential difficulties in learning and education (Stacey, Fortnum, Barton, & Summerfield, 2006), a risk of mental illness (Hindley, Hill, McGuigan, & Kitson, 1994), and restricted employment opportunities (Punch, Creed, & Hyde, 2005). As no child exists in isolation, an impairment also affects the family and systems supporting the child and family, whether they be statutory services or informal social networks (Hintermair, 2000). As such, childhood deafness and hearing impairment represents an important public health issue. The allocation of public resources to deafness and hearing impairment will depend on a number of interacting factors: public opinion; lobbying by pressure groups; local and national politics; and financial limitations. Major epidemiologic influences on the prioritization of services provided are:

1. the number of children having deafness or hearing impairment;
2. the degree of impairment and age of onset;
3. the predominant etiology of deafness; and
4. the potential quality, effectiveness, and cost of service provision, both in the prevention and amelioration of the limitations on the deaf by society (handicap).

Definitions

The two terms "prevalence" and "deafness" give potential for confusion. The term *prevalence* is used here to refer to the number of people in a defined population with a stated characteristic at a particular time, for example, the number of people who report a hearing problem in 2012. Sometimes the prevalence is stated as a percentage of the population. A term related to prevalence is *incidence*, which is defined as the number of new cases in a defined population with a stated characteristic over a particular time period, for example, the number of people with a new hearing problem arising between January 1, 2012 and December 31, 2012. The term *deafness* has many dimensions, some of which have unwanted connotations. From a practical point of view, it is often difficult to decide how and where to draw the line between who is deaf and who is not, particularly when carrying out a survey to determine prevalence. To overcome this terminological problem, in the rest of this chapter the more easily quantifiable term *childhood hearing impairment* (CHI) is used.

We shall refer to *congenital* hearing impairment, meaning that which is present and detectable using appropriate tests at or very soon after birth—the converse being *postnatal* hearing impairment. Where children experience *temporary* hearing impairment such as otitis media with effusion (OME or "glue ear"), the individual consequences are not as severe as *permanent* childhood hearing impairment (PCHI), but the greater numbers of children with OME mean that temporary hearing loss does have considerable impact on services (Higson & Haggard, 2005). Both congenital and acquired hearing impairments can be progressive in severity over time. The severity of hearing impairment in groups is usually categorized as *slight*, *mild*, *moderate*, *severe*, and *profound* based on hearing thresholds, with thresholds taken from the better ear to describe *bilateral* hearing impairment or the worse ear when also considering *unilateral* hearing impairment. Also, sometimes distinction is made between mechanisms of hearing impairment in terms of *sensorineural*, *conductive*, or *mixed*. Example definitions agreed on by the European Working Group on Genetics in Hearing (Stephens, 1996) are given in Table 5–1, but the exact definition has varied between countries and study groups.

Prevalence

Estimates for the prevalence of childhood hearing impairment worldwide are hindered by the great variation seen from study to study. These variations may be thought of as arising from three factors: how cases

Table 5–1. Proposed Definitions of Hearing Impairment

Pathology
Sensorineural: related to disease/deformity of the inner ear/cochlear nerve with an air-bone gap less than 15 dB HL averaged over 0.5, 1, and 2 kHz ∞ *Sensory:* a subdivision of sensorineural related to disease or deformity in the cochlea ∞ *Neural:* a subdivision of sensorineural related to a disease or deformity in the cochlear nerve ∞ *Central:* sensorineural hearing loss related to a disease or deformity central nervous system rostral to the cochlear nerve
Conductive: related to disease or deformity of the outer/middle ears. Audiometrically there are normal bone conduction thresholds (less than 20 dB) and an air-bone gap greater than 15 dB averaged over 0.5, 1, and 2 kHz
Mixed: related to combined involvement of the outer/middle ears and the inner ear/cochlear nerve. Audiometrically greater than 20 dB HL in the bone conduction threshold together with greater than or equal to 15 dB air-bone gap averaged over 0.5, 1 and 2 kHz
Severity
Average hearing level: the level of the thresholds (in dB HL) measured in the better hearing ear at 0.5, 1, 2, and 4 kHz ∞ *Mild:* average hearing level 20–39 dB ∞ *Moderate:* average hearing level 40–69 dB ∞ *Severe:* average hearing level 70–94 dB ∞ *Profound:* average hearing level +95 dB
Symmetry
Unilateral: one ear only has either a greater than 20 dB hearing impairment through 0.5, 1, and 2 kHz or one frequency exceeding 50 dB, with the other ear normal
Bilateral: greater than 20 dB hearing impairment through 0.5, 1, and 2 kHz or one frequency exceeding 50 dB in both ears
Asymmetric: greater than 10 dB difference between the ears in at least two frequencies, with the pure-tone average in the better ear exceeding 20 dB.

of hearing impairment are defined; how cases of hearing impairment are found; and the population from which the cases come. The prevalence of hearing impairment as an indicator of population need for hearing services should not be estimated by clinical performance indicators such as the number of hearing aids fitted last year, or the size of the waiting list for hearing aids, due to the hidden nature of hearing impairments and the substantial size of the existing unmet need. Prevalence may be estimated by population measures through epidemiological studies. Traditionally, studies have tended to be cross-sectional and based on retrospective ascertainment. One of the largest such studies, aiming at a calculation of prevalence of PCHI across the whole of the United Kingdom, was carried out by Fortnum and colleagues in 1998 (published as Fortnum, Summerfield, Marshall, Davis, & Bamford, 2001 and Fortnum, Marshall, & Summerfield, 2002). They approached both health professionals and the education professionals responsible for hearing impaired children around the country, requesting details on every child with PCHI under their care. Professionals (n = 486) replied with over 26,000 sets of details for 17,160 children, allowing an estimation of prevalence of between one and two per 1,000 children. The inclusion of such large numbers in the study allowed a breakdown into subgroups, demonstrating the variability of prevalence across age and severity. This study and other notification studies have some validity in the context of planning diagnostic and rehabilitative facilities for hearing-impaired children. Their weakness is that they include only those already identified, tending to underestimate the younger and milder cases, as well as the hard to reach populations such as the very poor and ethnic minorities.

An alternative is a cross-sectional survey, actively seeking children with a hearing impairment. An example of this was in the U.S. National Health and Nutritional Examination Survey III (NHANES; Niskar et al., 1998) in which a sample of 6,497 children aged 6 to 19 were screened using pure-tone audiometry in a mobile examination center. A hearing loss in at least one ear was present in 149 per 1,000 children (14.9%), most of which was unilateral and slight in severity. A bilateral hearing loss of at least mild severity at speech frequencies was present in four per 1,000. One disadvantage of survey-based studies, such as this, is that they are not able to comment on the likely progress of the hearing impairment, which is important as a slight temporary impairment has different implications to a permanent or progressive hearing impairment. They also are less able to comment accurately on the prevalence of relatively rarer, more severe impairments, as the numbers needed to screen would be prohibitively large. However, universal newborn hearing screening (UNHS) for early detection will pick up sufficiently large numbers in many countries, if linked up to a robust reporting system.

Results from universal newborn hearing screening (UNHS) programs provide a yield of hearing impairment detected per 1,000 babies screened. Depending on the coverage (percentage of babies screened out of the total babies born), the sensitivity of the test, and the numbers of families returning for the follow-up that will provide diagnosis, the prevalence of congenital hearing impairment can be made with increasing confidence. Results from the 21 pilot sites for the newborn hearing screening program (NHSP) in England between February 2002 and June 2004 were examined (Uus & Bamford, 2006). The program achieved 96% coverage with 169,487 babies screened; among the babies referred from the screen, 90% finished follow-up. A confirmed permanent bilateral hearing loss of moderate or greater severity was found in 169 cases. This leads to a rate of 1.00 (95% confidence interval 0.78 to 1.22) per 1,000 babies screened having a congenital hearing impairment ≥ 40 dB HL averaged over 0.5, 1, 2, and 4 kHz in the better ear. Prevalence estimates based on UNHS are in effect based on retrospective ascertainment, having the same limitations for milder cases and those not receiving health care as other notification studies.

Variations on Prevalence

Severity

As the severity of a hearing impairment will affect its impact on a child and family and be an indicator of the extra help needed, studies that have been large enough have divided cases by severity. Figure 5–1 shows two large notification studies (Fortnum et al., 2002; Maki-Torkko, Lindholm, Vayrynen, Leisti, & Sorri, 1998), along with the results of UNHS collated by the Centers for Disease Control (CDC) from the states across America for 2006 (CDC, 2008). These show that those with severe and profound deafness probably make up a minority of all cases.

Data from CDC (2008) also show newborns diagnosed with mild bilateral hearing impairment (not shown in Figure 5–1). If they are included, they make up 23% of the total. However, UNHS was not designed to detect mild hearing impairments, so these data are less robust. The decision to concentrate screening on

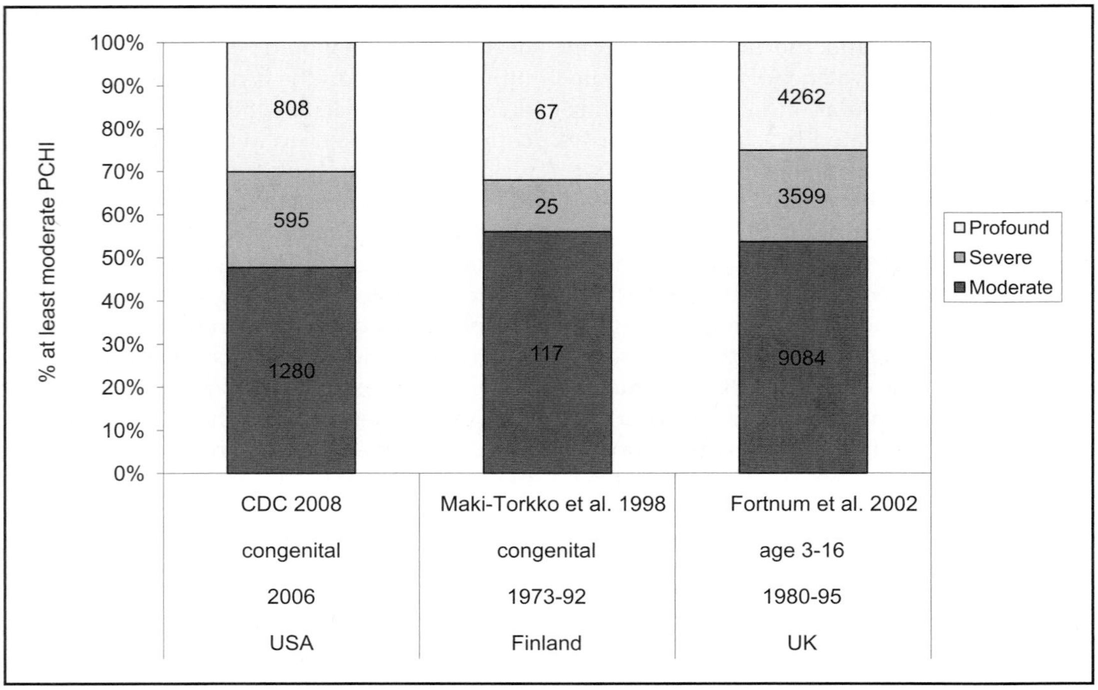

FIGURE 5–1. Distribution of severity of impairment moderate and greater.

moderate and greater hearing impairment rather than increase sensitivity for mild cases is partly because it is much less clear what the needs are, both in terms of numbers of children with mild PCHI or impact on a child's development (Wake, Hughes, Poulakis, Collins, & Rickards, 2004; Wake et al., 2006). In studies looking for sensorineural hearing loss (SNHL) averaging 16 to 40 dB bilaterally, Wake et al. (2006) found 8.8 per 1,000 school children in their sample of 7- and 11-year-olds from Australia affected, whereas NHANES III (Niskar et al., 1998) found over 24 per 1,000 cases in their sample of 6- to 19-year-olds (defining SNHL as loss at high frequencies where, they suggest, losses are unlikely to be conductive).

Site of Impairment

Some studies have published the distribution of conductive and sensorineural PCHI. With newborn hearing screening becoming more widespread, a subcategory of SNHL comprising neural and/or central hearing impairment, now known as auditory neuropathy spectrum disorders (ANSD), has become important. A child with ANSD will have an otoacoustic emission but no auditory brainstem response, thus they will not be picked up by newborn hearing screening protocols that discharge babies who have otoacoustic emission. The decision whether this should be changed depends on: (1) the prevalence of the disorder in the population and subgroups; and (2) the prognosis and management of children with ANSD. These have become topics of interest for research.

Figure 5–2 shows five sets of results: two from UNHS data (CDC, 2008; Uus & Bamford, 2006), one from diagnoses made at an ENT department over six years (Rodriguez Dominguez, Cubillana Herrero, Canizares Gallardo, & Perez Aguilera, 2007), and two from screening children with known PCHI for ANSD (Lotfi & Mehrkian, 2007; Tang, McPherson, Yuen, Wong, & Lee, 2004). Rodriguez Dominguez et al. found only half of the cases of auditory neuropathy were picked up by newborn screening, the rest being diagnosed later. This implies that the results taken from UNHS could be unrepresentative of the true prevalence.

Variations in Prevalence

Age

Prevalence of CHI is not even across the child population, but prevalence varies between studies for a variety of reasons, and it can sometimes be difficult to pick apart the variables having a true influence. Thus, it falls

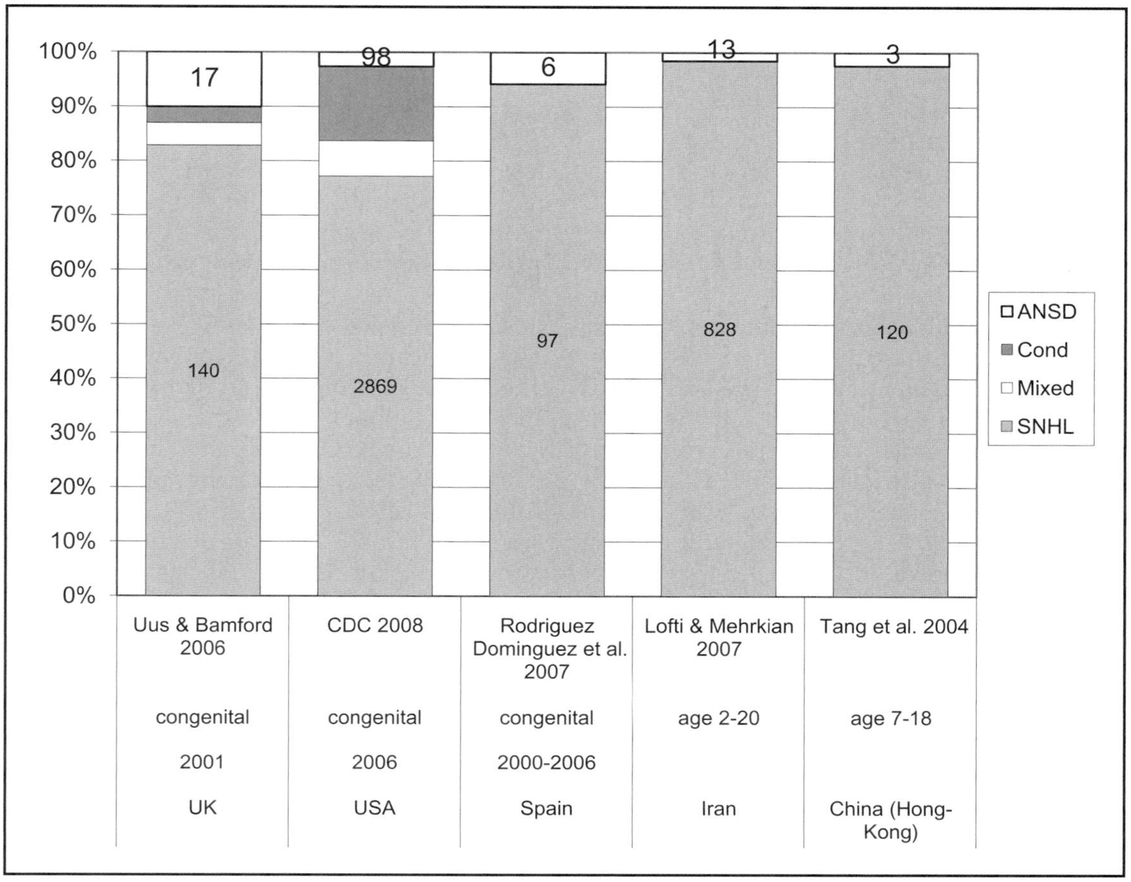

FIGURE 5–2. Distribution of type of impairment in a selection of populations: sensory (SNHL), conductive (Cond), mixed, auditory neuropathy spectrum disorder (ANSD).

to analysis within large studies to demonstrate the change in identified hearing loss between different age ranges. Fortnum and colleagues (Fortnum et al., 2001, 2002) found that the observed prevalence of PCHI increased with age until reaching a plateau at age 9 years, and that this was true at all studied severities: moderate, severe and profound. The adjusted prevalence of PCHI of moderate and greater severity at age 3 years was around 1.1 per 1,000, rising to 2.1 per 1,000 at aged 9 to 16, a rise of 92%. As this was a cross-sectional study, it is not ideal to confirm changes over time. Better ideas of change over time for cohorts of children come from longitudinal studies, such as those carried out by Watkin and colleagues in the East London borough of Waltham Forest (published in Bamford et al., 2007). The relevant cohorts were born between 1992 and 2000 and numbered around 29,000. Data were collected from educational and audiology services about the numbers of children diagnosed with PCHI (any severity) and the method of identification. These children were all offered UNHS and a school-entry sweep screen. Newborn screening identified 1.58 children with permanent hearing impairment per 1,000 live births; a further 0.24 per 1,000 were identified prior to 12 months of age; 1.30 between age 1 and 5 years old; and 0.34 by the school-entry screen. This gives a combined total prevalence of 3.47 per 1,000 children by primary school age identified as having PCHI, of which 1.89 (54%) was not detected at birth. This increase came partly from people moving into the area, but also from children who had not been offered, declined, or failed to complete the screening process. For the rest presenting postnatally, there are a number of possibilities:

- Some children acquire the cause of their impairment postnatally, for example, due to injury or illness (10% had a history of meningitis);

- Some children have the cause of their hearing impairment at birth but manifest it only postnatally;
- Confirmation of impairment is delayed in some children. This may be due to:
  - Lack of suspicion or testing;
  - Progressive or fluctuating impairment.

For the Waltham Forest group of children with PCHI, the severity as recorded in audiology data was bilateral moderate and greater severity in 43%, bilateral mild in 35% and unilateral (mild or above) in 22%. The screening used when these children were newborns was designed to pick up bilateral hearing losses of moderate and greater severity. They calculated that the sensitivity of the program (taking into account coverage, follow-up, and false negatives) was 83% for moderate and greater bilateral hearing impairment, 69% for unilateral and 46% for mild bilateral hearing impairment. Unless followed up owing to high risk of hearing loss, it is possible that children with mild or unilateral hearing loss are not suspected of such until speech is developing or they enter the classroom. This means that speech may be delayed or abnormal, and preschool opportunities for learning may have been compromised.

Sex Ratio

Boys make up a slight, but significant, majority of the cases from large research studies of PCHI around the world: Fortnum et al., 2002 (UK)—53%; Maki-Torkko et al., 1998 (Finland)—58%; Dunmade, Segun-Busari, Olajide, & Ologe, 2007 (Nigeria)—56%; Bener, Eihakeem, & Abdulhadi, 2005 (Qatar)—52%; Niskar et al., 1998 (USA)—57%; Wake et al., 2006 (Australia)—55%. Because most unmanipulated populations have an approximately even split of male and female babies, this excess is due either to a higher prevalence or higher detection. The consensus is that PCHI is more prevalent in boys. For poorly understood reasons, male babies have a higher incidence of perinatal problems and a higher prevalence of many congenital abnormalities (Di Renzo, Rosati, Sarti, Cruciani, & Cutuli, 2007; Kraemer, 2000), both of which correlate with hearing problems. They also are known to have more middle-ear disease (Bennett & Haggard, 1998).

Country

Findings from the study in the Trent region of the United Kingdom (Fortnum & Davis, 1997) can be compared with trials around the same time with similar methods and the same definitions of hearing impairment (permanent bilateral sensorineural or mixed impairment with better ear pure-tone average [PTA] 0.5 to 4k Hz of ≥ 40 dBHL). For example, preliminary data were compared with data from Denmark (Davis & Parving, 1994) showing comparable rates of PCHI, approximately 90% of which was presumed congenital. However, this headline figure disguised some more subtle differences. For instance, it seems that there were significantly more severely and profoundly hearing-impaired children in Denmark than in England. When risk factors were investigated it was found that significantly more congenitally hearing-impaired children had a neonatal intensive care unit (NICU) history in England (33%) than in Denmark (17%), whereas more hearing-impaired children had a family history of hearing impairment in Denmark (40%) than in England (27%). Data used in comparative studies is shown in Table 5–2. These results can also be compared against those from Atlanta, Georgia (Drews, Yeargin-Allsopp, Murphy, & Decoufle, 1994), although it is less similar in design and definition.

It is to be expected that differences in prevalence across more disparate countries is likely to be greater, and that data extrapolated from studies, such as the Trent study, may not be appropriate to plan services in non-Western countries. The World Health Organization (WHO) encourages countries to conduct random sample, population-based prevalence and cause surveys of hearing impairment in children (World Health Organization, 2008a). Importantly, it publishes a protocol to lay out good practice and make studies comparable. Survey protocol includes conductive and potentially reversible middle ear disease. This is appropriate in developing countries where the presence of middle ear disease is highly correlated with a long-term hearing loss. There seems to be an increased prevalence of middle ear disease in developing countries, and this can be aggressive becoming chronic supperative otitis media (CSOM) or leading to cholesteatoma, and complications are more likely where there is little access to health care and/or effective treatment (Alberti, 1999).

Table 5–3 shows the results from a selection of studies based on surveys of samples of school-aged children (the largest range was 4- to 19-year-old). Some use the WHO method of selecting from random households, and others have sampled from schools. The order of the studies is based upon on an objective measure of the development of the country—the human development index (HDI), a composite of indicators of life expectancy, educational attainment and income (United Nations Development Programme, 2008). The countries in Table 5–3 range from an index of 0.812 (Saudi

Table 5–2. Comparative Data Regarding Prevalence of PCHI from Europe and United States. Estimated prevalence per 1,000 live births (estimated 95% confidence intervals calculated for this table).

Cohort	*Reference*	*Moderate or greater*	*Profound *PTA > 90dB; †PTA ≥ 95dB*
Wales, UK (1975–1980)	Parving & Stephens, 1997	NA	0.41* (0.31–0.53)
Denmark (1975–1980)	Parving & Stephens, 1997	NA	0.45* (0.31–0.64)
Trent area, UK (1985–1990)	Fortnum & Davis, 1997	1.33 (1.22–1.45)	0.24† (0.20–0.30)
Denmark (1982–1988)	Davis & Parving, 1994	1.45 (1.25–1.68)	0.54† (0.42–0.69)
Oulu Area, Finland (1973–1992)	Maki-Torkko et al., 1998	1.19 (1.05–1.35)	0.36† (0.29–0.46)
Estonia (1985–1990)	Uus & Davis, 2000	1.72 (1.51–1.94)	NA
Glasgow, UK (1985–1994)	MacAndie et al., 2003	1.23 (1.03–1.46)	NA
Atlanta, USA (1985–1987)	Drews et al., 1994	1.1 (0.9–1.4)	0.5* (0.4–0.7)

Table 5–3. Estimated Prevalence of Bilateral Hearing Impairment in School-Aged Children Based on Survey Results

		Moderate or Greater		*Profound*	
Country	*Reference*	*Prev per 1,000*	*Threshold*	*Prev per 1,000*	*Threshold*
Saudi Arabia	Al-Shaikh et al., 2002	NA		7.1	> 75 dB
Brazil	Beria et al., 2007	33.5	> 30 dB	0.0	> 80 dB
Nicuragua	Saunders et al., 2007	NA		7.2	> 70 dB
Pakistan	Elahi et al., 1998	14.8	> 40 dB	1.6	> 80 dB
Swaziland	Swart et al., 1995	2.1	> 30 dB	NA	
Kenya	Hatcher et al., 1995	22.0	> 30 dB	2.4	> 80 dB
Zimbabwe	Westerberg et al., 2005	8.5	> 30 dB	2.7	> 70 dB
Nigeria	Olusanya et al., 2000	5.6	> 40 dB	0.0	> 70 dB
Sierra Leone	Seely et al., 1995	NA		4.0	> 80 dB

NA = not stated in paper.

Arabia) to 0.336 (Sierra Leone), all falling below the average index for a highly developed country (0.9).

For an overview of congenital hearing impairment, the results of pilot studies of UNHS could be useful. Unfortunately, the structure/quality of the programs and reporting/publishing of results have shown great variety. Table 5–4 shows the published results from a sample of UNHS studies or programs screening of newborns at both high and low risk of PCHI. Many study reports do not say what threshold they were using to define a "case," and where they have done so, the variation between them is such that an objective comparison is impossible. The results are also plotted in Figure 5–3, showing the large spread of yields, tending to be higher in smaller studies. This may reflect under-reporting of small studies with low yields, the increased case-finding in areas of research/excellence, or higher prevalence in less developed countries where implementing large-scale screening and research projects is more difficult.

Table 5–4. Selected Reports of Results of Universal Neonatal Screening

Citation	*Country (HDI)*	*Screened*	*Cases*	*Bilateral Cases*	*Flup Rate*	*Yield*	*Bilateral Yield*	*Corrected Bilateral Yield*
Bailey et al., 2002)	Australia (0.962)	12,708	12	9	90%	0.94	0.71	0.79
Fukushima et al., 2008	Japan (0.953)	47,346	40	40		0.84	0.84	0.84
Schmidt et al., 2007	France (0.952)	29,944	27	24	97%	0.90	0.80	0.83
Mehl & Thomson, 2002	USA, CO (0.951)	55,324	86	63	76%	1.55	1.14	1.50
Prieve et al., 2000	USA, NY (0.951)	43,311	85	49	72%	1.96	1.13	1.57
Vohr et al., 1998	USA, RI (0.951)	53,121	111	79	85%	2.09	1.49	1.75
Finitzo et al., 1998	USA, TX (0.951)	52,508	113	95	69%	2.15	1.81	2.64
Gonzalez de Aledo Linos et al., 2005	Spain (0.949)	8,836	12	11	85%	1.36	1.24	1.46
Welzl-Muller & Stephan, 2001	Austria (0.948)	37,543	91	91		2.42	2.42	2.42
Uus & Bamford, 2006	UK (0.946)	169,487	253	169	90%	1.49	1.00	1.10
Pastorino et al., 2005	Italy (0.941)	19,777	63	33		3.19	1.67	1.67
Neumann et al., 2006	Germany (0.935)	17,439	49	49		2.81	2.81	2.81
Attias et al., 2006	Israel (0.932)	8,400	40	19	97%	4.76	2.26	2.33
H. C. Lin et al., 2002	Taiwan (0.932)*	6,765	35	9	78%	5.17	1.33	1.71
Korres et al., 2008	Greece (0.926)	76,560	56	28	12%	0.73	0.37	3.05
Low et al., 2005	Singapore (0.922)	36,093	146	146	84%	4.05	4.05	4.84
Bener et al., 2005	Qatar (0.875)	2,227	119	78		53.44	35.02	35.02
Prpic et al., 2007	Croatia (0.850)	11,746	7	7		0.60	0.60	0.60
Yee-Arellano et al., 2006	Mexico (0.829)	3,066	5	5	100%	1.63	1.63	1.63
Khandekar et al., 2006	Oman (0.814)	21,387	9	9	65%	0.42	0.42	0.64
Habib & Abdelgaffar, 2005	Saudi Arabia (0.812)	11,986	22	20	100%	1.84	1.67	1.67
Mukari et al. 2006	Malaysia (0.811)	4,437	34	4	35%	7.66	0.90	2.56
Chapchap & Segre, 2001	Brazil (0.800)	4,196	10	10	82%	2.38	2.38	2.91
Nie et al., 2003	China (0.777)	10,501	62	29		5.90	2.76	2.76
Attias et al., 2006	Jordan (0.773)	8,251	113	90	81%	13.70	10.91	13.47
Olusanya et al., 2008a	Nigeria (0.470)	3,333	63	53	32%	18.90	15.90	49.69
Calculated totals		708,946	1,623	1,179		2.29	1.66	2.11

Country = country or state where screening based, although may have been limited only to one region or hospital. Cases = number with final diagnosis of PCHI (any severity). Yield = cases per 1,000 screened. Corrected bilateral yield = estimate of prevalence in the screened population by correcting for incomplete follow-up. *HDI for Taiwan calculated from government statistics (Directorate General of Budget, 2006).

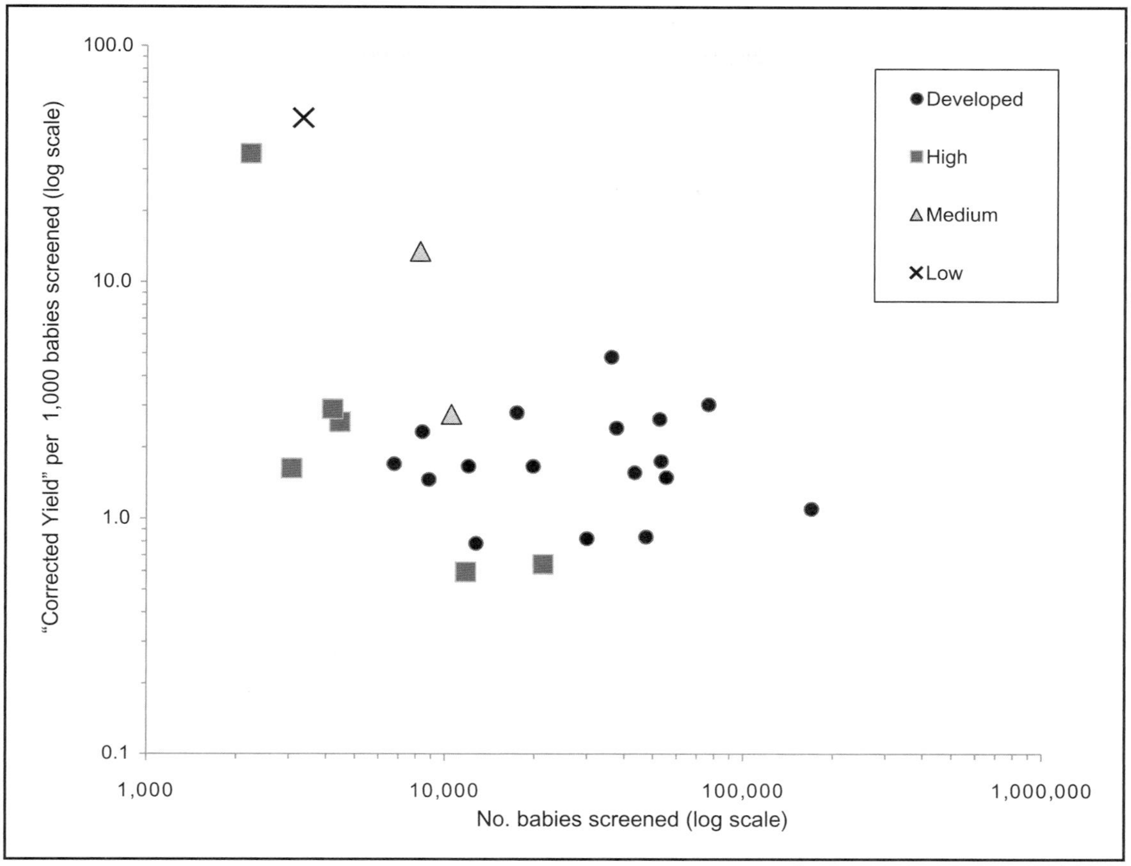

FIGURE 5–3. Worldwide UNHS Yields by study size. Studies from Table 5–4 stratified by developmental level of country where screening took place. Human development levels as per UN definitions (high/medium/low), with high human development split into "developed" (HDI ≥ 0.9) and "high" (0.9 > HDI ≥ 0.8). "Corrected yield" is the estimated number of bilateral cases of PCHI that could have been found with complete follow-up, assuming the same positive predictive value of first screen among those who did and did not attend follow-up.

The same factors that act to cause differences between countries will also act on communities within countries. There is some evidence to show that lower socioeconomic groups in developed countries have higher rates of hearing impairment. The U.S. Third National Health and Safety Examination Survey (NHANESIII: Niskar et al., 1998) found an overall prevalence of high frequency hearing impairment (PTA across 3, 4 and 6 kHz ≥ 16 dB HL) in 6- to 19-year-olds was 127 per 1,000 and did not differ significantly across racial groups, but ranged from 79 (95% CI 51–107) in the highest income bracket to 163 (95% CI 136–189) in the lowest. The nationwide notification study in the United Kingdom (Fortnum et al., 2002) examined the rates geographically, and found that the less affluent the area, the higher the rate of PCHI. A separate study in Glasgow, United Kingdom around the same time (Kubba, MacAndie, Ritchie, & MacFarlane, 2004) used a more sensitive measure of deprivation, and confirmed the finding. They found that as well as the higher rate of perinatal problems, the more deprived groups had more cases of familial PCHI, suggesting that although deprivation may increase the risk of PCHI, having hearing impairment (or having PCHI in a family) may also predispose to deprivation. The WHO in its report on chronic diseases (World Health Organization, 2005) views the process from poverty to chronic diseases as "interconnected in a vicious cycle." Poor people have a greater exposure to risks and decreased access to health services, predisposing them to disease and complications. People with disease have an increased burden of health expenditure and reduction in income, pushing them into poverty. This cycle can be envisaged in individuals, families, whole communities, and even countries.

Risk Factors

The identification of some risk factors have come from understanding the etiology of PCHI, conversely the etiology has sometimes been worked out after observational studies showed something as a risk factor. The study of the epidemiology of PCHI in the Trent region among children born from 1985 to 1993 (Fortnum & Davis, 1997) found that the majority of children with congenital PCHI of moderate or greater severity had one or more of just three risk factors: 29% had a stay in neonatal intensive care (NICU) ≥ 48 hours; 30% had a family history of PCHI; 12% had a craniofacial abnormality (CFA). By using these risk factors, they estimate a targeted newborn hearing screening program could detect 59% of congenital PCHI. A widely used list of risk factors comes from the Joint Committee on Infant Hearing (Joint Committee on Infant Hearing [JCIH], 2007), summarized in Table 5–5.

Even in places where universal screening is established, knowledge of risk factors helps to identify those for whom there is a risk of hearing impairment beyond the neonatal period, indicating the need for further observation of a child as they develop. In studies of children who developed hearing loss postnatally from London, United Kingdom (Bamford et al., 2007) and Austria (Weichbold, Nekahm-Heis, & Welzl-Mueller, 2006), data showed the vast majority had a risk factor. The Trent Study (Fortnum & Davis, 1997) found that 40% of those with hearing impairment had at least one other clinical or neurodevelopmental problem. Another way of looking at this is that congenital and developmental problems are risk factors that also bring children into contact with the health services. The authors of Bamford et al. (2007) suggest that around 30% of post-UNHS cases would have been found by routine hearing surveillance of those children attending a child development center. Children with disabilities are also a group in which active case-finding is needed due to the potential complexity of their needs.

TABLE 5–5. Risk Indicators Associated with Permanent Congenital, Delayed-Onset, or Progressive Hearing Loss in Childhood (Joint Committee on Infant Hearing, 2007)

Family history of permanent childhood hearing loss
In utero infections, such as CMV, herpes, rubella, syphilis, and toxoplasmosis
Neonatal intensive care of more than 5 days
Extracorporeal membrane oxygenation
Assisted ventilation
Exposure to ototoxic medications (Gentamicin, Tobramycin, Furosemide, etc.)
Hyperbilirubinaemia that requires exchange transfusion
Craniofacial abnormalities, including those that involve the pinna, ear canal, ear tags, ear pits, and temporal bone abnormalities
Diagnosis of a syndrome associated with hearing loss, or physical findings suggestive of such a syndrome, such as neurofibromatosis, osteoporosis, or a white forelock.
Neurodegenerative disorders
Culture-positive postnatal infections associated with sensorineural hearing loss, including bacterial and viral (especially herpes and varicella (chickenpox) viruses) meningitis
Head trauma, especially basal skull/temporal bone fracture that requires hospitalization
Chemotherapy

Perinatal Risk Factors

A history of significant perinatal problems appears prominently in studies of risk factors for PCHI. A paper from the Metropolitan Atlanta Developmental Disability Surveillance Program (MADDSP; Van Naarden & Decoufle, 1999) concentrates on PCHI among children who were of low and very low birth weight (LBW < 2500g but ≥ 1500g, and VLBW < 1500g) surviving to at least age 3 years. Of children born at normal birth weight, 0.37 per 1,000 had PCHI at age 3 years. Those with LBW had around 3.5 times this prevalence (1.27 per 1,000); those born at VLBW were 14 times more likely to have PCHI (5.1 per 1,000). Prematurity (birth before 27 weeks gestation) was not an independent risk factor once weight was controlled. The babies included in MADDSP were born in the 1980s, and since then developments in neonatal intensive care (NICU) have meant that younger and smaller babies can be helped to survive. These babies may have increased rates of neurodevelopmental and sensory problems, although studies have been inconclusive (for example, Wilson-Costello, Friedman, Minich, Fanaroff, & Hack, 2005). More recent estimates of hearing impairment in NICU graduates in highly developed countries include:

- A multicenter United States study on extremely low weight (ELBW < 1000g) babies born before 25 weeks (Hintz, Kendrick, Vohr, Poole, & Higgins, 2005) found that 27 out of 817 babies surviving to follow-up at 18 to 22 months (corrected age) needed bilateral hearing aids—33 per 1,000;
- A multicenter study in Hong Kong of ELBW babies (High Risk Follow-up Working Group, 2008) found four out of 49 available at 3 years of age had bilateral PCHI, two at moderate or greater severity—40 per 1,000;
- A Dutch nationwide cohort of NICU babies 1998–2002 born < 30 weeks gestation or ELBW (Hille, van Straaten, & Verkerk, 2007) found 71 out of 2,186 had PCHI in *either ear* at 3 months postbirth—32 per 1,000.

In the developing world, adverse perinatal conditions are also a prominent risk factor for developing PCHI. In Nigeria (innercity Lagos), parent reported "difficult delivery" was associated with attending a deaf school with odds ratio 20.5 (Olusanya & Okolo, 2006). In Mexico (Mexico City) a medical records review showed that 56% of children with prelingual SNHL had an "abnormal delivery" (Penazola-Lopez, Castillo-Maya, Garcia-Pedroza, & Sanchez-Lopez, 2004), and 11% were born weighing < 1500g. As part of a study of UNHS in Nigeria, risk factors were investigated in babies who had been born outside of hospital (Olusanya, Wirz, & Luxon, 2008); the finding of PCHI was positively associated with: (1) no skilled attendant at the birth (corrected odds ratio 4.2) and (2) severe neonatal jaundice (corrected odds ratio 19). Neonatal jaundice was also found to be important in Iran (Jafari, Malayeri, & Ashayeri, 2007), where of 86 children with profound PCHI studied, 40% had a history of jaundice.

Consanguinity as Risk Factor

Consanguinity is noted as a risk factor in a number of studies in the developing world and minority communities in developed countries, and some details are shown in Table 5–6. Although there is good reason to think consanguinity causes higher prevalence of hearing impairment, because of its link with disadvantage it is not easy to assess its true effects (Bajaj et al., 2009; Saggar & Bittles, 2008). The above-mentioned study in Nigeria (Olusanya & Okolo, 2006) found that consanguinity had as big an effect on the risk of hearing impairment as did a family history of deafness (odds risk of 6.7 for consanguineous parents and 6.3 for family history). Some authors point out that consanguinity

Table 5–6. Rates of First-Cousin Marriage in Parents of Children With and Without PCHI

Country (reference)	Method of Collecting Cases	Rate Consanguinity in Cases	Method of Calculating Background Rate	Background Rate
Oman (Al Khabori, 2004)	Etiology investigation of known cases	70%	Contemporary study (Rajab & Patton, 2000)	24%
Qatar (Bener et al., 2005)	UNHS pilot	61%	Children passing UNHS	25%
Saudi Arabia (Zakzouk, 2002a)	Cross-sectional hearing screening	30%	Children passing screening	19%

is a preventable risk factor that would be possible to reduce, but to do so would be no straightforward matter (World Health Organization, 2006).

Major Etiologic Factors From a "Worldwide" Perspective

We have categorized the etiology of hearing impairment as arising genetically or acquired pre-, peri-, or postnatally. A selection of recent etiologic studies is summarized in Table 5–7 and the accompanying Figure 5–4. Since different research teams use different definitions and categorization, their results are not directly comparable. Craniofacial abnormality (CFA) is not an etiological category, as hearing loss is rarely caused by the CFA itself, but due to the same cause as CFA: genetic, acquired, or multifactorial (Tapadia, Cordero, & Helms, 2005). In collecting the data together, there is likely to be some overlap between categories because of the complicated nature of congenital disorders and differing definitions in different studies. All of the studies in Table 5–7 and Figure 5–4 include children drawn from an area or department rather than special school in order to get a wide range of children with PCHI. It is possible to suggest some patterns along geographic lines—such as high rates from infectious diseases in Africa, a higher genetic load in the Middle East, or a higher relative contribution of perinatal causes in Western Europe—although caution should be taken not to draw conclusions due to the differing methodologies of the studies.

Unfortunately, it is common for a large percentage of cases to have an unknown etiology. The studies in Table 5–7 showed that 15 to 57% of PCHI was of unknown origin. Where a greater proportion of children have a known cause for their hearing loss, the largest proportion appears to be attributed to genetic causes. In the Trent study (Fortnum & Davis, 1997), 41% of children did not have a known etiology at identification. Nevertheless, it was possible to impute etiology from other data such as medical notes and this reduced the percentage of people who had no etiological information to approximately 25%. Taking this one step further, another study (Parker, Fortnum, Young, Davis, & Mueller, 2000) reported investigating 82 children from the Trent study using a questionnaire, home visit, and genetic test. They found eight children had a genetic syndrome not previously assigned, and seven additional cases had the most common genetic mutation causing hearing impairment in the United Kingdom, connexin-26 35delG. In Denmark (Parving, 1983), it was found that etiology was significantly more likely to be found if a child with PCHI had a nonaudiologic examination in addition to a standard audiologic exam (61% versus 52%). There are a number of guidelines now available for clinicians investigating the cause of hearing loss in individual children, for example, a good practice guideline used for the Newborn Hearing Screening Programme in the United Kingdom (National Newborn Hearing Screening Programme, 2009), and this type of systematic approach will also help in research.

The presence of one possible etiology does not exclude another. For example, it is increasingly recognized that some mutations do not cause permanent hearing loss, but lower the threshold for environmental insults pre-, peri-, and postnatally (Brent, 2004; Dyer, Strasnick, & Jacobson, 1998). Such mutations include the A1555G mitochondrial gene mutation, which predisposes to hearing loss when a child takes aminoglycoside antibiotics such as Gentamicin (Bitner-Glindzicz & Rahman, 2007). Children with a sensorineural hearing loss can be more at risk of conductive problems such as chronic otitis media (Das, 1996; Oghan, Harputluoglu, Ozturk, Guclu, & Mayda, 2008; Ozturk et al., 2005), something that can potentially be treated to improve functionality of hearing. Sometimes the number of potential causes for PCHI is increased due to the high prevalence of risk factors either on the level of the individual or population. For example, a study of PCHI in Nicaraguan children (Saunders et al., 2007) showed a high prevalence of PCHI (~180 per 1,000), with the majority (51%) of cases presenting with more than one potential etiology. Family history was present in 38%, prenatal infection found in over 30%, neonatal breathing problems in 28%, and aminoglycoside antibiotic (Gentamicin) use in 30%.

Changes Over Time

A school for deaf children in Copenhagen was used to study the causes of hearing loss in children attending in 1993 and 1994 (Parving & Hauch, 1994), and the results compared to cases evaluated 10 and 40 years previously in the same institution. They found that the frequency of congenital inherited hearing impairment increased steadily with time, whereas prenatal infections increased between the first two studies then decreased after 1983. A similar study in the Netherlands (Admiraal & Huygen, 2000) also showed a decrease in prenatal infectious causes from 1988 to 1998, whereas the proportion of PCHI thought to have perinatal causes increased. The changes in the developed world over the last few decades have shown the

Table 5–7. A Selection of Etiological Reports for Permanent Bilateral Hearing Loss (*including unilateral, limited to SNHL) in Areas Covered by ENT Departments, Clinic, or Study

1st Author, year	Dunmade, 2007	Westerberg, 2005	de Nobrega, 2005	Zakzouk, 2002b	Al Khabori, 2004	Uus, 2000	Levi, 2004	Morales-Angulo, 2004	Fortnum, 1997	Billings, 1999	Maki-Torkko, 1998	Walch, 2000
Location	Nigeria	Manicaland, Zimbabwe	Sao Paulo, Brazil	Saudi Arabia	Oman	Estonia	Jerusalem, Israel	Cantabria, Spain	Trent, UK	Boston, USA	North Norway	Austria
Severity	> 71 dB	> 30 dB*	Hearing loss	> 76 dB	> 60 dB	≥ 40 dB	≥ 56 dB	> 70 dB	≥ 40 dB	> 35 dB	≥ 40 dB	> 20 dB
N	115	56	442	302	1400	248	150	100	653	211	112	106
Prenatal	**3%**	**20%**	**26%**	**64%**	**46%**	**77%**	**54%**	**54%**	**45%**	**45%**	**36%**	**25%**
Genetic	0	18%	11%	52%	45%	36%	44%	46%	31%	23%	28%	18%
non-syndromic	0	0	11%	47%	42%	34%	39%	41%	26%	11%	24%	18%
syndromic	0	0	0	5%	3%	2%	5%	5%	5%	12%	4%	0
Acquired	1%	2%	15%	9%	1%	9%	7%	2%	4%	2%	1%	7%
rubella	1%	2%	15%	3%	1%	1%	-	2%	-	-	-	4%
other	0	0	0	5%	0	8%	-	0	-	-	-	3%
Unk inc CFA	3%	0	0	3%	0	20%	3%	6%	10%	20%	7%	1%
Perinatal	**8%**	**4%**	**13%**	**14%**	**12%**	**12%**	**9%**	**14%**	**25%**	**16%**	**12%**	**19%**
Postnatal	**54%**	**30%**	**12%**	**10%**	**8%**	**8%**	**5%**	**11%**	**16%**	**7%**	**3%**	**11%**
Systemic infection	32%	14%	12%	10%	1%	8%	5%	3%	-	4%	1%	11%
Toxic	3%	2%	0	0	0	0	0	8%	-	3%	2%	0
Trauma	0	2%	0	0	0	0	0	0	-	0	0	0
Other	18%	13%	0	0	7%	0	0	0	-	0	0	0
Missing	**35%**	**46%**	**48%**	**12%**	**34%**	**3%**	**33%**	**21%**	**13%**	**32%**	**50%**	**44%**

Some numbers have been calculated based on information in the respective study reports where the categorization differed. All have been rounded, meaning percentages may not add to unity. Unk inc CFA = prenatal onset with cause unknown, including children with congenital craniofacial abnormalities. Missing = etiology not placed in any of above categories.

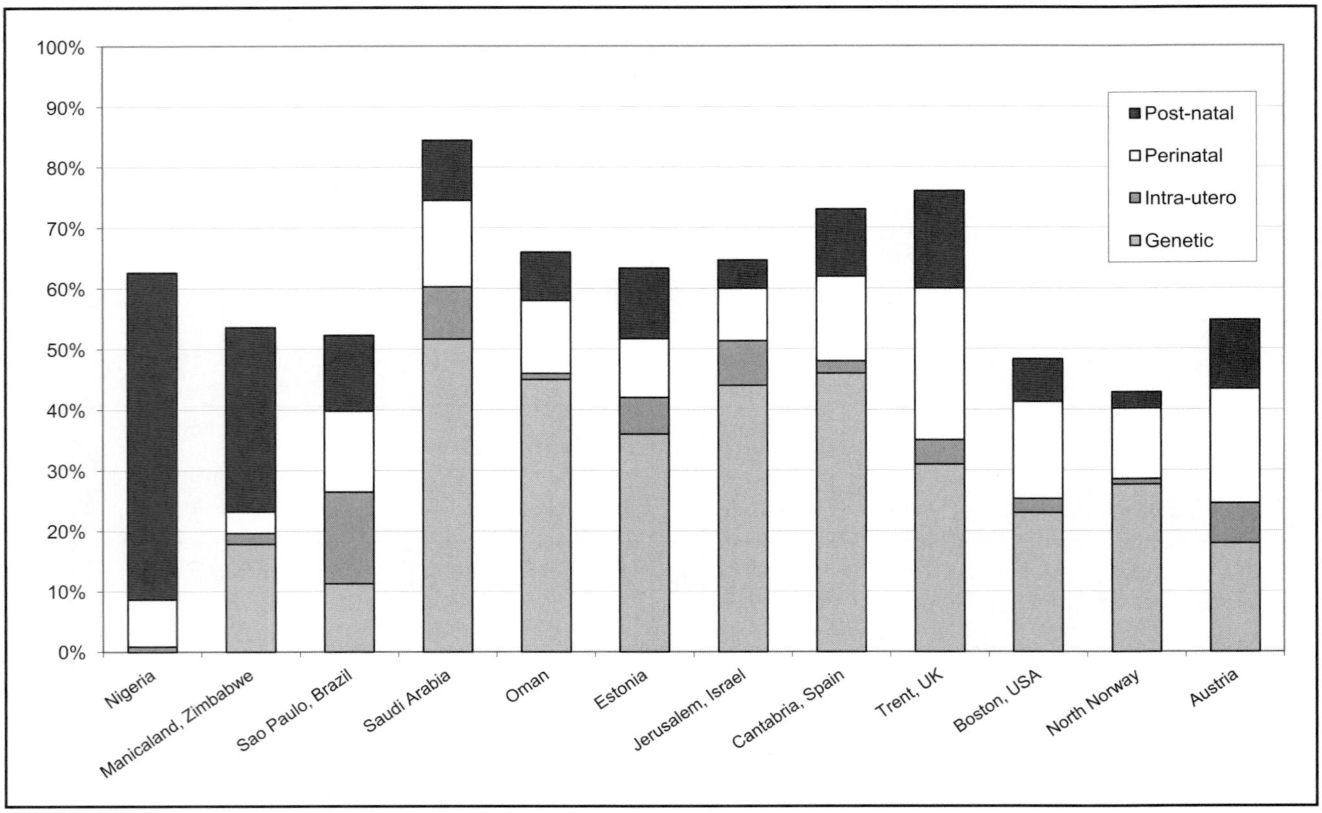

FIGURE 5–4. A selection of etiologic reports as in Table 5–7. Known causes only plotted, the remainder being unknown or missing, therefore bar height corresponds to the percentage of cases with an etiology attributed and is not related to sample size or prevalence.

success of primary prevention. Measles, mumps, rubella, and meningitis are all implicated in PCHI, and all have been the subject of immunization programs. Secondary prevention has also helped, with better nutrition and treatment leading to better outcomes from infections such as measles and meningitis. In contrast, comparing the etiology of sensorineural PCHI in Nigeria between 1980 and 2000 (Dunmade, Segun-Busari, Olajide, & Ologe, 2007), showed no significant change in infectious causes.

In developed countries there has been a rise, not just in the proportion of genetic cases, but in the actual numbers. In some cases this is due to better neonatal care leading to the survival of babies with life-threatening syndromes, in others it is due to the increase in prevalence of particular mutations. One paper suggests that the frequency of PCHI caused by connexin 26 or 30 mutations may have doubled in the last 200 years due to the establishment of a Deaf community leading to healthier hearing-impaired adults (Nance & Kearsey, 2004). These adults go on to have children, and this decreases genetic selection for the unmutated forms of the connexin gene.

Genetic Hearing Impairment

It is thought that at least half of all cases of PCHI have a genetic cause (Morton & Nance, 2006; Reardon, 1992) and the pattern shown in Figure 5–4 would seem to agree with this, at least in developed countries. Despite significant advances in the understanding of the molecular basis of hearing loss, identifying the precise genetic cause in an individual remains difficult. Hearing loss could result from a mutation in an estimated 300 to 500 genes, of which 120 have been identified so far. The majority of these genes are located on the autosomal chromosomes, up to 20% on the X-chromosome, and up to 20% in the maternally inherited mitochondrial DNA (Reardon, 1992).

Genetic disorders were thought to be syndromic or nonsyndromic, and recessive or dominant, but increasing knowledge about the human genome and genetic epidemiology has shown that these distinctions are not as simple in reality. Phenotype-genotype relationships do not strictly follow Mendelian patterns (McHugh & Friedman, 2006), such that mutations in the same gene can have different effects in different racial groups, families or individuals, probably due to gene-gene interactions and gene-environment interactions. Having acknowledged its limitations, the old nomenclature is sufficient for most clinical and epidemiologic purposes and will be used here.

Syndromic

Approximately 30% of genetic hearing impairment occurs as one of a number of developmental abnormalities—a syndrome (Morton & Nance, 2006). Over 400 syndromes featuring PCHI have been described and many of the genetic abnormalities responsible identified. Syndromal hearing impairment can be sensorineural, conductive or mixed. Many involve abnormalities of the temporal bone that can be seen on CT scan (McClay et al., 2002; Reardon, 1992). The presence of a genetic syndrome in children with PCHI should not be overlooked as it can be important in determining prognosis and intervention measures, as well as for estimating the recurrence risks in the family (Mueller, 1996; Parker, Fortnum, Young, & Davis, 1999).

Chromosomal syndromes including Down and Turner syndromes lead to increased risk of hearing impairment both temporary and permanent (Hultcrantz, 2003; Maatta, Kaski, Taanila, Keinanen-Kiukaanniemi, & Iivanainen, 2006). Autosomal dominant disorders tend to be caused by genes with a structural or developmental role leading to symptoms detectable at birth, and include Waardenburg, branchio-otorenal (BOS), and Stickler (STL) syndromes (Keats, 2002). The genetic craniofacial syndromes are also often dominantly inherited, such as velocardiofacial and CHARGE syndromes (Tapadia et al., 2005). Recessive disorders skip generations or occur where there is no close family history, especially where there is high interrelatedness. They tend to be caused by genes with metabolic or regulatory roles leading to symptoms that are late-onset or progressive. Usher and Pendred syndromes are autosomal recessive (Morton & Nance, 2006). Syndromes carried on the X-chromosome affect males predominantly because they have only one X chromosome. Females carry the mutated syndrome-causing gene but are unaffected when they have a normal copy on their other X chromosome. Examples of X-linked syndromes include a form of Alport syndrome and Mohr-Tranebjaerg syndrome, neither of which manifests at birth, but develops in early infancy (Keats, 2002). Mitochondrial syndromes are inherited from the mother and heterogeneous in expression (Kokotas, Petersen, & Willems, 2007).

The presence of syndromes is probably underestimated due to nonrecognition, as found in the follow-up to the Trent study (Parker et al., 2000). A recent meta-analysis of etiological studies (Morzaria, Westerberg, & Kozak, 2004) and results from other studies detailing individual syndromic etiology published since then are combined in Table 5–8. The mean prevalence of syndromal etiology is high compared to the mean in Table 5–7, suggesting selective reporting. The recent results agree with the meta-analysis that the most prevalent syndrome identified as causing PCHI is Waardenburg syndrome. Many of the other syndromes involve craniofacial abnormalities with involvement of hearing an inconsistent feature; other syndromes may manifest hearing loss at a later age than those studied. For example, it is elsewhere estimated that Pendred syndrome is the most common syndromal cause of hearing impairment (Morton & Nance, 2006), but since it causes PCHI of variable severity and age of onset, it comes out much lower in the observational studies that make up Table 5–8.

Nonsyndromic

Genetic hearing impairment that is not part of a syndromic presentation is inherited in an autosomal recessive pattern in around 70% of cases (Morton & Nance, 2006; Petersen & Willems, 2006). One gene whose mutations seem particularly important is *GJB2*—identified in 1997. This gene codes for a protein called connexin 26, a gap junction protein regulating the passage of ions in and out of human cells (OMIM 121011). An analysis of the *GJB2* gene from 52 people in a hearing loss clinic in Iowa (United States), who had congenital sensorineural hearing loss with no syndromic or environmental cause, no family history or consanguinity (Green et al., 1999) found that 22 had *GJB2* mutations (42%), 19 of whom had a mutation on both chromosomes. Of the 41 abnormal copies of *GJB2*, 29 (71%) had the same mutation—35delG. Pandya et al. (2003) in the United States compared the results of *GJB2* mutations for caucasian and noncaucasian children with hearing impairment, finding the prevalence of *GJB2* mutations was similar, 33% versus 23%, but the proportion of these mutations that were 35delG

Table 5–8. Prevalence of Syndromal Etiology in Children With PCHI

		Morzaria	*Morzaria*	*Totals*	
Year studies	**2003–2007**	**1990–2002**	**1966–1989**		
N	**1,616**	**1,131**	**12,380**	**15,127**	
Genetic etiology	**35%**	**32%**	**29%**	**30%**	
Syndromal etiology	**9%**	**3%**	**4%**	**4%**	
Cases of specific syndromes:					**Proportion of *syndromal* cases:**
Waardenburg	50	22	181	252	38%
Velocardiofacial	3	5	90	98	15%
Down	6	1	46	53	8%
Hemifacial micrsomia	1	1	22	25	4%
Branchio-oto-renal	7	0	9	16	2%
Usher	13	ns	ns	13	2%
Prendred	7	4	0	11	2%
Branchiooculofacial	9	ns	ns	9	1%
Klippel-Feil	8	ns	ns	8	1%
Stickler	6	ns	ns	6	1%
Other	73	4	104	181	27%
Total	**183**	**36**	**452**	**671**	

Based on data from meta-analysis (Morzaria et al., 2004) along with selected papers since its analysis (Deben et al., 2003; Egeli et al., 2003 Morales Angulo et al., 2004; Ozturk et al., 2005; Riga et al., 2005; Russ et al., 2003; Saunders et al., 2007). All syndromes shown that make ≥ 1% total syndromes; ns = number not stated in the paper (may be included in "other").

differed greatly, being 77% versus 42%. The most common mutation in the *GJB2* gene in China and Taiwan is 235delC (Chen et al., 2006; Hwa et al., 2003).

Mitochondrial genes differ from nuclear genes in two major ways that affect inheritance. First, as mitochondria for an embryo are from the oocyte, all mitochondrial genes come from the mother alone. Second, there are multiple copies of mitochondrial DNA (mDNA) in each mitochondrion, and therefore expression of a disease-causing gene is not inevitable, such that the clinical phenotype is extremely variable. The most common mutation causing PCHI worldwide is A1555G, which renders carriers susceptible to dramatic, profound deafness following standard doses of aminoglycoside antibiotics. This mutation is more common in individuals from Southeast Asia contributing to the high levels of antibiotic-induced hearing loss in some regions (Liu et al., 2008), but still has significant prevalence in European children. A study in the United Kingdom (Bitner-Glindzicz et al., 2009) showed that 18 of 9,371 children *without* hearing impairment had the A1555G mutation (1.9 per 1,000, 95% CI 1.0–2.8) and were therefore at risk.

Prenatal Infections

During the 1970 to 1980s, congenital rubella was the single most common reported cause of sensorineural hearing impairment in childhood, accounting for 16 to 22% of cases of hearing impairment in babies in Europe (Parving & Hauch, 1994). If a mother is infected with rubella during the first month of pregnancy there is a 50% chance of the fetus developing congenital rubella syndrome (CRS). Hearing impairment is the most common permanent manifestation and affects 68 to 93% of children with CRS (Anvar, Mencher, & Keet,

1984). The WHO estimates there are 110,000 cases per year (World Health Organization, 2008a). It considers the single rubella vaccine or a combination of mumps/measles/rubella (MMR) vaccine suitable for large-scale public health use, and reports that the number of countries using a rubella or conjugate vaccine in their national immunization strategy was 65 in 1996, rising to 125 in 2007 (World Health Organization, 2008b). In terms of population, this gives an estimated coverage of 31% of the global birth cohort in 2007, which will increase with the Chinese implementation of the rubella vaccination countrywide in 2010.

Cytomegalovirus (CMV) is a common chronic asymptomatic infection in adults, which can cross over the placenta to affect the developing fetus and child. CMV infection has been reported to occur in 2.2% of all newborns (Roizen, 1999), making it the most common intrauterine infection. A summary of seven studies between 1982 and 2004 (Fowler & Boppana, 2006) found that the risk of PCHI was 22 to 65% in those babies symptomatic at birth and 6 to 23% in those asymptomatic at birth. Among children affected, there were congenital, progressive, fluctuating and delayed-onset cases of PCHI. It is not yet established how much CMV infection contributes to the overall prevalence of PCHI. In the meta-analysis by Morzaria et al. (2004), the mean proportion of cases reportedly due to CMV in the studies from 1990 to 2002 was 0.92% (standard deviation 1.07) of the total, but separate studies show that within the group of children with hearing impairment of no obvious cause twice as many (13%) excrete CMV in their urine than hearing controls (Peckham, Stark, Dudgeon, Martin, & Hawkins, 1987) and 25% have CMV detectable in the Guthrie blood spot retained from birth (no control group; Barbi et al., 2003). Given the availability of an antiviral treatment for CMV (Kimberlin et al., 2003), there is an argument for screening newborn babies for CMV (Morton & Nance, 2006).

Toxoplasmosis is another prenatal infection that causes congenital abnormalities. In a study of 23,000 mothers and children from around 20 weeks gestation until 7 years of age (Sever et al., 1988), 38.7% of mothers had antibodies to toxoplasmosis during pregnancy, and children born to these mothers had double the risk of developing PCHI by age 7 years (0.4 versus 0.2%, $p = 0.01$).

Maternal Drug Exposure

Drugs such as alcohol, streptomycin, and quinine can destroy neural elements of the inner ear when the auditory system is developing, around 6 to 7 weeks postconception (Dyer et al., 1998). Toxins during gestation can cause ossicular malformations resulting in conductive PCHI. There are probably gene-environment/gene-toxin interactions involved in making particular drugs teratogenic in some mothers and pregnancies (Brent, 2004), such that it can be difficult to be definitive in identifying a drug as responsible for any individual case of PCHI, and difficult to advise mothers which medications are safe during pregnancy.

Perinatal Factors

Neonates admitted to NICU for any reason have a risk of developing PCHI many times higher than those who have not (Davis & Wood, 1992), and even if not hearing impaired, have worse high frequency hearing thresholds on average than children without perinatal complications (Razi & Das, 1994). There are many factors that seem to predispose to PCHI in these babies, and they probably interact, such that in any one infant it would be almost impossible to pick one cause. Along with perinatal problems being a cause of congenital disease such as PCHI, prenatally determined congenital abnormalities can in turn lead to perinatal difficulties (Newton, 2001), making a causal link between any of these factors and hearing loss even more difficult to demonstrate.

Postnatal Factors

It is possible for the cause of acquired PCHI to be genetic due to delayed onset of hearing impairment, but most acquired cases are probably caused postnatally by illness (primarily infection), ototoxic agents or trauma (Davidson, Hyde, & Alberti, 1989).

Infection

When discussing permanent hearing impairment, infection usually refers to systemic and neurological infections. But local infection, such as chronic supporative otitis media (CSOM) and otitis media with effusion (OME), is also included. It is not only a major cause of temporary hearing impairment, but may delay the detection of permanent hearing impairment, and also has the potential to lead to permanent impairment.

In the United Kingdom, those areas that monitor school-entry screening reported that around 2.6% of 5-year-olds are found to have temporary conductive hearing impairment, most likely to be OME (Fonseca, Forsyth, & Neary, 2005). Five is the peak age of presentation of OME in the United Kingdom (Bamford et al.,

2007). Comparison of point prevalence for conductive hearing loss from screening studies around the world, show:

- India, 10.9% of 284 individuals ages 6 to 10 years (Jacob, Rupa, Job, & Joseph, 1997);
- Nigeria, 5.0% of 359 individuals from ages 4 to 10 years (Olusanya, Okolo, & Ijaduola, 2000);
- Swaziland, 3.3% of 2480 individuals ages 5 to 15 years (Swart, Lemmer, Parbhoo, & Prescott, 1995).

Long-term complications of local infection are more common in developing countries (Davidson et al., 1989), but repeated otitis media can lead to some degree of permanent hearing impairment (sensorineural and conductive) even where health and health services are more robust (Dauman et al., 2000). The only study featured in Table 5–7 that mentioned local infection as a significant cause of permanent sensorineural hearing impairment was that from Zimbabwe (6/84 cases; Westerberg et al., 2005), possibly because it was the only study including unilateral hearing impairment.

Reports have indicated that bacterial meningitis is the most common cause of acquired permanent childhood hearing impairment (Davis, Wood, Healy, Webb, & Rowe, 1995). It can be caused by a variety of pathogens, most commonly *Haemophilus influenzae* type b (Hib), *Streptococcus pneumoniae* (pneumococcus), and *Neisseria meningitidis* (meningococcus). For children who survive meningitis sequelae can include learning disabilities, hydrocephalus, motor abnormalities, vestibular deficits, psychosis, hyperactivity, and visual and sensorineural hearing impairments (Bedford et al., 2001). The incidence of permanent postmeningitis hearing impairment in the literature varies from 2 to 31% depending on population characteristics, illness variables, and definition of hearing impairment included (Table 5–9). For non-neonatal bacterial meningitis, it appears that around one in ten will suffer permanent disabling hearing impairment. A vaccine against Hib was introduced in the United States in 1985, and is credited with a fall in the incidence of meningitis and subsequently reduced incidence of acquired hearing impairment (Woolley et al., 1999). This led to a relatively higher proportion of meningitis being caused by pneumococcal disease, which has higher complication rates, against which no pediatric vaccination was available until 2000 (Wellman, Sommer, & McKenna, 2003). One hopes that in countries where the new pneumococcal vaccine is used, it will substantially

Table 5–9. Selection Studies of Incidence of Hearing Impairment Related to Bacterial Meningitis

				Early			Permanent		
Study	**Country**	**Ages**	***N***	**Any**	**Bilateral at threshold**		**Any**	**Bilateral at threshold**	
Grimwood et al., 2000	Australia	0–14y	130	ns	ns		9%	3%	≥70 dB
Koomen et al., 2003*	Netherlands	0–9y	628	ns	ns		7%	4%	≥25 dB
Kutz et al., 2006	USA	0–17y	171	31%	7%	≥severe	ns	ns	
Woolley et al., 1999	USA	<5y	432	14%	10%	>25 dB	14%	10%	>25 dB
Bedford et al., 2001	UK	<1y	1717	ns	ns		6%	2%	≥severe
Richardson et al., 1997	UK	1m–16y	124	13%**	9%	≥50 dB	2%**	2%	≥50 dB
Kulahli et al., 1997	Turkey	children	50	52%	ns		28%	10%	≥severe
Cherian et al, 2002	India	1m–12y	32	28%	22%	≥30 dB	ns	ns	
Qazi et al., 1996	Pakistan	0–12y	69	53%	17%	≥severe	31%	4%	≥severe
Pitkaranta et al., 2007	Angola	0–15y	155	ns	26%	≥80 dB	ns	ns	
Melaku, 2003	Ethiopia	children	141	25%	13%	≥severe	ns	ns	

N = cohort size; number who had meningitis and were tested for hearing loss. *Excluded meningitis caused by *Haemophilus influenzae* type B Any = at least mild unilateral, except** = ≥50 dB. "Early" = Percentage of survivors with nonconductive hearing impairment at presentation, during treatment or before discharge from hospital. "Permanent" = Percentage of cohort followed-up with at nonconductive hearing impairment after discharge from hospital. ns = result not stated.

reduce the incidence of acquired PCHI due to meningitis. It may also reduce the burden of acute and chronic otitis media, which is associated with local pneumococcal infection (Lieu et al., 2000).

An episode of measles has a much lower probability of causing permanent hearing loss (SNHL) than meningitis. But, overall risk from measles is high due to the much greater incidence of the infection. In a recent epidemic in Germany (Wichmann et al., 2009), 19% of cases involved otitis media (rising to 22% among infants), three people developed encephalitis (0.6%, two children and one young adult), of whom two died; no mention is made of whether any child developed SNHL. Alarmingly, the incidence of measles in the United States and Europe in 2008 was the highest for 15 years, and this is linked to decreased levels of vaccination coverage among school-aged children who missed preschool immunization (Muscat et al., 2009).

Mumps can also cause SNHL, commonly unilateral (Davidson et al., 1989). In a survey of unilateral PCHI from Finland, the observed prevalence declined from the 1970s to the 1980s (Vartiainen & Karjalainen, 1998), with no cases of mumps or measles-related unilateral PCHI after 1979. This may have been related to the introduction of a vaccine in 1982. A demonstration of the epidemiology of mumps-related deafness in Japan (Kawashima et al., 2005) shows the relevance of vaccination for the control of this illness.

In countries without vaccination, the incidence of hearing loss due to preventable infection remains high. In Nigeria, a survey of etiology in teaching hospitals (Dunmade et al., 2007) showed that out of 115 cases of PCHI, those thought to be due to infection with measles was 16, meningitis 10, mumps 8, malaria 3, and "febrile illness" in 21—together accounting for 50% of all cases.

Toxicity

Children may be given a number of ototoxic treatments, one of the more important being aminoglycoside antibiotics. They cause dose-related renal toxicity and ototoxicity in almost everyone who receives a sufficiently high dose, but some people have an inherited predisposition that means that even a single dose could result in permanent hearing loss (Bitner-Glindzicz et al., 2009). A Japanese study of 459 unrelated individuals of all ages with SNHL found potential aminoglycoside-induced hearing loss in 43 (9%), with 20 of these testing positive for the A155G mitochondrial mutation (46%), compared to four mutations in individuals with SNHL not related to aminoglycoside injection (0.9%; Usami et al., 2000). Further studies on the prevalence of A155G are needed, and in the meantime, aminoglycosides should be used with caution, especially among those with family history of hearing loss (Bitner-Glindzicz et al., 2009).

Noise

Blast explosions can cause acoustic trauma due to dramatic damage to the structures of the ear (Mrena, Paakkonen, Back, Pirvola, & Ylikoski, 2004), and the delicate organ of corti also suffers trauma from the cumulative effects of loud sounds over prolonged periods in a dose related manner, termed noise-induced hearing loss (NIHL; Burns & Robinson, 1970). Whereas exposure to loud sounds has traditionally been as military- or occupation-related noise (that is, an unwanted sound), much of the exposure for the pediatric population comes from recreational sources, such as music played in clubs or through personal music players and regular attendance of major events (Godlee, 1992; SCENIHR, 2008; WHO-PDH, 1997). Concern over the rapid increase in use of personal music players led to the commissioning of a report by the European Commission Scientific Committee on Emerging and Newly Identified Health Risks (SCENIHR, 2008) that found conflicting evidence on the risks of NIHL in children who listen to loud music. There seem to be environmental and genetic factors leading to susceptibility to the detrimental effects of noise in adults, and presumably children as well (Ecob et al., 2008; Henderson, Subramaniam, & Boettcher, 1993).

What Services Does Evidence Indicate Are Needed for Children With Permanent Hearing Problems?

Aims

The vision for children who have permanent childhood hearing impairment (PCHI) is for them to be identified and assessed as early as possible (Department of Health [UK], 2008). It must be emphasized that identifying hearing loss through screening is not an end in itself, but requires good health and education services to be in place. For hearing-impaired children, this is an extremely important issue because early identification gives us a potential to work with parents and hearing impaired children to limit the impact of hearing impairment, but if handled inappropriately there is a greater potential for long-lasting damage to families and their children. An aspirational target should be to detect all hearing-impaired children with at least moderate impairments by the age of 2 months (adjusted for gestational age in NICU babies) and to begin habilitation, with or without amplification, by 3 months of age. There need to be clear referral criteria to specialist or subspecialist care as required. For the 40% of children with hearing impairment who have additional needs including mental health problems or a history of being abused (Hindley & Kitson, 2000), there should be close liaison with other specialist children's service networks.

Delivery

PCHI is a low-incidence condition, but newborn babies with PCHI require intensive professional support, including biweekly earmold changes, for example. The need for services can be highly variable, depending on social and economic circumstances. Service networks need to be organized across a sufficiently large population to absorb fluctuations in incidence, while enabling good local access. To maintain competence and improve accuracy in assessment and habilitation, individual audiologists probably need to assess 20 to 30 new cases per year to ensure best practice and improve expertise. This has a key impact on the quality of the service provided and is particularly important in low volume specialist activity such as early electrophysiological assessment of babies, early hearing aid fitting, and habilitation. Pediatric audiology services need to be planned to cover sufficient populations to generate the requisite critical mass of patients, and areas with low birth rates need to take account of this. The precise configuration of children's hearing service networks will vary, depending on local epidemiology, geography, and wider service configurations. The challenge is to provide an effective network of services that can treat the more common, milder hearing difficulties in facilities as close to a child's home as possible, while also ensuring rapid referral of the more serious cases to specialist centers, for which the use of expensive specialist equipment may inevitably require some centralization and physical concentration of facilities. Information technology (IT) can enable effective monitoring and is critical to the delivery of high quality continuous care, both in efficient record keeping for individual patients, and for the understanding of referral trends and patterns from which the capacity needed can be predicted.

Clinics that are known to be family and parent friendly have higher attendance rates, thus maximizing the efficiency of the service and reducing wait times. The components of a family-centered service include:

- Processes and structures to facilitate communication with families;
- Attractive clinics, toys and play areas for children and siblings;
- Clear information given to parents to facilitate attendance and reduce anxiety;
- Views of service users sought in annual surveys of families and children;
- Systems in place to manage transition to adult services.

Integration

The importance of effective multiagency working for high quality pediatric services cannot be overstated. A specific workforce development program may be required to ensure that all practitioners can work in this way. This will involve:

- The facilitation of peer support and networking between professional groups and teams;
- Participation in regional networks where they exist and the stimulation of new ones where they are not already established;
- Recognition of and participation in multiagency working practice (including interagency referral, information sharing, training, etc.);
- Regarding parents as full and equal partners in the team.

Summary

In this chapter we have looked at the epidemiology of childhood deafness and hearing impairment, particularly permanent (PCHI), as relevant to audiology service planning, clinical work and research. Estimates of the prevalence of PCHI vary depending on definitions and population. In most Westernized countries, the true prevalence of bilateral PCHI of at least moderate severity detectable very soon after birth is probably 1.2 to 1.7 per 1,000 live births, of which around 20 to 30% will have a profound hearing impairment. Around half again will be born with unilateral hearing loss. Many more will have milder hearing losses. The number of observed cases rises with age until around aged six, and this is due to a combination of acquired causes (mainly meningitis), delayed manifestation of hearing loss of pre/perinatal cause, and delayed detection of congenital PCHI. Universal newborn hearing screening (UNHS) implementation will cut the number of cases of moderate or greater hearing impairment who have a delayed diagnosis. It is hoped that through early intervention, handicap can be reduced for these children. From a research point of view, it means that longitudinal studies may be able to clarify how many children develop hearing loss after the neonatal period. UNHS may not detect children with auditory neuropathy spectrum disorders (ANSD), who may comprise up to 10% of congenital cases.

Comparing different populations shows that there are differences in the epidemiology in terms of overall prevalence, spread of severity, and etiology. Risk factors are the same across all populations, the main being family history, perinatal problems, and other congenital abnormality (especially craniofacial). Consanguinity, nonimmunization and poverty probably also predispose to PCHI. These latter tend to cluster together, which may explain the higher prevalence in certain areas. In these populations, infant mortality will also be above average, and this indicator may help to identify where PCHI is likely to be more prevalent.

Etiology is changing in developed countries, with infectious causes falling, and genetic and perinatal causes rising—meaning prevalence has stayed much the same. Genetic causes account for around half of cases in Western Europe, but more in the Middle East, possibly due to consanguinity. The increase in recreational noise exposure does not seem to have had an effect on childhood hearing, but may have the potential to accelerate age-related hearing loss that will affect these children as adults. In developing countries, acquired causes such as systemic infection, otitis media and aminoglycoside antibiotics still predominate. It is hoped that as their health care systems develop the prevention of childhood hearing impairment will be appropriately prioritized.

References

Admiraal, R. J., & Huygen, P. L. (2000). Changes in the aetiology of hearing impairment in deaf-blind pupils and deaf infant pupils at an institute for the deaf. *International Journal of Pediatric Otorhinolaryngology*, *55*(2), 133–142.

Al Khabori, M. (2004). Causes of severe to profound deafness in Omani paediatric population. *International Journal of Pediatric Otorhinolaryngology*, *68*(10), 1307–1313.

Al-Shaikh, A. H., Zakzouk, S. M., Metwalli, A. A., & Dasugi, A. A. (2002). Cochlear implants in deaf children. *Saudi Medical Journal*, *23*(4), 441–444.

Alberti, P. W. (1999). Pediatric ear, nose and throat services' demands and resources: A global perspective. *International Journal of Pediatric Otorhinolaryngology*, *49*(Suppl. 1), S1–S9.

Anvar, B., Mencher, G. T., & Keet, S. J. (1984). Hearing loss and congenital rubella in Atlantic Canada. *Ear and Hearing*, *5*(6), 340–345.

Attias, J., Al-Masri, M., Abukader, L., Cohen, G., Merlov, P., Pratt, H., . . . Noyek, A. (2006). The prevalence of congenital and early-onset hearing loss in Jordanian and Israeli infants. *International Journal of Audiology*, *45*(9), 528–536.

Bailey, H. D., Bower, C., Krishnaswamy, J., & Coates, H. L. (2002). Newborn hearing screening in Western Australia. *Medical Journal of Australia*, *177*(4), 180–185.

Bajaj, Y., Sirimanna, T., Albert, D. M., Qadir, P., Jenkins, L., Cortina-Borja, M., & Bitner-Glindzicz, M. (2009). Causes of deafness in British Bangladeshi children: A prevalence twice that of the UK population cannot be accounted for by consanguinity alone. *Clinical Otolaryngology*, *34*(2), 113–119.

Bamford, J., Fortnum, H., Bristow, K., Smith, J., Vamvakas, G., Davies, L., . . . Hind, S. (2007). Current practice, accuracy, effectiveness and cost-effectiveness of the school entry hearing screen. *Health Technology Assessment*, *11*(32), 1–168, iii–iv.

Barbi, M., Binda, S., Caroppo, S., Ambrosetti, U., Corbetta, C., & Sergi, P. (2003). A wider role for congenital cytomegalovirus infection in sensorineural hearing loss. *Journal of Pediatric Infectious Disease*, *22*(1), 39–42.

Bedford, H., de Louvois, J., Halket, S., Peckham, C., Hurley, R., & Harvey, D. (2001). Meningitis in infancy in England and Wales: Follow up at age 5 years. *British Medical Journal*, *323*(7312), 533–536.

Bener, A., Eihakeem, A. A., & Abdulhadi, K. (2005). Is there any association between consanguinity and hearing loss? *International Journal of Pediatric Otorhinolaryngology*, *69*(3), 327–333.

Bennett, K., & Haggard, M. (1998). Accumulation of factors influencing children's middle ear disease: Risk factor modeling on a large population cohort. *Journal of Epidemiology and Community Health*, *52*(12), 786–793.

Beria, J. U., Raymann, B. C., Gigante, L. P., Figueiredo, A. C., Jotz, G., Roithman, R., . . . Smith, A. (2007). Hearing impairment and socioeconomic factors: A population-based survey of an urban locality in southern Brazil. *Revista Panamericana de Salud Pública (Pan American Journal of Public Health)*, *21*(6), 381–387.

Billings, K. R., & Kenna, M. A. (1999). Causes of pediatric sensorineural hearing loss: Yesterday and today. *Archives of Otolaryngology-Head and Neck Surgery*, *125*(5), 517–521.

Bitner-Glindzicz, M., Pembrey, M., Duncan, A., Heron, J., Ring, S. M., Hall, A., . . . Rahman, S. (2009). Prevalence of mitochondrial 1555A→G mutation in European children. *New England Journal of Medicine*, *360*(6), 640–642.

Bitner-Glindzicz, M., & Rahman, S. (2007). Ototoxicity caused by aminoglycosides. *British Medical Journal*, *335*(7624), 784–785.

Brent, R. L. (2004). Environmental causes of human congenital malformations: The pediatrician's role in dealing with these complex clinical problems caused by a multiplicity of environmental and genetic factors. *Pediatrics, 113* (Suppl. 4), 957–968.

Burns, W., & Robinson, D. W. (1970). An investigation of the effects of occupational noise on hearing. In *Sensorineural hearing loss* (pp. 177–192). Ciba Foundation Symposium.

Centers for Disease Control and Prevention (CDC). (2008). *Annual EHDI data*. Retrieved September 29, 2008, from http://www.cdc.gov/NCBDDD/ehdi/data.htm

Chapchap, M. J., & Segre, C. M. (2001). Universal newborn hearing screening and transient evoked otoacoustic emission: New concepts in Brazil. *Scandinavian Audiology, Supplementum, 53*, 33–36.

Chen, D. Y., Chen, X. W., Cao, K. L., Jin, X., Zuo, J., Wei, C. G., & Feng, F. D. (2006). High prevalence of connexin-26 (*GJB2*) mutation in cochlear implant recipients [in Chinese]. *Zhonghua Yi Xue Za Zhi, 86*(44), 3114–3117.

Cherian, B., Singh, T., Chacko, B., & Abraham, A. (2002). Sensorineural hearing loss following acute bacterial meningitis in non-neonates. *Indian Journal of Pediatrics, 69*(11), 951–955.

Das, V. K. (1996). Aetiology of bilateral sensorineural hearing impairment in children: A 10 year study. *Archives of Disease in Childhood, 74*(1), 8–12.

Dauman, R., Daubech, Q., Gavilan, I., Colmet, L., Delaroche, M., Michas, N., . . . Debruge, E. (2000). Long-term outcome of childhood hearing deficiency. *Acta Oto-Laryngologica, 120*(2), 205–208.

Davidson, J., Hyde, M. L., & Alberti, P. W. (1989). Epidemiologic patterns in childhood hearing loss: A review. *International Journal of Pediatric Otorhinolaryngology, 17*(3), 239–266.

Davis, A., & Parving, A. (1994). Towards appropriate epidemiological data on childhood hearing disability: A comparative European study of birth cohorts 1982–1988. *International Journal of Audiological Medicine, 3*(1), 35.

Davis, A., & Wood, S. (1992). The epidemiology of childhood hearing impairment: Factor relevant to planning of services. *British Journal of Audiology, 26*(2), 77–90.

Davis, A., Wood, S., Healy, R., Webb, H., & Rowe, S. (1995). Risk factors for hearing disorders: Epidemiologic evidence of change over time in the UK. *Journal of the American Academy of Audiology, 6*(5), 365–370.

de Nobrega, M., Weckx, L. L., & Juliano, Y. (2005). Study of the hearing loss in children and adolescents, comparing the periods of 1990–1994 and 1994–2000. *International Journal of Pediatric Otorhinolaryngology, 69*(6), 829–838.

Deben, K., Janssens de Varebeke, S., Cox, T., & Van de Heyning, P. (2003). Epidemiology of hearing impairment at three Flemish institutes for deaf and speech defective children. *International Journal of Pediatric Otorhinolaryngology, 67*(9), 969–975.

Department of Health (UK). (2008). *Transforming services for children with hearing difficulty and their families: A good practice guide.* DH Publications policy and guidance. Retrieved June 17, 2010, from http://www.dh.gov.uk/en/Publicationsandstatistics/Publications/PublicationsPolicyAndGuidance/DH_088106

Di Renzo, G., Rosati, A., Sarti, R., Cruciani, L., & Cutuli, A. (2007). Does fetal sex affect pregnancy outcome? *Gender Medicine, 4*(1), 19–30.

Directorate General of Budget. (2006). *National Statistics, R.O.C. (Taiwan)* [in Chinese].

Drews, C. D., Yeargin-Allsopp, M., Murphy, C. C., & Decoufle, P. (1994). Hearing impairment among 10-year-old children: Metropolitan Atlanta, 1985 through 1987. *American Journal of Public Health, 84*(7), 1164–1166.

Dunmade, A. D., Segun-Busari, S., Olajide, T. G., & Ologe, F. E. (2007). Profound bilateral sensorineural hearing loss in Nigerian children: Any shift in etiology? *Journal of Deaf Studies and Deaf Education, 12*(1), 112–118.

Dyer, J. J., Strasnick, B., & Jacobson, J. T. (1998). Teratogenic hearing loss: A clinical perspective. *American Journal of Otology, 19*(5), 671–678.

Ecob, R., Sutton, G., Rudnicka, A., Smith, P., Power, C., Strachan, D., & Davis, A. (2008). Is the relation of social class to change in hearing threshold levels from childhood to middle age explained by noise, smoking, and drinking behaviour? *International Journal of Audiology, 47*(3), 100–108.

Egeli, E., Cicekci, G., Silan, F., Ozturk, O., Harputluoglu, U., Onur, A., . . . Yildiz, A. (2003). Etiology of deafness at the Yeditepe School for the deaf in Istanbul. *International Journal of Pediatric Otorhinolaryngology, 67*(5), 467–471.

Elahi, M. M., Elahi, F., Elahi, A., & Elahi, S. B. (1998). Paediatric hearing loss in rural Pakistan. *Journal of Otolaryngology, 27*(6), 348–353.

Finitzo, T., Albright, K., & O'Neal, J. (1998). The newborn with hearing loss: Detection in the nursery. *Pediatrics, 102*(6), 1452–1460.

Fonseca, S., Forsyth, H., & Neary, W. (2005). School hearing screening programme in the UK: Practice and performance. *Archives of Disease in Childhood, 90*(2), 154–156.

Fortnum, H., & Davis, A. (1997). Epidemiology of permanent childhood hearing impairment in Trent Region, 1985–1993. *British Journal of Audiology, 31*(6), 409–446.

Fortnum, H. M., Marshall, D. H., & Summerfield, A. Q. (2002). Epidemiology of the UK population of hearing-impaired children, including characteristics of those with and without cochlear implants—audiology, aetiology, comorbidity and affluence. *International Journal of Audiology, 41*(3), 170–179.

Fortnum, H. M., Summerfield, A. Q., Marshall, D. H., Davis, A. C., & Bamford, J. M. (2001). Prevalence of permanent childhood hearing impairment in the United Kingdom and implications for universal neonatal hearing screening: Questionnaire based ascertainment study. *British Medical Journal, 323*(7312), 536–540.

Fowler, K. B., & Boppana, S. B. (2006). Congenital cytomegalovirus (CMV) infection and hearing deficit. *Journal of Clinical Virology, 35*(2), 226–231.

Fukushima, K., Mimaki, N., Fukuda, S., & Nishizaki, K. (2008). Pilot study of universal newborn hearing screening in

Japan: District-based screening program in Okayama. *Annals of Otology, Rhinology and Laryngology, 117*(3), 166–171.
Godlee, F. (1992). Noise: Breaking the silence. *British Medical Journal, 304*(6819), 110–113.
Gonzalez de Aledo Linos, A., Bonilla Miera, C., Morales Angulo, C., Gomez Da Casa, F., & Barrasa Benito, J. (2005). Universal newborn hearing screening in Cantabria (Spain): Results of the first two years. *Anales de Pediatría (Barcelona), 62*(2), 135–140.
Green, G. E., Scott, D. A., McDonald, J. M., Woodworth, G. G., Sheffield, V. C., & Smith, R. J. (1999). Carrier rates in the midwestern United States for *GJB2* mutations causing inherited deafness. *Journal of the American Medical Association, 281*(23), 2211–2216.
Grimwood, K., Anderson, P., Anderson, V., Tan, L., & Nolan, T. (2000). Twelve year outcomes following bacterial meningitis: Further evidence for persisting effects. *Archives of Disease in Childhood, 83*(2), 111–116.
Habib, H. S., & Abdelgaffar, H. (2005). Neonatal hearing screening with transient evoked otoacoustic emissions in Western Saudi Arabia. *International Journal of Pediatric Otorhinolaryngology, 69*(6), 839–842.
Hatcher, J., Smith, A., Mackenzie, I., Thompson, S., Bal, I., Macharia, I., . . . Wanjohi, Z. (1995). A prevalence study of ear problems in school children in Kiambu district, Kenya, May 1992. *International Journal of Pediatric Otorhinolaryngology, 33*(3), 197–205.
Henderson, D., Subramaniam, M., & Boettcher, F. A. (1993). Individual susceptibility to noise-induced hearing loss: An old topic revisited. *Ear and Hearing, 14*(3), 152–168.
High Risk Follow-Up Working Group. (2008). Neurodevelopmental outcomes of extreme-low-birth-weight infants born between 2001 and 2002. *Hong Kong Medical Journal, 14*(1), 21–28.
Higson, J., & Haggard, M. (2005). Parent versus professional views of the developmental impact of a multi-faceted condition at school age: Otitis media with effusion ('glue ear'). *British Journal of Educational Psychology, 75*(Pt. 4), 623–643.
Hille, E. T., van Straaten, H. I., & Verkerk, P. H. (2007). Prevalence and independent risk factors for hearing loss in NICU infants. *Acta Paediatrica, 96*(8), 1155–1158.
Hindley, P., & Kitson, N. (Eds.). (2000). *Mental health and deafness.* London, UK: Whurr.
Hindley, P. A., Hill, P. D., McGuigan, S., & Kitson, N. (1994). Psychiatric disorder in deaf and hearing impaired children and young people: A prevalence study. *Journal of Child Psychology and Psychiatry, 35*(5), 917–934.
Hintermair, M. (2000). Hearing impairment, social networks, and coping: The need for families with hearing-impaired children to relate to other parents and to hearing-impaired adults. *American Annals of the Deaf, 145*(1), 41–53.
Hintz, S. R., Kendrick, D. E., Vohr, B. R., Poole, W. K., & Higgins, R. D. (2005). Changes in neurodevelopmental outcomes at 18 to 22 months' corrected age among infants of less than 25 weeks' gestational age born in 1993–1999. *Pediatrics, 115*(6), 1645–1651.
Hultcrantz, M. (2003). Ear and hearing problems in Turner's syndrome. *Acta Oto-Laryngologica, 123*(2), 253–257.
Hwa, H. L., Ko, T. M., Hsu, C. J., Huang, C. H., Chiang, Y. L., Oong, J. L., . . . Hsu, C. K. (2003). Mutation spectrum of the connexin 26 (*GJB2*) gene in Taiwanese patients with prelingual deafness. *Genetics in Medicine, 5*(3), 161–165.
Jacob, A., Rupa, V., Job, A., & Joseph, A. (1997). Hearing impairment and otitis media in a rural primary school in south India. *International Journal of Pediatric Otorhinolaryngology, 39*(2), 133–138.
Jafari, Z., Malayeri, S., & Ashayeri, H. (2007). The ages of suspicion, diagnosis, amplification, and intervention in deaf children. *International Journal of Pediatric Otorhinolaryngology, 71*(1), 35–40.
Joint Committee on Infant Hearing (JCIH). (2007). Year 2007 position statement: Principles and guidelines for early hearing detection and intervention programs. *Pediatrics, 120*(4), 898–921.
Kawashima, Y., Ihara, K., Nakamura, M., Nakashima, T., Fukuda, S., & Kitamura, K. (2005). Epidemiological study of mumps deafness in Japan. *Auris Nasus Larynx, 32*(2), 125–128.
Keats, B. J. (2002). Genes and syndromic hearing loss. *Journal of Communication Disorders, 35*(4), 355–366.
Khandekar, R., Khabori, M., Jaffer Mohammed, A., & Gupta, R. (2006). Neonatal screening for hearing impairment—The Oman experience. *International Journal of Pediatric Otorhinolaryngology, 70*(4), 663–670.
Kimberlin, D. W., Lin, C. Y., Sanchez, P. J., Demmler, G. J., Dankner, W., Shelton, M., . . . Whitley, R. J. (2003). Effect of ganciclovir therapy on hearing in symptomatic congenital cytomegalovirus disease involving the central nervous system: A randomized, controlled trial. *Journal of Pediatrics, 143*(1), 16–25.
Kokotas, H., Petersen, M. B., & Willems, P. J. (2007). Mitochondrial deafness. *Clinical Genetics, 71*(5), 379–391.
Koomen, I., Grobbee, D. E., Roord, J. J., Donders, R., Jennekens-Schinkel, A., & van Furth, A. M. (2003). Hearing loss at school age in survivors of bacterial meningitis: Assessment, incidence, and prediction. *Pediatrics, 112*(5), 1049–1053.
Korres, S., Nikolopoulos, T. P., Peraki, E. E., Tsiakou, M., Karakitsou, M., Apostolopoulos, N., . . . Ferekidis, E. (2008). Outcomes and efficacy of newborn hearing screening: Strengths and weaknesses (success or failure?). *Laryngoscope, 118*(7), 1253–1256.
Kraemer, S. (2000). The fragile male. *British Medical Journal, 321*(7276), 1609–1612.
Kubba, H., MacAndie, C., Ritchie, K., & MacFarlane, M. (2004). Is deafness a disease of poverty? The association between socio-economic deprivation and congenital hearing impairment. *International Journal of Audiology, 43*(3), 123–125.
Kulahli, I., Ozturk, M., Bilen, C., Cureoglu, S., Merhametsiz, A., & Cagil, N. (1997). Evaluation of hearing loss with auditory brainstem responses in the early and late period of bacterial meningitis in children. *Journal of Laryngology and Otology, 111*(3), 223–227.

Kutz, J. W., Simon, L. M., Chennupati, S. K., Giannoni, C. M., & Manolidis, S. (2006). Clinical predictors for hearing loss in children with bacterial meningitis. *Archives of Otolaryngology-Head and Neck Surgery, 132*(9), 941–945.

Levi, H., Tell, L., & Cohen, T. (2004). Sensorineural hearing loss in Jewish children born in Jerusalem. *International Journal of Pediatric Otorhinolaryngology, 68*(10), 1245–1250.

Lieu, T. A., Ray, G. T., Black, S. B., Butler, J. C., Klein, J. O., Breiman, R. F., . . . Shinefield, H. R. (2000). Projected cost-effectiveness of pneumococcal conjugate vaccination of healthy infants and young children. *Journal of the American Medical Association, 283*(11), 1460–1468.

Lin, H. C., Shu, M. T., Chang, K. C., & Bruna, S. M. (2002). A universal newborn hearing screening program in Taiwan. *International Journal of Pediatric Otorhinolaryngology, 63*(3), 209–218.

Liu, X. Z., Angeli, S., Ouyang, X. M., Liu, W., Ke, X. M., Liu, Y. H., . . . Yan, D. (2008). Audiological and genetic features of the mtDNA mutations. *Acta Oto-Laryngologica, 128*(7), 732–738.

Lotfi, Y., & Mehrkian, S. (2007). The prevalence of auditory neuropathy in students with hearing impairment in Tehran, Iran. *Archives of Iranian Medicine, 10*(2), 233–235.

Low, W. K., Pang, K. Y., Ho, L. Y., Lim, S. B., & Joseph, R. (2005). Universal newborn hearing screening in Singapore: The need, implementation and challenges. *Annals, Academy of Medicine, Singapore, 34*(4), 301–306.

Maatta, T., Kaski, M., Taanila, A., Keinanen-Kiukaanniemi, S., & Iivanainen, M. (2006). Sensory impairments and health concerns related to the degree of intellectual disability in people with Down syndrome. *Down Syndrome Research and Practice, 11*(2), 78–83.

MacAndie, C., Kubba, H., & McFarlane, M. (2003). Epidemiology of permanent childhood hearing loss in Glasgow, 1985–1994. *Scottish Medical Journal, 48*(4), 117–119.

Maki-Torkko, E. M., Lindholm, P. K., Vayrynen, M. R., Leisti, J. T., & Sorri, M. J. (1998). Epidemiology of moderate to profound childhood hearing impairments in northern Finland. Any changes in ten years? *Scandinavian Audiology, 27*(2), 95–103.

McClay, J. E., Tandy, R., Grundfast, K., Choi, S., Vezina, G., Zalzal, G., & Willner, A. (2002). Major and minor temporal bone abnormalities in children with and without congenital sensorineural hearing loss. *Archives of Otolaryngology, Head and Neck Surgery, 128*(6), 664–671.

McHugh, R. K., & Friedman, R. A. (2006). Genetics of hearing loss: Allelism and modifier genes produce a phenotypic continuum. *Anatomical Record. Part A—Discoveries in Molecular, Cellular and Evolutionary Biology, 288*(4), 370–381.

Mehl, A. L., & Thomson, V. (2002). The Colorado newborn hearing screening project, 1992–1999: On the threshold of effective population-based universal newborn hearing screening. *Pediatrics, 109*(1), E7.

Melaku, A. (2003). Sensorineural hearing loss in children with epidemic meningococcal meningitis at Tikur Anbessa Hospital. *Ethiopian Medical Journal, 41*(2), 113–121.

Morales Angulo, C., Gallo-Teran, J., Azuara, N., & Rama Quintela, J. (2004). Etiology of severe/profound, pre/perilingual bilateral hearing loss in Cantabria (Spain). *Acta Otorrinolaringologica Espanola, 55*, 351–355.

Morton, C. C., & Nance, W. E. (2006). Newborn hearing screening—a silent revolution. *New England Journal of Medicine, 354*(20), 2151–2164.

Morzaria, S., Westerberg, B. D., & Kozak, F. K. (2004). Systematic review of the etiology of bilateral sensorineural hearing loss in children. *International Journal of Pediatric Otorhinolaryngology, 68*(9), 1193–1198.

Mrena, R., Paakkonen, R., Back, L., Pirvola, U., & Ylikoski, J. (2004). Otologic consequences of blast exposure: A Finnish case study of a shopping mall bomb explosion. *Acta Oto-Laryngologica, 124*(8), 946–952.

Mueller, R. (1996). Genetic counselling for hearing impairment. In A. Martini, A. Read, & D. Stephens (Eds.), *Genetics and hearing impairment* (pp. 255–264). London, UK: Whurr.

Mukari, S. Z., Tan, K. Y., & Abdullah, A. (2006). A pilot project on hospital-based universal newborn hearing screening: Lessons learned. *International Journal of Pediatric Otorhinolaryngology, 70*(5), 843–851.

Muscat, M., Bang, H., Wohlfahrt, J., Glismann, S., Mølbak, K., & EUVAC.net group. (2009). Measles in Europe: An epidemiological assessment. *Lancet, 373*(9661), 383–389.

Nance, W. E., & Kearsey, M. J. (2004). Relevance of connexin deafness (DFNB1) to human evolution. *American Journal of Human Genetics, 74*(6), 1081–1087.

National Newborn Hearing Screening Programme, British Association of Audiological Physicians & Audiology (BAAP/BAPA). (2004). Medical management of infants with significant congenital hearing loss identified through the National Newborn Hearing Screening Programme—Best Practice. Retrieved June 17, 2010, from http://hearing.screening.nhs.uk/cms.php?folder=22

Neumann, K., Gross, M., Bottcher, P., Euler, H. A., Spormann-Lagodzinski, M., & Polzer, M. (2006). Effectiveness and efficiency of a universal newborn hearing screening in Germany. *Folia Phoniatrica et Logopaedica, 58*(6), 440–455.

Newton, V. (2001). Adverse perinatal conditions and the inner ear. *Seminars in Neonatology, 6*(6), 543–551.

Nie, W. Y., Gong, L. X., Liu, Y. J., Xiang, L. L., Lin, Q., Qi, Y. S., & Nie, Y. J. (2003). Hearing screening of 10,501 newborns [in Chinese]. *Zhonghua Yi Xue Za Zhi, 83*(4), 274–277.

Niskar, A. S., Kieszak, S. M., Holmes, A., Esteban, E., Rubin, C., & Brody, D. J. (1998). Prevalence of hearing loss among children 6 to 19 years of age: The Third National Health and Nutrition Examination Survey. *Journal of the American Medical Association, 279*(14), 1071–1075.

Oghan, F., Harputluoglu, U., Ozturk, O., Guclu, E., & Mayda, A. (2008). Does the prevalence of otolaryngological diseases in deaf children differ from children without hearing impairment? *European Archives of Oto-Rhino-Laryngology, 265*(2), 223–226.

Olusanya, B. O., & Okolo, A. A. (2006). Adverse perinatal conditions in hearing-impaired children in a developing country. *Paediatric and Perinatal Epidemiology, 20*(5), 366–371.

Olusanya, B. O., Okolo, A. A., & Ijaduola, G. T. (2000). The hearing profile of Nigerian school children. *International Journal of Pediatric Otorhinolaryngology, 55*(3), 173–179.

Olusanya, B. O., Somefun, A. O., & Swanepoel de, W. (2008a). The need for standardization of methods for worldwide infant hearing screening: A systematic review. *Laryngoscope, 118*(10), 1830–1836.

Olusanya, B. O., Wirz, S. L., & Luxon, L. M. (2008b). Non-hospital delivery and permanent congenital and early-onset hearing loss in a developing country. *British Journal of Obstetrics and Gynaecology, 115*(11), 1419–1427.

OMIM 121011. (2008). Gap Junction Protein, Beta-2; *GJB2*. Retrieved November 20, 2008, from http://www.ncbi.nlm.nih.gov/entrez/dispomim.cgi?id=121011

Ozturk, O., Silan, F., Oghan, F., Egeli, E., Belli, S., Tokmak, A., . . . Zafer, C. (2005). Evaluation of deaf children in a large series in Turkey. *International Journal of Pediatric Otorhinolaryngology, 69*(3), 367–373.

Pandya, A., Arnos, K. S., Xia, X. J., Welch, K. O., Blanton, S. H., Friedman, T. B., . . . Nance, W. E. (2003). Frequency and distribution of *GJB2* (connexin 26) and GJB6 (connexin 30) mutations in a large North American repository of deaf probands. *Genetics in Medicine, 5*(4), 295–303.

Parker, M. J., Fortnum, H., Young, I. D., & Davis, A. C. (1999). Variations in genetic assessment and recurrence risks quoted for childhood deafness: A survey of clinical geneticists. *Journal of Medical Genetics, 36*(2), 125–130.

Parker, M. J., Fortnum, H. M., Young, I. D., Davis, A. C., & Mueller, R. F. (2000). Population-based genetic study of childhood hearing impairment in the Trent region of the United Kingdom. *Audiology, 39*(4), 226–231.

Parving, A. (1983). Epidemiology of hearing loss and aetiological diagnosis of hearing impairment in childhood. *International Journal of Pediatric Otorhinolaryngology, 5*(2), 151–165.

Parving, A., & Hauch, A. M. (1994). The causes of profound hearing impairment in a school for the deaf—a longitudinal study. *British Journal of Audiology, 28*(2), 63–69.

Parving, A., & Stephens, D. (1997). Profound permanent hearing impairment in childhood: Causative factors in two European countries. *Acta Otolaryngologica, 117*(2), 158–160.

Pastorino, G., Sergi, P., Mastrangelo, M., Ravazzani, P., Tognola, G., Parazzini, M., . . . Grandori, F. (2005). The Milan project: A newborn hearing screening programme. *Acta Paediatrica, 94*(4), 458–463.

Peckham, C. S., Stark, O., Dudgeon, J. A., Martin, J. A., & Hawkins, G. (1987). Congenital cytomegalovirus infection: A cause of sensorineural hearing loss. *Archives of Disease in Childhood, 62*(12), 1233–1237.

Penazola-Lopez, Y. R., Castillo-Maya, G., Garcia-Pedroza, F., & Sanchez-Lopez, H. (2004). Hypoacusis-deafness related to perinatal adverse conditions. According to the register available in a specialized unit of Ciudad de Mexico. Analysis according to birth weight. *Acta Otorrinolaringologica Espanola, 55*(6), 252–259.

Petersen, M. B., & Willems, P. J. (2006). Nonsyndromic, autosomal-recessive deafness. *Clinical Genetics, 69*(5), 371–392.

Pitkaranta, A., Pelkonen, T., de Sousa, E. S. M. O., Bernardino, L., Roine, I., & Peltola, H. (2007). Setting up hearing screening in meningitis children in Luanda, Angola. *International Journal of Pediatric Otorhinolaryngology, 71*(12), 1929–1931.

Prieve, B., Dalzell, L., Berg, A., Bradley, M., Cacace, A., Campbell, D., & Stevens, F. (2000). The New York State universal newborn hearing screening demonstration project: Outpatient outcome measures. *Ear and Hearing, 21*(2), 104–117.

Prpic, I., Mahulja-Stamenkovic, V., Bilic, I., & Haller, H. (2007). Hearing loss assessed by universal newborn hearing screening—the new approach. *International Journal of Pediatric Otorhinolaryngology, 71*(11), 1757–1761.

Punch, R., Creed, P. A., & Hyde, M. (2005). Predicting career development in hard-of-hearing adolescents in Australia. *Journal of Deaf Studies and Deaf Education, 10*(2), 146–160.

Qazi, S. A., Khan, M. A., Mughal, N., Ahmad, M., Joomro, B., Sakata, Y., & Yamashita, F. (1996). Dexamethasone and bacterial meningitis in Pakistan. *Archives of Disease in Childhood, 75*(6), 482–488.

Rajab, A., & Patton, M. A. (2000). Short report: A study of consanguinity in the Sultanate of Oman. *Annals of Human Biology, 27*, 321–326.

Razi, M. S., & Das, V. K. (1994). Effects of adverse perinatal events on hearing. *International Journal of Pediatric Otorhinolaryngology, 30*(1), 29–40.

Reardon, W. (1992). Genetic deafness. *Journal of Medical Genetics, 29*(8), 521–526.

Richardson, M. P., Reid, A., Tarlow, M. J., & Rudd, P. T. (1997). Hearing loss during bacterial meningitis. *Archives of Disease in Childhood, 76*(2), 134–138.

Riga, M., Psarommatis, I., Lyra, C., Douniadakis, D., Tsakanikos, M., Neou, P., . . . Apostolopoulos, N. (2005). Etiological diagnosis of bilateral, sensorineural hearing impairment in a pediatric Greek population. *International Journal of Pediatric Otorhinolaryngology, 69*(4), 449–455.

Rodriguez Dominguez, F. J., Cubillana Herrero, J. D., Canizares Gallardo, N., & Perez Aguilera, R. (2007). Prevalence of auditory neuropathy: Prospective study in a tertiary-care center. *Acta Otorrinolaringologica Espanola, 58*(6), 239–245.

Roizen, N. J. (1999). Etiology of hearing loss in children. Nongenetic causes. *Pediatric Clinics of North America, 46*(1), 49–64, x.

Russ, S. A., Poulakis, Z., Barker, M., Wake, M., Rickards, F., Saunders, K., & Oberklaid, F. (2003). Epidemiology of congenital hearing loss in Victoria, Australia. *International Journal of Audiology, 42*(7), 385–390.

Saggar, A. K., & Bittles, A. H. (2008). Consanguinity and child health. *Paediatric and Child Health, 18*(5), 244–249.

Saunders, J. E., Vaz, S., Greinwald, J. H., Lai, J., Morin, L., & Mojica, K. (2007). Prevalence and etiology of hearing loss in rural Nicaraguan children. *Laryngoscope, 117*(3), 387–398.

SCENIHR (Scientific Committee on Emerging and Newly Identified Health Risks). (2008). *Scientific opinion on the potential health risks of exposure to noise from personal music players and mobile phones including a music playing function*. Brussels, Germany: European Commission.

Schmidt, P., Leveque, M., Danvin, J. B., Leroux, B., & Chays, A. (2007). Systematic hearing screening for newborns in the Champagne-Ardennes region: 32,500 births in 2 years of experience. *Annales d'oto-laryngologie et de chirurgie cervico faciale: bulletin de la Societe d'oto-laryngologie des hopitaux de Paris (Annals of Otolaryngology and Head-and-Neck Surgery), 124*(4), 157–165 (only available in French).

Seely, D. R., Gloyd, S. S., Wright, A. D., & Norton, S. J. (1995). Hearing loss prevalence and risk factors among Sierra Leonean children. *Archives of Otolaryngology-Head and Neck Surgery, 121*(8), 853–858.

Sever, J. L., Ellenberg, J. H., Ley, A. C., Madden, D. L., Fuccillo, D. A., Tzan, N. R., & Edmonds, D. M. (1988). Toxoplasmosis: Maternal and pediatric findings in 23,000 pregnancies. *Pediatrics, 82*(2), 181–192.

Stacey, P. C., Fortnum, H. M., Barton, G. R., & Summerfield, A. Q. (2006). Hearing-impaired children in the United Kingdom, I: Auditory performance, communication skills, educational achievements, quality of life, and cochlear implantation. *Ear and Hearing, 27*(2), 161–186.

Stephens, D. (1996). Audiological terms: European commission directorate, biomedical and health research programme (HEAR). In A. Martini (Ed.), *European group on genetics of hearing impairment—Infoletter 2*. Ferrara, Italy: European Commission.

Swart, S. M., Lemmer, R., Parbhoo, J. N., & Prescott, C. A. (1995). A survey of ear and hearing disorders amongst a representative sample of grade 1 schoolchildren in Swaziland. *International Journal of Pediatric Otorhinolaryngology, 32*(1), 23–34.

Tang, T. P., McPherson, B., Yuen, K. C., Wong, L. L., & Lee, J. S. (2004). Auditory neuropathy/auditory dys-synchrony in school children with hearing loss: Frequency of occurrence. *International Journal of Pediatric Otorhinolaryngology, 68*(2), 175–183.

Tapadia, M. D., Cordero, D. R., & Helms, J. A. (2005). It's all in your head: New insights into craniofacial development and deformation. *Journal of Anatomy, 207*(5), 461–477.

United Nations Development Programme. (2008). *Human Development Report 2007/2008*. New York.

Usami, S.-i., Abe, S., Akita, J., Namba, A., Shinkawa, H., Ishii, M., . . . Komune, S. (2000). Prevalence of mitochondrial gene mutations among hearing impaired patients. *Journal of Medical Genetics, 37*(1), 38–40.

Uus, K., & Bamford, J. (2006). Effectiveness of population-based newborn hearing screening in England: Ages of interventions and profile of cases. *Pediatrics, 117*(5), e887–893.

Uus, K., & Davis, A. C. (2000). Epidemiology of permanent childhood hearing impairment in Estonia, 1985–1990. *Audiology, 39*(4), 192–197.

Van Naarden, K., & Decoufle, P. (1999). Relative and attributable risks for moderate to profound bilateral sensorineural hearing impairment associated with lower birth weight in children 3 to 10 years old. *Pediatrics, 104*(4), 905–910.

Vartiainen, E., & Karjalainen, S. (1998). Prevalence and etiology of unilateral sensorineural hearing impairment in a Finnish childhood population. *International Journal of Pediatric Otorhinolaryngology, 43*(3), 253–259.

Vohr, B. R., Carty, L. M., Moore, P. E., & Letourneau, K. (1998). The Rhode Island Hearing Assessment Program: Experience with statewide hearing screening (1993–1996). *Journal of Pediatrics, 133*(3), 353–357.

Wake, M., Hughes, E. K., Poulakis, Z., Collins, C., & Rickards, F. W. (2004). Outcomes of children with mild-profound congenital hearing loss at 7 to 8 years: A population study. *Ear and Hearing, 25*(1), 1–8.

Wake, M., Tobin, S., Cone-Wesson, B., Dahl, H. H., Gillam, L., McCormick, L., . . . Williams, J. (2006). Slight/mild sensorineural hearing loss in children. *Pediatrics, 118*(5), 1842–1851.

Walch, C., Anderhuber, W., Kole, W., & Berghold, A. (2000). Bilateral sensorineural hearing disorders in children: Etiology of deafness and evaluation of hearing tests. *International Journal of Pediatric Otorhinolaryngology, 53*(1), 31–38.

Weichbold, V., Nekahm-Heis, D., & Welzl-Mueller, K. (2006). Universal newborn hearing screening and postnatal hearing loss. *Pediatrics, 117*(4), e631–636.

Wellman, M. B., Sommer, D. D., & McKenna, J. (2003). Sensorineural hearing loss in postmeningitic children. *Otology and Neurotology, 24*(6), 907–912.

Welzl-Muller, K., & Stephan, K. (2001). Examples of implemented neonatal hearing screening programs in Austria. *Scandinavian Audiology, Supplementum, 52*, 7–9.

Westerberg, B. D., Skowronski, D. M., Stewart, I. F., Stewart, L., Bernauer, M., & Mudarikwa, L. (2005). Prevalence of hearing loss in primary school children in Zimbabwe. *International Journal of Pediatric Otorhinolaryngology, 69*(4), 517–525.

WHO-PDH. (1997). *Prevention of noise-induced hearing loss—report of an informal consultation*. Retrieved March 20, 2009, from: http://www.who.int/pbd/deafness/en/noise.pdf

Wichmann, O., Siedler, A., Sagebiel, D., Hellenbrand, W., Santibanez, S., Mankertz, A., . . . Krause, G. (2009). Further efforts needed to achieve measles elimination in Germany: Results of an outbreak investigation. *Bulletin of the World Health Organization, 87*, 108–115.

Wilson-Costello, D., Friedman, H., Minich, N., Fanaroff, A. A., & Hack, M. (2005). Improved survival rates with increased neurodevelopmental disability for extremely low birth weight infants in the 1990s. *Pediatrics, 115*(4), 997–1003.

Woolley, A. L., Kirk, K. A., Neumann, A. M., Jr., McWilliams, S. M., Murray, J., Freind, D., . . . Wiatrak, B. J. (1999). Risk factors for hearing loss from meningitis in children: The Children's Hospital experience. *Archives of Otolaryngology-Head and Neck Surgery, 125*(5), 509–514.

World Health Organization (WHO). (2005). WHO global report. *Preventing chronic disease: A vital investment*. Retrieved June 17, 2010, from http://www.who.int/chp/chronic_disease_report/contents/en/index.html

World Health Organization (WHO). (2006). *Medical genetic services in developing countries: The ethical, legal and social implications of genetic testing and screening*. Retrieved June 17, 2010, from http://www.who.int/genomics/publications/GTS-MedicalGeneticServices-oct06.pdf
World Health Organization (WHO). (2008a). *Epidemiology and economic analysis*. Retrieved October 29, 2008, from http://www.who.int/pbd/deafness/activities/epidemiology_economic_analysis
World Health Organization (WHO). (2008b, 01/25/2008). *Rubella*. Retrieved December 30, 2008, from http://www.who.int/immunization/topics/rubella/en/index.html
Yee-Arellano, H. M., Leal-Garza, F., & Pauli-Muller, K. (2006). Universal newborn hearing screening in Mexico: Results of the first 2 years. *International Journal of Pediatric Otorhinolaryngology*, *70*(11), 1863–1870.
Zakzouk, S. (2002a). Consanguinity and hearing impairment in developing countries: A custom to be discouraged. *Journal of Laryngology and Otology*, *116*(10), 811–816.
Zakzouk, S. M., & Al-Anazy, F. (2002b). Sensorineural hearing impaired children with unknown causes: A comprehensive etiological study. *International Journal of Pediatric Otorhinolaryngology*, *64*(1), 17–21.

6

Genetics of Childhood Hearing Loss

Linda J. Hood and Bronya J. B. Keats

Introduction and Overview

Epidemiologic and Demographic Aspects of Genetic Hearing Loss

Congenital hearing loss occurs in approximately one to two of 1,000 births, and genetic factors account for at least 60% of childhood hearing loss. Genetic hearing loss is usually classified according to the presence (syndromic) or absence (nonsyndromic) of other clinical anomalies and the pattern of inheritance (autosomal, X-linked, dominant, recessive, mitochondrial). Over the past 10 to 15 years more than 80 hearing loss genes have been described, and the causal mutations in patients can often be identified through genetic testing. Most cases (> 70%) of childhood hearing loss are nonsyndromic with an autosomal recessive pattern of inheritance. Mutations in the gene (*GJB2*) encoding the protein known as connexin 26 explain as many as 50% of these cases in some populations.

A genetic etiology should be considered for every patient with a hearing problem. Even if a possible environmental cause is reported, a genetic cause cannot be ruled out. Conversely, if no obvious environmental insult or other cause can be determined, then the cause is most likely genetic. Also, it is important to realize that a family history of hearing loss is not necessary for the cause of a hearing loss to be related to a genetic defect. For example, a child with autosomal recessive hearing loss is often the only affected person in the family (see below). Not all inherited hearing loss is present at birth; hereditary loss can also have later onset. This is further discussed in the context of identification of hearing loss.

The Partnership of Geneticists and Audiologists

Because of the accumulating knowledge about genetic causes of hearing loss and the sophisticated auditory testing that is available, partnerships between audiologists and geneticists greatly enhance precise diagnosis and appropriate management of children with hearing loss. Additionally, expansion of newborn screening by both auditory and genetic diagnostic tests underscores the importance of this partnership.

Patterns of Inheritance

The human genome consists of 24 different types of chromosomes designated 1 to 22 (autosomes), X and Y (sex chromosomes). An offspring inherits one set of chromosomes from each parent, giving a total of 46 chromosomes (22 autosomal pairs plus XX or XY) in the nucleus of a cell. Each of these chromosomes consists of a single molecule of deoxyribonucleic acid (DNA), which has a double helical structure, and is composed of a sugar-phosphate backbone and four bases called adenine (A), guanine (G), thymine (T), and cytosine (C). The double helix is formed through the pairing of A with T, and C with G, and the bases are held together by hydrogen bonds. Thus, knowing the sequence of bases on one DNA strand automatically gives the sequence on the other strand. This precise pairing means that DNA can replicate by separation of the two strands followed by each strand serving as a template for a new complementary strand.

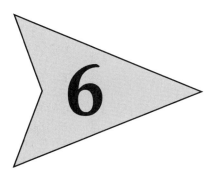

Chromosomes can be differentiated from one another by size, centromere location and the pattern of dark and light bands that is observed when various staining techniques are used. The arms on either side of the centromere are designated "p" and "q" for the shorter and longer arm, respectively. The bands are numbered from the centromere outwards to the end of the arm (known as the telomere), and have been subdivided numerous times as new banding methods were introduced. One of their uses is to give the approximate location of a gene. For example, a gene in the band numbered 2p11 is close to the centromere on the p arm of chromosome 2, whereas a gene in the band numbered 13q34 is toward the telomere on the q arm of chromosome 13.

Individuals inherit pairs of chromosomes and therefore, pairs of genes, which are known as the individual's genotype. Occasionally one or both copies of a gene may contain a mutation that prevents formation of the normal form of the protein encoded by that gene. When this happens, the individual may have a clinically abnormal phenotype, such as hearing loss. If there is a family history of hearing loss, then this information can be used to construct a pedigree and determine if it is consistent with autosomal or X-linked inheritance, which may be further categorized as dominant or recessive.

The pattern of inheritance of hearing loss is probably autosomal dominant if some of the individuals in each generation are hearing impaired, and both males and females are affected (Figure 6–1). The affected individuals usually have one normal (N) and one abnormal (D) copy of the gene for the hearing loss, meaning that each offspring of an affected individual has a 50% chance of inheriting the abnormal copy. Examples of dominantly inherited syndromes are Branchio-oto-renal (BOR), Waardenburg, and Treacher Collins. If all individuals who inherit the abnormal gene exhibit features of the disease, penetrance is said to be complete. However, with some disorders, individuals who must have the abnormal gene (because, for example, they have an affected parent and an affected child) show no phenotypic signs. In this case penetrance is said to be incomplete, perhaps due to the effect of other genetic factors or possibly environmental factors.

The mode of inheritance is autosomal recessive if the hearing loss is found only in individuals who have two copies of the abnormal gene (genotype DD). If both parents are carriers of an abnormal (D) copy (that is, both have the genotype ND), their child may inherit two copies of D, one from each parent (Figure 6–2). In this situation, the child is hearing impaired, but neither parent is affected. The probability that a child of carrier parents will be affected is one quarter. Note that family history is often negative with a recessive disorder because an abnormal form of the gene may be passed on from one (unaffected) carrier to the next for many generations before a couple, who by chance both carry an abnormal form, have a hearing-impaired child. Examples of recessively inherited syndromes are Jervell and Lange-Nielsen, Pendred, Usher, and Wolfram.

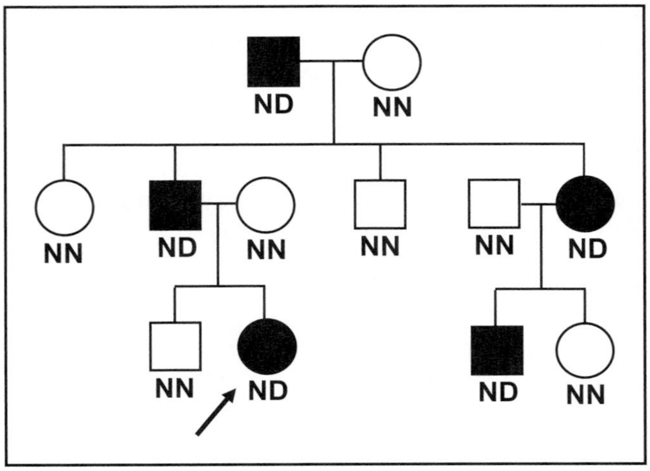

FIGURE 6–1. Three-generation pedigree depicting an autosomal dominant inheritance pattern. The arrow denotes the index case (or proband) for this pedigree.

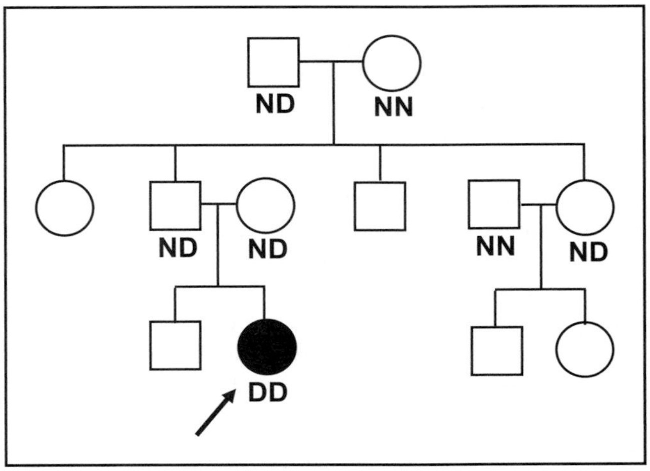

FIGURE 6–2. Three-generation pedigree depicting an autosomal recessive inheritance pattern. The arrow denotes the index case (or proband) for this pedigree.

Males have both an X and Y chromosome; females have two X chomosomes. For X-linked inheritance, father-to-son transmission is not possible because a son must receive his X chromosome from his mother. For an X-linked recessive trait, affected individuals are usually male because they have only one X chromosome, while females in the family may be carriers, but are unlikely to be affected. In contrast, all the daughters of affected fathers are affected for an X-linked dominant trait with complete penetrance, and each child (whether male or female) of an affected female has a 50% chance of being affected (assuming the mother has the ND genotype and the father is unaffected). Alport is an example of a syndrome for which the pattern of inheritance is usually X-linked.

Mitochondria are small organelles that are located within the cytoplasm of a cell. A process called oxidative phosphorylation (OXPHOS) takes place in the mitochondria and is responsible for energy (ATP) production in the cell. Mitochondria are maternally inherited and they have their own DNA (mtDNA). Thus, the expected family history for a disorder caused by a mtDNA mutation is that all children of an affected mother are affected whereas children of an affected father are never affected. However, each mitochondrion has multiple copies of mtDNA and each cell contains several hundred mitochondria. This means that cells may contain both mutant and normal copies of mtDNA, a condition known as heteroplasmy (as opposed to homoplasmy meaning that all the copies are the same). Also, children of an affected mother may inherit different percentages of mutant and normal mtDNA, which means that some may have more severe symptoms than others. If the normal copies can successfully provide the energy requirements of the cell, then normal function will be retained. But different cell types have differing energy requirements, so the effect of the mutant copies may vary from one organ to another. The organs with the most demand for energy are the skeletal muscle, heart, and brain. Thus, the typical symptoms found in mitochondrial disorders are muscle weakness, nervous system disorders, visual problems, hearing loss, and dementia.

Genetic hearing loss is not always the result of a mutation in a single gene. It may be one of the clinical findings associated with an anomaly involving one or more of the 46 chromosomes. All or a large segment of a chromosome may be deleted, duplicated or inverted, or one part of one chromosome may be attached to part of another chromosome, an event known as a translocation. Children with Down syndrome usually have an extra copy of chromosome 21 (Trisomy 21) giving them 47 chromosomes altogether, whereas those with Turner syndrome have 45 chromosomes because they have only one X chromosome and no Y. Hearing loss, particularly conductive hearing loss related to middle-ear anomalies, is often found in persons with Down syndrome.

In other situations a mutation in a single gene may contribute to the hearing loss, but additional genetic or environmental factors may be required for the hearing loss to be present. This type of hearing loss is usually familial, but the pattern of inheritance is unclear; it is called multifactorial inheritance. Also, in taking a family history and interpreting a pedigree, it is very important to remember that hearing loss is relatively common and the cause may not be the same for all affected members of a family.

Genes associated with hearing loss have been localized to all chromosomes, including the X and Y chromosomes. Genetic loci (locations on chromosomes) associated with autosomal dominant forms of hearing loss are conventionally denoted as DFNA followed by a number that was assigned when the locus was mapped to a chromosome (e.g., DFNA1, DFNA2). Similar nomenclature is used for other forms: DFNB(number) for recessive hearing loss, DFNX(number) for X-linked hearing loss, DFNY(number) for Y-linked hearing loss, and a locus for a gene that modifies the hearing loss phenotype associated with another gene is given the label DFNM(number). An excellent source of up to date information that includes a listing of current loci associated with various forms of hearing loss can be found at the Hereditary Hearing Loss Homepage (http://hereditaryhearingloss.org/) that was created and is maintained by G. Van Camp and R. J. H. Smith.

Nonsyndromic Hearing Loss

Genes associated with auditory function are involved in the creation of proteins that contribute to the development of the auditory system and underlie the many functions of specific structures of the external ear, middle ear, cochlea, vestibular system, and neural pathways. Many different genes associated with hearing and hearing loss have been identified across all human chromosomes. Furthermore, there are multiple specific mutations within individual genes that result in hearing loss.

An unexpected finding was that a high percentage of nonsyndromic hearing loss is associated with mutations in a gene named *GJB2,* which was the first identified form of recessive deafness, DFNB1 (Kelsell et al., 1997). *GJB2* maps to the chromosome position 13q11.12 and codes for the production of the protein connexin 26 (Cx26). Cx26 is one of a family of gap junction proteins that facilitate exchange of electrolytes, metabolites, and so forth, between cells. In the inner ear, Cx26 is widely expressed in the cochlea, in supporting cells and stria vascularis, and is thought to be important in endolymph equilibrium and maintaining high potassium levels in the scala media.

Although more than 80 mutations in *GJB2* have been reported, certain mutations account for many cases of hearing loss. The most common mutations are 35delG which is predominant in populations of European descent, 167delT found primarily in Ashkenazi Jewish persons, and 235delC in persons of Asian descent. Mutations in *GJB2* are usually associated with recessive hearing loss, but some mutations have been reported that result in dominant hearing loss (DFNA3) and also Vohwinkel syndrome (sensorineural hearing loss and keratoderma). A significant number of children with recessive hearing loss have one *GJB2* mutation together with a deletion on the other copy of chromosome 13 involving a gene, *GJB6,* which is very close to *GJB2* and codes for another gap junction protein, connexin 30. Thus, evaluation of *GJB6* is often recommended following testing for *GJB2* mutations, if results of *GJB2* testing alone are not definitive.

Some gene mutations are associated with more severe hearing losses than others, though this is not a clear-cut rule, and sometimes individuals with the same mutations have different degrees of hearing loss. The lack of consistency may be due to influences of other genes. A general observation of the relationship between gene mutations and characteristics of a hearing loss is that mutations having more severe effects on the protein tend to be associated with more severe hearing losses. For example, the 35delG mutation in the *GJB2* gene is a deletion of a G at position 35 of the DNA coding sequence. This sequence is read in sets of three bases (codons), which specify the addition of a particular amino acid to the protein (or a stop); thus, the 35delG mutation changes all of the following codons and creates a premature stop codon, which would result in a drastically truncated protein, if it is formed at all. Typically, children with two copies of this mutation have severe to profound hearing loss across all frequencies, although a few with mild or progressive loss have been reported.

Although the focus of this discussion has been recessive hearing loss and mutations in *GJB2*, mutations in many other genes are associated with nonsyndromic hearing loss. Adding to the complexity is the fact that mutations in the same gene may be associated with both nonsyndromic and syndromic deafness. Thus, the same gene can be associated with different phenotypes and different patterns of inheritance, which underscores the importance of obtaining thorough history, observational, and evaluation information from all patients and their families.

Syndromes Associated with Hearing Loss

Syndromic hearing loss is often classified by association with other system disorders (Konigsmark & Gorlin, 1976; Toriello, Reardon, & Gorlin, 2004) and genes have been identified for many syndromes that involve hearing loss. Some of the common syndromes that include hearing loss are shown in Table 6–1, along with the other systems involved.

Syndromes involving hearing loss probably share molecular mechanisms that are abnormal in both the ear and the other affected organ systems. Understanding the molecular defect in one system should help in understanding the other in most cases. Although unlikely, it is possible that the underlying causes are not the same in the two systems, which would confound analysis and understanding of the apparent syndrome.

The following sections provide brief summaries of phenotype and genotype information related to some of the more common syndromes that involve hearing loss (presented in alphabetical order). The reader is referred to the text *Hereditary Hearing Loss and Its Syndromes* (Toriello et al., 2004) for more detailed information about these and many other syndromes involving the auditory system. Up to date information is also available on the Hereditary Hearing Loss

Table 6-1. Classification of Syndromic Forms of Hearing Loss by Association With Other System Disorders

System	Syndrome
Eye disorders	Usher
Endocrine disorders	Pendred Wolfram
Cardiac disorders	Jervell and Lange-Nielsen
Pigmentary disorders	Waardenburg
Renal disorders	Alport Branchial-Oto-Renal (BOR)
Musculoskeletal disorders	Stickler

Homepage noted above and at the (National Institutes of Health) Web site, Online Mendelian Inheritance in Man (OMIM; http://www.ncbi.nlm.nih.gov/sites/entrez?db=omim).

Alport Syndrome

Alport syndrome is characterized by progressive loss of kidney function, sensorineural hearing loss, and sometimes visual defects. The inheritance pattern is usually X-linked, but about 15% is autosomal recessive and 5% is autosomal dominant, with an incidence of approximately one in 50,000 live births. The hearing loss is sensorineural in nature and high frequencies may be affected to a greater degree. Visual defects involve ocular lesions and maculopathy. Alport is the second most common inherited cause of kidney failure and approximately 0.2% of adults and 3% of children in the United States with end stage renal disease have been diagnosed with Alport syndrome.

Most cases of Alport syndrome are caused by mutations in the *COL4A5* gene on the q arm of the X chromosome. Carrier females may show signs of the disease but they are much less severely affected than males. The autosomal forms are associated with mutations in *COL4A3* and *COL4A4*, which are both on chromosome 2q. These three genes code for different chains of type IV collagen, which are major components of basement membranes, particularly in the glomerulus. In the inner ear they are present in the basilar membrane, parts of the spiral ligament, and the stria vascularis.

Branchio-Oto-Renal (BOR) Syndrome

Branchio-oto-renal (BOR) syndrome has an incidence of about one in 40,000 and may account for about 2% of profound deafness. BOR is characterized by sensorineural or mixed hearing loss and is often progressive. The branchial component of the syndrome name relates to anomalies involving the branchial arches in the structural development of the ear, and is present in about 50% of patients. Features of BOR include preauricular pits, branchial fistulae or cysts, and/or malformations of the external ear and middle ear. Patients with BOR syndrome have abnormalities in renal function that may be associated with extra kidney tissue.

The pattern of inheritance is autosomal dominant with extremely variable expression. Mutations in three genes, *EYA1*, *SIX5*, and *SIX1*, on chromosomes 8q13, 19q13, and 14q21, respectively, have been associated with this phenotype. Approximately 40% of patients have mutations in *EYA1* and more than 80 different mutations have been reported. The percentage with mutations in *SIX5* and *SIX1* is much smaller; additionally, for many affected individuals mutations are not found in any of these three genes, so more remain to be identified.

Jervell and Lange-Nielsen Syndrome

The hearing loss associated with Jervell and Lange-Nielsen syndrome is congenital and sensorineural. About 1 in 100 infants with profound sensorineural hearing loss may have this recessively inherited syndrome. The importance of identifying this syndrome is highlighted by the characteristics of electrocardiographic abnormalities, fainting spells, and sudden death. The electrocardiographic abnormality is a long QT interval and when identified, cardiac problems can be managed, making identification an important component of a workup of an infant or child identified with hearing loss. The importance of early identification of this syndrome also supports the value of newborn hearing screening programs.

Mutations in two genes, *KCNQ1* and *KCNE1* on chromosomes 11p and 21q, respectively, cause Jervell and Lange-Nielsen syndrome. They encode proteins that are required to form a potassium channel. Approximately 90% of affected individuals have mutations in both copies of *KCNQ1*; the remaining 10% have mutations in both copies of *KCNE1*. Those with a mutation in only one copy of either gene may have a dominant disorder called long QT syndrome, which does not include severe to profound hearing loss.

MELAS and MERRF

MELAS is the acronym for mitochondrial encephalomyopathy, lactic acidosis, strokelike episodes, and sensorineural hearing loss. Hearing loss is sensorineural in nature and typically severe. Characteristics of patients with MELAS are headaches, stroke-like episodes that can result in hemiparesis, seizures, growth deficiency, and lactic acidosis. Onset is typically in the first or second decade. Related pathology involves ragged-red fibers and other mitochondrial abnormalities observed in muscle.

MERRF denotes mitochondrial encephalomyopathy, myoclonus epilepsy, ragged-red fibers, and sensorineural hearing loss. MERRF is separated from other mitochondrial encephalomyopathies by the presence of myoclonic epilepsy. Onset occurs in the first decade or into adulthood and the early symptoms can include myoclonic jerks, ataxia, and sensorineural hearing loss.

Several different mutations in the mtDNA are associated with MELAS and MERRF. These mutations are usually heteroplasmic, with the highest levels being in nerves and muscles, which results in systemic neuromuscular dysfunction. The most common MELAS mutation, A3243G in the *MT-TL1* gene, has also been found in individuals with other clinical presentations, for example, sensorineural hearing loss and diabetes mellitus. A mutation, A8344G, in the *MT-TK* gene is the most common one found in patients with MERRF.

Pendred Syndrome

Pendred syndrome has an incidence of one in 7,500 and is one of the more common syndromes involving hearing loss. The pattern of inheritance is autosomal recessive, and hearing loss is characterized as profound, congenital, and sensorineural. This syndrome is thought to account for approximately 20% of the hearing losses in children with severe or profound hearing loss making it one of the most common forms of hearing loss. Other factors involved in Pendred syndrome are goiter (enlarged thyroid) and enlarged vestibular aqueduct (EVA).

Mutations in the *SLC26A4* gene explain about 50% of cases of Pendred syndrome. It is on chromosome 7q31 and encodes a protein called pendrin that functions as a chloride and iodide transporter. Although more than 170 mutations have been reported, three of them account for about 55% of those found in patients. Thus, genetic testing initially can be targeted to these three mutations. Another gene, *FOXI1*, on chromosome 5q35, codes for a protein that is involved in the regulation of *SLC26A4*, and mutations in *FOXI1* have recently been found in a small percentage of the Pendred patients who do not have *SLC26A4* mutations. It should be noted that some mutations in *SLC26A4* are associated with nonsyndromic autosomal recessive hearing loss (DFNB4). Additionally, carriers have a relatively high risk of having nonsyndromic EVA.

Stickler Syndrome

Stickler syndrome is one of the most common autosomal dominant disorders involving connective tissue. Incidence among neonates is estimated to be about one in 7,500 to 9,000. Characteristics include midfacial hypoplasia, flattened nasal bridge, abnormally small lower jaw, hearing loss, myopia, retinal detachment, joint hypermobility, and premature osteoarthritis. Three defined subtypes involve different genotypes and variable phenotypic characteristics. Hearing losses are typically sensorineural and progressive, affecting primarily the higher frequencies. Tympanometry may show hypermobile tympanic membranes. Cleft palate is seen in some cases.

Mutations in three collagen genes (*COL2A1*, *COL11A1*, and *COL11A2* on chromosomes 12q13, 1p21, and 6p21, respectively) are associated with autosomal dominant Stickler syndrome. If ocular anomalies are present, the mutation is likely to be in *COL2A1* or *COL11A1*; if the patient has craniofacial and joint abnormalities but no ocular findings, then genetic testing would usually begin with *COL11A2*. Mutations in *COL11A2* have also been found in individuals with nonsyndromic hearing loss (DFNA13). Collagen II is a major structural component of cartilaginous tissues; collagen XI is a minor constituent, but it is important for controlling the growth of collagen II fibrils.

Treacher Collins Syndrome

Treacher Collins syndrome is an autosomal dominant disorder that occurs in about one in 10,000 to 50,000 births. It is characterized by considerable phenotypic variability and, unlike usual autosomal dominant inheritance, family history may be negative due to failure to recognize the disorder in a parent, incomplete penetrance, or a new mutation. Patients with Treacher Collins syndrome have bones of the head and face that are under- or abnormally developed, such as an undersized jaw, undeveloped mandible, or cleft palate. Auditory characteristics typically relate to abnormalities of the external and middle ear, and inner ear structures are generally normal.

Mutations in the *TCOF1* gene that encodes a protein known as Treacle cause Treacher Collins syndrome. This gene is located on chromosome 5q32-q33.1 and more than 100 mutations have been described, most of which result in a premature stop codon. Approximately 60% of cases are due to new mutations, while in about 40% one of the parents has a mutation; however, because of incomplete penetrance or mild expression of the phenotype, the parent with the mutation may not have been diagnosed.

Usher Syndrome

Usher syndrome is characterized by hearing loss, retinitis pigmentosa (RP), a vision condition that involves progressive narrowing of the visual fields, and vestibular disorders. It is the most frequent cause of deafness accompanied by blindness in developed countries, accounting for greater than 50% of the deaf-blind population, about 18% of population with retinitis pigmentosa, and 3 to 6% of persons with congenital deafness. Usher syndrome is classified into three types based on clinical findings related to degree of hearing loss, vestibular responses, and onset of RP. Profound congenital hearing loss, earlier onset of RP (in the first decade of life) and absent vestibular responses are found in patients with Type I Usher syndrome. Patients with Type II also have congenital hearing loss though more moderate in degree, and vestibular responses are typically present. Type III has more variable characteristics including progressive hearing loss. Some forms of Usher syndrome are associated with certain populations, such as Usher Type IC, which is predominantly found in the Louisiana Acadian population (Keats, Nouri, Pelias, Deininger & Litt, 1994). Confirmation of Usher syndrome is difficult at birth and infants may be misdiagnosed with nonsyndromic congenital hearing loss until later determination of vision loss.

Nine different genes have so far been associated with Usher syndrome and at least three are yet to be identified. Many mutations in *MYO7A* (11q13), *USH1C* (11p15), *CDH23* (10q21-q22), *PCDH15* (10q21-q22), and *USH1G* (17q24-q25) cause Type I. An added complication is that mutations in the first four of these genes have also been associated with nonsyndromic hearing loss. However, targeted genetic testing for a specific mutation in *USH1C* or *PCDH15* is likely to be successful for Usher I patients of Acadian or Ashkenazi Jewish ancestry, respectively. Testing for these mutations in Acadian and Ashkenazi Jewish infants with profound hearing loss may enable Usher I to be diagnosed well before the onset of RP.

Mutations in *USH2A* on chromosome 1q are responsible for 80% of Usher Type II; two other genes, *GPR98* (5q14) and *DFNB31*(9q32-q34) are associated with about 15% and 5%, respectively. One Usher Type III gene, *USH3* (3q21-q25) has been identified and is relatively common in Finland. In addition to causing Usher II, *USH2A* mutations have also been found in 12% of patients with autosomal recessive RP. *DFNB31* mutations were first found in individuals with autosomal recessive nonsyndromic hearing loss (Mburu et al., 2003); more recently Ebermann et al. (2007) showed the association with Usher Type II.

The proteins encoded by the five Usher I genes and the three Usher II genes have been shown to interact with one another to form a large network that is necessary for normal function of the hair cells and stereocilia. A mutation in any one of these genes may disrupt the network.

Waardenburg Syndrome

Waardenburg syndrome is characterized by pigmentary abnormalities of the hair (white forelock), iris (heterochromia irides—different colored eyes) and skin. Another characteristic is wide-set eyes (dystopia canthorum). Hearing loss is sensorineural in nature and has variable presentation. Hearing can range from no hearing loss to profound unilateral or bilateral SNHL and is progressive in some types. Clinical classifications of Waardenburg involve several subtypes dependent on presence or absence of various phenotype characteristics. In particular, dystopia canthorum is present in Type I and absent in Type II. Estimates of the prevalence of Waardenburg syndrome range from one in 20,000 to one in 40,000.

The inheritance pattern for Waardenburg syndrome is usually autosomal dominant with variable expression. However, Type IV, which is a combination of Type II and Hirschsprung disease, has an autosomal recessive pattern of inheritance. Six different genes are associated with Waardenburg syndrome and there are probably at least two more. Mutations in the *PAX3* gene on chromosome 2q35 are found in patients with both Type I and Type III (Type I plus upper limb abnormalities), while Type II is associated with mutations in *MITF* (3p14-p12) and *SNAI2* (8q11), as well as deletion of *SOX10* (22q13). The autosomal recessive form, Type IV, is caused by mutations in both copies of three genes: *EDNRB* (13q22), *EDN3* (20q13), and *SOX10*.

Wolfram Syndrome

Wolfram syndrome involves diabetes insipidus, diabetes mellitus, optic atrophy, and sensorineural deafness and is also referred to as DIDMOAD (diabetes insipidus, diabetes mellitus, optic atrophy, deafness). The rate of occurrence is between 1 in 150 and 1 in 175 of patients with juvenile diabetes (Gunn et al., 1976). Individuals may be small in stature and underweight. Onset of bilateral progressive loss of visual acuity leading to blindness occurs most frequently in the first decade of life. Hearing losses associated with Wolfram syndrome are bilateral and progressive, most often leading to moderate to severe sensorineural losses with poorer hearing in the higher frequencies.

Wolfram syndrome has an autosomal recessive pattern of inheritance and is caused by mutations in the *WFS1* gene on chromosome 4p16.1, which encodes a protein known as wolframin. Over 70 different mutations associated with Wolfram syndrome have been reported. Mutations in this gene are also associated with autosomal dominant low-frequency nonsyndromic hearing loss (DFNA6/14/38).

Aminoglycoside-Induced Deafness

Some individuals are at increased risk of deafness as a result of sensitivity to low levels of aminoglycosides due to the presence of a mutation, A1555G, in the *MT-RNR1* gene of their maternally transmitted mtDNA. This mutation is usually homoplasmic in affected individuals, and exposure to aminoglycosides such as streptomycin and gentamicin is not always a prerequisite for deafness. It is the most common mtDNA mutation associated with deafness and probably explains up to one percent in Caucasians; higher prevalences have been reported in Asian and Spanish patients.

Auditory Neuropathy/Dys-synchrony (AN/AD; ANSD)

Patients ranging in age from infants to adults are identified with auditory neuropathy/dys-synchrony (AN/AD; Starr, Picton, Sininger, Hood, & Berlin 1996; Berlin, Hood, & Rose, 2001), which also is referred to as auditory neuropathy spectrum disorder (ANSD). AN/AD is characterized by the presence of responses associated with outer hair cells and functional cochlear amplification. This takes the form of otoacoustic emissions (OAEs) and/or cochlear microphonics and poor peripheral neural function at the level of the eighth nerve/brainstem, which is characterized by absent or highly abnormal auditory brainstem responses (Berlin et al., 1998) and absent or abnormal middle ear muscle and medial olivocochlear reflexes (ABR; Berlin et al., 2005; Hood, Berlin, Bordelon, & Rose, 2003). Most AN/AD patients show bilateral symptoms, though function may be asymmetric between ears, and cases of unilateral AN/AD have been documented. Speech recognition is quite variable, although generally much poorer than expected, particularly in noise. Some patients with AN/AD demonstrate timing problems (Zeng, Oba, Garde, Sininger, & Starr, 1999), which are suggestive of a disturbance in neural synchrony.

The mechanisms underlying AN/AD presently are unclear, and it is most likely that several mechanisms and etiologies exist. The mechanical transduction or other functional characteristics of the inner hair cells can be abnormal, the synaptic juncture between the inner hair cells and the cochlear branch of the vestibulocochlear (eighth) nerve may be affected, or the axons or cell bodies of the eighth nerve itself can be involved. Some patients, both children and adults, have no known etiology and no other identified neurological abnormalities. In other patients, the auditory findings may be associated with other peripheral neuropathies such as hereditary motor sensory neuropathy (HMSN; Charcot-Marie-Tooth disease). Infants with neonatal abnormalities, including exchange transfusion, prematurity, and anoxia, have been reported with AN/AD (e.g., Deltenre, Mansbach, Bozet, Clercx, & Hecox, 1997).

Autosomal dominant, autosomal recessive, X-linked and mitochondrial inheritance have all been reported for both syndromic and nonsyndromic AN/AD. Patients with syndromic AN/AD are often first diagnosed with peripheral neuropathy followed by the auditory neuropathy several years later, though this is not always the case. Mutations in HMSN genes such as *MPZ* are likely causes, particularly if the pattern of inheritance is autosomal dominant (Starr et al., 2003). Another gene that is highly expressed in nerves, *NDRG1*, was found to be associated with an autosomal recessive syndromic ANSD in the Gypsy population (Kalaydjieva et al., 2000). Also, patients with X-linked recessive Mohr-Tranebjaerg syndrome have auditory neuropathy, as do some patients with the mitochondrial disorder, Leber's hereditary optic neuropathy.

The majority of cases of nonsyndromic AN/AD are autosomal recessive, and the pure tone loss is generally severe to profound from infancy. Mutations in the gene *OTOF*, that encodes a protein known as otoferlin, have been found in some of these patients, but not in others (Varga et al., 2003). Thus, more AN/AD genes are yet to be identified. Delmaghani et al. (2006) studied an Iranian family and found a mutation in the gene for a protein they named pejvakin; however, this is unlikely to be a major cause of autosomal recessive AN/AD. Interestingly, *GJB2* mutations have been found in patients with nonsyndromic autosomal recessive AN/AD; thus, connexin 26 testing should be recommended even if the diagnosis is AN/AD.

Evaluation of Individuals With Hereditary Hearing Loss

Audiologists and geneticists are important partners in the evaluation and management of hereditary hearing loss. Thorough knowledge of a patient's family, medical and other history is critical in accurately characterizing a hearing loss and understanding the etiology. Knowing whether other members of the immediate or extended family have a hearing loss or other medical or physical characteristics in common helps in determining whether a condition might be inherited and the pattern of inheritance. This information is helpful in guiding geneticists, audiologists, and physicians toward appropriate recommendations for genetic testing and can be invaluable in counseling patients and their families.

Determining whether a hearing loss might be genetic involves obtaining a family history and constructing a pedigree to follow the inheritance of a trait. A family pedigree includes information about the patient, parents, grandparents, siblings, aunts, uncles and may extend to many generations and extended family members. Pedigrees utilize standardized symbols and include information about key disorders or conditions, as well as ethnicity information. A graphic record of family health history through a pedigree can provide a clearer picture than a simple case history by establishing the lineage of possible inherited conditions and patterns of transmission of familial disorders. Obtaining a pedigree also provides professionals with an opportunity to establish rapport with a patient and the family. Construction of a family pedigree requires care taken in obtaining personal and family information, as some instances may involve discussion of sensitive issues.

Recording physical characteristics of a patient is another important part of the evaluation process (Table 6–2). A dysmorphic evaluation includes examination of such factors as facial symmetry, the shape and size of the skull, ocular region, nose and midface, oral region and jaw, and external ears. Further evaluation involves the neck, chest, abdomen, limbs, skin, and hair. Medical follow-up testing may include an electrocardiogram (for example, to evaluate the QT interval which is affected in Jervell and Lange-Nielsen syndrome), ophthalmologic evaluation, imaging, and so forth, depending on the results of previous evaluations.

Table 6–2. Family and Health Information to Include in a Pedigree

Gender
Birthdate/age
Age of death
Cause of death
Pregnancy
Pregnancy complications (e.g., miscarriage, stillbirth, pregnancy termination)
Relevant health information
Known medical problems
Ethnic background
Consanguinity
Date pedigree was drawn
Name of person who provided the data

There are some additional factors in a family history that increase suspicion of an inherited trait. These factors can include another family member with a chromosome abnormality or genetic disorder, a family history of a genetic disorder, and couples who have had more than two miscarriages. Individuals of almost every ethnic group have increased risks for particular genetic conditions.

Audiologists have many tools available to them for the evaluation of hearing sensitivity and auditory function at suprathreshold levels. Pure-tone audiograms provide information about the degree, configuration and symmetry of a hearing loss, and comparison of air and bone conduction can help in defining the type of hearing loss as conductive, sensorineural, or mixed. In infants, ABR or auditory steady-state response (ASSR) methods can provide accurate estimates of threshold information via air and bone conduction.

It is fortunate that audiologists have many more sensitive methods available to characterize hearing loss beyond basic threshold measures. These tools serve two important purposes. First, methods such as OAEs and middle-ear muscle reflexes provide valuable diagnostic information that allows accurate differentiation among hearing losses. For example, changes in OAEs have been demonstrated in persons with Waardenburg syndrome before changes in pure tone thresholds are observed (Liu & Newton, 1997; see also Chapter 19 in this volume). Also, as we strive to better understand the relationships between genotype and phenotype, the more information that audiologists can obtain about auditory function, then the better geneticists can use this information to understand the role of various genes and functions of the proteins they encode.

Genetics and Newborn Hearing Screening

Molecular genetic testing has an important role in newborn hearing screening and diagnostic follow-up of identified hearing losses. When a hearing loss is identified, which hopefully occurs in the newborn period, then the inclusion of molecular genetic testing in the evaluation can contribute to establishing the etiology of the hearing loss. For example, identifying Jervell and Lange-Nielsen syndrome in infants identified with hearing loss has obvious value in facilitating intervention prior to a potentially tragic outcome.

According to Nance (2007), four tests in the newborn period could detect the major causes of deafness. These include testing for: (1) mutations in the connexin 26 (*GJB2*) gene and the connexin 30 (*GJB6*) gene; (2) the mtDNA A1555G mutation that increases susceptibility to aminoglycoside induced deafness; (3) *SLC26A4* mutations that are associated with Pendred syndrome and DFNB4, as well as an increased risk of nonsyndromic EVA in carriers; and (4) cytomegalovirus (CMV). Congenital CMV infection is a nongenetic cause for deafness at birth and in early childhood. Nance suggests that infants at risk could easily be detected by molecular testing of newborn blood spots for these traits.

Establishing the etiology of an identified hearing loss provides not only answers to parents, but also can be helpful in planning management appropriate to the characteristics of a particular genetic form. Furthermore, there are many questions related to hearing loss where genetic testing will likely have a future important role. For example, as the genetics of later onset hearing loss become known, then screening for genes related to these disorders in infants could avoid delays in identification.

Management of Patients and Families: A Team Approach

Partnering with geneticists and genetics counselors provides an important resource to audiologists, families, and all members of the health care team. Genetics and hereditary issues are not simple: questions and issues raised by gene testing can challenge family and other personal relationships. The genetics counseling process integrates: (1) collection and interpretation of family and medical histories to assess the chance of disease occurrence or recurrence, (2) education about inheritance, testing, management, prevention, resources and research, and (3) counseling to promote informed choices and adaptation to the risk or condition. The Web site of the National Society of Genetic Counselors provides information on locating a genetic counselor (http://www.nsgc.org/resourcelink.cfm).

The availability of genetics information clearly advances the ability to understand and focus appropriate management of individuals with hearing loss. Although genetic evaluation provides great benefit, there is also potential for harm in revealing information about individuals and families that they may not wish to know. Thus, it is important to understand the ramifications of obtaining and sharing information about an individual's genetic makeup. The need to understand the ethical, legal, and social issues was recognized early on in the development and work of the Human Genome Project. Efforts have focused on deciding how genetics information should be used in relation to the privacy of genetic information, safe and effective introduction of genetic information in the clinical setting, and fairness in use of genetic information. Additional work is directed toward preparing health professionals and society to use information effectively through professional and public education.

References

Berlin C. I., Bordelon, J., St. John, P., Wilensky, D., Hurley, A., Kluka, E., & Hood, L. J. (1998). Reversing click polarity may uncover auditory neuropathy in infants. *Ear and Hearing*, *19*, 37–47.

Berlin, C., Hood, L., & Rose, K. (2001). On renaming auditory neuropathy as auditory dys-synchrony: Implications for a clearer understanding of the underlying mechanisms and management options. *Audiology Today*, *13*, 15–17.

Berlin, C. I., Hood, L. J., Morlet, T., Wilensky, D., St. John, P., Montgomery, E., & Thibodeaux, M. (2005). Absent or elevated middle ear muscle reflexes in the presence of normal otoacoustic emissions: A universal finding in 136 cases of auditory neuropathy/dys-synchrony. *Journal of the American Academy of Audiology*, *16*, 546–553.

Delmaghani, S., del Castillo, F. J., Michel, V., Leibovici, M., Aghaie, A., Ron, U., . . . Petit, C. (2006). Mutations in the gene encoding pejvakin, a newly identified protein of the afferent auditory pathway, cause DFNB59 auditory neuropathy. *Nature Genetics*, *38*(7), 770–778.

Deltenre, P., Mansbach, A. L., Bozet, C., Clercx, A., & Hecox, K. E. (1997). Auditory neuropathy: A report on three cases with early onsets and major neonatal illnesses. *Electroencephalography and Clinical Neurophysiology*, *104*, 17–22.

Ebermann, I., Scholl, H. P., Charbel Issa, P., Becirovic, E., Lamprecht, J., Jurklies, B., . . . Bolz, H. (2007). Usher syndrome type 2: Mutations in the long isoform of whirlin are associated with retinitis pigmentosa and sensorineural hearing loss. *Human Genetics*, *121*, 203–211.

Gunn, T., Bortolussi, R., Little, J. M., Andermann, F., Fraser, F. C., & Belmonte, M. M. (1976). Juvenile diabetes mellitus, optic atrophy, sensory nerve deafness, and diabetes insipidus—a syndrome. *Journal of Pediatrics*, *89*(4), 565–570.

Hood, L. J., Berlin, C. I., Bordelon, J., & Rose, K. (2003). Patients with auditory neuropathy/dys-synchrony lack efferent suppression of transient evoked otoacoustic emissions. *Journal of the American Academy of Audiology*, *14*, 302–313.

Kalaydjieva, L., Gresham, D., Gooding, R., Heather, L., Baas, F., de Jonge, R., . . . Thomas, P. K. (2000). N-myc downstream-regulated gene 1 is mutated in hereditary motor and sensory neuropathy-Lom. *American Journal of Human Genetics*, *67*, 47–58.

Keats, B. J. B, Nouri, N., Pelias, M. Z., Deininger, P. L., & Litt, M. (1994). Tightly linked flanking microsatellite markers for the Usher syndrome type I locus on the short arm of chromosome 11. *American Journal of Human Genetics*, *54*, 681–686.

Kelsell, D. P., Dunlop, J., Stevens, H. P., Lench, N. J., Liang, J. N., Parry, G., . . . Leigh, I. M. (1997). Connexin 26 mutations in hereditary nonsyndromic sensorineural deafness. *Nature*, *387*, 80–83.

Konigsmark, B. W., & Gorlin, R. J. (1976). *Genetic and metabolic deafness*. Philadelphia, PA: WB Saunders.

Liu, X. Z., & Newton, V. E. (1997). Distortion product emissions in normal-hearing and low-frequency hearing loss carriers of genes for Waardenburg's syndrome. *Annals of Otology, Rhinology and Laryngology*, *106*(3), 220–225.

Mburu, P., Mustapha, M., Varela, A., Weil, D., El-Amraoui, A., Holme, R. H., . . . Brown, S. D. (2003). Defects in whirlin, a PDZ domain molecule involved in stereocilia elongation, cause deafness in the whirler mouse and families with DFNB31. *Nature Genetics*, *34*(4), 421–428.

Nance, W. (2007). How can newborn hearing screening be improved? *Audiology Today*, *19*, 14–19.

Starr, A., Michalewski, H. J., Zeng, F.- G., Fujikawa-Brooks, S., Linthicum, F., Kim, C. S., . . . Keats, B. J. B. (2003). Pathology and physiology of auditory neuropathy with a novel mutation in the *MPZ* gene (Tyr145→Ser). *Brain*, *126*, 1604–1619.

Starr, A., Picton, T. W., Sininger, Y., Hood, L. J., & Berlin, C. I. (1996). Auditory neuropathy. *Brain*, *119*, 741–753.

Toriello, H. V., Reardon, W., & Gorlin, R. J. (2004). *Hereditary hearing loss and its syndromes* (2nd ed.). Oxford, UK: Oxford University Press.

Varga, R., Kelley, P. M., Keats, B. J., Starr, A., Leal, S. M., Cohn, E., & Kimberling, W. J. (2003). Nonsyndromic recessive auditory neuropathy is the result of mutations in the otoferlin (OTOF) gene. *Journal of Medical Genetics*, *40*(1), 45–50.

Zeng, F-G., Oba, S., Garde, S., Sininger, Y., & Starr, A. (1999). Temporal and speech processing deficits in auditory neuropathy. *NeuroReport*, *10*, 3429–3435.

7

Medical Considerations for Infants and Young Children With Hearing Loss

A Pediatrician's Perspective

Betty R. Vohr

What Is the Medical Home?

The infant's pediatrician/primary health care provider is responsible for monitoring the general health, development, and well-being of the infant beginning in the newborn nursery. In 1999, the American Academy of Pediatrics (AAP) proposed the concept of a medical home for all children with special health care needs (AAP, 2002). The medical home provides health care that is accessible, family-centered, continuous, comprehensive, coordinated, compassionate, and culturally competent (AAP, 2002, 2010). The following sections describe the components of care required for infants and young children with permanent hearing loss, and the proposed role of the primary care provider and the medical home in coordinating and facilitating optimal care.

To maximize the outcome for infants with all degrees of congenital hearing loss, the hearing of all infants should be screened no later than 1 month of age. Every infant who does not pass the newborn screen should have a comprehensive audiologic diagnostic evaluation no later than 3 months of age, and infants with confirmed hearing loss should receive appropriate early intervention service by 6 months of age (AAP, 2007a). Figure 7–1 shows the algorithm developed to guide the pediatrician/ primary health care provider in the management of infants relative to hearing screening, diagnosis, and intervention. The primary care physician's proposed role in this process is reviewed (AAP, 2010).

The Medical Home and Newborn Hearing Screening

The Joint Committee on Infant Hearing (JCIH) recommends as a benchmark that 4% or less of infants fail the newborn hearing screen. The rate is usually higher for the neonatal intensive care unit (NICU) than for the well-baby nursery because of the risk factors for hearing loss associated with NICU care. Therefore, based on this benchmark, 40 of every 1,000 infants screened may fail the newborn screen. As the rate of congenital hearing loss (HL) is 2 per 1,000, there are approximately 38 infants with a false-positive screen. A false screen may be secondary to transient fluid in the middle ear, debris in the ear canal, upper airway congestion, excessive infant noise, background noise, or electrical noise. Since the cause of a fail is uncertain and may represent a true fail, it is important that the family return with the infant for the follow-up rescreen or diagnostic evaluation. Many states (in the United States) are currently achieving a 2% fail rate, which significantly reduces the false-positive rate.

It is currently recommended that families receive the results of the screen at the time of discharge from the birthing hospital and that physicians have access to the information, so that they may encourage the family to return for follow-up. Physicians must therefore be aware of the causes of a hearing screen fail and the types of permanent congenital hearing loss including sensorineural, permanent conductive, and neural/ auditory neuropathy.

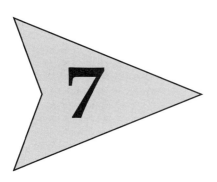

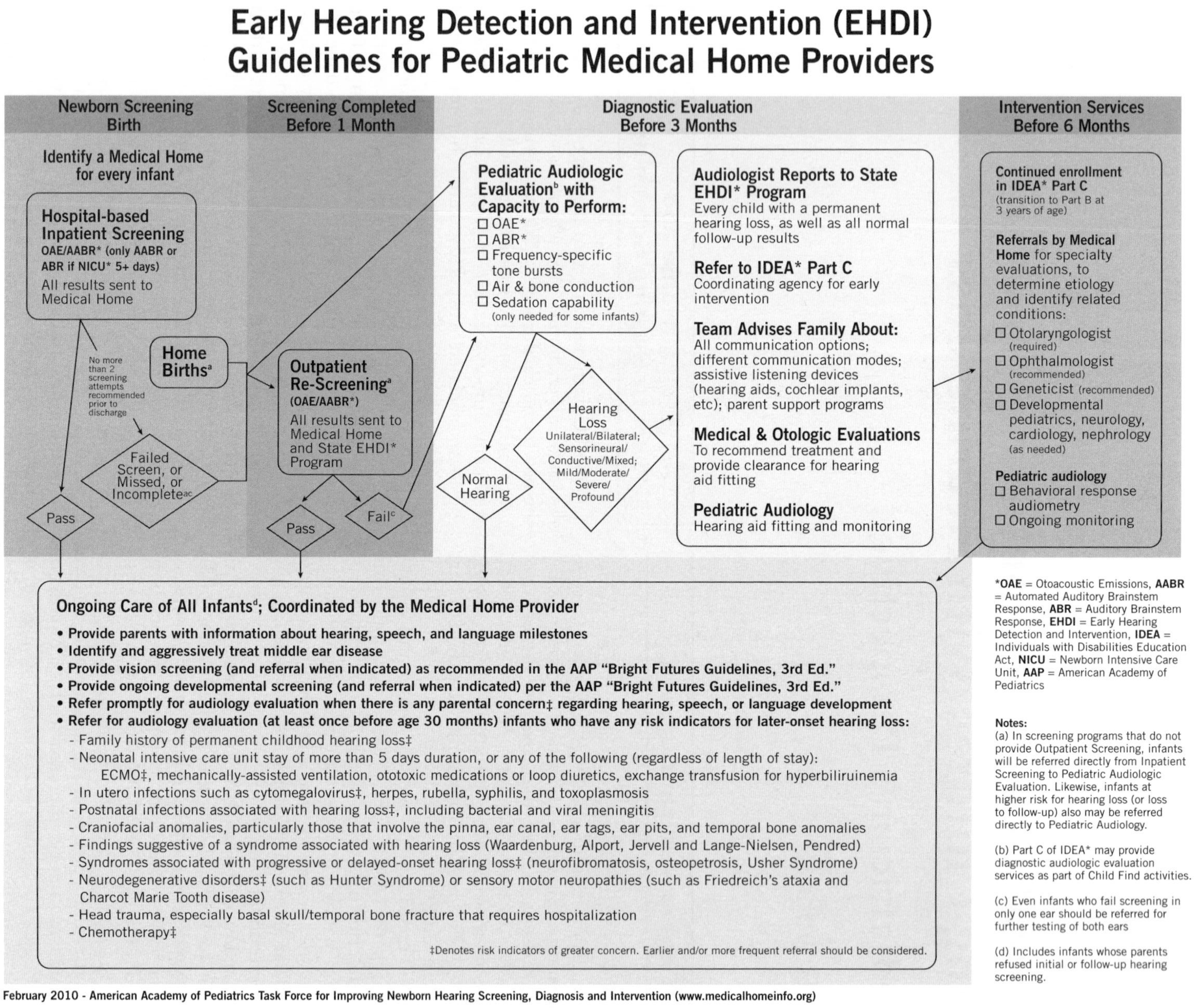

FIGURE 7–1. Universal newborn hearing screening, diagnosis, and intervention: guidelines for pediatric medical home providers. Reprinted with permission from the American Academy of Pediatrics.

The Medical Home and Risk Factors for Neonatal and Late Onset Hearing Loss

It is recommended that a history of risk factors be obtained or reviewed with the family at several time points: prior to delivery, during hospitalization, at discharge and after discharge. The pediatrician/primary health care provider may meet with the family prior to delivery to obtain a detailed family history of risk factors that includes neonatal or late onset hearing loss, syndromes or disorders associated with hearing loss. If this is not possible, a meeting with the parents should take place prior to hospital discharge. The pediatrician/primary health care physician needs to review every infant's medical record or discharge summary for the medical history and the presence of risk factors. Some risk factors are associated with hearing loss at birth, and some require monitoring for delayed onset or progressive hearing loss prior to discharge from the birthing hospital. The JCIH published an updated list of risk factors for hearing loss that we now review (2007).

Risk Factor 1

The first two recommendations depend on communication with the family. A family history of permanent childhood onset hearing loss, genetic disorders or syndromes associated with hearing loss (Cone-Wesson et al., 2000; Morton & Nance, 2006) are important predictors of both neonatal and late onset hearing loss. Recent studies have shown that at least 50% of congenital hearing loss is hereditary (Brookhouser, Worthington, & Kelly, 1994; Nance, 2003). It is recommended that a genetic consultation be offered to all families with a strong history of hearing loss or a newly identified infant with hearing loss. If appropriate, the evaluation should include genetic testing for nonsyndromic gene mutations such as *GJB2* (connexin-26) and syndromes commonly associated with early-onset childhood sensorineural hearing loss (Denoyelle et al., 1999; Nance, 2003; Nance & Kearsey, 2004; Santos et al., 2005).

Risk Factor 2

Caregiver concern regarding hearing, speech, language, or developmental delay in the first two to three years of life is associated with an increased risk of late onset hearing loss (Roizen, 1999). This is important, and professionals should not be complacent because of a passed newborn screen. The rate of permanent hearing loss in newborns is 2 to 3 per 1,000 and this rate rises to 7 per 1,000 at school age (Johnson et al., 2005).

Risk Factor 3

Recommendation 3 concerns infants admitted to the NICU. A new risk factor discussed in JCIH (2007) is for infants requiring neonatal intensive care or special care for greater than five days. This recommendation was added based on reports from the National Perinatal Research Center (NPIC) Quality Analytic Services (QAS). NPIC data indicated that approximately 25% of NICU and level 2 infants (i.e., those who are premature or ill) have low risk diagnoses, such as transient respiratory distress, temperature instability or negative sepsis work-up, and are discharged by 5 days of age. As specific risk factors are often difficult for paraprofessional screeners to identify in the medical record, establishing a more general time criterion (>5 days in the NICU) was felt to be easier for universal implementation (JCIH, 2007). The initial wording of Risk Factor 3 resulted in some confusion, and it was subsequently reworded and a clarification was added to the Joint Committee on Infant Hearing Web site (JCIH, http://jcih.org/posstatemts.htm) as follows:

> All infants requiring neonatal intensive care for greater than five days, *and any of the following regardless of length of stay:* extracorporeal membrane oxygenation (ECMO), assisted ventilation, exposure to ototoxic medications (gentamycin and tobramycin) or loop diuretics (furosemide/lasix) and hyperbilirubinemia requiring exchange transfusion, are considered risk factors for hearing loss. (Fligor, Neault, Mullen, Feldman, & Jones, 2005; Roizen, 1999, 2003)

Risk Factor 4

Risk Factor 4 is in utero infections, such as cytomegalovirus (CMV), herpes, rubella, syphilis, and toxoplasmosis (Fligor et al., 2005; Fowler et al., 1992, 1997; Madden et al., 2005; Nance, Lim, & Dodson, 2006; Rivera et al., 2002), which are important risk factors. Screening for these infections is not routine and is implemented if there is maternal history or the infant presents with signs or symptoms suggestive of disease. Workup is indicated for infants with a history or clinical signs of intrauterine infection. CMV remains the most common infectious cause of early or delayed onset hearing loss (Fowler et al., 1997).

Risk Factors 5 to 8

Risk Factors 5 to 8 are all associated with congenital abnormalities or syndromes. Risk Factor 5 includes craniofacial anomalies, including those involving the pinna, ear canal, ear tags, ear pits, and temporal bone anomalies (Cone-Wesson et al., 2000). These defects are common in both the well-baby nursery and the NICU. Risk Factor 6 includes physical findings such as a white forelock, which are associated with a syndrome known to include sensorineural or permanent conductive hearing loss. Risk factor 6 also includes atresias (Cone-Wesson et al., 2000). Risk Factor 7 includes syndromes associated with hearing loss or progressive or late onset hearing loss, such as neurofibromatosis, osteopetrosis, and Usher's syndrome (Roizen, 2003). Other frequently identified syndromes include Waardenburg, Alport, Pendred, and Jervell and Lange-Nielson (Nance, 2003). Risk Factor 8 consists of neurodegenerative disorders, such as Hunter syndrome, or sensory motor neuropathies such as Friedreich's ataxia and Charcot-Marie-Tooth disease (Roizen, 2003). Consultations with otolaryngology and genetics are indicated if a syndrome associated with hearing loss is suspected. In addition, these children need to be monitored longitudinally by a pediatric audiologist.

Risk Factor 9

Culture positive postnatal infections associated with sensorineural hearing loss including confirmed bacterial and viral (especially herpes viruses and varicella) meninigitis (Arditi et al., 1998; Bess, 1982; Biernath et al., 2006; Roizen, 2003) are important risk factors, and consultation with otolaryngology and audiology are indicated.

Risk Factors 10 and 11

Risk Factors 10 and 11 are essentially postdischarge risk factors. Serious head trauma, especially basal skull or temporal bone fractures requiring hospitalization, is a risk factor for hearing loss in childhood (Lew et al., 2004; Vartialnen, Karjalainen, & Karja, 1985; Zimmerman, Ganzel, Windmill, Nazar, & Phillips, 1993). Although rare in the pediatric population, chemotherapy for children with leukemia or cancer remains a risk factor, which in some cases is reversible (Bertolini, Lassalle, & Mercier, 2004).

The Medical Home and Continued Surveillance

Children with a documented risk factor for HL require close surveillance of hearing skills and language development and follow-up with audiology. For children with risk factors, the timing of hearing re-evaluations by an audiologist should be individualized depending on the likelihood of a subsequent delayed-onset hearing loss. JCIH (2007) currently recommends that infants who pass the neonatal screening but have a risk factor should have at least one diagnostic audiology assessment by 24 to 30 months of age. Early and more frequent assessment may be indicated for CMV infection, syndromes associated with progressive hearing loss, neurodegenerative disorders, trauma, or culture-positive postnatal infections associated with sensorineural hearing loss. Also children who have received ECMO or chemotherapy and children for whom there is caregiver concern or a family history of hearing loss should have more frequent assessments as clinically indicated (Fligor et al., 2005; Fowler et al., 1992; Madden et al., 2005; Rivera et al., 2002).

The Medical Home: The Medical Workup and Care Coordination

The primary care physician assumes responsibility for coordinating comprehensive health care and working as a team member with the family, all key professionals, and others identified by the family as members of the team. These efforts are initiated to ensure that no child is lost to follow-up, that all assessments occur in a timely fashion and that all appropriate and individualized services are provided (Figure 7–2).

Aside from the partnership of the family with the primary provider, other team members include the hospital hearing screening staff, the audiologist, the otolaryngologist, the geneticist, and specialized early intervention providers. Additional team members might include deaf services, the deaf community, interpreter services, parent support groups, and third-party payors. There is a sequence of events that occurs

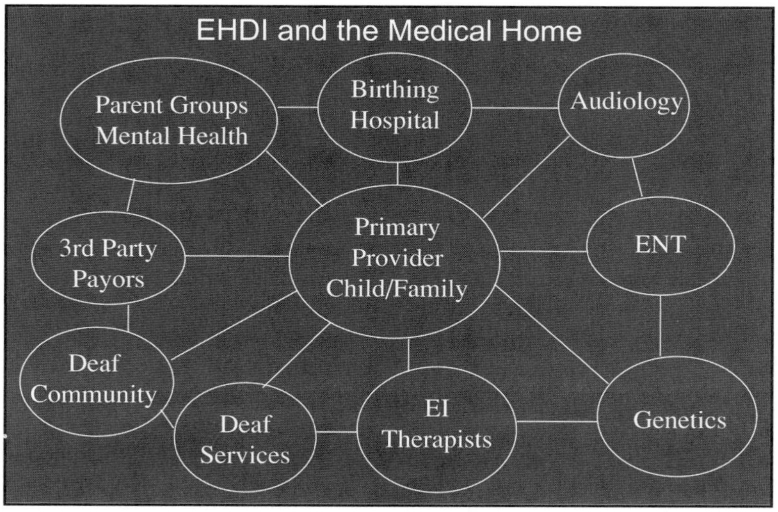

FIGURE 7–2. Potential members of the medical home team for the child and family. ENT = ear, nose, and throat physician; EI = early interventionist.

and not all members of the team may be active at any one time. Participation depends on the needs and wishes of the family.

Management of the Child Who Fails the Screen

The first step is for the hospital screening staff to share the results of the screen with the primary physician and family. The physician proceeds to discuss the results with the family either before discharge from the birthing hospital or at the time of the first office visit, and to encourage the family to return for a rescreen or diagnostic evaluation. The physician then checks with the family at each subsequent office visit to determine if the rescreen has been completed, to facilitate the visit if it has not occurred and to discuss the results with the family once the rescreen is completed.

Management of the Child Who Passes the Screen or Rescreen

For the child who passes the screen or rescreen the physician discusses the results with the family, shares that the screen pass does not mean that a subsequent hearing loss may not be identified, and informs the family that the child's hearing skills and development will be monitored. If the child has a risk factor for hearing loss, the primary care physician informs the family that a diagnostic audiologic evaluation will be completed at least once by 24 to 30 months of age.

In addition, the primary care physician is responsible for ongoing surveillance of parent concerns about language and hearing, auditory skills, and developmental milestones of all infants and children regardless of risk status, as outlined in the pediatric periodicity schedule published by the AAP (2000). This management approach permits the detection of children with either missed neonatal hearing loss or delayed onset hearing loss.

Management of the Child Who Fails the Rescreen and Is Referred for an Audiologic Diagnostic Evaluation

The physician ensures that the family takes the child for a diagnostic audiologic assessment at a center that has audiologists skilled in pediatric assessments as soon as possible. It is anticipated that the audiologist will call the pediatrician and send the test results for the child who does not pass. A complete report of the diagnostic assessment is sent to the primary care physician for all children evaluated whether they pass or fail. The pediatrician will then have a better understanding of the type and severity of hearing loss in order to support the recommendations of the audiologist and initiate the medical workup.

Management of the Child With a Failed Audiology Diagnostic Test

The pediatrician should schedule a meeting with the family as soon as possible to discuss the diagnosis, provide information, describe the next steps to be taken, and to be supportive of the family during a period of time in which they may experience significant stress. The benefits of active family participation in early intervention services and early amplification should be emphasized with the family. Communities may have a spectrum of pediatric diagnostic services and specialized early intervention programs. Families should be informed of programs appropriate for their infant. Many early hearing detection and intervention (EHDI) programs have developed guidebooks that are given to the family at the time of diagnosis that describe the available services. The primary care physician also should be aware of community resources and support the family choice of early intervention program and mode of communication.

Some components of the coordination may be implemented by different team members (see Figure 7–2). It is therefore important for the team members to communicate all interactions with the family and any actions taken with other team members. The audiologist in most cases will immediately facilitate a referral to the indicated specialized early intervention services chosen by the family. During the postdiagnosis appointment with the family, the physician reviews the family history again and re-examines the child for evidence of any craniofacial abnormalities or syndromes associated with hearing loss. It is important to emphasize to the family that their baby is still the same lovely baby, that the hearing loss was identified early, and that their baby will benefit from early intervention services and amplification.

The primary care physician must partner with the otolaryngologist. Every infant with confirmed hearing loss should be evaluated by an otolaryngologist with knowledge of pediatric hearing loss. Otolaryngologists who are skilled in childhood hearing loss will conduct a workup to determine the etiology of hearing loss and identify related risk indicators for hearing loss, including syndromes involving the head and neck. The otolaryngologist conducts a comprehensive assessment and provides recommendations and information to the family, audiologist, and primary health care provider on candidacy for amplification, assistive devices and surgical intervention, including reconstruction, bone-anchored hearing aids, and cochlear implantation.

Additional referrals may be made at that time for a developmental assessment, a genetics consultation, or other indicated specialist. The primary health care physician partners with other specialists to facilitate coordinated care for the infant and family. Because 30 to 40% of children with confirmed hearing loss will demonstrate developmental delays, comorbidities, or other disabilities, the primary care physician should closely monitor developmental milestones and initiate referrals related to suspected disabilities (Karchmer & Allen, 1999). The medical home algorithm for management of infants with either suspected or proven permanent hearing loss is seen in Figure 7–1 (AAP, 2010). Many families desire contact with another parent of a young child with a similar degree of hearing loss. Organizations such as Hands and Voices (www.handsandvoices.org/) are excellent in facilitating a family meeting. Middle-ear status should be monitored because the presence of middle-ear effusion can further compromise hearing.

The Academy of Pediatrics has realized the importance of just-in-time responses of physicians to a new diagnosis. In addition to assuming responsibility to ensure that the audiologic assessment is conducted on infants who do not pass screening, the physician must initiate referrals for medical specialty evaluations necessary to determine the etiology of the hearing loss.

Because of the association of hearing loss with other disabilities, including vision impairments, and the importance of vision for children with hearing loss, it is recommended that each child with a permanent hearing loss have at least one examination to assess visual acuity by an ophthalmologist experienced in evaluating infants.

It is estimated that at least 50% of congenital hearing loss is hereditary, and nearly 600 syndromes and 125 genes associated with hearing loss have already been identified (Brookhouser et al., 1994; Nance, 2003). The geneticist will review the family history for specific genetic disorders or syndromes, examine the child and complete genetic testing for syndromes or gene mutations for nondysmorphic hearing such as *GJB2* (connexin-26; Santos et al., 2005). Because of the prevalence of hereditary hearing loss, all families of children with confirmed hearing loss should be offered a genetics evaluation and counseling. This evaluation can provide families with information on etiology, prognosis, associated disorders, and the likelihood of hearing loss in future offspring.

The Medical Home and Surveillance

New recommendations for ongoing surveillance in the medical home for all infants with and without risk factors for hearing loss were published in JCIH (2007).

Regular surveillance of developmental milestones, auditory skills, parental concerns and middle ear status should be performed in the medical home, consistent with the AAP pediatric periodicity schedule (AAP, 2006). In addition, all infants should have an objective standardized screening of global development with a validated assessment tool at 9, 18, and 24 to 30 months of age or at any time if the health care professional or family has concern (JCIH, 2007). Infants who do not pass the speech-language portion of a medical home global screening or for whom there is a concern regarding hearing or language should be referred for speech-language evaluation and audiology assessment.

Table 7–1. Risk Factors for Developmental Difficulties*

Permanent hearing loss independent of OME
Suspected or diagnosed speech and language delay or disorder
Autism-spectrum disorder and other pervasive developmental disorders
Syndromes (e.g., Down) or craniofacial disorders that include cognitive, speech, and language delays
Blindness or uncorrectable visual impairment
Cleft palate with or without visual impairment
Developmental delay

*Sensory, physical, cognitive, or behavioral factors that place children who have OME at an increased risk for developmental difficulties (delay or disorder). Reprinted with permission from American Academy of Pediatrics and American Academy of Family Physicians. (2004). Diagnosis and management of acute otitis media. *Pediatrics*, *113*(5), 1451–1465. Copyright 2004.

The Medical Home and Middle Ear Disease

Middle Ear Effusion (OME)

The Agency for Healthcare Research and Quality clinical practice guidelines on otitis media with effusion (OME) were updated in 2004 to include all children 2 months to 12 years of age, including children with craniofacial abnormalities, neurologic abnormalities, and sensory deficits (AAP, 2004). The recommendations are based on the review of evidence and the collaborative efforts of the American Academy of Pediatrics, the American Academy of Family Medicine, and the American Academy of Otolaryngology, Head and Neck Surgery. OME is highly prevalent among young children, and approximately 90% of children have an episode of OME before starting school (Tos, 1984). OME is defined as the presence of middle ear fluid without acute signs or symptoms of acute ear infection. Recommendations related to diagnosis include: (1) pneumatic otoscope as the primary method to diagnose OME, and (2) physicians' documentation of laterality, duration of effusion and severity of symptoms. Although 40 to 50% of children are asymptomatic (Rosenfeld, Goldsmith, Tetlus, & Balzano, 1997), children may have associated hearing loss, balance problems (Golz, Angel-Yeger, & Parush, 1998), or delayed speech or language.

An important new recommendation concerns children with OME who are at risk of speech, language, or learning problems, and includes children with permanent hearing loss (Table 7–1). Medical management of children in these categories of risks may be expanded as needed to include hearing testing, speech and language evaluations, amplification or amplification adjustment, and tympanostomy tubes.

The management approach for children without risk factors, in contrast, is based on the fact that most OME is self limited (Rosenfeld & Kay, 2003), and 75 to 90% spontaneously resolves in 3 months. Therefore, a three-month period of observation is recommended. Evidence again suggests that no benefit is derived from the use of antihistamines or decongestants. In addition, no long-term benefits were identified for antimicrobial therapy or oral steroids. Children with persistent OME who are not at developmental risk are re-examined at 3- to 6-month intervals until either the OME resolves or a problem requiring intervention is identified.

Hearing testing is recommended for persistent OME when the child is considered at risk. Initial hearing testing is not appropriate in the primary care setting for children less than 4 years of age. Hearing screenings with earphones can be performed in a primary setting if equipment and space are available for the child 4 years or older. Children under 4 years need to be referred to an audiologist. Children who fail the diagnostic hearing assessment at 20 dB HL or more need to be referred for language testing, and subsequently any child with a language delay needs to be referred for intervention services. Language tests/screens that can be used in the primary care setting include the Early Language Milestone Scale (Coplan, 1993), the MacArthur Communicative Development Inventory (Fenson et al., 1993), the Language Development Survey (Rescoria, 1989), and Ages and Stages (Bricker & Squires, 1999).

Children with persistent OME should be referred for consultation to an otolaryngologist. Children who become candidates for surgical intervention with tympanostomy include those with OME at least 4 months duration with associated persistent hearing loss, recurrent or persistent OME in children at risk, and OME with associated structural injury to the tympanic membrane or middle ear. Tympanostomy is beneficial, and has been shown to be associated with decreases in middle ear effusion and improved hearing.

Acute Otitis Media

Updated recommendations for acute otitis media management for children 2 months to 12 years by the Agency for Health Care Research and Quality are reviewed (American Academy of Pediatrics and American Academy of Family Physicians, 2004). Acute otitis media continues to be the most common infection diagnosed in children in the United States. The definition of acute otitis media depends on the following characteristics: (1) a history of acute onset of signs and symptoms, (2) the presence of middle ear effusion, and (3) signs and symptoms of inflammation of the middle ear. The primary care physician must visualize the tympanic membrane for signs of middle ear effusion and inflammation to make the diagnosis. This is often challenging in uncooperative small infants and children with partially blocked ear canals or narrow ear canals.

Treatment includes pain management (acetaminophen or ibuprofen) as needed, and for children under 6 months of age, antibacterial treatment. For children older than 6 months, depending on severity of the illness, the options are antibacterial treatment or observation. Amoxicillin is currently the initial drug of choice. The recommendation of treatment for children with underlying permanent hearing loss and children at risk of language delays is antibacterial management.

The Medical Home and Children with Cochlear Implants

When cochlear implants first became available to children, the minimum age at implant was two years. Eligible children had to have bilateral, profound hearing loss. Studies, however, began to demonstrate that young congenitally deaf children with cochlear implants could learn to communicate orally. In addition, children with multiple disabilities could benefit from cochlear implants and develop auditory skills. As a result of these findings, candidacy criteria for pediatric cochlear implantation currently is 18 months or older for children with severe to profound bilateral sensorineural hearing loss and 12 to 18 months for children with profound hearing loss. In cases of deafness due to meningitis, implants may be placed early in the first year of life. A lack of benefit in the development of auditory skills with amplification needs to be demonstrated. Children up to 7 years of age appear to derive the greatest benefit (Sharma, Dorman, & Kral, 2005).

Pediatricians need to be aware of key management criteria for children with cochlear implants. The child will need the services of an audiologist skilled in fitting hearing aids and providing implant services including programming of the speech processer. The team at the implant center should include a skilled pediatric otolaryngologist and pediatric anesthesiologist. Finally, it is important that appropriate speech and language therapy services be provided to facilitate and optimize oral communication skills.

According to the Food and Drug Administration (FDA), 15,500 children in the United States had received cochlear implants at the end of 2006. Children with cochlear implants are at increased risk for bacterial meningitis compared to children in the general United States population (Reefhuis et al., 2003). Because of this risk, it is recommended that physicians monitor all patients with cochlear implants for meningitis and middle ear infections, but particularly children whose implants have a positioner (Biernath et al., 2006). *Streptococcus pneumoniae* is the most common pathogen causing bacterial meningitis in cochlear implant recipients of all ages (Manruqie, Cervera-Paz, Huarte, & Molina, 2004; Uchanski & Geers, 2003). Children less than 24 months of age with cochlear implants should receive PCV7, as recommended, and children ages 24 to 59 months with cochlear implants who have not received PCV7 should be vaccinated according to the high-risk schedule. The Centers for Disease Control and Prevention (CDC) recommends that children with implants also receive age-appropriate *Haemophilus influenzae* type b (Hib) vaccines (CDC, 2003).

Medical Home Stress and Impact on the Family

The Hearing Screen

Physicians need to be aware of the fact that parents perceive varying degrees of stress when they are informed that their infant has failed a newborn hearing screen. Although the possible cause may be either a false positive or a true fail, most parents will have some increase in worry until their infant is rescreened. NICU infants have higher false positive rates and higher fail rates than well-baby nursery infants. In one study of well-baby nursery infants, parents reported increased "worry" at 2 to 8 weeks of age when they returned for the rescreen (Vohr, Letourneau, & McDermott, 2001). Mothers who were more informed about hearing screening experienced decreased worry. Physicians who understand the screening process can support the family whose infant fails the screen, encourage the family to return for the rescreen, and follow-up with the family about the rescreen results. Stuart and colleagues (Stuart, Moretz, & Yang, 2000) administered the Parenting Stress Inventory at one month after discharge and found no differences in stress reported by mothers of infants who passed the screen and mothers of infants referred for further testing. This suggests that the stress and worry of a false positive is of short duration. A second study (Vohr et al., 2008) revealed that mothers of infants with a false positive screen result did not report increased levels of stress or impact at 12 to 16 or 18 to 24 months, and that older maternal age (perhaps more parenting and screening experience) and greater family resources were protective against persistent stress, whereas NICU stay contributed to prolonged stress (Vohr et al., 2008).

The Audiology Diagnostic Fail

It has been proposed that there is a continuum of increasing stress for families whose infants are identified with HL that increases as they progress through the hearing screen fail, rescreen fail, diagnostic fail, and intervention process (Kurtzer-White & Luterman, 2003). Abdala de Uzcategui and Yoshinaga-Itano (1997) conducted a study in which they sent mail interviews to families who had been referred for audiologic testing. Mothers reported feeling depressed, frustrated, and angry. Support and reassurance by the primary physician during this time is essential.

Parent perception of stress at the time of diagnosis varies significantly among parents. Parents who are culturally deaf may have anticipated the diagnosis and be totally accepting. Hearing parents of children diagnosed with a hearing loss perceive greater stress that is, in part, related to the fear of disability (Abdala deUzcategu & Yoshinaga-Itano, 1997; Barringer & Mauk, 1997; Bess & Paradise, 1994; Brand & Coetzer, 1994; Clemens, Davis, & Bailey, 2000; Gurian, Kinnamon, Henry, & Waisbren, 2006; Kurtzer-White & Luterman, 2003; Lee, Lee, Rankin, Alkon, & Weiss, 2005; Marhefka, Tepper, Brown, & Farley, 2006; Meadow-Orlans, 1990, 1995; Pal, Chaudhury, Das, & Sengupta, 2002; Thomas, Renaud, & Depaul, 2004; Tluczek et al., 1991; Vohr et al., 2001; Weichbold & Welzl-Mueller, 2001). Approximately 95% of children with congenital hearing loss are born to hearing parents. Hearing parents may not know someone with a significant hearing loss and may feel isolated. Meadow-Orlans (1995) reported that mothers of infants who were deaf or hard of hearing (HOH) perceived greater "life" stress (similar to that experienced with divorce, death in the family, moving, financial problems) than parents of hearing children. More recent studies have found similar "parenting" stress scores on the Parenting Stress Inventory for mothers of infants with HL and mothers of hearing infants (Meadow-Orlans, 1995). Prompt sharing of results with the family and physician and referral to early intervention by the audiologist on the day of diagnosis may facilitate the provision of needed information and support to parents to mediate stress. Both younger maternal age and lower level of maternal education have been associated with greater perception of maternal stress associated with hearing loss (Meadow-Orlans, 1990).

Impact on the family is a measure of how the child's condition (hearing loss) produces change in the family. Categories of impact include financial impact, family burden, caretaker burden and disruption of planning. In one study (Vohr et al., 2008), mothers of infants with hearing loss reported significantly greater financial impact at 12 to 16 months and greater financial and caretaker burden at 18 to 24 months compared to mothers infants who passed the screening process. This impact reflects "daily life" costs associated with hearing loss including amplification, speech and language therapy and transportation for visits to specialists. If physicians become aware of financial difficulties experienced by the family, the Early Intervention case manager should be alerted to assist and empower the family to identify resources such as a hearing aid loaner program, respite care, or eligibility for financial assistance programs.

Calderon and Greenberg (1999) reported that social support was an important predictor of maternal adjustment for hearing mothers of children who are deaf or HOH at school age. The physician can play an important role by informing and facilitating referral of the family to parent support groups such as Hands and Voices and Family Voices. As half of the children identified with congenital hearing loss are NICU graduates and approximately 40% of children with permanent hearing loss have other disabilities, these children may require the resources of a number of different medical and educational disciplines, adding to both the financial and emotional burden (Karchmer & Allen, 1999; Mitchell, 2004). As physicians become more informed about the needs of infants with hearing loss and their families, and community resources needed, they can become more effective members of the child/family EHDI team.

References

Abdala deUzcategu, C., & Yoshinaga-Itano, C. (1997). Parents' reactions to newborn hearing screening. *Audiology Today, 9*(1), 24–25.

American Academy of Pediatrics (AAP). (2000). Committee on practice and ambulatory medicine. Recommendations for preventive pediatric health care. *Pediatrics, 105*, 645–646.

American Academy of Pediatrics (AAP). (2002). Policy statement: The medical home. Medical home initiatives for children with special needs project advisory committee. *Pediatrics, 110*(1), 184–186.

American Academy of Pediatrics (AAP). (2010). *Task force on improving the effectiveness of newborn hearing screening, diagnosis, and intervention. Universal newborn hearing screening, diagnosis, and intervention: Guidelines for pediatric medical home providers.* Elk Grove Village, IL: Author. Available at http://www.medicalhomeinfo.org/how/clinical_care/hearing_screening/

American Academy of Pediatrics (AAP). (2004). Otitis media with effusion. *Pediatrics, 113*(5), 1412–1429.

American Academy of Pediatrics (AAP). (2006). Policy statement: Identifying infants and young children with developmental disorders in the medical home: An algorithm for developmental surveillance and screening. *Pediatrics, 118*(1), 405–420.

American Academy of Pediatrics (AAP). (2007a). Position statement: Principles and guidelines for early hearing detection and intervention programs. Joint Committee on Infant Hearing. *Pediatrics, 120*(4), 898–921.

American Academy of Pediatrics (AAP). (2007b). *Universal newborn hearing screening, diagnosis, and intervention: Guidelines for pediatric medical home providers.* Available at http://www.medicalhomeinfo.org/how/clinical_care/hearing_screening/

American Academy of Pediatrics and American Academy of Family Physicians. (2004). Diagnosis and management of acute otitis media. *Pediatrics, 113*(5), 1451–1465.

Arditi, M., Mason, E. O., Jr., Bradley, J. S., Tan, T. Q., Barson, W. J., Schutze, G. E., . . . Kaplan, S. L. (1998). Three-year multicenter surveillance of pneumococcal meningitis in children: Clinical characteristics, and outcome related to penicillin susceptibility and dexamethasone use. *Pediatrics, 102*(5), 1087–1097.

Barringer, D., & Mauk, G. (1997). Survey of parents' perspectives regarding hospital-based newborn hearing screening. *Audiology Today, 1*, 18–19.

Bertolini, P., Lassalle, M., & Mercier, G., Raquin, M. A., Izzi, G., Corradini, N., & Hartmann, O. (2004). Platinum compound-related ototoxicity in children: Long-term follow-up reveals continuous worsening of hearing loss. *Journal of Journal of Pediatric Hematology/Oncology, 26*, 649–655.

Bess, F. H. (1982). Children with unilateral hearing loss. *Journal of the Academy of Rehabilitative Audiology, 15*, 131–144.

Bess, F. H., & Paradise, J. L. (1994). Universal screening for infant hearing impairment: Not simple, not risk-free, not necessarily beneficial, and not presently justified. *Pediatrics, 93*(2), 330–334.

Biernath, K. R., Reefhuis, J., Whitney, C. G., Mann, E. A., Costa, P., Eichwald, J., & Boyle, C. (2006). Bacterial meningitis among children with cochlear implants beyond 24 months after implantation. *Pediatrics, 117*(2), 284–289.

Brand, H. J., & Coetzer, M. A. (1994). Parental response to their child's hearing impairment. *Psychological Report, 75*(3 Pt. 1), 1363–1368.

Bricker, D., & Squires, J. (1999). *Ages and stages questionnaires: A parent-completed, child-monitoring system.* Baltimore, MD: Paul H. Brookes.

Brookhouser, P. E., Worthington, D. W., & Kelly, W. J. (1994). Fluctuating and/or progressive sensorineural hearing loss in children. *Laryngoscope, 104*(8 Pt. 1), 958–964.

Calderon, R., & Greenberg, M. T. (1999). Stress and coping in hearing mothers of children with hearing loss: Factors affecting mother and child adjustment. *American Annals of the Deaf, 144*(1), 7–18.

Centers for Disease Control and Prevention (CDC). (2003). *Pneumococcal vaccination for cochlear implant candidates and recipients: Updated recommendations of the advisory committee on immunization practices.* Retrieved August 12, 2010, from http://www.cdc.gov/mmwr/preview/mmwrhtml/mm5231a5.htm

Clemens, C. J., Davis, S. A., & Bailey, A. R. (2000). The false-positive in universal newborn hearing screening. *Pediatrics, 106*(1), E7.

Cone-Wesson, B., Vohr, B. R., Sininger, Y. S., Widen, J. E., Folsom, R. C., Gorga, M. P., & Norton, S. J. (2000). Identification of neonatal hearing impairment: Infants with hearing loss. *Ear and Hearing, 21*(5), 488–507.

Coplan, J. (1993). *Early language milestone scale* (2nd ed.). Austin, TX: Pro-Ed.

Denoyelle, F., Marlin, S., Weil, D., Moatti, L., Chauvin, P., Garabédian, E. N., & Petit, C. (1999). Clinical features of the prevalent form of childhood deafness, DFNB1, due to a connexin-26 gene defect: Implications for genetic counselling. *Lancet, 353*(9161), 1298–1303.

Fenson, L., Dale, P. S., Reznick, J. S., Thal, D., Bates, E., Hartung, J. P., . . . Reilly, J. S. (1993). *The McArthur communicative development inventories: User's guide and technical manual.* San Diego, CA: Singular Thomson Learning.

Fligor, B. J., Neault, M. W., Mullen, C. H., Feldman, H. A., & Jones, D. T. (2005). Factors associated with sensorineural hearing loss among survivors of extracorporeal membrane oxygenation therapy. *Pediatrics, 115*(6), 1519–1528.

Fowler, K., Stagno, S., Pass, R., Britt, W., Boll, T., & Alford, C. (1992). The outcome of congenital cytomegalovirus infection in relation to maternal antibody status. *New England Journal of Medicine, 326*(10), 663–667.

Fowler, K. B., McCollister, F. P., Dahle, A. J., Boppana, S., Britt, W. J., & Pass, R. F. (1997). Progressive and fluctuating sensorineural hearing loss in children with asymptomatic congenital cytomegalovirus infection. *Journal of Pediatrics, 130*(4), 624–630.

Golz, A., Angel-Yeger, B., & Parush, S. (1998). Evaluation of balance disturbances in children with middle ear effusion. *International Journal of Pediatric Otorhinolaryngology, 43*(1), 21–26.

Gurian, E. A., Kinnamon, D. D., Henry, J. J., & Waisbren, S. E. (2006). Expanded newborn screening for biochemical disorders: The effect of a false-positive result. *Pediatrics, 117*(6), 1915–1921.

Joint Commission on Infant Hearing (JICH). (2007). www.jcih.org

Johnson, J. L., White, K. R., Widen, J. E., Gravel, J. S., Vohr, B. R., James, M., . . . Meyer, S. (2005). A multisite study to examine the efficacy of the otoacoustic emission/automated auditory brainstem response newborn hearing screening protocol: Introduction and overview of the study. *American Journal of Audiology, 14*(2), S178–S185.

Karchmer, M. A., & Allen, T. E. (1999). The functional assessment of deaf and hard of hearing students. *American Annals of the Deaf, 144*(2), 68–77.

Kurtzer-White, E., & Luterman, D. (2003). Families and children with hearing loss: Grief and coping. *Mental Retardation and Developmental Disabilities Research Reviews, 9*(4), 232–235.

Lee, S. Y., Lee, K. A., Rankin, S. H., Alkon, A., & Weiss, S. J. (2005). Acculturation and stress in Chinese-American parents of infants cared for in the intensive care unit. *Advances in Neonatal Care, 5*(6), 315–328.

Lew, H. L., Lee, E. H., Miyoshi, Y., Chang, D. G., Date, E. S., & Jerger, J. F. (2004). Brainstem auditory-evoked potentials as an objective tool for evaluating hearing dysfunction in traumatic brain injury. *American Journal of Physical Medicine and Rehabilitation, 83*(3), 210–215.

Madden, C., Wiley, S., Schleiss, M., Benton, C., Meinzen-Derr, J., Greinwald, J., & Choo, D. (2005). Audiometric, clinical and educational outcomes in a pediatric symptomatic congenital cytomegalovirus (CMV) population with sensorineural hearing loss. *International Journal of Pediatric Otorhinolaryngology, 69*(9), 1191–1198.

Manruqie, M., Cervera-Paz, F., Huarte, A., & Molina, M. (2004). Advantages of cochlear implantation in prelingual deaf children before 2 years of age when compared with later implantation. *Laryngoscope, 114*(8), 1462–1469.

Marhefka, S., Tepper, V., Brown, J., & Farley, J. (2006). Caregiver psychosocial characteristics and children's adherence to antiretroviral therapy. *AIDS Patient Care STDS, 20*(6), 429–437.

Meadow-Orlans, K. P. (1990). The impact of childhood hearing loss on the family. In D. F. Moores & K. P. Meadow-Orlans (Eds.), *Educational and developmental aspects of deafness* (pp. 11–23). Washington, DC: Gallaudet University Press.

Meadow-Orlans, K. P. (1995). Sources of stress for mothers and fathers of deaf and hard of hearing infants. *American Annals of the Deaf, 140*(4), 352–357.

Mitchell, R. E. (2004). National profile of deaf and hard of hearing students in special education from weighted survey results. *American Annals of the Deaf, 149*(4), 336–349.

Morton, C. C., & Nance, W. E. (2006). Newborn hearing screening—a silent revolution. *New England Journal of Medicine, 354*(20), 2151–2164.

Nance, W. E. (2003). The genetics of deafness. *Mental Retardation and Developmental Disabilities Research Reviews, 9*(2), 109–119.

Nance, W. E., & Kearsey, M. J. (2004). Relevance of connexin deafness (DFNB1) to human evolution. *American Journal of Human Genetics, 74*(6), 1081–1087.

Nance, W. E., Lim, B. G., & Dodson, K. M. (2006). Importance of congenital cytomegalovirus infections as a cause for pre-lingual hearing loss. *Journal of Clinical Virology, 35*(2), 221–225.

Pal, D. K., Chaudhury, G., Das, T., & Sengupta, S. (2002). Predictors of parental adjustment to children's epilepsy in rural India. *Child Care Health and Development, 28*(4), 295–300.

Reefhuis, J., Honein, M. A., Whitney, C. G., Chamany, S., Mann, E. A., Biernath, K. R., . . . Boyle, C. (2003). Risk of bacterial meningitis in children with cochlear implants. *New England Journal of Medicine, 349*(5), 435–445.

Rescoria, L. (1989). The language development survey: A screening tool for delayed language in toddlers. *Journal of Speech and Hearing Disorders, 54*, 587–599.

Rivera, L., Boppana, S., Fowler, K. B., Britt, W. J., Stagno, S., & Pass, R. (2002). Predictors of hearing loss in children with symptomatic congenital cytomegalovirus infection. *Pediatrics, 110*(4), 762–767.

Roizen, N. J. (1999). Etiology of hearing loss in children. Nongenetic causes. *Pediatric Clinics of North America, 46*(1), 49–64.

Roizen, N. J. (2003). Nongenetic causes of hearing loss. *Mental Retardation and Developmental Disabilities Research Reviews, 9*(2), 120–127.

Rosenfeld, R. M., Goldsmith, A. J., Tetlus, L., & Balzano, A. (1997). Quality of life for children with otitis media. *Archives of Otolaryngology-Head and Neck Surgery, 123*(10), 1049–1054.

Rosenfeld, R. M., & Kay, D. (2003). Natural history of untreated otitis media. *Laryngoscope, 113*(10), 1645–1657.

Santos, R. L., Aulchenko, Y. S., Huygen, P. L., van der Donk, K. P., de Wijs, I. J., Kemperman, M. H., . . . Cremers, C. W. (2005). Hearing impairment in Dutch patients with connexin 26 (GJB2) and connexin 30 (GJB6) mutations. *International Journal of Pediatric Otorhinolaryngology, 69*(2), 165–174.

Sharma, A., Dorman, M. F., & Kral, A. (2005). The influence of a sensitive period on central auditory development in children with unilateral and bilateral cochlear implants. *Hearing Research, 203*(1–2), 134–143.

Stuart, A., Moretz, M., & Yang, E. Y. K. (2000). An investigation of maternal stress after neonatal hearing screening. *American Journal of Audiology, 9*, 135–141.

Thomas, K. A., Renaud, M. T., & Depaul, D. (2004). Use of the parenting stress index in mothers of preterm infants. *Advances in Neonatal Care, 4*(1), 33–41.

Tluczek, A., Mischler, E. H., Bowers, B., Peterson, N. M., Morris, M. E., Farrell, P. M., . . . Fost, N. (1991). Psychological impact of false-positive results when screening for cystic fibrosis. *Pediatric Pulmonology Suppl, 7*, 29–37.

Tos, M. (1984). Epidemiology and natural history of secretory otitis. *American Journal of Otology, 5*(6), 459–462.

Uchanski, R., & Geers, A. (2003). Acoustic characteristics of the speech of young cochlear implant users: A comparisons with normal-hearing age-mates. *Ear and Hearing, 24*(1 Suppl.), 90S–105S.

Vartialnen, E., Karjalainen, S., & Karja, J. (1985). Auditory disorders following head injury in children. *Acta Oto-Laryngologica, 99*, 529–536.

Vohr, B. R., Jodoin-Krauzyk, J., Tucker, R., Johnson, M. J., Topol, D., & Ahlgren, M. (2008). Newborn hearing screen results: Impact on the family in the first two years of life. *Archives of Pediatrics and Adolescent Medicine, 162*(3), 205–211.

Vohr, B. R., Letourneau, K. S., & McDermott, C. (2001). Maternal worry about neonatal hearing screening. *Journal of Perinatology, 21*(1), 15–20.

Weichbold, V., & Welzl-Mueller, K. (2001). Maternal concern about positive test results in universal newborn hearing screening. *Pediatrics, 108*(5), 1111–1116.

Zimmerman, W. D., Ganzel, T. M., Windmill, I. M., Nazar, G. B., & Phillips, M. (1993). Peripheral hearing loss following head trauma in children. *Laryngoscope, 103*, 87–91.

8

Medical Considerations for Infants and Children With Hearing Loss: The Otologists' Perspective[1]

Craig A. Buchman, Oliver F. Adunka, Carlton J. Zdanski, and Harold C. Pillsbury

Background and Protocol

Hearing loss is common among newborn infants with an incidence rate of 3 to 4 per 1,000 live births per year. Approximately 25% of these children have a severe to profound hearing loss while the remaining is affected to a lesser degree. There also is a group of children who have passed their newborn hearing screen, only to later be identified as having a progressive type of hearing disorder. Untreated hearing loss reduces sound and environmental awareness. This may result in delayed speech and language acquisition and impaired communication abilities. These individuals frequently attain lower levels of educational achievement than the normal hearing population, thereby adversely affecting employment opportunities and quality of life.

In the United States, universal newborn hearing screening has been mandated by law for all children in 32 states and offered for all children in an additional 16 states. Currently, only Texas and California perform hearing screening selectively (http://genes-r-us.uthscsa.edu/nbsdisorders.pdf). Since the initiation of newborn infant hearing screening, a number of specialized programs have evolved to systematically evaluate and habilitate these children and provide a variety of resources for families. Many of these systems and processes have followed the recommendations of the 2007 Joint Committee on Infant Hearing (JCIH) statement that has been detailed elsewhere (American Academy of Pediatrics and Joint Committee on Infant Hearing 2007). Despite these efforts, late-onset hearing loss might not be identified by newborn screening protocols. Risk factors for identifying late-onset hearing loss have also been developed (American Academy of Pediatrics and Joint Committee on Infant Hearing, 2007).

Universal newborn hearing screening was mandated in North Carolina in 1999. The North Carolina program appears to be highly effective with 98.2% of the 133,823 infants born in 2007 receiving a hearing screening (personnel communication, North Carolina Early Hearing Detection and Intervention [EHDI] Program). Since the inception of screening in the state, there has been a dramatic increase in the number of children presenting for comprehensive hearing evaluation and management. The age at identification has decreased from 24 to 30 months down to 2 to 3 months (Harrison, Roush & Wallace, 2003). Currently, our center is serving more than 1300 children with hearing

---

[1]A version of this chapter was previously published as Buchman, C. A., Adunka, O. F., Zdanski, C. J. & Pillsbury, H. C. (2008) In R. Seewald & J. Bamford (Eds.), *A sound foundation through early amplification 2007: Proceedings of the fourth international conference* (pp. 95–105). Stäfa, Switzerland: Phonak AG. Reprinted with permission from Phonak A/G.

loss (roughly 650 using hearing aids and 650 using cochlear implants). To serve such a large population, we have developed a multidisciplinary approach and standardized protocols for the evaluation and treatment of these children. The multidisciplinary endeavor requires input from a diverse group of professionals with expertise in a variety of hearing-related disciplines. These areas are broadly depicted in Figure 8–1. It is common that certain disciplines might predominate during one phase of the process while others frequently become more active later. Cooperativity through mutual respect for one another's skills and opinions forms the backbone for successful collaboration for the child and family's benefit.

In an effort to create a timely diagnosis and early intervention, we have created a timeline for the events of the first year of life (Figure 8–2). Although not set in stone, we believe this serves as a rough guide for the events of the first year of life as it relates to hearing loss and its management. The cornerstone goals of the first year are:

1. *identification* of hearing loss and establishing precise auditory thresholds;
2. *diagnosis* of the etiology for the hearing impairment;
3. *intervention* through provision of appropriate treatment and/or technologies; and
4. *education* by providing information for families to help make decisions.

A comprehensive diagnostic hearing evaluation is the first required assessment following a confirmed "fail" or "refer" indication by the newborn infant hearing screening. At our center, this screening is carried out by a group of highly experienced audiologists with expertise in pediatric hearing testing. The initial follow-up testing for each child occurs under one of three environments: natural sleep, conscious sedation, or general anesthesia. Infants younger than about 3 months of age are tested in natural sleep, if possible. Babies older than this, without other medical contraindications, are sedated prior to testing. After medical clearance by a physician, a nurse from the hospital's pediatric sedation team administers a sedative and remains at bedside to monitor the entire session. Sedation typically is accomplished with chloral hydrate delivered orally or midazolam delivered intravenously. In cases where the infant is scheduled for a procedure under general anesthesia (e.g., surgery or imaging), the evoked potential testing is incorporated into the procedure sequence, if appropriate. Some children are not deemed candidates for safe monitored conscious sedation, and so testing is carried out under the supervision of an anesthesiologist (i.e., general anesthesia). The duration of

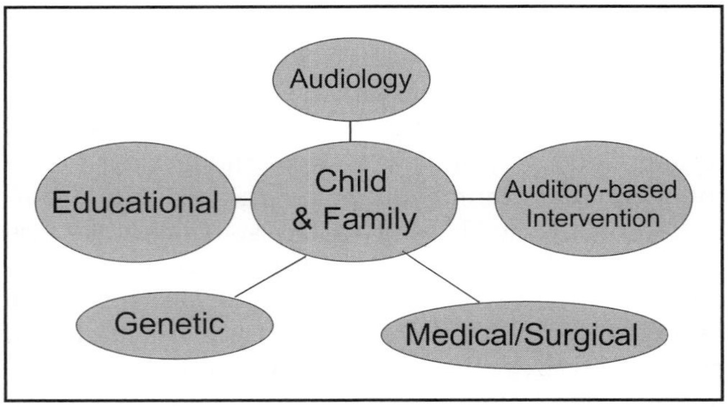

FIGURE 8–1. Schematic representation of the Hearing Loss Team at the University of North Carolina at Chapel Hill.

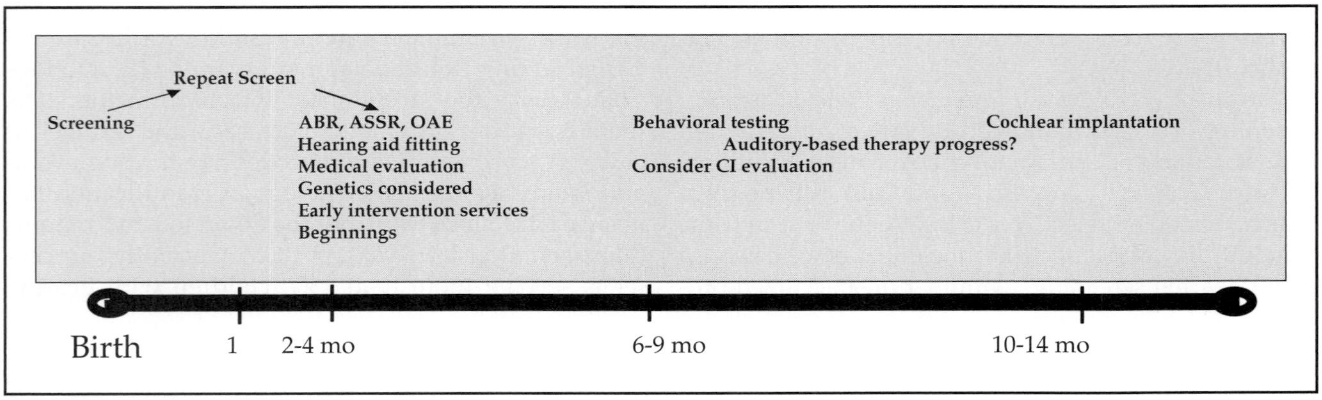

FIGURE 8–2. Time line for diagnostic and therapeutic interventions for infants that fail a newborn infant screen.

the test is usually dictated by the test environment, ranging from about 30 minutes in the operating room to over an hour under conscious sedation.

No single test modality is sufficient for precisely identifying the degree of hearing impairment in a baby (American Academy of Pediatrics and Joint Committee on Infant Hearing, 2007). Rather, a test battery is needed that might include a variety of measures such as: auditory brainstem response audiometry (ABR), auditory steady-state responses (ASSR), otoacoustic emissions (OAE), and tympanometry (immittance). Although reasonably accurate, each of these testing procedures has a variety of potential shortcomings. It is paramount that the individual administering the protocol be able to recognize and interpret the various tests results within the context of these shortcomings (American Academy of Pediatrics and Joint Committee on Infant Hearing, 2007).

ABR, OAEs, and tympanometry form the backbone of the diagnostic testing protocol at our institution for infants who fail newborn screening. Our protocols have been detailed previously (Buchman et al., 2006). ASSR has also been used at our institution, although we have found such testing adds very little diagnostic information beyond conventional ABR. In a manner similar to ABR, ASSR can over- or underestimate the degree of hearing loss with overestimation being more common (Ahn, Lee, Kim, Yoon, & Chung, 2007; Gorga et al., 2006; Stapells, Herdman, Small, Dimitrijevic, & Hatton, 2005). ASSR is notably less accurate in patients with lesser degrees of hearing loss and is unable to identify those ears with the auditory neuropathy/dyssynchrony (AN/AD) phenotype (Stapells et al., 2005; Tlumak, Rubinstein, & Durrant, 2007). In subjects with profound hearing loss, ASSR may produce artifactual responses that are recorded as auditory thresholds when, in fact, they are produced by nonauditory centers (Gorga et al., 2004; Small & Stapells, 2004). Thus, it is critical that clinicians understand that these electrophysiological modalities are useful for estimating thresholds for the purposes of amplification fitting in children. However, they are not precise enough for making decisions regarding surgical intervention when destruction of the underlying residual hearing may occur as a sequelae of that intervention.

The otologist's role in caring for the hearing impaired child is to:

1. *Diagnose* hearing loss by identifying:
   a. Etiology and severity;
   b. Specific anatomical relationships to functional findings;
   c. Identification of associated problems; and
   d. Referrals to related professionals.
2. *Treat* hearing loss by providing medical and/or surgical interventions;
3. *Refer* for amplification and/or speech therapy;
4. *Prevent* further hearing loss and other related complications through *education* of parents, children, and other health care providers; and
5. *Communicate with professionals* on the hearing loss team.

The otologist's role usually commences once a hearing disorder has been identified. One exception might be the child who requires diagnostic audiology, but is either unable to be tested under natural sleep or sedation because of associated medical conditions or when it is apparent that middle ear effusions need to be addressed in order to garner accurate test results. These children are taken to the operating room for general anesthesia. In this setting, the ears are examined using the operating microscope, and a determination regarding middle ear status is made. When fluid is present, we prefer to place tympanostomy tubes, and the audiological testing protocol is subsequently carried out. Ear canal bleeding must be avoided as this might negatively impact testing results. Placement of otic drops is deferred until after the auditory testing has been concluded. If a hearing impairment has been identified, ear canal impressions for future hearing aid molds are usually taken during the same setting for convenience. Findings are subsequently entered into the newborn infant hearing screening database.

Following the initial audiologic assessment, we have found that a search for a hearing loss etiology and associated medical conditions is critical and frequently impacts the treatment paradigm. In North Carolina, referrals are also made to BEGINNINGS (http://www.beginningssvcs.com) and the Early Intervention Services Program (http://www.ncei.org) from the State at this juncture. BEGINNINGS was established as a nonprofit organization, incorporated under the laws of North Carolina since 1987, to provide emotional support and access to impartial information as a central resource for families with deaf or hard of hearing children, ages birth through 21 years. Early Intervention Services refers to a variety of public state agencies working together to provide services for children with special needs age birth to 3 years. Early Intervention Services is usually the mechanism whereby assistive technologies (AT) are funded, and a speech-language pathologist (SLP) becomes involved in the child's care plan. In North Carolina, there are a growing number of

SLPs who are trained and certified in the methods of auditory verbal therapy (AVT). Emerging evidence suggests that in the setting of an adequate auditory signal (either through amplification or a cochlear implant), auditory-based intervention provides for better acquisition of spoken language in hearing-impaired children than communication modes that include sign language (Moog & Geers, 2003).

Medical Diagnostic Evaluation

The medical evaluation focuses on trying to identify an etiology for the hearing loss and associated problems that may negatively impact communication or other health issues. Implicit is the fact that a detailed understanding of the causes of hearing loss in children is needed to identify the salient issues in a particular patient. An excellent review of the potential etiologies of hearing loss has been previously published (Morton & Nance, 2006). In addition to searching for the etiology of hearing loss, careful evaluation must identify disorders in vision, craniofacial malformations, and primary speech and auditory processing disorders to allow a comprehensive approach to the communication needs of a child and the family. Referrals among a variety of medical professionals are often needed.

Currently, available data estimate the incidence of hearing loss at birth to be 186 per 100,000 while the prevalence is roughly 270 per 100,000 at 4 years of age (Morton & Nance, 2006). Genetic factors appear to play a greater role than acquired causes at birth, while acquired cases become more prevalent later in life. There are more than 300 distinct hearing loss syndromes that have been identified by their association with other clinical features. Syndromic forms of hearing loss are less common, accounting for only 10 to 20% of new cases. However, a thorough understanding of these syndromes allows for relatively simple and rapid identification of the genetics and associated comorbidities that might affect a particular child. Nonsyndromic (55%) and acquired (35%) forms of hearing loss are responsible for most of the newly identified cases emerging from the newborn hearing screening process, and the etiologies can be somewhat more difficult or even impossible to identify (Morton & Nance, 2006). For all types of hearing impairment in children, evaluation by a geneticist with expertise in pediatric hearing loss can provide additional information for families.

A careful history, physical examination and selective use of imaging studies and laboratory testing can identify the etiology of a child's hearing loss in many cases. In addition to knowing the details of the newborn infant screening and diagnostic auditory testing, the *medical history* should be thorough in the areas of pregnancy and complications, past medical/surgical history, and family history. Some of the details that should be extracted include:

1. Did the pregnancy progress to full term? Were there associated complications such as eclampsia, fetal distress, oligo- or polyhydramnios, bleeding, Rh incompatibility, premature rupture of membranes, preterm labor?
2. Was there perinatal infection such as toxoplasmosis, herpes simplex, rubella, syphilis, or cytomegalovirus (CMV) infection, group B streptococcus, or other infection (TORCHES)?
3. Was antibiotic treatment required? If yes, were aminoglycosides used?
4. Was perinatal hypoxia or meconium aspiration evident at the time of delivery?
5. Did the child spend time in the neonatal intensive care unit (NICU)? If so
   a. What was the birth weight? (Below 1500 grams?)
   b. Was the child on a ventilator? What duration?
   c. Were high oxygen concentrations needed?
   d. Were there blood transfusions?
   e. Intracranial hemorrhage?
   f. Necrotizing enterocolitis? This might be associated with the use of aminoglycoside antibiotics.
   g. Retinopathy of prematurity?
   h. Heart defects? If so what type?
6. Was the child jaundiced? If so, how high was the bilirubin concentration, for what duration and how was it treated?
7. Did the child have meningitis? Bacterial? If so, what organisms were present?
8. Did the infant require any surgeries?
9. What other medical disorders does the child have?
10. Are there difficulties with vision, feeding, or problems with other bodily functions?
11. In addition to the usual medical history regarding medicines, allergies, and past surgeries, it is important to assess other family members with hearing disorders and/or disorders related to hearing loss. Attempts should be made to uncover both first and second degree relatives who have or have had hearing loss.

The *physical examination* is focused on trying to identify syndromic features, associated ear-specific disorders, and anatomic situations that would adversely affect communication. Although a detailed listing of these issues is beyond the scope of this chapter, some specifics that are sought in the physical examination might include:

1. General appearance traits such as wide set eyes, pigmentary changes such as heterochromic irides and a white forelock of hair that are consistent with Waardenburg syndrome;
2. Cervical fistulas and pits with ear deformities suggesting branchio-oto-renal BOR. syndrome;
3. Cleft lip/palate, down-slanting eyes, coloboma, low-set small external ears, and mandible and maxillary hypoplasia in association with a conductive type of hearing loss that would possibly indicate Treacher Collins syndrome;
4. Palatal and lip clefts in association with choanal atresia, external ear deformity, and facial paralysis that might raise the suspicion for CHARGE association or similar syndromes;
5. Microcephaly that might be seen in association with perinatal CMV or rubella infection or other events such as birth asphyxia or brain underdevelopment;
6. The general neurologic status of the child should be assessed. Although this may not provide direct evidence for the etiology of the hearing loss, global neurologic, and cognitive impairment might clearly influence the effectiveness of a variety of interventions;
7. Otitis externa and otitis media should be assessed in all cases, as these can adversely affect precise hearing loss assessment and the institution of amplification.

Radiographic Imaging

Radiologic imaging is a critical aspect of the assessment of every child with newly identified hearing loss. In our program, it is recommended immediately after the diagnosis of hearing loss has been established by electrophysiologic measures. Early anatomic assessment of the temporal bones, auditory, vestibular, and facial nerves as well as brain may:

1. further characterize the hearing loss *etiology*,
2. identify anatomic markers for hearing loss *progression*,
3. predict *poor prognosis* from interventions such as amplification and/or cochlear implantation, and
4. *identify lesions of the central nervous system that require medical/surgical intervention* for the overall health of the patient.

Classical studies of temporal bone and ear morphology have been carried out using histologic/pathologic techniques in a variety of conditions (Schuknecht, 1993). Thus, the structural characteristics of many of the hearing loss syndromes have been described and can broadly be classified into those with or without radiographically detectable abnormalities. Patients with isolated inner ear cellular or membranous labyrinthine disorders are currently not identifiable based on current imaging resolution. Conversely, labyrinthine malformations of the external, middle, and inner ears and internal auditory canal (IAC) are clearly detectable using currently available imaging. Structural anomalies of the nerves of the IAC and brain are also resolvable in some cases. In general, high-resolution computed tomography (HRCT) is well suited for assessing the osseous structures (external auditory canal and middle ear), while magnetic resonance imaging (MRI) provides excellent soft tissue detail for looking at the cranial nerves and brain. The inner ear is well visualized using either MRI or HRCT. HRCT shows the osseous labyrinthine shell well, whereas MRI shows the fluids within the inner ear that conform to the otic capsule outline. The protocols that we use for these studies have been described previously (Adunka et al., 2006; Adunka, Jewells, & Buchman, 2007; Buchman et al., 2006).

There currently remains some debate regarding which of the various imaging modalities is most appropriate for assessing children with hearing loss (Adunka et al., 2006, 2007; Buchman et al., 2006; Parry, Booth, & Roland, 2005; Trimble, Blaser, James, & Papsin, 2007). This controversy stems mostly from otologists' and radiologists' familiarity in interpreting HRCT for inner ear morphological changes. For cases of aural atresia and other conductive hearing losses, HRCT remains superior to MRI for assessing bony detail. Conversely, we prefer MRI rather than HRCT in all children with newly identified sensorineural hearing loss as it allows direct imaging of the cochlear nerves and brain. The consequences of missing either isolated cochlear nerve deficiency or unsuspected retrocochlear/brain pathology could be profound and might ultimately result in inappropriate treatment of the child. For example, cochlear implantation in an ear without a cochlear nerve or in an ear affected by a tumor could be devastating for the child and family. In cases of sensorineural hearing loss, we use supplementary HRCT only in cases where: (1) semicircular canal defects are identified so that the anatomy of the facial nerve is determined, (2) inner ear obstruction is evident on MRI to further determine if the lesion is osseous or fibrous (postmeningitis), (3) the IAC is narrow to determine patency of the bony cochlear nerve canal, and (4) temporal bone pathology has been identified, such as in cases of tumors (Adunka et al., 2006, 2007; Buchman et al., 2006).

Inner ear malformations that are detectable on imaging studies are common in children with SNHL. Some studies have estimated that 20 to 30% of children with sensorineural hearing loss (SNHL) have some morphologic abnormality of their inner ear (Coticchia, Gokhale, Waltonen, & Sumer, 2006). They can be conveniently divided into abnormalities of the cochlear and/or vestibular apparatus or abnormalities of the neural structures. Cochlear abnormalities can take the form of aplasia (absence or Michel aplasia; Figure 8–3), hypoplasia (small cochlea; Figure 8–4), or dysplasia. Cochlear dysplasias are usually characterized as an incomplete partitioning as in the classical Mondini malformation (Figure 8–5) or modiolar deficiency as in X-linked stapes gusher syndrome (Figure 8–6). Vestibular morphologic variants can also have aplasia, hypoplasia or dysplasias and can affect the semicircular canals, otolithic organs, and the vestibular aqueduct. Vestibular aplasia is shown in Figure 8–7.

Children with inner ear or neural malformations may have no identifiable clinical syndrome. For instance, absent semicircular canals (see Figure 8–7) with or without cochlear hypoplasia and cochlear nerve deficiency are very common in children with CHARGE association, VATER complex, as well as BOR syndrome. An enlarged vestibular aqueduct (and endolymphatic duct) when seen in isolation or in association with an incompletely partitioned cochlea (Mondini's deformity; see Figure 8–5) might indicate that Pendred's syndrome is present. Children with Waardenburg's syndrome might also have inner ear malformations along the Mondini spectrum of findings as well. A bulbous or dilated IAC that widely communicates with a deficient cochlear modiolus is suggestive of the X-linked stapes gusher syndrome (see Figure 8–6; Morton & Nance, 2006).

Children with hearing loss can also have a variety of congenital and acquired changes to the central nerv-

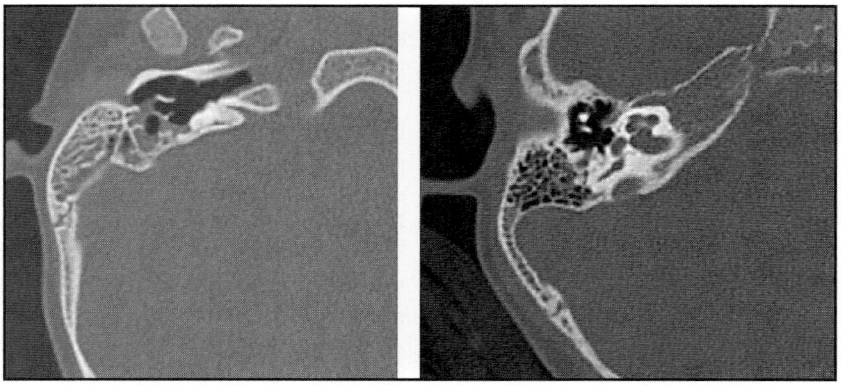

FIGURE 8–3. Michel aplasia (inner ear aplasia) on the left and normal inner ear on the right.

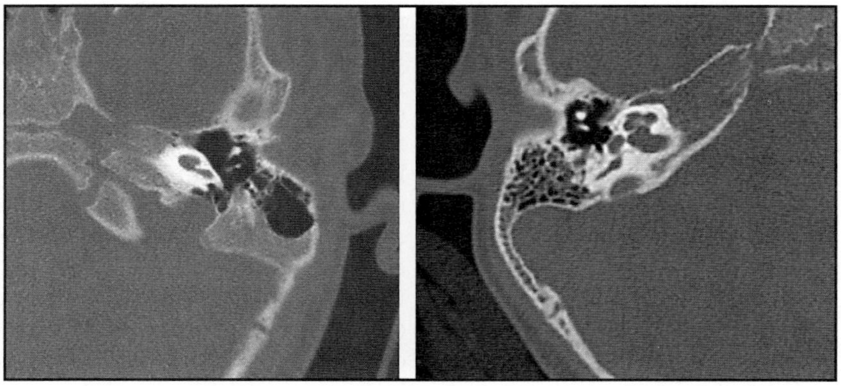

FIGURE 8–4. Cochlear hypoplasia (small cochlea) on the left as compared to normal on the right.

ous system that are evident on imaging. Dandy-Walker syndrome is a congenital, developmental abnormality involving the cerebellum and posterior cranial fossa. The key features of this syndrome are enlargement of the fourth ventricle, a partial or complete absence of the cerebellar vermis, and cyst formation near the base of the skull. An increase in the size of the fluid spaces surrounding the brain as well as an

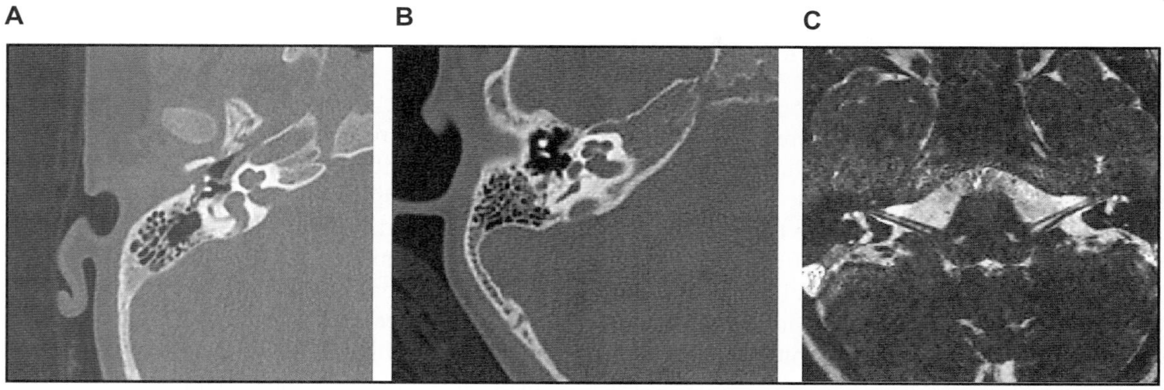

FIGURE 8–5. Mondini malformation (cochlear dysplasia, large vestibule, small horizontal canal and enlarged vestibular aqueduct) as seen on HRCT **(A)**, and MRI **(C)**. A normal HRCT is shown in **(B)** for comparison.

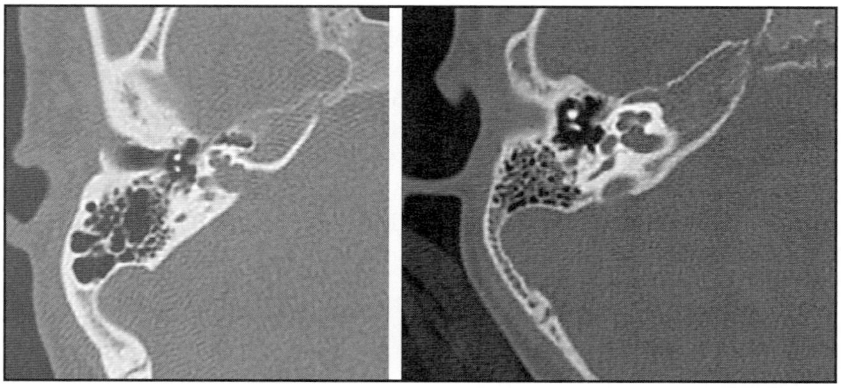

FIGURE 8–6. Cochlear dysplasia (modiolus deficiency) on the left from X-linked stapes gusher syndrome compared to normal on the right.

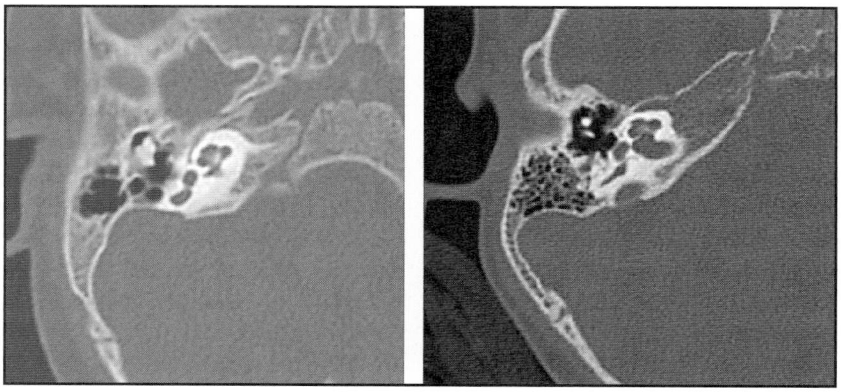

FIGURE 8–7. Vestibular aplasia (*left*) and normal inner ear (*right*).

increase in pressure may also be present (Parisi & Dobyns, 2003). Congenital CMV may result in microcephaly and/or cerebral calcifications and gliosis, which can be prominent in the temporal lobes. However, imaging findings can be difficult to distinguish from other viral infections of the central nervous system (Baskin & Hedlund, 2007). Meningitis from a variety of organisms can acutely result in varying degrees of brain edema, infarction, hydrocephalus, subdural pathology and brain abscess that commonly leads to gliosis (Jan et al., 2003). Inner ear involvement by inflammation and infection can result in labyrinthine obstruction from fibrosis and ultimate neo-ossification (Young, Hughes, Byrd, & Darling, 2000). Children with neurofibromatosis type II can have bilateral acoustic neruomas that can present very early in life as well. In children born prematurely, radiographic sequelae from intraventricular hemorrhages and hydrocephalus can occur. Moreover, children with kernicterus and associated auditory neuropathy/dyssynchrony (AN/AD) resulting from hyperbilirubinemia frequently have changes in the basal ganglia secondary to bilirubin staining (Katar, Akay, Taskesen, & Devecioglu, 2008).

In addition to changes in the brain, anatomic deficiency of the cochlear nerve can be identified on MRI (Adunka et al., 2006, 2007; Buchman et al., 2006; Roche, Huang, Bassim, Adunka, & Buchman, 2010). While this disorder was originally described in children with inner ear malformations and very narrow IACs on HRCT, it has more recently been identified in children with normal inner ears and IACs. Moreover, it has been associated with a variety of conditions such as CHARGE and VATER and can present in ears with electrophysiological evidence of AN/AD on ABR testing. Figure 8–8 shows such an example (Adunka et al., 2006, 2007; Buchman et al., 2006; Roche et al., 2010).

Laboratory Assessment

Laboratory assessment is dictated, in part, by the patient's presenting situation. For children who have failed a newborn screening and have undergone confirmatory testing that documents a SNHL, testing might include:

1. electrocardiogram (EKG) for Jervell and Lange-Nielsen syndrome;
2. Guthrie card polymerase chain reaction (PCR) for CMV infection;
3. connexin 26 and 30 mutation testing;
4. Venereal Disease Research Laboratory (VDRL; syphilis);
5. erythrocyte sedimentation rate (ESR), complete blood count (CBC);
6. rheumatoid factor (RF), antinuclear cytoplasmic antibody (ANCA), antinuclear antibody (ANA), anticardiolipin antibody;
7. renal ultrasound (BOR) and urinalysis (Alport's);
8. eye examination/electroretinography (Usher).

In general, an EKG, CMV assessment, and connexin testing are offered to all families while an eye examination with an ophthalmologist should be considered. Although the Jervell and Lange-Nielsen syndrome is exceedingly rare, a properly performed EKG can identify some cases. Since there are treatments for this disorder that can be life saving, this simple and cheap test appears justified for all children with SNHL (Morton & Nance, 2006). For Usher's syndrome, the hearing loss usually presents prior to the onset of visual changes making detection as an infant difficult without an electroretinography (ERG). The VDRL is offered to families of children that have been adopted, where the background of the parents might be unknown or when a concern regarding syphilis exists. Tests listed in #5 and 6 (above) are considered in older children or adults with progressive hearing loss when autoimmune disorders might occur. Finally, the renal ultrasound is used in children with the clinical stigma of BOR where pits, ear tags, and microtia/atresia exist. Routine screening for Alport's currently is not carried out as the proteinuria/hematuria usually occurs later (Morton & Nance, 2006).

Protocol Variation: Auditory Neuropathy/Dyssynchrony (AN/AD)

AN/AD is a clinical syndrome characterized by the presence of OAEs and/or cochlear microphonics (CM) suggesting normal hair cell function in conjunction with absent or grossly abnormal ABRs (Starr, Picton, Sininger, Hood, & Berlin, 1996). AN/AD is thought to account for up to 10% of newly diagnosed cases of hearing loss in children (Madden, Rutter, Hilbert, Greinwald, & Choo, 2002). Less than 10% of AN/AD cases are thought to involve only one ear. With bilateral presentation, patients exhibit a wide range of auditory capabilities. Hearing thresholds for pure tone detection can range from normal to profound levels (Madden et al., 2002; Rance, Cone-Wesson, Wunderlich, & Dowell, 2002). Recent studies in older children and adults suggest that these patients' perceptual abilities can be severely impaired for both pitch discrimination

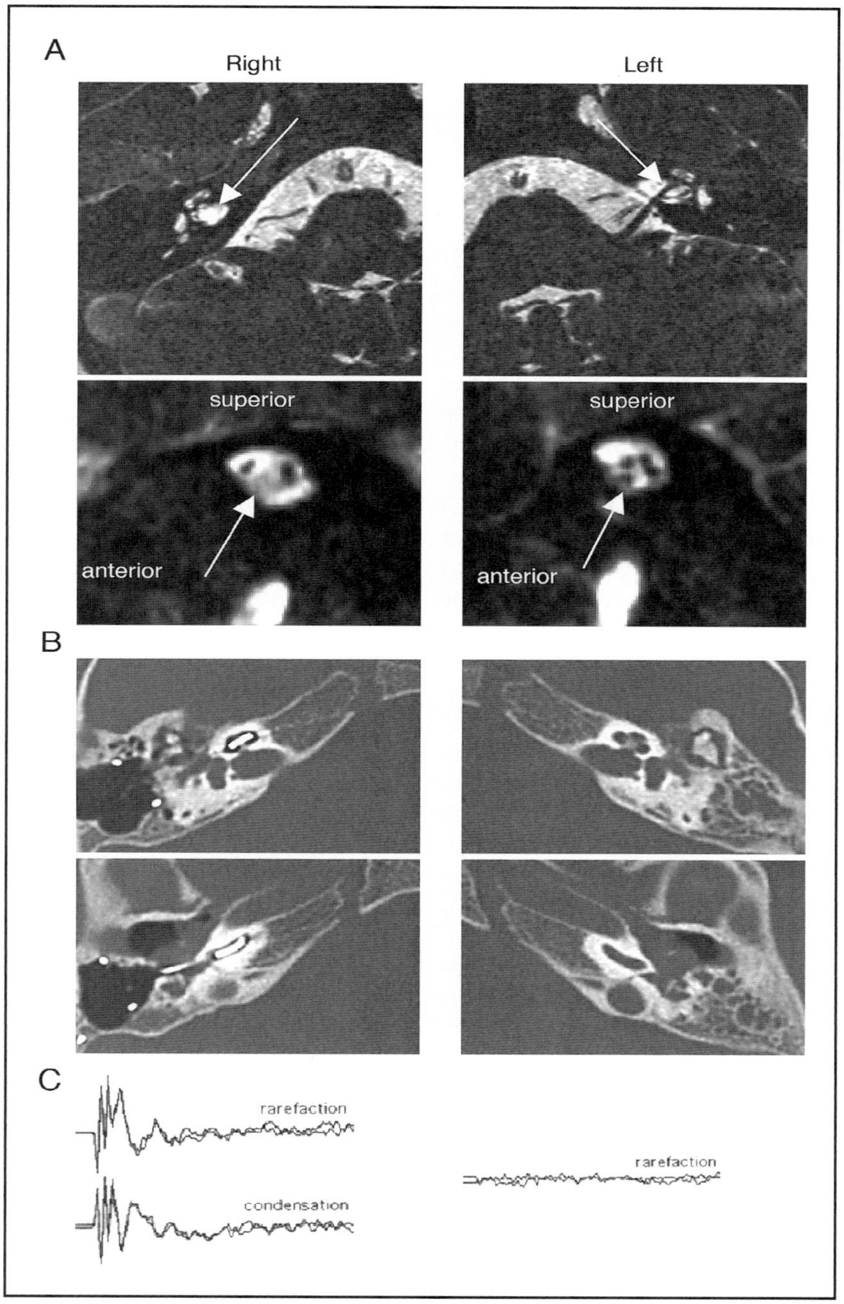

FIGURE 8–8. Cochlear nerve deficiency (*right ear*) in a child that experienced sudden hearing loss. MRI **(A)** shows axial and parasaggital reconstructed images in a plane perpendicular to the IAC. In the left ear, four nerves (superior and inferior vestibular, facial and cochlear) are well-visualized. In the right ear, the cochlear nerve is absent. The arrow points to the normal cochlear nerve on the left and the region of the absent cochlear nerve on the right. HRCT **(B)** shows normal inner ear morphology and a satisfactorily placed cochlear implant in the ear without a cochlear nerve. The ABR shows a distinct cochlear microphonic in the right ear and no response in the ear with a normal nerve. The cochlear implant in the right ear provided limited perceptual abilities and left cochlear implantation resulted in normal, open-set speech perception.

in the low frequencies as well as temporal processing tasks (Rance, McKay, & Grayden, 2004; Zeng, Kong, Michalewski, & Starr, 2005). It has been hypothesized that lesions in the inner hair cells, the synapse between the inner hair cell and the auditory nerve, and the auditory nerve itself may account for the clinical findings (Berlin, Morlet, & Hood, 2003; Berlin, Hood, Morlet, Rose, & Brashears, 2003; Fuchs, Glowatzki, & Moser, 2003; Starr et al., 1996).

The etiology of AN/AD appears to be multifactorial. Rather than a single lesion, it is plausible that the AN/AD phenotype can result from a variety of lesions throughout the auditory pathway. Mutations in a number of genes (*MPZ, NDRG1, PMP22, OTOF, AUNA1*) have now been characterized in hereditary cases of AN/AD (Varga et al., 2006). Associations have also been made between infectious (measles, mumps), metabolic (diabetes, hyperbilirubinemia, hypoxia), and neoplastic processes (acoustic neuroma), as well as prematurity (Rance et al., 1999; Starr et al., 2001). In most children with AN/AD, the cochlear nerve is known to be anatomically present because residual hearing abilities exist. Many of these affected individuals have varying levels of pure tone thresholds with disproportionately poor speech perception abilities. Since some children with AN/AD who have received cochlear implants have had robust electrically-evoked intracochlear compound action potentials (ECAPs) and good performance (Buss et al., 2002; Madden et al., 2002; Mason, De Michele, Stevens, Ruth, & Hashisaki, 2003), the abnormal hearing that some of these children have is thought to be due to disordered signal transduction at the inner hair cells, hair cell-dendrite synapse, or the cochlear neurons (i.e., auditory dys-synchrony; Berlin, Hood, Morlet, Rose, & Brashears, 2003; Berlin, Morlet, & Hood, 2003; Fuchs et al., 2003; Starr et al., 1996).

Opinions regarding management of children with AN/AD vary widely. When hearing loss has been documented, conservative amplification has been proposed (Rance et al., 2002). On the contrary, other investigators believe that the distorted speech perception abilities resulting from AN/AD precludes effective use of amplification (Berlin, Hood, Morlet, Rose, & Brashears, 2003). Regarding the utility of cochlear implantation in children with AN/AD, limited data have demonstrated efficacy in many cases, implying that electrical stimulation may restore neural synchrony in some of these patients (Buss et al., 2002; Madden et al., 2002; Mason et al., 2003; Peterson et al., 2003; Sininger & Trautwein, 2002).

At University of North Carolina-Chapel Hill, we established a prospective, institutional review board (IRB)-approved protocol five years ago to study the clinical characteristics and outcomes of children with newly identified AN/AD. The protocol was based on the premise that children with AN/AD can have a diversity of clinical characteristics and auditory abilities, suggesting that some might benefit from certain interventions while others may not. We believed that some children with AN/AD might have severely distorted perceptual abilities, as described above, while others may not. Thus, we chose to approach children with AN/AD individually, assessing their perceptual abilities with and without amplification prior to considering cochlear implantation. Although this assessment and management paradigm sounds remarkably similar to that previously described for children without AN/AD, some modifications were made in an attempt to better understand each child's perceptual abilities prior to instituting amplification or cochlear implantation. This management paradigm has been discussed in previous publications (Teagle et al., 2010; Zdanski, Buchman, Roush, Teagle, & Brown, 2006).

In our program, when a child is identified with the electrophysiological characteristics of AN/AD, the parents are told that their child has clear evidence of an auditory disorder. We also tell them that we cannot predict their child's auditory thresholds or speech perceptual abilities, and thus a period of careful observation ensues until an age when auditory thresholds can be determined. With highly experienced audiologists, thresholds are usually attainable using visual reinforcement audiometry (VRA) around 7 to 9 months corrected age. Should VRA demonstrate a significant hearing loss, a trial of amplification is instituted, based on real ear measures and Desired Sensation Level (DSL) targets (Scollie et al., 2005; see Chapter 25 for additional information). Should amplification prove fruitless in the setting of ongoing diagnostic and therapeutic speech and language therapy, cochlear implantation is then considered. While this protocol does result in minor delays, we believe the approach is justified, so that children who can benefit from amplification are identified and inappropriate cochlear implantation is avoided.

In multiply handicapped children, VRA can frequently be impossible to obtain. For these children and their families, as well as the clinicians who care for them, rehabilitative decision-making can be very difficult (see Chapter 36 for additional information).

We currently are following approximately 185 children with AN/AD, all of whom had diagnostic electrophysiological testing carried out at our institution similar to that described previously. What is clear from looking at this group of children is that AN/AD is a very heterogeneous group of disorders that presents with a common electrophysiological profile. Some children are profoundly affected by global and progressive neurological disease while others are otherwise completely normal. Some children have a genetic form that is similar among affected siblings whereas others have an association with prematurity, a stay in the NICU, hyperbilirubinemia, and so forth. When behavioral audiometry becomes possible, some children have near normal pure tone thresholds while others have a profound hearing loss. Following identification of pure tone thresholds, some children benefit from appropriately fitted amplification similar to those children with "typical sensorineural hearing loss" whereas others go on to cochlear implantation. Most of the children who have gone on to cochlear implantation have had a severe to profound hearing loss and have met criteria for implantation based on conventional parameters. Very few children with AN/AD and less than a severe to profound hearing loss have received implants at our institution. Of this very select group of children with substantial residual hearing and AN/AD, decision-making on their behalf was very challenging for both the families and clinicians. In general, cochlear implantation has been very successful for most children with AN/AD, although exceptions do exist. One group of children that provided significant insight into this disorder was that with anatomic cochlear nerve deficiency as detailed above (Buchman et al., 2006; Roche et al., 2010).

Medical Management of Hearing Loss in Children

The medical intervention for children with hearing loss depends on the type of hearing loss (conductive, sensorineural, mixed) and the functional-anatomic (or pathologic) correlations that exist. Moreover, the desires and wishes of the family and child (in older children) are paramount. Patients and families not committed or interested in auditory-oral communication are by no means coerced into hearing restorative interventions unless medical necessity dictates such treatment. Although the details of every medical intervention for every type of hearing loss are beyond the scope of this work, some generalizations can be made that may act as a rough guide for families and professionals.

Behavioral Audiometry

In our program, behavioral audiometric testing continues to form the backbone for decision-making when medical/surgical intervention is being contemplated for a child. The shortcomings of both ABR and ASSR have been detailed previously. Although these tests are clearly useful for estimating initial thresholds for the purposes of fitting amplification, the published literature and our experiences suggest that they are not precise enough for making decisions regarding irreversible procedures. Specifically, as cochlear implantation usually results in a loss of the native or residual hearing, we believe that an ear-specific behavioral audiogram using VRA is essential prior to considering cochlear implantation or other major ear interventions, although rare exceptions exist.

Hearing restorative medical interventions can be broadly classified into those that are disease-specific or those that are not disease-specific. Some examples of interventions that are not disease-specific include referral for hearing aid evaluation and fitting or surgical placement of hearing devices such as cochlear implants, bone conduction devices, or auditory brainstem implants.

Cochlear implants are reserved for those children with a severe-to-profound sensorineural hearing loss (> 90 dB) in the presence of an anatomically intact cochlea and cochlear nerve. These children should also be enrolled in an educational program committed to an auditory-oral approach and demonstrate limited progress with speech and language development while using appropriately fitted amplification (http://www.nidcd.nih.gov/health/hearing/coch.asp). As the hearing loss is severe to profound, high-gain amplification is required and these devices must be fitted using real ear measurements and according to DSL targets for prescribed hearing aid performance (Scollie et al., 2005). In addition to the auditory and speech criteria listed above, participation in such a program requires significant commitment by family members. In the best scenario, children are identified following birth by a newborn infant hearing screening program. Following verification in the first month of life, the diagnosis is confirmed by way of electrophysiological testing methods described above and the trial of amplification is instituted. At the same time, the child is followed by a trained speech-language pathologist with experience in auditory-oral approaches. By 6 to 9 months of age, behavioral audiometry confirms the degree of hearing loss, and the therapist can provide feedback regarding auditory awareness and the development of the earliest vocalizations such as canonical babbling. When progress is evident, continued observation and therapy occurs. Conversely, when the child is making limited progress, cochlear implantation is considered with the goal of getting the device implanted around the end of the first year of life (see Figure 8–2). Factors that might delay cochlear implantation beyond the first year of life include: (1) delayed or inaccurate diagnosis, (2) delayed, underfitted, or nonuse of prescribed amplification, (3) lack of or inappropriate participation in a speech/language therapy trial, (4) medical comorbidities that delay diagnosis or preclude surgical intervention, (5) severe motor or cognitive developmental delays that hinder accurate auditory assessment, (6) diagnosis of AN/AD, and (7) lack of commitment by the family. Later ages at implantation are also expected in children with progressive hearing loss, since these children achieve the severe-to-profound benchmark later in life and usually have better speech and language development because of their residual hearing.

Cochlear implant surgery takes roughly 90 minutes to 2 hours to perform at our institution. Following placement, intraoperative electrical telemetry is used to interrogate the device for integrity and to roughly estimate a starting point for programming in the postoperative period. Although complications are possible, they remain very unusual (Francis et al., 2008). Most children are implanted on an outpatient basis with anesthesia provided by a pediatric anesthesiologist. The children wear a head bandage for 3 to 5 days and return for a check approximately 1 week postoperatively. The device is usually activated 3 to 4 weeks postoperatively.

Outcomes following cochlear implantation in children are truly remarkable. Most children demonstrate significant closed-set (using visual cues) speech perception ability after one year of usage. Open-set (without visual cues) speech perception skills are usually evident after 2 to 3 years of device experience. Figure 8–9 demonstrates the results of open-set speech perception testing using the phonetically-balanced kindergarten (PBK; Haskins 1949) word test for a group of 315 prelinguistic children implanted in our program as a function of years of implant usage and age at implantation. It is evident from the graph that earlier implantation is better for developing this skill.

Are bilateral cochlear implants better than unilateral implants in children? Recent evidence suggests that binaural implantation in postlinguistically deafened adults provides significant improvements for hearing in noise and sound localization abilities (Buss et al., 2008; Grantham, Ashmead, Ricketts, Labadie, & Haynes, 2007). In children, the data are only recently starting to emerge, but similar conclusions seem evident (Litovsky et al., 2006; Peters, Litovsky, Parkinson,

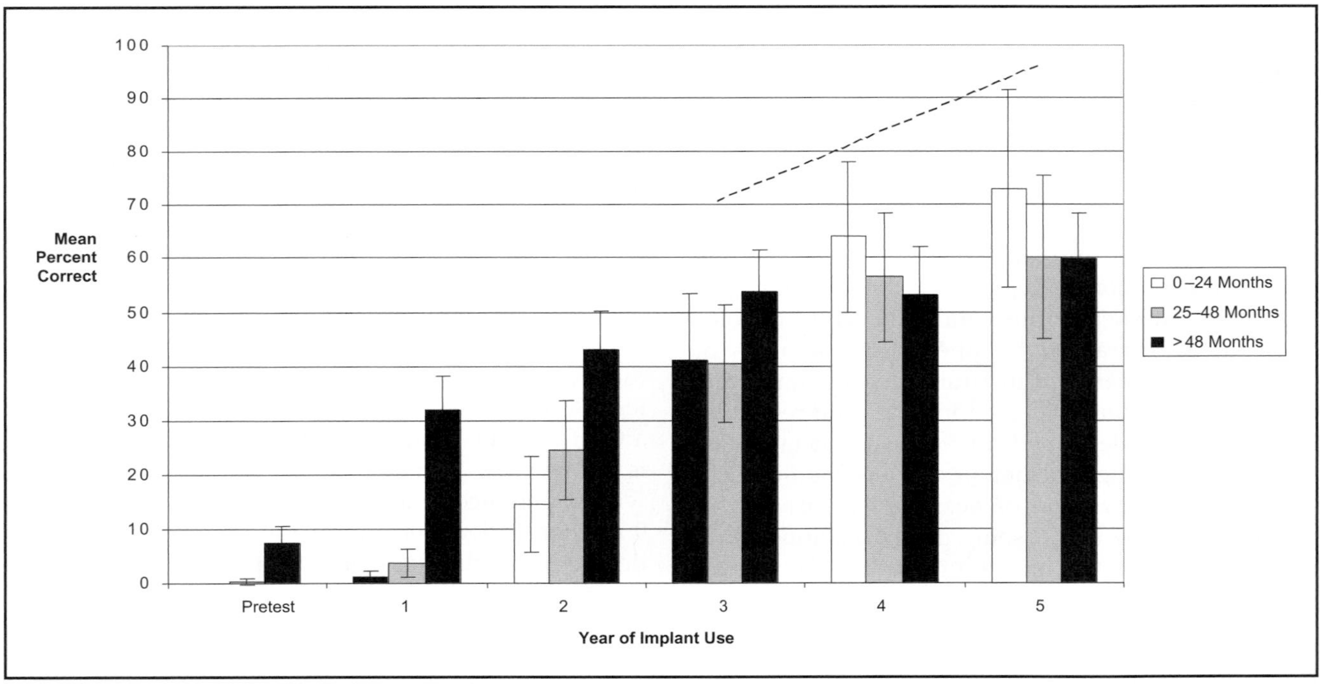

FIGURE 8–9. Phonetically balanced kindergarten (PBK) word scores as a function of duration of implant usage by age at implantation for 315 children with prelinguistic hearing loss. The dashed line indicates the scores for a group of children with normal hearing. In general, children implanted earlier ultimately achieve better scores at an earlier age than those children implanted later in life.

& Lake, 2007). Only further research will determine whether there is a critical time window for developing these binaural skills in prelinguistic infants. Whether binaural implants will allow children to develop speech and language faster and to a higher level remains the critical unanswered question. What is clear regarding binaural implantation is that having a second device provides a backup should there be trouble with the equipment in one ear. Should the device problems require surgery, having the backup or second side device will prevent unwanted time "off the air."

Recent evidence suggests that children with sensorineural hearing loss with or without cochlear implants are at a higher risk for developing bacterial meningitis than the population in general (Biernath et al., 2006; Parner et al., 2007). It does appear from these data that cochlear implants impart an additional risk for contracting meningitis beyond that of having hearing loss alone. Although the factors responsible for this increased risk have not been completely elucidated, one particular model of cochlear implant device that used a separate electrode positioner was implicated as predisposing to meningitis at a much greater rate than other models. This model has been removed from the market. The findings of these studies also prompted the U.S. Food and Drug Administration (FDA) and the Centers for Disease Control and Prevention (CDC) to recommend routine vaccination against the common bacteria implicated in cases of meningitis for all cochlear implantees. Thus, *Streptococcus pneumoniae* (i.e., pneumococcus) and *Hemophilus influenzae* type B vaccination are indicated in all children with cochlear implants. The pneumococcal vaccines include the heptavalent conjugate vaccine (Prevnar®, Wyeth, Madison NJ) for children less than age 2 years and the 23-valent polysaccharide vaccine (Pneumovax®, Merck & Co, Whitehouse Station, NJ) after age 2 years and again five years later (before age 10). The precise recommendations of the CDC and FDA vaccine programs are available on their website. Currently, this is required prior to cochlear implantation in all children and adults in our program.

Implantable bone conduction devices are used in children when significant conductive or mixed hearing loss exists and direct reconstruction of the hearing apparatus is either not feasible or not desired. This is relatively common in children with unilateral or poorly developed aural atresia. The current U.S. FDA-approved system for this application is the bone anchored hearing aid (Baha®; Cochlear Corp. Englewood, CO, USA). It is based on the concept of implanting an osseointegrated fixture into the skull to provide direct access to bone conduction of sound without the detrimental effects of soft tissue attenuation by the scalp. Low gain amplification via osteo-oscillation is highly effective and very well tolerated. Implicit in the placement of such an implant is the need for a percutaneous connection, thus skin tolerance issues can be significant. Moreover, the skull of young children can be very thin precluding effective osseointegration. The BAHA is approved for use in children after age 5 years and is possible when skull thickness is sufficient (> 3 to 4 mm). A preoperative CT scan can be useful in assessing skull thickness. The operation takes approximately 1 hour to perform and is usually outpatient surgery, although in children the operation is frequently performed in two stages. The device must heal for roughly 3 months prior to activation. It can be expected to provide auditory detection in the range of the bone conduction thresholds present on preoperative audiometric testing. The binaural benefits are only now becoming evident in congenitally affected patients (Kunst et al., 2008).

Auditory brainstem implants (ABIs) are currently only approved for usage in the U.S. for children with cochlear nerve deficiency resulting from neurofibromatosis type II (NF2). Although the initial results of ABIs in children without NF2 are interesting, further data regarding the risks and potential benefits are needed (Colletti, 2007).

Certain ear diseases that result in hearing loss can or must be addressed by way of disease-specific treatment of the underlying disorder. Examples of these disorders include: otitis externa and otitis media, congenital ossicular malformations and atresia, sensorineural hearing losses resulting from inflammatory conditions, and tumors of the temporal bone and brain.

Otitis externa is defined as inflammation of the external auditory canal and commonly results from bacterial or fungal infection. The hallmark signs and symptoms of this disorder are pain with auricular motion, minimal discharge, and conductive hearing loss when canal swelling is substantial. These findings should prompt a visit to a physician with experience treating ear disorders. It may follow ear canal trauma or contamination, such as that which occurs from swimming pools or bathtubs. In some instances, a poorly fitted hearing aid mold might cause pressure on the ear canal skin, thereby predisposing to infection. Treatment requires removal of the offending agent (foreign body or hearing aid ear mold) when present and application of an otic drop preparation containing either an acidifying or antimicrobial agent. When skin infection occurs outside of the ear canal, involving the pinna or surrounding soft tissues, an oral antimicrobial agent is also indicated. Patients with an immunocompromised state need to be treated particularly aggressively to prevent systemic infection and complications. Prevention in recurrent cases can usually be accomplished through careful cleaning and drying of hearing aid molds, removal of ear canal wax buildup, and prophylactic usage of drying agents (e.g., 50:50 mix of white vinegar and isopropyl alcohol) when the tympanic membrane is known to be intact (Buchman & Wambach, 2002).

Otitis media is a primary inflammation of the middle ear space and commonly results from a bacterial and/or viral infection. Otitis media represents the most common ailment following the common cold for which a child will visit the doctor's office with a peak occurrence between the ages of 6 months and 2 years. Otitis media is commonly associated with episodes of upper respiratory tract infection and thus, day care is a significant risk factor (Buchman & Das, 2003). The signs and symptoms of otitis media include some degree of conductive hearing loss with or without associated ear pain, fever, nausea, irritability, cold symptoms, and ear drainage if the tympanic membrane has ruptured. During episodes, fluid is evident behind the intact tympanic membrane and signs of inflammation might be present. While the natural resolution rate is high, treatment is instituted to resolve pain more quickly, clear middle ear fluid, and prevent complications that at times can be severe and life threatening. Treatment of acute otitis media requires an oral antimicrobial agent and analgesics with follow up to insure the clearance of middle ear fluid. In otherwise uncomplicated cases, persistent middle ear fluid can take more than 3 months to resolve. Thus, associated conductive hearing loss should be expected. Tympanostomy tubes are considered for middle ear ventilation and drainage in an effort to decrease or eliminate the duration and severity of otitis media episodes, as well as to treat fluid related hearing loss. Tympanostomy tubes are not routinely indicted for otherwise healthy children unless middle ear fluid persists for a prolonged period (> 3–4 months) and is associated with significant hearing loss (> 30 dB) or when the severity of otitis media episodes are severe and disabling. However, when children have other associated communication disorders such as permanent hearing loss, developmental delays in speech and language, craniofacial disorders, immune system disorders, or anatomic changes in the tympanic membrane that can predispose to complications, tube placement is considered earlier (Paradise & Bluestone, 2005).

Congenital conductive hearing loss can occur as a result of an isolated ossicular malformation or when external auditory canal atresia is present. For children with an isolated conductive loss with otherwise normal ear findings, stapes fixation represents the most common form of the disorder. Management of these children as infants is similar to those children with sensorineural hearing loss. That is, thresholds are determined and amplification is fitted as early as possible. When an ear canal lumen is not present bilaterally, a bone conduction hearing aid is applied to take advantage of the excellent speech discrimination abilities that these children usually have. When the child is older, reconstructive surgical options versus BAHA can be considered.

For a child with a congenital conductive hearing loss, a nonspecific approach to the restoration of audition in the affected ear includes implantation of the BAHA device as described above (Kunst et al., 2008). For some families and children, the necessity for a percutaneous connector is unacceptable. Some payors will also not support this intervention because the price is considered prohibitive.

Another option for children with congenital conductive hearing loss is direct, surgical reconstruction. For the ear with an intact external auditory canal, this can be accomplished either through the canal or from a postauricular approach. When stapes fixation is identified, a stapedectomy or stapedotomy is possible with excellent hearing results anticipated. When the malleus or incus is involved, hearing outcomes may be slightly worse. Prior to considering middle ear exploration for congenital conductive hearing loss, preoperative imaging is needed to rule out an inner ear malformation that might predispose to intraoperative cerebrospinal fluid leakage and further hearing loss. This usually occurs around the age of 8 or older (Welling, Merrell, Merz, & Dodson, 2003).

Reconstruction can also be considered for children with external auditory canal atresia. Indications for this procedure might include: (1) bilateral involvement, (2) the presence of a developmental temporal bone cholesteatoma in the affected ear, or (3) when observation or the BAHA is unacceptable to the family for the previously mentioned reasons. This procedure is major otological surgery and requires a very cooperative patient in the postoperative period. The operation can take more than 4 hours and requires, in addition to an ear incision, a split thickness skin graft harvested from a site other than the head or neck (such as the leg or arm). Atresiaplasty is usually carried out after the time when the associated microtia surgery has been performed. Thus, most children undergo this surgery after the age of 7 or 8 years.

The results of atresiaplasty are quite variable and are dependent on the operating surgeon's experience, the healing of the patient, and the patient's anatomy.

In general, roughly 75% of patients achieve a postoperative air bone gap of less than 30 dB. In those with a patent ear canal that is dry, a conventional hearing aid is also possible, thereby obviating the need for a bone conductor (McKinnon & Jahrsdoerfer, 2002).

Inner ear malformations are present in 20 to 30% of children with congenital sensorineural hearing loss. These children can present in a variety of ways. Although most will fail a newborn screen, some may not. Children with these anomalies clearly have a higher incidence of progressive hearing loss. It has been posited that sudden drops in hearing may be related to minor degrees of head trauma in these children. Many of these children will ultimately go on to cochlear implantation, which has a number of special considerations in this population (Buchman et al., 2004).

Although there currently is no available method to repair developmental anomalies of the inner ear, a few facts are important for managing these children. First, it important for families to recognize that progressive hearing loss is common in these children. Moreover, children with inner ear malformations are at a higher risk for developing meningitis than children without malformations. Families need to be educated regarding the signs and symptoms of meningitis and about aggressive treatment of otitis media. In this regard, these children should also be considered for preventive vaccination similar to those children with cochlear implants. Finally, because of the association of sudden hearing changes and head trauma in these children, families are cautioned regarding the participation in contact sports and activities.

Acknowledgments. We would like to thank those individuals who work with us on a daily basis, to provide care for the hearing-impaired children that we are so privileged to serve. Their efforts are no less than spectacular. I would especially like to acknowledge Patricia Roush, Corrine Macpherson, Sarah Martinho, Paula Johnson, Jill Rich, Marcia Adunka, Holly Teagle, Carolyn Brown, Lisa DiMaria, Jennifer Woodard, Deborah Hatch, Hannah Eskridge, Tom Page, Jori Thomas, and BJ Squires for their caring efforts and diligence.

References

Adunka, O. F., Jewells, V., & Buchman, C. A. (2007). Value of computed tomography in the evaluation of children with cochlear nerve deficiency. *Otology and Neurotology, 28*(5), 597–604.

Adunka, O. F., Roush, P. A., Teagle, H. F., Brown, C. J., Zdanski, C. J., Jewells, V., & Buchman, C. A. (2006). Internal auditory canal morphology in children with cochlear nerve deficiency. *Otology and Neurotology, 27*(6), 793–801.

Ahn, J. H., Lee, H. S., Kim, Y. J., Yoon, T. H., & Chung, J. W. (2007). Comparing pure-tone audiometry and auditory steady state response for the measurement of hearing loss. *Otolaryngology-Head and Neck Surgery, 136*(6), 966–971.

American Academy of Pediatrics and Joint Committee on Infant Hearing. (2007). Year 2007 position statement: Principles and guidelines for early hearing detection and intervention programs. *Pediatrics, 120*(4), 898–921.

Baskin, H. J., & Hedlund, G. (2007). Neuroimaging of herpesvirus infections in children. *Pediatric Radiology, 37*(10), 949–963.

Berlin, C. I., Hood, L., Morlet, T., Rose, K., & Brashears, S. (2003). Auditory neuropathy/dys-synchrony: Diagnosis and management. *Mental Retardation and Developmental Disability Research and Reviews, 9*(4), 225–231.

Berlin, C. I., Morlet, T., & Hood, L. J. (2003). Auditory neuropathy/dyssynchrony: Its diagnosis and management. *Pediatric Clinics of North America, 50*(2), 331–340.

Biernath, K. R., Reefhuis, J., Whitney, C. G., Mann, E. A., Costa, P., Eichwald, J., & Boyle, C. (2006). Bacterial meningitis among children with cochlear implants beyond 24 months after implantation. *Pediatrics, 117*(2), 284–289.

Buchman, C. A., Copeland, B. J., Yu, K. K., Brown, C. J., Carrasco, V. N., & Pillsbury H. C. III. (2004). Cochlear implantation in children with congenital inner ear malformations. *Laryngoscope, 114*(2), 309–316.

Buchman, C. A., & Das, S. (2003). Prevention of acute otitis media during the common cold. In Alper, Bluestone, Casselbrant, Dohar, & Mandel (Eds.), *Advanced therapy of otitis media* (pp. 152–157). Ontario, Canada: BC Decker.

Buchman, C. A., Roush, P. A., Teagle, H. F., Brown, C. J., Zdanski, C. J., & Grose, J. H. (2006). Auditory neuropathy characteristics in children with cochlear nerve deficiency. *Ear and Hearing, 27*(4), 399–408.

Buchman, C. A., & Wambach, B. A. (2002). Otitis externa. In R. E. Rakel & E. T. Bope (Eds.), *Conn's current therapy* (pp. 114–117). Philadelphia, PA: W.B. Saunders Co.

Buss, E., Labadie, R., Brown, C., Gross, A., Grose, J., & Pillsbury, H. (2002). Outcome of cochlear implantation in pediatric auditory neuropathy. *Otology and Neurotology, 23*, 328–332.

Buss, E., Pillsbury, H. C., Buchman, C. A., Pillsbury, C. H., Clark, M. S., Haynes, D. S., . . . Barco, A. L. (2008). Multicenter U.S. bilateral MED-EL cochlear implantation study: Speech perception over the first year of use. *Ear and Hearing, 29*(1), 20–32.

Centers for Disease Control and Prevention. (2006). *Continued risk of bacterial meningitis in children with cochlear implants with a positioner beyond twenty-four months post-implantation.* Retrieved May 16, 2010, from www.fda.gov/cdrh/safety/101007-cochlear.html

Colletti, L. (2007). Beneficial auditory and cognitive effects of auditory brainstem implantation in children. *Acta Otolaryngologica, 127*(9), 943–946.

Coticchia, J. M., Gokhale, A., Waltonen, J., & Sumer, B. (2006). Characteristics of sensorineural hearing loss in children with inner ear anomalies. *American Journal of Otolaryngology, 27*(1), 33–38.

Francis, H. W., Buchman, C. A., Visaya, J. M., Wang, N. Y., Zwolan, T. A., Fink, N. E., Niparko, J. K. & The CDaCI Investigative Team. (2008). Surgical factors in pediatric cochlear implantation and their early effects on electrode activation and functional outcomes. *Otology and Neurotology, 29*(4), 502–508.

Fuchs, P. A., Glowatzki, E., & Moser, T. (2003). The afferent synapse of cochlear hair cells. *Current Opinion in Neurobiology, 13*(4), 452–458.

Gorga, M. P., Johnson, T. A., Kaminski, J. R., Beauchaine, K. L., Garner, C. A., & Neely, S. T. (2006). Using a combination of click- and tone burst-evoked auditory brain stem response measurements to estimate pure-tone thresholds. *Ear and Hearing, 27*(1), 60–74.

Gorga, M. P., Neely, S. T., Hoover, B. M., Dierking, D. M., Beauchaine, K. L., & Manning, C. (2004). Determining the upper limits of stimulation for auditory steady-state response measurements. *Ear and Hearing, 25*(3), 302–307.

Grantham, D. W., Ashmead, D. H., Ricketts, T. A., Labadie, R. F., & Haynes, D. S. (2007). Horizontal-plane localization of noise and speech signals by postlingually deafened adults fitted with bilateral cochlear implants. *Ear and Hearing, 28*(4), 524–541.

Harrison, M., Roush, J., & Wallace, J. (2003). Trends in age of identification and intervention in infants with hearing loss. *Ear and Hearing, 24*(1), 89–95.

Haskins, H. (1949). *A phonetically balanced test of speech discrimination for children.* Unpublished master's thesis. Evanston, IL: Northwestern University.

Jan, W., Zimmerman, R. A., Bilaniuk, L. T., Hunter, J. V., Simon, E. M., & Haselgrove, J. (2003). Diffusion-weighted imaging in acute bacterial meningitis in infancy. *Neuroradiology, 45*(9), 634–639.

Katar, S., Akay, H. O., Taskesen, M., & Devecioglu, C. (2008). Clinical and cranial magnetic resonance imaging (MRI) findings of 21 patients with serious hyperbilirubinemia. *Journal of Child Neurology, 23*(4), 415–417.

Kunst, S. J., Leijendeckers, J. M., Mylanus, E. A., Hol, M. K., Snik, A. F., & Cremers, C. W. (2008). Bone-anchored hearing aid system application for unilateral congenital conductive hearing impairment: Audiometric results. *Otology and Neurotology, 29*(1), 2–7.

Litovsky, R. Y., Johnstone, P. M., Godar, S., Agrawal, S., Parkinson, A., Peters, R., & Lake, J. (2006). Bilateral cochlear implants in children: Localization acuity measured with minimum audible angle. *Ear and Hearing, 27*(1), 43–59.

Madden, C., Rutter, M., Hilbert, L., Greinwald, J. H. Jr., & Choo, D. I. (2002). Clinical and audiological features in auditory neuropathy. *Archives Otolaryngology-Head and Neck Surgery, 128*(9), 1026–1030.

Mason, J. C., De Michele, A., Stevens, C., Ruth, R. A., & Hashisaki, G. T. (2003). Cochlear implantation in patients with auditory neuropathy of varied etiologies. *Laryngoscope, 113*(1), 45–49.

McKinnon, B. J., & Jahrsdoerfer, R. A. (2002). Congenital auricular atresia: Update on options for intervention and timing of repair. *Otolaryngologic Clinics of North America, 35*(4), 877–890.

Moog, J. S., & Geers, A. E. (2003). Epilogue: Major findings, conclusions and implications for deaf education. *Ear and Hearing, 24*(1 Suppl.), 121S–125S.

Morton, C. C., & Nance, W. E. (2006). Newborn hearing screening—a silent revolution. *New England Journal of Medicine, 354*(20), 2151–2164.

Paradise, J. L., & Bluestone, C. D. (2005). Consultation with the specialist: Tympanostomy tubes: A contemporary guide to judicious use. *Pediatric Reviews, 26*(2), 61–66.

Parisi, M. A., & Dobyns, W. B. (2003). Human malformations of the midbrain and hindbrain: Review and proposed classification scheme. *Molecular Genetics and Metabolism, 80*(1–2), 36–53.

Parner, E. T., Reefhuis, J., Schendel, D., Thomsen, J. L., Ovesen, T., & Thorsen, P. (2007). Hearing loss diagnosis followed by meningitis in Danish children, 1995–2004. *Otolaryngology-Head and Neck Surgery, 136*(3), 428–433.

Parry, D. A., Booth, T., & Roland, P. S. (2005). Advantages of magnetic resonance imaging over computed tomography in preoperative evaluation of pediatric cochlear implant candidates. *Otology and Neurotology, 26*(5), 976–982.

Peters, B. R., Litovsky, R., Parkinson, A., & Lake, J. (2007). Importance of age and postimplantation experience on speech perception measures in children with sequential bilateral cochlear implants. *Otology and Neurotology, 28*(5), 649–657.

Peterson, A., Shallop, J., Driscoll, C., Breneman, A., Babb, J., Stoeckel, R., & Fabry, L. (2003). Outcomes of cochlear implantation in children with auditory neuropathy. *Journal of the American Academy of Audiology, 14*(4), 188–201.

Rance, G., Beer, D., Cone-Wesson, B., Shepard, R. K., Dowell, R. C., King, A. M., . . . Clark, G. M. (1999). Clinical findings for a group of infants and young children with auditory neuropathy. *Ear and Hearing, 20*(3), 238–263.

Rance, G., Cone-Wesson, B., Wunderlich, J., & Dowell, R. (2002). Speech perception and cortical event related potentials in children with auditory neuropathy. *Ear and Hearing, 23*(3), 239–253.

Rance, G., McKay, C., & Grayden, D. (2004). Perceptual characterization of children with auditory neuropathy. *Ear and Hearing, 25*(1), 34–46.

Roche, J., Huang, B., Bassim, M., Adunka, O., & Buchman, C. A. (2010). Radiological assessment of children with auditory neuropathy spectrum disorder. *Otology and Neurotology, 31*(5), 780–788.

Schuknecht, H. F. (1993). *Pathology of the ear* (2nd ed.). Philadelphia, PA: Lea and Febiger.

Scollie, S. D., Seewald, R. C., Cornelisse, L. C., Moodie, S. T., Bagatto, M. P., Laurnagaray, D., . . . Pumford, J. M. (2005). The Desired Sensation Level multistage input/output algorithm. *Trends in Amplification, 9*(4), 159–197.

Sininger, Y. S., & Trautwein, P. (2002). Electrical stimulation of the auditory nerve via cochlear implants in patients with auditory neuropathy. *Annals of Otology, Rhinology, and Laryngology Suppl*, *189*, 29–31.

Small S. A., & Stapells D. R. (2004). Artifactual responses when recording auditory steady-state responses. *Ear and Hearing*, *25*(6), 611–623.

Stapells, D. R., Herdman, A., Small, S. A., Dimitrijevic, A., & Hatton, J. (2005). Current status of the auditory steady-state responses for estimating an infant's audiogram. In R. C. Seewald & J. Bamford (Eds.), *A sound foundation through early amplification 2004: Proceedings of the third international conference* (pp. 43–59). Stäfa, Switzerland: Phonak AG.

Starr, A., Picton, T., Sininger, Y., Hood, L., & Berlin, C. (1996). Auditory neuropathy. *Brain*, *119*, 741–753.

Starr, A., Sininger, Y., Nguyen, T., Michalewski, H. J., Oba, S., & Abdala, C. (2001). Cochlear receptor (microphonic and summating potentials, otoacoustic emissions) and auditory pathway (auditory brain stem potentials) activity in auditory neuropathy. *Ear and Hearing*, *22*(2), 91–99.

Teagle, H. F. B., Woodard, J., Hatch, D., Roush, P., Zdanski, C., Buss, E., & Buchman, C. A. (2010). Cochlear implantation for children with auditory neuropathy spectrum disorder. *Ear and Hearing*, *31*(3), 325–335.

Tlumak, A. I., Rubinstein, E., & Durrant, J. D. (2007). Meta-analysis of variables that affect accuracy of threshold estimation via measurement of the auditory steady-state response (ASSR). *International Journal of Audiology*, *46*(11), 692–710.

Trimble, K., Blaser, S., James, A. L., & Papsin, B. C. (2007). Computed tomography and/or magnetic resonance imaging before pediatric cochlear implantation? Developing an investigative strategy. *Otology and Neurotology*, *28*(3), 317–324.

Varga, R., Avenarius, M. R., Kelley, P. M., Keats, B. J., Berlin, C. I., Hood, L. J., . . . Kimberling, W. J. (2006). OTOF mutations revealed by genetic analysis of hearing loss families including a potential temperature sensitive auditory neuropathy allele. *Journal of Medical Genetics*, *43*(7), 576–581.

Welling, D. B., Merrell, J. A., Merz, M., & Dodson, E. E. (2003). Predictive factors in pediatric stapedectomy. *Laryngoscope*, *113*(9), 1515–1519.

Young, N. M., Hughes, C. A., Byrd, S. E., & Darling, C. (2000). Postmeningitic ossification in pediatric cochlear implantation. *Otolaryngology-Head and Neck Surgery*, *122*(2), 183–188.

Zdanski, C. J., Buchman, C. A., Roush, P. A., Teagle, H. F. B., Brown, C. J. (2006). Cochlear implantation in children with auditory neuropathy. *Perspectives on Hearing and Hearing Disorders in Childhood*, *16*(1), 12–20.

Zeng, F. G., Kong, Y. Y., Michalewski, H. J., & Starr, A. (2005). Perceptual consequences of disrupted auditory nerve activity. *Journal of Neurophysiology*, *93*(6), 3050–3063.

III

Auditory Disorders

9

Conductive Hearing Loss in Children: Otitis Media With Effusion and Congenital Impairments

Lisa L. Hunter and Kathleen A. Daly

Introduction

Conductive hearing loss in all its various forms presents as the most common clinical scenario faced on a daily basis by pediatric audiologists, from the newborn period through to adolescence. In the case of an infant presenting for the first time to the audiology clinic, usually on referral from a newborn screening program, it becomes an important diagnostic goal to distinguish between transient and permanent forms of conductive or mixed hearing loss, distinct from sensorineural hearing loss. Congenital, permanent conductive hearing loss also presents a classic genetic quest to distinguish between syndromic and nonsyndromic forms of the disorder. A carefully considered stepwise protocol of diagnostic tests with adequate levels of clinical evidence, as detailed in other chapters within this handbook, can assist audiologists in making the determination about type, degree, and configuration of the hearing loss as early as possible. Coupled with case history information and interdisciplinary consultation by otology, audiology, radiology, pediatrics, neurology, genetics, and orthopedics as indicated, determination of etiology can be made at an earlier age. In the case of the older child (defined as beyond the first 6 months of age and assuming that newborn screening was passed), the question of whether conductive loss is congenital or acquired is generally more clear, and the ubiquitous nature of otitis media with effusion means that most infants and children will present with transient as opposed to permanent conductive hearing loss. In this chapter, we discuss various types of congenital and acquired conductive hearing loss and the underlying epidemiologic, etiologic, diagnostic, and referral implications, taking an international perspective where supportive literature is available.

Congenital Aural Atresia and Microtia

It is important for audiologists to develop the habit of examining a child's pinna for size, shape, landmarks, and position on the head. Each of the features may be directly related to hearing function and to the presence of certain congenital anomalies or syndromes. Figure 9–1 illustrates facial structural landmarks of which one should be aware (after Brent, 2006). Although there are no hard and fast rules for measurement of facial structure, landmarks as classically described by Leonardo da Vinci are still appropriate today. The top of the auricle should line up with the lateral eye brow; the nasal collumella-labial junction should approximately line up with the inferior earlobe; the longitudinal axis of the auricle should be parallel with the nasal dorsum; the infraorbital rim should line up with the superior ear canal, and because the auricle is a paired structure on the face, symmetry is key.

The mildest and most common anomalies are ear tags, in which rudimentary soft tissue is present in front of the ear, and pits, which may be shallow or

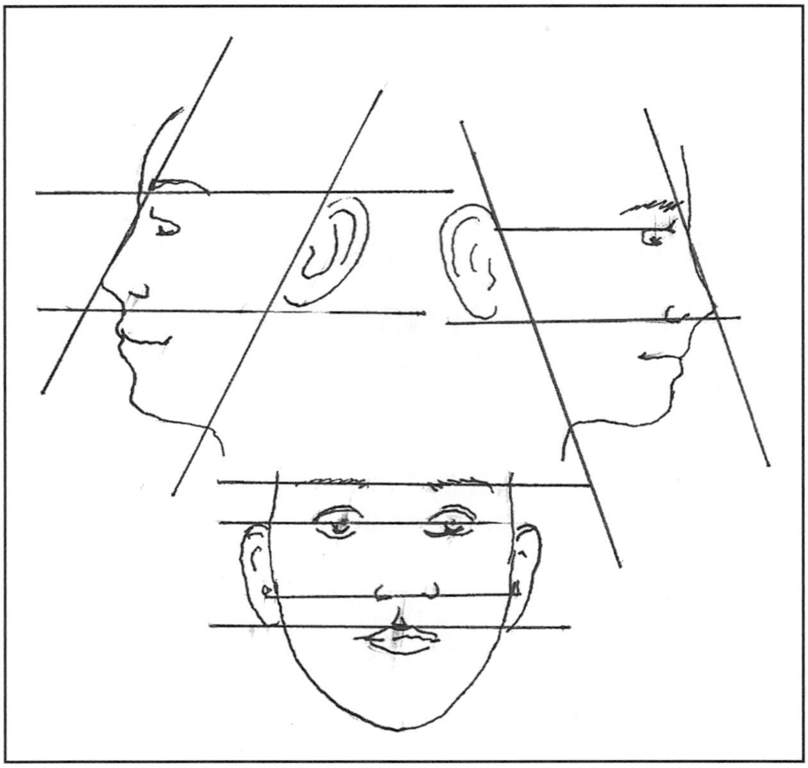

FIGURE 9–1. Illustration of facial structures in relation to the auricle.

deep, and may be associated with branchial clefts. Ears may be low-set or set too far posteriorly, and these features are commonly seen in a number of craniofacial syndromes. Congenital aural microtia and atresia are serious and complex birth malformations in which the auricle, the external auditory canal (EAC), the ossicles, and sometimes the cochlea fail to develop completely. Microtia refers to underdevelopment of the auricle ("micro" means small and "otia" means ear), and can range from a normally shaped but smaller pinna to complete absence of the pinna with rudimentary soft tissue ear tags. Classification of microtia severity into three subtypes was originally proposed by Marx (1926). Examples of the three subtypes are shown in Figure 9–2, which illustrates anomalies of the EAC and pinna varying from normal to a narrowed canal to complete atresia or absence of the canal. Severity of EAC stenosis has been described by Schuknecht (1989) and Jahrsdoerfer, Yeakley, Aguilar, Cole, and Gray (1992). In Grade I microtia, the pinna is smaller than normal but the external canal is patent, and all of the normal ear structures are present. In Grade II, the external ear is malformed, the external canal is present but stenotic, and the middle-ear space is small and the ossicles are malformed or fused. Grade III, the most severe, involves severe malformation or absence of the pinna, absence or complete stenosis of the external canal and absence or near absence of the middle-ear space and ossicles. Anomalies of the middle-ear structure may include stapes deformity, absence of the oval and/or round windows, facial nerve absence or anomalous development, poor pneumatization of the middle-ear cells and space, and fusion of the malleus and incus into a columella-type of structure. The incidence of inner ear abnormalities associated with microtia is estimated to be between 10% and 47% (Swartz & Faerber, 1985). The principle that "better developed outer ears go with better developed middle ears" has been demonstrated with high resolution CT scanning (Ishimoto, Ito & Yamasobo, 2005). As expected, this adage also holds true for hearing—better developed pinnas and ear canals correlate with better hearing function.

A single genetic cause for microtia has not been identified, but there is evidence that it is associated with multifactorial genetic risk coupled with prenatal or intrauterine factors. The familial recurrence risk is

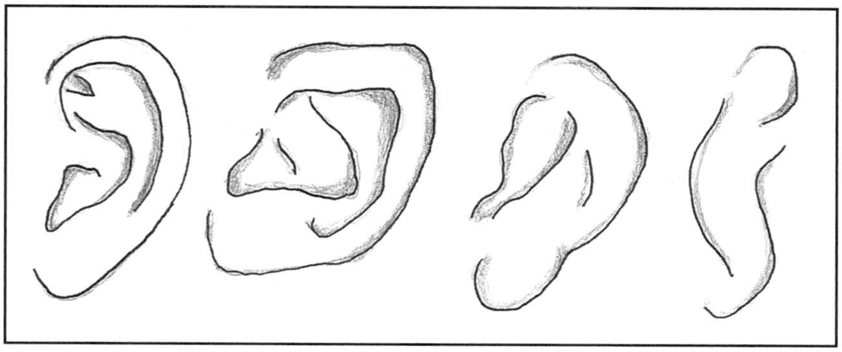

FIGURE 9–2. Grades of auricular malformations described by Marx (1926). Normal auricle. I. Slightly smaller auricle, mild deformity but each part can be clearly distinguished. II. Auricle is one-half to two-thirds of normal size; its structure is only partially retained. III. Severely malformed structure, often peanut shaped.

estimated to be 5.7% (Takahashi & Maeda, 1982), but increases to 25% when all branchial arch abnormalities are considered (Tanzer, 1971). Known risk factors include rubella and prenatal use of teratogenic drugs, including thalidomide, accutane, retinoic acid and clomid. While the overall incidence of microtia is estimated at 1 in 6,000 births, the risk appears to be greater in Japanese populations (1:4000) and in Native American populations (1:2000), especially in Navajos (1:1000) Grabb, (1965). Unilateral microtia is thought to be a mild variant of hemifacial microsomia, which is underdevelopment of half of the face. Microtia occurs in males twice as often as in females and occurs unilaterally in 70 to 90% of cases (Jafek, Nager, Strife, & Gayler, 1975; Schuknecht, 1989). Interestingly, microtia occurs in the right ear 55% to 65% of the time, possibly due to blood flow and growth signaling asymmetries. Evidence for the blood flow theory has been reported by McKenzie and Craig (1955) and Poswillo (1973), who theorize that tissue ischemia (decreased blood flow) resulting from an obliterated artery is the cause of developmental auricular abnormalities. Many cases of microtia have been reported in patients who have normal ears, with identical or fraternal twins. More support for the blood flow hypothesis comes from pediatric dysmorphologists, who observe that many types of birth deformities are more common in multiple births due to a phenomenon called "placental steal syndrome" in which the blood flow to the larger twin is greater than to the smaller twin owing to asymmetric placental development and resultant circulatory asymmetries.

Congenital Conductive Hearing Loss Associated with External Ear Malformations

In general, the degree of conductive hearing loss corresponds to the severity (Grades I–III) of external and middle-ear microtia. Sensorineural hearing loss is more common in Grade III microtia, and is due to cochlear malformations. Approximately 40 hereditary hearing loss syndromes associated with external ear malformations and conductive hearing loss have been described (Allanson, 2004). In many of these syndromes, the auditory ossicles may be absent or malformed as well. For example, Treacher Collins syndrome includes malformation or absence of the malleus, incus and stapes, mastoid, absence of the external auditory canal, and occasional complete absence of the middle-ear and epitympanic space. Bilateral hearing loss occurs in approximately half of cases, and the degree of conductive hearing loss corresponds to the degree of external ear stenosis (Pron, Galloway, Armstrong, & Posnick, 1993). Most of the known syndromes associated with external and middle-ear malformations have been described in only sporadic cases or in a few families, and most are of autosomal recessive inheritance, sometimes associated with consanguinity. Table 9–1 details the most common syndromes associated with external ear malformations, the known hearing loss characteristics, and other associated congenital malformations.

Table 9–1. Syndromes Associated With External Ear Anomalies and Congenital Conductive Hearing Loss

Syndrome, Incidence, Genetics	*Ear Malformations*	*Hearing Loss Characteristics*	*Other Associated Malformations*
Treacher Collins syndrome (Mandibulofacial dysostosis) Incidence 1:50,000 (Jahrsdoerfer & Jacobson, 1995). Autosomal dominant inheritance with variable expressivity. New mutations in 60% associated with paternal age.	Agenesis or hypoplasia of the mastoid and antrum; external ear canal atresia or stenosis; middle-ear agenesis, agenesis or malformation of the malleus, incus, stapes and oval wndow; cochlea and vestibular organs usually normal but also may be malformed.	Bilateral conductive hearing loss (55%); generally moderate to severe and associated with degree of external canal malformation.	Hypoplastic midface, coloboma of lower eyelid (75%), choanal atresia (few reports), macrostomia (cleft palate (35%).
Goldenhar syndrome (Oculo-auriculo-vertebral spectrum or hemofacial microsomia) Incidence 1:3500 to 1:5600 (Bayraktar et al., 2005) Mostly sporadic but autosomal dominant inheritance in 1–2%.	Usually unilateral; malformation varies from anotia to malformed auricular tissue displaced ant/inf to a mildly dysmorphic auricle. Preauricular tags common. Occasional isolated microtia.	Conductive and sensorineural hearing loss (50%) due to diverse anomalies of external and middle-ear; including ossicular hypoplasia, patulous eustachian tube, skull base abnormalities.	Mild to marked facial asymmetry (65%), cleft lip/palate (7%–15%), eye anomalies (esp. epibulbar dermoids, unilateral colobomas); facial nerve weakness, cranial nerve involvement, intracranial brain malformations, developmental delay, heart anomalies, renal, GI and musculoskeletal anomalies.
Branchio-oto-renal (BOR) syndrome or ear-pit hearing loss syndrome Incidence 1:40,000 (Fraser et al., 1980) Autosomal dominant with variable expressivity; linkage to chromosome 8q.	External ear anomalies (30–60%), ranging from severe microtia to minor pinna anomalies (cup-shaped, lopped, or hypoplastic). Stenosis, malformation or upward slanting of ear canal. Preauricular ear pits (70–80%).	Hearing loss reported in 75%, including conductive (30%), sensorineural (20%), and mixed types (50%).	Long narrow face shape, facila nerve paralysis (10%), branchial cyst/fitulas (60%), structural renal anomalies (75%), functional renal anomalies (33%), ossicular malformations, congenital cholesteatoma, cochlear malformations including Mondini dysplasia.
CHARGE association (**C**oloboma, **H**eart defects, **A**tresia of choanae, **R**etarded growth and development, **G**enital hypoplasia, **E**ar anomalies and deafness) Heterogeneous, 6% recurrence risk; may be dominant in some cases.	Characteristic short, wide pinna missing features such as tragus, helix. Prominent anthelix and triangular concha. Small or absent earlobes. Ear canal stenosis and atresia rare.	Hearing loss in 85%, ranging from mild to profound sensorineural or mixed hearing loss due to ossicular and cochlear anomalies, distinctive wedge-shaped hearing loss due to middle-ear disease and sensorineural loss.	Choanal atresia (blockage of the nasal passage), congenital heart disease (60–70%), developmental, renal abnormalities (15%), tracheoesophageal problems, minor skeletal defects.
Congenital aural atresia Incidence 1–5:10,000 Sporadic, no known inheritance patterns (Lambert, 2001).	Congenital atresia without other anomalies; microtia or anotia in 95% of cases. Male: female ratio is 2:1, right ears affected more often (65%). More common in Native Americans (1:2000).	Conductive hearing loss, generally moderate to severe depending on degree of stenosis and ossicular/middle-ear abnormalities.	No other associated anomalies.

Treatment for Aural Atresia

Treatment for congenital atresia includes a traditional bone conduction hearing aid, a bone anchored hearing aid (BAHA) system, or atresiaplasty to create an ear canal/middle ear. There are few evidence-based studies published to assist parents, otologists, and audiologists in objectively making these choices based on outcome data. An evidence-based review was recently completed (Riemer et al., 2008) comparing results of atresiaplasty with BAHA. Included in this review, De Alarcon and Choo (2007) published an expert opinion on the current controversies in the treatment of aural atresia, citing studies that have shown positive outcomes for good surgical candidates. Candidacy was determined by using the Jahrsdoerfer scale (Jahrsdoerfer et al., 1992), along with high-resolution computed tomography (HRCT), to predict the outcome from atresiaplasty. Patients with a score of 7 or greater (Choo, personal communication) have a higher degree of good audiometric outcome with a resulting speech reception threshold of 30 dB hearing level or less than those with scores below 7. Patel and Shelton (2007) investigated 64 atresiaplasty cases and showed that stable short-term hearing results occurred after 32 surgeries and stable long-term hearing results occurred after 48 procedures. A retrospective study by Evans and Kazahaya (2007) compared both the outcomes and the costs of external auditory canal (EAC) reconstruction and the BAHA system. Twenty-nine pediatric patients underwent EAC reconstruction and six pediatric patients underwent BAHA system surgery. BAHA system patients had more positive hearing outcomes (average hearing gain of 31.8 dB versus 17.3 dB for EAC reconstruction), lower costs ($826 per dB hearing gain versus $2,910 per dB for EAC reconstruction), and 93% of patients receiving EAC reconstruction required some form of amplification postoperatively. There are other articles in the otology literature that report the results of experienced surgeons who demonstrate improved hearing postoperatively for atresiaplasty, but the definitions of success vary considerably. Reducing the air-bone gap by 20 to 30 dB while showing improvement over preoperative hearing levels generally failed to improve hearing to the level of normal (Chang, Choi, & Hur, 2006; De La Cruz & Teufert, 2003; Digoy & Cueva, 2007; Lambert, 1998; Patel & Shelton, 2007). Success is defined in these studies by improved hearing and stable hearing levels, rather than complete resolution of the air-bone gap or speech reception thresholds (SRT) and pure tone averages that fall within the normal range. If the goal of atresiaplasty is to "reliably create an ear canal and middle ear system that allows normal hearing without assistive devices" (Evans & Kazahaya, 2007), then there is insufficient evidence in the literature to support this option. If audiologists define success for children as having an average 15 dB hearing level for speech reception threshold or better in order to function in a classroom without amplification, then atresiaplasty is unlikely to achieve this goal.

Studies of the BAHA system in achieving hearing outcomes within the normal range are also very few. Yellon (2007) reported on 13 children, 11 of whom had no complications and are using their devices. The mean postoperative SRT was 18.5 dB (with a range of 14–25 dB). Evans and Kazahaya (2007) reported on six children who received surgery to implant the BAHA system but had audiometric postoperative data on only three of those children. The observed average gain was 31.8 dB, with an average SRT of 17.5 dB. There clearly is a need for studies with greater numbers of subjects that compare hearing outcomes from the use of an osseointegrated BAHA system and atresiaplasty.

Recommendations of the Joint Committee on Infant Hearing for Middle-Ear Conditions

The Joint Committee on Infant Hearing (JCIH) 2007 Position Statement identifies craniofacial anomalies as a risk factor for permanent congenital, delayed onset, or progressive loss in childhood, including anomalies of the pinna, ear canal, ear tags, ear pits, and temporal bone anomalies. The JCIH recommends that:

> A complete head and neck examination for craniofacial anomalies should document defects of the auricles, patency of the external ear canals, and status of the eardrum and middle-ear structures. Atypical findings on eye examination, including irises of two different colors or abnormal positioning of the eyes, may signal a syndrome that includes hearing loss. Congenital permanent conductive hearing loss may be associated with craniofacial anomalies that are seen in disorders such as Crouzon disease, Klippel-Feil syndrome, and Goldenhar syndrome. The assessment of infants with these congenital anomalies should be coordinated with a clinical geneticist. (pp. 15–16)

For all children, JCIH recommends assessment of middle-ear status (using pneumatic otoscopy and/or tympanometry) at all well-child visits and referral of children with persistent middle-ear effusion lasting for three months or longer for otologic evaluation. As noted by the JCIH, with regard to universal newborn hearing screening, both otoacoustic emission (OAE) and auditory brainstem response (ABR) screening technologies can be used to detect sensory (cochlear) hearing loss; however, both technologies may be affected by outer or middle-ear dysfunction. Consequently, transient conditions of the outer and middle-ear may result in a "failed" screening-test result in the presence of normal cochlear and/or neural function.

Middle-Ear Assessment in the Newborn

ABR and OAE tests, the primary tests used in Universal Newborn Hearing Screening (UNHS) programs are sensitive to the condition of the middle ear. For example, Hall, Smith, and Popelka (2004) found that conductive hearing loss can persist for several weeks after birth. Stuart, Yang and Green (1994) reported elevated (> 10 dB) air-conducted ABR thresholds in neonates during the initial 48 hours after birth, whereas bone-conducted ABR thresholds changed by less than 1 dB. Doyle, Burggraaff, Fujikawa, Jim, and MacArthur (1997) reported that newborn hearing screening pass rates in ears with occluding vernix were 66% for ABR, but only 38% for OAEs. Transient middle ear conditions may result in a "referred" test result regardless of the presence of normal cochlear function due to decreased forward transmission of the stimulus and reverse transmission of the OAE signal through the middle-ear.

Assessment of middle ear function is not currently part of UNHS guidelines for well babies and graduates of neonatal intensive care units (NICU) for several reasons (JCIH, 2007). First, pneumatic otoscopy and bone-conducted ABR are impractical in a UNHS protocol due to the use of ancillary screening personnel rather than audiologists or otologists. Tympanometry using a low-frequency probe tone is insensitive to middle ear dysfunction in newborns (Hunter & Margolis, 1992; Paradise, Smith, & Bluestone 1976; Sprague, Wiley, & Goldstein, 1985). Anatomical differences in the infant ear, such as a more compliant ear-canal wall (Holte, Margolis, & Cavanaugh, 1991), smaller ear canal and middle-ear space, and a more horizontal orientation of the tympanic membrane with respect to the axis of the ear canal contribute to developmental differences in tympanometry (Ikui, Sando, & Fujita, 1997; Ruah, Schachern, Zelterman, Paparella, & Yoon, 1991; Saunders, Kaltenback, & Relkin, 1983).

As discussed in Chapter 18, tympanometry using higher probe-tone frequencies (up to 1 kHz) is currently recommended for diagnostic testing by JCIH guidelines. Tympanometry using a 1-kHz probe tone is more sensitive to changes in middle-ear status in infants younger than 4 months old compared to 0.226-kHz tympanometry (Alaerts, Lutz, & Woulters, 2007; Calandruccio, Fitzgerald, & Prieve 2006). Margolis, Bass-Ringdahl, Hanks, Holte, and Zapala (2003) reported that 1-kHz tympanometry is 91% specific in predicting distortion product (DP) OAE passes, but only 50% sensitive for DPOAE fails. Kei and colleagues (2003) reported 1-kHz tympanograms in 106 infants (1–6 days old) who passed a click-evoked otoacoustic emission (CE) OAE hearing screening. Single-peaked tympanograms were present in 92.3% of their sample; six tympanometric variables were measured, but no procedure for choosing among these variables was described. Baldwin (2006) reported sensitivity of 0.99 and specificity of 0.89 for 1 kHz tympanometry for infants with a mean age of 10 weeks but findings may not apply to neonates, as the youngest infant was 2 weeks old.

Wideband energy reflectance (ER) is an alternative test to assess middle-ear status. Ambient-pressure ER and other acoustic transfer functions (ATFs) have been reported in children and infants (Hunter, Tubaugh, Jackson, & Propes, 2008; Keefe, Bulen, Arehart, & Burns, 1993; Vander Werff, Prieve & Georgantas, 2007), and neonates (Abdala et al., 2007; Keefe et al., 2000; Keefe & Abdala, 2007). ER is sensitive to middle ear disorders including otitis media with effusion (OME; Feeney, Keefe, & Marryott, 2003; Piskorski, Keefe, Simmons, & Gorga, 1999), otosclerosis, ossicular discontinuity and perforation of the tympanic membrane (Feeney et al., 2003). Because ER can assess middle ear function in young infants, it could potentially be a useful tool in UNHS and early hearing detection and intervention (EHDI) programs. For example, Keefe, Zhao, Neely, Gorga, and Vohr (2003b) analyzed a subset of data obtained from two-stage UNHS protocols (OAE/ABR) that produced a 5% false positive rate. They reported significant correlations between two ambient-pressure ER variables and CEOAE responses, suggesting that ER may help to interpret CEOAEs. Applying ER factors identified in Keefe et al. (2003b) to a predictive test of middle-ear dysfunction in infants, Keefe, Gorga, Zhao, Neely, and Vohr (2003a) showed that these factors decreased the false positive rate from 5% to 1%. Thus, ER detects transient middle-ear dysfunction in newborns. Infants failing an OAE screening had significantly higher ER (exceeding test-retest variability) for frequencies between 0.63 to 2 kHz than infants who passed (Vander Werff et al., 2007). Test-retest reliability has high interclass correlation coefficients in infants and children (Hunter et al., 2008), and ER was significantly higher in infants and children with clinically diagnosed OME in the same study.

Keefe and Simmons (2003) investigated the test performance of 226 Hz admittance tympanometry, ambient-pressure ER, and wideband (WB) tympanometry as predictors of conductive hearing loss (CHL) in children 10 years of age or older. Data were obtained from 42 normal-functioning ears and 18 ears with CHL. For a fixed specificity of 0.90, the sensitivity of these measures to detect CHL was 0.28 for static acoustic admittance (226 Hz), 0.72 for ambient-pressure ER, and 0.94 for WB tympanometry. These studies further demonstrate that WB tympanometry may be a reliable and sensitive diagnostic tool in newborns as well as older infants and children.

Due to the use of ancillary screening personnel in many settings, a physiologic middle-ear test such as wideband ER that does not rely on subjective interpretation would improve UNHS programs. A need exists to understand whether infants referred by an UNHS exam have a sensorineural hearing loss (SNHL) or CHL associated with middle-ear dysfunction. The development of cost-effective tools to separate CHL from SNHL will allow systems for UNHS and diagnosis to accurately categorize type of hearing loss, so that appropriate intervention can be initiated as soon as possible after birth. Development of improved infant middle-ear tests are needed to improve the management and follow-up care of infants referred from NHS programs.

Assessment of Children with Craniofacial Anomalies

Children with cranial-facial anomolies who are at highest risk for chronic OME and CHL present special challenges for pediatric audiologists and craniofacial teams. As highlighted in the clinical practice guideline for otitis media with effusion by Rosenfeld, Culpepper, Doyle, Grundfast, and Hoberman (2004), children at risk for speech or language delay would likely be further affected by hearing problems from OME, even though definitive studies are lacking. Small comparative studies of children with Down syndrome show poorer articulation and receptive language associated with a history of early otitis media. Children with craniofacial anomalies have a higher prevalence of chronic OME, hearing loss (conductive and sensorineural), and speech or language delay than do children without these anomalies.

The associated cognitive problems in children with Down syndrome make behavioral assessment problematic, and available studies in populations such as Down syndrome have found a 38 to 78% incidence of hearing loss, but if treated aggressively, hearing levels improve to the normal range for 98% (Shott, Joseph, & Heithaus, 2001). In the United States, approximately 3% of babies are born with some type of birth defect, including craniofacial anomalies, Down syndrome (1.4 per 1,000) or cleft palate (1 per 1,000; Centers for Disease Control and Prevention [CDC], 2006). Often, these children have an associated problem of OME (JCIH, 2007). These children are more difficult to test if intellectual disability is present, and they typically require more frequent visits and routine use of physiologic measures, including ABR with sedation in order to determine hearing levels with certainty.

Although middle ear effusion is common in healthy infants, it is nearly universal in infants with cleft lip and/or palate. Prior to palate closure, 92 to 99% of infants with cleft palate have OME due to eustachian tube dysfunction (Dhillon, 1988; Paradise & Bluestone, 1974; Schönweiler, Lisson, Schonweiler, Eckard, Ptok, et al., 1999). Hearing loss due to OME has been found to be substantial in a study of 40 infants 0 to 3 months old with cleft palate (Andrews, Chorbachi, Sirimanna, Sommerlad, Hartley, et al., 2004). In that study, thresholds measured with auditory brainstem evoked responses averaged 49 and 53 dB in the right and left ears, respectively. The conductive component was approximately 25 dB, and 83% of the infants with cleft palate had flat high frequency tympanograms, consistent with middle ear effusion. Thus, it appears that middle ear effusion and conductive hearing losses occur at an extremely high rate in children with cleft palate.

Incidence and Prevalence of Acute Otitis Media and Otitis Media with Effusion (USA)

Acute otitis media (AOM) has rapid onset, characteristic symptoms, and is of short duration. Otitis media with effusion (OME) is middle-ear fluid that remains after the acute infection is gone, or it can arise de novo. Both can produce conductive hearing loss. Incidence and prevalence rates are useful in reporting and following changes in the impact of AOM and OME in the pediatric population. The two rates provide different information. Prevalence conveys information about OM burden in a population at a given point in time, and depends on both disease development and duration. Incidence measures new episodes of AOM/OME, that is, the probability of OM-free individuals developing OM over a specified time period.

AOM and OME have been studied internationally, and rates vary widely around the globe. Variation in these two measures may be related to: (1) demographic characteristics of the group studied, (e.g., age, race, ethnicity, socioeconomic status); (2) frequency and type of ascertainment (e.g., physician exam versus parent or self report); and (3) the criteria used to diagnosis these two conditions. Population-based studies provide better estimates than convenience samples (such as daycare centers and schools) because they represent the broader community. Some of these studies have included hearing as a study factor in participants.

There are several sources of incidence data. Information from over 8,000 parents of preschoolers collected in National Health and Nutrition Examination Survey (NHANES) III showed a nonsignificant 3% increase in reported rates of OM between 1988 and 1994 (Auringer, Lanphear, Kalkwarf, & Mansour, 2003). Significant increases of 5% in OM onset by 12 months and 6% in recurrent OM were also demonstrated. Children from low income families and those with less educated parents showed the greatest increase in these two measures. The Early Childhood Longitudinal Study Birth Cohort included over 8,000 children representative of 2001 United States births. Based on parent report of physician diagnosis, OM incidence was 39% by 9 months and 62% by 2 years of age (Hoffman, Park, Losonczy, & Chiu, 2007).

A clinical trial compared prevalence of tympanic membrane (TM) sequelae at age 5 years among three groups of children with chronic OME: immediate tube treatment, delayed tube treatment, and an observation group not meeting the study surgical criterion for the duration of middle-ear effusion (Johnston et al., 2004). TM sequelae rates exceeded 80% in the tube treated groups, but were 19% or lower in the nontreated group. Pure tone average (PTA) hearing thresholds did not vary between the treatment groups (PTA ~6 dB for both), but thresholds in both treatment groups were significantly higher than in the nontreatment group (PTA ~4 to 4.5 dB).

Since the licensure and routine use of the 7-valent pneumococcal conjugate vaccine (PCV-7) in 2000, important trends have emerged in OM incidence and prevalence. Prior to routine immunization with this vaccine in the United States, *S. pneumoniae* was the most prevalent otitis media pathogen (Bluestone, Stephenson, & Martin, 1992; Del Beccaro et al., 1992). Early randomized controlled trials revealed that the vaccine was effective in reducing OM rates. Black showed a 7% decrease in all OM (Black et al., 2000) and Eskola showed a reduction in type-specific incidence of 25 to 87% for vaccine serotypes, and an increase of 33% in replacement serotypes during follow-up (Eskola et al., 2001). Since routine use of PCV-7 in infants and children, overall OM incidence and prevalence rates have declined, particularly among young children (Grijalva et al., 2006; Zhou, Shefer, Kong, & Nuorti, 2008). Parent-reported recurrent OM incidence among children younger than 18 years also declined from 335 in 1,000 in 1997 to 214 in 1,000 in 2004 (United States Department of Health and Human Services [USDHHS], 2008). Similarly, physician office visits with an OM diagnosis declined from 118 to 78 per 100 children younger than 3 years old from 1997 to 2005, a 34% decrease (USDHHS, 2008).

Mirroring the decrease in OM episodes, a decline in recurrent OM (three in 6 months or four in 12 months) and tympanostomy tube prevalence was noted in two large birth cohorts (Poehling et al., 2007). Between 1998 to 1999 and 2000 to 2001, recurrent OM rates declined 17% and 28%, respectively, and tube treatment declined 16% and 23% in the two birth cohorts. Although the decrease in overall OM is encouraging, other less promising changes have occurred. Although middle-ear fluid cultures have shown a decrease in *S. pneumoniae* organisms, particularly for vaccine serotypes (Block et al., 2004; Casey & Pichichero, 2004), prevalence of persistent ear infections caused by vaccine-related pneumococcal serotypes rose from 8% pre PCV-7 to 32% post PCV-7. OM caused by *H. influenzae* increased 36 to 50% pre- to post-PCV-7 (Block et al., 2004; Casey & Pichichero, 2004). Surveillance of replacement organisms should continue, but declining rates of OM may reduce the occurrence of conductive hearing loss in young children.

Treatment of OME and AOM

Guidelines for treatment of AOM and OME draw on the expertise of the Agency for Healthcare Research and Quality (AHRQ). The guidelines use common resources for literature review and incorporate similar criteria for recommendations. Recognizing that inappropriate diagnosis, treatment and management of AOM and OME can prolong disease course and attendant conductive hearing loss, primary care and specialist physician groups published evidence-based clinical practice guidelines for both OME and AOM in 2004 (Rosenfeld, Culpepper, Doyle, Grundfast, & Hoberman, et al., 2004). Using levels of recommendation from "strongly recommended" to "no recommendation," the OME panel graded the quality of evidence from published research from A (randomized controlled trials) to D (expert opinion, case reports). The panel recommended identifying children at risk for speech, language and learning problems for prompt assessment and early hearing evaluation. Watchful waiting for three months is recommended for the low-risk child with OME because of the likelihood of resolution in the majority of children. A child would be considered low risk unless he or she has one or more of the following: permanent hearing loss, suspected or diagnosed speech and/or language delay, autism spectrum disorder, other developmental disorders, Down syndrome, craniofacial anomalies associated with cognitive or speech and language delay, blindness, cleft palate, developmental delay. The panel also advocated hearing testing for children who have OME for 3 months or longer, language delay, or speech problems, and limiting surgical treatment to tympanostomy tubes unless findings indicate that additional procedures (e.g., adenoidectomy with or without tonsillectomy) are needed. The panel discourages population-based screening programs for OME among asymptomatic children, and routine treatment of OME with antihistamines, decongestants, antibiotics, and corticosteroids. The guidelines made no recommendations about complementary medicine or allergy management as OME treatment based on a lack of scientific evidence.

Guidelines for AOM (American Academy of Pediatrics and American Academy of Family Physicians, 2004) focus on diagnosis and initial treatment based on age and severity. The Committee advocates for judicious use of antibiotics. Their concern arises from inappropriate use of antibiotics, which results in high rates of resistance and multiply-resistant organisms, leading to the societal expense of developing and marketing new antimicrobials. The committee provided a detailed description of recommended diagnostic criteria for AOM: acute onset of signs and symptoms, presence of middle-ear fluid, and symptoms of middle-ear inflammation. Diagnosis in young children may be uncertain because middle-ear fluid cannot be accurately ascertained (cerumen in the canal, narrow canal, lack of a proper seal for pneumatic otoscopy and/or tympanometry). Other recommendations include assessment and treatment of pain, observation as an option to treatment for uncomplicated AOM taking into account age, severity of illness, ability to follow-up and diagnostic certainty. Antibacterial therapy was recommended for infants younger than 6 months, and for those 6 months or older to 2 years with severe illness and certain diagnosis. In this age group, if illness is not severe and diagnosis is uncertain, "watchful waiting" is an option. Children 2 years or older should be observed and receive pain medication if needed, but antibiotics should not be given unless OM is severe. Another recommendation is to prevent AOM by reducing risk factors. Complementary or alternative medicines were not recommended for AOM treatment because of inadequate data on effectiveness. Guidelines stress that observation is appropriate only when follow-up is possible and treatment can be provided if the illness worsens.

A Cochrane Systematic Review of randomized controlled trials of tympanostomy tube placement for OME studied effects on hearing and a variety of other outcomes (e.g., quality of life, preventing adverse developmental outcomes; Lous et al., 2005). These authors concluded that the duration of effusion was reduced 32% and hearing level was improved by 9 dB after six months, and 6 dB by 12 months. No effect of tubes on speech and language was detected.

International OM Rates

In the Netherlands, a retrospective cohort study of children younger than 13 years used data from the University Medical Center Utrecht Primary Care Network collected in 1995 to 2003. (Plasschaert, Rovers, Schilder, Verheij, & Hak, 2006). Among those under 2 years, AOM and OME incidence increased by 46% and 66% respectively, whereas antibiotic prescription rates for AOM and OME increased by 45% and 25%. The contrast of declining rates in the United States and increasing rates in the Netherlands is most likely due to the later introduction of universal pneumococcal conjugate vaccination in the Netherlands in 2006 (M. Rovers, personal communication). A database of over 2 million patients of 291 general practitioners in the United Kingdom was used to evaluate middle-ear disease workload between 1991 and 2001 (Williamson, Benge, Mullee, & Little, 2006). AOM visits for 2 to 10 year olds decreased from 105.3 to 34.7 per 1,000 over this period, whereas chronic OME visits were relatively stable (15.2 to 16.7 per 1,000 each year). In a study of Chinese kindergartners 3 to 6 years ($n = 3{,}013$), overall prevalence of OM diagnosed by a senior otolaryngologist using pneumatic otoscopy and tympanometry was 9.8%, rates were higher in 3 to 5 year olds (11–12%) and lower in the 6 year olds (6%; Chen, Lin, Hwang, & Ku, 2003).

Longitudinal data on early AOM in the Oslo Birth Cohort revealed a 5% incidence before 6 months of age and 28% incidence by 12 months (Bentdal, Karevold, Nafstad, & Kvaerner, 2007). Thirteen percent of 10-year-olds were reported to have AOM in the previous 12 months (Karevold, Kvestad, Nafstad, & Kvaerner, 2006).

High-Risk Populations

Indigenous populations continue to suffer a considerable OM burden, but not all studies have evaluated hearing. A systematic review of population-based studies of OM incidence and prevalence in children under 18-year-olds included over 250,000 children (Gunasekera, Hayson, Morris, & Craig, 2007). Results showed that OM prevalence in Inuits and Australian aboriginals exceeded 80%. Hearing impairment ranged from less than 1% in Greek children to 23% in Australian aboriginal children. Hearing loss was more common if OM was present. Five and six–year-old Inuit children had a hearing screening fail rate of 19% (Ayukawa, Lejeune, & Proulx, 2004), and one-third of Australian aboriginal children had hearing losses of 30 dB or greater (Thorne, 2003). American Indian children in Minnesota had early OM onset: 63% had OM and 30% failed OAE by 6 months of age (Daly, Pirie, Rhodes, Hunter, & Davey, 2007; Hunter, Davey, Kohtz, & Daly, 2007).

Nigerian children with chronic suppurative OM (CSOM) are at high risk for conductive hearing loss. Study subjects were identified from three hospitals and two primary care centers. Controls were school children, children of hospital workers, and hospital visitors (age range of 4 months to 12 years). Among children with chronic suppurative OM, 47% had hearing loss, 72% of those with hearing loss had OM onset by age one, and 82% with hearing loss had conductive loss. Only social class was related to hearing loss (Lasisi et al., 2007a). Bottle feeding as well as poverty related indices (lower socioeconomics status, crowding, malnutrition) were associated with CSOM (Lasisi, Sulaiman, & Afolabi, 2007b).

In a Canadian indigenous population, children under 2 years old had 2,300 outpatient AOM visits per 1,000 child-years (Dallaire, Dewailly, Vezina, Bruneau, & Ayotte, 2006). Among Australian aboriginal children, 41% had OME, 33% had AOM, and 40% had tympanic membrane perforations by 18 months (Morris et al., 2005). In another study of 280 western Australian children followed from birth to age 2 years, 74% of aboriginal children and 45% of nonaboriginal children had OM (Jacoby et al. 2008). Of New Zealand Pacific Islander 2-year-olds (n = 1,001) who participated in a screening program, 75% failed the initial tympanometry screening. Of the 502 who attended the second screening at home or clinic, 51% failed. Of those failing two or three screens, 73% and 82% were determined to have OME or AOM. Because less than 50% of those referred to the clinic complied, the authors' population estimate was 27% for AOM or OME (Paterson et al., 2006). Chronic suppurative OM was experienced by 12% of children in a Bangladesh study (Biswas, Joarder, & Siddiquee, 2005) and 2.5% in a Nigerian study (Amusa, Ijadunola, & Onayade, 2005).

Special Populations at High Risk

Cleft Palate (CP) and Other Craniofacial Syndromes

A questionnaire sent to parents of children in a cleft palate registry in Ireland revealed that rates of middle-ear disease were similar in children with cleft palate and cleft lip and palate, with considerably lower rates observed in children with cleft lip only (Sheahan, Miller, Sheahan, Earley, & Blayney, 2003). Rates of otitis media history, tube treatment, and current hearing loss were highest in 10- to 12-year-olds (65%, 83%, and 46%, respectively). OM onset typically was in the first year of life. Hearing was significantly poorer among those who had multiple tube surgeries, no doubt a marker for ongoing and recurrent middle-ear disease.

Compared to children without CP, affected children are predisposed to persistent OM, which often persists into school age (Shah et al., 2004). Children with cleft palate have poor eustachian tube (ET) function due to a number of possible abnormalities (e.g., ET obstruction, narrow opening, and abnormal muscular control of the ET). Abnormal tubal function may persist even after palate repair. CP is also a common characteristic in many craniofacial conditions, including fetal alcohol, velocardiofacial, DiGeorge, CHARGE, and Down syndrome. These syndromes predispose affected children to recurrent ear infections and persistent middle-ear effusion.

Immunocompromise

Maternal antibody is transferred in utero during pregnancy and to the infant at delivery (Englund, 2007), but maternal antibodies do not persist. Infants do not begin to produce their own antibodies until 6 to 12 months of age (Glezen, 2003). Thus, otitis media incidence is high in the first year of life as a result of low levels of passive antibody, coupled with the infant's exposure to pathogens carried by siblings and children in day care. Besides low levels of antibody that affect all infants in early life, infants and children may have specific immunodeficiencies that increase the risk of OM and associated hearing loss. Primary specific immunodeficiency, the most common immune abnormality, results in defective antibody production, making individuals susceptible to respiratory diseases, including acute OM (Rynnel-Dagöö, 2004). Other less common deficiencies include selective IgA deficiency, which may result in chronic and recurrent OM; selective IgG subclass deficiency, often associated with IgA deficiency, results in frequent upper respiratory infections; and transient hypogammaglobulinemia, which affects premature infants disproportionately. Low IgG concentrations, coupled with delayed antibody production may result in low antibody levels for up to 3 years of age. Hereditary and congenital conditions (e.g., Down syndrome, Turner syndrome) may also result in recurrent OM (Rynnel-Dagöö, 2004).

Children requiring organ or bone marrow transplants become immunocompromised as a result of treatments to reduce the likelihood of graft rejection. Other chronic conditions (e.g., diabetes, cancer) may increase the likelihood of immunodeficiency. A chart review of infectious diseases in 92 pediatric patients with primary immunodeficiencies revealed that 24% of those with antibody deficiency had OM, compared to 9 to 14% of those with cellular deficiency, combined deficiency or phagocyte defect (Chang, Yang, & Chiang, 2006).

Effects of Genes and Environment on AOM/OME

Both environmental and host factors contribute to making infancy the period of greatest OM susceptibility. OM pathogens in the nasopharynx have ready access to the middle-ear via the shallow angle of the infant ET. Levels of passive antibody transferred to the fetus during pregnancy decline, and the infant's immune system lacks the ability to mount an effective antibody response to infections that are commonly acquired in group child care.

Exploration of genetic influences in otitis media is in its early stages, but animal studies provide evidence that may be relevant to human OM. Eya4-/- mice have hearing deficits and abnormal middle-ear and eustachian tube morphology resulting in middle-ear effusion (Depreux et al., 2008). The homologue of this gene could be important in human middle-ear disease, but has not yet been studied The *Jeff* gene was first reported to be associated with eustachian tube dysfunction and middle-ear effusion in mice (Hardisty-Hughes et al., 2006), followed by reports of association of its human homologue, the FBOX11 gene, to affected status among members of Minnesota families participating in a study of chronic OME/recurrent OM (COME/ROM; Segade et al., 2006). In the same study, individuals in families with two or more affected members were phenotyped using data from ear examinations, tympanograms, medical records, and reported OM histories. Analysis provided evidence for linkage of COME/ROM to areas on chromosomes 10q (LOD = 3.78) and 19q (LOD = 2.61). In addition, an interaction between these two chromosomes and chromosome 3p was demonstrated, suggesting that COME/ROM may be caused by gene interactions as well as environmental risk factors (Daly et al., 2004). Fine mapping increased evidence for linkage on both chromosomes (Sale et al., 2007).

A Norwegian study of 4,247 twin pairs reported that genes involved in OM risk do not vary by gender (Kvestad et al., 2004). A five-year follow-up of the Pittsburgh twin and triplet cohort (Casselbrant et al., 2004) reported that heritability of total time with OME by age 5 years was 0.72. Heritability refers to the proportion of variation in time with OME that can be attributed to genetic factors.

Researchers have explored genes related to functions and processes that may be involved in OM etiology. Children undergoing tube surgery for chronic/recurrent OM and control children without OM histories had middle-ear epithelium biopsies. Cases had mean mucin 2 (MUC2) expression six times greater than control levels (Ubell, Kerschner, Wackym, & Burrows, 2008). MUC2, which is a mucus-forming protein active in the middle ear and gut, plays a major role in chronic middle-ear effusion, which often results in conductive hearing loss. In a study of relationships between single nucleotide polymorphisms (SNPs) of proinflammatory cytokines ($TNF\alpha^{-308}$, $IL6^{-174}$, and $IL1b^{+3953}$) and OM susceptibility, Patel and colleagues (2006) reported that $TNF\alpha^{-308}$ and $IL6^{-174}$ were both related to OM susceptibility and tube treatment. Children with $TNF\alpha^{-308}$ exposed to tobacco smoke were more susceptible to OM than unexposed children. Alper, Winther, Hendley, and Doyle (2008) explored genotypes involved in OM concurrent with rhinovirus and other respiratory infections. In logistic regression, younger age (OR = .61), OM history (OR = 2.87), care outside the home (OR = 1.54), longer duration of breastfeeding (OR = 4.78), high production phenotypes of TNFα and IL10 (OR = 2.47, 1.63 respectively), and low production IL-6 (OR = 0.41) were significantly related to OM incidence during a rhinovirus upper respiratory infection. A Dutch study explored the relationship between mannan binding lectin (MBL2) haplotypes and MBL serum levels of children (Wiertsema et al., 2006). LXPA haplotype carriers with SNP 3130G had lower MBL levels than those with SNP 3130C (0.19 versus 070 mcg/mL, p = .03). Between ages 1 and 2 years, children with nonwild type MBL2 had more OM episodes per year than wild-type carriers (p = .03), but this relationship did not persist beyond age 2 years.

Environmental and Other Risk Factors

Pacfier use in a study of 495 children less than 4 years was related to recurrent OM, but not to AOM (Rovers et al., 2008). A National Institute of Child Health and Human Development (NICHD) study was conducted among more than 11,000 children who entered daycare after 3 years of age. Those in settings with over six children had a 50% higher rate of OM from 3 to 4.5 years than those in daycare with fewer children. Daycare entry before age 3 years was somewhat less likely to result in OM from age 3 to 4.5 years, but earlier daycare entry was not protective against OM (NICHD and Early Child Care Network, 2003). In Mozambique, overcrowding, exposure to tobacco and wood smoke and short duration of breastfeeding increased the risk of OM (da Costa, Navarro, Neves, & Martin, 2004).

A 2003 study of more than 3,000 infants reported that supine sleeping decreased risk of OM by 30 to 40% by age 6 months compared to prone sleeping (Hunt et al., 2003), but these findings have not yet been replicated. Jacoby's study of western Australian children reported that those exposed to tobacco smoke (64%) were 3.5 times more likely to have OM than those not exposed (Jacoby et al., 2008). Although 40% of nonaboriginal children were exposed to tobacco smoke, this exposure did not significantly increase OM risk. Nonaboriginal children were twice as likely to be diagnosed with OM if there were other children in the home, while very few aboriginal children were in daycare and daycare did not increase their risk of OM. Among 6- to 12-year-olds identified with OME in a Greek screening program, exposure to tobacco smoke did not increase risk of OME 16 months later (Xenellis et al., 2005). Earlier extrusion of tympanostomy tubes was also reported in children whose parents smoked compared to children of nonsmokers (Praveen & Terry, 2005). A novel study in Germany and the Netherlands reported a slight but significant increase in OM by age 2 years in children with higher exposure to traffic-related pollutants identified by home address (Brauer et al., 2006). In a study of Pacific Islander children, predictive factors for OME included child care for 20 hours per week or more (OR 5.21), attending church events (OR 2.78), and a variety of respiratory and airway conditions in the prior year: draining ears (OR 2.10), more than 5 cough or cold illnesses (OR 1.91), frequent snoring (OR 2.60) and home treatment for breathing symptoms (OR 2.61; Paterson et al., 2007).

Researchers in Pennsylvania and Virginia studied middle-ear effusion in 148 1- to 8-year-olds during the North American respiratory disease season (Mandel, Doyle, Winther, & Alper, 2008). Parents recorded information on onset and duration of respiratory illnesses throughout the study, and validated otoscopists performed ear exams weekly. Overall incidence of new OM episodes was about one per 100 child-days. Factors significantly related to respiratory disease (including OM) burden were young age, history of frequent colds, and parent occupation. Forty percent of OM episodes resolved within one week, and 75 to 90% by one month, whereas daily prevalence of OM ranged from 20 to 35% with peak prevalence in March.

Analyses of NHANES data collected in 1988 to 1994 revealed that shorter exclusive breast-feeding (≤ 4 to 6 months compared > 6 months) increased the risk of recurrent OM among children younger than 2 years about two-fold, whereas exposure to both pre- and postnatal passive smoke increased ROM risk about 50% (Chandy, Howard, & Auringer, 2006).

Summary

It is vitally important for the pediatric audiologist to be well acquainted with the causes of conductive hearing loss in infants and children, and to understand the best clinical practices for assessment and intervention for these children. Often, it seems that conductive hearing loss is disregarded or downplayed since it is nearly a universal occurrence at some point in all children due to otitis media. Knowledge of craniofacial characteristics to be alert for during ear examinations and history can assist the audiologist in making appropriate referrals to other medical professionals such as otology, genetics, and developmental pediatrics to assess the child for the presence of a syndrome. Understanding the special issues related to assessment of the neonatal ear allows us to be more accurate in diagnoses of conductive hearing loss, be it temporary or permanent. Finally, understanding the complexity of risk factors associated with recurrent and chronic otitis media can assist the audiologist in counseling parents on ways to reduce or prevent otitis media.

References

Abdala, C., Keefe, D. H., & Oba, S. I. (2007). Distortion product otoacoustic emission suppression tuning and acoustic admittance in human infants: Birth through 6 months. *Journal of the Acoustical Society of America*, *121*, 3617–3627.

Alaerts, J., Lutz, H., & Woulters, J. (2007). Evaluation of middle ear function in young children: Clinical guidelines for the use of 226- and 1,000-Hz tympanometry. *Otology and Neurotology*, *28*, 727–732.

Allanson, J. (2004). Genetic hearing loss associated with external ear abnormalities. In H. V. Toriello, W. Reardon, & R. J. Gorlin (Eds.), *Hereditary hearing loss and its syndromes* (Chap. 6). Oxford, New York: University Press.

Alper, C. M., Winther, B., Hendley, J. O., & Doyle, W. J. (2008). Cytokine polymorphisms predict the frequency of otitis media as a complication of rhinovirus and RSV infections in children. *European Archives of Otorhinolaryngology*. E pub June 17, 2008.

American Academy of Pediatrics and American Academy of Family Physicians. (2004). Clinical practice guideline: Diagnosis and management of acute otitis media. *Pediatrics*, *113*, 1451–1465.

Andrews, P. J., Chorbachi, R., Sirimanna, T., Sommerlad, B., & Hartley, B. E. J. (2004). Evaluation of hearing thresholds in 3 month-old children with a cleft palate: The basis for a selective policy for ventilation tube insertion at the time of palate repair. *Clinics in Otolaryngology*, *29*, 10–17.

Amusa, Y. B., Ijadunola, I. K., & Onayade, O. O. (2005). Epidemiology of otitis media in a local tropical African population. *West African Journal of Medicine*, *24*, 227–230.

Auringer, P., Lanphear, B. P., Kalkwarf, H. J., & Mansour, M. E. (2003). Trends in otitis media among children in the United States. *Pediatrics*, *112*, 514–520.

Ayukawa, H., Lejeune, P., & Proulx, J. F. (2004). Hearing screening outcomes in Inuit children in Nunavik, Quebec, Canada. *International Journal of Circumpolar Health*, *63*(Suppl. 2), 309–311.

Baldwin, M. (2006). Choice of probe tone and classification of trace patterns in tympanometry undertaken in early infancy. *International Journal of Audiology*, *45*, 417–427.

Bayraktar, S., Bayraktar, S. T., Ataoglu, E., Ayaz, A., & Elevli, M. (2005). Goldenhar's syndrome associated with multiple congenital abnormalities. *Journal of Tropical Pediatrics*, *51*, 377–379.

Bentdal, Y., Karevold, A., Nafstad, P., & Kvaerner, K. J. (2007). Early acute otitis media. Predictor for AOM and respiratory infections in childhood? *International Journal of Pediatric Otorhinolaryngology*, *71*, 1251–1259.

Biswas, A. C., Joarder, A. H., & Siddiquee, B. H. (2005). Prevalence of CSOM among rural school going children. *Mymensingh Medical Journal*, *14*, 152–155.

Black, S., Shinefield, H., Fireman, B., Lewis, E., Ray, P., Hansen, J. R., Elvin, L., . . . Edwards K. (2000). Efficacy, safety and immunogenicity of heptavalent pneumococcal conjugate vaccine in children. Northern California Kaiser Permanente Vaccine Study Center Group. *Pediatric Infectious Disease Journal*, *19*, 187–195.

Block, S. L., Hedrick, J., Harrison, C. J., Tyler, R., Smith, A., Findlay, R., & Keegan, E. (2004). Community-wide vaccination with the heptavalent pneumococcal conjugate significantly alters the microbiology of acute otitis media. *Pediatric Infectious Disease Journal*, *2*, 829–833.

Bluestone, C. D., Stephenson, J. S., & Martin, L. M. (1992). Ten-year review of otitis media pathogens. *Pediatric Infectious Disease Journal*, *11*(8 Suppl.), S7–S11.

Brauer, M., Gehring, U., Brunekreef, B., de Jongste, J., Gerritsen, J., Rovers, M., . . . Heinrich, J. (2006). Traffic-related air pollution and otitis media. *Environmental Health Perspectives*, *114*, 1414–1418.

Brent, B. (2006). Reconstruction of the auricle. In S. Mathes (Ed.), *Plastic surgery* (p. 643). Philadelphia, PA: Saunders Elsevier.

Calandruccio, L., Fitzgerald, T. S., & Prieve, B. A. (2006). Normative multifrequency tympanometry in infants and toddlers. *Journal of the American Academy of Audiology*, *17*, 470–480.

Casey, J. R., & Pichichero, M. E. (2004). Changes in frequency and pathogens causing acute otitis media in 1995–2003. *Pediatric Infectious Disease Journal*, *23*, 824–828.

Casselbrant, M. L., Mandel, E. M., Rockette, H. E., Kurs-Lasky, M., Fall, P. A., & Bluestone, C. D. (2004). The genetic component of middle ear disease in the first 5 years of life. *Archives of Otolaryngology-Head and Neck Surgery*, *130*, 273–278.

Centers for Disease Control (CDC). (2006). Improved national prevalence estimates for 18 selected major birth defects—United States, 1999–2001. *Morbidity and Mortality Weekly Report*, *54*, 1301–1305.

Chandy, C. J., Howard, C. R., & Auringer, P. (2006). Full breastfeeding duration and associated decrease in respiratory tract infection in US children. *Pediatrics*, *117*, 425–432.

Chang, S. H., Yang, Y. H., & Chiang, B. L. (2006a). Infectious pathogens in pediatric patients with primary immunodeficiencies. *Journal of Microbiology, Immunology and Infection*, *39*, 503–515.

Chang, S. O., Choi, B. Y., & Hur, D. G. (2006b). Analysis of the long-term hearing results after the surgical repair of aural atresia. *Laryngoscope*, *166*(10), 1835–1841.

Chen, C. H., Lin, C. J., Hwang, Y. H., & Ku, C. J. (2003). Epidemiology of otitis media in Chinese children. *Clinics in Otolaryngology*, *28*, 442–445.

da Costa, J. L., Navarro, A., Neves, J. B., & Martin, M. (2004). Household wood and charcoal smoke increases risk of otitis media in childhood in Maputo. *International Journal of Epidemiology, 33*, 573–578.

Dallaire, F., Dewailly, E., Vezina, C., Bruneau, S., & Ayotte, P. (2006). Portrait of outpatient visits and hospitalizations for acute infections in Nunavik preschool children. *Canadian Journal of Public Health, 97*, 362–368.

Daly, K. A., Brown, W. M., Segade, F., Bowden, D. W., Keats, B. J., Lindgren, B. R., . . . Rich, S. S. (2004). Chronic and recurrent otitis media: A genome scan for susceptibility loci. *American Journal of Human Genetics, 75*, 988–997.

Daly, K. A., Pirie, P. L., Rhodes, K. L., Hunter, L. L., & Davey, C. S. (2007). Early otitis media among Minnesota American Indians: The little ears study. *American Journal of Public Health, 97*, 317–322.

De Alarcon, A., & Choo, D. I. (2007). Controversies in aural atresia repair. *Current Opinions in Otolaryngology and Head and Neck Surgery, 15*, 310–314.

De La Cruz, A., & Teufert, K. B. (2003). Congenital aural atresia surgery: Long-term results. *Otolaryngology–Head and Neck Surgery, 129*(1), 121–127.

Del Beccaro, M. A., Mendelman, P. M., Inglis, A. F., Richardson, M. A., Duncan, N. O., Clausen, C. R., & Stull, T. L. (1992). Bacteriology of acute otitis media: A new perspective. *Journal of Pediatrics, 120*, 81–84.

Depreux, F., Darrow, K., Conner, D., Eavey, R., Liberman, M., Seidman, C., & Seidman, J. (2008). Eya4-deficient mice are a model for heritable otitis media. *Journal of Clinical Investigation, 118*, 651–658.

Dhillon, R. S. (1988). The middle ear in cleft palate children pre and post palatal closure. *Journal of the Royal Society of Medicine, 81*, 710–713.

Digoy, G. P., & Cueva, R. A. (2007). Congenital aural atresia: Review of short- and long-term surgical results. *Otology and Neurotology, 28*, 54–60.

Doyle, K. J., Burggraaff, B., Fujikawa, S., Jim, J., & MacArthur, C. J. (1997). Neonatal hearing screening with otoscopy, auditory brain stem response, and otoacoustic emissions. *Otolaryngology-Head and Neck Surgery, 116*, 597–603.

Englund, J. A. (2007). The influence of maternal immunization on infant immune responses. *Journal of Comparative Pathology, 137*, S16–S19.

Eskola, J., Kilpi, T., Palmu, A., Jokinen, J., Haapakoski, J., Herva, E., . . . Mäkelä, P. H. (2001). Finnish Otitis Media Study Group, Efficacy of a pneumococcal conjugate vaccine against acute otitis media. *New England Journal of Medicine, 344*, 403–409.

Evans, A. E., & Kazahaya, K. (2007). Canal atresia: Surgery or implantable hearing devices? The expert's question is revisited. *International Journal of Pediatric Otorhinolaryngology, 71*, 367–374.

Feeney, M. P., Keefe, D. H., & Marryott, L. P. (2003). Contralateral acoustic reflex threshold for tonal activators using wideband reflectance and admittance. *Journal of Speech, Language, and Hearing, Research, 46*, 128–136.

Fraser, F. C., Sproule, J. R., & Halal, F. (1980). Frequency of the branchio-oto-renal (BOR) syndrome in children with profound hearing loss. *American Journal of Medical Genetics, 7*, 341–349.

Glezen, W. P. (2003). Effect of maternal antibodies on the infant immune response. *Vaccine, 28*, 3389–3392.

Grabb W. (1965). The first and second bronchial arch syndrome. *Plastic and Reconstructive Surgery, 36*, 485.

Grijalva, C. G., Poehling, K. A., Nuorti, J. P., Zhu, Y., Martin, S. W., Edwards, K. M., & Griffin, M. R. (2006). National impact of universal childhood immunization with pneumococcal conjugate vaccine on outpatient medical care visits in the United States. *Pediatrics, 118*, 865–873.

Gunasekera, H., Hayson, L., Morris, P., & Craig, J. (2007). *The global burden of childhood otitis media and hearing impairment (HI): A systemic review*. Paper presented at the 9th International Symposium on Recent Advances in Otitis Media. St. Petersburg Beach, FL.

Hall, J. W., III., Smith, S. D., & Popelka, G. R. (2004). Newborn hearing screening with combined otoacoustic emissions and auditory brainstem responses. *Journal of the American Academy of Audiology, 15*, 414–425.

Hardisty-Hughes, R. E., Tateossian, H., Morse, S. A., Romero, M. R., Middleton, A., Tymowska-Lalanne, Z., . . . Brown, S. D. (2006). A mutation in the F-box gene, Fbxo11, causes otitis media in the jeff mouse. *Human Molecular Genetics, 15*, 3273–3279.

Hoffman, H. J., Park, J., Losonczy, K. G., & Chiu, M. S. (2007). *Risk factors, treatments, and other conditions associated with frequent ear infections in US children through 2 years of age: The Early Childhood Longitudinal Study Birth Cohort (ECLS-B)*. Paper presented at the 9th International Symposium on Recent Advances in Otitis Media. St. Petersburg Beach, FL.

Holte, L., Margolis, R. H., & Cavanaugh, R. M. (1991). Developmental changes in multifrequency tympanograms. *Audiology, 30*, 1–24.

Hunt, C. E., Lesko, S. M., Vezina, R. M., McCoy, R., Corwin, M. J., & Mandell, F. (2003). Infant sleep position and associated health outcomes. *Archives of Pediatric Adolescent Medicine, 157*, 469–474.

Hunter, L. L., Davey, C. S., Kohtz, A., & Daly, K. A. (2007). Hearing screening and middle ear measures in American Indian infants and toddlers. *International Journal of Pediatric Otorhinolaryngology, 71*, 1429–1438.

Hunter, L. L., & Margolis, R. H. (1992). Multifrequency tympanometry, current clinical application. *American Journal of Audiology, 1*, 33–43.

Hunter, L. L., Tubaugh, L., Jackson, A., & Propes, S. (2008). Wideband middle ear power measurement in infants and children. *Journal of the American Academy of Audiology, 19*, 309–324.

Ikui, A., Sando, I., & Fujita, S. (1997). Postnatal change in angle between the tympanic annulus and surrounding structures: Computer-aided three-dimensional reconstruction study. *Annals of Otolaryngology, Rhinology and Laryngology, 106*, 33–36.

Ishimoto, S., Ito, K., Yamasoba, T., Kondo, K., Karino, S., Takegoshi, H., & Kaga, K. (2005). Correlation between microtia and temporal bone malformation evaluated using grading systems. *Archives of Otolaryngology-Head and Neck Surgery, 131*, 326–329.

Jacoby, P. A., Coates, H. L., Arumgaswamy, A., Elsbury, D., Stokes, A., Monck, R., . . . Lehman, D. (2008). The effect of passive smoking on the risk of otitis media in Aboriginal and non-Aboriginal children in the Kalgoorlie-Boulder region of Western Australia. *Medical Journal of Australia, 188*, 599–603.

Jafek, B. W., Nager, G. T., Strife, J., & Gayler, R. W. (1975). Congenital aural atresia: An analysis of 311 cases. *Transactions of the Section Otolaryngology of the American Academy of Opthamology and Otolaryngology, 80*, 588–595.

Jahrsdoerfer, R. A., & Jacobson, J. T. (1995). Treacher Collins syndrome: Otologic and auditory management. *Journal of the American Academy of Audiology, 6*, 93–102.

Jahrsdoerfer, R. A., Yeakley, J. W., Aguilar, E. A., Cole, R. R., & Gray, L. C. (1992). Grading system for the selection of patients with congenital aural atresia. *American Journal of Otology, 13*, 6–12.

Johnston, L. C., Feldman, H. M., Paradise, J. L., Bernard, B. S., Colborn, D. K., Casselbrant, M. L., & Janosky, J. E. (2004). Tympanic membrane abnormalities and hearing levels at the ages of 5 and 6 years in relation to persistent otitis media and tympanostomy tube insertion in the first 3 years of life: A prospective study incorporating a randomized clinical trial. *Pediatrics, 114*, e58–67.

Joint Committee on Infant Hearing (JCIH). (2007). Year 2007 Position statement: Principles and guidelines for early hearing detection and intervention programs. *Pediatrics, 120*, 898–921.

Karevold, G., Kvestad, E., Nafstad, P., & Kvaerner, K. J. (2006). Respiratory infections in schoolchildren: Co-morbidity and risk factors. *Archives of Diseases in Childhood, 91*, 391–395.

Keefe, D. H., & Abdala, C. (2007). Theory of forward and reverse middle-ear transmission applied to otoacoustic emissions in infant and adult ears. *Journal of the Acoustical Society of America, 121*, 978–993.

Keefe, D. H., Bulen, J. C., Arehart, K. H., & Burns, E. M. (1993). Ear-canal impedance and reflection coefficient in human infants and adults. *Journal of the Acoustical Society of America, 94*, 2617–2638.

Keefe, D. H., Folsom, R., Gorga, M. P., Vohr, B. R., Bulen, J. C., & Norton, S. (2000). Identification of neonatal hearing impairment: Ear-canal measurements of acoustic admittance and reflectance in neonates. *Ear and Hearing, 21*, 443–461.

Keefe, D. H., Gorga, M. P., Zhao, F., Neely, S. T., & Vohr, B. (2003a). Ear-canal acoustic admittance and reflectance effects in human neonates. II. Predictions of middle-ear dysfunction and sensorineural hearing loss. *Journal of the Acoustical Society of America, 113*, 407–422.

Keefe, D. H., & Simmons, J. L. (2003). Energy transmittance predicts conductive hearing loss in older children and adults. *Journal of the Acoustical Society of America, 114*, 3217–3238.

Keefe, D. H., Zhao, F., Neely, S. T., Gorga, M. P., & Vohr, B. (2003b). Ear-canal acoustic admittance and reflectance effects in human neonates. I. Predictions of otoacoustic emission and auditory brainstem responses. *Journal of the Acoustical Society of America, 113*, 389–406.

Kei, J., Allison-Levick, J., Dockray, J., Harrys, R., Kirkegard, C., Wong, J., . . . Tudehope, D. (2003). High-frequency (1000-Hz) tympanometry in normal neonates. *Journal of the American Academy of Audiology, 14*, 20–28.

Kvestad, E., Kvaerner, K. J., Roysamb, E., Tambs, K., Harris, J. R., & Magnus, P. (2004). Otitis media: Genetic factors and sex differences. *Twin Research, 7*, 239–244.

Lambert, P. R. (1998). Congenital aural atresia: Stability of surgical results. *Laryngoscope, 108*(12), 1801–1805.

Lambert, P. R. (2001). Congenital aural atresia. In B. J. Bailey, (Ed.), *Head and neck surgery: Otolaryngology* (pp. 1745–1757). Philadelphia, PA: Lippincott Williams and Wilkins.

Lasisi, A. O., Olaniyan, F. A., Muibi, S. A., Azeez, I. A., Abulwasiu, K. G., Lasisi, T. J., . . . Olayemi, O. (2007a). Clinical and demographic risk factors associated with chronic suppurative otitis media. *International Journal of Pediatric Otorhinolaryngology, 71*; 1549–1554.

Lasisi, A. O., Sulaiman, O. A., & Afolabi, O. A. (2007b). Socioeconomic status and hearing loss in chronic suppurative otitis media in Nigeria. *Annals of Tropical Paediatrics, 27*, 21–26.

Lous, J., Burton, M. J., Felding, J. U., Ovesen, T., Rovers, M. M., & Williamson, I. Grommets (ventilation tubes) for hearing loss associated with otitis media with effusion in children. *Cochrane Database of Systematic Reviews*. 2005, Issue 1. Art. No. CD001801.

Mandel, E. M., Doyle, W. J., Winther, B., & Alper, C. (2008). The incidence, prevalence and burden of OM in unselected children aged 1–8 year followed by weekly otoscopy through the "common cold" season. *International Journal of Pediatric Otorhinolaryngology, 72*, 491–499.

Margolis, R. H., Bass-Ringdahl, S., Hanks, W. D., Holte, L., & Zapala, D. A. (2003). Tympanometry in newborn infants —1 kHz norms. *Journal of the American Academy of Audiology, 14*, 383–392.

Marx, H. (1926). Die missbildungen des ohres. In F. Henke, & O. Lubarsh (Eds.), *Handbuch der spez path anatomie histology* (pp. 620–625). Berlin, Germany: Springer.

McKenzie, J., & Craig, J. (1955). Mandibulo-facial dysotosis (Treacher-Collins syndrome). *Archives of Diseases in Childhood, 30*, 391.

Morris, P. S., Leach, A. J., Silberberg, P., Mellon, G., Wilson, C., Hamilton, E., & Beissbarth, J. (2005). Otitis media in young Aboriginal children from remote communities in Northern and Central Australia: A cross-sectional survey. *BMC Pediatrics, 5*, 27.

NICHD and Early Child Care Network. (2003). Child care and communicable illness in children aged 37 to 54 months. *Archives of Pediatrics and Adolescent Medicine, 157*, 196–200.

Paradise, J. L., & Bluestone, C. D. (1974). Early treatment of the universal otitis media of infants with cleft palate. *Pediatrics, 53*, 48–54.

Paradise, J. L., Smith, C. G., & Bluestone, C. D. (1976). Tympanometric detection of middle ear effusion in infants and young children. *Pediatrics, 58*, 198–210.

Patel, J. A., Nair, S., Revai, K., Grady, J., Saeed, K., Matalon, R., . . . Chonmaitree, T. (2006). Association of proinflammatory cytokine gene polymorphisms with susceptibility to otitis media. *Pediatrics, 118*, 2273–2279.

Patel, N., & Shelton, C. (2007). The surgical learning curve in aural atresia surgery. *Laryngoscope, 117*(1), 67–73.

Paterson, J. E., Carter, S., Wallace, J., Ahmad, Z., Garett, N., & Silva, P. A. (2006). Pacific Island family study: The prevalence of chronic middle ear disease in 2-year old Pacific Island children living in New Zealand. *International Journal of Pediatric Otorhinolaryngology, 70*, 1771–1778.

Paterson, J. E., Carter, S., Wallace, J., Ahmad, Z., Garett, N., & Silva, P. A. (2007). Pacific Island Families Study: Risk factors associated with otitis media with effusions among Pacific 2-year old children. *International Journal of Pediatric Otorhinolaryngology, 71*, 1047–1054.

Piskorski, P., Keefe, D. H., Simmons, J., & Gorga, M. P. (1999). Prediction of conductive hearing loss based on acoustic ear-canal response using a multivariate clinical decision theory. *Journal of the Acoustical Society of America, 105*, 1749–1764.

Plasschaert, A. I., Rovers, M. M., Schilder, A. G., Verheij, T. J., & Hak, E. (2006). Trends in doctor consultations, antibiotic prescription, and specialist referrals for otitis media in children: 1995–2003. *Pediatrics, 17*, 1879–1886.

Poehling, K. A., Szilagyi, P. G., Grijalva, C. G., Martin, S. W., LaFleur, B., Mitchell, E., . . . Griffin, M. R. (2007). Reduction in frequent otitis media and pressure equalizing tube insertions after introduction of pneumococcal conjugate vaccine. *Pediatrics, 119*, 1394–1402.

Poswillo, D. E. (1973). The pathogenesis of first and second branchial arch syndrome. *Oral Surgery, 35*, 302.

Praveen, C. V., & Terry, R. M. (2005). Does passive smoking affect the outcome of grommet insertion in children? *Journal of Laryngology and Otology, 119*, 448–454.

Pron, G., Galloway, C., Armstrong, D., & Posnick, J. (1993). Ear malformation and hearing loss in patients with Treacher Collins syndrome. *Cleft Palate Craniofacial Journal, 30*, 97–103.

Riemer, G., Castiglione, M., Ferrall-Pack, A., Staudigel, H., Summers, L., & Choo, D. (2008). *Best evidence statement on aural atresia*. Cincinnati Children's Hospital Medical Center unpublished evidence statement.

Rosenfeld, R. M., Culpepper, L., Doyle, K. J., Grundfast, K. M., & Hoberman, A. (2004). American Academy of Pediatrics Subcommittee on Otitis Media with Effusion; American Academy of Family Physicians; American Academy of Otolaryngology-Head and Neck Surgery. *Clinical Practice Guideline: Otitis media with effusion, 130* (5 Suppl.), S95–S118.

Rovers, M. M., Numans, M. E., Langenback, E., Grobee, D. E., Verheij, T. J., & Schilder, A. G. (2008). Is pacifier use a risk factor for acute otitis media? A dynamic cohort study. *Family Practice, 25*, 233–236.

Ruah, C. B., Schachern, P. A., Zelterman, D., Paparella, M. M., & Yoon, T. H. (1991). Age-related morphologic changes in the human tympanic membrane. A light and electron microscopic study. *Archives of Otolaryngology-Head and Neck Surgery, 117*, 627–634.

Rynnel-Dagöö, B. (2004): Acute otitis media and otitis media with effusion in the immunocompromised child. In C. Alper, C. Bluestone, M. Casselbrant, J. Dohar, & E. Mandel (Eds.), *Advanced therapy of otitis media* (pp. 462–464). Hamilton, ON: B.C. Decker Inc.

Sale, M. M., Perlegas, P., Marion, M., Hicks, P. J., Rich, S. S., & Daly, K. A. (2007). *Fine mapping of two loci for chronic otitis media with effusion and recurrent otitis media*. Paper presented at the 9th international symposium on recent advances in otitis media. St. Petersburg Beach, FL.

Saunders, J. C., Kaltenback, J. A., & Relkin, E. M. (1983). The structural and functional development of the outer and middle ear. In R. Romand & M. R. Romand (Eds.), *Development of auditory and vestibular systems* (pp. 3–25). New York, NY: Academic.

Schönweiler, R., Lisson, J. A., Schönweiler, B., Eckardt, A., Ptok, M., Tränkmann, J., & Hausamen, J. E. (1999). A retrospective study of hearing, speech and language function in children with clefts following palatoplasty and veloplasty procedures at 18–24 months of age. *International Journal of Pediatrics in Otorhinolaryngology, 50*, 205–217.

Schuknecht, H. F. (1989). Congenital aural atresia. *Laryngoscope, 99*, 908–917.

Segade, F., Daly, K. A., Allred, D., Hicks, P. J., Cox, M., Brown, M., . . . Bowden, D.W. (2006). Association of the FBXO11 gene with chronic otitis media with effusion and recurrent otitis media: The Minnesota COME/ROM Family Study. *Archives of Otolaryngology-Head and Neck Surgery, 132*, 729–733.

Shah, U. K. (2004). Otitis media with effusion in craniofacial syndromes. In C. M.Alper, C. D.Bluestone, M. L. Casselbrant, J. E. Dohar, & E. M. Mandel, (Eds.), *Advanced therapy of otitis media* (pp. 468–473). Hamilton, Ontario: B.C. Decker.

Sheahan, P., Miller, I., Sheahan, J. N., Earley, M. J., & Blayney, A. W. (2003). Incidence and outcome of middle ear disease in cleft lip and palate. *International Journal of Pediatric Otorhinolaryngology, 67*, 785–793.

Shott, S. R., Joseph, A., & Heithaus, D. (2001). Hearing loss in children with Down syndrome. *International Journal of Pediatric Otorhinolaryngology, 61*, 199–205.

Sprague, B. H., Wiley, T. L., & Goldstein, R. (1985). Tympanometric and acoustic-reflex studies in neonates. *Journal of Speech Hearing Research, 28*, 265–272.

Stuart, A., Yang, E. Y., & Green, W. B. (1994). Neonatal auditory brain-stem response thresholds to air- and bone-conducted clicks. *Journal of the American Academy of Audiology, 5*, 163–172.

Swartz, J. D., & Faerber, E. N. (1985). Congenital malformations of the external and middle ear: high-resolution CT findings of surgical import. *American Journal of Roentgenology, 144*, 501–506.

Takahashi, H., & Maeda, K. (1982). Survey of familial occurrence in 171 microtia cases. *Japanese Journal Plastic Surgery, 15*, 310.

Tanzer, R. (1971). Total reconstruction of the auricle. The evolution of a plan of treatment. *Plastic and Reconstructive Surgery, 47*, 523.

Thorne, J. A. (2003). Middle ear problems in Aboriginal school children cause developmental and educational concerns. *Contemporary Nurse, 16*, 145–150.

Ubell, M. L., Kerschner, J. E., Wackym, P. A., & Burrows, A. (2008). MUC2 expression in human middle ear epithelium of patients with otitis media. *Archives of Otolaryngology-Head and Neck Surgery, 134*, 39–41.

U.S. Department of Health and Human Services (DHHS). (2008). Vision and hearing. In *Healthy people 2010 mid-course review* (pp. 28–25). Washington, DC: U.S. Government Printing Office, December 2006.

Vander Werff, K. R., Prieve, B. A., & Georgantas, L. M. (2007). Test-retest reliability of wideband reflectance measures in infants under screening and diagnostic test conditions. *Ear and Hearing, 28*, 669–681.

Wiertsema, S. P., Herpers, B. L., Veenhoven, R. H., Salimans, M. M., Ruven, H. J., & Sanders, E. A. (2006). Functional polymorphisms in the mannan-binding lectin 2 gene: Effect on MBL levels and otitis media. *Journal of Allergy and Clinical Immunology, 117*, 1344–1350.

Williamson, I., Benge, S., Mullee, M., & Little, P. (2006). Consultations for middle ear disease, antibiotic prescribing and risk factors for reattendance: A case-linked cohort study. *British Journal of Genetic Practice, 56*, 170–175.

Xenellis, J., Paschalidis, J., Georgalas, C., Davilis, D., Tzagaroulakis, A., & Ferekidis, E. (2005). Factors influencing the presence of otitis media with effusion 16 months after initial diagnosis in a cohort of school-age children in rural Greece: A prospective study. *International Journal of Pediatric Otorhinolaryngology, 69*, 1641–1647.

Yellon, R. F. (2007). Bone anchored hearing aid in children—prevention of complications. *Pediatric Otorhinolaryngology, 71*, 823–826.

Zhou, F., Shefer, A., Kong, Y., & Nuorti, J. P. (2008). Trends in acute otitis media-related health care utilization by privately insured young children in the US, 1997–2004. *Pediatrics, 121*, 253–260.

10

Children With Unilateral Hearing Loss

Heather Porter and Fred H. Bess

Introduction

A time-honored maxim among physicians, educators, and many audiologists has been that children with a loss of hearing in one ear generally experience few, if any, communicative or psychoeducational difficulties. Historically, the typical management strategy for this population has been relatively incomprehensive. Once the unilateral hearing loss (UHL) has been identified, the parents are told that the hearing loss exists, and they are often assured that no problems will occur as a result of the loss. Preferential seating in the classroom is recommended and occasionally some type of amplification (e.g., CROS, FM) is recommended on a trial basis. Because of the long-standing belief that UHL is without significant consequence, many of these children are not always considered educationally handicapped, and in many schools they are not eligible for special services. Despite the widespread impression that UHL is not a serious problem there is a lack of experimental evidence to support such an assumption.

To the contrary, available research conducted on both adults and children suggests that individuals with only one good ear experience a variety of communicative, educational, and psychosocial problems (Bess, Dodd-Murphy, & Parker, 1998; Culbertson & Gilbert, 1986; Priwin, Jönsson, Hultcrantz, & Granström, 2007). In fact, the findings of early research, conducted mostly with adults, show that persons with hearing loss in one ear experience a variety of listening difficulties. Predictably, the greatest problem in hearing and understanding speech occurs when the spoken message originates on the impaired side while a competing message or noise originates from the side with better hearing. However, adults with UHL have also noted difficulty understanding speech originating from the impaired side even when the ear with better hearing is not receiving competing signals. Localizing a signal source is also difficult for adults with UHL. Moreover, adults with UHL have reported feelings of embarrassment, annoyance, confusion and helplessness (Giolas & Wark, 1967).

Based on findings from adults with UHL, it is not surprising to learn that children with UHL also encounter similar listening difficulties, particularly in the school setting. Such listening problems could very well inhibit the development of language, discrimination of individual speech sounds, and other communicative skills—skills considered essential for learning in school. Indeed, early research suggests that children with UHL may experience a variety of educational, auditory and psychosocial difficulties (Boyd, 1974; Quigley & Thomure, 1969; Simon, 1977). In a landmark study on the topic, Quigley and Thomure (1969) identified school-aged children with hearing loss who were not receiving support services (n = 116). The majority of children identified were children with hearing threshold levels of less than 26 dB HL (82.7%) —a number of these students had UHL. As a group, the identified children scored below expected levels on subtests of the Sanford Achievement Test (i.e., word meaning, paragraph meaning, and language) and on average, were one grade behind expected levels based on age. Similar findings have been reported by others (Bess, 1982; Bess & Tharpe, 1984, 1986; Boyd, 1974; Oyler, 1988; Simon, 1977).

Indeed, a contemporary review of UHL in children leads one to several realities. First, the majority of studies on children with UHL have reported a variety of auditory, educational, and psychoeducational complications (e.g., Bess, Dodd-Murphy, & Parker, 1998;

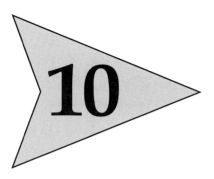

Bess & Tharpe, 1984; Boyd, 1974; Culbertson & Gilbert, 1986; Jenson, Johansen, & Børre, 1989; Oyler, 1988; Quigley & Thomure, 1969; Simon, 1977). A few studies, however, have reported no such difficulties for children with UHL (Hallmo, Moller, Lind, & Tonning, 1986; Stein, 1983; Tieri, Masi, Ducci, & Marsella, 1988). Second, definitions of normal hearing sensitivity vary, and one consequence of this variation in definition is confusion and indecision regarding intervention (Gravel, Knightly, & McKay, 2008). Third, nomenclature within our profession appears to promote a lack of importance for certain hearing loss categories. That is, UHL is often categorized as minimal hearing loss (MHL) and as such, carries a connotation of minimal consequence. Finally, but not without significant influence, is the adherence of educational support and health care specialists to a failure-based model of intervention which includes "wait-and-see" policies that support monitoring a child's development and intervening only at the point of academic failure.

This chapter presents a contemporary overview on children with UHL. To this end, topic areas to be covered include definitions, etiology, prevalence, advantages of binaural hearing, auditory deprivation, auditory performance, real-world outcomes, and audiologic considerations such as hearing screening, age of identification, and diagnosis. The chapter also includes a section on future directions and research needs. The management of children with UHL is covered in Chapter 34 of this volume.

Definition of UHL

The most commonly accepted definition of UHL has been proposed by the Centers for Disease Control Early Hearing Detection Intervention Program (2005). This definition specifies an average pure tone threshold at 500, 1000, and 2000 Hz of any level greater than or equal to 20 dB HL or pure tone threshold greater than 25 dB HL at two or more frequencies above 2000 Hz in the affected ear and an average pure tone threshold in the good ear less than or equal to 15 dB HL. Unfortunately, many broad definitions of UHL are used by clinicians ranging from "two or more thresholds greater than 20 dB HL in one ear" to "difference in ears greater than 15 dB across three frequencies" (Gravel et al., 2008).

Etiology

Information about the etiology of UHL has been limited. In fact, estimates have suggested that etiology of UHL is unknown for 35 to 60% of cases in children (Brookhouser, Worthington, & Kelly, 1991; English & Church, 1999). A summary of major etiologic factors associated with UHL is shown in Table 10–1.

Congenital cytomegalovirus (CMV) is the most common cause of nongenetic hearing loss and the leading cause of UHL in children (Nance, 2007). CMV infection occurs in 0.2 to 2.5% of all live births; however, it does not always present with symptoms (Leung, Sauve, & Davies, 2003). By age 6 years, 35% of infants with symptomatic CMV and 11% of infants with nonsymptomatic CMV have hearing loss (Fowler, Dahle, Boppana, & Pass, 1999). Nance, Lim, and Dodson (2006) found congenital CMV and genetic mutations related to connexin[1] to be two major causes of deafness at birth and enlarged vestibular aqueduct syndrome (EVAS) and congenital CMV as the major causes for late onset prelingual hearing loss.

Other infections can also be responsible for UHL. Prior to 1967 when the mumps vaccine was introduced, mumps was the leading cause of acquired UHL. Since that time, there has been a 90 to 95% decrease in the incidence of the pathology; however, recent outbreaks have been noted in the United States and the United Kingdom (Cohen et al., 2007; Dayan et al., 2008). Bacterial and viral meningitis can also cause hearing loss. Although viral meningitis is more common than bacterial meningitis, hearing loss is often associated with the bacterial form of this condition. Hearing loss, ranging from mild unilateral to profound bilateral, is the most common complication of bacterial meningitis among children (Baraff, Lee, & Schriger, 1993). Approximately 30% of cases of hearing loss resulting from bacterial meningitis are unilateral (Kutz, Simon, Chennupati, Giannoni, & Manolidis, 2006).

Enlarged vestibular aqueduct syndrome (EVAS) is the most common form of inner ear malformation associated with sensorineural hearing loss (Boston et al., 2007). In the majority of cases, hearing loss associated with EVAS is bilateral, but cases of UHL have been reported (Govaerts et al., 1999). Additional malformations shown to cause hearing loss, such as Chiari malformation, may occur unilaterally more often than bilaterally (Simons, Ruscetta, & Chi, 2008).

[1]Connexin is a subunit of connexon, a protein that forms a gap junction between cells. These junctions are essential to the function of the inner ear as they permit intercellular exchange of potassium and calcium.

Table 10–1. Summary of Etiologic Factors Associated With UHL

Cause	*Frequency of Occurrence*	*Reference*
Congenital Cytomegalovirus (CMV)	The leading cause of unilateral hearing loss in children. Occurs in 0.2 to 2.5% of all live births.	(Leung et al., 2003; Nance, 2007)
Bacterial Meningitis	Approximately 30% of cases result in at least a unilateral hearing loss.	(Kutz et al., 2006)
Viral/Bacterial Mumps	Approximately 80 to 95% of cases of hearing loss caused by viral or bacterial mumps are unilateral.	(Unal et al., 1998)
Enlarged Vestibular Aqueduct Syndrome (EVAS)	Approximately 20% of cases of EVAS are unilateral.	(Govaerts et al., 1999)
Chiari Malformation	Majority of cases (~65%) are unilateral.	(Simons et al., 2008)
Auditory Neuropathy Spectrum Disorder (ANSD)	Most cases of ANSD are bilateral, though some cases of unilateral hearing loss have been reported.	(Podwall et al., 2002)
Sudden Sensorineural Hearing Loss (SNHL)	Approximately 85% of cases of sudden SNHL in children are unilateral.	(Roman et al., 2001)
Atresia	Congenital atresia or microtia occurs in approximately 1 out of 10,000 live births. Approximately 70% of cases of atresia are unilateral.	(Schuknecht, 1989)
Gap Junction Beta 2 (*GJB2*)	Over 80 mutations of GJB2 are responsible for hearing loss. Some cases of UHL have been reported, but most cases are profound.	(Kenna et al., 2001; Wilcox et al., 2000)
Prematurity	Approximately 5% of premature infants have minimal bilateral or unilateral hearing loss.	(Herrgård, Karjalainen, Martikainen, & Heinonen, 1995)

Other less common causes of UHL in children include auditory neuropathy spectrum disorder (ANSD), sudden idiopathic hearing loss, and congenital aural atresia and microtia. Though ANSD is typically bilateral, unilateral cases have been reported (Podwall, Podwall, Gordon, Lamendola, & Gold, 2002). Sudden idiopathic hearing loss typically occurs unilaterally; however, the prevalence is lower in children than adults (Roman, Aladio, Paris, Nicollas, & Triglia, 2001). Approximately 3.5% occurs in patients under 14 years of age (Nakashima & Yanagita, 1993). Congenital aural atresia or microtia occurs in approximately 1 per 10,000 live births as part of syndromic or nonsyndromic disorders (Melnick & Myrianthopoulos, 1979). The severity of anomaly can range from mild to more severe symptoms that could include absence of the middle ear structures in combination with anotia. Unilateral aural atresia occurs in approximately 70% of cases of atresia (Schuknecht, 1989). Other possible causes of UHL, not referenced in Table 10–1, include noise-induced hearing loss and head trauma (Brookhouser et al., 1991).

About 200 genes that contribute to hearing loss have been isolated (Griffith & Friedman, 2002). Mutations involving the Gap Junction Beta 2 (*GJB2*) gene[2]

[2]Also known as connexin 26 (*Cx26*), this gene codes for proteins that form gap junctions between cells. Recall that these junctions are essential to the function of the inner ear as they permit intercellular exchange of potassium and calcium. Mutations of *GJB2/Cx26* are responsible for 30 to 40% of genetic deafness (Pandya et al., 2003).

are the most frequent cause of deafness in many populations (Nance & Kearsey, 2004). More than 80 mutations of *GJB2* are involved with the phenotypic presentation of hearing loss including deletions, insertions, nonsense, and missense anomalies (Cohn & Kelley, 1999). Most reports of hearing loss related to *GJB2* have been profound, but associations with less severe and UHL have been reported (Kenna, Wu, Cotanche, Korf, & Rehm, 2001; Wilcox et al., 2000).

As we learn more about genetic testing and as we identify children with hearing loss at an earlier age, we should become better able to identify the causes of UHL. Currently, identification of etiology at birth may be accomplished in approximately 60% of late onset prelingual cases of hearing loss (Nance et al., 2006). Although this is an improvement over past estimates; there is room for even more. Morton and Nance (2006) suggest an etiologic focus on newborn hearing screening—a focus that also identifies infants at risk for late onset hearing loss. By screening for four causes of hearing loss, the majority of children with congenital deafness and late-onset prelingual deafness could be identified shortly after birth: *GJB2* deafness, mitochondrial *A1555G*[3] mutations, Pendred's syndrome, and congenital CMV (Nance et al., 2006). Recent studies continue to document etiology for approximately 50% of patients (Declau, Boudewyns, Van den Ende, Peeters, & van den Heyning, 2008). This type of large-scale early etiologic work not only helps to identify children with, and those at risk for, prelingual hearing loss, but also helps to better define the causes of early onset UHL in children.

Progression of UHL to Bilateral Hearing Loss

UHL may progress to bilateral hearing loss (BHL). Neault (2005) investigated 159 infants who were found to have hearing loss following a unilaterally failed newborn hearing screening; 64% were diagnosed with UHL, 36% had BHL. Approximately half of the children with UHL had CT scans that demonstrated abnormalities. Of those cases with abnormalities, 60% were associated with progressive hearing loss. In at least two other studies, universal newborn hearing screening provided information regarding the possibility of progression from UHL to BHL. Edwards (2008) investigated the hearing status of 110 newborn infants who exhibited a unilateral fail on the newborn hearing screening. Of these infants, 26% were eventually diagnosed with UHL and 4.5% were diagnosed with BHL; other studies have also demonstrated the possibility of a progression from UHL to BHL. Declau and colleagues (2008) confirmed permanent hearing loss in 68.2% consecutive referrals for failed UNHS. In these cases, 8.3% of infants with UHL from universal newborn hearing screening were ultimately diagnosed with BHL. It is reasonable to assume for at least some of these infants that the hearing loss progressed from UHL to BHL.

Prevalence

In 2006, 92.3% of infants were screened for hearing loss in the United States (3,555,223 per 3,852,148 live births; CDC, 2006). Of the 46 states and territories offering epidemiological data, hearing loss was diagnosed in approximately 1.2 per 1,000 infants screened. Similar prevalence has been reported by others (Dalzell et al., 2000; Finitzo, Albright, & Neal, 1998; Prieve et al., 2000). Of those infants screened for hearing loss, 0.03% are reported to have ultimately been diagnosed with UHL. Interestingly, studies on the prevalence of UHL in school-aged children suggest a much higher prevalence within the general population relative to infancy. For example, Bess and coworkers (1998) reported UHL in 37/1218 (3.0%) of children in 3rd, 6th, and 9th grades. Additionally, Niskar et al. (1998) investigated 6,166 children aged 6 to 19 years and noted that 14.2% of these children had low-frequency or high-frequency UHL.

The aforementioned data suggest that by the time children reach school-age, the prevalence of UHL increases from 0.03% to approximately 3%, a 100-fold increase. Why is there such a large discrepancy in prevalence rates from birth to school-age children with UHL? Possible explanations include: (1) cases of progressive or late-onset hearing losses; (2) variability as a result of differing definitions/inclusion criteria; (3) low follow-up rates in newborn screening programs which results in underestimation of true prevalence; and (4) a large percentage of cases missed to follow-up.

[3]Mutations of A1555G are associated with sensitivity to aminoglycosides and account for 10% of hearing loss attributed to ototoxicity in the United States (Nance et al., 2006).

The Advantages of Binaural Hearing

There are some situations in which two ears provide a listening advantage over one ear alone. Improvements in threshold, localization, and speech understanding in adverse listening conditions are all improved when binaural listening is utilized. These improvements are facilitated by the processes of binaural summation, the head shadow effect, binaural release from masking, and the precedence effect. In addition, binaural cues are the dominant cues utilized for localization in the horizontal plane.

Binaural Summation

A sound presented to two ears is perceived louder than if the same sound were presented monaurally. At threshold, sound presented binaurally provides up to a 3 dB advantage over monaural presentation. This translates into an 18% improvement in monosyllable word recognition scores and a 30% improvement in sentence scores. At suprathreshold levels, up to a 6 dB improvement in detection can be seen. Binaural gains can be as large as 10 dB for stimuli presented at 90 dB SL (Fletcher & Munson, 1933; Hirsh, 1948).

Localization

Localization of sounds along the horizontal plane is facilitated by the use of two ears. Sounds originating from a single location in space will arrive at each ear at a different time and at a different intensity. The interaural time difference (ITD) of a sound can vary from 0 ms for sound originating at 0° azimuth to 0.6 ms for sounds generated at 90° or 270° azimuth. For frequencies below approximately 1500 Hz, the ITD can also be encoded into an interaural phase difference (IPD). Interaural intensity differences (IID) are most prominent for high-frequency sounds. The maximum IID for a 500-Hz tone is 4 dB compared to the maximum IID for a 6000-Hz tone, which is nearly 20 dB (for review see Grantham, 1995). Difficulties with localization increase as the degree of hearing loss in the poorer ear increases (Bess, Tharpe, & Gibler, 1986; Bovo et al., 1988; Humes, Allen, & Bess, 1980; Newton, 1983). The combined use of ITD at low frequencies and IID at high frequencies is known as the duplex theory of sound localization. Although additional monaural and binaural cues are included in this theory, interaural time and intensity differences are considered to be the most prominent cues.

Head Shadow Effect

The head shadow effect provides a reduction of sound intensity between ears of 6 to 12 dB for complex signals. Those with normal hearing can attend to the ear with the better signal-to-noise ratio. The most salient condition for this effect occurs when a signal is presented at 45° azimuth. The most profound effect for those with UHL occurs in conditions when the signal and noise are separate. That is, the most salient listening condition for those with UHL occurs when the signal of interest is presented toward the better hearing ear and noise is presented toward the poorer hearing ear. Conversely, the most difficult listening condition for those with UHL occurs when the signal of interest is presented toward the poorer hearing ear and noise is presented toward the better hearing ear.

Studies have shown that those with UHL perform more poorly than those with normal hearing on speech perception in noise. As you would expect, this effect is greater when speech is directed to the poorer hearing ear and the noise is directed to the better hearing ear (Bess et al., 1986; Kenworthy, Klee, & Tharpe, 1990; Ruscetta, Arjmand, & Pratt, 2005). In this case, the head shadow effect can present problems with speech understanding for those with UHL. Recall that IID are most pronounced for high frequencies. Considering that high-frequency consonants carry approximately 60% of speech intelligibility, it is clear the head shadow effect can have a negative impact on speech understanding for those with UHL under some circumstances.

Precedence Effect

Sound reflects from multiple surfaces and at different rates and intensities throughout reverberant rooms. Only some of these sounds are useful for localizing the source of the signal or understanding speech. Another benefit of binaural hearing is that it provides the central auditory system with information to suppress early reflections contained within reverberations. This assists listeners who are attempting to attend to a direct source of sound in a reverberant room. This is known as the precedence effect and its benefits are not enjoyed by people with UHL. Reverberation can degrade the quality of sound in a large room setting.

The primary effect of excessive reverberation on speech understanding is that vowel sounds mask the lower intensity consonants thereby degrading speech intelligibility (Berg, Blair, & Benson, 1996).

Binaural Release from Masking

Many individuals experience difficulty attending to a single speaker in a room full of many sources of sound. This problem is improved by binaural information for listeners with normal hearing. These improvements are related to the spatial separation of the signal of interest and those that interfere. Spatial separation creates spectral and/or temporal differences between the target and the interference. This phenomenon is studied under headphones in the laboratory and is known as binaural release from masking or masking level difference.

In general, the ability to hear a unilaterally presented signal is adversely affected when noise is presented to the same ear. Interestingly, adding contralateral noise to this configuration improves threshold by 6 dB. However, the addition of an identical signal to the contralateral noise, so that the listener has identical signal and noise conditions bilaterally, once again adversely affects threshold. An improvement in threshold is seen, however, when the phase of one of the signals is presented 180° out of phase compared to its contralateral counterpart. The improvement to the threshold of a target signal improves up to 15 dB in cases when the target signal is presented out of phase and noise is presented binaurally. A person with UHL is unable to take advantage of this phenomenon. Several studies have demonstrated the positive effects of binaural release from masking on speech recognition in adverse listening situations (Carhart, 1965; Harris, 1965; MacKeith & Coles, 1971; Moncur & Dirks, 1967). Binaural speech recognition is also better than monaural speech recognition in reverberant conditions. Up to a 3 dB signal-to-noise ratio (SNR) advantage can be observed for binaural over monaural listening conditions.

Auditory Deprivation

Early auditory experiences shape the way the brain processes and perceives sound. As such, the potential effects of auditory deprivation are another important consideration with regard to the difficulties experienced by children with UHL. In general, auditory deprivation has been described as a systematic decrease over time in performance associated with the reduced availability of acoustic information (Palmer, 1999). Detrimental effects of auditory deprivation on speech understanding have been shown for adults. Silverman, Silman, Emmer, Schoepflin, and Lutolf (2006) reported that word recognition performance of adults with asymmetric hearing loss declined in the poorer ear of adults who did not utilize amplification compared to a group of adults with asymmetric hearing loss who wore amplification.

Neural changes also occur within the anatomic structure of the brain in cases of UHL. For example, congenitally deaf individuals have reduced activation in the left lateral temporal cortex when compared to normal hearing controls during speech-reading tasks (MacSweeney et al., 2001). In cases of monaural stimulation, people with normal hearing display contralateral activation on fMRI (Jäncke, Wüstenberg, Schulze, & Heinze, 2002); however, people with UHL display bilateral activation patterns (Scheffler, Bilecen, Schmid, Tschopp, & Seelig, 1998; Tschopp, et al., 2000). Schmithorst and coworkers (2005) recently demonstrated cortical reorganization in children with UHL such that children with left UHL and right UHL had varying responses to random tonal stimuli when compared using fMRI. Although robust activation was seen in the auditory cortex bilaterally for both groups, children with left UHL displayed increased activation in the superior temporal areas and those with right UHL showed increased activation in the inferior frontal areas. These results suggest a differing cortical reorganization that is dependent on the laterality of hearing loss.

The anatomic and physiologic asymmetry for speech perception in the brain provides a theoretical framework for poorer outcomes for children with right ear hearing loss than left ear hearing loss. Limited data have been published to support this notion. Future research is needed in addition to a reanalysis of existing research that has analyzed children with UHL as a whole rather than differentiating between ears.

Structural changes have also been demonstrated in animal models. Animal studies have shown reorganization of the auditory brainstem (Illing, Kraus, & Meidinger, 2005) as well as cortical reorganization (Hutson, Durham, Imig, & Tucci, 2007) following unilateral deafness in rats and gerbils. Unilateral ablations tend to cause reorganization of the auditory pathway resulting in a strengthening of the functional role of the intact ear. Independent of whether unilateral ablation occurs in a developing or adult animal, the pathway from the intact ear to the ipsilateral cortex is strengthened (Syka, 2002).

Auditory Performance of Children with UHL

Localization

Children with UHL experience significantly greater problems localizing sounds on the horizontal plane than normal hearing listeners. Bess and coworkers (1986) reported significantly greater errors in localizing 500-Hz and 3000-Hz pure tones in children with UHL compared to their peers with normal hearing. Localization scores were positively correlated with degree of hearing loss; localization errors increased as the degree of hearing loss in the impaired ear worsened. With regard to right ear versus left ear, no difference in localization skills were observed in children with UHL at 500 Hz; however, children with right ear UHL had greater difficulty localizing at 3000 Hz compared to children with left ear UHL. Results from other studies also illustrate the detrimental effect of UHL on localization. For example, Priwin and colleagues (2007) reported poor localization skills in a broad study of children and adults aged 3 to 80 years with UHL. In addition, Morrongiello (1988) noted significant negative effects of localization in 28 infants aged 6 to 18 months of age during the time at which they had an active case of unilateral otitis media. Although this study used only otoscopy and did not verify middle ear function or hearing loss, improvements in localization were observed two weeks following treatment for otitis media.

It is noteworthy that though the negative effects of localization have been documented in research studies, they may go unnoticed by children in real-world situations. In a study of sound localization in children with severe UHL, 57% of the participants were unaware of problems prior to the study (Newton, 1983). This suggests that children may not have reliable self-report, at least for sound localization—such a finding has implications for safety considerations.

Speech Understanding

Children with UHL exhibit considerable difficulty understanding speech stimuli especially under adverse listening conditions (Bess et al., 1986). The mean syllable recognition scores for a group of children with UHL and their normal hearing counterparts is shown in Figure 10–1. Children with UHL exhibit poorer speech recognition scores in both monaural direct (speech to good ear, noise to impaired ear) and monaural indirect (noise to good ear, speech to impaired ear) conditions. In addition, the more adverse the listening condition, that is, the lower the SNR, the greater the discrepancy between children with UHL and children with normal hearing. Children with UHL performed significantly poorer than normal hearing children in the monaural indirect condition. Even in situations where the signal of interest is directed to the good ear with noise directed to the hearing impaired ear, children with UHL did not perform as well as their peers with normal hearing.

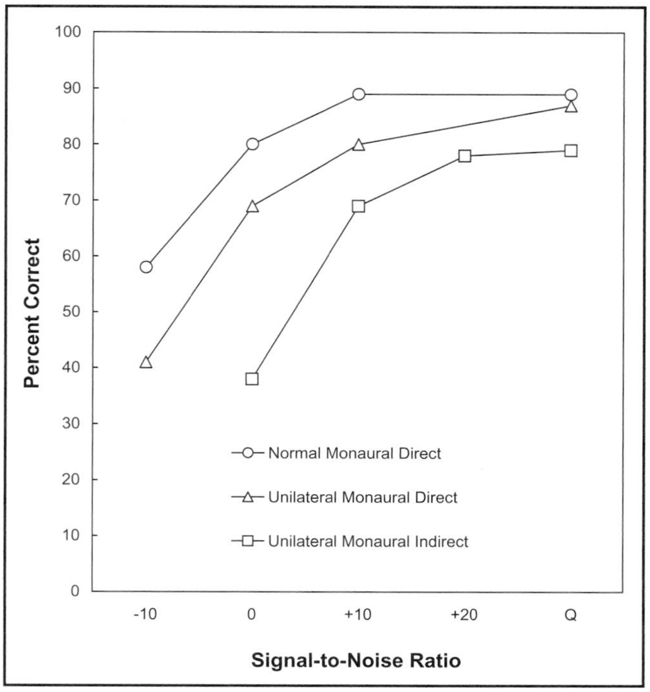

FIGURE 10–1. Mean sound field composite scores (in percent) on the Nonsense Syllable Test (NST) across several signal-to-noise ratio (SNR) conditions for normal-hearing children and children with UHL. The children were assessed in the monaural direct and monaural indirect conditions (data adapted from Bess, Tharpe & Gibler, 1986). Children with normal hearing were assessed with speech in the right ear and noise in the left ear.

The ability to perform well on speech-in-noise tasks is also affected by degree of impairment. Ruscetta et al. (2005) found that children aged 6 to 14 years with severe to profound UHL required a significantly greater SNR to perform as well as children with normal hearing on sentence and syllable recognition tasks. Other research has also demonstrated that some children and adults with UHL have difficulty understanding speech in noise (Priwin et al., 2007; Welsh, Welsh, Rosen, & Dragonette, 2004).

Some research has shown an effect of side of impairment on speech in noise tasks. Bess and colleagues (1986) demonstrated that children with right ear UHL tended to perform more poorly than children with normal hearing and left ear UHL on speech recognition tasks across SNR conditions. The more adverse the listening condition, the greater the discrepancy between ears (Figure 10–2).

Jensen, Johansen, and Børre (1989) supported the findings of Bess and coworkers, that is, children with right ear UHL exhibited poorer performance on speech in noise tests than children with left ear UHL; children with left ear UHL performed similarly to children with normal hearing. Jensen and coworkers also investigated ear effects on nonverbal tests and reported that children with right ear UHL perform significantly poorer than children with left ear UHL. Such information sheds some light on the findings that show children with right ear hearing loss are more likely to have failed a grade in school than children with left ear hearing loss (Bess & Tharpe, 1986; Oyler, 1988). It should be mentioned, however, that at least one study has suggested that children with right ear UHL and left ear UHL perform similarly on language performance measures (Lieu, Tye-Murray, Karzon,& Piccirillo, 2010).

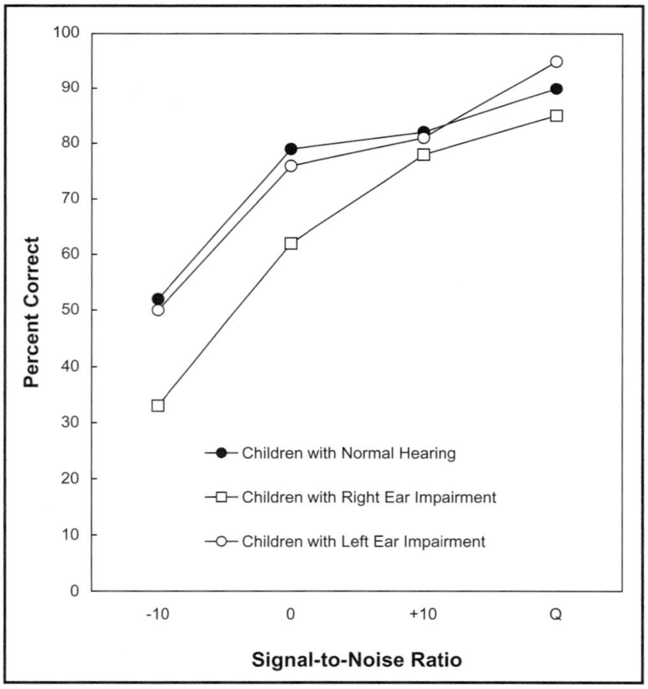

FIGURE 10–2. Mean sound field composite scores (in percent) on the NST in the monaural direct condition as a function of side of impairment (data adapted from Bess, Tharpe & Gibler, 1986).

Finally, research suggests that children with UHL who exhibit poor speech perception abilities are more likely to struggle academically. Bess and colleagues (1986) examined speech recognition abilities of children with UHL who had failed a grade and those who had not failed a grade. There is a tendency for children who perform more poorly in certain listening conditions to experience more difficulty in school.

Real-World Outcomes for Children With UHL

Learning and Educational Issues

In general, many children with significant UHL experience educational, social, emotional, and behavioral problems in school (Bess & Tharpe, 1984; Culbertson & Gilbert, 1986; Stein, 1983). Importantly, degree of hearing loss alone may not be a good predictor of a child's language or educational performance (Davis, Elfenbein, Schum, & Bentler, 1986; Moeller, 2007). Brookhouser and coworkers (1991) demonstrated that 59% of 172 children with UHL experienced academic or behavioral problems. They found no correlation between degree of impairment and amount of academic difficulty. Degree of hearing loss often acts in accord with other variables that contribute to development. Age of identification, family motivation, intervention plans, and the presence of additional disabilities, among other factors contribute to the overall development of the hearing-impaired child.

Not all children with UHL experience functional difficulties; however, some are clearly at risk for problems. Approximately 35% of children with UHL will fail at least one grade; an additional 15 to 60% will be in need of resource assistance in the schools. A distribution of grades failed by a group of 60 children with UHL is shown in Figure 10–3. Note that many children with UHL failed at the first grade level, however, one-half of the subjects failed grades above the first grade.

In another study of 1,218 children with mild sensorineural hearing loss, two-thirds of whom had UHL, 37% failed at least one grade and exhibited significantly greater dysfunction than normal hearing children on subtests of a screening tool for functional status such as behavior, energy, stress, social support,

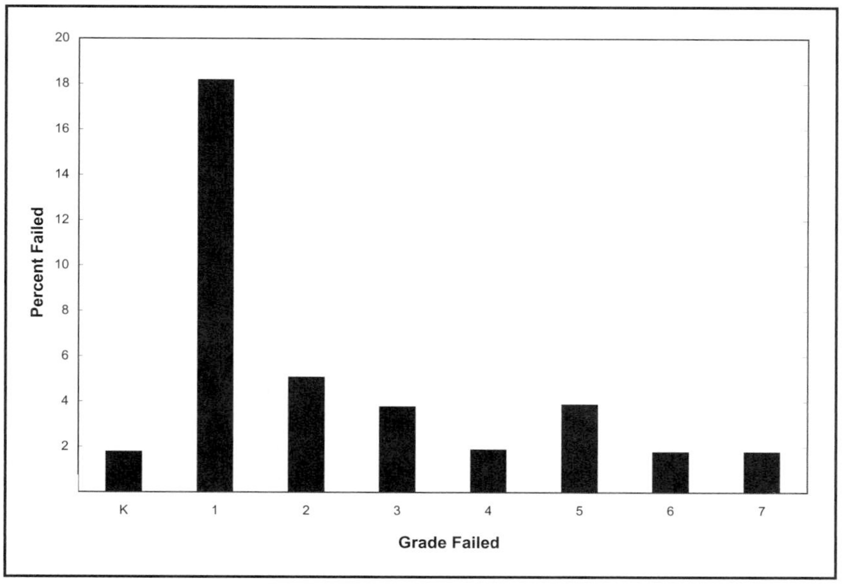

FIGURE 10–3. Distribution (in percent) of grade failed by children with UHL (data adapted from Bess & Tharpe, 1984).

and self-esteem (Bess et al., 1998). Interestingly, there were significant differences between children with bilateral minimal hearing loss and those with UHL. Children with UHL reported poorer communication with family members and greater difficulty getting along well with others than children with bilateral minimal hearing loss. Other studies have shown similar results. For example, excessive behavior problems have been shown in 20 to 42% of children with UHL (Brookhouser et al., 1991; Stein, 1983).

It is informative to examine these statistics in view of the general population. Oyler (1988) collected teacher survey data and found 24% of students with UHL failed at least one grade compared to an overall district rate of 2%. Children with right ear hearing loss were more likely to have failed a grade than children with left ear hearing loss and children with severe to profound hearing loss were more likely to have failed a grade than children with lesser degrees of impairment. Overall, 41% of children with UHL had received additional educational services compared to an average district rate of 8.6%. Interestingly, teacher ratings of behavior were similar for children with UHL and children with normal hearing. Although UHL does not always have obvious repercussions on speech and language acquisition, children with UHL should be monitored for subtle speech and language problems. Some screening tests for speech and language problems might not be sensitive to the types of problems the children with UHL experience. Discussions with teachers and parents regarding the child's performance at home and in school can provide valuable information on the child's developmental progress.

Importantly, not everyone has found that children with UHL are at risk for communicative and psychoeducational difficulties. For instance, Keller and Bundy (1980) reported no differences on standardized test scores between children with UHL, siblings used as a control group, and national norms. Lack of statistical power (limited sample size) has been suggested as the possible reason no differences were seen between groups (Lieu, 2004). Tieri and colleagues (1988) found parental report of academic difficulty in the majority of cases of a cohort of 280 children with UHL; they did not, however, identify any specific speech or language problems. Additionally, Hallmo and colleagues (1986) reported no differences in linguistic development or academic progress in children with UHL; however, these inferences were not based on a standardized test measure nor did they include a control group. Finally, Stein (1983) noted that of 19 children with UHL, only one student needed to repeat a grade. Within this group, however, 42% were reported to have excessive behavior problems. Hence, even if educational difficulties are not noted in some children with hearing loss, behavioral problems can exist.

Language and Cognitive Skills

Mixed evidence also exists regarding specific implications for language development in children with UHL (Borg et al., 2002; Kiese-Himmel, 2002; Klee & Davis-Dansky, 1986; Peckham & Sheridan, 1976). Some evidence has shown differences in early word usage between children with UHL and children with normal hearing. Kiese-Himmel (2002) reported that children with UHL were delayed in using two-word phrases, but not in acquisition and use of their first words. Further evidence for an adverse effect of UHL on language development was shown by Borg and colleagues (2002) who found that a group of 58 children with UHL had significantly delayed language development compared to peers with normal hearing. Recently, Lieu et al. (2010) demonstrated that school-aged children with UHL had worse language skills than their siblings with normal hearing. Persistent negative effects of UHL were seen on language scores after adjustment for confounding variables such as IQ, family income, and maternal level of education. Children with UHL also were more likely to have received speech therapy and have individualized education plans (IEP) or Section 504c accommodations suggesting academic difficulty.

Studies have also suggested that children with UHL might not be at high risk for language and cognitive skills. Peckham and Sheridan (1976) reported a higher proportion of speech difficulties in a longitudinal study of 44 children with severe UHL, however, only four children still had poor speech intelligibility at 11 years. In addition, Klee and Davis-Dansky (1986) found no differences between children with UHL and children with normal hearing on six standardized language tests. Within the group of children studied, however, it was noted that children with UHL of 60 dB HL or greater had lower full scale IQ scores as measured by the WISC-R compared to children with less severe losses. Additionally, eight children who failed a grade in elementary school had significantly lower verbal IQ scores than children with UHL who were academically successful. From these data, the authors suggest that children with UHL may have language difficulties, but that the tests they chose to use in this study were not sensitive enough to measure them.

Psychosocial Skills

It has been well documented that a percentage of children with significant UHL experience social, emotional, and behavioral problems in school (Bess et al., 1998; Bess & Tharpe, 1984; Brookhouser et al., 1991; Culbertson & Gilbert, 1986; Keller & Bundy, 1980). To illustrate, behavior rating data by teachers on several behavioral dimensions for both unilaterally hearing-impaired children and normal children is shown in Figure 10–4. Note that children with UHL had a higher percentage of negative teacher ratings than children with normal hearing. The group of children with UHL received more negative ratings on attention to task, peer relations, dependence/independence, emotional lability, and total negative responses. The only behavioral category in which no differences were found between the two groups was organization skills.

Poor behavior ratings and dysfunction in the areas of self-esteem, energy, and social support have also been documented for some children with UHL (Bess et al., 1998; Brookhouser et al., 1991; Culbertson & Gilbert, 1986). Children with hearing loss experience difficulty following communication in conversations with multiple talkers, following most conversations in noise, and hearing from a distance. These difficulties have implications for language and psychosocial development (Moeller, 2007). In addition, it has been reported that some children with hearing loss experience self-esteem detriment, increased stress, increased energy expenditure, strained peer relations, and decreased social support (Bess et al., 1998; Stinson, Whitmire, & Kluwin, 1996).

Even though many children with UHL experience no difficulties, UHL must be considered a risk factor given that at least one-third of the population experience educational and psychoeducational problems. Recent research supports findings of psychosocial difficulties in those with UHL. Priwin and colleagues (2007) noted a moderate to high degree of self-assessed hearing problems in children and adults aged 3 to 80 years. Borton (2007) also quantitatively demonstrated that children with UHL had lower reported quality of life and psychosocial functioning than children with normal hearing, even though these differences were less apparent in parent reports versus child reports; none of the differences, however, were statistically significant. This suggests that although problems may not be noted in observable behaviors, children with UHL may experience problems with socialization and self-perceived quality of life that might not be apparent to their parents.

Teacher expectations of students with UHL might be lower for children with hearing loss compared to peers with normal hearing. Dancer, Burl, and Waters (1995) reported that Screening Tool for Targeting Educational Risk (SIFTER) scores were significantly lower for children with UHL compared to children with normal hearing suggesting increased risk for academic

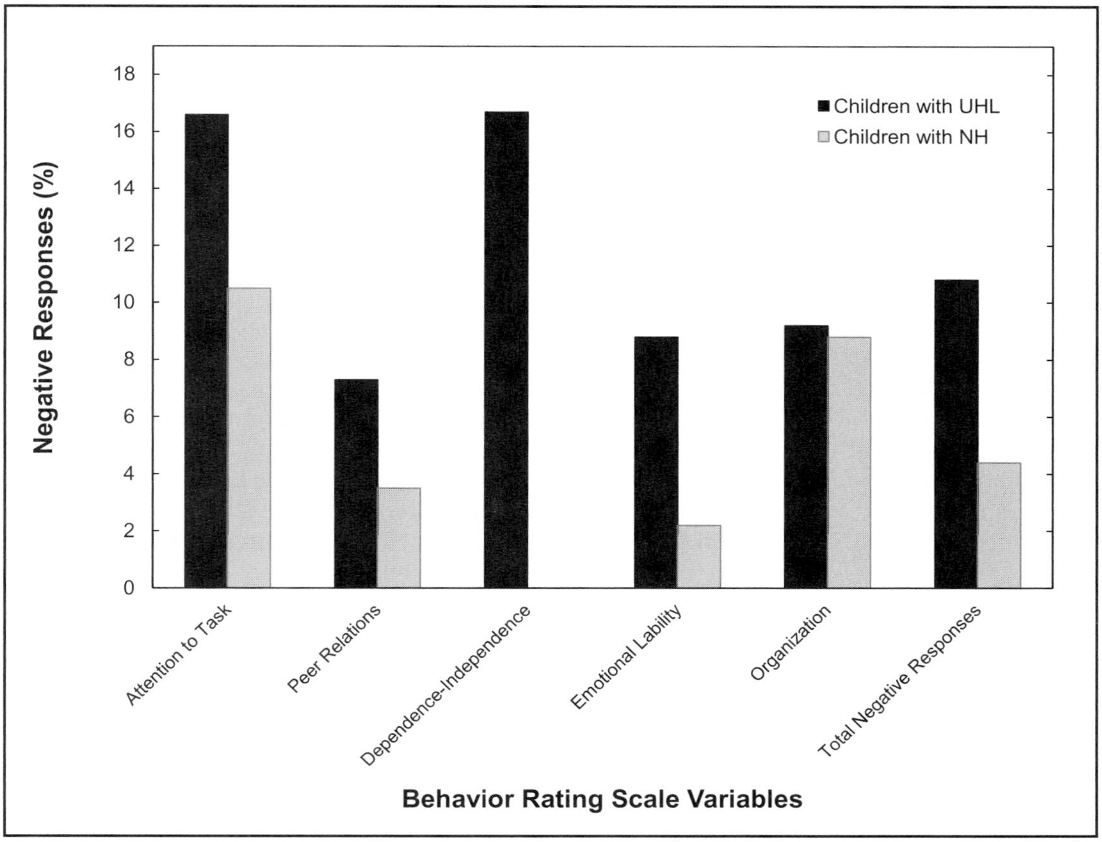

FIGURE 10–4. Behavioral characteristics of children with UHL and children with normal hearing. Data reflects teachers negative ratings of children across several different domains (data adapted from Culbertson & Gilbert, 1986).

difficulty; no differences were found, however, between groups in terms of teacher ratings of whether students were working to expectations. This may suggest that teachers had lower expectations for children with hearing loss. It may be reasonable to consider that lower expectations may affect students' willingness to challenge themselves and the teachers' willingness to challenge these students academically.

Audiologic Considerations

Hearing Screening

The identification of UHL can be confounded by current universal hearing screening protocols. In order to identify children with hearing loss, a screening test must be sensitive enough to identify hearing loss; however, highly sensitive tests are prone to contamination of results such as myogenic noise and residual vernix at the time of testing. Newborns who fail a hearing screening typically are referred for follow-up testing and these costs rise as more children are referred. Universal newborn hearing screening programs must utilize protocols that identify an acceptable number of children with hearing loss yet maintain cost effectiveness (Porter, Neely, & Gorga, 2009).

One way to evaluate the efficacy of current newborn hearing screening protocols is to invite infants who have participated in a newborn hearing screening program to return for diagnostic hearing testing. Johnson and colleagues (2005) reported data from 973 infants known to have failed the first stage of a newborn hearing screening protocol, which included otoacoustic emissions (OAE) screening, and then subsequently passed automated auditory brainstem response (A-ABR) testing. Infants in this study were tested behaviorally between 8 and 12 months of age. Permanent hearing loss was identified in 21 infants who passed their newborn hearing screening at the second stage, nine of whom were found to have UHL. Other studies have also shown that infants and children with UHL are likely to remain undetected unless special efforts are made to identify their losses (Bess et al., 1998; Brookhouser et al., 1991).

The demonstrated increase in prevalence of UHL from newborn to school-ages suggests at least some cases of late-onset UHL. This is an important area in need of exploration. Efforts to identify UHL in the preschool-aged population might be a more effective approach for detecting late onset cases than concentrating on newborn hearing screenings. Eiserman et al. (2007) screened over 3,000 preschool children (i.e., 0–3 years of age) and reported that some children were identified with hearing loss within this group of children who had not been identified at birth. Early data from another ongoing study has shown similar results: 0.5% of children screened at preschool ages were identified with permanent bilateral or UHL (Gravel et al., 2008).

In addition to issues inherent in attempting to screen for congenital hearing loss, concerns arise about follow-up testing once an infant has failed initial screening. Approximately 50% of children who refer universal newborn hearing screening are not seen for follow-up testing (CDC, 2006). It is reasonable to assume that unilateral referral results on newborn hearing screening do not cause as much concern as bilateral referrals and therefore make up a larger percentage of those infants lost to follow-up.

Age of Identification

Prior to universal newborn hearing screening, the mean age of identification of UHL was 5½ years (Bess & Tharpe, 1984; Watkin, 1991). Bess and Tharpe (1984) found that only 23% of children were identified before the age of 5 years, suggesting that the losses were identified as the children entered school (Figure 10–5).

Brookhouser and colleagues (1991) reported the age of identification of UHL was identical to the age of the first audiologic evaluation in most cases of chil-

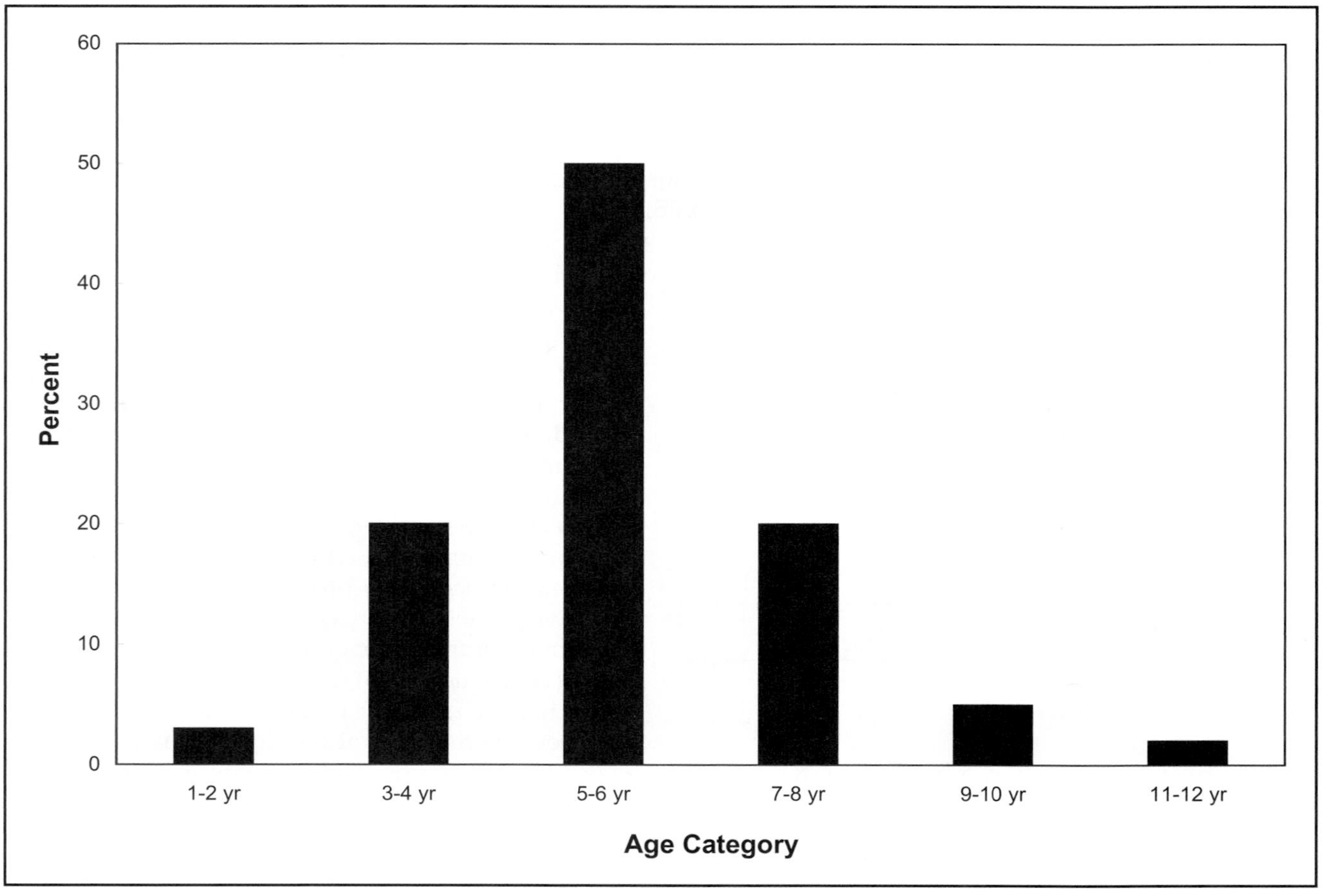

FIGURE 10–5. Average age of identification for children with UHL (data adapted from Bess & Tharpe, 1984).

dren with sensorineural hearing loss, however, approximately 50% of all children with UHL were identified by 7.75 years of age.

With the advent of universal newborn hearing screening one would think that age of identification would improve—this is not necessarily the case, at least for those children with milder unilateral losses. To explain, Ruscetta and Arjmand (2003) demonstrated that children with mild UHL were diagnosed by approximately 6 years of age and children with moderate or greater hearing loss were diagnosed earlier, by approximately 4 years of age. Thus, the average age of diagnosis of UHL decreases with severity of impairment. As such, current data suggest that the average age of diagnosis of UHL has not changed dramatically since the implementation of universal newborn hearing screening.

Diagnosis

Current American Speech-Language-Hearing Association (ASHA) guidelines for audiologic assessment of children from birth to 4 months include frequency specific ABR, click ABR using rarefaction and condensation stimuli, OAE testing, high-frequency typmanometry, and developmental screening and functional auditory assessments in addition to an extensive child and family history. Acoustic immittance measures including acoustic reflex thresholds should also be obtained. As infants develop to acquire the skills necessary to sit upright unassisted, the guidelines broaden to include the use of behavioral measures including speech and frequency specific stimuli (ASHA, 2004). Information obtained from sound field testing is not adequate, and ear specific testing must be performed in order for a complete evaluation of auditory abilities to occur. Currently, the Joint Commission on Infant Hearing (JCIH, 2007) recommends developmental monitoring at 6-month intervals for special populations of children with hearing loss, noting that approximately one third of children with permanent UHL can experience significant language and academic delays.

When a child is identified with a UHL, additional evaluations are recommended including otologic, vestibular, ophthalmologic, and genetic. Identification of etiology is crucial in determining any risk for additional underlying pathology, such as enlarged vestibular aqueduct syndrome, Usher syndrome, or Jervell-Lange-Nielsen syndrome, which require early identification to alert parents and professionals to the possibility of progressive vision and vestibular difficulty or heart arrhythmia. Middle ear status should be monitored for children with UHL, particularly in young children susceptible to pathology and unable to self-monitor auditory abilities. A conductive overlay secondary to otitis media with effusion can cause significant problems for children with unilateral sensorineural hearing loss.

It has been suggested that the problems children with UHL experience with speech and language development and psychoeducational delay may be secondary to the causal agent of the hearing loss. In a significant percentage of children with UHL who exhibit speech and language or educational deficits, the suspected etiology of the loss has been associated with neurological damage (e.g., bacterial meningitis or viral infection). These data highlight the importance of a thorough case history when assessing the child with UHL and evaluating risk for developing academic, psychosocial, or speech and language difficulty. These factors are important to consider when designing intervention strategies for the child.

Future Research Directions

The overview on UHL presented in this chapter raises a number of research questions that are worthy of investigation. For example, although not every child with UHL experiences problems with communication or pschoeducational achievement, it is known that many of these children will indeed have difficulties, difficulties that have the potential to compromise social emotional learning and educational progress. The challenge is to identify early on children with UHL who are at-risk for problems so that a timely intervention strategy can be implemented. Developmental issues concerned with attention, memory, listening effort, and fatigue are undefined for children with UHL. To this end, future research is needed to delineate the specific deficits that underlie the academic and psychosocial adversity seen in this population. Moreover, it is important to establish whether the problems seen in these children will lessen over time, that is, will the children eventually learn to compensate for the adversities imposed by the UHL?

Another important area of research includes the social and emotional correlates of UHL in children. Psychosocial skills are known to play an important role in an individual's receipt of social, academic and emotional rewards. Emotional-behavior functioning of children with hearing loss is thought to be a significant predictor of educational performance. In addition, it is well documented that problems in social and emotional development are linked to peer status, school maladjustment, school dropout, and juvenile delinquency. Because social emotional competence is important to later emotional health and development, it is essential for us to develop a better understanding of the underlying psychosocial factors that contribute to poor social development. Future research should define the peer relationships of children and adolescents with UHL and seek to answer the following questions: (1) what factors underlie poor peer relationships for some children with UHL? and (2) do children with UHL experience transient periods of poor function or are the social/emotional problems present over the long term?

Questions also remain regarding the benefit of intervention for children with UHL. Though it is not apparent that all children with UHL need intervention to avoid academic and psychosocial problems, it is possible that all children with UHL may receive benefit from some type of intervention. Children with UHL may not fail a grade or require additional academic assistance, but it is not unreasonable to consider that children who receive intervention have a better chance of reaching their full potential. Outcomes associated with various types of amplification (i.e., traditional air-conduction hearing aids, BAHA, ear-level, and sound field FM systems) for children with UHL are undefined and merit future study. Future research is also needed to outline evidence-based practices concerning general management, support, and intervention for children with UHL and their families. Longitudinal studies are needed as they could begin to delineate the effects of early intervention on academic achievement and psychosocial constructs for older school-aged children.

Efforts should be made to improve early identification of UHL, including improvements to technology for early identification and diagnosis. Future research must include systematic etiologic evaluations. By understanding the causes of UHL we may be better able to identify children at risk for progressive loss or other developmental disabilities that may be associated with the etiology of the hearing loss. To this effect, prevalence data in newborns and school-aged children also reflect a need for further investigation. This information will be useful when making policy decisions relative to school-aged children, establishing newborn hearing screening protocols, and justifying funding for intervention and future research.

Afterword

It is generally believed that UHL in children does not produce handicapping conditions. An evidence-supported case is made that children with UHL experience a variety of auditory, linguistic, and cognitive problems that appear to be compromising, in some unknown way, educational progress. The major conclusion from this chapter, is that a growing body of scientific-based research exists to support the premise that UHL can indeed compromise social and emotional behaviors, success in school, and ultimately, life learning. Clearly, a need exists to develop a better understanding of UHL in children—research is needed in such areas as identification, diagnosis, prevalence, etiology, educational and social risk factors, and management strategies. Indeed, we cannot afford to do less.

References

American Speech-Language-Hearing Association (ASHA). (2004). *Guidelines for the audiologic assessment of children from birth to 5 years of age* [Guidelines], from http://www.asha.org/docs/pdf/GL2004-00002.pdf.

Baraff, L., Lee, S., & Schriger, D. (1993). Outcomes of bacterial meningitis in children: A meta-analysis. *Pediatric Infectious Disease Journal, 12*(5), 389–394.

Berg, F., Blair, J., & Benson, P. (1996). Classroom acoustics: The problem, impact, and solution. *Language, Speech, and Hearing Services in Schools, 27*(1), 16–20.

Bess, F. (1982). Children with unilateral hearing loss. *Journal of the Academy of Rehabilitative Audiology, 15*, 131–143.

Bess, F., Dodd-Murphy, J., & Parker, R. (1998). Children with minimal sensorineural hearing loss: Prevalence, educational performance, and functional status. *Ear and Hearing, 19*(5), 339–354.

Bess, F., & Tharpe, A. (1984). Unilateral hearing impairment in children. *Pediatrics, 74*(2), 206–216.

Bess, F., & Tharpe, A. (1986). Case history data on unilaterally hearing-impaired children. *Ear and Hearing, 7*(1), 14–19.

Bess, F., Tharpe, A., & Gibler, A. (1986). Auditory performance of children with unilateral sensorineural hearing loss. *Ear and Hearing, 7*(1), 20–26.

Borg, E., Risberg, A., McAllister, B., Undemar, B., Edquist, G., Reinholdson, A., . . . Willstedt-Svensson, U. (2002). Language development in hearing-impaired children. Establishment of a reference material for a 'Language test for hearing-impaired children,' LATHIC. *International Journal of Pediatric Otorhinolaryngology, 65*(1), 15–26.

Borton, S. (2007). *Quality of life in children with unilateral hearing loss: A pilot study.* Washington DC: Washington University School of Medicine.

Boston, M., Halsted, M., Meinzen-Derr, J., Bean, J., Vijayasekaran, S., Arjmand, E., . . . Greinwald, J. (2007). The large vestibular aqueduct: A new definition based on audiologic and computed tomography correlation. *Otolaryngology-Head and Neck Surgery, 136*(6), 972–977.

Bovo, R., Martini, A., Agnoletto, M., Beghi, A., Carmignoto, D., Milani, M., & Zangaglia, A. M. (1988). Auditory and academic performance of children with unilateral hearing loss. *Scandinavian Audiology* (Suppl), *30*, 71–74.

Boyd, S. (1974). *Hearing loss: Its educationally measurable effects on achievement*. Masters Degree research requirement, Department of Education, Southern Illinois University.

Brookhouser, P., Worthington, D., & Kelly, W. (1991). Unilateral hearing loss in children. *Laryngoscope, 101*(12), 1264–1272.

Carhart, R. (1965). Monaural and binaural discrimination against competing sentences. *International Journal of Audiology, 4*, 5–10.

CDC. (2006). *Directors of Speech and Hearing Programs in State and Health and Welfare Agencies (DSHPSHWA) data summary: Reporting year 2006, Version 3.* Retrieved March, 2010, from: http://www.cdc.gov

Centers for Disease Control and Prevention, E. H. D. a. I. P., & Center, M. D. H. (2005). *National Workshop of Mild and Unilateral Hearing Loss.* Breckenridge, Colorado.

Cohen, C., White, J., Savage, E., Glynn, J., Choi, Y., Andrews, N., . . . Ramsay, M. E. (2007). Vaccine effectiveness estimates, 2004–2005 mumps outbreak, England. *Emerging Infectious Diseases, 13*(1), 12–17.

Cohn, E. S., & Kelley, P. M. (1999). Clinical phenotype and mutations in connexin 26 (DFNB1/GJB2), the most common cause of childhood hearing loss. *American Journal of Medical Genetics, 89*(3), 130–136.

Culbertson, J., & Gilbert, L. (1986). Children with unilateral sensorineural hearing loss: Cognitive, academic, and social development. *Ear and Hearing, 7*(1), 38–42.

Dalzell, L., Orlando, M., MacDonald, M., Berg, A., Bradley, M., Cacace, A., . . . Prieve, B. (2000). The New York state universal newborn hearing screening demonstration project: Ages of hearing loss identification, hearing aid fitting, and enrollment in early intervention. *Ear and Hearing, 21*(2), 118–130.

Dancer, J., Burl, N., & Waters, S. (1995). Effects of unilateral hearing loss on teacher responses to the SIFTER. Screening Instrument for Targeting Educational Risk. *American Annals of the Deaf, 140*(3), 291–294.

Davis, J., Elfenbein, J., Schum, R., & Bentler, R. (1986). Effects of mild and moderate hearing impairments on language, educational, and psychosocial behavior of children. *Journal of Speech and Hearing Disorders, 51*(1), 53–62.

Dayan, G., Quinlisk, M., Parker, A., Barskey, A., Harris, M., Schwartz, J., . . . Seward, J. F. (2008). Recent resurgence of mumps in the United States. *New England Journal of Medicine, 358*(15), 1580–1589.

Declau, F., Boudewyns, A., Van den Ende, J., Peeters, A., & van den Heyning, P. (2008). Etiologic and audiologic evaluations after universal neonatal hearing screening: Analysis of 170 referred neonates. *Pediatrics, 121*(6), 1119–1126.

Edwards, M. (2008). *Follow-up of unilateral failures in a newborn hearing screening program.* Nashville, TN: Vanderbilt.

Eiserman, W. D., Shisler, L., Foust, T., Buhrmann, J., Winston, R., & White, K. R. (2007). Screening for hearing loss in early childhood programs. *Early Childhood Research Quarterly, 22*(1), 105–117.

English, K., & Church, G. (1999). Unilateral hearing loss in children: An update for the 1990s. *Language, Speech, and Hearing Services in Schools, 30*(1), 26–31.

Finitzo, T., Albright, K., & Neal, J. O. (1998). The newborn with hearing loss: Detection in the nursery. *Pediatrics, 102*(6), 1452–1460.

Fletcher, H., & Munson, W. (1933). Loudness, its definition, measurement and calculation. *Journal of the Acoustical Society of America, 5*, 82–108.

Fowler, K. B., Dahle, A. J., Boppana, S. B., & Pass, R. F. (1999). Newborn hearing screening: Will children with hearing loss caused by congenital cytomegalovirus be missed? *Journal of Pediatrics, 135*(1), 60–64.

Giolas, T., & Wark, D. (1967). Communication problems associated with unilateral hearing loss. *Journal of Speech and Hearing Disorders, 32*(4), 336–343.

Govaerts, P. J., Casselman, J., Daemers, K., De Ceulaer, G., Somers, T., & Offeciers, F. E. (1999). Audiological findings in large vestibular aqueduct syndrome. *International Journal of Pediatric Otorhinolaryngology, 51*(3), 157–164.

Grantham, D. (1995). Spatial hearing and related phenomena. in B. C. J. Moore (Ed.), *Hearing* (pp. 297–345). New York, NY: Academic.

Gravel, J., Knightly, C., & McKay, S. (2008). *Minimal hearing loss in infants and young children.* Unpublished RO1 grant work; presented by Carol Knightly. The Children's Hospital of Philadelphia.

Griffith, A. J., & Friedman, T. B. (2002). Autosomal and X-linked auditory disorder. In B. Keats, A. N. Popper, & R. R. Fay (Eds.), *Genetics and auditory disorders* (pp. 121–227). New York, NY: Springer.

Hallmo, P., Moller, P., Lind, O., & Tonning, F. M. (1986). Unilateral sensorineural hearing loss in children less than 15 years of age. *Scandinavian Audiology, 15*(3), 131–137.

Harris, J. (1965). Monaural and binaural speech intelligibility and the stereophonic effect based upon temporal cues. *Laryngoscope, 75*, 428–446.

Herrgård, E., Karjalainen, S., Martikainen, A., & Heinonen, K. (1995). Hearing loss at the age of 5 years of children born preterm—a matter of definition. *Acta Paediatrica, 84*, 1160–1164.

Hirsh, I. (1948). Binaural summation—a century of investigation. *Psychological Bulletin, 45*, 193–206.

Humes, L., Allen, S., & Bess, F. (1980). Horizontal sound localization skills of unilaterally hearing-impaired children. *International Journal of Audiology, 19*(6), 508–518.

Hutson, K., Durham, D., Imig, T., & Tucci, D. (2007). Consequences of unilateral hearing loss: Cortical adjustment to unilateral deprivation. *Hearing Research, 237*(1–2), 19–31.

Illing, R., Kraus, K., & Meidinger, M. (2005). Reconnecting neuronal networks in the auditory brainstem following unilateral deafening. *Hearing Research, 206*(1–2), 185–199.

Jäncke, L., Wüstenberg, T., Schulze, K., & Heinze, H. (2002). Asymmetric hemodynamic responses of the human auditory cortex to monaural and binaural stimulation. *Hearing Research, 170*(1–2), 166–178.

Jensen, J., Johansen, P., & Børre, S. (1989). Unilateral sensorineural hearing loss in children and auditory performance with respect to right/left ear differences. *British Journal of Audiology, 23*(3), 207–213.

Johnson, J., White, K., Widen, J., Gravel, J., James, M., Kennalley, T., . . . Holstrum, J. (2005). A multicenter evaluation of how many infants with permanent hearing loss pass a two-stage otoacoustic emissions/automated auditory brainstem response newborn hearing screening protocol. *Pediatrics, 116*(3), 663–672.

Joint Committee on Infant Hearing (JCIH). (2007). Year 2007 position statement: Principles and guidelines for early hearing detection and intervention programs. *Pediatrics, 120*(4), 898–921.

Keller, W., & Bundy, R. (1980). Effects of unilateral hearing loss upon educational achievement. *Child: Care Health Development, 6*, 93–100.

Kenna, M. A., Wu, B.-L., Cotanche, D. A., Korf, B. R., & Rehm, H. L. (2001). Connexin 26 studies in patients with sensorineural hearing loss. *Archives of Otolaryngology-Head and Neck Surgery, 127*(9), 1037–1042.

Kenworthy, O., Klee, T., & Tharpe, A. (1990). Speech recognition ability of children with unilateral sensorineural hearing loss as a function of amplification, speech stimuli and listening condition. *Ear and Hearing, 11*(4), 264–270.

Kiese-Himmel, C. (2002). Unilateral sensorineural hearing impairment in childhood: Analysis of 31 consecutive cases: Problemas auditivos sensorineurales unilaterales en niños: Análisis de 31 casos consecutivos. *International Journal of Audiology, 41*(1), 57–63.

Klee, T., & Davis-Dansky, E. (1986). A comparison of unilaterally hearing-impaired children and normal-hearing children on a battery of standardized language tests. *Ear and Hearing, 7*(1), 27–37.

Kutz, J., Simon, L., Chennupati, S., Giannoni, C., & Manolidis, S. (2006). Clinical predictors for hearing loss in children with bacterial meningitis. *Archives of Otolaryngology, Head and Neck Surgery, 132*(9), 941–945.

Leung, A., Sauve, R., & Davies, H. (2003). Congenital cytomegalovirus infection. *Journal of the National Medical Association, 95*(3), 213–218.

Lieu, J. (2004). Speech-language and educational consequences of unilateral hearing loss in children. *Archives of Otolaryngology-Head and Neck Surgery, 130*(5), 524–530.

Lieu, J., Tye-Murray, N., Karzon, R., & Piccirillo, J. (2010). Unilateral hearing loss is associated with worse speech-language scores in children. *Pediatrics, 125*(6) 1348–e1355.

MacKeith, N. W., & Coles, R. R. A. (1971). Binaural advantages in hearing of speech. *Journal of Laryngology and Otology, 85*(03), 213–232.

MacSweeney, M., Campbell, R., Calvert, G., McGuire, P., David, A., Suckling, J., . . . Brammer, M. J. (2001). Dispersed activation in the left temporal cortex for speech-reading in congenitally deaf people. *Proceedings of the Royal Society of London, 268*(1466), 451–457.

Melnick, M., & Myrianthopoulos, N. (1979). External ear malformations: Epidemiology, genetics and natural history. *Birth Defects: Original Article Series* (Vol. XV, pp. 1–140). New York, NY: Alan R. Liss, Inc.

Moeller, M. (2007). Current state of knowledge: Psychosocial development in children with hearing impairment. *Ear and Hearing, 28*(6), 729–739.

Moncur, J., & Dirks, D. (1967). Binaural and monaural speech intelligibility in reverberation. *Journal of Speech, Language and Hearing Research, 10*(2), 186–195.

Morrongiello, B. (1988). Infants' localization of sounds along the horizontal axis: Estimates of minimum audible angle. *Developmental Psychology, 24*(1), 8–13.

Morton, C., & Nance, W. (2006). Newborn hearing screening —A silent revolution. *New England Journal of Medicine, 354*(20), 2151–2164.

Nakashima, T., & Yanagita, N. (1993). Outcome of sudden deafness with and without vertigo. *Laryngoscope, 103*, 1145–1149.

Nance, W. E. (2007). Marion Downs lecture: How can newborn hearing screening be improved? *Audiology Now*. Denver, CO.

Nance, W. E., & Kearsey, M. J. (2004). Relevance of connexin deafness (DFNB1) to human evolution. *American Journal of Human Genetics, 74*, 1081–1087.

Nance, W. E., Lim, B., & Dodson, K. (2006). Importance of congenital cytomegalovirus infections as a cause for prelingual hearing loss. *Journal of Clinical Virology, 35*(2), 221–225.

Neault, M. (2005). *Progression from unilateral to bilateral loss*. In National Workshop on Mild and Unilateral Hearing Loss: Workshop Proceedings. Breckenridge, CO: Centers for Disease Control and Prevention.

Newton, V. (1983). Sound localisation in children with a severe unilateral hearing loss. *International Journal of Audiology, 22*(2), 189–198.

Niskar, A., Kieszak, S., Holmes, A., Esteban, E., Rubin, C., & Brody, D. (1998). Prevalence of hearing loss among children 6 to 19 years of age. The third national health and nutrition examination survey. *American Medical Association, 279*, 1071–1075.

Oyler, R. (1988). Unilateral hearing loss: Demographics and educational impact. *Language, Speech, and Hearing Services in the Schools, 19*(2), 201–210.

Palmer, C. (1999). Deprivation and acclimatization in the human auditory system: Do they happen? Do they matter? *Hearing Journal, 52*, 23–25.

Pandya, A., Arnos, K., Xia, X., Welch, K., Blanton, S., Friedman, T., . . . Nance, W. E. (2003). Frequency and distribution of GJB2 (connexin 26) and GJB6 (connexin 30) mutations in a large North American repository of deaf probands. *Genetics in Medicine, 5*(4), 295–303.

Peckham, C., & Sheridan, M. (1976). Follow-up at 11 years of 46 children with severe unilateral hearing loss at 7 years. *Child: Care, Health and Development, 2*(2), 107–111.

Podwall, A., Podwall, D., Gordon, T., Lamendola, P., & Gold, A. (2002). Unilateral auditory neuropathy: Case study. *Journal of Child Neurology, 17*(4), 306–309.

Porter, H., Neely, S., & Gorga, M. (2009). Using benefit-cost ratio to select universal newborn hearing screening test criteria. *Ear and Hearing, 30*(4), 447–457.

Prieve, B., Dalzell, L., Berg, A., Bradley, M., Cacace, A., Campbell, D., . . . Stevens, F. (2000). The New York State universal newborn hearing screening demonstration project: Outpatient outcome measures. *Ear and Hearing, 21*(2), 104–117.

Priwin, C., Jönsson, R., Hultcrantz, M., & Granström, G. (2007). BAHA in children and adolescents with unilateral or bilateral conductive hearing loss: A study of outcome. *International Journal of Pediatric Otorhinolaryngology, 71*(1), 135–145.

Quigley, S., & Thomure, F. (1969). *Some effects of hearing impairment upon school performance*. Retrieved June 18, 2010, from http://www.eric.ed.gov/ERICDocs/data/ericdocs2sql/content_storage_01/0000019b/80/36/7a/fa.pdf

Roman, S., Aladio, P., Paris, J., Nicollas, R., & Triglia, J. (2001). Prognostic factors of sudden hearing loss in children. *International Journal of Pediatric Otorhinolaryngology, 61*(1), 17–21.

Ruscetta, M., & Arjmand, E. (2003). *Unilateral hearing impairment in children: Age of diagnosis*. Retrieved February 27, 2010, from http://www.audiologyonline.com.

Ruscetta, M., Arjmand, E., & Pratt, S. (2005). Speech recognition abilities in noise for children with severe-to-profound unilateral hearing impairment. *International Journal of Pediatric Otorhinolaryngology, 69*(6), 771–779.

Scheffler, K., Bilecen, D., Schmid, N., Tschopp, K., & Seelig, J. (1998). Auditory cortical responses in hearing subjects and unilateral deaf patients as detected by functional magnetic resonance imaging. *Cerebral Cortex, 8*(2), 156–163.

Schmithorst, V., Holland, S., Ret, J., Duggins, A., Arjmand, E., & Greinwald, J. (2005). Cortical reorganization in children with unilateral sensorineural hearing loss. *NeuroReport, 16*(5), 463–467.

Schuknecht, H. (1989). Congenital aural atresia. *Laryngoscope, 99*(9), 908–917.

Silverman, C., Silman, S., Emmer, M., Schoepflin, J., & Lutolf, J. (2006). Auditory deprivation in adults with asymmetric, sensorineural hearing impairment. *Journal of the American Academy of Audiology, 17*(10), 747–762.

Simon, B. (1977). *Unilateral hearing impairment and the question of learning disability*. Paper presented at the Illinois Speech and Hearing Association.

Simons, J. P., Ruscetta, M. N., & Chi, D. H. (2008). Sensorineural hearing impairment in children with Chiari I malformation. *Annals of Otology, Rhinology and Laryngology, 117*(6), 443–447.

Stein, D. M. (1983). Psychosocial characteristics of school-aged children with unilateral hearing loss. *Journal of the Academy of Rehabilitative Audiology, 16*, 12–22.

Stinson, M. S., Whitmire, K., & Kluwin, T. N. (1996). Self-perceptions of social relationships in hearing-impaired adolescents. *Journal of Educational Psychology, 88*(1), 132–143.

Syka, J. (2002). Plastic changes in the central auditory system after hearing loss, restoration of function, and during learning. *Physiological Reviews, 82*(3), 601–636.

Tieri, L., Masi, R., Ducci, M., & Marsella, P. (1988). Unilateral sensorineural hearing loss in children. *Scandinavian Audiology Suppl., 30*, 33–36.

Tschopp, K., Schillinger, C., Schmid, N., Rausch, M., Bilecen, D., & Scheffler, K. (2000). Detection of central auditory compensation in unilateral deafness with functional magnetic resonance tomography. *Laryngo-rhino-otologie, 79*(12), 753–757.

Unal, M., Katircioglu, S., Can Karatay, M., Suoglu, Y., Erdamar, B., & Aslan, I. (1998). Sudden total bilateral deafness due to asymptomatic mumps infection. *International Journal of Pediatric Otorhinolaryngology, 45*(2), 167–169.

Watkin, P. (1991). The age of identification of childhood deafness—improvements since the 1970s. *Public Health, 105*(4), 303–312.

Welsh, L., Welsh, J., Rosen, L., & Dragonette, J. (2004). Functional impairments due to unilateral deafness. *Annals of Otology, Rhinology, and Laryngology, 113*(12), 987–993.

Wilcox, S. A., Saunders, K., Osborn, A. H., Arnold, A., Wunderlich, J., Kelly, T., . . . Dahl, E. E. (2000). High frequency hearing loss correlated with mutations in the GJB2 gene. *Human Genetics, 106*(4), 399–405.

11

Permanent Minimal and Mild Bilateral Hearing Loss in Children

Implications and Outcomes

Anne Marie Tharpe

Background

In the one-year period between 1964 and 1965, a rubella epidemic resulted in approximately 12.5 million cases of rubella leading to almost 12,000 babies being born deaf in the United States. As such, the following decade was one in which audiologists found themselves focused on the management of children with severe-to-profound degrees of hearing loss. Considering those circumstances, it is not surprising that the profession of audiology gave little consideration to mild degrees of hearing loss at that time. After all, when compared to children with severe-to-profound hearing loss, many of whom had additional handicapping conditions, the potential impact of mild degrees of hearing loss on children seemed of little consequence. However, for the last several decades, children with mild degrees of hearing loss have garnered the interest of audiologists, especially since the 1980s when studies were expanded to include what was termed minimal hearing loss (Bess & Tharpe, 1986). It was then that the negative impact of minimal hearing loss on child development was widely realized, and educational policy changes were implemented in an attempt to improve outcomes.

A starting point in our discussion of this topic should reasonably be the definition of minimal and mild hearing loss. Because of the importance of acute hearing for the normal development of speech and language, some have suggested that "normal" hearing for children should be defined more conservatively than for adults; specifically, a pure tone threshold average (PTA) between −10 and 15 dB (Clarke 1981; Diefendorf & Gravel, 1996). Mild hearing loss is typically defined as between 25 to 40 dB HL, which suggests that minimal loss is defined as a PTA ≥ 15 and ≤ 25 dB HL. However, even the term "minimal" is controversial as it might imply that these losses are not important or are inconsequential. In fact, a survey of parental impressions of commonly used terms to describe degrees of hearing loss suggested that specific terminology (e.g., slight, mild, minimal) might result in an underestimation of the potential magnitude of the disability (Haggard & Primus, 1999). As you can see from the definitions of minimal hearing loss proffered by Bess, Dodd-Murphy and Parker (1998), the term is as much about configuration of hearing loss as it is about degree of loss:

- unilateral sensorineural hearing loss—average air-conduction thresholds (.5, 1.0, 2.0 kHz) ≥ 20 dB HL in the impaired ear and an average air-bone gap no greater than 10 dB at 1.0, 2.0, and 4.0 kHz and average air-conduction thresholds in the normal hearing ear ≤ 15 dB HL;
- bilateral sensorineural hearing loss—average pure-tone thresholds between 20 and 40 dB HL bilaterally with average air-bone gaps no greater than 10 dB at frequencies 1.0, 2.0, and 4.0 kHz;

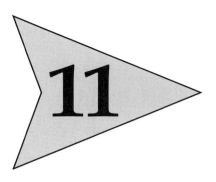

- high-frequency sensorineural hearing loss—air-conduction thresholds greater than 25 dB HL at two or more frequencies above 2 kHz (i.e., 3.0, 4.0, 6.0, or 8.0 kHz) in one or both ears with air-bone gaps at 3.0 and 4.0 kHz no greater than 10 dB.

Others have used different definitions (Ross, Visser, Holstrum, & Kenneson, 2005) but regardless of the definition used, an effort should be made for standardized terminology to enable meaningful comparisons of data across studies. Our attempts to evaluate data on the impact of minimal and mild hearing loss on children obtained across studies are compromised when we are not using uniform definitions. Commonly accepted examples of minimal degrees of hearing loss are shown in Figure 11–1.

This chapter reviews what we know about the impact of bilateral minimal and mild degrees of permanent hearing loss on children. Although unilateral hearing loss is considered a minimal hearing loss by definition, the specific impact of unilateral hearing loss in children is addressed in Chapter 10. Management of all types of permanent minimal and mild hearing losses, including unilateral loss, is addressed in Chapter 34.

Identification and Prevalence

Numerous changes have taken place over the past 40 to 50 years with regard to the characteristics of children with hearing loss. Specifically, a shift has occurred in the incidence and prevalence of certain causative factors and degrees of hearing loss. Disorders that resulted in severe-to-profound sensorineural hearing loss in the 1950s and 1960s, such as rubella and menengitis, are no longer as prevalent as they once were. This is because of improvements in health care—we have a better understanding of the pathogenesis of disease and we have developed new and effective immunizations. In addition, our ability to manage the complications associated with premature delivery has resulted in dramatically improved infant survival rates. Although we are grateful for the lowered limit of viability, these small and fragile babies face high morbidity. Those born weighing less than 750 grams are at highest risk of lifelong morbidity, including hearing loss. These hearing losses tend to be milder in degree than what we were seeing decades ago. Hence, today, we as pediatric audiologists are being asked to serve a distinctively different group of children than we served in the past;

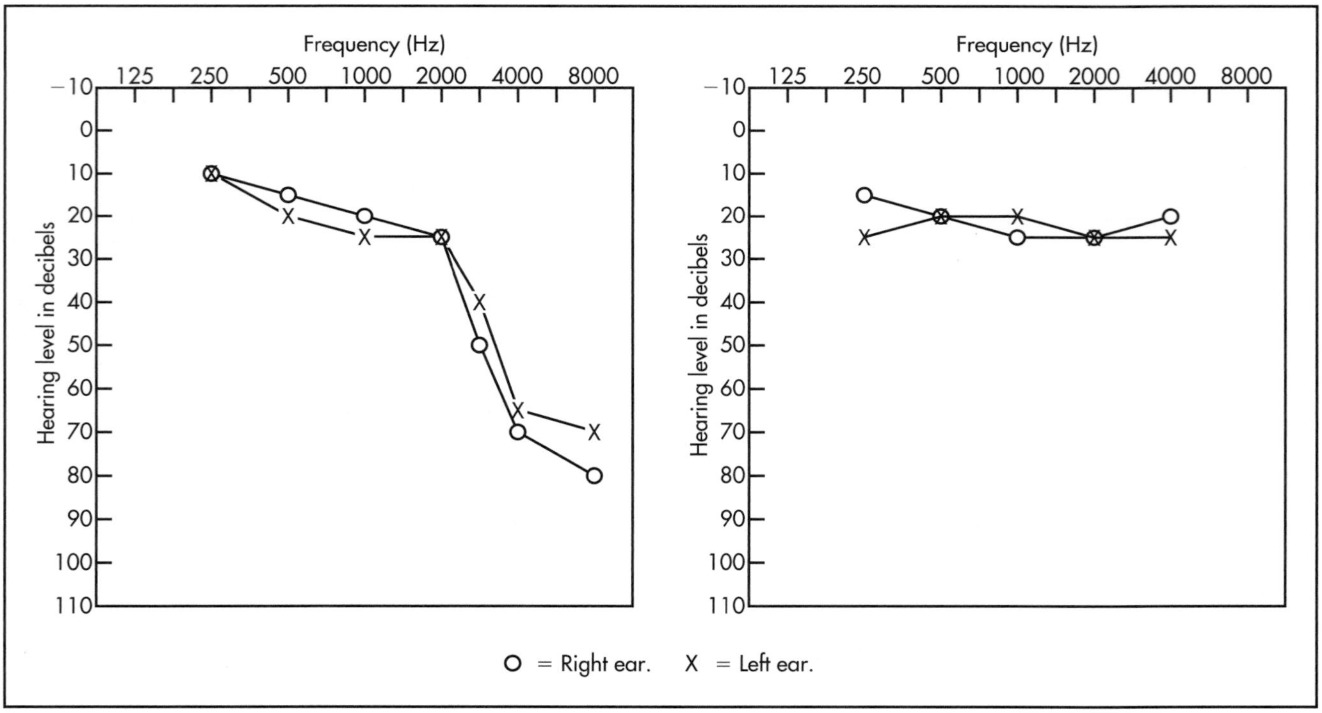

FIGURE 11–1. Two examples of minimal degrees of hearing loss. The left-hand panel illustrates a high-frequency hearing loss, and the right-hand panel represents a flat, minimal hearing loss.

children with milder degrees of hearing loss. Moreover, these milder hearing losses are more prevalent than the severe-to-profound losses we used to see.

Prevalence estimates of mild and minimal degrees of permanent hearing loss in newborns vary widely. As alluded to previously, prevalence rates are uncertain because of the differences in defining the audiometric thresholds of these categories. Furthermore, the Joint Committee on Infant Hearing (JCIH) whose charge it is to make recommendations concerning newborn hearing screening processes, does not recommend targeting minimal and mild degrees of hearing loss with our newborn hearing screening programs (JCIH, 2007). Therefore, we can only estimate prevalence of such losses in the newborn period and it is assumed that the numbers of children with minimal to mild degrees of hearing loss are significantly underidentified and/or underreported in the United States (Gravel, 2005). Current estimates of minimal to mild hearing loss in newborns range from 0.36 to 1.3:1000 (Johnson et al., 2005; Watkin & Baldwin, 1999).

The prevalence of minimal to mild losses appears to be much higher by the time children reach school age. This is not totally unexpected as prevalence typically increases with age. Bess and colleagues (1998) estimated 2.4:100 school-age children had permanent minimal to mild bilateral hearing loss, or about 2.5 million school-age children in the United States. In addition to possible underestimation of these losses in the newborn period, the increase in estimated prevalence rates by school age can be attributed to several different factors including:

- misses by the early hearing detection and intervention systems (EHDI);
- high lost-to-follow-up rates by newborn screening programs;
- progressive or late-onset hearing loss.

Keep in mind that, in part, because minimal to mild hearing losses are not targeted by our newborn screening programs, these losses are identified considerably later than more severe losses. One reason for not targeting these losses is because the lower the target degree of hearing loss, the greater the number of false alarms and the more expensive the program. This late age of identification can complicate our ability to determine the causes of these losses. For example, tests for one of the most common causes of hearing loss in children, congenital cytomegalovirus, must be performed early in the newborn period for accurate interpretation. That is, because of the high prevalence of acquired cytomegalovirus in the general population, the virus must be isolated in the newborn period for confirmation of congenital infection. Furthermore, parental memory for causative factors such as maternal viral or bacterial illnesses or other teratogenic exposures can be compromised over time. Primary contributors to permanent minimal and mild bilateral hearing loss in children include noise exposure, viral/bacterial insult, genetics, enlarged vestibular aqueduct, and prematurity, among others (see Tharpe & Sladen, 2008, for a review of causative factors for minimal and mild hearing loss).

Screening and Diagnostic Challenges

Screening principles and methods are thoroughly addressed in Chapter 16 and will not be repeated here. However, a brief mention of screening and diagnostic factors relevant specifically to minimal and mild degrees of hearing loss is warranted.

Most children with hearing loss ≥ 35 to 40 dB will be identified through newborn hearing screening programs. But, as noted previously, those with lesser degrees of loss or with progressive or late-onset losses will not. Even if newborn hearing screening programs wanted to target these losses, a number of technical barriers to early identification of minimal and mild hearing loss in the newborn period have been suggested (Gravel, 2005):

- Current otoacoustic emissions (OAE) and auditory brainstem response audiometry (ABR) technologies do not reliably distinguish between normal and mild hearing loss (Norton et al., 2000). Because of the variability in ear canal volume and geometry, the intensity of the ABR stimulus level varies somewhat from infant to infant. At this time, screening instruments do not automatically calibrate the stimulus levels for each ear.
- The configuration of loss in some hearing-impaired ears could result in ABR and OAE results that are indistinguishable from normal hearing ears (i.e., significant loss at some frequencies but normal hearing over a range of frequencies; Norton et al., 2000);
- There is insufficient manufacturer supporting evidence to allow for the determination of the validity of specific pass-fail criteria and automated screening algorithms.

Therefore, identifying permanent minimal and mild hearing loss in the newborn period is likely to remain problematic for the foreseeable future. Our ability to distinguish minimal to mild permanent hearing loss from temporary conductive loss is also a significant challenge and impacts our financial resources dedicated to hearing screening follow-up. A common cause of temporary conductive hearing loss in children, otitis media, is discussed in more detail later in this chapter. Furthermore, beyond the newborn period, there is no systematic hearing screening program for children prior to school entry. Given the documented increase in prevalence of minimal and mild hearing loss between the newborn period and school age, and the potential impact of such losses on psychoeducational development, this is a public health need that requires further examination and action.

Because our newborn hearing screening programs do not target minimal to mild permanent losses, these children are not likely to be referred for diagnostic evaluations during infancy. Without the usual indicators pointing to a possible hearing loss, such as obvious speech or language deficits, or academic difficulties, suspicion of minimal to mild hearing loss in infancy and early childhood based on parental observation is not likely. However, even if hearing loss is suspected, the accuracy of current diagnostic methods used to define minimal and mild losses in infants and young children might be suboptimal (Cone-Wesson, Sininger, & Widen, 2005; Rance & Rickards, 2002). Specifically, the variability in electrophysiologic (i.e., ABR and auditory steady-state response [ASSR]) and behavioral tests (i.e., visual reinforcement audiometry [VRA]) is felt to limit one's ability to differentiate minimal and mild losses from normal hearing sensitivity.

All pediatric hearing evaluations should incorporate a test battery approach as opposed to the use of only one test to determine hearing status. As discussed in Chapter 16, the 2007 JCIH recommended that assessments include a child and family history and a combination of both physiological and behavioral tests appropriate for a child's developmental age. The following discussion focuses on specific testing strategies that can be employed by audiologists to decrease the likelihood of missing or misdiagnosing minimal to mild hearing loss in children.

Behavioral Testing

Starting at approximately 6 months developmental age, behavioral testing can be included as a reliable component in the pediatric test battery. Whenever possible, ear-specific testing, as opposed to sound field testing, should be employed. Insert earphones are recommended unless contraindicated, and bone conduction should be utilized if air-conduction responses are not within normal range. Although audiologic standards for pediatric testing recommend inclusion of 500 Hz and 2000 Hz at a minimum (ASHA, 2004; Pediatric Working Group, 1996), testing this limited frequency range will preclude one's ability to identify some high-frequency hearing loss. More detail on methods of pediatric behavioral hearing testing can be found in Chapters 22 and 23.

Accuracy in estimating thresholds, whether using electrophysiological or behavioral tests, is directly linked to the bracketing characteristics (i.e., step size, stopping rules). That is, to detect a minimal or mild hearing loss, using a small step size of, for example, 5 dB would be more accurate than a larger step size of 10 dB. Likewise, a stopping level of, for example, 10 dB would be better able to detect a minimal loss than a stopping level of 25 dB. However, utilization of small step sizes and low stopping levels requires additional testing time that might not be available with restless children. Furthermore, young children with normal hearing often respond only to suprathreshold signals between +15 and 30 dB, making it difficult to ascertain a minimal or mild hearing loss. It is important to remember that if one uses large step sizes and high stopping levels, minimal hearing loss will likely be missed.

Physiologic Testing

Frequency-specific testing is recommended when utilizing auditory brainstem responses (ABR) for purposes of threshold estimation. Unlike wideband, click-evoked responses, frequency-specific stimuli are better predictors of audiometric thresholds and will assist in identifying varying hearing loss configurations, such as high frequency losses. Clicks, on the other hand, merely test for responses in the 1 to 4-kHz range. As with behavioral testing, if one is attempting to identify all types and degrees of hearing loss, testing should include high-frequency stimuli (e.g., 3000 or 4000 Hz) in addition to lower frequencies.

Another limitation of using ABR to identify minimal or mild degrees of loss is that we do not know the actual sound pressure level of the stimulus at the eardrum of the baby being tested. That is, even when using a signal of, for example, 35 dB nHL the sound pressure level at the eardrum will vary from baby to baby depending on the volume of the ear canal and the age of the baby; the smaller the ear canal volume, the larger the SPL at the eardrum, thus often exceeding the 35 dB that we thought we were using. Therefore, one might obtain normal ABR recordings from a child with minimal to mild hearing loss. Additional discussion of ABR testing can be found in Chapter 20.

Evoked otoacoustic emissions (EOAEs) are a useful contribution to our pediatric test battery. Transient EOAEs (TEOAEs) are typically evoked from all normal hearing ears and are absent if losses exceed approximately 30 dB HL (Norton, 1993). Distortion product EOAEs (DPOAEs) are also typically present in normal hearing ears but absent if hearing loss exceeds 40 to 50 dB HL (Gorga, Neely, & Dorn, 1999). Therefore, although EOAEs are a quick and relatively inexpensive indicator of gross hearing status, they are likely to miss minimal and mild degrees of hearing loss.

Another diagnostic challenge is the presence of otitis media with effusion, which is often accompanied by minimal to mild, conductive hearing loss in the speech frequency range. Distinguishing between a transient loss secondary to otitis media with effusion and a permanent hearing loss requires the convergence of several diagnostic indicators including bone-conduction thresholds, immittance audiometry, and pneumatic otoscopy. The presence of an abnormal tympanogram is an excellent predictor of otitis media with effusion. Acoustic stapedial reflex testing can also supply information about the functional status of the middle ear and cochlea. However, acoustic stapedial reflexes can be present within the normal range even in the presence of minimal or mild hearing loss (see Chapter 18 for additional information on immittance testing in children).

Audiologic uncertainty about either the type or degree of hearing loss can delay definitive diagnosis and intervention. As noted previously, we have known for decades that children with milder hearing losses are identified later than children with more severe losses (e.g., Elssman, Matkin, & Sabo, 1987). In a more recent survey of pediatric audiology practices in the United States and the United Kingdom, Bamford and colleagues (2001) shed additional light on why we might be seeing that delay. They queried audiologists about the age at which they thought they would achieve "audiologic certainty" in young children defined as reliable estimates of hearing thresholds for low, mid and high frequencies, and clarity on whether the loss was sensorineural, conductive or mixed, for children with varying degrees of hearing loss with no risk factors and no other obvious disabilities. Eighty percent or more of the respondents indicated that they reached audiologic certainty about three months sooner for children with severe or profound hearing loss than for those with mild hearing losses.

Functional Auditory Assessment

If it is the case that audiologists are not as confident in their ability to diagnose minimal to mild losses with our current audiologic test battery as they are with greater degrees of loss, functional auditory measures might provide an enhancement to the battery and thus, add a degree of confidence to the diagnosis. Furthermore, although some of these assessments are designed to supplement the diagnostic test battery, others are used to determine the degree of handicap that might be associated with the hearing loss and can guide professionals towards appropriate intervention options. Note that handicap is defined as the loss or limitation of opportunities to take part in the life of the community on an equal level with others (World Health Organization, 1980). By assessing listening behaviors in real world settings, outside the confines of the soundproof booth where most formal audiologic testing takes place, functional assessments can contribute information about what a child hears and, perhaps more importantly, how the child uses what is heard in everyday situations. Typically, these assessments consist of parent or teacher questionnaires. Some of these tools are designed specifically to identify the subtle differences in listening behavior by those with minimal and mild degrees of hearing loss. A summary of functional auditory assessments that are designed to identify or assist in managing minimal to mild losses can be found in Table 11–1.

Developmental Outcomes

Evidence has accumulated over the past several decades to suggest that many school-age children with permanent bilateral minimal and mild hearing loss are at an elevated risk for developmental problems. However, it is not clear whether these problems are initiated during infancy or early childhood, whether etiology of the hearing loss is a contributing factor to these problems, whether children can outgrow these deficits over time, and whether early intervention is effective with these children. The following section reviews our current state of knowledge about the developmental outcomes of children with permanent bilateral minimal and mild hearing loss.

Table 11–1. Functional Auditory Assessment Measures for Use With Children With Minimal to Mild Hearing Losses

ABEL: Auditory Behavior in Everyday Life (Purdy, Farrington, Moran, Chard, & Hodgson, 2002)	
Age range:	2 to 12 years
Purpose:	Twenty-four item questionnaire with three subscales (aural-oral, auditory awareness, social/conversational skills) which evaluates auditory behavior in everyday life.
CHILD: Children's Home Inventory for Listening Difficulties (Anderson & Smaldino 2000)	
Age range:	3 to 12 years
Purpose:	Parent and child questionnaire with 15 situations that rate how well the child understood speech.
COW: Children's Outcome Worksheets (Williams, 2003)	
Age range:	4 to 12 years
Purpose:	Three worksheets (child, parent, and teacher) are requested to specify five situations where improved hearing is desired.
ELF: Early Listening Function (Anderson, 2000)	
Age range:	5 months to 3 years
Purpose:	Twelve listening situations in which the parent and audiologist observe the child and record the distance the child responds to the auditory stimuli.
LIFE: Listening Inventory for Education (Anderson & Smaldino, 1996)	
Age range:	6 years and up.
Purpose:	Questionnaire which identifies classroom situations which are challenging for the child. There are two formats of the questionnaire: a teacher questionnaire with 16 items and a child questionnaire with 15 items.
Little Ears (Küehn-Inacker, Weichbold, Tsiakpini, Coninx, & D'Haese, 2003)	
Age range:	0 years and up
Purpose:	Questionnaire for the parent with 35 age-dependent questions that assesses auditory development.
LSQ: Listening Situations Questionnaire (Grimshaw, 1996)	
Age range:	7 years and up
Purpose:	Questionnaire for the parent and child with eight situations. Responses focus on help of amplification, difficulty of understanding, and satisfaction of amplification.
PEACH: Parents' Evaluation of Aural/oral performance of Children (Ching, Hill, & Psarros, 2000)	
Age range:	Preschool to 7 years
Purpose:	Interview with parent with 15 questions targeting the child's everyday environment. Includes scoring for 5 subscales (use, quiet, noise, telephone, environment)
Preschool SIFTER: Preschool Screening Instrument For Targeting Educational Risk (Anderson & Matkin, 1996)	
Age range:	3 to 6 years
Purpose:	Questionnaire with 15 items completed by the teacher which identifies children at risk for educational failure with five subscales (academics, attention, communication, participation, behavior).
SIFTER: Screening Instrument for Targeting Educational Risk (Anderson, 1989)	
Age range:	6 years and above.
Purpose:	Questionnaire with 15 items completed by the teacher which identifies children at risk for educational failure with five subscales (academics, attention, communication, participation, behavior).
TEACH: Teachers' Evaluation of Aural/oral performance of Children (Ching, Hill, & Psarros, 2000)	
Age range:	preschool to 7 years
Purpose:	Interview with teacher with 13 questions targeting the child's everyday environment. Includes scoring for five subscales (use, quiet, noise, telephone, environment).

Note. Age refers to child's developmental, as opposed to chronologic, age level.

Impact on Speech-Language, Educational, and Social-Emotional Abilities

When compared to children with normal hearing, children with minimal and mild degrees of permanent hearing loss appear to be more likely to experience academic difficulties. A few studies have concluded that there are no adverse academic outcomes associated with these losses (Briscoe, Bishop, & Norbury, 2001; Norbury, Bishop, & Briscoe, 2001; Wake et al., 2006), but there is a collective body of evidence to suggest otherwise. In fact, most studies suggest that children with minimal to mild permanent hearing losses are significantly more likely than their normal hearing peers to have to repeat a grade in school or access resource assistance for a variety of academic and/or cognitive deficits (Bess et al., 1998; Blair, Peterson, & Viehweg, 1985; Davis, Elfenbein, Schum, & Bentler, 1986; Most, 2004; Ross et al., 2005; Yoshinaga-Itano, Johnson, Carpenter, & Brown, 2008). Specifically, when compared to children without hearing loss, children with minimal to mild losses have been shown to score more poorly on standardized academic tests including those of reading vocabulary, language mechanics, phonologic short-term memory, phonologic discrimination, word analysis, spelling, and science.

When teacher questionnaires have been utilized to document classroom performance of children with minimal to mild degrees of hearing loss, teachers observe higher levels of dysfunction in classroom settings for these children as compared to their normal hearing peers (Bess et al., 1998; Dodd-Murphy & Murphy, 2007; Most, 2004; Tharpe, Ricketts, & Sladen, 2004). Areas queried have included academics, attention, communication, class participation, and behavior. It has been speculated that these deficits are the result of later identification of this degree of hearing loss and fewer available support services for these children as compared to those for children with more severe degrees of hearing loss.

Self-perception inventories of emotional and physical health by school-age children with minimal to mild hearing losses have also revealed a perception of greater dysfunction as compared to their normal-hearing peers. Specifically, children with hearing loss perceived themselves as having more difficulty in areas of stress, self-esteem, and behavior than their normal hearing peers (Bess et al., 1998). In addition, younger children with hearing loss rated themselves as having less energy than their peers. Along those lines, there is some evidence to suggest that children with minimal to mild degrees of hearing loss might have less energy because increased listening effort is required relative to normal hearing children (Hicks & Tharpe, 2002). To the extent that this is true, effort expended to listen in the classroom setting might be a contributing factor to academic difficulties.

Despite a recent focus on management of minimal and mild hearing losses by the audiology and education communities, studies within the last 10 years have persisted in revealing academic difficulties encountered by these children. It appears that enhanced awareness by teachers, audiologists, and other professionals of the high risk status associated with minimal to mild hearing loss has not been sufficient to thwart its effects.

Impact on Auditory Skills

For children with hearing loss to understand speech optimally, the signal ideally should be 30 dB more intense than the room noise. Any ratio less than +30 dB has been shown to produce a degradation in word recognition among individuals with impaired hearing. Unfortunately, the ambient noise levels in typical classroom environments are often too high to produce an appropriate signal-to-noise ratio. Numerous studies over several decades have documented the poor acoustic conditions of classrooms (see, for example, Knecht, Nelson, Whitelaw, & Feth, 2002; Picard & Bradley, 2001). Likewise, if a child has a minimal or mild degree of hearing loss, this ideal signal-to-noise ratio is difficult, if not impossible, to attain. This situation is compounded by the fact that individuals with hearing loss exhibit greater difficulty in speech recognition than normal hearers under the same noise conditions. Other factors that contribute to the adversity of the listening condition and can possibly produce a synergistic effect include reverberation (persistent reflection of sound); speaker-listener distance; the degree, configuration, and type of hearing loss; type of amplification; age of the child; linguistic abilities of the child; the complexity of the message; classroom acoustics properties; and classroom lighting (see American Speech-Hearing-Language [ASHA], 2009, for a review of classroom listening challenges for children with hearing loss).

Conventional wisdom would lead us to conclude that the acoustic environment can have a significant effect on speech perception and learning in children. That is, the poorer the acoustic environment, the more difficult it is to hear clearly, resulting in academic difficulties. Furthermore, there is an abundance of evidence demonstrating that children, regardless of hearing status, require more favorable acoustic environments than adults to achieve equivalent speech recognition scores (e.g., Elliott, 1979; Nabelek & Robinson, 1982).

The effect of speaker-to-listener distance on speech recognition is of particular concern when considering children with minimal to mild degrees of hearing loss. After all, these children often do not use hearing technology that can assist them in listening. The most important factor in determining the signal-to-noise ratio is the distance between the speaker and the listener. According to the inverse square law, sound pressure decreases by 6 dB when the distance between the speaker and receiver is doubled. Thus, if the sound pressure of a signal is 70 dB at two feet, it will be 64 dB at four feet, 58 dB at eight feet, 52 dB at 16 feet, and so forth. This loss of distance hearing can impact incidental learning. Issues related to the development of speech and language include the ability to hear word-sound distinctions that form important morphological markers and difficulty with word recognition and spelling. For example, a child with minimal or mild hearing loss might miss indicators of plurality, tense and possession.

Examinations of speech perception ability of children with minimal to mild degrees of hearing loss have consistently demonstrated adverse effects of noise and reverberation on the perception of consonant, vowel, word, and sentence materials. Many of these studies simulate the noise and reverberation levels that are typical of those found in classroom settings (Boney & Bess, 1984; Crandall, 1993). Collectively, these studies provide evidence that children with permanent minimal to mild bilateral hearing loss experience greater difficulty understanding speech than their normal-hearing peers under acoustic conditions that simulate those typically found in school classrooms.

Conclusion

As stated over 30 years ago, " . . . hard-of-hearing children are not easily recognizable and often are mistaken for children with vague, sometimes exotic, always bewildering 'problems.' Thus, in many educational systems they are invisible children" (Davis, 1977, p. 1). We have come a long way since then in learning about the potential difficulties that children with minimal to mild hearing loss might face and making them more "visible" to audiologists, educators, and other professionals. However, we still have a long way to go. Certainly, in the context of hearing loss, we have learned that the term "minimal" does not mean "inconsequential" (Bess, 2004). Still there is much yet to learn about diminishing the effects of these losses and assessing the suitability of our current educational and management approaches.

Acknowledgment. The author appreciates the graphic services of the Vanderbilt Kennedy Center for Research on Human Development, supported in part by NICHD Grant P30 HD15052.

References

American Speech-Language-Hearing Association (ASHA). (2004). *Guidelines for the audiologic assessment of children from birth to 5 years of age*. Retrieved from: http://www.asha.org/docs/html/GL2004-00002.html

American Speech-Hearing-Language Association (ASHA). (2009). *Classroom acoustics*. Retrieved from http://www.asha.org/public/hearing/classroom.htm

Anderson, K. L. (1989). *Screening Instrument for Targeting Educational Risk (SIFTER)*. Retrieved from http://www.hear2learn.com

Anderson, K. L. (2000). *Early Listening Function (ELF)*. Retrieved from http://www.hear2learn.com

Anderson, K. L., & Matkin, N. (1996). *Screening Instrument for Targeting Educational Risk in Preschool Children (Preschool SIFTER)*. Retrieved from http://www.hear2learn.com

Anderson, K. L., & Smaldino, J. J. (1996). *Listening Inventory for Education: An efficacy tool (LIFE)*. Retrieved from http://www.hear2learn.com

Anderson, K. L, & Smaldino J. J. (2000). *Children's Home Inventory for Listening Difficulties (CHILD)*. Retrieved from http://www.hear2learn.com

Bamford, J., Beresford, D., Mencher, G., DeVoe, S., Owen, V., & Davis, A. (2001). Provision and fitting of new technology hearing aids: Implications from a survey of some "good practice services" in UK and USA. In R. C. Seewald & J. S. Gravel (Eds.), *A sound foundation through early amplification: Proceedings of the second international conference* (pp. 213–219). Stäfa, Switzerland: Phonak AG.

Bess, F. H. (2004, May). *Children with minimal sensorineural hearing loss*. Paper presented at Children with Hearing Loss Workshop, Casper, WY.

Bess, F. H., Dodd-Murphy, J., & Parker, R. A. (1998). Children with minimal sensorineural hearing loss: Prevalence, educational performance, and functional status. *Ear and Hearing, 19*, 339–354.

Bess, F. H., & Tharpe, A. M. (1986). Case history data on unilateral sensorineural hearing loss in children. *Ear and Hearing, 7*, 14–19.

Blair, J., Peterson, M. E., & Viehweg, S. H. (1985). The effects of mild sensorineural hearing loss on academic performance of young school-age children. *Volta Review, 93*, 87–93.

Boney, S., & Bess, J. H. (1984, November). *Noise and reverberation effects on speech recognition in children with minimal hearing loss*. Paper presented at the American Speech-Language-Hearing Association. San Francisco, CA.

Briscoe, J., Bishop, D. V., & Norbury, C. F. (2001). Phonological processing, language, and literacy: A comparison of children with mild-to-moderate sensorineural hearing loss and those with specific language impairment. *Journal of Child Psychology and Psychiatry*, *42*, 329–340.

Ching, T. C., Hill, M., & Psarros, C. (2000, August). *Strategies for evaluation of hearing aid fitting for children.* Paper presented at the International Hearing Aid Research Conference. Lake Tahoe, CA (www.nal.gov.au).

Clark, J. G. (1981). Uses and abuses of hearing loss classification. *ASHA*, *23*, 493–500.

Cone-Wesson, B., Sininger, Y., & Widen, J. (2005). *Issues associated with conducting diagnostic audiologic evaluations in children with suspected mild and unilateral hearing loss.* Proceedings from a National Workshop on Mild and Unilateral Hearing Loss. Breckenridge, CO. Retrieved from http://www.cdc.gov/ncbddd/ehdi/documents/unilateralhl/Mild_Uni_2005%20Workshop_Proceedings. pdf

Crandall, C. (1993). Speech recognition in noise by children with minimal degrees of sensorineural hearing loss. *Ear and Hearing*, *14*, 210–216.

Davis, J. (1977). *Our forgotten children: Hard-of-hearing pupils in the schools*. Minneapolis, MN: University of Minnesota.

Davis, J. M., Elfenbein, J., Schum, R., & Bentler, R. A. (1986). Effects of mild and moderate hearing impairments on language, educational, and psychosocial behavior of children. *Journal of Speech and Hearing Disorders*, *51*, 53–62.

Diefendorf, A., & Gravel, J. (1996). Behavioral observation and visual reinforcement audiometry. In S. Gerber (Ed.), *The handbook of pediatric audiology* (pp. 55–83). Washington, DC: Gallaudet University Press.

Dodd-Murphy, J., & Murphy, W. (2007, November). *Educational risk and perception of hearing difficulty in school children.* Paper presented at American Speech-Language-Hearing Association National Convention, Boston, MA.

Elliott, L. (1979). Performance of children aged 9 to 17 years on a test of speech intelligibility in noise using sentence material with controlled word predictability. *Journal of the Acoustical Society of America*, *66*, 651–653.

Elssmann, S. F., Matkin, N. D., & Sabo, M. P. (1987). Early identification and habilitation of hearing impaired children: Fact or fiction. *Proceedings of a symposium in audiology.* Conducted at Rochester Methodist Hospital, Rochester, MN.

Gorga, M. P., Neely, S. T., & Dorn, P. A. (1999). Distortion product otoacoustic emission test performance for a priori criteria and for multifrequency audiometric standards. *Ear and Hearing*, *20*, 345–362.

Gravel, J. S. (2005). Prevalence and screening in newborns. *Proceedings of a National Workshop on Mild and Unilateral Hearing Loss*. Breckenridge, CO. Retrieved from http://www.cdc.gov/ncbddd/ehdi/documents/unilateralhl/Mild_Uni_2005%20Workshop_Proceedings.pdf

Grimshaw, S. (1996). *The extraction of listening situations which are relevant to young children, and the perception of normal-hearing subjects of the degree of difficulty experienced by the hearing impaired in different types of listening situations*. Nottingham: MRC Institute of Hearing Research.

Haggard, R. S., & Primus, M. A. (1999). Parental perceptions of hearing loss classification in children. *American Journal of Audiology*, *8*, 83–92.

Hicks, C. B., & Tharpe, A. M. (2002). Listening effort and fatigue in school-age children with and without hearing loss. *Journal of Speech, Language, and Hearing Research*, *45*, 573–584.

Joint Committee on Infant Hearing (JCIH). (2007). Year 2007 Position Statement: Principles and guidelines for early hearing detection and intervention programs. *Pediatrics*, *120*(4), 898–921.

Johnson, J. L., White, K. R., Widen, J. E., Gravel, J. S., James-Trychel, M., Kennalley, T., . . . Holstrum, J. (2005). A multicenter evaluation of how many infants with permanent hearing loss pass a two-stage OAE/A-ABR newborn hearing screening protocol. *Pediatrics*, *116*, 663–672.

Knecht, H., Nelson, P., Whitelaw, G., & Feth, L. (2002). Background noise levels and reverberation times in unoccupied classrooms: Predictions and measurements. *American Journal of Audiology*, *11*, 65–71.

Küehn-Inacker, H., Weichbold, V., Tsiakpini, L., Coninx, S., & D'Haese, P. (2003). *Little ears: Auditory questionnaire*. Innsbruck, Switzerland: MED-EL.

Most, T. (2004). The effects of degree and type of hearing loss on children's performance in class. *Deafness and Education International*, *6*(3), 154–166.

Nabelek, A., & Robinson, P. (1982). Monaural and binaural speech perception in reverberation for listeners of various ages. *Journal of the Acoustical Society of America*, *71*, 1242–1248.

Norbury, C. F., Bishop, D. V. M., & Briscoe, J. (2001). Production of English finite verb morphology: A comparison of SLI and mild moderate hearing impairment. *Journal of Speech, Language, Hearing Research*, *44*, 165–178.

Norton, S. J. (1993). Applications of transient evoked otoacoustic emissions to pediatric populations. *Ear and Hearing*, *14*, 64–73.

Norton, S. J., Gorga, M. P., Widen, J. E., Folsom, R. C., Sininger, Y., Cone-Wesson, B., . . . Fletcher, K. (2000). Identification of neonatal hearing impairment: Evaluation of transient evoked otoacoustic emission, distortion product otoacoustic emission, and auditory brain stem response test performance. *Ear and Hearing*, *21*(5), 508–528.

Pediatric Working Group. (1996). Amplification for infants and children with hearing loss. *American Journal of Audiology*, *5*(1), 53–68.

Picard, M., & Bradley, J. (2001). Revisiting speech interference in classrooms. *Audiology*, *40*, 221–244.

Purdy, S., Farrington, D. R., Moran, C. A., Chard, L. L., & Hodgson, S. A. (2002). ABEL: Auditory behavior in everyday life. *American Journal of Audiology*, *11*, 72–82.

Rance, G., & Rickards, F. (2002). Prediction of hearing threshold in infants using auditory steady-state evoked potentials. *Journal of the American Academy of Audiology*, *13*(5), 236–245.

Ross, D. S., Visser, S., Holstrum, J., & Kenneson, A. (2005). Minimal hearing loss and cognitive performance in children: Brief update. *Proceedings from a National Workshop on Mild and Unilateral Hearing Loss*, Breckenridge, CO. Retrieved from: http://www.cdc.gov/ncbddd/ehdi/documents/unilateralhl/Mild_Uni_2005%20Workshop Proceedings.pdf

Tharpe, A. M., Ricketts, T., & Sladen, D. P. (2004). FM systems for children with minimal to mild hearing loss. In D. Fabry, C. D. Johnson (Eds.), *Access conference proceedings* (pp. 191–197). Chicago, IL: Phonak AG.

Tharpe, A. M., & Sladen, D. P. (2008). Causation of permanent unilateral and mild bilateral hearing loss in children. *Trends in Amplification*, *12*, 17–25.

Wake, M., Tobin, S., Cone-Wesson, B., Hans-Henrik, D., Gillam, L., McCormick, L., . . . Williams, J. (2006). Slight/mild sensorineural hearing loss in children. *Pediatrics*, *118*, 1842–1851.

Watkin, P. M., & Baldwin, M. (1999). Confirmation of deafness in infancy. *Archives of Disease in Childhood*, *81*, 380–389.

Williams, C. (2003, January). The children's outcome worksheets—an outcome measure focusing on children's needs. *News from Oticon*. Retrieved from http://www.oticon. com

World Health Organization. (1980). *International classification of impairments, disabilities, and handicaps*. Geneva, Switzerland: Author.

Yoshinaga-Itano, C, Johnson, C. D., Carpenter, K., & Brown, A. S. (2008). Outcomes of children with mild bilateral hearing loss and unilateral hearing loss. *Seminars in Hearing*, *29*, 196–211.

12

Moderate to Profound Sensory Hearing Loss in Children

Karen C. Johnson, Laurie S. Eisenberg, and Amy S. Martinez

Introduction

In this chapter, we discuss the impact of moderate to profound bilateral hearing loss (HL) on auditory abilities in young children, specifically those related to speech perception and production, which are intrinsically linked in development. In considering the two, we are dealing with a moving and complex target. Much of what has been reported in the past is based on outcomes in older children, often identified at ages well beyond one year. With the implementation of early hearing detection and intervention (EHDI) programs, many more children with hearing loss are being diagnosed under one year of age. Although outcome data on language development (and speech production to a lesser degree) are beginning to emerge in this population, studies regarding speech perception abilities in early-identified children have lagged far behind. In large part, this is due to the challenges of testing very young children (i.e., the motor, attentional, linguistic, and cognitive skills required to participate in testing) and the lack of appropriate clinical tools. In audiology, there is a long tradition of evaluating speech perception at the level of word identification and recognition. However, performance on such tasks requires not only a basic level of lexical knowledge, but also the ability to demonstrate that knowledge through pointing, speaking, or sometimes signing a response. With the advent of pediatric cochlear implantation, increasing attention is being given to approaches for assessing the ability of young children to perceive phonetic and phonemic contrasts in ways that minimize the influence of extra-auditory skills and cognitive/linguistic development.

Finally, many studies of speech perception in children with hearing loss have been conducted with sensory devices (acoustic amplification, tactile devices, and cochlear implants) in place, particularly in the case of children with severe and profound hearing losses. Other studies have been conducted through earphones or other transducers as opposed to the child's personal sensory device. Thus, reported outcomes have reflected not only children's auditory capabilities, but also the type and bandwidth of the transducer, the nature and generation of sensory device if used, and the sophistication of any strategies to fit and set that device.

In an attempt to delineate some of these issues, we have organized this chapter around a conceptual framework of perceptual development to describe speech perception and production in young children with hearing loss. We also report some speech perception data collected in our laboratory on young children with varying degrees of hearing loss. Finally, we discuss more recent outcomes for children with severe and profound hearing losses in the context of the changing criteria for cochlear implantation and the contribution of multimodal processing.

Classification of Hearing Loss

Remarkably, 50 years after the National Research Council proposed a scale by which to categorize hearing loss (Davis, 1960), there remains no universally applied classification scheme for describing hearing loss by degree (cf., Centers for Disease Control [CDC], 2006; National Institute on Deafness and Other Communication Disorders [NIDCD], 2006; World Health

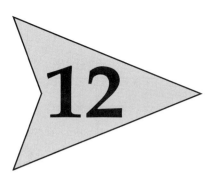

Organization [WHO], 2002). Thus, the boundaries between hearing loss categories referred to in the literature vary somewhat, even among studies conducted within the United States. For the purpose of this chapter we consider children whose auditory detection thresholds in both ears average 40 dB HL (re: pure tone average, or PTA, at 500, 1000, and 2000 Hz) or greater. Unless otherwise specified, we are using the following hearing loss categories to describe degree of loss: moderate, 40-to-55 dB HL; moderately severe, 56-to-69 dB HL; severe, 70-to-89 dB HL; profound, 90 dB HL and greater.

Because much of the literature concerning auditory abilities in children with hearing loss does not distinguish among clinical subtypes (e.g., conductive versus sensorineural), our discussion will include children with permanent conductive and mixed losses, as well as those with primarily sensory (cochlear) disorders. Nevertheless, it is assumed that most children with permanent loss described herein have some degree of cochlear involvement and the perceptual consequences that typically accompany sensory loss.

Prevalence of Moderate to Profound Hearing Loss

Large-scale population studies in the United States (Bhasin, Brocksen, Avchen, & Braun, 2006; Van Naarden, Decoufle & Caldwell, 1999) and the United Kingdom (Fortnum & Davis, 1997; MacAndie, Kubba, & MacFarlane, 2003) have put the estimated annual prevalence of permanent childhood hearing loss ≥ 40 dB at around 1.1 to 1.3 cases per 1,000. In these studies, degree of hearing loss has been almost equally divided between those categorized as "moderate" and "moderately-severe" (approximately 40 to 70 dB HL) versus those categorized as "severe" or "profound" (approximately 71 dB HL or greater). Although congenital and perinatal hearing loss is estimated to occur in 0.68 to 0.94 cases per 1,000 live births (Prieve & Stevens, 2000; Thompson et al., 2001; Wessex Universal Hearing Screening Trial Group, 1998), progressive and acquired losses are estimated to account for 11% (MacAndie et al., 2003) upward to 30% (Fortnum, Summerfield, Marshall, Davis, & Bamford, 2001; Van Narden et al., 1999) of permanent hearing loss in children 9 to 10 years of age. Thus, the impact of hearing loss on child development will depend not only on its degree, but also on its age of onset and progression (along with other numerous child, family, and intervention-related factors).

Conceptual Framework

A framework that we have found useful in considering the effects of early childhood hearing loss is Aslin and Smith's (1988) model of perceptual development. This model is organized around three levels assumed to underlie development in all perceptual systems: sensory primitives, perceptual representation, and cognitive/linguistic processing. These levels reflect not only the stages in perceptual processing from sensory reception at the periphery to assignment of relevance and meaning at higher cortical centers, but also the transition from less to more complex processing of sensory stimuli made possible with neuromaturation and auditory/linguistic experience.

Carney (1996) and Moeller and Carney (1993) adopted and extended Aslin and Smith's three-tiered model to describe the development of both speech perception and production, which typically emerge in parallel in normal-hearing infants and young children. Level I, sensory/production primitives, corresponds to the most basic stage of auditory perception (sound detection) and production (primitive vocalizations). Level II, perceptual/production representation, involves the coding at higher levels within the neural system that underlies phonetic discrimination and complex vocal utterances at the pre-word stage. Level III involves the cognitive/linguistic processing that allows for word recognition and phonemic-syllabic representation.

Sensory Primitives (Level I)

Speech Perception

At the most basic level of auditory perception, sound is transformed into a pattern of neural stimulation, reflecting the frequency, intensity, and temporal characteristics of the auditory stimulus. The structures responsible for encoding these parameters (cochlea, auditory nerve, and brainstem) are morphologically mature by the end of the second trimester of gestation (Moore & Linthicum, 2007), and the onset of auditory function is evident by 26 to 28 weeks of gestation (Birnholtz & Bencerraf, 1983; Starr, Amlie, Martin, & Sanders, 1977). Thus, at birth, the typically hearing and developing child has been detecting and responding to sound in utero for two to three months (Lecanuet & Schaal, 1996; Querleu, Renard, Versyp, Paris-Delrue, & Crepin, 1988). It has been suggested that this experience may assist infants in attending to specific sounds or speech features shortly following birth, especially those related to prosody and stress (DeCasper & Spence, 1986; Moon & Fifer, 2000; Lecanuet & Schaal, 1996). Nevertheless, it is only after birth that infants are exposed to the full range of sound in their environment (Werner, 2007).

Impact of Hearing Loss. The primary impact of hearing loss is to reduce or eliminate the sensory primitive, and it is at this level that sensory intervention is targeted (Carney, 1996; Moeller & Carney, 1993). Without sensory assistance, children with hearing losses of moderate or greater severity will have inconsistent, incomplete, or possibly no access to speech produced by themselves or others (re: average speech spectra; Cornelisse, Gagné, & Seewald, 1991; Pittman, Stelmachowicz, Lewis, & Hoover, 2003). For most of these children appropriately fitted hearing aids (HAs) are likely to bring much of the speech spectrum into the audible range. Still, depending on the configuration of the hearing loss and/or bandwidth of the sensory device, some components of speech (e.g., low amplitude, high frequency) may continue to be inaudible (Stelmachowicz, Pittman, Hoover, & Lewis, 2001, 2002). For some children with profound loss it may not be possible to provide sufficient gain to access much beyond the temporal envelop of speech signals, available in the lower frequencies. As hearing loss increases beyond 110 dB HL, any response to sound using acoustic amplification is likely to be based more on vibration than actual audition (Boothroyd & Cawkwell, 1970; Erber, 1972). For these children, cochlear implants (CIs) may provide access to acoustic signals across a broader frequency range.

Beyond the issue of audibility, the broadened frequency tuning and poorer temporal resolution that often accompany cochlear dysfunction will alter the pattern of neural activation sent forward to the next stage of perception processing. In addition, the necessity for listening to signals processed through acoustic amplification is likely to further impact speech perception, given the intrastimulus masking (i.e., upward spread of masking, backward masking) that may occur at high intensity levels (Boothroyd, 1978; Moore, 1996). Any or all of these factors may play a role in the reduced speech perception abilities demonstrated by individuals with cochlear involvement. For excellent summaries concerning cochlear processing and the perceptual consequences of cochlear impairment, the reader is referred to two publications by Moore (1996, 2008).

Speech Production

The most basic level of speech output is represented by the cries, vegetative sounds (associated with feeding and protection of the airway), undifferentiated vocalizations, and vocal play characteristic of infants during the first half year of life. Due to anatomic and neuromuscular immaturities of the vocal tract, these early sound productions are, for the most part, qualitatively distinct from those characteristic of adults in terms of frequency, resonance, and duration (Kent & Murray, 1982; Oller, 1980; Stark, 1980). Nevertheless, there is recent evidence that babies only a few days old are able to coordinate enough respiratory-laryngeal control to produce cries reflective of the prosody of the ambient language (Mampe, Friederici, Christophe, & Wermke, 2009). Analyzing the cries produced by newborns born to French versus German-speaking families, Mampe and colleagues (2009) found that the babies born to French-speaking families tended to produce cries with a rising melodic contours, whereas babies born to German-speaking families tended to produce cries with falling contours; intonation patterns consistent with each of the parent languages. These data also provide evidence of the very early influence of the language to which an infant is exposed, not only on speech perception, but vocal production as well.

Development at this stage continues to reflect the infant's emerging laryngeal and articulatory motor control. Beginning around 3 months of age, infants are able to produce vocalizations that perceptually match the vowels produced by an adult speaker (Kuhl & Meltzoff, 1996). Around 4 months of age, the infant begins to combine vowel-like and consonant-like productions, during what has been referred to as "marginal babbling" by Oller (1980) and "vocal play" by Stark (1980). Although the consonant and vocalic elements in these utterances do not yet match those of adult speech in duration, formant transitions, or vowel space, the developmental progression toward adultlike targets over the first six months provides further evidence that the infant's early auditory experience with the ambient language, combined with maturation, helps to shape subsequent vocal and speech production.

Impact of Hearing Loss. Until fairly recently, vocal development over the first few months of life has been considered to be constrained largely by anatomical and maturational factors. Thus, little difference has been reported in production primitives between infants with and without hearing loss, apart from the protracted period of time infants with hearing loss tend to remain in this stage (Carney, 1996; Koopmans-van Beinum, Clement, & van den Dikkenberg-Pot, 2001; Oller, Eilers, Bull, & Carney, 1985). This prolongation in time spent at the production primitive stage has been attributed to delays in attaining subsequent vocal milestones compared to normal hearing age-mates. However, recent evidence of the impact of auditory experience on the melodic characteristics of the cries of newborns only 2 to 5 days of age (Mampe et al., 2009), coupled with the implementation of universal early hearing detection programs, is likely to generate renewed interest in the impact of hearing loss on vocal production at the earliest stages of vocal development.

Perceptual Representation (Level II)

Speech Perception

Although sensory primitives are necessary for perception, an intermediate stage of processing is required to encode the neural stimulation patterns generated at the sensory periphery into perceptual units that are directly relevant to real world objects and events (Aslin & Smith, 1988). In auditory perception, this stage corresponds to the prelinguistic encoding of complex acoustic features that underlies discrimination at the phonemic level. Nearly 40 years of research have demonstrated that infants are born with an astonishing array of abilities for differentiating and categorizing the sounds of speech (For reviews, see: Jusczyk & Luce, 2002; Houston, Chapter 3 in this volume; Werker & Tees, 1999). Newborns are able to recognize and show preference for their mother's voice (DeCasper & Fifer, 1980). Infants a few days old have been shown to distinguish between their mother's native language and another language (Moon, Cooper, & Fifer, 1993), even when spoken by the same (bilingual) woman (Mehler et al., 1988). Furthermore, the now classic experiments conducted by investigators in the 1970s and 1980s demonstrated that infants within the first 6 months of life are able to discriminate the majority of phonetic contrasts underlying perception of most segmental features of importance in the ambient language, along with those found in non-native languages (e.g., Eimas, 1974; Eimas, Siqueland, Jusczyk, & Vigorito, 1971; Kuhl & Miller, 1975; Morse, 1972; Trehub, 1973). In addition, infants have demonstrated the ability to manage the variability introduced into speech by different talkers (Kuhl, 1983; Jusczyk, Pisoni, & Mullennix, 1992) and speaking rates (Eimas & Miller, 1980; Miller & Eimas, 1983).

Impact of Hearing Loss. In contrast to the vast literature regarding discriminative abilities in normal-hearing infants and children, this intermediate stage of perceptual processing has received comparatively limited attention in children with hearing loss. Until relatively recently, much of what we know about this level of representation in deaf and hard of hearing children came from seminal studies conducted in older children by pioneering investigators more than 30 years ago (Boothroyd, 1984; Erber 1972, 1979; Erber & Alencewicz, 1976; Hack & Erber, 1982; Smith, 1975). The aim of this research was to determine which speech features were available to children with different degrees of loss, in order to identify those acoustic and prosodic cues that might be made more accessible through focused auditory training. A second goal was to investigate the contribution of nonauditory sources of information (e.g., visual, tactile) to children who had little or no access to acoustic information with amplification, for the purpose of suggesting supplementary or alternative approaches to sensory intervention (e.g., lip-reading, vibrotactile devices).

In a series of investigations in school-aged children, Erber and colleagues determined that, in general, those with hearing loss in the severe range (approximately 70 to 95 dB HL) were able to discriminate between consonants on the basis of voicing and manner (e.g., plosive versus nasal; Erber, 1972, 1979; Erber & Alencewicz, 1976). Place of articulation (e.g., bilabial, alveolar, velar) was discriminated with less consistency through listening alone (Erber, 1972). Importantly, the ability to perceive most consonants meant that children with severe hearing loss typically were able to identify the number of syllables within words (Erber, 1971; Zeiser & Erber, 1977), although words containing voiced continuant consonants (e.g., /m/, /n/) at syllable boundaries were more difficult to segment than those marked by stops or plosives (Erber, 1971, 1979). In contrast, children with hearing losses greater than 95 dB HL tended to have access only to the gross temporal and intensity cues (waveform envelope) available in the lower frequency regions and through vibrotactile reception (Cramer & Erber, 1974; Zeiser & Erber, 1977). The inability to access the spectral information underlying consonant perception meant that these children also had difficulty identifying syllabic boundaries and thus the pattern of speech (Erber, 1971).

Boothroyd (1984) used pairs of consonant-vowel-consonants (CVCs) to examine contrast perception in 120 orally educated children with hearing losses ranging from moderate to profound (55 to 130 dB HL). Using a four-alternative forced choice paradigm (Speech Pattern Contrast test; SPAC), eight contrasts were assessed, including: vowel height, vowel place, consonant voicing, consonant continuance (manner), consonant place, temporal (syllabic) pattern, pitch variation, and talker gender. Testing was conducted monaurally (better ear) under earphones at the listener's most comfortable listening level. Performance decreased with increasing hearing loss. Children with hearing losses averaging 55 to 74 dB HL (moderate to severe) were able to perceive all contrasts with 66% or greater accuracy. Children with hearing losses in the 75 to 89 dB HL range (severe) scored above chance on all contrasts except consonant place. Children with hearing losses in the profound range (90 dB HL and greater) showed systematic decreases in the ability to discriminate segmental contrasts as hearing loss increased from 90 to 130 dB HL. In this group of subjects, temporal pattern (number of syllables) and vowel height were the contrasts that remained most perceivable with increasing degrees of hearing loss.

With the advent of pediatric cochlear implantation, there was renewed interest in the acoustic-phonemic level of perceptual representation. Drawing largely on the work of Erber and Boothroyd, a number of tools were compiled to assess a hierarchy of discrimination skills below the level of word recognition in children with profound hearing loss and limited verbal skills. These tools included: the Discrimination After Training (DAT) test (Thielemeir, Brimacombe, & Eisenberg, 1982), the Minimal Pairs test (Robbins, Renshaw, Miyamoto, Osberger, & Pope, 1988), the Early Speech Perception test (ESP)-Pattern Perception Subtest (Geers & Moog, 1989; Moog & Geers, 1990), the Screening Inventory of Perception Skills (Osberger et al., 1991a), and the Change-No Change procedure (Carney et al., 1993; Robbins, Osberger, Miyamoto, Renshaw & Carney, 1988). Researchers used such measures to examine outcomes in profoundly deaf children using early generations of CI devices and to compare rate of change in speech perception abilities across children using different types of sensory devices (single-channel versus multichannel CIs; CIs versus HAs versus tactile aids). In general, it was demonstrated that the single-channel implant (3M/House) primarily provided enhanced suprasegmental information (timing, intensity, stress, duration) compared to that provided by power-gain HAs being used at the time, with some limited encoding of low-frequency segmental (speech feature) cues (Eisenberg, Berliner, Thielemeir, Kirk, & Tiber, 1983; Eisenberg, Kirk, Thielemeir, Luxford, & Cunningham, 1986). Nevertheless, a small subset of children (primarily those with acquired hearing loss) obtained enough segmental information to discriminate between spondees in closed-sets and obtain "nonzero" open-set recognition (Berliner, Tonokawa, Brown, & Dye, 1988; Thielemeir, Tonokawa, Petersen, & Eisenberg, 1985). Children using the multichannel Nucleus-22 demonstrated, on average, better vowel and consonant perception than those using either the single-channel implant (Chute, Hellman, Parisier, & Selesnick, 1990; Miyamoto et al., 1991, 1992; Osberger, Robbins, Todd, Riley, Kirk, & Carney, 1996) or tactile aids (Carney et al., 1993; Geers & Brenner, 1994; Osberger et al., 1996; Robbins et al., 1988). Furthermore, speech feature discrimination for children using multichannel devices tended to be comparable to those demonstrated by children with PTA's in the 90 to 100 dB HL range using HAs (Geers & Brenner, 1994; Osberger et al., 1991b; Osberger et al., 1996). The significance of this comparison was that, at the time, children with PTAs in the range of 90 to 100 or 105 dB HL were still generally considered to have functional hearing for the purpose of developing oral communication (Boothroyd, 1985a; Geers & Moog, 1994; Miyamoto et al., 1991; Osberger et al., 1996; Smith, 1975).

In recent years we have been working with Arthur Boothroyd to develop a test battery for the purpose of assessing speech pattern contrast perception in young children, ages 6 months to 5 years (Eisenberg, Boothroyd, & Martinez, 2007). Derived from the Speech Pattern Contrast Test (SPAC; Boothroyd, 1984), this progressive test battery is comprised of four measures: Visual Reinforcement Assessment of the Perception of Speech Pattern Contrast (VRASPAC), Play Assessment of Speech Pattern Contrasts (PLAYSPAC), Online Imitative Test of Speech Feature Contrast Perception (OLIMSPAC), and Video Speech Pattern Contrast Test (VIDSPAC). All of the measures examine the same six phonetic contrasts: vowel height (e.g., /aa/ versus /oo/), vowel place (e.g., /ee/ versus /oo/), consonant voicing (e.g., /d/ versus /t/), consonant continuance or manner (e.g., /t/ versus /s/), consonant place in the front (alveolar versus bilabial position, e.g., /d/ versus /b/), and consonant place in the rear position (alveolar versus velar, e.g., /d/ versus /g/). However, each measure employs a different behavioral response task, based on the child's age and developmental abilities, to determine whether phonetic change has been perceived.

For example, VRASPAC (Martinez, Eisenberg, Visser-Dumont, & Boothroyd, 2007) uses a visually reinforced head turn to indicate that a child has detected phonetic change in a series of replicated syllables. Figure 12–1 shows VRASPAC results obtained over a 9-month period from a child with profound hearing loss. For each phonetic contrast, results are plotted according to the confidence level that the child's head turn responses are not random. Diagnosed at 1 month of age, this child was fitted with amplification by the age of 2 months. He was implanted bilaterally (Nucleus 24) in sequential surgeries at 12 months (right ear) and 14 months (left ear) of age, with device activation at 13

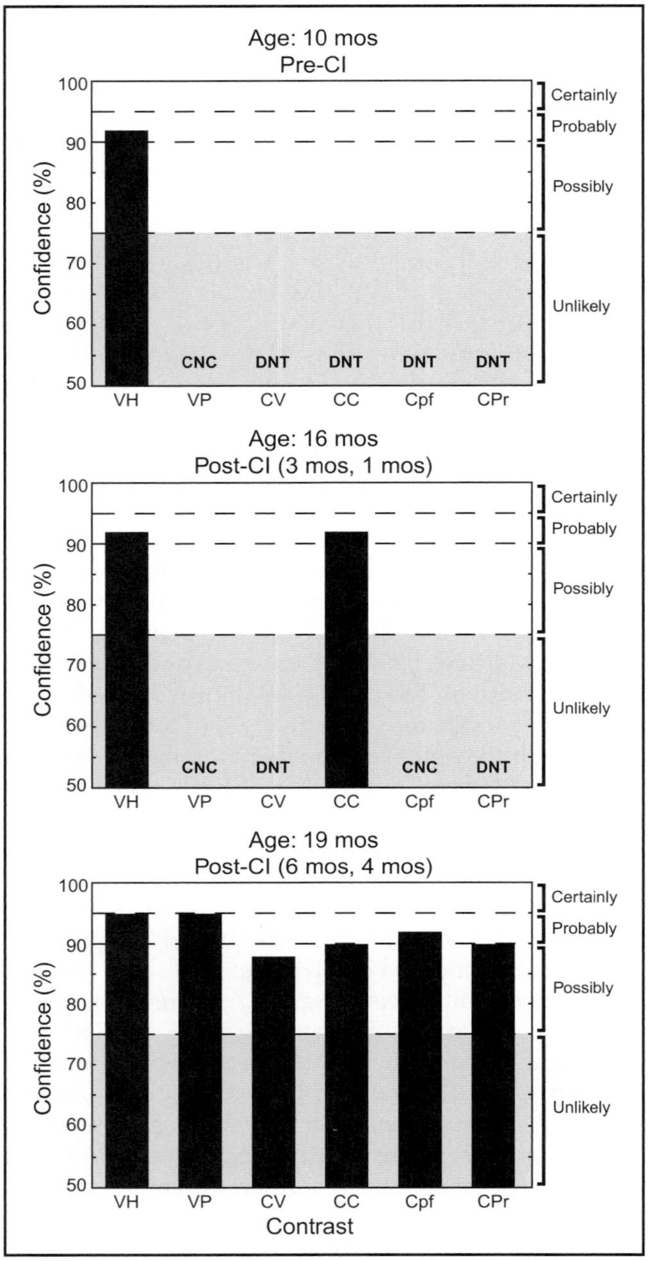

FIGURE 12–1. VRASPAC results for a young child with profound hearing loss at three test intervals: prior to sequential bilateral cochlear implantation (*top*), and at 3 months (*middle*) and 6 months (*bottom*) following activation of the first implanted ear. Trials to which the child could not be conditioned are indicated by "CNC." Contrast conditions that were not tested are indicated by "DNT." The six speech pattern contrasts tested were: vowel height (VH), vowel place (VP), consonant voicing (CV), consonant continuance/manner (CC), consonant place in the front position (CPf), and consonant place in the rear position (CPr).

and 15 months, respectively. The top graph shows results obtained from this child at 10 months of age, prior to implantation. With amplification, this child was able to detect a change in vowel height with greater than 90% confidence, but could not be conditioned to respond to a change in vowel place. The consonant contrasts were not attempted. The middle graph shows this child's results at the age of 16 months, 1 and 3 months following activation of his first and second implants, respectively. At this test interval, he demonstrated the ability to detect consonant continuance, as well as vowel height, at a confidence level of over 90%. Again, however, he could not be conditioned to respond consistently to vowel place nor to consonant place in the frontal position. Consonant voicing and consonant place in the rear position were not tested. The bottom graph shows results obtained only 3 months later, 6 months following activation of his first CI and 4 months following the second CI. At this interval, he met or exceeded the 90% confidence level for detection for five of the six contrasts.

The OLIMSPAC (Boothroyd, Eisenberg, & Martinez, 2010) differs from the other tests in the battery because it requires the child to imitate the syllable heard. "On-line" refers to fact that the child's responses are scored by an examiner while the test is in progress, as opposed to off-line by a panel of judges in the earlier IMSPAC version (Boothroyd, 1985b). Figure 12–2 shows results obtained using OLIMSPAC in 12 children, ages 32 months to 50 months (mean age: 40 months) with hearing losses ranging from mild to profound. All 12 children were using HAs at the time of assessment. The individual scores (percent correct) for each of the six contrasts are displayed in separate panels. Also shown on the left side of each panel is the mean (open circle) and two standard errors obtained for that contrast in 17 normal-hearing children, ages 34 months to 49 months (mean age: 42 months). The horizontal dashed line at 60% within each panel corresponds to chance performance after correction for guessing. Scores below this line are considered random responses. Among the six contrasts, vowel height (panel A, upper left) was the easiest to perceive for all children, normal hearing and those with hearing loss, scoring 100%. All 17 of the normal-hearing children and eight children with hearing loss achieved 100% on vowel place (panel B, upper right). The four children who scored below chance on this contrast included one child of the two with profound loss (who went on to get a cochlear implant) and three children with mild and moderate hearing losses who were relatively late identified and had been using amplification for shorter periods of time. In general, consonant contrasts were more difficult for all children, regardless of hearing status.

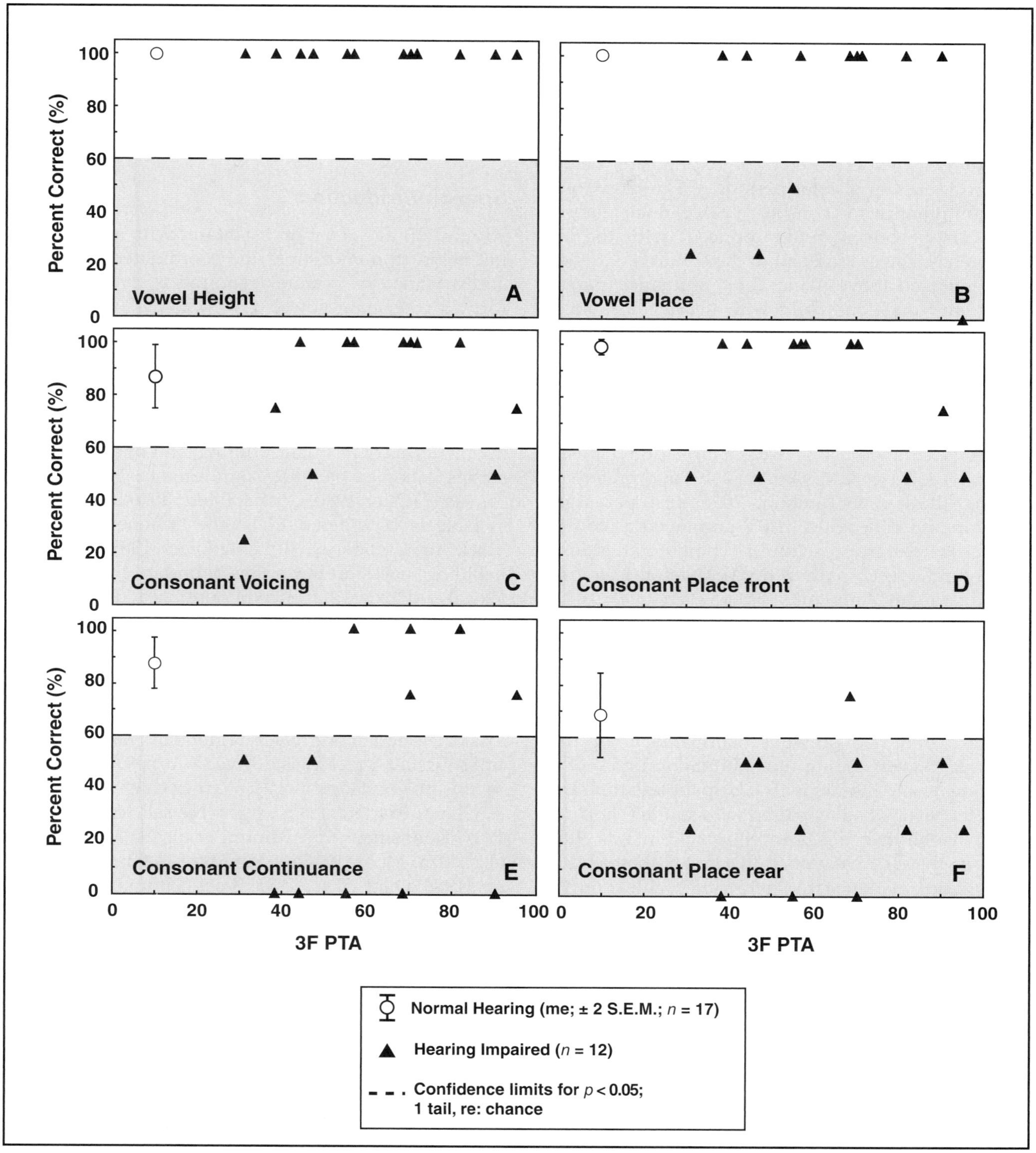

FIGURE 12–2. OLIMSPAC results for each of six speech pattern contrasts (panels A-F) for 12 young children with hearing losses ranging in degree from mild to profound. For each contrast, scores (percent correct) are plotted as a function of their unaided three-frequency pure tone average (3F PTA) at 500, 1000, and 2000 Hz in their better hearing ear. The open circle in each panel represents mean performance for the contrast obtained in a group of 17 children with normal hearing. The shaded area below the dashed line represents chance performance, corrected for guessing.

Consonant voicing (panel C, middle left) and place in the front position (panel D, middle right) were correctly perceived by all of the children with normal hearing and more than half of the children with hearing loss. Again, children scoring below chance on these two contrasts tended to be those with greater degrees of hearing loss or shorter periods of HA use. Consonant continuance and consonant place in the rear position were perceived (and produced) with the least consistency. Fewer than half of the children with hearing loss scored above chance for continuance (panel E, lower left); only one child with hearing loss scored above chance for consonant place in the rear (panel F, lower right). A number of normal-hearing children scored below chance on place in the rear position, as well.

The ability of infants and young children with cochlear implants to discriminate speech contrasts also has been examined using visual habituation (Houston, Pisoni, Kirk, Ying, & Miyamoto, 2003) and preferential looking (Barker & Tomblin, 2004) test paradigms. Houston and colleagues (2003) employed a modified visual habituation procedure to compare attention to speech and speech pattern discrimination in a group of 16 deaf infants implanted at less than 2 years of age with those of 48 normal-hearing infants, ages 6 months ($n = 24$) and 9 months ($n = 24$). Normal hearing infants and those with CIs both spent significantly longer periods of time looking at a visual display paired with a novel sound stimulus ("ahhh") compared to the one to which they had previous habituated ("hop, hop, hop"). However, during the habituation phase of the experiment, the infants with CIs spent less time looking at the visual display paired with sound ("hop, hop, hop") overall than did normal-hearing infants. Taken together, these investigators interpreted their findings as providing evidence that following cochlear implantation, deaf infants are able to detect and discriminate some sound patterns, although their attention to sound may be weaker than that displayed by normal-hearing infants.

Barker and Tomblin (2004) used a preferential looking procedure to examine the ability of 10 toddlers with CIs (mean age at activation: 1 year, 3 months) to match phonetic information between the face and voice. Video still images of a female talker articulating /a/ and /i/ were presented side-by-side on a split screen during a series of trials. For each trial, an audio file of either /a/ or /i/ produced by the same talker was played. The amount of time an infant spent looking at the picture matching to the phoneme presented (target) versus the picture matching the other phoneme (nontarget) was assessed at 2, 4, 6, and 9 months postactivation. On average, the mean looking times toward the target versus nontarget reached statistical significance at 9 months postactivation, suggesting that improved audibility and experience with listening with the device enabled these children to begin matching phonetic information.

Speech Production

Around the age of 6 months, infants with normal hearing begin to demonstrate the coordinated phonation and articulatory gestures required to produce well-formed consonant-vowel (CV) syllables (Oller, 1980). The combining of CV or VC syllables in repetitive sequences ("reduplicated" or "canonical" babbling), which typically emerges between the ages of 6 to 10 months of age, marks an important milestone in the child's vocal development. Its onset is quite sudden and, in terms of its quality, timing, and frequency transitions, canonical babbling sounds noticeably like adult "speech" (Oller, 1980; Oller & Eilers, 1988). Because the syllable is considered to be the "phonetic building block" of adult speech (Oller & Eilers, 1988), canonical babbling marks an important boundary between prelexical and lexical stages of phonological development (Gillis, Schauwers, & Govaerts, 2002) and is a necessary precursor for the first spoken words (Oller, Wieman, Doyle, & Ross, 1975; Vihman, Ferguson, & Elbert, 1986).

Impact of Hearing Loss. In the presence of hearing loss of moderate or greater degree the onset of canonical babbling typically is delayed (Carney, 1996; Davis, Morrison, von Hapsburg, & Warner Czyz, 2005; Eilers & Oller, 1994; Kent, Osberger, Netsell, & Hustedde, 1987; Koopsmans-van Beinum et al., 2001; Moeller et al., 2007a; Moore & Bass-Ringdahl, 2002; Oller & Eilers, 1988; Oller et al., 1985; Stoel-Gammon & Otomo, 1986; von Hapsburg & Davis, 2006). The extent of the delay is variable, with reports of some children (usually, but not always, those with more residual hearing) demonstrating canonical babbling within the age range of normal hearing peers (Koopmans-van Beinum et al., 2001; Moeller et al., 2007a). Most children with hearing loss do not start babbling, however, until well after their normal hearing age-mates, and the delay tends to lengthen as degree of hearing loss increases from moderate to profound (Carney, 1996; Moeller et al., 2007a). This pattern of delay was observed even among the majority of infants who were early identified and amplified (Davis et al., 2005; Moeller et al., 2007a). Furthermore, some children with severe and profound hearing losses do not produce enough canonical syllables within their ongoing vocalizations to be considered "consistent" (canonical babbling ratios, or CBRs, of 0.20 or greater; Davis et al., 2005; Eilers & Oller, 1994; Oller & Eilers, 1988; Oller et al., 1985; von Hapsburg & Davis, 2006).

Notable exceptions to these trends have been described for infants with profound hearing loss who have received cochlear implants. A number of young children with CIs have been reported to begin babbling 1 to 6 months after device activation (Colletti et al., 2005; Ertmer & Mellon, 2001; Moeller et al., 2007a; Moore & Bass-Ringdahl, 2002). Further advancement in vocal behavior and expansion of phonetic inventories following cochlear implantation have also been reported, with some CI children attaining vocal and verbal milestones with fewer months of auditory experience than typically hearing children (Ertmer & Mellon, 2001; Ertmer, Young, & Nathani, 2007; Moore & Bass-Ringdahl, 2002).

Cognitive/Linguistic Processing (Level III)

Speech Perception

Beginning at about six months, the normally hearing infant shows an increasing ability to recognize those sounds (Werker & Lalonde, 1988; Werker & Tees, 1984), sound sequences (Juscyzk, Friederici, Wessles, Svenkerud, & Juscyzk, 1993), and rhythmic/stress patterns (Juscyzk, Cutler, & Redanz, 1993) that are likely to appear in the words of the ambient language. This knowledge underlies the infant's developing ability to segment words from fluent speech, which in turn provides the basis for the building of a lexicon. Processing begins to take place at the level of the whole word rather than the phonemes that comprise it (Carney, 1996).

Speech perception skills continue to develop throughout childhood and adolescence with further maturation of the auditory pathways and other cortical centers, accumulating exposure to and experience with the ambient language, and expansion of the child's own receptive and expressive language skills. In addition, a number of more generalized cognitive factors and information processing skills are likely to play an important role in the child's developing abilities to comprehend spoken language. These include selective attention, lexical access, working memory, verbal rehearsal, and multimodal processing (Pisoni, 2000).

Impact of Hearing Loss. In the presence of hearing loss, the output at the perceptual representation stage is reduced, incomplete, or absent. This inconsistent or lack of access to the sound patterns of the ambient language is likely to delay the development of lexical representation underlying word recognition (Moeller & Carney, 1993; Moeller et al., 2007b; Nott, Cowan, Brown, & Wigglesworth, 2009). Likely delays in language development further restrict a child's ability to "fill in the blanks" in complex or difficult listening situations.

Despite the number of cognitive, linguistic, and other nonauditory influences on word and sentence recognition, it is at this level that speech perception is typically assessed for clinical purposes. In many instances, an attempt is made to control for such influences by restricting the response set to a fixed number of alternatives (i.e., "closed-set"). This approach is often used to assess young children or other individuals who may have limited vocabularies and/or verbal abilities (e.g., Elliot & Katz, 1980; Jerger, Lewis, Hawkins, & Jerger, 1980; Moog & Geers, 1990; Ross & Lerman, 1970). As described previously, a closed-set format also is commonly used for tasks involving discrimination between specific speech features and prosodic cues (e.g., Boothroyd, 1984; Erber & Alencewicz, 1976; Moog & Geers, 1990). In other instances, no attempt is made to limit responses to a set of predetermined alternatives (i.e., "open-set"; e.g., Bench, Doyle, & Greenwood, 1987; Gelnett, Sumida, Nilsson, & Soli, 1995; Haskins, 1949; Kirk, Pisoni, & Osberger, 1995), so as to better reflect the demands of "real-world" listening (Kirk, French, & Choi, 2009). In doing so, open-set measures also tap into the listener's linguistic and cognitive processing skills as well as auditory-perceptual capabilities.

In general, children with hearing losses in the moderate and severe hearing range (roughly < 90 dB HL) achieve open-set recognition for speech that is made audible (i.e., amplified under earphones or via personal hearing aids; Blamey et al., 2001b; Eisenberg, Kirk, Martinez, Ying, & Miyamoto, 2004; Hicks & Tharpe, 2002). Nevertheless, word and sentence recognition scores tend to decrease systematically as degree of hearing loss increases (e.g., Blamey et al., 2001b; Snik, Vermeulen, Brokx, Beijk, & van der Broek, 1997). As part of a larger study comparing speech perception, speech production, and language outcomes in children using HAs versus CIs, Blamey and colleagues (2001b) conducted a series of regression analyses on open-set word recognition scores as a function of child age and degree of loss. For the 40 children using HAs with hearing losses ranging from moderate to profound, consonant-nucleus-consonant (CNC) word scores (Peterson & Lehiste, 1962) decreased by approximately 5% for every 10 dB of threshold change across a range of 40 to 103 dB HL, after accounting for child age (age range: 4.3 to 13.0 years; see Blamey et al., 2001b, Table 2, p. 271). The rate of change was slightly shallower for

CNC phoneme scores (i.e., percentage of correct phonemes within CNC words, regardless of position within word or any other phoneme errors within same response), which decreased by approximately 4% per 10 dB of hearing loss, and slightly steeper for BKB sentences scored for key words (Bench-Kowal-Bamford Sentence Test; Bench et al., 1987), which decreased by approximately 6% for every dB of loss.

Children with profound hearing loss (≥ 90 dB HL) also exhibit a range of speech perception abilities (Boothroyd 1985a; Boothroyd, Geers, & Moog, 1991; Erber & Alencewicz, 1976). Erber and Alencewicz (1976, see Figure 4, p. 262) provided early evidence regarding the range of speech perception abilities of children with profound loss using a newly developed speech perception battery that subsequently became known as the Monosyllable-Trochee-Spondee (MTS) test. Stimuli consisted of four monosyllables, four trochees, and four spondees presented in a closed-set format using picture card depictions of the word items. Each of the 12 words was presented twice and scored in two ways. The first score was for correct identification of syllabic stress pattern, regardless of whether the word was correctly identified; the second score was for correct identification of the word itself. Presenting data obtained on 126 ears (67 children), these investigators showed that children with average hearing thresholds less than 110 dB HL achieved a wide range of scores for closed-set word identification. Analyzing these same word scores further, Boothroyd et al. (1991, see Figure 2, p. 82S) showed that most subjects with hearing losses less than 90 dB HL were able to identify words within syllable categories with 70 to 100% accuracy. Those with hearing losses greater than 110 dB HL tended to score at chance (25%) or below and thus, according to Boothroyd and colleagues, appeared to be guessing within syllabic categories. Children with hearing losses between 90 and 110 dB HL demonstrated the wide range of scores reported by Erber and Alencewicz (1976), from a little above 0% to over 90% correct identification. Nevertheless, most subjects within this hearing loss range scored above chance, suggesting at least some ability to use spectral information to identify words in a closed set.

The early CI studies comparing sensory aid benefit for deaf children using various devices also provide relevant data with regard to the aided speech perception abilities of children with profound loss (Meyer, Svirsky, Kirk, & Miyamoto, 1998; Osberger et al., 1996). In these studies, children with unaided thresholds between 90 and 105 dB HL served as "control groups," or the standard against which deaf children using other sensory devices were to be compared. Children with hearing aids who had unaided thresholds below 105 dB HL were observed to achieve modest recognition for Common Phrases (Osberger et al., 1996; Meyer et al., 1998). The Common Phrases test included familiar phrases used in everyday situations with young children and thus were considered to be more easily recognizable than monosyllabic words (Osberger et al., 1991b). Although children with unaided PTAs between 90 and 100 dB HL demonstrated better phrase recognition than those whose hearing losses fell between 100 and 105 dB HL, variability was high and there was significant overlap between the two groups. Nevertheless, when presented in the auditory-visual modality, scores for Common Phrases improved dramatically for both groups, suggesting that in combination with the visual cues available under "real-life" listening conditions, children with profound hearing losses averaging less than 110 dB HL could perceive enough spectral information through their hearing aids to function in an auditory world. In contrast, children with losses averaging greater than 110 dB HL were not able to achieve any auditory-only recognition for Common Phrases using hearing aids or tactile devices, although with tactile cues a modicum of improvement was noted.

Children with CIs using contemporary signal processing strategies are likely to achieve open-set word recognition similar to that exhibited by children with severe hearing loss who use HAs (Blamey et al., 2001b; Eisenberg et al., 2004). Two studies assessing outcomes in children implanted for 10 years or longer reported that the majority of CI children ultimately were able to understand conversational speech without the use of visual cues and use the telephone with a familiar talker (Beadle et al., 2005; Uziel et al., 2007). Although the most speech perception skill growth tends to occur within the first 3 to 5 years postimplant, continued improvement has been observed beyond 5 years (Beadle et al., 2005; Tyler et al., 2000; Uziel et al., 2007). Furthermore, the time course over which different skills (e.g., pattern perception, closed-set identification, open-set recognition) emerge varies considerably across CI children (Fryauf-Bertschy, Tyler, Kelsay, Gantz, & Woodworth, 1997). Nevertheless, a small subset of children does not develop functional open-set speech recognition, even after five years or more of CI use (Geers, Brenner, & Davidson, 2003; Tyler et al., 2000; Uziel et al., 2007).

Adverse Listening Conditions. Speech perception scores obtained in quiet, under the controlled conditions of the laboratory or clinic, belie the amount of difficulty that children, with or without hearing loss, may experience under everyday listening conditions. It is well established that even among normal-hearing children the ability to detect and understand speech under adverse or degraded conditions is not equivalent to that demonstrated by adults (Elliot, 1979; Eisenberg, Shannon, Martinez, Wygonski, & Boothroyd, 2000; Fallon, Trehub, & Schneider, 2000; Hall, Grose, Buss, & Dev, 2002; Johnson, 2000; Nozza, Rossman, Bond, & Miller, 1990; Trehub, Bull, & Schneider, 1981). These are skills that continue to develop throughout childhood, not reaching adultlike performance until well into adolescence (Elliot, 1979; Eisenberg et al., 2000; Fallon et al., 2000; Johnson, 2000; Neuman & Hochberg, 1983)

Children with hearing loss experience greater difficulty understanding speech under degraded or complex listening conditions than their normal-hearing peers (e.g., Crandell, 1993; Erber, 1971; Finitzo-Hieber & Tillman, 1978; Hicks & Tharpe, 2002). In general, when tested under the same noise conditions, younger children demonstrate poorer speech recognition than older children (Gravel, Fausel, Liskow, & Chobot, 1999), and children with greater degrees of hearing loss show poorer speech recognition than those with milder degrees of loss (Davis, Elfenbein, Schum, & Bentler, 1986; Erber, 1971). Still, children with minimal hearing loss may demonstrate significant decrements in performance compared to normal-hearing children, as listening conditions become increasingly adverse (Crandell, 1993). Furthermore, even when relatively high levels of performance can be maintained in noise, it is likely to require more effort on the part of children with hearing loss compared to their normally hearing peers (Hicks & Tharpe, 2002).

Figure 12–3 illustrates the impact of listening in competition on two groups of 3- to 4-year-old children. Shown are mean percent correct identification scores obtained on a closed-set sentence identification test for 10 children with normal hearing and 10 children with hearing loss. For the children in the hearing loss group, PTAs ranged from 30.0 to 78.3 dB HL; all were fitted with bilateral amplification. Stimuli were sentences from the Pediatric Speech Identification (PSI) test (Jerger et al., 1980), presented at 70 dB(A) from a loudspeaker located in front of the child (0° azimuth). The child's task was to point to the picture depicting the sentence heard from a set of five alternatives. In the competing conditions, single-talker competition was introduced from a speaker located behind the child (180° azimuth) and varied in 10 dB steps relative to the target to generate a range of message-to-competition ratios (MCRs), from relatively easy (+10 MCR) to difficult (–10 MCR). At +10 MCR, the easiest condition, both groups of children scored at or near ceiling. As the listening difficulty increased, performance decreased for both groups. However, the rate of decline was more pronounced for the hearing loss group. At 0 MCR, mean performance for the hearing loss group (85%) was slightly below that of the normal hearing group (95%). At –10 MCR, the most difficult listening condition, sentence identification for the children with hearing loss was markedly poorer (10%) than that shown by the majority of children with normal hearing (57%).

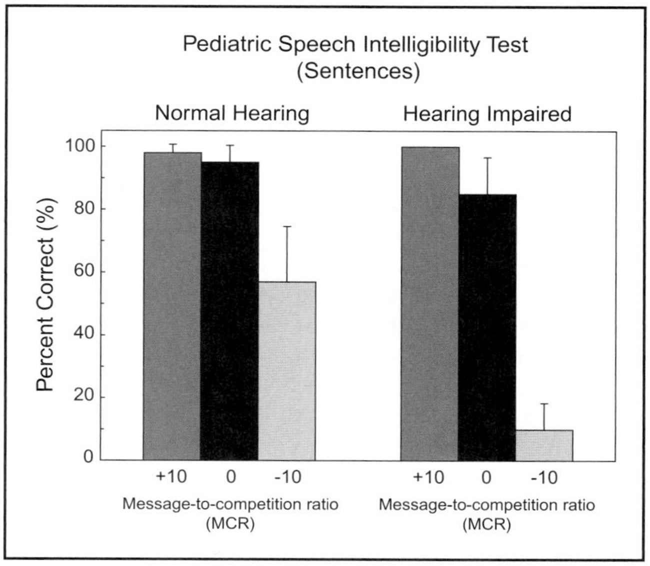

FIGURE 12–3. Performance on the Pediatric Speech Intelligibility Test (PSI; Sentences) at three message-to-competition ratios (MCRs; +10, 0, –10) for 10 children with normal hearing and 10 children with hearing loss.

Speech Production

At about 10 months of age, the infant's vocalizations and syllabic patterns begin to shift from universal forms that are easiest to produce toward those that are used in the ambient language (de Boysson-Bardies & Vihman, 1991; Werker & Tees, 1999). By 12 to 15 months of age, normal-hearing infants and toddlers begin to produce their first recognizable words (Kent & Bauer, 1985; Stoel-Gammon, 1985; Vihman, Ferguson, & Elbert, 1986).

Normal-hearing children continue to develop and master their phonological skills over the course of childhood. Ages 1 to 4 years are characterized by an orderly progression in speech sound acquisition that includes vowels, diphthongs, stops, nasals, and glides (Kent, 2004; Stoel-Gammon, 1985). Among vowels, central, low-mid-front and low-front vowels precede high vowels in order of acquisition (Kent & Bauer, 1985). Among consonants, voiced stop consonants precede voiceless stops and stop consonants produced in the frontal position precede those produced in the rear position (Stoel-Gammon, 1988). Fricatives, liquids, and initial consonant clusters are finally mastered during ages 5 to 9 years (Kent, 2004; Smit, Hand, Freilinger, Bernthal, & Bird, 1990). Despite the fact that not all speech sounds have yet been acquired, 3-year-old children typically are judged to be 50 to 80% intelligible by unfamiliar listeners (Vihman, 1988); 4-year-olds are judged to be roughly 70 to 100% intelligible (Gordon-Brannan, 1994).

Impact of Hearing Loss. During the transition from prelexical vocalization to first words, infants and toddlers with hearing loss exhibit a more restricted range of phonetic elements compared to normal-hearing children the same age (Kent et al., 1987; Moeller et al., 2007a; Stoel-Gammon, 1988). They also tend to be slower in moving from production of simpler to more complex syllabic forms (Koopmans-van Beinum et al., 2001; Moeller et al., 2007a, 2007b; Stoel-Gammon, 1988). The extent of hearing loss plays a significant role in early speech sound acquisition; children with milder degrees of hearing loss tend to demonstrate larger phonetic and syllabic repertoires than children with more severe losses (Davis et al., 2005; Moeller et al., 2007a; Stoel-Gammon & Otomo, 1986; Yoshinaga-Itano & Sedey, 2000). Nevertheless, acquisition of first true words is likely to be delayed even among infants who were early identified and fitted with sensory devices within the first year of life (Moeller et al., 2007b, Nott et al., 2009).

In general, the overall pattern of phonologic development in most children with hearing loss follows that demonstrated by normal-hearing children, albeit somewhat delayed (Moeller et al., 2007a; Stoel-Gammon, 1983). Furthermore, a number of investigators report that many of the production errors observed in older children with hearing loss are those characteristic of younger children with normal hearing (McDermott & Jones, 1984; Oller et al., 1985; Stoel-Gammon, 1983). The pattern of production errors appears to be similar across children, with the number and types of errors increasing as degree of loss increases (Gordon, 1987; Markides, 1970; McDermott & Jones, 1984; Smith, 1975; Stoel-Gammon, 1983).

Fricatives and affricates appear to be particularly vulnerable to omission and substitution across children with all degrees of hearing loss (Elfenbein, Hardin-Jones, & Davis, 1994). In a recent longitudinal study of phonetic development, Moeller and colleagues (2007a) observed different developmental trajectories for fricatives/affricates versus nonaffricates between children with early identified hearing loss and normal-hearing controls. Not only did the group with hearing loss produce fewer fricative/affricates than the group with normal hearing at a comparable age, but the gap in usage between the two widened with age. Relevant to these findings are previous studies from the same laboratory showing the peak energy of /s/ to be outside the bandwidth of current hearing aids (Stelmachowicz et al., 2001, 2002). In addition, fricatives tend to be low in amplitude, particularly in connected speech and in the final position in words. Thus, children with hearing loss, even of milder degrees, may not have consistent access to phonemes within this class in the course of daily listening across a number of environments.

Most children with moderate and severe hearing losses develop intelligible speech (Boothroyd, 1984; Elfenbein et al., 1994; Jesnema, Karchmer, & Trybus, 1978; Monson, 1978). Children with profound loss vary widely in their production skills (Boothroyd, 1984; Ling & Milne, 1981; Monson, 1978; Smith, 1975; Svirsky, Chin, Miyamoto, Sloan, & Caldwell, 2002). Amount of residual hearing appears to be the key factor in development of intelligible speech among children with profound loss (Boothroyd, 1984; Svirsky et al., 2002).

Many children with profound loss using CIs develop intelligible speech (e.g., Blamey et al., 2001a; Tobey, Geers, Brenner, Altuna, & Gabbert, 2003; Tomblin, Peng, Spencer, & Lu, 2008). Although speech skill development in children with CIs tends to lag behind that of normal-hearing children, as a group they tend to perform within one standard deviation of their normal-hearing peers (Blamey et al., 2001a). The most rapid progress typically is observed over the first 6 years of device use (Blamey et al., 2001a; Tomblin et al., 2008).

However, not all children using CIs develop intelligible speech, even after many years of implant use (Beadle et al., 2005; Uziel, 2007). One factor observed to correlate with communication outcomes in children with profound hearing loss is mode of communication. Specifically, children whose educational settings emphasize an oral-aural approach consistently have shown better speech perception and production outcomes than children from settings using total communication, whether using a CI or hearing aids. (Boothroyd, 1984; Svirsky et al., 2002; Tobey et al., 2003).

Sensory Device Use in Children With Severe and Profound Hearing Loss

Data from a number of studies conducted with early generations of multichannel cochlear implants suggested that children with profound losses in excess of 100 dB HL derive greater benefit from CIs than from HAs (Geers & Brenner, 1994; Meyer et al., 1998; Osberger et al., 1996; Svirsky & Meyer, 1999; Zwolan et al., 1997). More recent studies suggest that a CI enables the child with profound hearing loss to function more like a child with severe loss (Blamey et al., 2001b; Boothroyd & Boothroyd-Turner, 2002; Dettman et al., 2004; Eisenberg et al., 2004; Gantz et al., 2000). Nevertheless, it is still important that each child considered for cochlear implantation be evaluated on an individual basis in order to assess the potential for HA benefit before recommending a CI. This is especially true with regard to infants, for whom decisions about implantation are sometimes made before behavioral testing and hearing aid trials are instituted. In such cases, there may be over reliance on electrophysiologic measures to predict auditory function. However, absent auditory brainstem responses do not necessarily indicate lack of aidable residual hearing (e.g., see Luxford, Eisenberg, Johnson, & Mahnke, 2004). Furthermore, some children with severe or profound hearing loss using contemporary HAs may perform at levels comparable to or better than what might be expected with CI use.

Complicating the picture is asymmetric hearing loss, with a profound loss in one ear and a moderately severe or severe hearing loss in the other ear. In the early years of pediatric cochlear implantation, even the better hearing ear was required to be in the profound hearing loss range before an implant would be recommended. This created a hardship for some children with severe loss in their better hearing ear, but who were not progressing with HAs to the extent typically demonstrated by children with bilateral profound loss who use a CI. Today, many centers implant children with significant residual hearing in one ear, thereby pairing acoustic amplification in the better hearing ear and electrical stimulation in the poorer hearing ear. However, even implant users with fairly symmetric hearing loss (whether severe or profound) are often encouraged to keep an HA on the ear opposite to the implant so that they might benefit from low-frequency acoustic cues. The combination of a CI in one ear and an HA in the other ear is referred to as a bimodal fitting.

There also is a growing trend for the implantation of both ears, referred to as bilateral cochlear implantation. Children are either implanted sequentially (requiring two different surgeries) or simultaneously (two devices implanted during the same surgery). For both bimodal and bilateral device configurations, the goal is the same as for the fitting of two HAs—to provide binaural hearing for enhanced sound localization and improved speech recognition in noise. Results to date suggest that some, but not all, children who use CIs are better able to localize sound with bimodal or bilateral listening (Ching, Psarros, Hill, Dillon, & Incerti, 2001; Litovsky et al., 2006b; Litovsky et al., 2004). In addition, many children demonstrate improved speech recognition in noise using a bimodal or bilateral device configuration relative to that achieved under a monaural CI condition. Other children, however, show no difference or even poorer performance in noise using two devices compared to one CI alone (Ching et al., 2001; Holt, Kirk, Eisenberg, Martinez, & Campbell, 2005; Litovsky, Johnstone, & Godar, 2006a). The reader is referred to Ching, van Wanrooy, and Dillon (2007) for an excellent summary of the results from bimodal and bilateral fittings in both children and adults.

A word of caution is in order when comparing auditory access through acoustic amplification versus cochlear implantation. Whereas real-ear measures can be used to determine the spectral information available to the child through the HA, no corresponding measure exists for CIs. Thus, access to sound across the frequency region important for speech perception is frequently (and crudely) estimated through a sound field detection audiogram. It is important to note that although detection levels using the implant may be brought to within what generally is considered the "mild hearing loss" range, electrical stimulation is not equivalent to acoustic stimulation and the child will still be required to map meaning onto these sensations. Therefore, a child with profound hearing loss who demonstrates sound field thresholds of 15 dB HL using a CI cannot be expected to have comparable suprathreshold performance as a child with similar aided or unaided thresholds. It can be assumed only that the implant processor has been adjusted in such a way that the child is able to detect soft sounds at different frequencies. In fact, it has been demonstrated that children with CIs who have detection thresholds in the "mild loss" range function more like children with moderately severe and severe hearing losses using amplification in terms of their speech perception and speech production (Blamey et al., 2001b; Boothroyd & Boothroyd-Turner, 2002; Eisenberg et al., 2004).

Multimodal Perception

Speech communication is multimodal in that both auditory and visual cues provide complementary information to the listener. With greater degrees of hearing loss, the visual modality is likely to play an increasingly important role in providing access to the sensory primitives and perceptual representations upon which speech perception at the cognitive/linguistic level develops (Moeller & Carney, 1993).

In early infancy, children are sensitive to the associations between auditory and visual speech sounds, and it has been suggested that auditory-visual integration plays a role in the development of articulation (Kuhl & Meltzoff, 1982; Patterson & Werker, 1999). Children with hearing loss rely on the combination of auditory and visual cues to maximize comprehension of spoken language. With assistance from their sensory devices, many children with hearing loss learn to perceive and produce vowels and consonants (Eisenberg et al., 2003). Much of the acoustic information that enables differentiation among vowels or processing of consonant voicing and manner features is found in the time/intensity domain, cues that are generally accessible across a wide range of frequencies. Place of articulation is restricted to the frequency/time domain, and listeners with hearing loss often experience difficulty differentiating between speech sounds that are most reliant on the higher frequency spectral cues (e.g., /i/ versus /u/, or /b/ versus /d/). The addition of the visual modality can resolve perceptual ambiguities in the acoustic signal, particularly in adverse listening conditions (Erber, 1971; Sumby & Pollack, 1954).

A number of investigators have compared auditory-visual versus auditory-only and/or visual-only perception of speech in children with hearing loss. Early studies were aimed at assessing children with severe-to-profound hearing loss (Erber, 1971, 1972; Hack & Erber, 1982), although more recent investigators have evaluated children with a broad range of hearing losses (Eisenberg et al., 2003; Seewald, Ross, Giolas, & Yonovitz, 1985; Tillberg, Ronnberg, Svard, & Ahlner, 1996). After CIs became commercially available for children with profound hearing loss, a number of studies were conducted to evaluate the multimodal benefits with this sensory device (Bergeson, Pisoni, & Davis, 2005; Geers & Brenner, 1994; Kirk, Hay-McCutcheon, Holt, Gao, Qi, & Gerlein, 2007; Lachs, Pisoni, & Kirk, 2001; Schorr, Fox, van Wassenhove, & Knudsen, 2005). Despite the use of different speech materials with children of different ages, degree of hearing loss and sensory device type, results across studies have been generally consistent; speech recognition is more accurate when assessed via the auditory-visual modality relative to auditory-only or visual-only modalities. In addition, children with greater amounts of residual hearing have been shown to benefit more from both auditory-visual and auditory-only delivery of speech than children with little residual hearing (Erber, 1972; Seewald et al., 1985). Children with CIs who demonstrate higher language skills also perform more accurately on measures of speech recognition presented in auditory-visual and auditory-only formats than those with poorer language skills (Kirk et al., 2007). Moreover, children with CIs who derive greater benefit from visual enhancement of the auditory speech signal have more intelligible speech than children who receive little or no benefit from the addition of visual speech cues (Lachs et al., 2001). Lastly, children implanted at earlier ages (2.5 years and younger) have been shown to develop better auditory-visual integrative skills than children implanted at later ages (Schorr et al., 2005).

In view of the fact that auditory-visual processing of speech is reflective of real-world communication and demonstrates underlying perceptual skills, it is rather interesting that standard audiologic practice focuses almost exclusively on the administration of speech recognition tests in the auditory-only modality. Audiologic assessment of speech recognition in auditory-visual, auditory-only, and visual-only modalities would provide a more complete glimpse of how a child with hearing loss is performing with their sensory device. Thus, it is quite promising that new directions in test development are starting to emphasize multimodal speech processing and that such tests may be available for future clinical use (see Kirk et al., 2009).

Impact of Early Identification and Intervention

Prior to the widespread implementation of universal newborn hearing screening, the delay in the identification and confirmation of hearing loss in young children with no recognized risk factors ranged between 13 to 24 months for those with severe and profound loss and 22 months to 4 years for those with mild to moderate loss (Harrison & Roush, 1996; Nelson, Bougatsos & Nygren, 2008; Thompson et al., 2001). With the implementation of universal hearing screening, the average age at which hearing loss is confirmed has finally begun to decrease. In a recent study (Sininger et al., 2009), the median age of diagnosis was 3.03 months for infants who were screened at birth, compared to 27.83 months for infants who were not screened. More importantly, the median ages for the initiation of amplification and early intervention service among screened infants in this sample were 5.59 and 10.58 months, respectively, compared to 31.07 and 37.33 months for nonscreened infants.

To date, studies reporting outcomes in children in EHDI programs have focused primarily on language outcomes (Kennedy et al., 2006; Mayne, Yoshinaga-Itano, Sedey, & Carey, 2000b; Mayne, Yoshinaga-Itano, & Sedey, 2000a; Moeller, 2000; Moeller et al., 2007b, Nott et al., 2009; Watkin et al., 2007; Yoshinaga-Itano, Sedey, Coulter, & Mehl, 1998). Studies regarding speech perception and production outcomes, especially very early vocal behavior, in children in EHDI programs are beginning to emerge (e.g., Moeller et al., 2007a). Although these initial reports do not as yet point to a clear advantage of early identification and intervention on developing speech production abilities (except among children with cochlear implants), links between early vocal behavior and subsequent language development in early-identified infants have been established and are encouraging (Wallace, Menn, & Yoshinaga-Itano, 2000; Yoshinaga-Itano & Sedey, 2000).

Conclusions

In this chapter we attempted to highlight important research findings relating to the speech perception and production abilities of children with moderate to profound hearing loss. In reviewing the early literature, one can point to a general trend for performance to decrease with increasing severity of hearing loss. However, confounding variables impacting past outcome data include the duration and degree of auditory deprivation experienced by the child and the quality of the sensory assistance available at the time.

More recent evidence suggests that differences among groups categorized by hearing loss may become obscured due to a number of factors, including: technologic innovations in cochlear implants and digital hearing aids, improved assessment and device fitting protocols, and widespread implementation of EHDI programs. Thus, as suggested at the beginning of this chapter, the children we describe today may not be "representative" of children with hearing loss a few years hence, as the influence of these factors are more fully realized. Future reports based on longitudinal studies currently tracking early identified infants fitted with current technologies are expected to delineate the impact of hearing loss per se versus the confounding effects of long-term auditory deprivation that have clouded our picture in the past.

Acknowledgments. This work was supported, in part, by grants R01 DC006238, R01 DC004433, R01 DC R01004797, DC008875, and R01 DC009561 from the National Institutes on Deafness and Other Communication Disorders (NIDCD) of the National Institutes of Health (NIH).

References

Aslin, R. N., & Smith, L. B. (1988). Perceptual development. *Annual Review of Psychology, 39*, 435–473.

Barker, B. A., & Tomblin. J. B. (2004). Bimodal speech perception in infant hearing aid and cochlear implant users. *Archives of Otolaryngology-Head and Neck Surgery, 130*, 582–587.

Beadle, E. A. R., McKinley, D. J., Nikolopoulos, T. P., Brough, J., O'Donoghue, G. M., & Archbold, S. M. (2005). Long-term functional outcomes and academic-occupational status in implanted children after 10 to 14 years of cochlear implant use. *Otology & Neurotology, 26*, 1152–1160.

Bench, J., Doyle, J., & Greenwood, K. M. (1987) A standardization of the BKB/A Sentence Test for children in comparison with the NAL-CID Sentence Test and CAL-PBM Word Test. *Australian Journal of Audiology, 9*, 39–48.

Bergeson, T. R., Pisoni, D. B., & Davis, R. A. O. (2005). Development of audiovisual comprehension skills in prelingually deaf children with cochlear implants. *Ear and Hearing, 26*, 149–164.

Berliner, K. I., Tonokawa, L. L., Brown, C. J., & Dye, L. M. (1988) Cochlear implants in children: Benefits and concerns. *American Journal of Otology, 9*(Suppl.), 86–92.

Bhasin, T. K., Brocksen, S., Avchen, R. N., & Braun, K. V. N. (2006). *Prevalence of four developmental disabilities among children aged 8 years—Metropolitan Atlanta Developmental Disabilities Surveillance Program, 1996 and 2000.* MMWR Surveillance Summaries, 55(SS01), 1–9. Retrieved January 6, 2008, from: http://www.cdc.gov/mmwR/preview/mmwr html/ss5501a1.htm

Birnholtz, J., & Benacerraf, B. (1983). The development of human fetal hearing. *Science, 222*, 516–518.

Blamey, P. J., Barry, J., Bow, C., Sarant, J., Paatsch, L., & Wales, R., (2001a). The development of speech production following cochlear implantation. *Clinical Linguisitcs and Phonetics, 15*, 363–382.

Blamey, P. J., Sarant, J. Z., Paatsch, L. E., Barry, J. G., Bow, C. P. & Wales, R. J., . . . Tooher, R. (2001b). Relationships among speech perception, production. language, hearing loss and age in children with impaired hearing. *Journal of Speech, Language, and Hearing Research*, *44*, 264–285.

Boothroyd, A. (1978). Speech perception and sensorineural hearing loss. In M. Ross & T. G. Giolas (Eds.), *Auditory management of hearing-impaired children; Principles and prerequisites for intervention* (pp. 117–144). Baltimore, MD: University Park Press.

Boothroyd, A. (1984). Auditory perception of speech contrasts by subjects with sensorineural hearing loss. *Journal of Speech and Hearing Research*, *27*, 134–144.

Boothroyd, A. (1985a). Auditory capacity and the generalization of speech skills. In J. Lauter (Ed.), *Speech planning and production in normal and hearing-impaired children. ASHA Reports 1985*, *15*, 8–14.

Boothroyd, A. (1985b). Evaluation of speech production in the hearing-impaired: Some benefits of forced-choice testing. *Journal of Speech and Hearing Research*, *28*, 185–196.

Boothroyd, A., & Boothroyd-Turner, D. (2002). Post-implantation audition and educational attainment in children with pre-lingually acquired profound deafness. *Annals of Otology, Rhinology, & Laryngology*, *111*, 79–84.

Boothroyd, A., & Cawkwell, S. (1970). Vibrotactile thresholds in pure-tone audiometry. *Acta Otolaryngologica*, *69*, 384–387.

Boothroyd, A., Eisenberg, L. S., & Martinez, A. S. (2010). An On-Line Imitative Test of Speech Pattern Contrast Perception (OLIMSPAC): Developmental effects in normally hearing children. *Journal of Speech, Language, and Hearing Research*, *53*, 531–542.

Boothroyd, A., Geers, A. E., & Moog, J. S. (1991). Practical implications of cochlear implants in children. *Ear and Hearing*, *12*(Suppl.), 81S–89S.

Carney, A. E. (1996). Audition and the development of oral communication competency. In F. E. Bess, J. S. Gravel, & A. M. Tharpe (Eds.), *Amplification for children with auditory deficits* (pp. 29–53). Nashville, TN: Bill Wilkerson Press.

Carney, A. E., Osberger, M. J., Carney, E., Robbins, A. M. Renshaw, J. J., & Miyamoto, R. T. (1993). A comparison of speech discrimination with cochlear implants and tactile aids. *Journal of the Acoustical Society of America*, *94*, 2036–2049.

Centers for Disease Control [CDC]. (2006). *Frequently asked questions (FAQS) on general information on hearing loss.* Early Hearing Detection & Intervention (EHDI) Program. Retrieved May 7, 2009, from http://www.cdc.gov/ncbddd/ehdi/FAQ/questionsgeneralHL.htm

Ching, T. Y. C., Psarros, C., Hill, M., Dillon, H., & Incerti, P. (2001). Should children who use cochlear implants wear hearing aids in the opposite ear? *Ear and Hearing*, *22*, 365–380.

Ching, T. Y. C., van Wanrooy, E., & Dillon, H. (2007). Binaural-bimodal fitting or bilateral implantation for managing severe to profound deafness: A review. *Trends in Amplification*, *11*, 161–192.

Chute, P. M., Hellman, S. A., Parisier, S. C., & Selesnick, S. H. (1990). A matched-pairs comparison of single and multichannel cochlear implants in children. *Laryngoscope*, *100*(1), 25–28.

Colletti, V., Carner, M., Miorelli, V., Guida, M., Colletti, L., & Fiorino, F. G. (2005). Cochlear implantation at under 12 months: Report on 10 patients. *Laryngoscope*, *115*, 445–449.

Cornelisse, L. E., Gagné, J-P., & Seewald, R. C. (1991). Ear level recordings of the long-term average spectrum of speech. *Ear and Hearing*, *12*, 47–54.

Cramer, K. D., & Erber, N. P. 1974). A spondee recognition test for young hearing-impaired children. *Journal of Speech and Hearing Disorders*, *39*(3), 304–311.

Crandell, C. C. (1993). Speech recognition in noise by children with minimal degrees of sensorineural hearing loss. *Ear and Hearing*, *14*, 210–216.

Davis, B. L., Morrison, H. M., Von Hapsberg, D., & Warner-Czyz, A. (2005). Early vocal patterns in infants with varied hearing levels. *Volta Review*, *105*, 7–27.

Davis, H. (1960). Miltiary standards and medicolegal rules. In H. Davis & S. R. Silverman (Eds.), *Hearing and deafness* (pp. 242–246). New York, NY: Holt, Rinehart, & Winston.

Davis, J. M., Elfenbein, J., Schum, R., & Bentler, R. (1986). Effects of mild and moderate hearing impairments on language, educational, and psychosocial behavior of children. *Journal of Speech and Hearing Disorders*, *51*, 53–62.

de Boysson-Bardies, B., & Vihman, M. M. (1991). Adaption to language: Evidence from babbling and first words in four languages. *Language*, *67*, 297–319.

DeCasper, A. J., & Fifer, W. P. (1980). Of human bonding: Newborns prefer their mothers' voices. *Science*, *208*, 1174–1176.

DeCasper, A. J., & Spence, M. J. (1986). Prenatal maternal speech influences newborns' perception of speech sounds. *Infant Behavior and Development*, *9*, 133–150.

Dettman S. J., D'Costa, W. A., Dowell, R. C., Winton, E. J., Hill, K. L., & Williams, S. S. (2004). Cochlear implants in children with significant residual hearing. *Archives of Otolaryngology-Head and Neck Surgery*, *130*, 612–618.

Eilers, R. E., & Oller, D. K. (1994). Infant vocalizations and the early diagnosis of severe hearing impairment. *Journal of Pediatrics*, *12*, 199–203.

Eimas, P. D. (1974). Auditory and linguistic processing of cues for place of articulation by infants. *Perception & Psychophysics*, *16*, 513–521.

Eimas, P. D., & Miller, J. L. (1980). Contextual effects in infant speech perception. *Science*, *209*, 1140–1141.

Eimas, P. D., Siqueland, E. R., Jusczyk, P., & Vigorito, J. (1971). Speech perception in infants. *Science*, *171*, 303–306.

Eisenberg, L. S., Berliner, K. I., Thielemeir, M. A., Kirk, K. I., & Tiber, N. (1983). Cochlear implants in children. *Ear and Hearing*, *4*, 41–50.

Eisenberg, L. S., Boothroyd, A., & Martinez, A. S. (2007). Assessing auditory capabilities in young children. *International Journal of Pediatric Otorhinolaryngology*, *71*, 1339–1350.

Eisenberg, L. S., Kirk, K. I., Martinez, A. S., Ying, E. A., & Miyamoto, R. T. (2004). Communication abilities of children with aided residual hearing: Comparison with cochlear implant users. *Archives of Otolaryngology-Head and Neck Surgery*, *130*, 563–569.

Eisenberg, L. S., Martinez, A. S., & Boothroyd, A. (2003). Auditory-visual and auditory-only perception of phonetic contrasts in children. *Volta Review*, *103*, 327–346.

Eisenberg, L. S., Shannon, R. V., Martinez, A. S., Wygonski, J., & Boothroyd, A. (2000). Speech recognition with reduced spectral cues as a function of age. *Journal of the Acoustical Society of America*, *107*, 2704–2710.

Elfenbein, J. L., Hardin-Jones, M. A., & Davis, J. M. (1994). Oral communication skills of children who are hard of hearing. *Journal of Speech and Hearing Research*, *37*, 216–226.

Elliot, L. L. (1979). Performance of children aged 9 to 17 years on a test of speech intelligibility in noise using sentence material with controlled word predictability. *Journal of the Acoustical Society of America*, *66*, 651–653.

Elliot, L. L., & Katz, D. R. (1980). *Northwestern University Children's Perception of Speech (NU-CHIPS): Technical manual.* St. Louis, MO: Auditec of St. Louis.

Erber, N. P. (1971). Auditory and audiovisual reception of words in low-frequency noise by children with normal hearing and by children with impaired hearing. *Journal of Speech and Hearing Research*, *14*, 496–512.

Erber, N. P. (1972). Auditory, visual, and auditory-visual recognition of consonants by children with normal and impaired hearing. *Journal of Speech and Hearing Research*, *15*, 413–422.

Erber, N. P. (1979). Speech perception by profoundly hearing-impaired children. *Journal of Speech and Hearing Disorders*, *44*, 255–270.

Erber, N. P., & Alencewicz, C. M. (1976). Audiologic evaluation of deaf children. *Journal of Speech and Hearing Disorders*, *41*, 256–267.

Ertmer, D. J., & Mellon, J. A. (2001). Beginning to talk at 20 months: Early vocal development in a young cochlear implant recipient. *Journal of Speech, Language and Hearing Research*, *44*, 192–206.

Ertmer, D. J., Young, N., & Nathani, S. (2007). Profiles of vocal development in young cochlear implant recipients. *Journal of Speech, Language, and Hearing Research*, *50*, 393–407.

Fallon, M., Trehub, S. E., & Schneider, B. A. (2000). Children's perception of speech in multi-talker babble. *Journal of the Acoustical Society of America*, *108*, 3023–3029.

Finitzo-Hieber, T., & Tillman, T.W. (1978). Room acoustics effects on monosyllabic word discrimination ability for normal and hearing-impaired children. *Journal of Speech and Hearing Research*, *21*, 440–456.

Fortnum, H., & Davis, A. (1997). Epidemiology of permanent hearing loss in Trent Region, 1985–1993. *British Journal of Audiology*, *31*, 409–446.

Fortnum, H. M., Summerfield, Q., Marshall, D. H., Davis, A. C., & Bamford, J. M. (2001). Prevalence of permanent childhood hearing impairment in the United Kingdom and implications for universal neonatal hearing screening: Questionnaire based ascertainment study. *British Medical Journal*, *323*, 536–540.

Fryauf-Bertschy, H., Tyler, R. S., Kelsay, D. M. T., Gantz, B. J., & Woodworth, G. G. (1997). Cochlear implant use by prelingually deafened children: The influence of age at implant and length of device use. *Journal of Speech, Language, and Hearing Research*, *40*, 183–199.

Gantz, B. J., Rubinstein, J. T., Tyler, R. S., Teagle, H. F. B., Cohen, N. L., Waltzman, S. B., Miyamoto, R. T., & Kirk, K. I. (2000). Long-term results of cochlear implants in children with residual hearing. *Annals of Otology, Rhinology, & Laryngology*, *109*(Suppl. 185), 33–36.

Geers, A., & Brenner, C. (1994). Speech perception results: Auditory and lipreading enhancement. *Volta Review*, *5*, 97–108.

Geers, A., Brenner, C., & Davidson, L. (2003). Factors associated with development of speech perception skills in children implanted by age five. *Ear and Hearing*, *24*, 24S-35S.

Geers A., E., & Moog, J. S. (1994). Description of the CID sensory aids study. *Volta Review*, *5*, 1–11.

Gelnett, D., Sumida, A., Nilsson, M., & Soli, S. D. (1995). *Development of the Hearing in Noise Test for Children (HINT-C).* Presented at the Annual Meeting of the American Academy of Audiology, Dallas, TX.

Gillis, S., Schauwers, K., & Govaerts, P. J. (2002). Babbling milestones and beyond: Early speech development in CI children. In K. Schauwers, P. J Govaerts, & S. Gillis (Eds.), *Language acquisition in very young children with a cochlear implant* (pp. 23–39). Antwerp Papers in Linguistics (102). Retrieved July 9, 2009, from http://webh01.ua.ac.be/apil/apil102/apil102.pdf

Gordon-Brannan, M. (1994). Assessing intelligibility: Children's expressive phonologies. *Topics in Language Disorders*, *14*, 17–25.

Gordon, T. G. (1987). Communication skills of mainstreamed hearing-impaired children. In H. Levitt, N. C. McGarr, & D. Geffner (Eds.), *Development of language and communication skills in hearing-impaired children, ASHA Monographs Number 26* (pp. 108–122). Rockville, MD: American Speech-Language-Hearing Association.

Gravel, J. S., Fausel, N., Liskow, C., & Chobot, J. (1999). Children's speech recognition in noise using omni-directional and dual-microphone hearing aid technology. *Ear and Hearing*, *20*, 1–11.

Hack, Z. C., & Erber, N. P. (1982). Auditory, visual, and auditory-visual perception of vowels by hearing-impaired children. *Journal of Speech and Hearing Research*, *25*, 100–107.

Hall, J. W., Grose, J. H., Buss, E., & Dev, M. (2002). Spondee recognition in a two-talker masker and a speech-shaped noise masker in adults and children. *Ear and Hearing*, *23*, 159–165.

Harrison, M., & Roush, J. (1996). Age of suspicion, identification and intervention for infants and young children with hearing loss: A national study. *Ear and Hearing*, *17*, 55–62.

Haskins, H. (1949). *A phonologically balanced test of speech discrimination for children.* Unpublished master's thesis, Evanston, IL: Northwestern University.

Hicks, C. B., & Tharpe, A. M. (2002). Listening effort and fatigue in school-age children with and without hearing loss. *Journal of Speech, Language, and Hearing Research, 45*, 573–584.

Holt, R., Kirk, K. I., Eisenberg, L. S., Martinez, A. S., & Campbell, W. (2005). Spoken word recognition development in children with residual hearing aids using cochlear implants and hearing aids in opposite ears. *Ear and Hearing, 26*(4 Suppl.), 82S-91S.

Houston, D. (2002). What infants learn about native language sounds organization during their first year, and what may happen if they don't. In K. Schauwers, P. J Govaerts, & S. Gillis (Eds.), *Language acquisition in very young children with a cochlear implant. Antwerp Papers in Linguistics (102).* Retrieved July 9, 2009, from http://webh01.ua.ac.be/apil/apil102/apil102.pdf

Houston, D. M., Pisoni, D. B., Kirk, K. I., Ying, E. A., & Miyamoto, R. T. (2003). Speech perception skills of deaf infants following cochlear implantation: A first report. *International Journal of Pediatric Otorhinolaryngology, 67*, 479–495.

Jensema, C., Karchmer, M., & Trybus, R. (1978). *The rated speech intelligibility of hearing-impaired children: Basic relationships and a detailed analysis* (Series R, No. 6). Washington, DC: Gallaudet College, Office of Demographic Studies.

Jerger, S., Lewis, S., Hawkins, J., & Jerger, J. (1980). Pediatric Speech Intelligibility Test. I. Generation of test materials. *International Journal of Pediatric Otorhinolaryngology, 2*, 217–230.

Johnson, C. E. (2000). Children's phoneme identification in reverberation and noise. *Journal of Speech, Language and Hearing Research, 43*, 144–157.

Juscyzk, P. W., Cutler, A. & Redanz, N. (1993). Preferences for the predominant stress patterns of English words. *Child Development, 64*, 675–687.

Juscyzk, P. W., Friederici, A. D., Wessles, J., Svenkerud, V. Y., & Juscyzk, A. M. (1993). Infants' sensitivity to sound patterns of native language words. *Journal of Memory and Language, 32*, 402–420.

Jusczyk, P. W., & Luce, P. A. (2002). Speech perception and spoken word recognition - Past and present. *Ear and Hearing, 23*, 2–40.

Juszyck, P. W., Pisoni, D. B., & Mullennix, J. (1992). Some consequences of stimulus variability on speech processing by 2–month old infants. *Cognition, 43*, 253–291.

Kennedy, C. R., McCann, D. M., Campbell, M. J., Law, C. M., Mullee, M., Petrou, S., . . . Stevenson, J. (2006). Language ability after early detection of permanent childhood hearing impairment. *New England Journal of Medicine, 354*(20), 2131–2141.

Kent, R. D. (2004). Development, pathology and remediation of speech. In J. Slifka, S. Manuel, & M. Matthies (Eds.), *From sound to sense: 50+ years of discoveries in speech.* Conference Proceedings. Cambridge, MA: Massachusetts Institute of Technology.

Kent, R. D., & Bauer, H. (1985). Vocalizations of one-year olds. *Journal of Child Language, 12*, 491–526.

Kent, R. D., & Murray, A. D. (1982) Acoustic features of infant vocalic utterances at 3, 6 and 9 months. *Journal of the Acoustical Society of America, 72*, 353–365.

Kent, R. D., Osberger, M. J., Netsell, R., & Hustedde, C G. (1987). Phonetic development in identical twins differing in auditory function. *Journal of Speech and Hearing Disorders, 52*, 64–75.

Kirk, K. I., French, B. F., & Choi, S. (2009). Assessing spoken word recognition in children with cochlear implants. In L. S. Eisenberg (Ed.), *Clinical management of children with cochlear implants* (pp. 217–250). San Diego, CA: Plural.

Kirk, K. I., Hay-McCutcheon, M. J., Holt, R. F., Gao, S., Qi, R., & Gerlain, B. L. (2007). Audiovisual spoken word recognition by children with cochlear implants. *Audiological Medicine, 5*, 250–261.

Kirk, K. I., Pisoni, D. B., & Osberger, M. (1995). Lexical effects on spoken word recognition by pediatric cochlear implant users. *Ear and Hearing, 16*, 470–481.

Koopmans-van Beinum, F. J., Clement, C. J., & van den Dikkenberg-Pot, I. (2001). Babbling and the lack of auditory speech perception: A matter of coordination? *Developmental Science, 4*, 61–70.

Kuhl, P. K. (1983). Perception of auditory equivalence classes for speech in early infancy. *Infant Behavior and Development, 6*, 263–285.

Kuhl, P. K., & Meltzoff, A. N. (1982). The bimodal perception of speech in infancy. *Science, 218*, 1138–1141.

Kuhl, P. K., & Meltzoff, A. N. (1996). Infant vocalizations in responses to speech: Vocal imitation and developmental change. *Journal of the Acoustical Society of America, 100*, 2425–2438.

Kuhl, P. K., & Miller, J. D. (1975). Speech perception in early infancy: Discrimination of speech-sound categories. *Journal of the Acoustical Society of America, 58*(Suppl. 1), S56.

Lachs, L., Pisoni, D. B., & Kirk, K. I. (2001). Use of audiovisual information in speech perception by prelingually deaf children with cochlear implants: A first report. *Ear and Hearing, 22*, 236–251.

Lecanuet, J.-P., & Schaal, B. (1996). Fetal sensory competencies. *European Journal of Obstetrics & Gynecology and Reproductive Biology, 68*, 1–23.

Levitt, A., Jusczyk, P. W., Murray, J., & Carden, G. (1988). Context effects in two-month-old infants' perception of labiodental/interdental fricative contrasts. *Journal of Experimental Psychology: Human Perception and Performance, 14*(3), 361–368.

Ling, D., & Milne, M. (1981). The development of speech in hearing-impaired children. In F. H. Bess, B. A. Freeman, & J. S. Sinclair (Eds.), *Amplification in education* (pp. 99–108). Washington, DC: Alexander Graham Bell Association for the Deaf.

Litovsky, R. Y., Johnstone, P.M., & Godar, S. P. (2006a). Benefits of bilateral cochlear implants and/or hearing aids in children. *International Journal of Audiology, 45*(Suppl. 1), 78–91.

Litovsky, R. Y., Johnstone, P. M., Godar, S., Agrawal, S., Parkinson, A., Peters, R., & Lake, J. (2006b). Bilateral cochlear implants in children: Localization acuity measured with minimum audible angle. *Ear and Hearing, 27*, 43–59.

Litovsky, R. Y., Parkinson, A., Arcaroli, J., Peters, R., Lake, J., Johnstone, P., & Yu, G. (2004). Bilateral cochlear implants in adults and children. *Archives of Otolaryngology-Head and Neck Surgery, 130*, 648–655.

Luxford, W. M., Eisenberg, L. S., Johnson, K.C., & Mahnke, E. (2004). Cochlear implantation in infants younger than 12 months. In R. Miyamoto (Ed.), *Proceedings of the 8th international cochlear implant conference. International Congress Series, Vol. 1273* (pp. 376–379). The Netherlands: Elsevier.

MacAndie, C., Kubba, H., & MacFarlane, M. (2003). Epidemiology of permanent childhood hearing loss in Glasgow, 1985–1994. *Scottish Medical Journal, 48*, 117–119.

Mampe, B., Friederici, A. D., Christophe, A., & Wermke, K. (2009). Newborns' cry melody is shaped by their native language. *Current Biology, 19*, 1994–1997.

Markides, A. (1970). The speech of deaf and partially-hearing children with special reference to factors affecting intelligibility. *British Journal of Disorders of Communication, 5*, 126–140.

Martinez, A., Eisenberg, L., Visser-Dumont, L., & Boothroyd, A. (2007). Assessing speech pattern contrast perception in infants: Early results on VRASPAC. *Otology & Neurotology, 29*, 183–180.

Mayne, A. M., Yoshinaga-Itano, C., & Sedey, A. L. (2000a). Receptive vocabulary development of infants and toddlers who are deaf or hard of hearing. *Volta Review, 100*, 29–52.

Mayne, A. M., Yoshinaga-Itano, C., Sedey, A. L., & Carey, A. (2000b). Expressive vocabulary development of infants and toddlers who are deaf or hard of hearing. *Volta Review, 100*, 1–28.

McDermott, R., & Jones, T. (1984). Articulation characteristics and listeners' judgments of the speech of children with severe hearing loss. *Language, Speech, and Hearing Services in Schools, 15*, 110–126.

Mehler, J., Jusczyk, P., Lambertz, G., Halsted, N., Bertoncini, J., & Amiel-Tison, C. (1988). A precursor of language acquisition in young infants. *Cognition, 29*, 143–178.

Meyer, T. A., Svirsky, M. A., Kirk, K. I., & Miyamoto, R. T. (1998). Improvements in speech perception by children with profound prelingual hearing loss: Effects of device, communication mode, and chronological age. *Journal of Speech, Language, and Hearing Research, 41*, 846–858.

Miller, J. L., & Eimas, P. D. (1983). Studies on the categorization of speech by infants. *Cognition, 13*, 135–165.

Miyamoto, R., T., Osberger, M. J., Robbins, A. M., Myers, W. A., Kessler, K., & Pope, M. L. (1991). Comparison of speech perception abilities in deaf children with hearing aids or cochlear implants. *Otolaryngology-Head and Neck Surgery, 104*, 42–46.

Miyamoto, R. T., Osberger, M. J., Robbins, A. M., Myers, W. A., Kessler, K., & Pope, M. L. (1992). Longitudinal evaluation of communication skills of children with single- or multichannel cochlear implants. *American Journal of Otology, 13*, 215–222.

Moeller, M. P. (2000). Early intervention and language development in children who are deaf and hard of hearing. *Pediatrics, 106*(3), 1–9.

Moeller, M. P., & Carney, A. E. (1993). Assessment and intervention with preschool hearing impaired children. In J. Alpiner & P. McCarthy (Eds.), *Rehabilitative audiology children and adults* (2nd ed., pp. 106–135). Baltimore, MD: Williams & Wilkins.

Moeller, M. P., Hoover, B., Putman, C., Arbataitis, K., Bohnenkamp, G., Peterson, B., . . . Stelmachowicz, P. (2007a). Vocalizations of infants with hearing loss compared with infants with normal hearing: Part I—Phonetic development. *Ear and Hearing, 28*, 605–627.

Moeller, M. P., Hoover, B., Putman, C., Arbataitis, K., Bohnenkamp, G., Peterson, B., . . . Stelmachowicz, P. (2007b). Vocalizations of infants with hearing loss compared with infants with normal hearing: Part II—Transition to words. *Ear and Hearing, 28*, 628–642.

Monson, R. B. (1978). Toward measuring how well hearing-impaired children speak. *Journal of Speech and Hearing Research, 21*, 197–219.

Moog, J. S., & Geers, A. E. (1990). *Early speech perception test for profoundly hearing-impaired children*. St. Louis, MO: Central Institute for the Deaf.

Moon, C., Cooper, R. P., & Fifer, W. P. (1993). Two-day-olds prefer their native language. *Infant Behavior and Development, 16*, 495–500.

Moon, C. M., & Fifer, W. P. (2000). The fetus: Evidence of transnatal auditory learning. *Journal of Perinatology, 20*(8 Pt. 2), S37–S44.

Moore, B. C. J. (1996). Perceptual consequences of cochlear hearing loss and their implications for the design of hearing aids. *Ear and Hearing, 17*, 133–161.

Moore, B. C. J. (2008). Basic auditory processes involved in the analysis of speech sounds. *Philosophical Transactions of the Royal Society B. 363*, 947–963.

Moore, J. A., & Bass-Ringdahl, S. (2002). Role of infant vocal development in candidacy for and efficacy of cochlear implantation. *Annals of Otology, Rhinology, & Laryngology, 111*, 52–55.

Moore, J. K., & Linthicum, F. H. (2007). The human auditory system: A timeline of development. *International Journal of Audiology, 46*, 460–478

Morse, P. (1972). The discrimination of speech and non-speech stimuli in early infancy. *Journal of Experimental Child Psychology, 14*, 477–492.

National Institute on Deafness and Other Communication Disorders (NICDC). (2006). *NIDCD Outcomes research in children with hearing loss*. December 12 and 13, 2006, Bethesda, Maryland. Retrieved May 7, 2009, from http://www.nidcd.nih.gov/funding/programs/hb/outcomes/report.htm

Nelson, H. D., Bougatsos, C., & Nygren, P. (2008). Universal newborn hearing screening: Systematic review to update the 2001 U.S. Preventative Services Task Force recommendations. *Pediatrics, 116*, 205–209.

Neuman, A. C., & Hochberg, I. (1983). Children's perception of speech in reverberation. *Journal of the Acoustical Society of America, 73*, 2145–2149.

Nott, P., Cowan, R., Brown, M., & Wigglesworth, G. (2009). Early language development in children with profound hearing loss fitted with a device at a young age. Part I—The time taken to acquire first words and first word combinations. *Ear and Hearing, 30*(5), 526–540.

Nozza, R. J., Rossman, R. N. F., Bond, L. C., & Miller, S. L. (1990). Infant speech-sound discrimination in noise. *Journal of the Acoustical Society of America*, *87*, 339–350.

Nozza, R. J., Wagner, E. F., & Crandall, M. A. (1988). Binaural release from masking for a speech sound in infants, preschool children and adults. *Journal of Speech and Hearing Research*, *31*, 212–218.

Oller, D. K. (1980). The emergence of the sounds of speech in infancy. In G. H. Yeni-Kromshian, J. F. Kavanaugh, & C. A. Ferguson (Eds.), *Child phonology, Vol. 1: Production* (pp. 93–112). New York, NY: Academic Press.

Oller, D. K., & Eilers, R. E. (1988). The role of audition in infant babbling. *Child Development*, *59*, 441–449.

Oller, D. K., Eilers, R. E. Bull, D. H., & Carney, A. E. (1985). Prespeech vocalizations of a deaf infant: Comparison with normal meta-phonological development. *Journal of Speech and Hearing Research*, *28*, 47–63.

Oller, D. K., Wieman, L. A., Doyle, W., & Ross, C. (1975). Infant babbling and speech. *Journal of Child Language*, *3*, 1–11.

Osberger, M. J., Miyamoto, R. T., Zimmermen-Phillips, S., Kemink, J., Stroer, B. S., Firszt, J., & Novak, M. (1991a). Independent evaluation of the speech perception abilities of children with the Nucleus 22–channel cochlear implant system. *Ear and Hearing*, *12*(Suppl.), 66–80.

Osberger, M. J., Robbins, A. M., Miyamoto, R. T., Berry, S. W., Myers, W. A., Kessler, K., & Pope, M. L. (1991b). Speech perception abilities of children with cochlear implants, tactile aids, or hearing aids. *American Journal of Otology*, *12*(Suppl.), 105–115.

Osberger, M. J., Robbins, A. M., Todd, S. L., Riley, A. I., Kirk, K. I., & Carney, A. E. (1996). Cochlear implants and tactile aids for children with profound hearing impairment. In F. E. Bess, J. S. Gravel, & A. M. Tharpe (Eds.), *Amplification for children with auditory deficits* (pp. 283–308). Nashville, TN: Bill Wilkerson Press.

Patterson, M. L., & Werker, J. F. (1999). Two-month old infants match phonetic information in lips and voice. *Developmental Science*, *6*, 191–196.

Peterson, G. E., & Lehiste, I. (1962). Revised CNC lists for auditory tests. *Journal of Speech and Hearing Disorders*, *27*, 62–70.

Pisoni, D. (2000). Cognitive factors and cochlear implants: Some thoughts on perception, learning, and memory in speech perception. *Ear and Hearing*, *21*, 70–78.

Pittman, A. L., Stelmachowicz, P. G., Lewis, D. E., & Hoover, B. M. (2003). Spectral characteristics of speech at the ear: Implications for amplification in children. *Journal of Speech, Language and Hearing Research*, *46*, 649–657.

Prieve B. A., & Stevens, F. (2000). The New York State universal newborn hearing screening demonstration project: Introduction and overview. *Ear and Hearing*, *21*, 85–91.

Querleu, D., Renard, X., Versyp, F., Paris-Delrue, L., & Crepin, G. (1988). Fetal hearing. *European Journal of Obstetrics, Gynecology and Reproductive Biology*, *28*, 191–212.

Robbins, A. M., Osberger, M. J., Miyamoto, R. T., Renshaw, J. J., & Carney, A. E. (1988). Longitudinal study of speech perception by children with cochlear implants and tactile aids: Progress report. *Journal of the Academy of Rehabilitative Audiology*, *21*, 11–28.

Robbins, A. M., Renshaw, J. J., Miyamoto, R. T., Osberger, M. J., & Pope, M. L. (1988) *Minimal pairs test*. Indianapolis, IN: Indiana University School of Medicine.

Ross, M., & Lerman, J. (1970). A picture identification test for hearing impaired children. *Journal of Speech and Hearing Research*, *13*, 44–53.

Schorr, E. A., Fox, N. A., van Wassenhove, V., & Knudsen, E. I. (2005). Auditory-visual fusion in speech perception in children with cochlear implants. *Proceedings of the National Academy of Sciences*, *102*, 18748–18750.

Seewald, R. C., Ross, M., & Giolas, T. G. (1985). Primary modality for speech perception in children with normal and impaired hearing. *Journal of Speech, Language, and Hearing Research*, *28*, 36–46.

Sininger, Y. S., Martinez, A. S., Eisenberg, L. E., Christensen, E., Grimes, A., & Hu, J. (2009). Newborn hearing screening speeds diagnosis and access to intervention by 20–25 months. *Journal of the American Academy of Audiology*, *20*, 49–57.

Smit, A. B., Hand, L., Freilinger, J. J., Bernthal, J. E., & Bird, A. (1990). The Iowa Articulation Norms Project and its Nebraska replication. *Journal of Speech and Hearing Disorders*, *55*, 779–789.

Smith, C. R. (1975). Residual hearing and speech production in deaf children. *Journal of Speech and Hearing Research*, *18*, 795–811.

Snik, A. F. M., Verneulen, A. M., Brokx, J. P. L., Beijk, C., & van der Broek, P. (1997). Speech perception performance of children with a cochlear implant compared to that of children with conventional hearing aids. I. The "equivalent hearing loss" concept. *Acta Otolarygologica (Stockh)*, *117*, 750–754.

Stark, R. E. (1980). Stages of speech development in the first year of life. In G. H. Yeni-Kromshian, J. F. Kavanaugh, & C. A. Ferguson (Eds.), *Child phonology, Vol. 1: Production* (pp. 73–92). New York, NY: Academic Press.

Starr, A., Amlie, R., Martin, W., & Sanders, S. (1977). Development of auditory function in newborn infants revealed by auditory brainstem potentials. *Pediatrics*, *60*, 831– 839.

Stelmachowicz, P. G., Pittman, A. L., Hoover, B. M., & Lewis, D. E. (2001). Effect of stimulus bandwidth on the perception of /s/ in normal- and hearing-impaired children and adults. *Journal of the Acoustical Society of America*, *110*, 2183–2190.

Stelmachowicz, P. G., Pittman, A. L., Hoover, B. M., & Lewis, D. E. (2002). Aided perception of /s/ and /z/ by hearing impaired children. *Ear and Hearing*, *23*, 316–324.

Stoel-Gammon, C. (1983). The acquisition of segmental phonology by normal and hearing-impaired children (pp. 267–280). In I. Hochberg, H. Levitt, & M. J. Osberger (Eds.), *Speech of the hearing impaired: Research, training, and personnel preparation*. Baltimore, MD: University Park Press.

Stoel-Gammon, C. (1985). Phonetic inventories: 15 to 24 months: A longitudinal study. *Journal of Speech and Hearing Research*, *28*, 505–512.

Stoel-Gammon, C. (1988). Prelinguistic vocalizations of hearing-impaired and normally hearing subjects: A comparison of consonantal inventories. *Journal of Speech and Hearing Disorders, 53*, 505–512.

Stoel-Gammon, C., & Otomo, K. (1986). Babbling development of hearing-impaired and normally hearing subjects. *Journal of Speech and Hearing Disorders, 51*, 33–41.

Sumby, W. H., & Pollack, I. (1954). Visual contributions to speech intelligibility in noise. *Journal of the Acoustical Society of America, 26*, 212–215.

Svirsky, M. A., Chin, S. B., Miyamoto, R. T., Sloan, R. B., & Caldwell, M. D. (2002). Speech intelligibility of profoundly deaf pediatric hearing aid users. *Volta Review, 102*, 175–198.

Svirsky, M. A., & Meyer, T. A. (1999). Comparison of speech perception in pediatric Clarion cochlear implant and hearing aid users. *Annals of Otology, Rhinology, & Laryngology, 108*, 104–109.

Thielemeir, M. A., Brimacombe, J. A., & Eisenberg, L. S. (1982). Audiological results with the cochlear implant. *Annals of Otology, Rhinology, & Laryngology, 91*(Suppl.) 27–34.

Thielemeir, M. A., Tonokawa, L. L., Petersen, B., & Eisenberg, L. S. (1985). Audiological results in children with a cochlear implant. *Ear and Hearing, 6*(Suppl.), 27S–35S.

Thompson, D. C., McPhillips, H., Davis, R. L., Lieu, T. A., Homer, C. J., & Helfand, M. (2001). Universal newborn hearing screening: Summary of evidence. *Journal of the American Medical Association, 286*, 2000–2010.

Tillberg, I., Ronnberg, J., Svard, I., & Ahlner, B. (1996). Audiovisual speech reading in a group of hearing aid users: The effects of onset age, handicap age and degree of hearing loss. *Scandinavian Audiology, 25*, 267–272.

Tobey, E. A., Geers, A. E., Brenner, C. B., Altuna, D., & Gabbert, G. (2003). Factors associated with development of speech production skills in children implanted by five years of age. *Ear and Hearing, 24*, 36S-45S.

Tomblin, J. B., Peng, S-C., Spencer, L. J., & Lu, N. (2008). Long-term trajectories of the development of speech sound production in pediatric cochlear implants. *Journal of Speech, Language, and Hearing Research, 51*, 1353–1368.

Trehub, S. E. (1973). Infants' sensitivity to vowel and tonal contrasts. *Developmental Psychology, 9*, 91–96.

Trehub, S. E., Bull, D., & Schneider, B. A. (1981). Infants' detection of speech in noise. *Journal of Speech and Hearing Research, 24*, 202–206.

Tyler, R. S., Kelsay, D. M. R., Teagle, H. F. B., Rubenstein, J. T., Gantz, B. J., & Christ, A. M. (2000). 7–year speech perception results and the effects of age, residual hearing, and pre-implant speech perception in prelingually deaf children using the Nucleus and Clarion Cochlear Implants. *Advances in Otorhinolaryngology, 57*, 305–310.

Uziel, A. S., Sillon, M., Vieu, A., Artieres, F., Prion, J-P., Daures, J. P., & Mondain, M. (2007). Ten-year follow-up of a consecutive series of children with multichannel cochlear implants. *Otology & Neurotology, 28*, 615–628.

Van Naarden, K. V., Decoufle, P., & Caldwell, K. (1999). Prevalance and characteristics of children with serious hearing impairment in metropolitan Atlanta, 1991–1993. *Pediatrics, 103*, 570–575.

Vihman, M. M. (1988). Early phonological development. In J. Bernthal & N. Bankson (Eds.), *Articulation and phonological disorders* (2nd ed., pp. 60–109). Baltimore, MD: Williams & Wilkins.

Vihman, M., Ferguson, C. A., & Elbert, M. (1986). Phonological development from babbling to speech: Common tendencies and individual difference. *Applied Psycholinguistics, 7*, 3–40.

von Hapsburg, D., & Davis, B. L. (2006). Auditory sensitivity and the prelinguistic vocalizations of early-amplified infants. *Journal of Speech, Language, and Hearing Research, 49*, 809–822.

Wallace, V., Menn, L., & Yoshinaga-Itano, C. (2000). Is babble the gateway to speech for all children? A longitudinal study of children who are deaf and hard of hearing. *Volta Review, 100*, 121–148.

Watkin, P., McCann, D., Law, C., Mullee, M., Petrou, S., Stevenson, J., . . . Kenney, C. (2007). Language ability in children with permanent hearing impairment: The influence of early management and family participation. *Pediatrics, 120*, e694–e701. Accessed May 7, 2009 from www.pediatrics.org/cgi/content/full/120/3/e694

Werker, J. F., & Lalonde, C. E. (1988). Cross-language speech perception: Initial capabilities and developmental change. *Developmental Psychology, 24*, 672–683.

Werker, J. F., & Tees, R. C. (1984). Cross-language speech perception: Evidence for perceptual reorganization during the first year of life. *Infant Behavior and Development, 7*, 49–63.

Werker, J. F., & Tees, R. C. (1999). Influences on infant speech processing: Toward a new synthesis. *Annual Review of Psychology, 50*, 509–535.

Werner, L. A. (2007). Issues in human auditory development. *Journal of Communication Disorders, 40*, 275–283.

Wessex Universal Hearing Screening Trial Group. (1998). Controlled trial of universal neonatal screening for early identification of permanent childhood hearing impairment. *Lancet, 352*, 1957–1964.

World Health Organization (WHO). (2002). *Grades of hearing impairment*. Retrieved July 7, 2009, from http://www.who.int/pdh/Docs/GRADESTABLE-DEFs.pdf

Yoshinaga-Itano, C., & Sedey, A. (2000). Early speech development in children who are deaf or hard of hearing: Interrelationships with language and hearing. *Volta Review, 100*, 181–211.

Yoshinaga-Itano, C., A. L., Sedey, Coulter, D. K., & Mehl, A. L. (1998). Language of early- and later-identified children with hearing loss. *Pediatrics, 102*, 1161–1171.

Zeiser, M. L., & Erber, N. P. (1977). Auditory/vibratory perception of syllabic structure in words by profoundly hearing-impaired children. *Journal of Speech and Hearing Research, 20*, 430–436.

Zwolan, T. A., Zimmerman-Phillips, S., Ashbaugh, C. J., Hieber, S. J., Kileny, P. R., & Telian, S. A. (1997). Cochlear implantation of children with minimal open-set speech recognition skills. *Ear and Hearing, 18*, 240–251.

13

Auditory Neuropathy/Dys-Synchrony Type Hearing Loss

Gary Rance and Arnold Starr

Introduction

The recent development of objective measures of function of cochlear receptor elements (inner and outer hair cells), auditory nerve and auditory brainstem pathways now allow the opportunity to define the site(s) of disorder at the level of the auditory nerve and inner hair cells (IHCs) responsible for "sensorineural" deafness. Disordered auditory nerve function affects the processing of auditory temporal cues and interferes with language comprehension, localization of the sources of sound, and binaural perceptions (Zeng, Kong, Michalewski, & Starr, 2005). Attention to clinical features such as age of onset, associated medical findings, imaging results, and family history are essential for defining the likely sites of the disorder as being "preneural" (affecting receptor elements and the formation or release of neural transmitters) and "neural" (affecting the function of auditory nerve and its brainstem connections). The nosology of disordered auditory temporal processing include auditory neuropathy (Starr, Picton, Sininger, Hood, & Berlin, 1996) attributable to postsynaptic or presynaptic auditory nerve disorder (Starr et al., 2004), auditory neuropathy/dys-synchrony (AN/AD) (Berlin, Hood, & Rose, 2001), and auditory synaptopathy (Moser et al., 2006). Differentiating the site(s) affected in an individual subject is an area of considerable research interest and remains a clinical challenge. What is clear is that the perceptual effects of this form of auditory disorder in both children and adults are quite different from those typically seen with sensory (cochlear) hearing loss. As up to 10% of children with permanent hearing deficit show the AN/AD result pattern, every pediatric audiologist must be able to identify it in children of all ages and have some insight into their particular management questions. This chapter addresses each of these issues and provides a neurologic overview of auditory inner hair cell, auditory nerve, and auditory central pathway disorders.

Identification of AN/AD

The clinical audiologic findings that suggest the presence of disrupted auditory nerve activity are the demonstration of cochlear (outer hair cell) integrity by cochlear microphonic and/or otoacoustic emission recordings, in conjunction with absence or marked abnormality of the auditory brainstem response (ABR) beyond that expected for the degree of hearing loss. The demonstration of impaired auditory temporal perceptions independent of audibility changes is also a cardinal feature of the disorder but is currently not possible to demonstrate in newborns or infants.

Auditory Brainstem Response

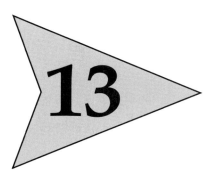

The ABR arises from neural activity occurring in the 10 to 15 ms immediately following an abrupt auditory stimulus (see Chapter 20 for details). In ears with significant peripheral (middle ear or cochlear) hearing loss the threshold for detecting ABRs may be elevated or the response absent because the stimuli are not sufficiently intense to elicit the chain reaction of neural activity in the auditory brainstem. In contrast, subjects with AN/AD show absent or severely distorted ABRs at maximum presentation levels, not because the stimuli are insufficient to generate a response, but because the neural activities of auditory nerve and brainstem pathways are disrupted. Establishing ABR abnormality in such cases is relatively straightforward when the brainstem potentials are "absent" (or at least unrecordable). A present but "severely disrupted" response is more problematic, particularly when assessing premature infants who commonly display abnormal ABRs (prolonged latency, reduced amplitude, etc.) based on incomplete myelination of auditory nerve and brainstem structures (Starr, Amlie, Martin, & Sanders, 1977). A commonly used definition (Sininger & Oba, 2001) for ABR abnormality consistent with AN/AD is that the ABR be of low amplitude, prolonged latency and only discernable to high level stimuli (≥ 70 dB nHL). Some of the mechanisms by which the ABR may be disrupted in AN/AD are described in the following sections.

Tests of Cochlear (Outer Hair Cell) Function

Evoked Otoacoustic Emissions (EOAE)

An otoacoustic emission (OAE) is a release of sound energy produced within the cochlea that can be recorded in the ear canal (Kemp, 1978). This signal is thought to be the byproduct of the mechanical activity of the outer hair cells (see Chapter 19 for further details). EOAEs, in providing an indirect measure of this process, offer a means of distinguishing between sensory hearing loss and AN/AD. Ears with absent or significantly elevated ABRs due to sensory hearing loss typically show audiometric thresholds in the severe/profound range. Cochlear insult sufficient to produce a hearing loss of this degree typically disrupts the active mechanisms that produce the OAE resulting in nonresponse (Collet, Levy, & Veuillet, 1993; Lonsbury-Martin, Harris, Stagner, & Hawkins, 1990). EOAE presence in conjunction with significant ABR disruption therefore suggests AN/AD rather than sensory-type hearing loss.

Cochlear Microphonic (CM)

The cochlear microphonic is a receptor potential produced by the polarization and depolarization of cochlear hair cells. The response is preneural and appears as an alternating current potential providing a bioelectric analogue of the stimulus (Dallos & Cheatham, 1976). The potential therefore is unlike those produced by neural activity (such as the ABR), showing a direct phase relationship to the acoustic waveform. This relationship can be seen in Figure 13–1 where the CM reverses polarity as the stimuli are changed from rarefaction to compression clicks.

When recorded from extra-tympanic sites (such as the scalp) the CM is dominated by the activity of the outer hair cells because their numbers are three times the numbers of inner hair cells (Dallos, 1973; Norton, Ferguson, & Mascher, 1989). As such, in the same way as OAE responses, this potential can be used in conjunction with the ABR to identify AN/AD. As discussed previously, sensory hearing loss severe enough to prevent an ABR would be expected to affect cochlear OHC function. Hence, AN/AD is indicated when the CM is present but the ABR is disrupted. The reader is referred to Berlin et al. (1998), Rance et al. (1999), and Starr et al. (1991) for description of clinical CM recording procedures.

Possible Mechanisms Producing the AN/AD Result Pattern

The absence of ABRs in subjects who can clearly "hear" the clicks was disturbing when the phenomenon was first noticed in the 1970s and 1980s. That was the time when ABRs seemed on the verge of providing a means for the long sought goal of having an objective measure of "hearing" and even "threshold." A number of investigators described the paradox (Davis & Hirsh, 1979; Hildesheimer, Muchnik, & Rubinstein, 1985; Kraus, Ozdamar, Stein, & Reed, 1984) but could not realize the mechanisms. One of the authors (AS) saw such a child in 1989 and defined that, in spite of absence of ABRs, the cochlear microphonic receptor potentials were present. Clearly, the disordered function was in the nerve due either to a disorder of the nerve itself, the inner hair cell, or in their synapses. The child's hearing provided a clue to the type of disordered function of the nerve. She had relatively normal pure tone thresholds but impaired perceptions dependent on auditory temporal cues. Thus, both monaural processes of speech discrimination and thresholds for gap detection as well as binaural processes for masking level differences and perception of binaural beats were markedly abnormal. In contrast the difference limens for high (but not low) frequencies and intensity were normal. The child had a disorder of auditory temporal process-

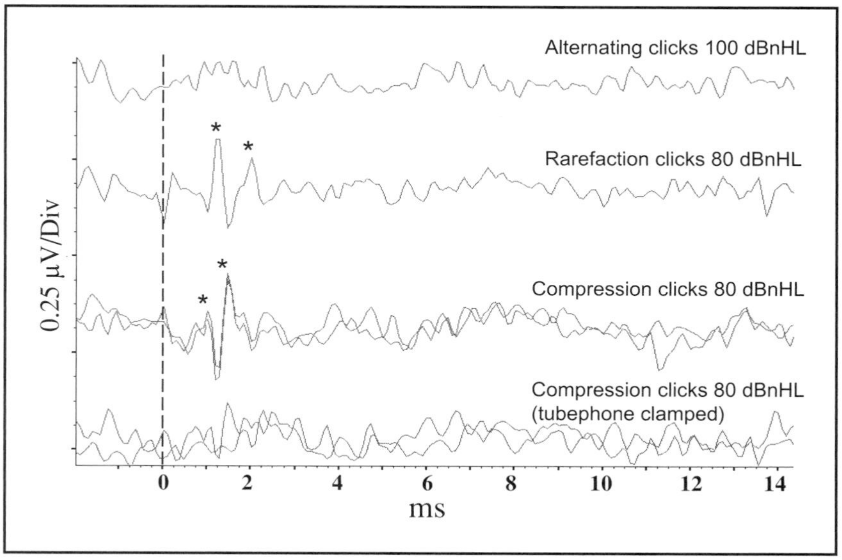

FIGURE 13–1. Averaged EEG tracings for Subject A. The dotted line represents the point of stimulus generation (at the transducer). The top tracing shows no recordable potentials to alternating acoustic clicks presented at 100 dB nHL. The middle tracings show cochlear microphonic responses but absent ABRs to unipolar stimuli at 80 dB nHL. Asterisks denote the positive peaks in the CM waveform. The bottom tracings were obtained to compression clicks presented with the tubephone clamped (no stimulus trials).

ing affecting both evoked potentials and auditory perceptions. Just before publication (Starr et al., 1991) OAEs were demonstrated to be present.

A physiologic model for this phenomenon is that auditory nerve input is not temporally precise to the repetitions of the same stimulus such that an averaged ABR can be absent or severely distorted even though "hearing" the signals may not be affected. The distortion of the temporal processes is reflected in the inability to normally use temporal cues for life's daily perceptions.

The peripheral auditory system encodes temporal cues both at onset of the stimulus and during the stimulus, the latter particularly for low frequencies. The nerve and brainstem tracts discharge at a preferential phase of the low frequency tones and produce a potential at the frequency of the tone recordable by scalp electrodes. These potentials are known as frequency-following responses (FFR) and are absent in AN/AD. A second mechanism that would disrupt ABRs and auditory temporal perceptions would be a loss of the magnitude of the afferent input due to abnormal nerve fibers, abnormal neurotransmitter release, or abnormal synaptic function. Deafferentation can be actual loss of fibers or functional loss due to failure to activate the fibers.

Temporal bone analyses in eight patients with different etiologies of AN/AD have been published. They have all shown loss of nerve fibers, abnormal myelin formation in some of the remaining nerve fibers and preserved inner and outer hair cells. There is need for defining temporal bone in patients or animal models of inner hair cell disorders accompanying, for example, otoferlin gene mutations, which affect neurotransmitter release by inner hair cells. We do not expect that the inner hair cells are lost or have abnormal potentials in this condition. Rather, the defect in neurotransmitter release will likely lead to atrophy and morphologic changes of the nerve terminals, a trans-synaptic degeneration.

The definition of physiologic processes responsible for the clinical picture of AN/AD are difficult to address using auditory brainstem potential measures, since these responses are typically absent and when present consist of a wave V generated by brainstem auditory structures. The registration of cochlear potentials from an electrode passed through the tympanic membrane and placed directly on the bony promontory or round window of the cochlea can reveal neural and cochlear receptor potentials not apparent in the ABR. Both children (McMahon, Patuzzi, Gibson, & Sanli, 2008) and adults (Santarelli, Starr, Michalewski, & Arslan, 2008) have been studied using these electrocochleographic methods (ECochG). Receptor summating potentials generated primarily by inner hair cells and cochlear microphonics generated primarily by outer hair cells appear normal. In contrast, auditory nerve compound action potentials (CAPs) are absent or present with low amplitudes consistent with disordered function of auditory nerve. Abnormally prolonged neural negative potentials are also evident in many AN/AD subjects. This negative potential has been suggested to reflect activity of auditory nerve terminal dendrites accompanying abnormal generation of CAPs, and/or abnormal synaptic function (transmitter release, transmitter binding) between inner hair cells and auditory nerve.

Medical Aspects of AN/AD

Auditory neuropathy/dys-synchrony is most common in the newborn population, particularly the premature population and those who have medical illness. The risk factors for AN/AD include hyperbilirubinemia, hypoxia and accompanying metabolic acidosis, and exposure to antibiotics that are toxic to hair cells. Bilirubin excess occurring alone will be deposited in auditory brainstem and auditory ganglion cells. In such a circumstance, nerve death or dysfunction will result. But the inner hair cells will not be affected.

Genetic causes of AN/AD acting at the inner hair cells and their synapses with the auditory nerve include mutations of connexin 26 and of otoferlin and are expressed early in infancy. A variant of otoferlin mutation can be accompanied by a temperature sensitive deafness (Starr et al., 1998) that is readily treated with Tylenol that reduces body temperature.

Congenital disorders such as atresia of the auditory nerve can produce the picture of AN/AD, and the diagnosis will be established with a high definition MRI (Buchman et al., 2006). When should an MRI be done? We suggest that in all infants correct diagnosis is important for parents and should be separated from therapeutic considerations such as decisions on cochlear implantation.

The etiologies described below occur as part of a general medical disorder, and these patients need to be evaluated by appropriate specialists such as neurologists, pediatricians, radiologists, and otologists. Infectious diseases due to bacterial involvement most commonly affect cochlear functions by involvement of both the auditory nerve and the arterial blood vessels supplying the cochlea. When the nerve is primarily affected the clinical picture is of AN/AD. If the arterial supply is not affected, ABR wave I and CM and OAEs can be defined. When the arterial supply is compromised, both neural and cochlear receptor elements will be affected.

Infectious disorders due to viral involvement can have sequelae of hearing impairment due to auditory nerve involvement. Mumps and measles seem to have this association. The auditory nerve involvement in such cases may be unilateral.

Tumors of the brainstem and auditory vestibular nerve schwannomas can affect auditory nerve function by compression, and if the blood supply is compromised, the ABR will be abnormal (absent or delayed components after a normal wave I with preserved CMs and/or OAEs). Brain imaging and clinical examination will reveal such tumors, and clinical neurological examination will define disorders of cranial nerves such as III, IV, and VI controlling eye movements, VII controlling facial movements, and V controlling facial sensations.

Genetic disorders affecting the auditory nerve as part of more general peripheral and/or cranial nerve involvement is common. The age of onset typically is after 8 years and can include mitochondrial disorders due to both the nuclear genes, such as Friedreich's ataxia and dominant optic atrophy, and mitochondrial genetic disorders, such as Leber's hereditary optic neuropathy.

Immune disorders can be accompanied by deafness typical of AN/AD. The site of the disorder is not known. For instance, deafness is reported in Guillain-Barré syndrome, an immune disorder affecting the proximal nerve roots and the proximal portions of the auditory nerve. Patients may be deaf and paralysed, and yet the prognosis for recovery typically is excellent though lengthy in time.

In summary, AN/AD is a medical disorder affecting the output of the cochleae and their connections in the brainstem. Patients must be evaluated by a clinician skilled in neurology to define the site of affection as being in the central portions of the auditory nerve. Audiologists can be suspicious of central auditory nerve problems when they detect either an absent or severely distorted ABR or a waveform complex associated with normal latency wave I. Wave I is generated by the auditory nerve close to the cochlea and wave II by the auditory nerve close to the brainstem. Waves III, IV, and V are generated by central auditory brainstem structures in the regions of cochlear nucleus (wave III), superior olive and lateral lemniscus (waves IV and V).

Screening for AN/AD

As discussed above, adult and early childhood onset forms of AN/AD can be associated with progressive sensory motor neuropathies such as Friedreich's ataxia. The majority of pediatric AN/AD cases do, however, involve congenital or perinatal presentation (Sininger & Oba, 2001; Starr, Sinninger, & Pratt, 2000), and most diagnoses are made following infant-hearing screening. This raises questions concerning the ways in which universal screening procedures should be configured to capture affected babies. Clearly, programs employing only the OAE technique will miss a high proportion of AN/AD cases as most affected infants show normal emissions.[1] For this reason, the Joint Committee on Infant Hearing (JCIH, 2007) has recommended that ABR be used as the screening measure for NICU babies, arguing that most affected children suffer a rocky neonatal course and hence are graduates of the special care nursery (Rance et al., 1999; Sininger & Oba, 2001).

OAE screening in the well-baby population may be less of an issue, as the incidence of AN/AD in this group is much lower. Furthermore, most babies who have a normal neonatal course and yet still suffer AN/AD will have a genetic cause, so it should be possible to identify those in need of ABR screening on the basis of family history (hearing loss and/or sensory neuropathy). For screening programs employing OAE assessment, Berlin et al. (2005) have also suggested that middle ear muscle reflex (MEMR) testing can identify children in need of referral for ABR assessment (see later section in this chapter for details).

Prevalence

The prevalence of AN/AD in adult, and well-baby populations is yet to be determined. Data describing the proportion of affected children in high-risk populations is also sketchy, and estimates range from 0.23% to 9.63% (Table 13–1). The high variability reflects some methodological differences between studies and raises some important issues regarding the criteria for diagnosis of AN/AD in early infancy. In particular, the age

Table 13–1. Prevalence of Auditory AN/AD in "At-Risk" Infant Populations

Study	Population	No. of Subjects	No. of AN/AD Subjects	% of Total
Stein et al. (1996)	Special care nursery	100	4	4.00
Psarommatis et al. (1997)	Intensive care unit	102	2	1.96
Rance et al. (1999)	"at-risk" infants	5199	12	0.23
Berg et al. (2005)	Intensive care unit	1194	115*	9.63
Psarommatis et al. (2006)	Intensive care unit	1150	25**	2.17

*ABR assessment in this study was only at screening levels (35 dBnHL)

**12 of these 25 subjects subsequently showed recovery of neural synchrony (ABRs of normal morphology with response threshold ≤ 40 dB nHL) when reviewed at 4 to 6 months of age.

[1]A number of studies, in fact, have indicated that in a high proportion (30–50%) of AN/AD cases the OAE can disappear over time (Rance et al., 1999; Starr et al., 2000). Most reports of OAE deterioration, however, have occurred in the postneonatal period.

at which evoked potential assessments are carried out also will affect the AN/AD diagnosis rate in high-risk babies. Rance et al. (1999), for example, only included children who showed no ABR on repeated measures through the first year of life. Psarommatis et al. (2006), in contrast, considered that ≈1 in 50 of their ICU babies fit the AN/AD pattern when assessed in the neonatal period, but subsequently found that in more than half of their AN/AD cohort (12/20 cases) the ABR abnormalities had "resolved" when testing was repeated at 4 to 6 months of age.[2]

The proportion of children with permanent hearing disability showing the AN/AD result pattern has been considered in a number of studies over the past decade. Estimates vary (again probably reflecting methodological differences), but it appears that one in every 10 to 20 children with educationally significant hearing impairment will show evidence of normal cochlear (OHC) function and auditory pathway disorder (Table 13–2). It is likely that undiagnosed AN/AD has always accounted for a proportion of permanent hearing loss. The high prevalence rates in recent studies (and anecdotal reports from neonatal screening programs), may however reflect an increase in the condition due to decreased mortality rates in very premature/low birth weight babies and the relatively high incidence of neurologic consequences in those who survive (Rance et al., 1999).

Management (at Diagnosis)

Medical/Developmental Workup

All recommendations for initial management of children with sensorineural-type hearing loss by the Joint Committee on Infant Hearing (JCIH, 2007) are appropriate for babies with AN/AD. These assessments include:

1. Pediatric and developmental evaluation and history;
2. Otologic evaluation with imaging of the cochlear and auditory nerves (CT/MRI) and vestibular assessment;
3. Medical genetics evaluation;
4. Ophthalmologic assessment;
5. Communication development assessment and ongoing monitoring.

In addition, referral for neurologic evaluation to assess peripheral and cranial nerve function is also warranted in children with the AN/AD result pattern.

Audiologic Follow-Up

As described in a previous section, diagnosing a baby with AN/AD is relatively straightforward. Determin-

Table 13–2. Prevalence of AN/AD in Children With Permanent Hearing Loss

Study	*Population*	*No. of Cases Permanent Hearing Loss*	*No. of AN/AD Cases*	*% of Total*
Kraus et al. (1984)	Hg. Impaired children	48	7	14.58
Park & Lee (1998)	Hg. Impaired children	139	7	5.04
Vohr et al. (1998)	Universal Screening	111	2	1.80
Rance et al. (1999)	"at-risk" infants	109	12	11.01
Berlin et al. (2000)	Hg. Impaired children	1000	87	8.70
Cone-Wesson et al. (2000)	Universal Screening	56	3	5.36
Lee et al. (2001)	Hg. Impaired children	67	2	2.98
Madden et al. (2002)	Hg. Impaired children	428	22	5.14
Tang et al. (2004)	Hg. Impaired children	56	1	1.78
Rance et al. (2005)	"at-risk" infants	290	19	6.55

[2]These authors now recommend that diagnosis of AN/AD be delayed in NICU graduates until 3 to 6 months corrected age.

ing the child's auditory capacity in the infant period is rather more of a challenge. One of the particular difficulties associated with early management of AN/AD children relates to the inability of brainstem-evoked potential measures to predict the behavioral audiogram.[3] While sound detection in this population does not predict the degree of functional disability (to the extent that peripheral hearing loss does), access to sound, in particular speech at conversational levels, still forms the basis of early intervention strategies (such as hearing aid fitting). In AN/AD listeners with complete ABR absence, behavioral hearing thresholds can vary from normal to profound levels (Rance et al., 1999). Children with present but abnormal ABR, tend to present with lesser degrees of loss, but in this group, ABR threshold still shows no relation to hearing level.

Auditory steady-state response (ASSR) thresholds also show no correlation with sound detection in listeners with AN/AD. When stimuli modulated at high rates (70–100 Hz) are employed, responses can be obtained, suggesting that the ASSR requires a lesser degree of neural synchrony in the auditory brainstem (Rance et al., 1999). High level signals (≥ 80 dB HL), however, are typically required to elicit the potential even in children who show subsequently normal behavioral audiograms (Attias, Buller, Rubel, & Raveh, 2006; Rance & Briggs, 2002; Rance, Dowell, Rickards, Beer, & Clark, 1998). The possibility of using lower modulation rates (e.g., 40 Hz) to elicit ASSRs from the auditory cortex in children with AN/AD is yet to be fully explored.

Establishing sound detection levels in infants with AN/AD requires careful evaluation of auditory behavior. Conditioned audiometric techniques (visual reinforcement audiometry/conditioned orientation audiometry) can be used in developmentally normal children from 6 months of age onwards. In younger or delayed children, some information can be obtained using "behavioral observation audiometry" (BOA) techniques. To date there are no published findings describing BOA results in AN/AD populations, but data from our laboratory suggests that minimum response levels obtained at < 6 months of age to speech and noisemaker stimuli can at least differentiate between those cases with normal to near normal, and those with elevated sound detection levels. Parental observation beyond the clinic including formal assessment tools (questionnaires) can also inform this process.

A number of recent reports have demonstrated that some children presenting with the AN/AD result pattern in infancy can show "recovery" of the ABR and/or improvement in hearing thresholds (Attias & Raveh, 2007; Madden, Rutter, Hilbert, Greinwald, & Choo, 2002; Psarommatis et al., 2006; Stein et al., 1996). In most cases this improvement has involved children with either hyperbilirubinemia or very low birthweight and has occurred in the first year of life. These findings highlight a need for repeat ABR assessment and careful audiometric monitoring of infants with AN/AD, particularly those who are NICU graduates. Long-term monitoring of children who have shown recovery is also warranted, as it is not yet clear if restored neural synchrony in the auditory brainstem guarantees normal auditory processing.

The proportion of AN/AD youngsters demonstrating ABR recovery is yet to be determined. In our laboratory, and the Australia-wide population, the proportion of babies showing improvement is relatively small. In fact, less than 5% of cases with the AN/AD result pattern in the neonatal period have shown ABR improvement on repeat assessments over the first two years of life. Establishing the likelihood of ABR development and its' time course are clearly important clinical questions, potentially impacting infant assessment protocols (e.g., at what age should screening occur for high risk populations? for how long should ABR status be monitored?) and both short and long term management decisions (e.g., when should amplification be provided or cochlear implantation considered?).

Audiologic Clinical Profile

Sound Detection

While some children (< 10%) show audiograms within the normal audiometric range (Berlin, Morlet, & Hood, 2003; Rance et al., 1999), most present with impaired sound detection. Behavioral hearing thresholds range from normal to profound levels and in most subjects, are essentially the same in both ears. Average hearing levels are evenly distributed across the audiometric range (Madden et al., 2002; Rance et al., 1999; Sininger & Oba, 2001; Starr et al., 2000).

Audiograms with a low frequency (reverse slope) configuration are common. Approximately 30 to 40% of reported AN/AD children have shown poorest

[3]The use of cortical auditory evoked potentials to predict audiometric threshold is yet to be explored but may offer insights in some cases.

detection for stimuli in the 250 Hz to 500 Hz range. In contrast, the high frequency configuration typical of sensory hearing loss only occurs in ≈ 10% of cases (Madden et al., 2002; Rance et al., 1999; Sininger & Oba, 2001; Vinay & Moore, 2007). This may reflect that low frequencies are encoded by both a place and temporal code, whereas high frequencies are encoded only by cochlear place of activation.

Fluctuation in sound detection has been a consistently reported feature of AN/AD. Day-to-day variations in audiometric threshold (without directional trend) of 20 dB or more have been reported to affect up to 30% of pediatric cases (Rance et al., 1999; Sininger & Oba, 2001). In some instances, these fluctuations can be related to clinical changes in the subjects. Gorga, Stelmachowicz, Barlow, and Brookhauser (1995) and Starr et al. (1998), for example, have described a temperature-sensitive form of neuropathy where core body temperature increases of as little as 1° can result in dramatic auditory evoked potential changes and temporary drops in both sound detection and speech understanding. In most AN/AD cases, however, the cause of hearing level fluctuation is unknown.

Middle Ear Muscle Reflex

The middle ear muscle reflex (MEMR) is one of the two efferent reflexes modulated by the inner hair cell, eighth nerve, and auditory brainstem pathways and is consistently abnormal in cases of AN/AD regardless of the subject's behavioral hearing levels[4] (Berlin et al., 2005; Sininger & Oba, 2001; Starr et al., 1996). In the most comprehensive study of the MEMR in AN/AD patients, Berlin et al. (2005) found that the reflex was absent at all test frequencies and in all test conditions (ipsilateral/contralateral) in 88.3% of cases and that none of the 128 subjects showed a normal response pattern. As such, these authors recommend that tympanometry and MEMR testing be used as a triage procedure for all audiology patients and that MEMR testing be carried out to identify AN/AD infants in screening programs that use only OAEs.[5]

Cortical Auditory Evoked Potentials

Despite the absence or severe disruption of ABRs in ears with AN/AD, potentials from the auditory cortex including the middle latency response (Kraus et al., 1984; Starr et al., 1996), the cortical auditory evoked potentials (Kraus et al., 2000; Kumar & Vanaja, 2008; Michalewski, Starr, Nguyen, Kong, & Zeng, 2005; Rance, Cone-Wesson, Wunderlich, & Dowell, 2002; Starr et al., 1996), mismatch negativity (Cone-Wesson, Rance, & Wunderlich 2003) and the P300 cognitive potential (Starr et al., 1996) are recordable in some affected adults and children. That these potentials can be observed on occasion may reflect the fact that they are less dependent on synchronous neural firing than the ABR (Rance, 2005) and as such, may offer a broad measure of the degree of neural disruption in the central auditory pathways. Rance et al. (2002) for example recorded obligatory cortical potentials (P_1-N_1-P_2) in a group of school-aged children with AN/AD and found a high correlation between auditory processing ability (open-set speech understanding) and the presence or absence of the response. Similarly, Kumar and Vanaja (2008) have shown a relationship between N_1/P_2 amplitude and speech identification in a group of adolescent and young adult subjects. These findings suggest that cortical-AEPs may be useful indicators of the neural capacity to support speech perception. The clinical application of these responses is yet to be fully explored, but early reports suggest that they can be used to inform early management decisions (Pearce, Golding, & Dillon, 2007).

Speech Perception

Speech understanding difficulties are a consistently reported feature of AN/AD. Almost all affected adults have shown perceptual deficits greater than predicted from their audiogram (Rance et al., 2008; Starr et al., 1996; Starr et al., 2000; Zeng, Oba, & Starr, 2001). Results in children have been more variable. At best, young AN/AD listeners show speech perception test results comparable to their peers with sensory-type hearing loss. At worst, they show no functional hearing at all despite (in many cases) enjoying complete access to the normal speech spectrum. Figure 13–2 shows this broad spread of perceptual performance and reflects the lack of relationship between and speech understanding and sound detection in children with AN/AD.

The presence of background noise poses a particular problem for many AN/AD listeners (Kraus et al.,

[4]The other is the medial olivocochlear reflex, which is responsible for suppression of the OAE by ipsilateral or contralateral masking and absent in ears with AN/AD (Hood, Berlin, Bordelon, & Rose, 2003).

[5]Immaturity of the neonatal ear canal and middle ear, may however complicate MEMR recording in this population (Margolis, Bass-Ringdahl, Hnaks, Holte, & Zapala, 2003).

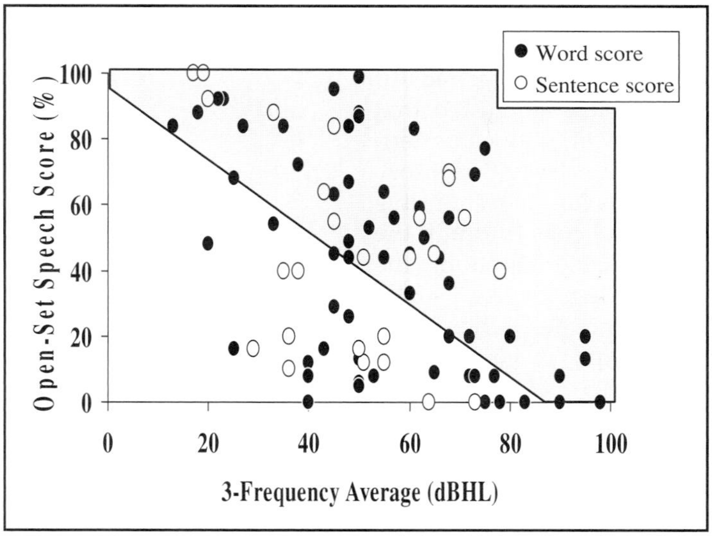

FIGURE 13–2. Open-set speech perception score/average hearing level comparisons for 110 children with AN/AD type hearing loss. The filled data points represent findings from open-set word tests and the open points show open-set sentence test results. The gray area represents the expected performance range for ears with sensorineural hearing loss (Yellin, Jerger, & Fifer, 1989). Data for this meta-analysis were obtained from the following studies: Berlin, Hood, Hurley, and Wen, 1996; Konradsson, 1996; Kumar and Jayaram, 2005; Lee et al., 2001; Michalewski et al., 2005; Miyamoto, Iler Kirk, Renshaw, and Hussain, 1999; Narne and Vanaja, 2008; Picton et al., 1998; Rance et al., 2004; Rance et al., 2007; Sininger, Hood, Starr, Berlin, and Picton, 1995; Starr et al., 1991; Starr et al., 1998; Vinay and Moore, 2007; Zeng et al., 2005; Zeng and Liu, 2006.

2000; Rance et al., 2008; Shallop, 2002; Starr et al., 1998). Figure 13–3 shows an example of these extreme figure-ground difficulties presenting open-set speech perception results for a child with essentially normal hearing thresholds. Despite demonstrating normal scores in quiet (+20 dB SNR), this subject showed negligible speech understanding in listening conditions typical of the average school classroom (0-5 dB SNR) (Crandell & Smalldino, 2000). The mechanisms underlying figure-ground problems in AN/AD are not yet understood. Psychophysical studies, however, have shown similarly exaggerated noise effects in both simultaneous (where the signal is presented within the noise) and nonsimultaneous (where the signal occurs immediately before or after the noise) masking experiments (Kraus et al., 2000; Vinay & Moore, 2007; Zeng et al., 2005).

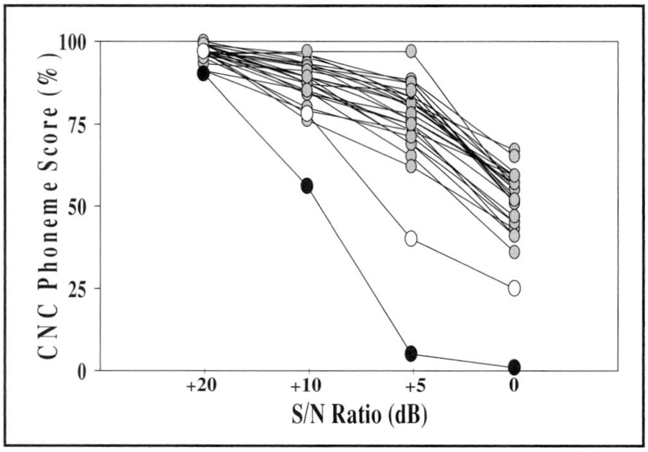

FIGURE 13–3. CNC-phoneme scores plotted as a function of listening condition. Results for Subject A are represented by the white (left ear) and black (right ear) circles. Findings for a control group of school-aged children are shown in gray (Rance et al., 2007).

Auditory Processing

The mismatch between audibility and speech understanding in listeners with AN/AD suggests that distortion of suprathreshold cues is the limiting factor in perceptual performance (Rance et al., 1999, 2002; Starr et al., 2000). Speech perception ability, in fact, appears more closely related to the degree of neural disruption in the central auditory pathways than sound detection

(Kraus et al., 2000; Rance et al., 2002). Psychophysical studies investigating the ways in which this disruption affects basic auditory processing have been carried out over the past two decades and have suggested that both children and adults with AN/AD show a pattern of effects that is distinct from that seen with sensory hearing loss. For example, as the cochlea is responsible for the initial processing of spectral cues (through the precise tonotopic arrangement of signals along the basilar membrane), sensory hearing loss is usually associated with impaired "frequency resolution" (the ability to perceive [resolve] the frequency components of a complex sound; Moore, 1995). Listeners with AN/AD type hearing loss on the other hand, who typically show evidence of normal cochlear (outer hair cell) function, usually enjoy normal cochlear frequency processing (Cacace, Satya-Murti, & Grimes, 1983; Rance, McKay, & Graydon, 2004; Vinay & Moore, 2007).

In contrast, by disrupting the timing of neural signals in the auditory pathway, AN/AD affects perception based upon temporal cues.[6] In particular, temporal resolution (the ability to perceive rapid changes in auditory signals over time) and the temporal aspects of pitch discrimination (such as neural phase locking) can be severely compromised. Temporal resolution deficits have been demonstrated both in "gap detection" tasks where AN/AD listeners typically require a silent period 2 to 5 times longer than normal controls before they become aware of a change in a continuous signal (Starr et al., 1991; Zeng et al., 2005) and in "amplitude modulation detection" experiments where they show an impaired ability to track rapid amplitude envelope changes (Rance et al., 2004; Zeng et al., 2005). Figure 13–4 demonstrates this inability to cope with rapidly varying stimuli. In this experiment, many of the AN/AD subjects struggled to detect amplitude changes occurring relatively slowly (10 Hz) and some could not detect the variations at all when they occurred at a rapid rate (150 Hz; Rance et al., 2004).

Temporal processing limitations can also affect frequency discrimination in children with AN/AD (Rance et al., 2004; Starr et al., 1991; Zeng et al., 2005). The ability to perceive pitch differences between stimuli is primarily determined by the spatial arrangement of excitation along the basilar membrane (Sek & Moore, 1995). Pitch perception in the low frequency range, however, is enhanced by temporal cues through "phase locking" where the frequency of the stimulus waveform is reflected in neural firing patterns. Phase locking requires a high degree of temporal precision

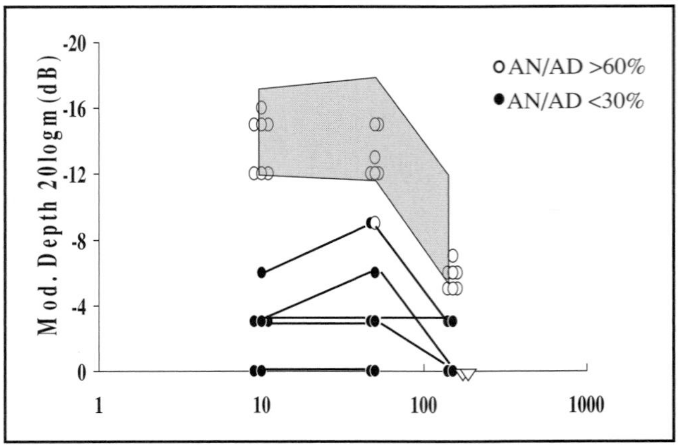

FIGURE 13–4. Amplitude modulation detection thresholds in children with AN/AD (*circles*). The shaded area represents the mean ± 2 SD range for a control group of children with normal hearing (Rance et al., 2004).

and so, not surprisingly, children and adults with AN/AD typically show an impaired ability to use this cue and demonstrate low frequency difference limen (the smallest detectable frequency difference between sounds) approximately 10 times that of normally hearing listeners.

Processing of binaural temporal cues is also affected by AN/AD type hearing loss. Masking difference level (MDL) testing for example, which measures the release of masking obtained when phase-inverted inputs are presented to the two ears, has consistently shown abnormal results (Starr et al., 1991, 1996). Furthermore, localization based on interaural timing differences is impaired, even in individuals who can accurately judge sound direction using interaural intensity differences (Zeng et al., 2005).

In summary, disruption of neural activity in the auditory pathways of children with AN/AD can significantly affect the processing of timing cues. The severity of this temporal disruption is highly correlated with the overall level of functional disability (Rance et al., 2004; Zeng et al., 2005). The degree of temporal disruption, however, is not consistent across subjects. In Figure 13–4, for example, those subjects with reasonable (> 60%) open-set speech perception scores tended to show relatively normal amplitude modulation detection ability, whereas those with severely impaired temporal processing showed negligible speech understanding. Clearly, the ability to quantify

[6]In most cases temporal processing is unimpaired by sensory loss.

temporal processing in youngsters with AN/AD offers a key to predicting their long-term capacity to use auditory cues.

Case Study (Auditory Processing)

Subject A was born at 32 weeks post conceptual age weighing 2.25 kg. Despite his prematurity, the infant presented with no neonatal risk factors for permanent hearing loss apart from hyperbilirubinemia (peak serum bilirubin level: 400 μmol/L) for which he received blood transfusion.

Click-ABR assessment was carried out at 1 month corrected age. Findings for the right ear showing a repeatable CM but absent ABR at maximum presentation levels are shown in Figure 13–1. Identical results were obtained for the left ear.[7] Transient otoacoustic emissions were present bilaterally. On the basis of these findings, Subject A was referred for medical (pediatric, neurologic, otologic) workup, and was enrolled for early intervention support. Audiologic monitoring over the next 8 months showed consistent behavioral responses to speech and noisemaker stimuli at levels within the normal developmental range. As such, amplification was not recommended. Subsequent conditioned audiometric testing showed sound detection within normal limits for the left ear, and mild low-frequency threshold elevation in the right ear (Figure 13–5).

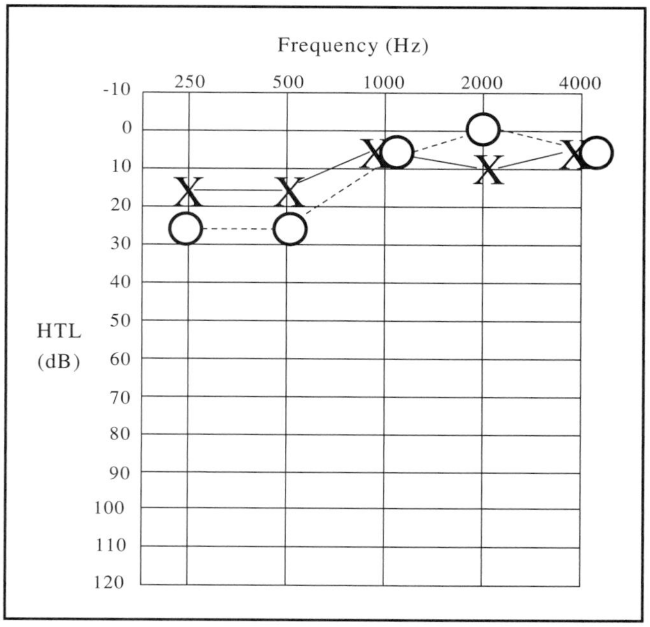

FIGURE 13–5. Conditioned audiometric thresholds for subject A obtained at 8 months of age. Open circles represent hearing levels for the right ear, and Xs show findings for the left ear.

Subject A's speech, language and general developmental progress were monitored, and were considered normal at primary school entry (5 years of age). At this point he underwent a detailed speech perception and psychophysical assessment to evaluate his auditory processing ability.

Figure 13–6 shows gap detection thresholds for Subject A and for a control cohort of children of equivalent age (5–7 years). In the left ear, his gap threshold was mildly elevated, suggesting only slightly impaired temporal resolution on this side. Temporal processing for stimuli presented to the right ear, however, was significantly affected. This pattern was repeated on amplitude modulation detection testing (Figure 13–7) where Subject A's ability to detect rapid amplitude changes in stimuli presented to the left ear was only mildly impaired, but results for the right ear were grossly abnormal.

Open-set speech perception results for Subject A reflected his temporal processing limitations. Figure 13–3 shows CNC-phoneme scores in four listening conditions. Speech understanding in quiet (+20 dB SNR) was relatively normal in both ears, but the introduction of background noise resulted in greater than typical deterioration in performance, particularly in the psychophysically poorer (right) ear. These speech-in-noise difficulties were subsequently reflected in Subject A's school progress where both he and his teacher reported significant communication problems in the classroom. As such, he has recently been fit with an FM listening device. At the time of writing we cannot comment on long-term device outcome, but free-field testing (CNC words at +3 dB SNR) at the time of fitting did show significant perceptual improvement from 28% phonemes correct in the unaided condition to 96% correct in the aided.

Case Summary

Findings for Subject A highlight the fact that it is possible for a child to have normal speech/language development, reasonably normal auditory temporal

[7]Absent ABRs were also obtained on repeat assessment at 6 months, 12 months, and 5 years of age.

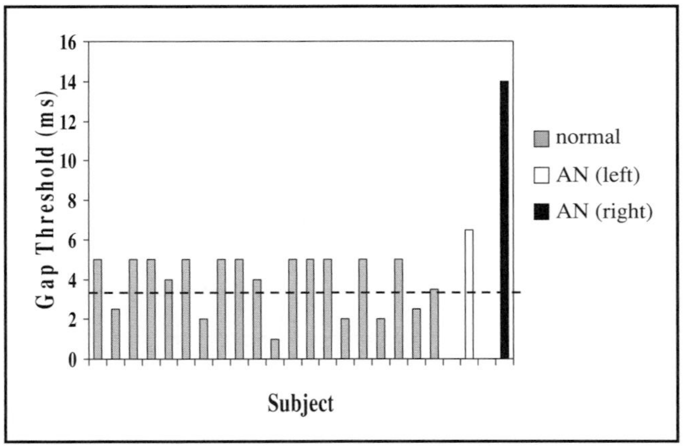

FIGURE 13–6. Threshold levels for gap detection in white noise presented at 70 dB SPL. Results for Subject A are represented by the white (*left ear*) and black (*right ear*) columns. The dashed line represents the mean detection threshold for a control group of school-aged children (5–7 years).

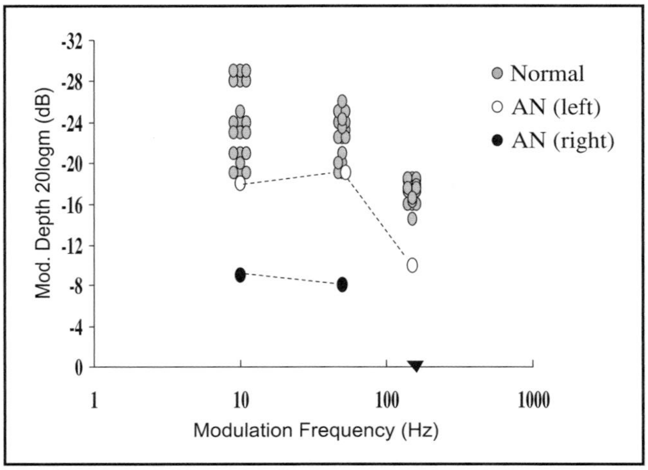

FIGURE 13–7. Amplitude modulation detection thresholds for white noise stimuli modulated at 10, 50, and 150 Hz. Findings for Subject A are represented by the white and black circles. Results for a control group of school aged children are shown in gray (Rance et al., 2004).

processing and normal speech perception (at least in quiet) despite the absence of a recordable ABR. Comparing result patterns for the two ears also demonstrates the relationship between basic auditory processing abilities (measured psychophysically) and functional disability.

Management of AN/AD

Amplification

Fitting hearing aids to children with AN/AD has been a controversial issue since the condition was first identified. There are two main arguments against the use of conventional amplification in this population. The first is that the amplified signal may cause damage to cochlear structures in ears with outer hair cell function. The evidence for amplification-related damage actually occurring is weak. In our Australian cohort where children have been routinely fitted to National Acoustic Laboratories (NAL) prescribed levels for over 15 years, there have been no obvious cases of noise-related threshold shift. Nonetheless, a number of authors have recommended that serial OAE assessments be carried out in amplified ears to monitor cochlear (outer hair cell) function. This seems a reasonable precaution although the possibility of spontaneous OAE loss (which can occur in both amplified and unamplified AN/AD ears; Deltenre et al., 1999; Starr et al., 2000) could complicate interpretation.

The second major argument against amplification in children with AN/AD relates to the fact that conventional hearing aids are not designed to overcome temporal processing disorders. As such, the aided AN/AD child may simply be presented with a loud, but equally incomprehensible signal.

The only way in which hearing aids can help a child with AN/AD is by improving the audibility of the speech spectrum. This is no small thing as many affected children present with significantly elevated hearing thresholds and cannot detect speech signals at normal levels without amplification. As such, it is not surprising that conservative (low-gain) aiding strategies have proven unsuccessful (Hood, 1998).

Outcomes for AN/AD children managed with conventional amplification have been mixed. Most have shown little or no benefit (according to anecdotal reports and formal speech perception testing) despite being afforded complete access to the amplified speech spectrum (Lee et al., 2001; Rance et al., 1999, 2002). A significant proportion (≈40%) of children in the Australian cohort, however, has progressed well with amplification. These children (typically those with lesser degrees of temporal processing disruption) have shown aided speech perception ability (Rance et al., 2002) and overall speech and language development (Rance et al., 2007) consistent with their peers with sensory hearing loss.

The possibility of AN/AD specific hearing devices is an area of current investigation (Narne & Vanaja, 2008; Zeng et al., 2001). Clinically applicable systems are (at the time of writing) not yet available, but speech processing algorithms designed to accentuate temporal and/or amplitude differences, or transpose spectral information into regions where frequency discrimination is optimal, offer some possibility for AN/AD listeners in the future.

Recommended Amplification Approach

1. Amplification should be offered if sound detection levels indicate that access to conversational level speech will be limited.
2. Affected children should be fitted using amplification targets based on the behavioral audiogram.
3. Where appropriate, amplification should be provided as early as possible.

Cochlear Implant

Cochlear implantation is currently the management option of choice for AN/AD children with limited auditory capacity. Most of the 200+ CI cases reported thus far have shown normal device function (mapping levels) and perceptual outcomes consistent with expectations for young implantees with sensorineural hearing loss (Jeong, Kim, Kim, Bae, & Kim, 2008; Madden et al., 2002; Mason, DeMichele, Stevens, Ruth, & Hashisaki, 2003; Rance & Barker, 2008; Shallop, Peterson, Facer, Fabry, & Driscoll, 2001; Trautwein, Shallop, Fabry, & Friedman, 2001). Some recently presented data, however, have suggested that the auditory processing disorder may not entirely be overcome by cochlear implantation in all cases (Gibson & Sanli, 2007; Rance & Barker, 2008; Zeng & Liu, 2006) similar to the situation with CI in "sensorineural" hearing loss.

The ways in which cochlear implants improve perception in individuals with AN/AD is a current area of investigation. The fact that in most cases auditory brainstem potentials can be recorded to electrical stimulation suggests either an increase in the number of neural elements contributing to the ABR (perhaps as a result of bypassing abnormality of the cochlear IHCs or IHC/auditory nerve synapse) or an improvement in the synchrony of neural firing (perhaps reflecting the fact that cochlear implants stimulate the auditory pathway with series of discrete electric pulses rather than analog signals).

Recommended CI Selection Approach

1. Cochlear implantation should be considered for all AN/AD children with limited access to the normal speech spectrum (i.e., detection thresholds in the severe/profound range).[8] The audiometric selection criteria should be the same as for candidates with sensory hearing loss.[9]
2. In addition, candidates with audiograms in the normal-moderate range should be considered for implantation if significant speech perception/auditory processing deficit is established (i.e., those children with limited capacity to benefit from amplification).

Case Study (Management)

Child B suffered birth asphyxia when born at 38 weeks post conceptual age. Apart from severe oxygen deprivation, she presented with no risk factors for permanent hearing loss. Neonatal OAE screening showed normal responses bilaterally. Severe/profound hearing loss, however, was identified when she was reviewed at 8 months of age, after her parents expressed concerns about her lack of auditory responsiveness (Figure 13–8). When transient OAE assessment again showed robust responses, she was referred for ABR assessment, which showed the AN/AD result pattern (Figure 13–9a).

Child B also underwent cortical auditory evoked potential (CAEP) testing (Figure 13–10). Results of this assessment indicated that both speech and tonal stimuli could elicit electrical responses of normal latency and morphology at the level of the auditory cortex, if presented at high enough levels (100 dB SPL).

After an initial trial with low-gain hearing aids (which elicited no consistent response to sound), Child B was amplified to the degree of her hearing loss (NAL

[8]Special care should be taken to ensure the presence of an adequate cochlear nerve in cases of profound hearing loss (Buchman et al., 2006; Walton, Gibson, Sanli, & Prelog, 2008).

[9]Families however, should be made aware of the possibility of "hearing" recovery in infancy (Madden et al., 2002; Psarromatis et al., 2006).

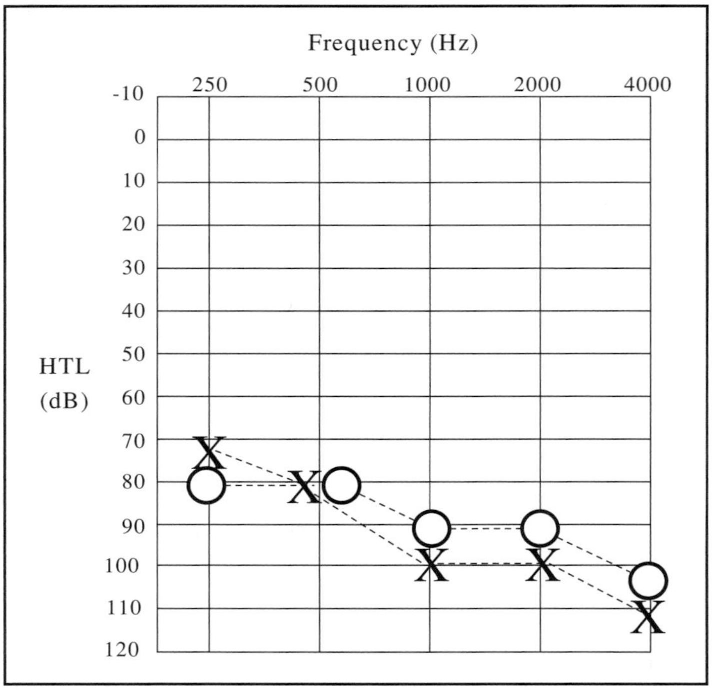

FIGURE 13–8. Conditioned audiometric thresholds for Subject B obtained at 8 months of age. Open circles represent hearing levels for the right ear, and X's show findings for the left ear.

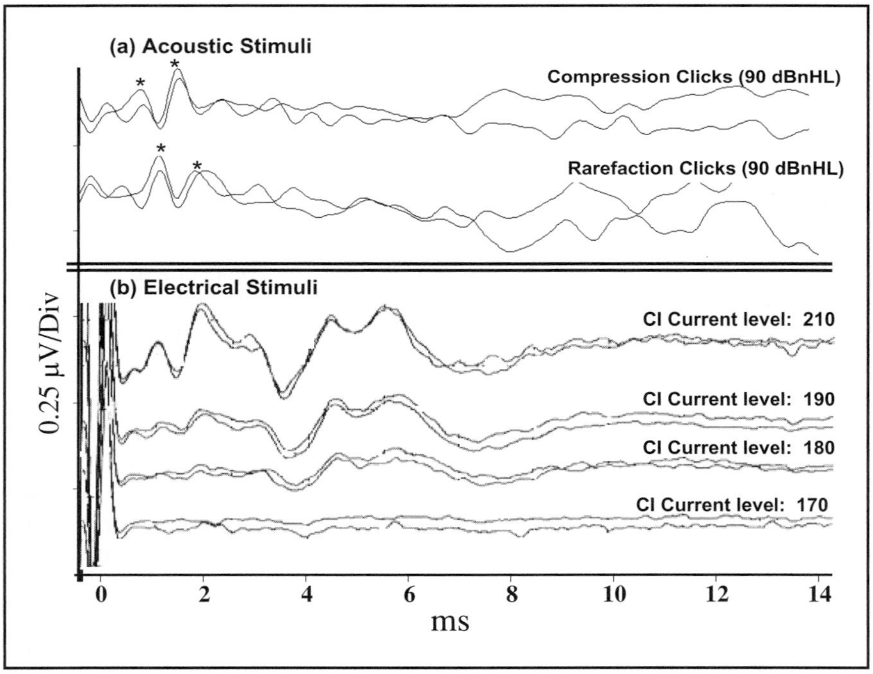

FIGURE 13–9. Averaged EEG tracings for Subject B. Section (a) shows potentials elicited by acoustic click stimuli at 90 dB nHL. Cochlear microphonic responses (represented by the asterisks) are present but brainstem potentials are absent. Section (b) shows repeatable ABRs to electrical (cochlear implant generated) stimuli.

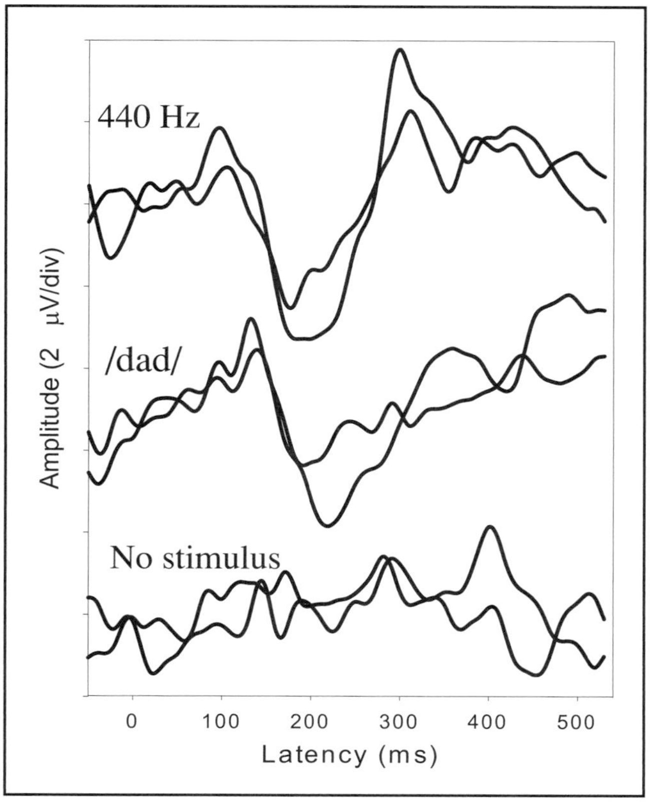

FIGURE 13–10. Cortical auditory evoked potential (CAEP) responses for Subject B to 440-Hz tones (*top tracings*) and synthetic speech stimuli - /dad/ (*middle tracings*) presented at 100 dB SPL.

prescribed levels). She subsequently showed a capacity to use the amplified signal. Functional survey data (Meaningful Auditory Integration Scale; IT-MAIS) were used to track her auditory progress from 15 months of age when she began to show increased vocalization rates when aided, through to 2½ years of age, at which point she had developed an expressive vocabulary of ≈ 45 words. Formal speech perception testing (at 3½ years) however, did highlight Child B's auditory limitations. Open-set word assessment showed perceptual levels below those expected for the typical young implantee (left ear aided: 34%; right ear aided: 40%; binaural aided: 40%). As such, it was recommended that she receive a cochlear implant in the left ear.

Child B was implanted with the CI-24 device at 4 years of age. Intraoperative electric ABR testing showed repeatable potentials to electrical pulses presented at typical current levels. The result suggested the presence of synchronized neural firing in the auditory brainstem (Figure 13–9b).

Postoperatively, Child B has performed well with her cochlear implant.[10] At 14 years of age she scores at close to 100% on open-set speech perception tests in quiet, and in background noise understands more than the average implantee. Receptive and expressive language measures show only mild delay, and she has been successfully integrated into her local school.

Case Summary

Clearly, this child has had a successful outcome with her CI and as such, resembles most of the reported AN/AD cases that have followed this management path. She did receive her device relatively late (4 years) and we might expect an even better outcome had she been implanted earlier (although she did show some progress with amplification). Child B in fact was identified reasonably early in our series (early 1990s) and if seen now would probably be implanted younger (based on her limited access to the amplified speech spectrum). The question however, does remain in children (like Child B) who show some ability to use their residual hearing: how do we predict whether amplification or implantation will provide the best perceptual outcome?

Summary

A constant theme running through this chapter (and the literature on children with AN/AD) is that "hearing" as typically quantified in the audiology clinic and auditory "perception" are not the same thing. If our experience with AN/AD hearing loss has taught us anything, it is that auditory function as measured by behavioral sound detection or electrophysiologic potentials do not necessarily reflect function. Children with AN/AD present with a common pattern of electrophysiologic and electroacoustic results, but their auditory capacity varies enormously. Developing methods that can quantify this capacity, predict long-term outcomes and inform the management process is a significant challenge for the future.

[10]She originally wore the implant and hearing aid in concert, but rejected the aid after only 6 months of CI use.

References

Attias, J., Buller, N., Rubel, Y., & Raveh, E. (2006). Multiple auditory steady-state responses in children and adults with normal hearing, sensorineural hearing loss or auditory neuropathy. *Annals of Otology, Rhinology and Laryngology, 115*(4), 268–276.

Attias, J., & Raveh, H. (2007). Transient deafness in young cochlear implant candidates. *Audiology and Neuro-Otology, 12*, 325–333.

Berg, A. L., Spitzer, J. B., Towers, H. M., Bartosiewicz, C., & Diamond, B. E. (2005). Newborn hearing screening in the NICU: Profile of failed auditory brainstem response/passed otoacoustic emission. *Pediatrics, 116*, 933–938.

Berlin, C. I., Bordelon, J., St. John, P., Wilenski, D., Hurley, A, Kluka, E., & Hood, L. J. (1998). Reversing click polarity may uncover auditory neuropathy in infants. *Ear and Hearing, 19*, 37–47.

Berlin, C. I., Hood, L. J., Hurley, M. S., & Wen, H. (1996). Hearing aids: Only for hearing impaired patients with abnormal otoacoustic emissions. In C. I. Berlin (Ed.), *Hair cells and hearing aids* (pp. 99–111). San Diego, CA: Singular.

Berlin, C. I., Hood, L. J., & Morlet, T. (2000). The search for auditory neuropathy patients and connexin 26 patients in schools for the deaf. *Association for Research in Otolaryngology Abstract, 23*, 23–24.

Berlin, C. I., Hood, L. J., Morlet, T., Wilenski, D., St. John, P., Montgomery, E., & Thibadaux, M. (2005). Absent or elevated middle ear muscle reflexes in the presence of normal otoacoustic emissions: A universal finding in 136 cases of auditory neuropathy/dys-synchrony. *Journal of the American Academy of Audiology, 16*, 546–553.

Berlin, C. I., Hood, L. J., & Rose, K. (2001). On renaming auditory neuropathy as auditory dys-synchrony. *Audiology Today, 13*, 15–17.

Berlin, C. I., Morlet, T., & Hood, L. J. (2003). Auditory neuropathy/dys-synhcrony: Its diagnosis and management. *Pediatric Clinics of North America, 50*, 331–340.

Buchman, C. A., Roush, P. A., Teagle, H. F. B., Brown, C., Zdanski, C. J., & Grose, J. H. (2006). Auditory neuropathy characteristics in children with cochlear nerve deficiency. *Ear and Hearing, 27*, 399–408.

Cacace, A. T., Satya-Murti, S., & Grimes, C. T. (1983). Frequency selectivity and temporal processing in Friedreich's Ataxia. *Annals of Otology, Rhinology and Laryngology, 92*, 276–280.

Collet, L., Levy, V., & Veuillet, E. (1993). Click-evoked otoacoustic emissions and hearing threshold in sensorineural hearing loss. *Ear and Hearing, 14*(2), 141–143.

Cone-Wesson, B., Rance, G., & Wunderlich, J. L. (2003). Mismatch negativity in children with auditory neuropathy and sensorineural hearing loss. *Association for Research in Otolaryngology Abstracts, 26*, 191.

Cone-Wesson, B., Vohr, B. R., Sininger, Y. S., Widen, J. E., Folsom, R. C., Gorga, M. P., & Norton, S. J. (2000). Identification of neonatal hearing impairment: Infants with hearing loss. *Ear and Hearing, 21*, 488–507.

Crandell, C. C., & Smaldino, J. J. (2000). Classroom acoustics for children with normal hearing and with hearing impairment. *Language, Speech and Hearing Services in Schools, 31*, 362–370.

Dallos, P., (1973). *The auditory periphery: Biophysics and physiology*. New York, NY: Academic Press.

Dallos, P., & Cheatham, M. A. (1976). Production of cochlear potentials by inner and outer hair cells. *Journal of the Acoustical Society of America, 60*, 510–512.

Davis, H., & Hirsh, S. K. (1979). The audiometric utility of the brain stem response to low frequency sounds. *Audiology, 15*, 181–195.

Deltenre, P., Mansbach, A. L., Bozet, C., Christiaens, F., Barthelemy, P., Paulissen, D., & Renglet, T. (1999). Auditory neuropathy with preserved cochlear microphonics and secondary loss of otoacoustic emissions. *Audiology, 38*(4), 187–195.

Gibson, W. P. R., & Sanli, H. (2007) Auditory neuropathy: An update. *Ear and Hearing, 28*, 102–106S.

Gorga, M. P., Stelmachowicz, P. G., Barlow, S. M., & Brookhouser, P. E. (1995). Case of recurrent, sudden sensorineural hearing loss in a child. *Journal of the American Academy of Audiology, 6*, 163–172.

Hildesheimer, M., Muchnik, C., & Rubinstein, M. (1985). Problems in interpretation of brainstem-evoked response audiometry. *Audiology, 24*(5), 374–379.

Hood, L. J. (1998). Auditory neuropathy: What is it and what can we do about it? *Hearing Journal, 51*(8), 10–18.

Hood, L. J., Berlin, C. I., Bordelon, J., & Rose, K. (2003). Patients with auditory neuropathy/dys-synchrony lack efferent suppression of transient evoked otoacoustic emissions. *Journal of the American Academy of Audiology, 14*, 302–313.

Jeong, S-W., Kim, L-S., Kim, B-Y., Bae, W-Y., & Kim, J-R. (2008). Cochlear implantation in children with auditory neuropathy: Outcomes and rationale. *Acta Oto-Laryngologica, Suppl., 558*, 36–43.

Joint Committee on Infant Hearing (JCIH). (2007). Position statement: Principles and guidelines for early hearing detection and intervention programs. *Pediatrics, 120*, 898–921.

Kemp, D. T. (1978). Stimulated acoustic emission from the human auditory system. *Journal of the Acoustical Society of America, 64*, 1386–1391.

Konradsson, K. S. (1996). Bilaterally presented otoacoustic emissions in four children with profound idiopathic unilateral hearing loss. *Audiology, 35*, 217–227.

Kraus, N., Bradlow, A. R., Cheatham, J., Cunningham, C. D., King, D. B., Koch, T. G., . . . Wright, B. A. (2000). Consequences of neural asynchrony: A case of auditory neuropathy. *Journal of the Association for Research in Otolaryngology, 1*(1), 33–45.

Kraus, N. A., Ozdamar, O., Stein, L., & Reed, N. (1984). Absent auditory brainstem response: Peripheral hearing loss or brainstem dysfunction? *Laryngoscope, 94*, 400–406.

Kumar, A. U., & Jayaram, M. (2005). Auditory processing in individuals with auditory neuropathy. *Behavioral and Brain Functions, 1*, 21.

Kumar, V., & Vanaja, C. S. (2008). Speech identification and cortical potentials in individuals with auditory neuropathy. *Behavioral and Brain Functions, 4*, 15.

Lee, J. S. M., McPherson, B., Yuen K. C. P., & Wong, L. L. N. (2001). Screening for auditory neuropathy in a school for hearing impaired children. *International Journal of Pediatric Otorhinolaryngology, 61*, 39–46.

Lonsbury-Martin, B. L., Harris, F. P., Stagner, B. B., & Hawkins, M. D. (1990). Distortion product emissions in humans: I. Basic properties in normally hearing subjects. *Annals of Otology, Rhinology and Laryngology, 147*, 3–14.

Madden, C., Rutter, M., Hilbert, L., Greinwald, J., & Choo, D. (2002). Clinical and audiological features in auditory neuropathy. *Archives of Otolaryngology-Head and Neck Surgery, 128*, 1026–1030.

Margolis, R. H., Bass-Ringdahl S., Hnaks, W. D., Holte, L., & Zapala D. A. (2003). Tympanometry in newborn infants—1 kHz norms. *Journal of the American Academy of Audiology, 14*(7), 383–392.

Mason, J. C., De Michele, A., Stevens, C., Ruth, R., & Hashisaki, G. (2003). Cochlear implantation in patients with auditory neuropathy of varied etiologies. *Laryngoscope, 113*(1), 45–49.

McMahon, C. M., Patuzzi, R. B., Gibson, W. B., & Sanli, H. (2008). Frequency-specific electrocochleography indicates that presynaptic and postsynaptic mechanisms of auditory neuropathy exist. *Ear and Hearing, 29*, 314–325.

Michalewski, H. J., Starr, A., Nguyen, T. T., Kong, Y-Y., & Zeng, F-G. (2005). Auditory temporal processes in normal-hearing individuals and in patients with auditory neuropathy. *Clinical Neurophysiology, 116*, 669–680.

Miyamoto, R. T., Iler Kirk, K., Renshaw, J., & Hussain, D. (1999). Cochlear implantation in auditory neuropathy. *Laryngoscope, 109*, 181–185.

Moore, B. C. J. (1995). Speech perception in people with cochlear damage. In *Perceptual consequences of cochlear damage* (pp. 147–172). Oxford, NY: Oxford University Press.

Moser, T., Strenzke, N., Meyer, A., Lesinski-Shiedat, A., Lenarz, T., Beutner, D., . . . Strutz, J. (2006). Diagnosis and therapy of auditory synaptopathy/neuropathy. *HNO, 54*(11), 833–839.

Narne, V. K., & Vanaja, C. S. (2008). Effect of envelope enhancement on speech perception in individuals with auditory neuropathy. *Ear and Hearing, 29*, 45–53.

Norton, S. J., Ferguson, R., & Mascher, K. (1989). Evoked otoacoustic emissions and extratympanic cochlear microphonics recorded from human ears. *Abstracts of the Twelfth Midwinter Research Meeting of the Association for Research in Otolaryngology, 227*(A).

Park, M. S., & Lee, J. H. (1998). Diagnostic potential of distortion product otoacoustic emissions in severe or profound sensorineural hearing loss. *Acta Otolaryngologica (Stockh), 118*, 496–500.

Pearce W., Golding M., & Dillon, H. (2007). Cortical auditory evoked potentials in the assessment of auditory neuropathy: Two case studies. *Journal of the American Academy of Audiology, 18*, 380–390.

Picton, T. W., Durieux-Smith, A., Champagne, S. C., Whittingham, J., Moran, L. M., Giguere, C., & Beauregard, Y. (1998). Objective evaluation of aided thresholds using auditory steady-state responses. *Journal of the American Academy of Audiology, 9*, 315–331.

Psarommatis, I. M., Riga, M., Douros, K., Koltsidopolous, P., Douniadakis, D., Kapetanakis, I., & Apostolopolous, N. (2006). Transient infantile auditory neuropathy and its clinical implications. *International Journal of Pediatric Otorhinolaryngology, 70*, 1629–1637.

Psarommatis, I. M., Tsakanikos, M. D., Kontorgianni, A. D., Ntouniadakis, D. E., & Apostolopoulos, N. K. (1997). Profound hearing loss and presence of click-evoked otoacoustic emissions in the neonate: A report of two cases. *International Journal of Pediatric Otorhinolaryngology, 39*, 237–243.

Rance, G. (2005). Auditory neuropathy/dys-synchrony and its perceptual consequences. *Trends in Amplification, 9*(1), 1–43.

Rance, G., & Barker, E. (2008). Speech perception in children with auditory neuropathy/dys-synchrony managed with either hearing aids or cochlear implants. *Otology and Neurotology, 29*, 179–182.

Rance, G., Barker, E., Mok, M., Dowell, R., Rincon, A., & Garratt, R. (2007). Speech perception in noise for children with auditory neuropathy/dys-synchrony type hearing loss. *Ear and Hearing, 28*(3), 351–360.

Rance, G., Beer, D. E., Cone-Wesson, B., Shepherd R. K., Dowell, R. C., King, A. K., . . . Clark, G. M. (1999). Clinical findings for a group of infants and young children with auditory neuropathy. *Ear and Hearing, 20*, 238–252.

Rance, G., & Briggs, R. J. S. (2002). Assessment of hearing level in infants with significant hearing loss: The Melbourne experience with steady-state evoked potential threshold testing. *Annals of Otology, Rhinology and Laryngology, 111*(5), 22–28.

Rance, G., Cone-Wesson, B., Wunderlich, J., & Dowell, R. C. (2002). Speech perception and cortical event related potentials in children with auditory neuropathy. *Ear and Hearing, 23*, 239–253.

Rance, G., Dowell, R. C., Rickards, F. W., Beer, D. E., & Clark, G. M. (1998). Steady-state evoked potential and behavioral hearing thresholds in a group of children with absent click-evoked auditory brainstem response. *Ear and Hearing, 19*, 48–61.

Rance, G., Fava, R., Baldock, H., Chong, A., Barker, E., Corben, L., & Delatycki, M. (2008). Speech perception ability in individuals with Friedeich ataxia. *Brain, 131*, 2002–2012.

Rance, G., McKay, C., & Grayden, D. (2004). Perceptual characterization of children with auditory neuropathy. *Ear and Hearing, 25*, 34–46.

Rance, G., Roper, R., Symonds, L., Moody, L. J., Poulis, C., Dourlay, M., & Kelly, T. (2005). Hearing threshold estimation in infants using auditory steady state responses. *Journal of the American Academy of Audiology, 16*, 293–302.

Santarelli, R., Starr, A. Michalewski, H. J., & Arslan, E. (2008). Neural and receptor cochlear potentials obtained by transtympanic electrocochleography in auditory neuropathy. *Clinical Neurophysiology, 119*(5), 1028–1041.

Sek, A., & Moore, B. C. J. (1995). Frequency discrimination as a function of frequency, measured in several ways. *Journal of the Acoustical Society of America, 97*, 2479–2486.

Shallop, J. K. (2002). Auditory neuropathy/dys-synchrony in adults and children. *Seminars in Hearing, 23*(3), 215–223.

Shallop, J. K., Peterson, A., Facer, G. W., Fabry, L. B., & Driscoll, C. L. (2001). Cochlear implants in five cases of auditory neuropathy: Postoperative findings and progress. *Laryngoscope, 111*, 555–562.

Sininger, Y. S., Hood, L. J., Starr, A., Berlin, C. I., & Picton, T. W. (1995). Hearing loss due to auditory neuropathy. *Audiology Today, 7*, 10–13.

Sininger, Y. S., & Oba, S. (2001). Patients with auditory neuropathy: Who are they and what can they hear? In Y. S. Sininger & A. Starr (Eds.), *Auditory neuropathy* (pp. 15–36). San Diego, CA: Singular.

Starr, A., Amlie, R. N. Martin, W. H., & Sanders, S. (1977). Development of auditory function in newborn infants revealed by auditory brainstem potentials. *Pediatrics, 60*(6), 831–840.

Starr, A., Isaacson, B., Zeng, F-G., Kong, Y-Y., Beale, P., Paulson, G. W., . . . Lesperence, M. M. (2004). A dominantly inherited progressive deafness affecting distal auditory nerve and hair cells. *Journal of the Association for Research in Otolaryngology, 5*(4), 411–426.

Starr, A., McPherson, D., Patterson, J., Don, M., Luxford, W., Shannon, R., . . . Waring, M. (1991). Absence of both auditory evoked potentials and auditory percepts dependent on timing cues. *Brain, 114*, 1157–1180.

Starr, A., Picton, T. W., Sininger, Y. S., Hood, L. J., & Berlin, C. I. (1996). Auditory Neuropathy. *Brain, 119*(3), 741–753.

Starr, A., Sininger, Y. S., & Pratt, H. (2000). The varieties of auditory neuropathy. *Journal of Basic and Clinical Physiology and Pharmacology, 11*(3), 215–230.

Starr, A., Sininger, Y. S., Winter, M., Derebery, M. J., Oba, S., & Michalewski, H. J. (1998). Transient deafness due to temperature-sensitive auditory neuropathy. *Ear and Hearing, 19*, 169–179.

Stein, L., Tremblay, K., Pasternak, J., Banerjee, S., Lindermann, K., & Kraus, N. (1996). Brainstem abnormalities in neonates with normal otoacoustic emissions. *Seminars in Hearing, 17*(2), 197–213.

Tang, T. P. Y., McPherson, B., Yuen, K. C. P., Wong, L. L. N., & Lee, J. S. M. (2004). Auditory neuropathy/auditory dyssynchrony in school children with hearing loss: Frequency of occurrence. *International Journal of Pediatric Otorhinolaryngology, 68*, 175–183.

Trautwein, P., Shallop J., Fabry, L., & Friedman, R. (2001). Cochlear implantation of patients with auditory neuropathy. In Y. S. Sininger & A. Starr (Eds.), *Auditory neuropathy* (pp. 203–232). San Diego, CA: Singular.

Vinay, & Moore, B. C. J. (2007). Ten(HL)-test results and psychophysical tuning curves for subjects with auditory neuropathy. *International Journal of Audiology, 46*(1), 39–46.

Vohr, B. R., Carty, L. M., Moore, P. E., & Letourneau, K. (1998). The Rhode Island hearing assessment program: Experience with statewide hearing screening (1993–1996). *Journal of Pediatrics, 133*(3), 353–357.

Walton, J., Gibson, W. P. R., Sanli, H., & Prelog, K. (2008). Predicting cochlear implant outcomes in children with auditory neuropathy. *Otology and Neurotology, 29*, 302–309.

Yellin, M. W., Jerger, J., & Fifer, R. C. (1989). Norms for disproportionate loss in speech intelligibility. *Ear and Hearing, 10*(4), 231–234.

Zeng, F.-G., Kong, Y.,-Y., Michalewski, H. J., & Starr, A. (2005). Perceptual consequences of disrupted auditory nerve activity. *Journal of Neurophysiology, 93*, 3050–3063.

Zeng, F.-G. & Liu, S. (2006). Speech perception in individuals with auditory neuropathy. *Journal of Speech-Language and Hearing Research, 49*, 36.

Zeng, F.-G., Oba, S., & Starr, A. (2001). Supra threshold processing deficits due to desynchronous neural activities in auditory neuropathy. In D. J. Breebaart, A. J. M. Houstma, A. Kohlrausch, V. F. Prijs & R. Schoonhoven (Eds.), *Physiological and psychophysical bases of auditory function* (pp. 365–372). Maastricht, The Netherlands: Shaker Publishing BV.

14

(Central) Auditory Processing Disorders in Children

Prudence Allen

What Is Auditory Processing?

For many children the understanding of complex sounds, particularly in difficult listening situations, is extremely difficult even though they have normal hearing sensitivity. They find it difficult to listen in noise, ignore competing signals, learn new sounds, or understand sounds that have been distorted in some way. This may lead to difficulty following orally-presented directions, learning from what they hear, achieving well in school, and developing good communication skills. These children likely suffer from an auditory processing disorder.

The discussion of auditory processing disorders and the clinical evaluation and treatment of these disorders are probably some of the most controversial areas of contemporary audiology. In spite of over 50 years of research and discussion on the topic there remains today no standard protocol for assessment or intervention. Our professional organizations have published recommendations (e.g., American Speech-Language, Hearing Association [ASHA], 1996, 2005a; British Society for Audiology [BSA], 2007; Jerger & Musiek, 2000), but the selection of clinical protocols remains under the discretion of the individual clinician. Test selection is difficult because there is no gold standard against which to evaluate the effectiveness of diagnostic tools. Most clinicians use a battery of tests for evaluation, but many of them report being unhappy with the contents of the battery (Chermak, Silva, Nye, Hasbrouck, & Musiek, 2007; Chermak, Traynham, Seikel, & Musiek, 1998; Emanuel, 2002; Noel, 2003). Rehabilitation protocols are not standardized and a clear link between diagnostic outcomes and treatment recommendations does not exist. Yet there is nearly unanimous agreement on the existence of the problem and that the care of individuals suffering from an auditory processing disorder falls within the scope of practice of audiologists (e.g., ASHA, 2005b; Canadian Academy of Audiology [CAA], 2002; BSA, 2007).

Auditory processing is the hearing that takes place beyond the ability to sense or detect the presence of a sound. It includes the ability to perceive, interpret, and ultimately understand a sound, even when the sound is presented in less than optimal conditions. It allows a listener to recognize familiar sounds and learn new ones, to make meaningful associations between what is heard and what is known, to be selective and vigilant in listening, and to be able to monitor and understand multiple sounds at once. Familiarity and sound quality play important roles in the efficiency of auditory processing. Perceiving familiar sounds, especially in a quiet environment, is relatively effortless. Links to memory and language representations are made easily and rapidly even if signal clarity is reduced. When the signals are unfamiliar, substantially degraded, or presented in a background of noise or other competition, significantly greater processing resources and effort may be required for understanding. There is often a greater need for clear acoustic features under such conditions and as new sounds are learned. For a person with an auditory processing disorder, understanding unfamiliar sounds or those presented in noise may be very difficult, especially if his or her encoding skills are impaired. The consequences of difficulty understanding these sounds can be debilitating when the listener is a child trying to learn from what they hear and when much of what they are learning includes new words that are presented in a noisy classroom.

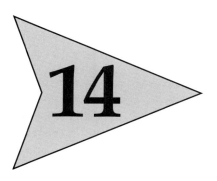

Learning from our perceptions is a complex process. Early theories suggested that perception is constructive, that sensory experiences are impoverished and that the mind is charged with the task of building mental representations from this impoverished information (see Gibson & Pick, 2003, for review). Children were thought to build their perceptions from their experiences and the emphasis was not on the information from the sensory system but on that which the child brought to the experience, that is, their prior knowledge. Perception was thought to be very much a top down, constructive process. Later theories argued that the sensory information and the environment in which it occurs are actually rich in detail and intimately linked (Gibson, 1991, 2000). During development a child learns to perceive and appreciate a much finer level of that detail. Perception is achieved within the context of a vast array of multisensory information coming from the environment in which the perception is taking place. Therefore, to understand perceptual development and the learning that results from it, consideration must be made of the quality of the sensory encoding, of the ability to attend to and explore the information as it is encoded, of the prior experience and knowledge the individual brings to the experience, and of the environment in which the perception occurs. It is because of the intricate links between sensation, attention and prior knowledge occurring within an environmental context that makes assessment of complex auditory processes challenging.

What are the processes used by a child as perceptual ability is developed and as the (auditory) world is organized? There are several principles by which perceptual development unfolds (e.g., Goldstone, 1998). These principles are useful as we consider whether a child has the proper auditory skills to serve perceptual development. At the neural level, patterns of activation are developed and reinforced in response to frequently occurring stimuli. This allows the recognition of familiar stimuli to be rapid and resistant to degradation. It underlies auditory learning and the plasticity observed in response to auditory training and the introduction of assistive listening devices. With repeated exposure the recognition of a stimulus is easier and quicker. The details become increasingly better perceived. As children mature they become more adept at focusing attention on stimuli that are of interest to them and on the detail within a stimulus. Children are active and selective in their perception, and this skill improves with maturation. Because of the integration of information with that from the other senses and prior knowledge, the sensory experience strengthens such that when the stimulus occurs again only some of the components may be necessary to bring about the perception of the entire event. This makes stimulus recognition and identification fast and efficient. It is more reliable, even in the face of noise or stimulus degradation.

A stimulus will be most easily recognized or learned when it is clear. Signal clarity is governed by the quality with which it is produced, the media in which it is transmitted to the listener, and the integrity of the auditory system that receives it. A signal may lose clarity through interference from ambient noise or distortion as could occur from poor room acoustics or because the transmission medium has limited bandwidth, reduced dynamic range, or produces harmonic distortion. The stimulus, when it is speech, may also appear to be distorted because the speaker has an unfamiliar accent, articulates poorly, or speaks at a very fast rate. Individuals with normal hearing are usually much less affected by reduced signal clarity than are individuals with auditory processing disorders. In fact, one way that audiologists traditionally test for the presence of an auditory processing disorder is to look for reduced recognition of noisy or distorted signals. Clinical tests have been developed that distort speech signals by adding noise, filtering, and time altering.

Signal clarity also will be affected by how well the auditory system of the listener receives and processes the stimulus. It is with this aspect of signal clarity that we are most concerned during clinical assessment. The processing of acoustic features generally occurs effortlessly through the responses and connections of brainstem nuclei (For a thorough review of the auditory system the reader is referred to the excellent material available in the Springer Handbook of Auditory Research, e.g., Popper & Fay, 1992; Webster, Popper, & Fay, 1992). Ascending from the cochlea, which has already coded the complex spectral and temporal qualities of the stimulus, the tonotopic information is transmitted to multiple nuclei where it is further analyzed, and information about the frequency, phase, and level relations of the components is coded. For example, the cochlear nucleus codes fine structure and envelope cues thus facilitating localization, aiding in signal-to-noise enhancement, and playing a role in pattern recognition, auditory attention and learning. The superior olive, the first site of binaural convergence of information, codes interaural time, phase, and level differences essential for placing sounds in space. The inferior colliculus, as an obligatory relay, sees the convergence of auditory information from the lower brainstem nuclei. It also receives input from the visual, somatosensory, auditory and motor areas of the cortex, making it a complex integrating center important for processing multisensory information, facilitating spectral coding and sound localization. The medial geniculate body of the thalamus transmits information from the brainstem to the cortex. It is significant for its role in attention, behavioral readiness, gain control, and selective signal amplification or suppression. The medial geniculate body preserves tonotopic and binaural representation coded at lower nuclei and receives input from the superior colliculus enabling coordination of visual, motor, and acoustic representation of images in three dimensional space. Furthermore, it aids in visual pursuit and plays a role in arousal through its links with the limbic system. At the level of the cortex the integrated signal links to memory, and associations and meaning is deter mined. The auditory system is thus highly complex.As signals progress from the cochlea to the cortex, multiple aspects of their features are coded and integrated with information from other senses and from the cortex, as ecologic theories of perception suggest. What ultimately reaches the cortex is actively determined by attentive mechanisms working through the efferent system. The process of perceiving sound is rich and active.

In the assessment of auditory processing disorders, we are interested in how the encoding of auditory signals takes place as a sound proceeds through the system and how encoding preserves the richness of information contained in those signals. Encoding can be evaluated through behavioral tests that measure discrimination and resolution abilities and through objective tests that measure the physiologic integrity of the neural pathways. A detailed review of auditory system anatomy and physiology as it relates to clinical pathology can be found in Musiek and Baran (2007). However, it is unlikely that with auditory processing disorders we will see a strong relationship between auditory skills and a specific locus within the central nervous system. Consideration of how the auditory system processes information should serve as a guide in how to think about auditory evaluation and what abilities are important, not as a way to determine a site of lesion. There is not a simple link between behavioral deficiencies and processing at specific levels of the auditory system.

Stimulus Encoding: Discrimination and Resolution of Acoustic Features

As with any audiologic assessment, one of the first areas to be examined is *detection*. It is critical to know what sounds are and are not audible. Assessment of detection typically includes the estimation of thresholds at octave intervals between 250 and 8000 Hz. Most children suspected of having disorders of auditory processing have normal pure tone thresholds in this range. High frequency thresholds (above 8 kHz) can be used to evaluate the effects of ototoxic drugs, noise, and other conditions (e.g., Goldstein, Shulman, & Kisiel, 1987) but thresholds in this range have not been studied in children with auditory processing disorders (APD) and the contribution of high frequency hearing to auditory function is not well understood. It has been suggested that adults with poor high-frequency thresholds report more difficulty hearing in noise than do individuals with good high frequency hearing (Liddell, Campbell, de Placido, Owens, & Wolters, 2007), but whether the reduced high frequency thresholds cause the difficulty hearing in noise or are comorbid with it is not clear. Although it is important that audibility be evaluated prior to any central auditory assessment, the presence of a peripheral hearing loss should not preclude an assessment of central auditory abilities if the child experiences difficulties that seem incommensurate with the degree of hearing loss.

Beyond the ability to detect signals, it is important to know how well stimulus features are discriminated or resolved. Discrimination of acoustic features can be measured by evaluating the smallest difference that can be perceived in an acoustic dimension. This is usually done by asking a listener to compare successively presented stimuli that vary in only one acoustic dimension. Resolution of features within a complex sound is slightly more complicated but also can be measured through discrimination tasks.

The minimum discriminable difference for frequency, level, and duration, vary with the base value of the stimulus and with the age of the listener. In the region where the ear is most sensitive, the 1000- to 4000-Hz range, and at a comfortable listening level, adults generally are able to perceive frequency differences of about 1 to 2% (Sek & Moore, 1995), level differences of less than 1 dB for signals above 40 dB HL (Florentine, Buus, & Mason, 1987), and durational increments of 15 ms for a 100-ms signal (e.g., Abel, 1972). Young, normal hearing children show improvements in basic discrimination abilities throughout the first few years of life, but large individual differences are seen (e.g., Jensen & Neff, 1993; Maxon & Hochberg, 1982). Improvements in the discrimination of intensity differences are fairly rapid with the discrimination of frequency and duration lagging behind and continuing to show variability into the school-aged years.

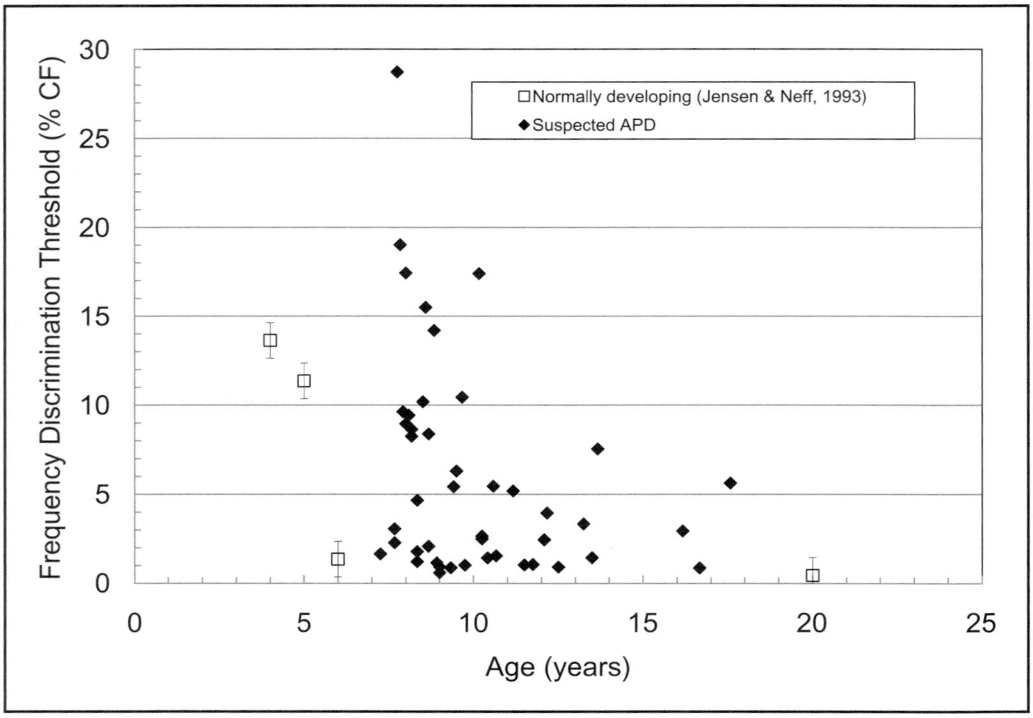

FIGURE 14–1. The frequency discrimination thresholds in normally developing children and in those suspected of having an auditory processing disorder. Open squares show averaged thresholds obtained from normal hearing preschool-aged children for a base frequency of 440 Hz (Jensen & Neff, 1993). Error bars show ±1 standard deviation. Filled diamonds show *individual* data obtained from children seen in our laboratory for auditory processing disorder assessment. Note the large variability in the performance of the children in the clinical sample. Many of the children performed at adultlike levels but many did not, performing consistently with younger children or much worse.

Poor *basic discrimination ability* has been observed in children with specific language impairment (Hill, Hogben, & Bishop, 2005), auditory neuropathy (Zeng, Oba, Garde, Sininger, & Starr, 1999) and those with cortical damage (Thompson & Abel, 1992). Preliminary data from our laboratory with children suspected of having auditory processing disorders suggest they may require much larger differences for discrimination of simple features than normally developing children of the same age. Frequency and discrimination data from these individual children are shown by the filled diamonds in Figures 14–1 and 14–2, respectively. Open squares show data from normally developing children averaged within age groups (Jensen & Neff, 1993). Error bars show ±1 standard deviation. Note the large variability in the clinical group. Many children perform at age-expected levels, but many perform more like younger normally developing children or worse. Unfortunately, there are as yet no clinical procedures available for estimating frequency or intensity discrimination thresholds.

Most natural sounds are perceived as temporally changing spectral patterns. It is not the absolute energy at any one frequency that predicts a sound's identity, but the relative distribution of energy across frequencies, the spectral shape, and how it changes over the signal duration that is important. Green (1988) suggests that even simple tasks such as intensity increment detection are likely perceived by analysis of spectral content within, not between, sounds.

Spectral resolution can be investigated using a variety of psychometric procedures. Two common ways include evaluation of psychoacoustic tuning curves (Zwicker & Fastl, 1999) and estimates of detection thresholds in flat and notched-spectrum noises (Patterson, 1976). These measures tend to reflect the integrity

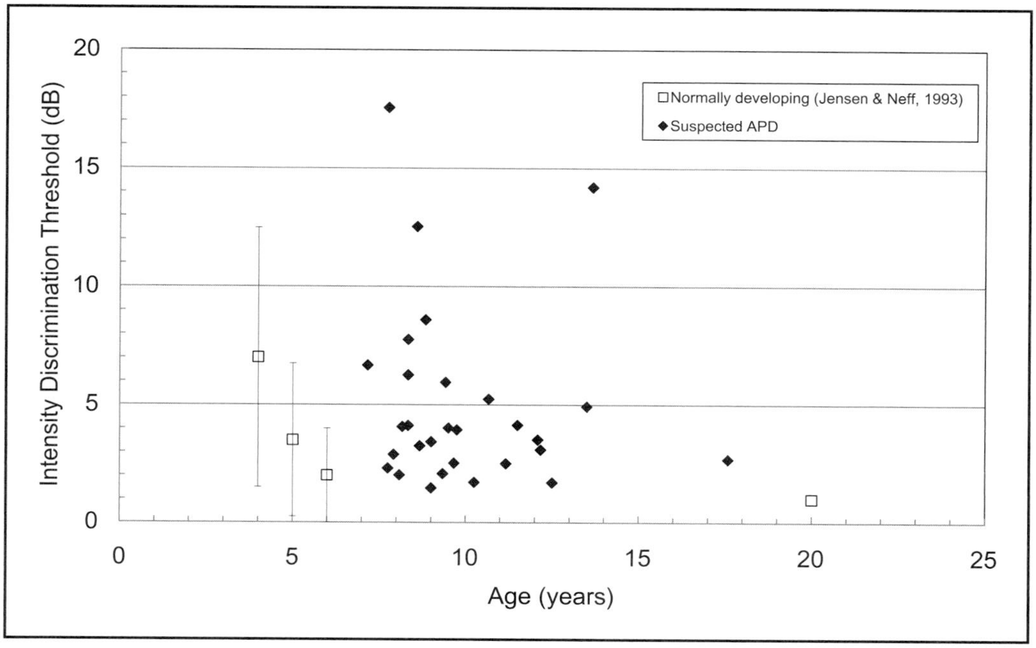

FIGURE 14–2. The intensity discrimination thresholds in normally developing children and in those suspected of having an auditory processing disorder. Open squares show data from 4- to 6-year-old children detecting an increment in a 440-Hz pure tone (Jensen & Neff, 1993). Error bars show one standard deviation. Filled diamonds show *individual* data from a group of children referred for testing for suspected auditory processing disorders. Note the large variability in performance with some children performing at close to age-appropriate levels and some performing very poorly or consistent with the performance of younger children.

of the auditory periphery, specifically the function of the basilar membrane mechanics and outer hair cells. Both give an estimate of auditory filter bandwidth and efficiency. Bandwidth reflects the sharpness of tuning arising from basilar membrane mechanics and outer hair cell function, and efficiency reflects the signal-to-noise ratio at which detection occurs arising from a variety of likely more central factors. Psychoacoustic tuning curves are measured by presenting a tonal signal at near threshold levels and measuring threshold shifts in the presence of narrowband noise maskers placed slightly above or below the signal. As the frequency of the masker moves away from the signal, more masker energy is required to eliminate signal audibility. The rate at which thresholds improve as the masker moves spectrally away from the signal can be used to estimate the tuning characteristics of the inner ear. Data from infants suggest that frequency resolution matures fairly rapidly although efficiency remains immature for a prolonged period (Olsho, 1985). Data obtained from notched-noise masking procedures show a more protracted period of immaturity in frequency resolution extending through the preschool-aged years (Allen, Wightman, Kistler, & Dolan, 1989). With this procedure, the listener is asked to detect a signal in a broadband noise masker. A spectral notch is then placed in the masker around the signal frequency. The presence of the notch should improve audibility of the signal. The amount of improvement is thought to reflect the tuning characteristics of the periphery. Greater improvement reflects sharper tuning.

Figure 14–3, panel A shows frequency resolution data obtained using the notched-noise masking procedure. Diamonds show data from the suspected APD population seen in our laboratory, and squares show data of normal-developing children from Allen et al. (1989). Filled symbols show threshold estimates in a

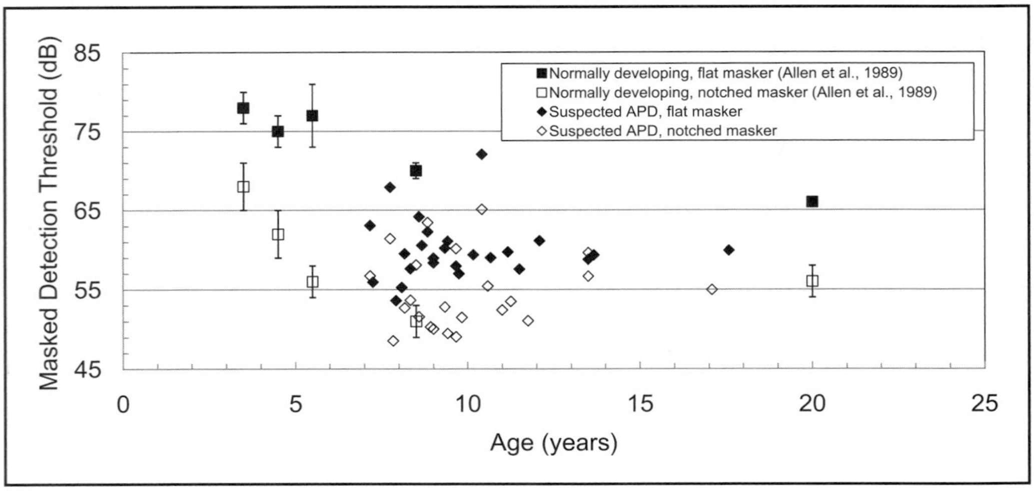

A

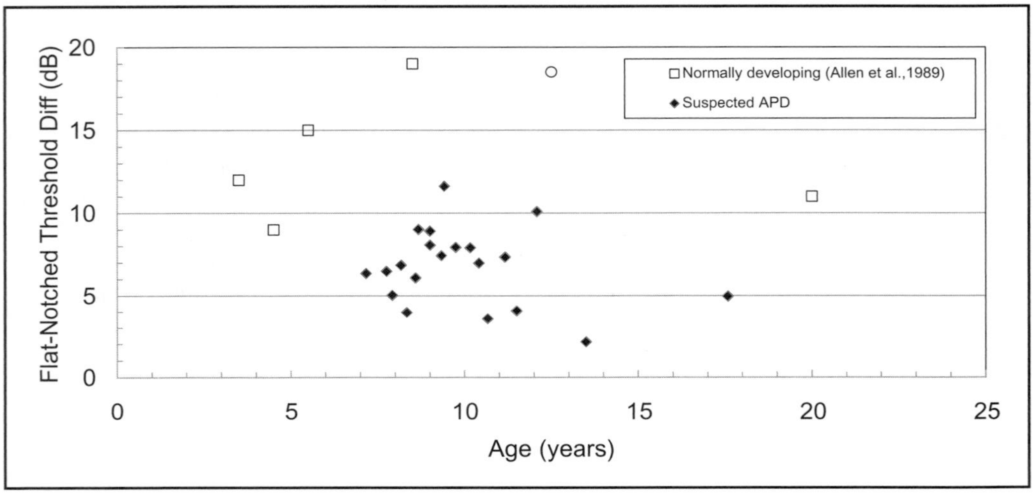

B

FIGURE 14–3. The frequency resolution data from normally developing children and those suspected of having an APD. (**A**) shows thresholds in the flat noise masker (*filled symbols*) and in the notched-noise masker (*open symbols*). Squares show averaged data from normally developing children at 2000 Hz (Allen et al., 1989) Filled diamonds show *individual* data at 1000 Hz from our laboratory obtained from children suspected of suffering from an auditory processing disorder. (**B**) shows the difference in thresholds in the flat versus notched noise masker. Open squares show averaged data from the normally developing children (Allen et al., 1989) and filled diamonds show individual data from the suspected APD children in our laboratory.

flat spectrum masker, and open symbols show thresholds estimated in the presence of a notched spectrum masker. Panel B shows threshold differences (flat versus notched noise thresholds). Averaged data from normally developing preschool-aged children are shown by the open squares (Allen et al., 1989) and filled diamonds show individual data from the suspected APD population.

As Figure 14–3, panel A shows, with increasing age thresholds for both conditions improve but the effect is more dramatic for the notched-noise masking condition, suggesting a greater amount of frequency selective listening in the older subjects. For the children with suspected APD, there is a trend for better thresholds in the notched noise masker than in the flat noise. However, as can be seen in panel B, the difference in two thresholds is in many cases smaller than for younger children, possibly suggesting reduced frequency resolution. This procedure has not been used extensively with clinical populations. However, Rosen and Manganari (2001) reported adultlike frequency resolution data using the notched-noise procedure with a group of children with reading problems. Because thresholds in these masking conditions for younger children may be affected by attentional factors including the acoustic cues to which the child attends (Allen & Korpela, 1999), additional research using other procedures may be warranted before the APD data are interpreted. However, it remains that this clinical population, for whatever reason, does seem to do more poorly on this task than normally developing children.

Temporal resolution has been studied extensively owing to the perceived importance to speech perception of the ability to perceive rapid changes in a stimulus. It is most frequently measured via gap detection thresholds. In this procedure listeners are asked to discriminate between brief duration signals (usually noise samples) that are either continuous or that have a temporal gap in them. The ability to detect a gap of various durations is measured. A broadband background noise is usually presented to limit any cues provided by spectral splatter resulting from the sharp rise and fall times around the gap.

Normal hearing adults can, with practice, generally discriminate temporal gaps of less than two milliseconds at higher frequencies. Children up to 6 years require much longer gaps for the same level of detection accuracy as adults (Irwin, Ball, Kay, Stillman, & Rosser, 1985; Wightman, Allen, Dolan, Kistler, & Jamieson, 1989). There is not only a change in gap detection threshold with age, but also a reduction in the variability between subjects.

Many individuals with auditory and learning disorders have been studied using gap detection tasks. Poor performance has been shown in children who have difficulties with reading or language (e.g., Wright et al., 1997) and in adults with auditory neuropathy spectrum disorders (ANSD; Zeng et al., 1999). Data from children with auditory processing disorders seen in our laboratory also show larger gap detection thresholds as can be seen in the filled diamonds of Figure 14–4. Also shown are averaged data from groups of normally-developing children from three different studies (Davis & McCroskey, 1980; Irwin et al., 1985; Wightman et al., 1989). Note the large developmental trend in performance and the large between-subject differences in the children with suspected APD. Many children perform at or near age-appropriate levels, but many perform much more poorly suggesting temporal processing deficits.

Because of the perceived importance of temporal resolution in speech processing, several tests of temporal resolution are available clinically, most assessing gap detection thresholds. These include, for example, the Auditory Fusion Test–Revised (McCroskey & Keith, 1996), the Random Gap Detection Test (Keith, 2000), the Gaps-in-Noise test (Musiek et al., 2005), and the Adaptive Test of Temporal Resolution (Lister, Roberts, Shackelford, & Rogers, 2006).

Temporal resolution is likely a much more complex construct than is exemplified in a simple gap detection threshold estimate. Other measures that assess the ability of the auditory system to code sounds rapidly in time include nonsimultaneous masking (e.g., forward and backward masking) and estimation of the temporal modulation transfer function. Nonsimultaneous masking procedures have suggested abnormal temporal processing in children with language impairments (e.g., Marler, Champlin, & Gillam, 2002; Wright et al., 1997) and reading disorders (Rosen & Manganari, 2001). Abnormal temporal modulation transfer functions have been observed in cases of ANSD (Kumar & Jayaram 2005; Zeng et al., 1999). More data examining these temporal processing abilities in children referred for auditory processing assessment are warranted.

Binaural Processing

Once auditory features are encoded at each ear, the information is combined to form a single image. This allows the listener to place the sound in space creating a three-dimensional listening environment and facilitating the separation of real-world sound sources. There are many ways to study binaural hearing in the laboratory, and the effect of hearing impairment on performance has been of interest among researchers for some time (see Durlach, Thompson, & Colburn, 1981). Some assess the way interaural differences in time and level are perceived and how they affect perceived position or loudness. These studies can be done using headphones. Other tasks assess the way sounds are perceived in three dimensional environments, asking listeners to discriminate between positions, detect perceived motion in a sound source, identify the sound source location, or perceive signals presented in noise that is spatially segregated from the signal. These free field studies take into account the frequency and location-dependent spectral changes that occur as a result of

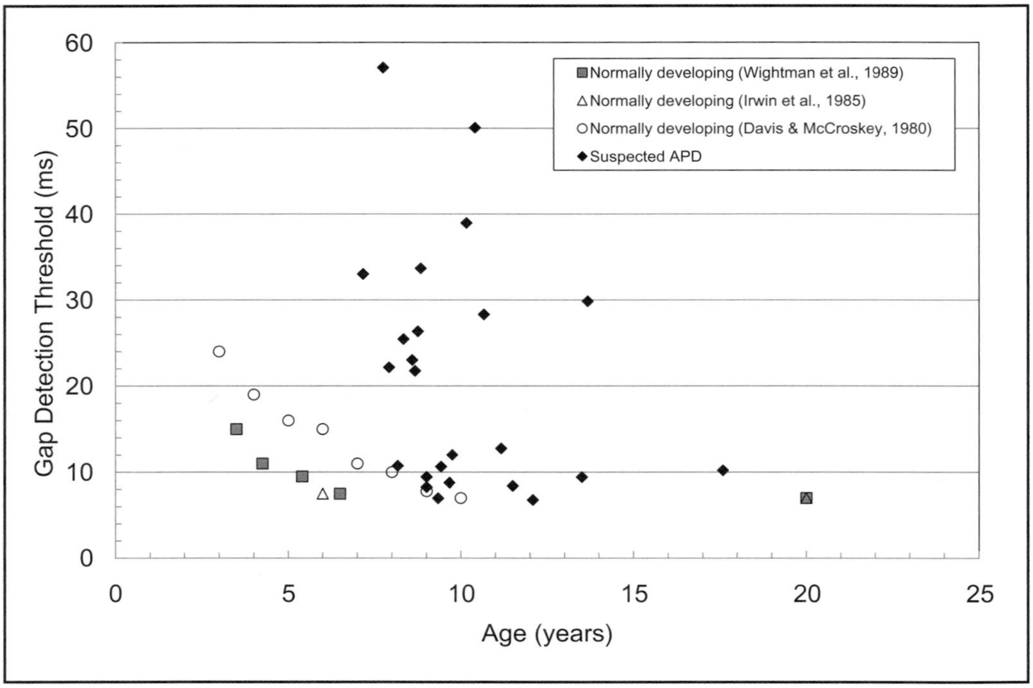

FIGURE 14–4. The gap detection thresholds in normally developing children and those who are suspected of having an auditory processing disorder. Open symbols show averaged data from normally developing children. Open squares show data from Wightman et al. (1989) made using a 2000-Hz signal. Open triangles show data from Irwin et al. (1985). Open circles show data from Davis and McCroskey (1980). Filled diamonds show *individual* thresholds at 1000 Hz from children seen in our laboratory. Many of the children show thresholds falling with age-expected ranges but many do not.

the outer ear resonance. These cues can be modeled to create simulated three-dimensional sensations under headphones. The spectral transforms are the head-related transfer functions (HRTFs). Although a great deal is now known about how the adult auditory system functions in a binaural environment, somewhat less is known about children's capabilities (see Litovsky & Ashmead, 1997) and how children with auditory processing disorders perform.

Most of what is currently possible in clinic is done under headphones. One method through which we can gain clinical information on how the binaural system functions is through estimation of the masking level difference (MLD). In this procedure the threshold for the detection of a binaural signal is estimated in the presence of a binaural masker. The signal can be speech or low-frequency pure tones. The masker is noise. Threshold is measured when the signal and masker are presented in phase at the two ears (S_0N_0) and when either the signal ($S_\pi N_0$), or the masker (S_0N_π), is 180 degrees out of phase at the two ears. Thresholds may improve 10 to 15 dB with a shift in the binaural phase of the signal or the masker.

Developmentally, the MLD to speech stimuli has been shown to be adultlike in preschool-aged children (Nozza, 1987; Nozza, Wagener, & Crandell, 1988), whereas the MLD elicited to narrow band stimuli showed a developmental trend until the age of 5 to 6 years (Grose, Hall, & Dev, 1997). The MLD in children with auditory processing disorders has been reported to be somewhat reduced (Sweetow & Reddell, 1978) possibly suggesting difficulties in the binaural integration of information between the two ears at the level of the brainstem (Olsen & Noffsinger, 1976). Data from children with suspected APD seen in our laboratory are shown in the filled diamonds of Figure 14–5. Open squares show averaged data from groups of normally developing children (Grose et al., 1997). Many of the

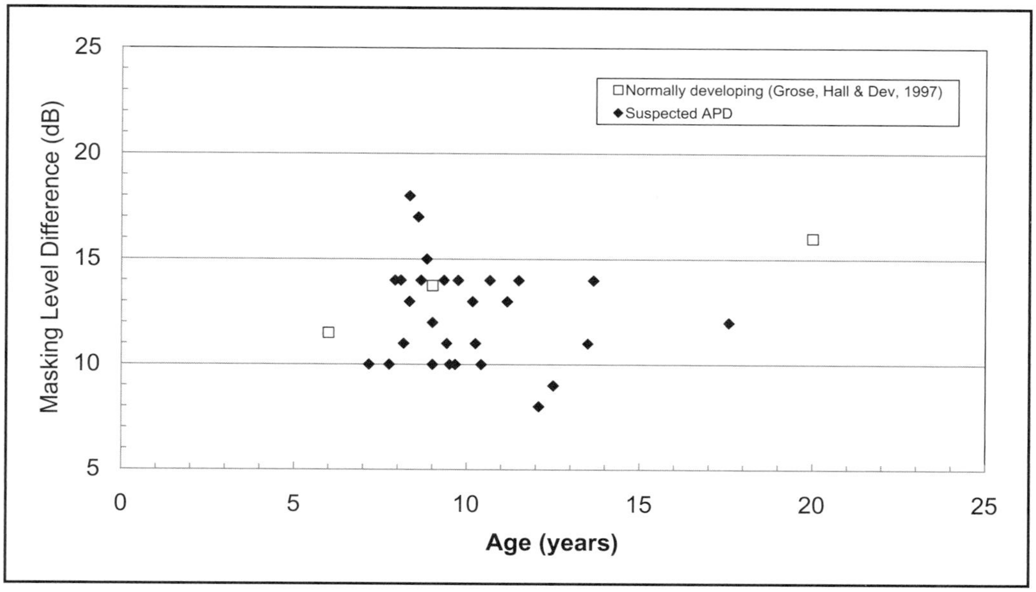

FIGURE 14–5. The average masking level differences for normally developing children in the open symbols (Grose, Hall, & Dev, 1997) and individual thresholds for children with suspected auditory processing disorders in the filled diamonds.

children with suspected APD children show an improvement of thresholds when the signal is out of phase at the two ears suggesting good MLDs, others do not.

More recently, studies have begun to test children in simulated three dimensional environments. In the Listening in Spatialized Noise-Sentence Test (LISN-S; Cameron & Dillon, 2008) speech reception thresholds are measured in the presence of competing noise that can be spatially separated from the signal allowing an estimate of the binaural advantage. The test creates a spatial perception through the use of head-related transfer functions and allows a perceived separation of speech and noise sources. Preliminary work with children having auditory processing disorders suggests this procedure may be useful in measuring a child's ability to benefit from binaural cues in the perception of speech in noise and has shown that many children with APD fail to derive a binaural advantage.

Binaural integration has also been measured through the presentation of speech signals that are spectrally or temporally split between the two ears. In the test of binaural fusion (Matzger, 1959) a speech signal is filtered into two narrow frequency bands. A low-pass band, 500 to 800 Hz, is presented to one ear and a high-pass band, 1815 to 2500 Hz, is presented to the other. Each band when presented alone does not permit good recognition of the signal. However, when both bands are presented, one to each ear, the signal is much more readily identified if the binaural system is intact. With central auditory processing disorders, specifically those originating in the brainstem, performance is reduced (Smith & Resnick, 1972). Recently, it has been shown that younger children require slightly wider frequency bands for the same level of speech recognition accuracy as adults, but that their ability to integrate the information from the two bands is similar to that of adults (Mlot, Buus, & Hall, 2010). Improvement in binaural fusion continues into the early school-aged years (Stollman, van Velzen, Simkens, Snik, & van den Broek, 2004). The speech stream may also be temporally split between the two ears using alternating segments (Bocca & Calearo, 1953). In the test of rapidly alternating speech perception (RASP; Willeford, 1976a), the speech signal is rapidly alternated between the two ears, often at a rate of 300 ms. The information arriving to one ear alone is unintelligible, but when both streams are presented to the intact system, the speech is easily understood. Adults with auditory processing deficits sometimes performed very poorly on these tests (e.g., Lynn & Gilroy, 1977; Musiek, 1983), and this is taken to suggest underlying difficulty at the level of the brainstem (Musiek & Geurking, 1982). Binaural fusion tests are available for clinical use through Auditec of St. Louis, although their use is falling out of favor as their sensitivity in detecting disorders is questionable.

Once signals reach the auditory cortex they can be recognized, and associations between what is heard and what is known can be made. Making these associations has a strong language and cognitive component. It is for this reason that central auditory evaluation should include a team of professionals and should include a pediatric speech-language specialist. There are numerous excellent tools available for assessing the phonologic and semantic aspects of hearing, the complete review of which is outside the scope of this chapter. Consultation with a qualified speech language pathologist is an invaluable tool in APD assessments.

The discrimination and resolution skills discussed so far are meant to provide a representative, though not exhaustive, sample of encoding abilities that can be used to assess (central) auditory function. With recent advances in testing capabilities, it is likely that psychophysical procedures will become an important part of our diagnostic battery in the future. Interpreting the results will require a greater understanding of normal variability and developmental changes. The advantage of these procedures is that they use non-speech signals that are easily calibrated and useful regardless of the child's first language. The procedures require relatively minimal language skills and therefore are useful even in cases of language problems. It should be noted, however, that individual differences are common in complex listening tasks and particularly so when children and/or clinical populations are tested. These differences most likely reflect characteristics of the listener, not error in the measurement. In some children, performance on a discrimination task, such as that described in these sections, may vary with their attention and motivation. In a study of masked detection thresholds for example, Allen and Wightman (1994) showed individual differences in psychometric functions that persisted across conditions and over several months. Approximately one-third of the preschool-aged children produced data with adultlike psychometric function slopes but elevated thresholds, one-third showed poor thresholds and shallower slopes, and the final third showed variability between conditions and between repetitions (Allen & Wightman, 1994). Similar results were reported by Moore and colleagues in a study of discrimination learning. In the examination of performance changes over time they found that children were likely to fall into one of three general categories, those with consistently good performance, those with consistently poor performance, and those who showed more variability with a tendency to do well initially and more poorly thereafter, possibly because of lost motivation over time (Moore, Ferguson, Halliday, & Riley, 2007). It also has been suggested that a child with an untreated attention disorder may do poorly on an auditory discrimination task suggesting, perhaps falsely, the existence of a hearing related disorder (e.g., Sutcliffe, Bishop, Houghton, & Taylor, 2006). Because attention and motivation can affect performance, it is important that in any psychophysical measurement of performance, repeated measures be taken, especially when performance is not at age expectations.

Auditory Attention: Listening as an Active Process

Normal hearing individuals generally are able to choose to what they will listen, at what level of detail, and for what duration. The ability to hear and understand signals in the presence of noise, the ability to concentrate on auditory information for extended periods, the ability to attend to multiple sources of information and to switch attention quickly and efficiently between sources are important aspects of how individuals hear and listen. These abilities are frequently reported areas of difficulty for individuals suffering from auditory processing disorders. We cannot evaluate complex hearing abilities without consideration of auditory attention.

What is attention? According to William James (1890, reprinted in 1966):

> Everyone knows what attention is. It is the taking of possession by the mind, in clear and vivid form, of one out of what seem several simultaneously possible objects or trains of thought. Focalization and concentration of consciousness are of its essence. It implies withdrawal from some things in order to deal effectively with others. (p. 5)

What causes a stimulus to take our attention? Familiar signals often do so, such as when we hear someone call out our name. Very strong signals or components of signals will also capture our attention, as will unusual or unexpected signals. Once something has taken our attention, how well can we sustain it over time, and can we explore it with an increasing level of detail? Can we continue to focus on something of interest and with what ease and for how long? Can we focus on multiple items simultaneously? What causes us to lose our attention? How distractible are we and under what circumstances? Regardless of how well an auditory signal is encoded, the ability to listen to it can be greatly influenced by our auditory attention abilities. As such, auditory attention has occupied a major place in central auditory assessment. Auditory attention includes the ability to intentionally attend to a signal or portion of a signal in the presence of another stimulus (selective attention), the ability to monitor multiple messages and to switch between them at will (divided attention and executive control), and the ability to maintain focus on an auditory signal of interest (sustained attention).

Selective Attention

Signals of interest in everyday life are seldom presented in isolation. Instead, we are most often asked to attend to signals in the presence of irrelevant signals that are considered to be noise or competition, largely because we deem them to be of no or lesser importance than the signal of interest. Similarly, we sometimes wish to listen to more detail in a signal, an important aspect of perceptual learning. Our ability to attend to the signal of interest, or a portion of that signal, is termed selective or focused attention. When noise interferes with the perception of the signal of interest it is deemed to be distracting, especially when there is unlikely to be peripheral masking from spectral and/or temporal overlap. Technologies that require a listener to repeat words as soon as they are heard (shadowing), retain the content of a message in the presence of competition, and avoid distraction (or intrusions) from a competing source, suggest that auditory selective attention matures throughout the school-aged years (Davies, Jones, & Taylor, 1984).

One method used to study auditory selective auditory attention is the probe-tone method (Greenburg & Larkin, 1968). In this procedure, a listener is led to expect a signal of a given frequency. On a random, small portion of the trials, the signal frequency is different. Highly selective attention would allow a listener to detect the expected signal very well but detection of the unexpected signal would be less reliable as attention is focused on the expected signal frequency. If the listener is not listening selectively, but using a broader auditory filter, the expected and unexpected signals would be perceived with equal proficiency. Very young children appear to listen broadly and not in a frequency selective manner (Allen, Spencer, & Eskritt, 2001). It is not until school age that children listen with good frequency selectivity (Greenburg, Bray, & Beasley, 1970). Listening in a frequency selective manner can also be evaluated using a distraction paradigm. In this procedure a signal at an off-frequency is presented simultaneously with a signal at an expected frequency. Frequency selective listening would eliminate any influence of the off-frequency distracter. As with attention band studies, distracter procedures also show that young children do not listen selectively. They are less able to "filter out" distraction, and detection accuracy for a signal that is otherwise readily detectable suffers in the presence of a distracter (Allen & Wightman, 1995; Bargones & Werner, 1994).

Direct measures of attention typically are not part of an audiologic battery. But some tests are included that indirectly assess selective attention. These include auditory figure ground tasks. In these tasks, recognition of a signal, usually speech, is measured in the presence of a masker, which may be broadband noise, multitalker babble or continuous discourse. The disruption that occurs, which cannot be attributed to simple masking of the signal (limiting audibility of some or all of the components), is called "informational masking." Tests of auditory figure ground for which the signal and masker are presented in the same ear include the Speech Perception in Noise (SPIN; Kalikow, Stevens, & Elliott, 1977), the Speech-in-Noise Test (Quick-SIN; Killion, Niquette, Gudmundsen, Revit, & Banerjee, 2004), the Hearing-in-Noise Test (HINT; Nilsson, Soli, & Sullivan, 1994), the Synthetic Sentence Identification with Ipsilaterally Competing Message (SSI-ICM; Speaks & Jerger, 1965), the Auditory Figure Ground subtest of the Screening Test for Auditory Processing Disorders for Children (SCAN-C; Keith, 2002), the Selective Attention Test of the Goldman-Fristoe-Wookcock Auditory Skills Test Battery (GFW; Goldman, Fristoe, & Woodcock, 1970), an optional subtest on the Test of Auditory Processing Skills (TAPS-3; Martin & Brownell, 2005), the Words in Ipsilateral Competition test (WIC; Ivey, 1987), and the Selective Auditory Attention Test (SAAT; Cherry, 1980).

Selective attention also can be assessed with the noise masker presented to the opposite ear. For example, the Pediatric Speech Intelligibility test presents word and sentence length material to the listener with competition that can be presented in the contralateral as well as the ipsilateral ear (PSI; Jerger, 1987). Poor performance on these various tests of auditory figure-ground perception frequently are observed in children with auditory processing disorders.

Divided Attention

Hearing in the natural world is dichotic. That is, there are slight differences in the phase, level, time of arrival, and spectral shape of a signal arriving at the two ears. This is in contrast to diotic stimulation in which both ears receive identical stimuli. Dichotic listening has occupied a central position in central auditory assessments for over 50 years. Early dichotic listening work originated in the development of filter theories of attention (e.g., Broadbent, 1958; Cherry, 1958) that postulated that the system had a limited capacity for processing information requiring a filter that could switch between the various available stimulus inputs. In these studies, the stimuli in the two ears are very different (e.g., different consonant-vowel pairs, digits, words, or sentences). The application to auditory processing disorders began with the work of Kimura (1961) who used dichotic consonant–vowel stimuli to study processing in individuals with brain lesions. She noted that patients with cortical lesions had difficulty perceiving the syllable presented in the ear contralateral to the lesion but did well with that presented to the ipsilateral ear. Since then, many tests of dichotic listening have gained popularity in clinical use. These include, for example, the Staggered Spondaic Word Test (Katz, 1962), which uses dichotic spondees tested in both noncompeting and competing conditions, dichotic consonant vowel syllables (Berlin, Hughes, Lowe-Bell, & Berlin, 1973) and digits (Musiek, 1983). These tasks require stimuli in both ears to be reported. Children with APD show large reductions in dichotic listening tests.

Sustained Attention

Another important aspect of attention is the ability to attend consistently over time. This aspect is less frequently tested in the clinic but may be important in children with auditory processing disorders. The question is whether children have problems simply attending to auditory information or if they cease to attend to information that is hard to understand (as would be the case if auditory processing were reduced). Most tasks that assess sustained attention require the individual to detect or identify signals in a very boring task that lasts for an extended period of time. Identification accuracy over time in these vigilance tasks is taken as an estimate of sustained attention ability. Studies using vigilance procedures suggest that performance improves during the early school years (see Davies et al., 1984). Sustained attention can also be studied by measuring how long a listener or observer will focus on a stimulus at will. Studies with infants have shown that inspection of an unfamiliar visual stimulus is longer than for a familiar one (Richards, 2004). This suggests that the ability to sustain attention at will is an important element of perceptual processing.

Some common tests of auditory attention that assess sustained and selective listening include the Auditory Continuous Performance Test (ACPT; Keith, 1994) and the Test of Everyday Attention for Children (TEA-Ch; Manly, Robertson, Anderson, & Nimmo-Smith, 1998). The ACPT asks a child to listen to words over a 10-minute period and indicate when a target word occurs. The TEA-Ch has nine subtests that evaluate auditory and visual attention in simple and complex tasks, some of which are timed. It tests not only selective and sustained attention but also the extent to which a child can regulate their attention, switching between tasks and inhibiting responses. Performance across the subtests is different for individuals with a primary attention disorder (e.g., ADD, ADHD) and those with traumatic brain injury (TBI). The TBI pattern shows general depression across all subtests examining selective and sustained attention as well as executive control. Interestingly, most children in our laboratory suspected to have an APD perform similarly to those with TBI, showing general depression across all subtests. Upper, middle, and lower panels of Figure 14–6, respectively, show individual composite scores on subtests examining sustained, selective attention, and executive control, respectively. Note that many children fall more than one standard deviation below expectations.

Note on Behavioral Indicators of Attention Disorders and Auditory Processing Deficits

Clinical identification of attention deficit disorder is made by addressing behavioral manifestations as indicated by the DSM-IV (American Psychiatric Association, 2000). The indicators identify behavioral symptoms of inattention or hyperactivity-impulsivity. Presence of these symptoms is evaluated within the context of onset, severity, and persistence before a diagnosis is made. One tool that is often used to delineate problem behaviors consistent with an attentional disorder and the DSM-IV classification criteria is the Conners' Rating Scales–Revised (Conners, 2000). Interestingly, some of these behaviors are very like those used to describe children with auditory processing disorders (e.g., fails to give close attention to detail, difficulty sustaining attention, does not seem to listen to what is being said, and gets distracted when given instructions to do something). It also is interesting that when children meeting the diagnostic classification for inattention or impulsivity are evaluated on cognitive tests that assess these constructs, the correlations are not convincing, the performance is not predictable, and the perform-

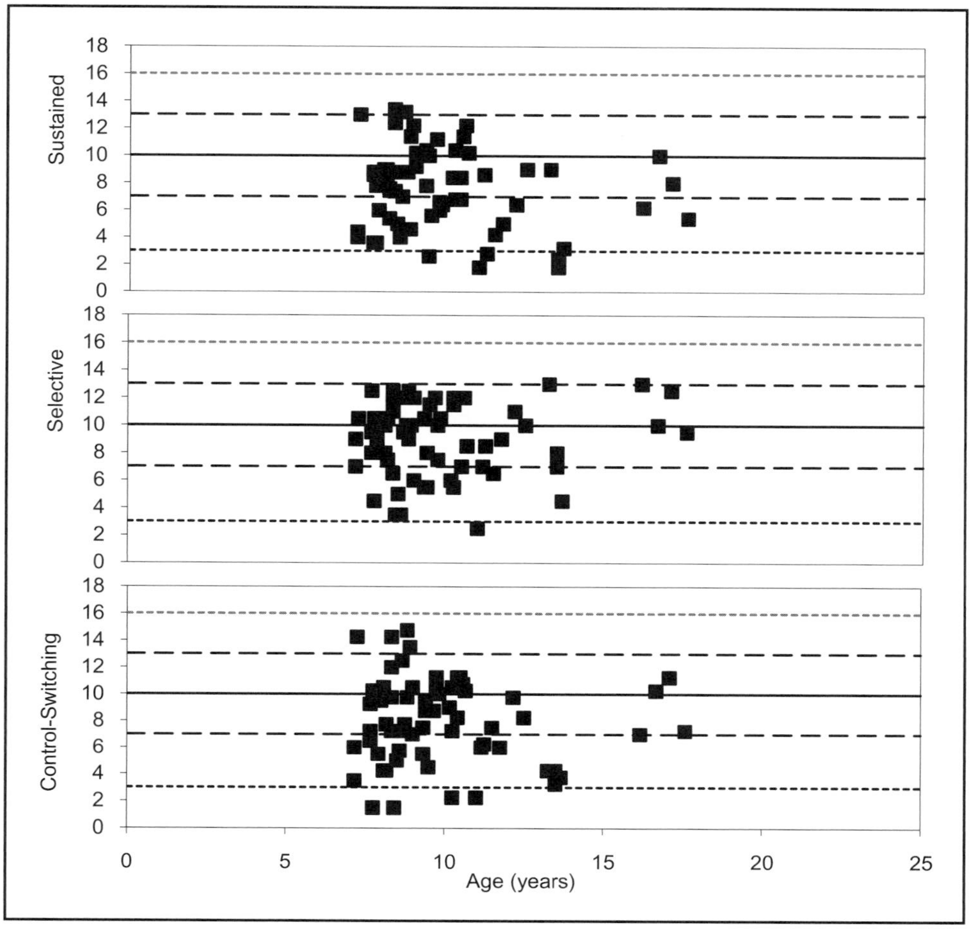

FIGURE 14–6. The composite scores on TEA-Ch subtests measuring sustained (*top*), selective (*middle*), and execute control (*lower*) in our group of children with suspected APD. Note that performance often falls one or more standard deviations below expectations on all types of attention.

ance deficits are not unique to children thought to suffer from attention disorders but are also seen in other clinical populations (see Swanson, Casey, Nigg, Castellanos, Volkow, & Taylor, 2004). This speaks to the importance of attention to most cognitive and learning abilities, including auditory processing.

Neural Integrity of the Auditory System Pathways

The ability of a listener to perceive subtle differences between sounds and hear the detail in complex sounds and attend to them will be a function of the underlying neurobiology of the auditory periphery and central mechanisms. Assessment of the neural integrity of the auditory pathways is therefore important in confirming the possible origins of the behavioral difficulties, in predicting difficulties in young children or others who may not be able to perform behavioral tasks and advancing earlier diagnosis of potential problems. For a more thorough review of how objective techniques can be used to assess auditory system integrity the reader is referred to Chapters 19 through 21 of this text. This section only reviews some areas of objective testing that may be particularly useful in assessing central auditory integrity.

Because of the significant encoding that takes place in the cochlea and brainstem pathways, it is important to conduct a thorough evaluation of the integrity of these structures. One useful measure is the acoustic reflex threshold, particularly when ipsilaterally and contralaterally stimulated and measured reflexes are compared. Elevated or absent reflexes can be seen in cases of disruption of low brainstem pathways. When ipsilateral reflexes are intact but contralateral reflexes are abnormal, it is an indication of pathology in the intra-axial brainstem, whereas a pattern of abnormalities both ipsi- and contralaterally more often are associated with extra-axial lesions (Jerger & Jerger, 1975, 1977). Although reflex abnormalities are common in cases of confirmed lesions, they have been reported to be less so in cases of suspected APD (Jerger, Johnson, & Loiselle, 1988). However, in our laboratory we have observed a large proportion of the children showing abnormal crossed reflexes in the presence of normal ipsilateral responses. Figure 14–7 shows data from the children with suspected APD seen in our laboratory (Allen & Allan, 2007). Average reflexes at 500, 1000, and 2000 Hz stimulated and recorded ipsilaterally are plotted against the average at those same frequencies stimulated in one ear and recorded in the contrateral ear. Individual data for right and left ears are shown by the circles and diamonds, respectively. Note the large numbers of children for whom ipsilateral thresholds are elicited at normal levels but contralateral responses are not. These children also tend to do quite poorly on clinical tests of central auditory processing disorders suggesting a possible link between efferent system dysfunction and APD.

Another excellent measure of auditory brainstem integrity is the auditory brainstem response (ABR). Although auditory processing disorders are believed to be diffuse in locus with peripheral function likely to be normal (e.g., Hood, 2007) we have observed a large number of abnormal ABRs in children referred for central auditory testing. This suggests poor neural integrity of the auditory nerve and brainstem in at least a portion of the children suffering from these dis-

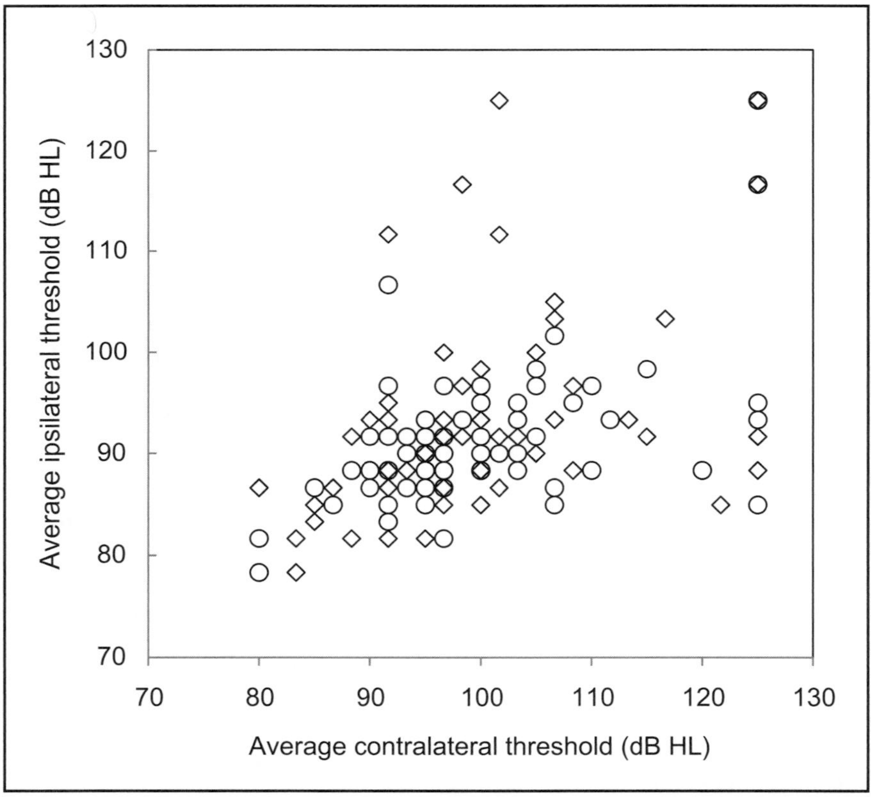

FIGURE 14–7. The average ipsilateral reflex threshold for 500, 1000, and 2000 Hz plotted against the same three frequency average for reflexes elicited with contralateral stimulation. Diamonds and circles represent data for left and right ear stimulation, respectively. Each data point represents data from one child. Reprinted with permission from Allen and Allan, 2007, Figure 2. Copyright 2007 Phonak AG.

orders (Allen & Allan, 2007). Abnormalities include poor replicability, missing waves, low V/I amplitude ratios, and delayed latencies. Figure 14–8 shows ABR wave V latencies in a group of children with suspected APD seen in our laboratory. Symbols show individual wave V latencies from right and left ears plotted for both slow and fast repetition rates. Several of the children show latencies more than two standard deviations beyond expectations even at a slow repetition rate with rate dependent abnormalities common. Figure 14–9 shows sample waveforms from two of the children (Allen & Allan 2007). The top panel shows responses with prolonged wave V latencies and low V/I amplitude ratios. The bottom panel shows responses with only wave V present and at a delayed latency. These results suggest that the neural integrity of the ABR may be reduced in children with APD. For a more detailed description of these two children and their other test results see Allen and Allan (2007).

The auditory steady-state response (ASSR) may be one of the more useful potentials for evaluating neural correlates to suprathreshold hearing processes. The ASSR is an evoked response to stimuli that are frequency or amplitude modulated. The response is evaluated in the frequency domain rather than in the time domain. It has been used to estimate psychophysical tuning curves (Markessis et al., 2009), temporal acuity (Purcell, John, Schneider, & Picton, 2004), and complex stimuli such as speech (e.g., Aiken & Picton, 2006; Banai, Abrams, & Kraus, 2007; Dimitrijevic, John, van Roon, & Picton, 2001). It may prove to be a very useful tool for the clinical estimation of such processing skills in young children or those who cannot complete behavioral testing. To date, there is still only a small amount of data on children with suspected auditory problems and these potentials.

Integrity of the binaural pathways may also be measured using the ABR. The Binaural Interaction

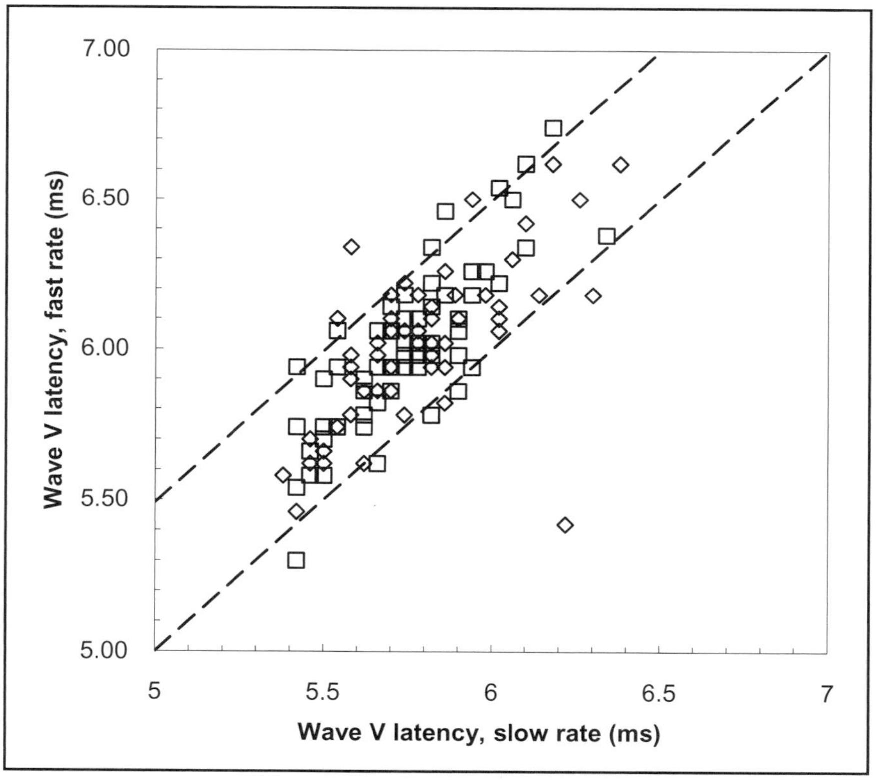

FIGURE 14–8. Wave V ABR latencies for individual children elicited to click stimuli at a faster repetition rate (57.7/sec) plotted against wave V latencies measured for a slower stimulation rate (11.1–31.1/sec). Data for left and right ears are shown by diamonds and squares, respectively. Reprinted with permission from Allen and Allan, 2007, Figure 4. Copyright 2007 Phonak AG.

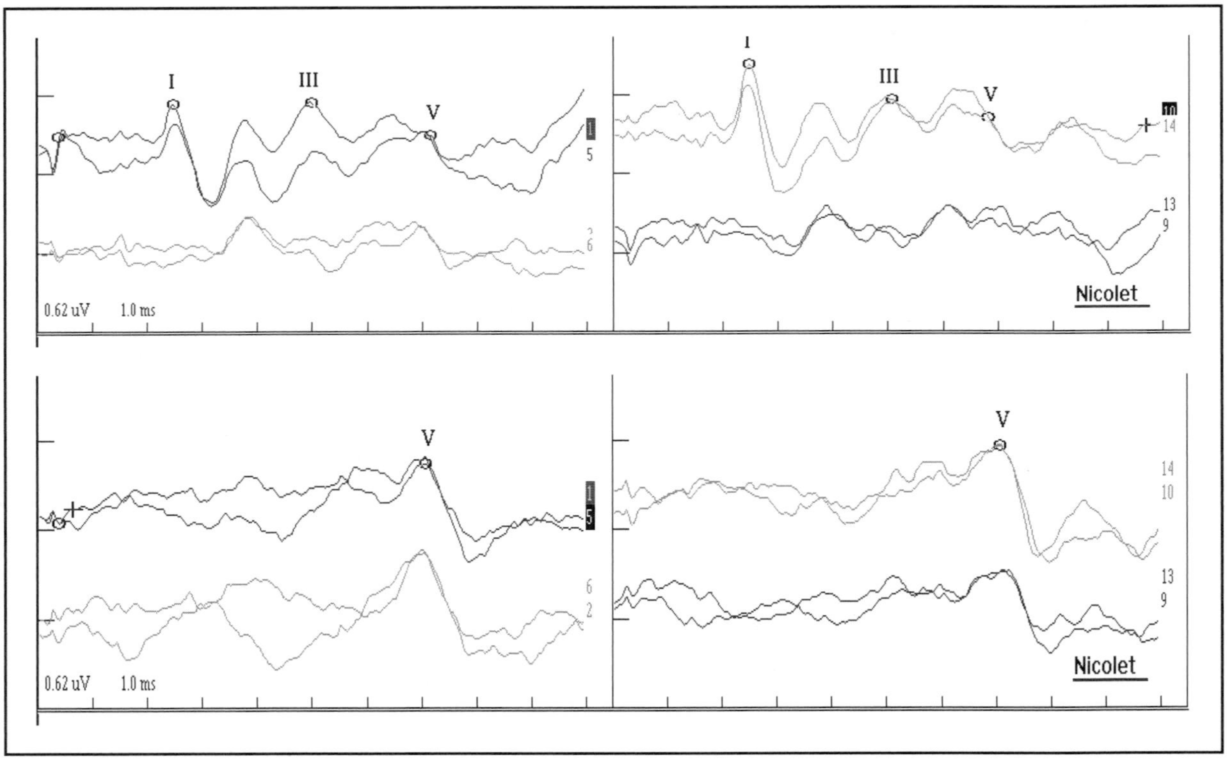

FIGURE 14–9. Auditory brainstem responses for two children with suspected APD seen at our laboratory. Left-most panels show left ear stimulation; right panels show right ear stimulation. Upper and lower traces show ipsilateral and contralateral recordings, respectively. *Top:* Auditory brainstem responses for subject CAFH show slightly delayed wave III (4.18 and 4.10 for right and left ears, respectively) and V (5.94 and 6.27 for right and left ears, respectively) latencies producing a prolongated I–III and I–V interwave interval. The amplitude of wave V relative to wave I is also quite low. *Bottom:* Auditory brainstem testing with subject CACN using a slow rate of stimulation (27.7/sec) shows significantly abnormal responses. Waves I–III are missing and wave V is significantly delayed in latency (6.18 bilaterally). Reprinted with permission from Allen and Allan, 2007, Figures 12 and 13. Copyright 2007 Phonak AG.

Component (Dobie & Berlin, 1979; Dobie & Norton, 1980) is obtained through a subtractive technique comparing the summed responses to monaural stimulation with the response elicited from binaural stimulation. A small negative going potential in the 7- to 9-ms range likely reflects the binaural activity in the brainstem (Polyakov & Pratt, 1994). A binaural response also occurs in the 20- to 40-ms range when evaluating middle latency responses (Berlin, Hood, & Allen, 1984). Neither procedure has enjoyed widespread clinical use although there is a strong potential for yielding data on the integrity of the binaural auditory system. For example, reduced amplitudes of the binaural interaction component of the brainstem have been observed in children with suspected APD when compared to those of age-matched normal-hearing children (Delb, Strauss, Hohenberg, Plinkert, & Delb, 2003; Gopal & Pierel, 1999). The ASSR may also be useful in the evaluation of binaural processing (Schwarz & Taylor, 2005).

Because we know that damage to higher auditory centers, such as the cortex, also have been known to produce abnormal discrimination abilities, it is important to examine auditory potentials evoked primarily from these regions. The middle and late evoked potentials are candidates for this analysis. Also, there have been several studies examining discrimination correlates in the cortex via event related potentials, most notably the P300 response for which an infrequent stimulus is presented in a train of more frequent stimuli. The response to the different stimulus, when compared to the expected stimuli, can give an indication of discrimination for that change. Due to its variability between subjects, the P300 has not enjoyed a great deal of success in clinical application. The mismatch negativity response (Näätänen, Gaillard, & Mantysalo, 1978) is a cortical evoked potential that may have some applicability to auditory attention as it appears to represent a pre-attentive response to discrimination. The potential is measured using an oddball paradigm in which an odd stimulus is interspersed in a train of expected stimuli. The response to this odd stimulus represents neural activity occurring prior to discrimination. It is measured using subtractive techniques but, like the P300, clinical use has been limited due to high between- and within-subject variability.

Professional Practice

ASHA, the American Academy of Audiology (AAA) and the BSA have published position papers on Auditory Processing Disorders (ASHA, 1996, 2005a; BSA, 2007; Jerger & Musiek, 2000). The Canadian professional associations are in the process of preparing a statement. It is clear from these initiatives that the associations are trying to meet the needs of their members in providing rigorous, evidenced-based solutions to the understanding, diagnosis, and treatment of hearing disorders that fall beyond sensitivity losses.

The documents from ASHA are noteworthy for their excellent review of scientific and professional issues surrounding auditory processing and its disorders as well as their treatment of clinical issues. ASHA suggests that central auditory processing refers to the " . . . perceptual processing of auditory information in the CNS and the neurobiological activity that underlies that processing . . . " (ASHA 1996, p. 145). It involves those mechanism that underlie " . . . sound localization and lateralization, auditory discrimination, auditory pattern recognition, temporal aspects of audition including temporal integration, temporal discrimination, temporal ordering, and temporal masking; auditory performance in competing acoustic signals (including dichotic listening); and auditory performance decrements with degraded acoustic signals" (ASHA 2005a, p. 2). A disorder is deemed to be present when there is an observed deficiency in any of these areas. Similarly, the BSA (2007) acknowledges the neural underpinnings of APD in their statement that an APD " . . . results from impaired neural function and is characterized by poor recognition, discrimination, separation, grouping, localization, or ordering of nonspeech sounds" (p. 1). Their statement acknowledges that an APD may impact on speech sounds but that the label of APD should be applied only when nonspeech sound perception is impaired, in an attempt to avoid confusing language-based problems from those that arise from auditory processing deficits. The presenting problems of APD noted include " . . . understanding when listening to speech, reading, remembering instructions or staying focussed while listening" (p. 3).

The test battery approach is universally recommended for assessment although the specific tests are not named and the categories of tests are somewhat varied across recommendations. For some categories (e.g., localization and lateralization, basic discrimination) there are few tests commercially available. It generally is accepted that an evaluation begins with a thorough case history and information, and it is also important to obtain a description of the problem the child is experiencing. Issues such as understanding speech in difficult listening situations or noise, problems understanding and receiving auditory information, problems with auditory attention, and difficulties learning songs, reading, and spelling must be determined. A good way to get at these issues is through the use of behavioral checklists and questionnaires. These can help delineate the types of situations in which the child experiences difficulty and can guide the assessment protocol. Possible checklists include, for example, the Children's Auditory Performance Scale (CHAPS; Smoski, Brunt, & Tannahill, 1992), the Fisher Auditory Problems Checklist (Fisher, 1976), or the Screening Identification for Targeting Educational Risk (SIFTER; Anderson, 1989). These tools have normative data for children of various ages and grade levels. They also are useful for flagging the situations in which the child may have the most difficulty.

It also is clinical practice to begin an APD evaluation with a thorough evaluation of peripheral hearing status. This includes pure tone thresholds, speech discrimination in quiet, otoacoustic emissions, and immittance testing. The goal primarily is to rule out a middle ear or cochlear problem, although comorbidity between peripheral and central auditory problems may exist. Acoustic reflex thresholds are also included in assessment recommendations although interpretation of abnormal results is not addressed in the various task force or professional association reports other than in their use in evaluating peripheral system integrity and possibly ruling out ANSD. In the several surveys of professional practice in APD assessment mentioned earlier, acoustic reflex thresholds were used by the majority of clinicians in their assessment battery.

It is further recommended that evaluation include assessment of the reception of both speech and nonspeech signals. Many speech type tests are available for APD evaluation. In one category there are speech tests that attempt to degrade the signal in some way, such as by filtering, time altering, or presenting background noise or competition, either monaurally or dichotically.

Also, it generally is agreed that tests of basic discrimination be included in any APD assessment. ASHA recommends tests that evaluate frequency and intensity discrimination, frequency resolution and temporal processes including gap detection, and forward and backward masking. Adaptive procedures embedded in a rigorous psychoacoustic paradigm generally are not available at this time but given the improvements in signal processing capabilities it is likely that such testing will be available in the future (e.g., Meng, 2009; Park, 2008).

Pattern recognition tests also figure quite prominently in test recommendations. Commercially available tests that are most popular include the Pitch Pattern Sequencing Test (Pinheiro & Musiek, 1985) and the Duration Pattern Sequencing Test (Musiek, Baran, & Pinheiro, 1990). In these tests, the listener is presented with a series of three tones and must report back the pattern they heard. In the Pitch and Duration Pattern test, the tones differ in frequency or duration, respectively. Children with APD tend to have a great deal of difficulty perceiving the patterns correctly. One of the interesting aspects of these patterning tests is their possible relationship to the processing of envelope information and the slower changing acoustic features of a signal so important to the perception of prosody, an area we have found difficult for many children with auditory processing disorders (McFaddden, 2006).

For the clinical interpretation of test results it is recommended that performance be evaluated against age expectations to determine if a deficiency represents a clinical problem or a maturational delay and to examine performance within a child to determine areas of relative strength and weakness. This requires that a test have good normative data. It is recommended that for a diagnosis of APD, performance on at least two tests should be two standard deviations or more below expectations. Performance at least three standard deviations below age expectations on only one test also may be considered significant if there are significant behavioral indicators consistent with an APD (ASHA, 2005a). The specific tests to be used and the number of tests are not specified.

Objective measures are also strongly encouraged in APD assessment although there is some controversy about how to interpret the results (Katz et al., 2002). Among the recommended procedures are OAEs and acoustic reflexes with decay, and evoked responses such as the ABR, middle and late responses, the 40-Hz response, ASSR, frequency-following responses, and event related potentials. Such tests are thought to prove most useful in the testing of young children for whom behavioral testing may be difficult, when a neurologic disorder is suspected, or to confirm behavioral findings that may be inconclusive. These tests likely are very important given the strong belief stated by our professional associations that the neurobiologic processes that underlie auditory processing are critical for proper functioning.

Because auditory processing difficulties most likely do not occur in isolation, and because success in academics and communication depends upon multiple skills, it is strongly encouraged that other areas of processing be evaluated when a child is referred for APD assessment. Specifically, the assessment of language, cognition, and memory are recommended.

Screening

The issue of screening is not addressed extensively in the documents by ASHA (1996, 2005a) however it is addressed in some detail in the document from the AAA (Jerger & Musiek, 2000). This latter report suggests a screening tool is required and acknowledges that in seeking high sensitivity there will be a tradeoff with specificity. However, the importance of a suitable screening test is emphasized. The document suggests that screening can be done via a behavioral checklist and/or by testing. In agreement with ASHA, the suggestion is made that the behavioral checklists should tap the functions of interest in auditory processing, that is, perception of speech in noise or other difficult listening situations, the ability to follow oral instructions, discriminate between and identify speech sounds, and auditory inattention. A screening test, they state, should include one measure of dichotic perception, specifically, the perception of dichotically presented digits, and a test of gap detection to assess temporal processing. In a more recent editorial, Jerger (2009) noted that the search for a " . . . simple, quick, and easy to score screening test for APD . . . " (p. 160) may be inappropriate. He argues for a more thorough and systematic approach to assessment of this complex disorder even though it may be more time consuming.

As a minimal test battery, the AAA recommends (Jerger & Musiek, 2000) evaluation of pure tone thresholds, speech discrimination testing over a range of presentation levels, dichotic listening, duration pattern sequencing, and gap detection thresholds. Supporting this minimal battery is a recommendation for immittance including tympanometry, acoustic reflex thresholds and otoacoustic emissions to rule out problems in the middle and inner ears. To evaluate the status of the brainstem and cortex, auditory brainstem and middle latency evoked responses are recommended.

Current Practice Patterns

What audiologists actually do in clinical assessment varies greatly between individuals and clinics and has changed over time. Chermak et al. (1998) reported the results of a survey taken in the United States just after the first ASHA task force report was published in 1998. Responses were received from 183 audiologists. This same survey was also sent to audiologists in Canada to which 101 registered audiologists responded (Noel, 2003). Chermak's group reported that 48% of the audiologists responding conducted central auditory assessments and most used a test battery approach but were unhappy with their choice of battery. The most common tests used included two objective procedures: acoustic reflexes and ABR. The behavioral test most frequently used varied by location of practice. Audiologists practicing in the school system used the SCAN (Keith, 2002), a screening test that samples the perception of filtered speech, speech in noise, competing words and competing sentences. Audiologists practicing in medical settings were most likely to use the Staggered Spondaic Word Test (SSW; Katz, 1962). Also used frequently were the Low-Pass Filtered Speech Test (FS; Willeford, 1976b) and the Synthetic Sentence Identification with Ipsilateral Competing Message (SSI-ICM; Speaks & Jerger, 1965). Binaural hearing was evaluated, although not frequently, using a test of binaural fusion (Calearo & Antonelli, 1973). Noel's results in Canada (2003) showed that the two most frequently used tests were acoustic reflexes and the SCAN. Infrequently audiologists reported using frequency patterns, dichotic digits, and the SSW. As with their American colleagues, most were dissatisfied with their protocols.

Emanuel (2002) reported the results of a survey a few years later suggesting that most clinicians continued to use the SCAN or the SSW as their primary behavioral assessment tool. Electrophysiologic measures remained in common use and included the ABR and acoustic reflexes. One change since 1998 was an increase in the use of systematic behavior questionnaires such as the Children's Auditory Performance Scale (CHAPS; Smoski et al., 1992), the Fisher Auditory Problems Checklist (Fisher, 1976), or the Screening Identification for Targeting Educational Risk (SIFTER; Anderson, 1989), a practice that had been suggested in the Task Force Report of 1998 (ASHA, 1998). An additional change in practice was the use of tests of auditory attention and memory, such as the Auditory Continuous Performance Test (Keith, 1994) or the Screening Auditory Abilities Test (SAAT; Cherry, 1980). In the category of monaural degraded speech tests clinicians reported two subtests of the Test of Auditory Processing Disorders in Children–Revised (SCAN; Keith, 2000)-Filtered Words and Auditory Figure Ground. Other low redundancy speech tests used included filtered speech, time compressed speech, and speech presented in the presence of ipsilateral noise or competing messages. Slightly less commonly used were tests of temporal processing in spite of their endorsement. The most commonly used test in that category was the Pitch Pattern Sequence Test (PPS; Pinheiro & Musiek, 1985). A few reported use of the duration pattern test and the Auditory Fusion Test (AFT-R; McCroskey & Keith, 1996), which tests gap detection. Few respondents reported using binaural tests, unlike the previous survey report. Of those that did, the Rapidly Alternating Speech Test (RASP; Willeford, 1976a) and the masking level difference (MLD) were the most common.

In a follow-up to their 1998 survey, Chermak and colleagues (Chermak et al., 2007) found that acoustic reflexes remained the most frequently used test but that the ABR had fallen in popularity. Some of the same procedures remained in use including dichotic tests (competing sentences, the SSW, dichotic digits) and filtered speech. However, pitch and duration pattern testing, speech in noise testing, and the Fisher's questionnaire emerged as more common procedures and the use of reflex decay and middle latency responses became more popular.

Summary

It is unfortunate that in spite of so many years of interest and concern and volumes of research, we are still in a state of questioning over how to assess (and even what to call) auditory processing disorders. As the proceeding sections have attempted to show, the auditory system is extremely complex and the unraveling of acoustic signals and the derivation of meaning from them that takes place holds many opportunities for disruption. Perhaps part of the problem in APD assessment lies in this complexity and our inability to easily define patient populations that are similar enough to allow us to establish definitive tests that evaluate hearing and listening skills. Perhaps one of the most promising changes in audiologic assessment has come with the recognition of ANSD. In these individuals, we are able to see a wide range of hearing sensitivity levels with hearing problems that far exceed these thresholds. Through our study of these disorders, we are beginning to find new ways to assess hearing and new ways to understand auditory system pathology. Some of the behaviors seen in children with APD are not unlike those presented by individuals with ANSD. It is possible that some of our children with APD may be suffering from some form of neural disorder that is similar to ANSD, either in kind or in neural location. Still others may be suffering from similar neural disruptions that are occurring more central in the auditory nervous system, beyond the auditory nerve and lower brainstem.

It is clear from these reports that clinicians use a test battery approach and that they try to adhere to the recommendations of their professional associations. Limiting factors included the poor availability of materials for adaptive discrimination testing, the lack of standardization in most available tests, limited access to electrophysiologic test equipment in some practices, lack of materials suitable for many different first languages, and poor availability of suitable procedures for very young children.

As is noted in our professional association reports (ASHA 1996, 2005a; Jerger & Musiek, 2000), much research is needed in the area of APD assessment. It is suggested that tests be developed that use rigorous psychophysical principles, validate these tests against individuals with known central nervous system problems, and make these tests commercially available. Techniques that use rigorous, adaptive psychophysical procedures to examine basic discrimination and resolution abilities in children with APD are much needed before they will be useful clinically. Laboratory psychometric measures have been used for a number of years with very young children (e.g., Allen & Wightman, 1992, 1994; Allen et al., 1989; Wightman et al., 1989) and coupled with new advancements in technology these procedures may be adapted for clinical use in the very near future (Meng, 2009; Park, 2008). This will certainly enhance the ability of clinicians to evaluate the manner in which the child's auditory system preserves signal clarity.

Rehabilitation

Auditory processing disorders must not be thought of as a specific disease entity. The term more appropriately describes the types of problems an individual with a hearing loss may experience when there is difficulty hearing, but the cause cannot be attributed to a loss of audibility. Until such time as we have greater knowledge of the underlying causes of the problems, treatment will be limited to the amelioration of behavioral issues. This requires that we find ways to make listening easier, to help build the child's cognitive abilities so as to minimize the difficulties they experience, and to help them manage their hearing and learning more effectively through metacognitive strategies. The literature on aural rehabilitation for APD is vast and there are many good texts giving strategies, treatment plans, and theories (Bellis, 1996; Chermak & Musiek, 2007; Katz, 2009; Masters, Stecker, & Katz, 1998; Sloan, 1991). Unfortunately, there is a relative paucity of efficacy research in most areas.

Categories of intervention strategies can be placed into a few broad areas. These include improving the quality of the signal, training the auditory system to recognize signals more effectively by taking advantage of neural plasticity, teaching the child to know when they will have difficulty and providing strategies to improve coping, and facilitating speech and language processing skills to enable better proficiency in general communication abilities. As with any treatment plan, the beginning is a comprehensive assessment protocol that will delineate the child's pattern of strengths and weaknesses. The treatment plan must be individualized and the child's progress with any recommendations must be carefully monitored.

Improving Signal Quality

If the auditory system is compromised such that degraded signals or those presented in noise or competition are poorly perceived, one intervention is to improve the quality and clarity of the signal. This can be accomplished by improving the acoustics in the room such that signal transduction is better. Rooms in which there is significant noise and/or reverberation will degrade the quality of the signal. Allowing instruction to take place in rooms that are acoustically treated and quiet can help not only children with auditory processing disorders, but all children who are learning new or unfamiliar material. Recommendations for improving the acoustics of learning spaces have been published (ANSI, 2002). In many cases it is difficult to achieve the recommended levels for noise, particularly since the children themselves will create a large amount of noise in any active learning environment. For children with APD it may be useful to fit them with an FM device that will transmit to their ear a clear sound with a better signal-to-noise ratio (Rosenberg, 2002).

Auditory Training

Taking advantage of auditory plasticity and improving neural connections and efficiency is a key concept underlying another category of rehabilitative techniques. Generally, auditory training programs are intensive, requiring the child to work at them for extended periods of time several days each week. The difficulty of the tasks is generally presented in graded difficulty and most often target specific stimulus features or dimensions. Chermak and Musiek (2002) provide a fairly comprehensive review of remedial techniques in the area of auditory training for children based on their primary area of difficulty. For those whose primary problems are in basic discrimination they recommend training in speech and nonspeech discrimination tasks in graded difficulty. For difficulties in temporal processing they recommend sequencing tasks, prosody training, poetry reading, and following directions. For problems with the perception of speech in noise or degraded conditions, vocabulary building and practice listening in degraded or noisy conditions is recommended, and for those with binaural hearing deficits a variety of dichotic listening tasks may be appropriate.

Speech and Language Training

Perhaps as much, or more, than any other area of pediatric audiology, the speech-language pathologist will be a valued asset in the intervention team for children with auditory processing disorders. A child will rely less on acoustic features when the sounds and words to which they listen are familiar and well learned. Exercises aimed at building the child's vocabulary, improving their knowledge of language structures, and predicting vocabulary content, will be key in minimizing the impact of an auditory processing disorder.

Metacognitive Strategies, Self-Advocacy, and Compensatory Strategies

It is important that we find ways to help children to cope with hearing difficulties. Tools to help them predict what situations will be most difficult and to aid them in minimizing the impact of being asked to work in difficult situations or tasks is very important. It is critical that intervention consider the child's self esteem and minimize failures. To do so will require the involvement of parents, guardians, and teachers. Chermak (1998) outlines a management approach that is designed to allow children to help themselves. Key features include attribution training that motivates the child to continue to try to do well, cognitive behavior modification that is designed to promote active and self-regulatory listening behavior, reciprocal teaching that is aimed at promoting flexibility in the selection of appropriate strategies, and assertiveness training that is designed to build self-confidence and self-esteem.

Summary and Conclusions

Auditory assessment for auditory processing should consider the child's auditory skills within the context of adequacy for perceptual development and in support of learning and language development. The goal should be to assess the behavioral and neurologic integrity of the auditory system. What skills does the child have or not have? Can the child identify and discriminate between sounds and resolve features within sounds? Are acoustic components properly integrated into useful wholes that can be positioned in a three-dimensional space? Can the child selectively attend to sounds of interest and do so in a sustained manner even when the sounds are unfamiliar or presented in a difficult listening situation? Is the underlying neural integrity such that auditory skills are functional and mature according to age-matched peers or is neural integrity showing reduced synchrony and transmission delays that could be expected to impair auditory processing? If we can answer these questions then, as audiologists, we will have made a useful contribution to the team of professionals who are supporting the child's academic and social growth and development. We can then better prepare audiologic rehabilitation programs that are not general to all children with hearing difficulties, but that speak to the areas of strength and weakness in the individual child.

References

Abel, S. M. (1972). Duration discrimination of noise and tone bursts. *Journal of the Acoustical Society of America, 51*, 1219–1223.

Aiken, S., & Picton, T. W. (2006). Envelope following response to natural vowels. *Audiology and Neuro-Otology, 11*, 213–232.

Allen, P., & Allan, C. (2007). Putting the "neural" back into sensorineural hearing loss. In R. C. Seewald & J. M. Bamford (Eds.), *A sound foundation through early amplification 2007: Proceedings of the fourth international conference* (pp. 221–233). Stäfa, Switzerland: Phonak AG.

Allen, P., & Korpela, L. (1999). Notched-noise measures of frequency resolution in children revisited: What acoustic cues are available at children's threshold levels? Proceedings of the Joint meeting of Acoustical Society of America and the European Acoustical Association, Berlin, Germany. *Journal of the Acoustical Society of America, 105,* 1152(A).

Allen, P., Spencer, D., & Eskritt, K. (2001). Frequency selective listening in children as indicated by the measurement of auditory attention bands. *Association for Research in Otolaryngology*, St Petersburg, Florida.

Allen, P., & Wightman, F. (1992). Spectral pattern discrimination by children. *Journal of Speech and Hearing Research, 35,* 222–233.

Allen, P., & Wightman, F. (1994). Psychometric functions for children's detection of tones in noise. *Journal of Speech and Hearing Research, 37,* 205–215.

Allen, P., & Wightman, F. (1995). Effects of signal and masker uncertainty on children's detection. *Journal of Speech and Hearing Research, 38,* 503–511.

Allen, P., Wightman, F., Kistler, D., & Dolan, T. (1989). Frequency resolution in children. *Journal of Speech and Hearing Research, 32,* 317–324.

American National Standards Institute (ANSI). (2002). *Acoustical performance criteria, design requirements, and guidelines for schools.* New York, NY: Author.

American Psychiatric Association. (2000). *Diagnostic and statistical manual of mental disorders (DSM-IV-TR)* (4th ed., text revision). Washington, DC: Author.

American Speech-Language-Hearing Association. (ASHA). (1996). Central auditory processing: Current status of research and implications for clinical practice. *American Journal of Audiology, 5,* 41–54.

American Speech-Language-Hearing Association (ASHA). (2005a). *(Central) Auditory processing disorders* [Technical report]. Available from http://www.asha.org/policy

American Speech-Language-Hearing Association (ASHA). (2005b). *Scope of practice.* Available from http://www.asha.org/policy

Anderson, K. L. (1989). *S.I.F.T.E.R: Screening Instrument for Targeting Educational Risk in children identified by hearing screening or who have known hearing loss.* Danvill, IL: The Interstate Printers and Publishers.

Banai, K., Abrams, D., & Kraus, N. (2007). Sensory based learning disability: Insights from brainstem processing of speech sounds. *International Journal of Audiology, 46,* 524–532.

Bargones, J. Y., & Werner, L. A. (1994). Adults listen selectively; Infants do not. *Journal of the American Psychological Society, 5,* 170–174.

Bellis, T. J. (1996). *Assessment and management of central auditory processing disorders in the educational setting: From science to practice.* San Diego, CA: Singular.

Berg, K. M. & Boswell, A. E. (2000). Noise increment detection in children 1 to 3 years of age. *Perception and Psychophysics, 62,* 868–873.

Berlin, C., Hood, L., & Allen, P. (1984). Asymmetries in evoked potentials. In C. I. Berlin (Ed.), *Hearing science.* San Diego, CA: College-Hill Press.

Berlin, C., Hughes, L. F., Lowe-Bell, S. S., & Berlin, H. L. (1973). Dichotic right ear advantage in children 5–13. *Cortex, 9,* 394–403.

Bocca, E., & Calearo, C. (1953). Central hearing processes. In J. Jerger (Ed.), *Modern development in audiology* (pp. 337–370). New York, NY: Academic Press.

British Society for Audiology (BAS). (2007). *Position statement final draft.* Retrieved June 24, 2010, from http://www.thebsa.org.uk/apd/BSA_APD_Position_statement_Final_Draft_Feb_2007.pdf

Broadbent, D. E. (1958). *Perception and communication.* London, UK: Pergamon.

Calearo, M. D., & Antonelli, A. R. (1973). Disorders of the central auditory nervous system. In M. Paparella & D. Shumrick (Eds.), *Otolaryngology* (pp. 407–425). Philadelphia, PA: Saunders.

Cameron, S., & Dillon, H. (2008). The listening in spatialized noise-sentences test (LISN-S): Comparison to the prototype LISN and results from children with either a suspected (central) auditory processing disorder or a confirmed language disorder. *Journal of the American Academy of Audiology, 19,* 377–391.

Canadian Academy of Audiology (CAA). (2002). *Position statement on audiology scope of practice.* Available at: http://www.canadianaudiology.ca/professionals/position_statements/ scope_of_practice.html#scope

Chermak, G. D. (1998). Metacogntive approaches to managing central auditory processing disorders. In M. G. Masters, N. A. Stecker, & J. Katz (Eds.), *Central auditory processing disorders: Mostly management.* Boston, MA: Allyn and Bacon.

Chermak, G. D., & Musiek, F. E. (2002). Auditory training: Principles and approaches for remediating and managing auditory processing disorders. *Seminars in Hearing, 23,* 297–308.

Chermak, G. D., & Musiek, F. E. (Eds.). (2007). *Handbook of (central) auditory processing disorder: Comprehensive intervention, Vol II.* San Diego, CA: Plural.

Chermak, G. D., Silva, M. E., Nye, J., Hasbrouck, J., & Musiek, F. E. (2007). An update on professional education and clinical practices in central auditory processing. *Journal of the American Academy of Audiology, 52,* 428–452.

Chermak, G. D., Traynham, W. A., Seikel, J. A., & Musiek, F. E. (1998). Professional education and assessment practices in central auditory processing. *Journal of the American Academy of Audiology, 9,* 452–465.

Cherry, E. C. (1958). Some experiments on the recognition of speech with one and two ears. *Journal of the Acoustical Society of America, 25,* 975–979.

Cherry, R. (1980). *Selective Auditory Attention Test (SAAT).* St. Louis, MO: Auditec.

Conners, C. K. (2000). *Conners' Rating Scales-Revised.* North Tonawanda, NY: Multi-Health Systems.

Davies, D. R., Jones, D. M., & Taylor, A. (1984). Selective- and sustained-attention tasks: Individual and group differences. In R. Parasuraman & D. R. Davies (Eds.), *Varieties of attention.* New York, NY: Academic Press.

Davis, S. M., & McCroskey, R. L. (1980). Auditory fusion in children. *Child Development, 51,* 75–80.

Delb, W., Strauss, D., Hohenberg, G., Plinkert, P. K., & Delb, W. (2003). The binaural interaction component (BIC) in children with central auditory processing disorders (CAPD). *International Journal of Audiology, 7,* 401–412.

Dimitrijevic, A., John, M. S., van Roon, P., & Picton, T. W. (2001). Human auditory steady-state responses to tones independently modulated in both frequency and amplitude. *Ear and Hearing, 22,* 100–111.

Dobie, R., & Berlin, C. (1979). Binaural interaction in brainstem evoked responses. *Archives of Otolaryngology, 105,* 391–398.

Dobie, R., & Norton, S. (1980). Binaural interaction in human auditory evoked potentials. *Electroechphalography and Clinical Neurophysiology, 49,* 303–313.

Durlach, N. I., Thompson, C. L., & Colburn, H. S. (1981). Binaural interaction in impaired listeners: A review of past research. *Audiology, 20,* 181–211.

Emanuel, D. C. (2002). The auditory processing battery: Survey of common practices. *Journal of the American Academy of Audiology, 13,* 93–117.

Fisher, L. (1976). *Fisher's auditory problems checklist.* Bemidji, MN: Life Products.

Florentine, M., Buus, S., & Mason, C. R. (1987). Level discrimination as a function of level for tones from 0.25 to 16 kHz. *Journal of the Acoustical Society of America, 81,* 1528–1541.

Gibson, E. J. (1991). *An odyssey in learning and perception.* Cambridge, MA: The MIT Press.

Gibson, E. J. (2000). Perceptual learning in development: Some basic concepts. *Ecological Psychology, 12,* 295–302.

Gibson, E. J., & Pick, A. D. (2003). *An ecological approach to perceptual learning and development.* New York, NY: Oxford University Press.

Goldman, R., Fristoe, M., & Woodcock, R. (1970). *Goldman-Fristoe-Woodcock test of auditory discrimination.* San Antonio, TX: Pearson, Psychological Corporation.

Goldstein, B., Shulman, A., & Kisiel, D. (1987). Electrical high frequency audiometry: Preliminary medical audiologic experience. *Audiology, 26,* 321–331.

Goldstone, R. (1998). Perceptual learning. *Annual Review Psychology, 49,* 585–612.

Gopal, K. V., & Pierel, K. (1999). Binaural interaction component in children at risk for central auditory processing disorders, *Scandanavian Audiology, 28,* 77–84.

Green, D. M. (1988). *Profile analysis: Auditory intensity discrimination.* New York, NY: Oxford University Press.

Greenberg, G. Z., Bray, N. W., & Beasley, D. S. (1970). Children's frequency- selective detection of signals in noise. *Perception and Psychophysics, 8,* 173–175.

Greenberg, G. Z., & Larkin, W. D. (1968). Frequency-response characteristic of auditory observers detecting signals of a single frequency in noise: The probe-signal method. *Journal of the Acoustical Society of America, 44,* 1513–1523.

Grose, J. H., Hall, J. W., & Dev, M. B. (1997). MLD in children: Effects of signal and masker bandwidths. *Journal of Speech, Language, and Hearing Research, 40,* 955–959.

Hill, P. R., Hogben, J. H., & Bishop, D. M. (2005). Auditory frequency discrimination in children with specific language impairment: A longitudinal study. *Journal of Speech, Language and Hearing Research, 48,* 1136–1146.

Hood, L. J. (2007). Auditory neuropathy and dys-synchrony. In R. F. Burkard, J. J. Eggermont, & M. Don (Eds.), *Auditory evoked potentials: Basic principles and clinical application.* Philadelphia, PA: Lippincott Williams and Wilkins.

Irwin, R. J., Ball, A. K. R., Kay, N., Stillman, J. A., & Rosser, J. (1985). The development of auditory temporal acuity in children. *Child Development, 56,* 614–620.

Ivey, R. G. (1987). *Words in ipsilateral competition (WIC)–Version 2.* Unpublished Normative Study.

James, W. (1966). Attention. In P. Bakan (Ed.), *Attention.* Princeton, NJ: D. Van Norstrand.

Jensen, J. K., & Neff, D. L. (1993). Development of basic auditory discrimination in preschool children. *Psychological Science, 4,* 104–107.

Jerger, J. (2009). Editorial: On the diagnosis of auditory processing disorder. *Journal of the American Academy of Audiology, 20,* 160.

Jerger, J., & Jerger, S. (1975). Extra- and intra-axial brainstem auditory disorders. *Audiology, 14,* 93–117.

Jerger, J., & Jerger, S. (1977). Diagnostic value of cross vs. uncrossed acoustic reflexes: Eighth nerve and brainstem disorders. *Archives of Otolaryngology, 103,* 445–453.

Jerger, J., & Musiek, F. (2000). Report of the consensus conference on the diagnosis of auditory processing disorders in school-aged children. *Journal of the American Academy of Audiology, 11,* 467–474.

Jerger, S. (1987). Validation of the pediatric speech intelligibility test in children with central nervous system lesions. *Audiology, 26,* 298–311.

Jerger, S., Johnson, K., & Loiselle, L. (1988). Pediatric central auditory dysfunction: Comparison of children with confirmed lesions versus suspected processing disorders. *American Journal of Otology, 9,* 63–71.

Kalikow, D. N., Stevens, K. N., & Elliott, L. L. (1977). Development of a test of speech intelligibility in noise using sentence materials with controlled word predictability. *Journal of the Acoustical Society of America, 61,* 1337–1351.

Katz, J. (1962). The use of staggered spondaic words in assessing the integrity of the central auditory system. *Journal of Auditory Research, 2,* 327–337.

Katz, J. (2009). *Therapy for auditory processing disorders: Simple effective procedures.* Westminster, CO: Educational Audiology Association.

Katz, J., Johnson, C. D., Tillery, K. L., Brander, S., Delagrange, T. N., Ferre, J. M., . . . Stecker, N. A. (2002). *Clinical and research concerns–Regarding Jerger & Musiek (2000) APD recommendations.* Retrieved June 24, 2010, from www.audiologyonline.com/articles/pf_article_detail.asp?article_id=341

Keith, R. W. (1994). *The Auditory Continuous Performance Test.* San Antonio, TX: Psychological Corp.

Keith, R. W. (2000). *Random Gap Detection test.* St. Louis, MO: Auditec.

Keith, R. W. (2002). *SCAN-C Revised. A Screening test for auditory processing disorders.* San Antonio, TX: Psychological Corp.

Killion, M. C., Niquette, P. A., Gudmundsen, G. I., Revit, L. J., & Banerjee, S. (2004). Development of a quick speech-in-noise test for measuring signal-to-noise ratio loss in normal-hearing and hearing-impaired listeners. *Journal of the Acoustical Society of America, 116*, 2395–2405.

Kimura, D. (1961). Cerebral dominance and the perception of verbal stimuli. *Canadian Journal of Psychology, 15,* 166–171.

Kumar, A. U., & Jayaram, M. (2005). Auditory processing in individuals with auditory neuropathy. *Behavioral and Brain Functions, 1,* 1–21.

Liddell, A., Campbell, P., DePlacido, C., Owens, D., & Wolters, M. (2007). *Can extended high frequency hearing thresholds be used to detect auditory processing difficulties in an ageing population?* Proceedings of the European Federation of Audiology, Heidelberg, Germany.

Lister, J. J., Roberts, R. A., Shackelford, J., & Rogers, C. L. (2006). An adaptive clinical test of temporal resolution. *American Journal of Audiology, 15,* 133–140.

Litovsky, R., & Ashmead, D. (1997). Development of binaural and spatial hearing in infants and children. In R. H. Gilkey & T. R. Anderson (Eds.), *Binaural and spatial hearing* (pp. 571–592). Hillsdale, NJ: Lawrence Erlbaum Associates.

Lynn, G. E., & Gilroy, J. (1977). Evaluation of central auditory dysfunction in patients with neurological disorders. In R. W. Keith (Ed.), *Central auditory dysfunction.* New York, NY: Grune and Stratton.

Manly, T., Robertson, I. H., Anderson, V., & Nimmo-Smith, I. (1998). *Test of Everyday Attention for Children (TEA-Ch).* Toronto, Cananda: Pearson Assessment, PsychCorp.

Markessis, E., Poncelet, L., Colin, C., Coppens, A., Hoonhorst, I., Kadhim, H., & Deltenre, P. (2009). Frequency tuning curves derived from auditory steady state evoked potentials: A proof-of-concept study. *Ear and Hearing, 30,* 43–53.

Marler, J. A., Champlin, C. A., & Gilliam, R. B. (2002). Auditory memory for backward masking signals in children with language impairment. *Psychophysiology, 39,* 767–780.

Martin, N., & Brownell, R. (2005). *Test of auditory processing skills* (3rd ed). Novato, CA: Academic Therapy.

Masters, M. G., Stecker, N. A., & Katz, J. (1998). *Central auditory processing disorders: Mostly management.* Boston, MA: Allyn and Bacon.

Matzker, J. (1959).Two methods for the assessment of central auditory functions in cases of brain disease. *Annals of Otolaryngology, Rhinology and Laryngology, 68,* 1155–1197.

Maxon, A. B., & Hochberg, I. (1982). Development of psychoacoustic behavior: Sensitivity and discrimination. *Ear and Hearing, 3,* 301–308.

McCroskey, R. L., & Keith, R. W. (1996). *Auditory fusion threshold test-revised.* St. Louis, MO: Auditec.

McFadden, M. (2006). *The receptive prosodic abilities of children with auditory processing disorders: A comparative study.* Unpublished master's thesis, University of Western Ontario.

Meng, Q. (2009). *Design and evaluation of portable psychoacoustic testing systems.* M.E.Sc. thesis. Dept. of Electrical and Computer Engineering, University of Western Ontario, London, ON.

Mlot, S., Buus, E., & Hall, J. W. (2010). Spectral integration and bandwidth effects on speech recognition in school-aged children and adults. *Ear and Hearing, 31,* 56–62.

Moore, D. R., Ferguson, M. A., Halliday, L. F., & Riley, A. (2007). Frequency discrimination in children: Perception, learning and attention. *Hearing Research, 238,* 147–154.

Musiek, F. E. (1983). Assessment of central auditory dysfunction: The dichotic digit test revisited. *Ear and Hearing, 4,* 79–83.

Musiek, F., & Baran, J. A. (2007). *The auditory system: Anatomy, physiology, and clinical correlates.* Boston, MA: Allyn and Bacon.

Musiek, F., Baran, J. A., & Piniheiro, M. (1990). Duration pattern recognition in normal subjects and in patients with cerebral and cochlear lesions. *Audiology, 29,* 304–313.

Musiek, F. E., & Geurking, N. A. (1982). Auditory brainstem response (ABR) and central auditory test (CAT) findings for patients with brainstem lesions: A preliminary report. *Laryngoscope, 92,* 891–900.

Musiek, F. E., Shinn, J. B., Jirsa, R., Bamiou, D. E., Baran, J. A., & Zaida, E. (2005). GIN (Gaps-In-Noise) test performance in subjects with confirmed central auditory nervous system involvement. *Ear and Hearing, 26,* 608–618.

Näätänen, R., Gaillard, A. W. K., & Montysalo, S. (1978). Early selective-attention effect on evoked potential reinterpreted. *Acta Psychologica, 42,* 313–329.

Nilsson, M., Soli, S. D., & Sullivan, J. A. (1994). Development of the Hearing in Noise Test for the measurement of speech reception thresholds in quiet and in noise. *Journal of the Acoustical Society of America, 95,* 1085–1099.

Noel, G. (2003). *Professional education and assessment practices in central auditory processing.* Canadian Academy of Audiology, Pre-conference workshop on Central Auditory Processing Disorders, Vancouver, CA.

Nozza, R. J. (1987). The binaural masking level difference in infants and adults: Developmental change in binaural hearing. *Infant Behavior and Development, 10,* 105–110.

Nozza, R., Wagener, E. F., & Crandell, M. A. (1988). Binaural release for masking for speech sounds in infants, preschoolers, and adults. *Journal of Speech and Hearing Research, 31,* 212–218.

Olsen, W. O., & Noffsinger, D. (1976). Masking level differences for cochlear and brainstem lesions. *Annals of Otology, Rhinology and Laryngology, 85,* 820–825.

Olsho, L. W. (1985). Infant auditory perception: Tonal masking. *Infant Behavior and Development, 8,* 371–384.

Park, S. (2008). *The effectiveness of a handheld pocket PC in psychoacoustic measurements.* Seniors honors thesis. Dept. of Psychology, University of Western Ontario, London, ON.

Patterson, R. (1976). Auditory filter shapes derived with noise stimuli. *Journal of the Acoustical Society of America, 59,* 640–654.

Pinheiro, M. L., & Musiek, F. E. (1985). Sequencing and temporal ordering in the auditory system. In M. L. Pinheiro & F. E. Musiek (Eds.), *Assessment of central auditory dysfunction: Foundations and clinical correlates* (pp. 219–238). Baltimore, MD: Williams and Wilkins.

Polyakov, A., & Pratt, H. (1994). Three-channel Lissajous' Trajectory of the binaural interaction components in human auditory brainstem evoked potentials. *Electroencephalography and Clinical Neurology, 92,* 396–404.

Popper, A. N., & Fay, R. R. (Eds.). (1992). The mammalian auditory pathway: Neurophysiology. *Springer handbook of auditory research* (Vol. 2). Berlin, Germany: Springer.

Purcell, D. W., John, M. S., Schneider, B. A., & Picton, T. W. (2004). Human temporal auditory acuity as assessed by envelope following responses. *Journal of the Acoustical Society of America, 116,* 3581–3593.

Rosen, S., & Manganari, E. (2001). Is there a relationship between speech and nonspeech auditory processing in children with dyslexia? *Journal of Speech, Language, and Hearing Research, 44,* 720–736.

Rosenberg, G. G. (2002). Classroom acoustics and personal FM technology in the management of auditory processing disorder. *Seminars in Hearing, 23,* 309–317.

Richards, J. E. (2004). The development of sustained attention in infants. In M. I. Posner (Ed.), *Cognitive neuroscience of attention.* New York, NY: The Guilford Press.

Schwarz, D. W. F., & Taylor, P. (2005). Human auditory steady-state responses to binaural and monaural beats. *Clinical Neurophysiology, 116,* 658–668.

Sek, A., & Moore, B. C. (1995). Frequency discrimination as a function of frequency, measured in several ways. *Journal of the Acoustical Society of America, 97,* 2479–2486.

Sloan, C. (1991). *Treating auditory processing difficulties in children.* San Diego, CA: Singular.

Smith, B. B., & Resnick, D. M. (1972). An auditory test for assessing brain stem integrity: Preliminary report. *Laryngoscope, 82,* 414–424.

Smoski, W. J., Brunt, M. A., & Tannahill, J. C. (1992). Listening characteristics of children with central auditory processing disorders. *Language, Speech and Hearing Services in Schools, 23,* 145–152.

Speaks, C., & Jerger, J. (1965). Method for measurement of speech identification. *Journal of Speech and Hearing Research, 8,* 185–194.

Stollman, M. H. P., van Velzen, E. C. W., Simkens, H. M. F., Snik, A. F. M., & van den Broek, P. (2004). Development of auditory processing in 6–12 year old children: A longitudinal study. *International Journal of Audiology, 43,* 34–44.

Sutcliffe, P. A., Bishop, D. V. M, Houghton, S., & Taylor, M. (2006). Effect of attentional state on frequency discrimination: A comparison of children with ADHD on and off medication. *Journal of Speech and Hearing Research, 49,* 1072–1084.

Swanson, J. M., Casey, B. J., Nigg, J., Castellanos, F. X., Volkow, N. D., & Taylor, E. (2004). Clinical and cognitive definitions of attention deficits in children with attention-deficit/hyperactivity disorder. In. M. I. Posner (Ed.), *Cognitive neuroscience of attention.* New York, NY: Guilford Press.

Sweetow, R., & Reddell, R. (1978). The use of masking level differences in the identification of children with perceptual problems. *Journal of the Acoustical Society of America, 4,* 52–56.

Thompson, M. E., & Abel, M. (1992). Indices of hearing in patients with central auditory pathology. *Scandanavian Audiology, 34*(Suppl.), 3–22.

Webster, D. B., Popper, A. N., Fay, R. R. (Eds.). (1992). *The mammalian auditory pathway: Neuroanatomy. Springer handbook of auditory research* (Vol. 1). Berlin, Germany: Springer.

Wightman, F., Allen, P., Dolan, T., Kistler, D., & Jamieson, D. (1989). Temporal resolution in children. *Child Development, 60,* 611–624.

Willeford, J. (1976a). Differential diagnosis of central auditory dysfunction. In L. Bradford (Ed.), *Audiology: An audio journal for continuing education* (Vol. 2). New York, NY: Grune and Stratton.

Willeford, J. (1976b). Central auditory function in children with language disabilities. *Audiology and Hearing Education, 2,* 12–20.

Wright, B. A., Lombardino, L. D., King. W. M., Puranik, C. S., Leonard, C. M., & Merzenich, M. M. (1997). Deficits in auditory temporal and spectral resolution in language-impaired children. *Nature, 387,* 176–178.

Zeng, F-G., Oba, S., Garde, S., Sininger, Y., & Starr, A. (1999). Temporal and speech processing deficits in auditory neuropathy. *NeuroReport, 10,* 3429–3435.

Zwicker, E., & Fastl, E. (1999). *Psychoacoustics: Facts and models.* Berlin, Germany: Springer.

15

Pseudohypacusis: False and Exaggerated Hearing Loss

James E. Peck

Introduction

Interest in pseudohypacusis has decreased in the last quarter century, even though its prevalence most likely has not. Childhood pseudohypacusis is almost certainly more common than, say, auditory processing disorders, or auditory neuropathy/dys-synchrony. In addition, there is ample evidence of widespread psychosocial problems among children with pseudohypacusis. Yet, audiologists receive little background in how to check for such problems, how to discuss and explain them, or how to approach making a referral for further management. Beyond determining genuine hearing status, audiologists can play a key role in identifying the possibility of psychosocial problems and referring for evaluation of any underlying problems.

The several terms used in regard to pseudohypacusis need scrutiny. "Nonorganic" and "functional" hearing loss are essentially synonymous, meaning apparent hearing deficit in the absence of anatomic and/or physiologic explanation (Mendel, Danhauer, & Singh, 1999; Stach, 2003). Note that, in medical usage, "nonorganic" and "functional" do not mean the absence of any physical problem. Yet, audiologists use these terms to mean that there is no hearing problem. "The loss either does not exist at all or does not exist to the degree that is indicated" (Roeser, Buckley, & Stickney, 2000, p. 237). Thus, it is illogical to say that a hearing loss is nonorganic or functional, when the "essential quality is precisely that it is *not* a hearing loss" (Noble, 1978, p. 228).

Two other words are "malingering" and "psychogenic." Malingering means intentionally producing false or exaggerated symptoms for external gain (e.g., money or avoiding undesired activity; American Psychiatric Association, 2000). Psychogenic refers to producing or causing a symptom or illness by mental factors as opposed to organic ones (Shahrokh & Hales, 2003). The term "psychogenic" has been replaced by "conversion disorder," in which psychological stresses are converted into symptoms (American Psychiatric Association, 2000). Malingering and psychogenic are not terms synonymous with pseudohypacusis, and since no audiologic test can determine what is in the patient's mind, are not appropriate audiologically.

"Pseudohypacusis" means erroneous hearing test results or untrue complaint of hearing loss in that a person responds "to stimuli only at levels well above their true organic thresholds" but without "implying an underlying causal factor" (Olsen, 1991, p. 40). Perhaps, equally logical and more straightforward would be the plain English "false and exaggerated hearing loss" or FEHL. In the reality of the clinic, audiologists define the problem operationally as inconsistencies in tests or behavior. This author offers this definition for pseudohypacusis or for false and exaggerated hearing loss:

> A supposed hearing loss that does not exist or not to the degree presented, typically characterized by inconsistencies and discrepancies that have no medical or historical explanation and with no implication regarding psychological factors.

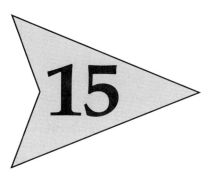

Characteristics

Demographics

Data on prevalence of FEHL are sparse. Beagley and Knight (1968) felt that prevalence was substantially less than 1% in children seen for hearing evaluations. Leshin (1960) reported 2.5% of 1,900 children failing a state hearing screening exhibited false hearing loss. Campanelli (1963) found 41 cases or 1.7% out of 2,300 screened in one year. Also in a year, Pracy, Walsh, Mepham, and Bowdler (1996) saw 10 children with FEHL out of approximately 1,000 for a rate of 1 per 100 children (1%).

The gender ratio of FEHL is about 2:1 in favor of females (Aplin & Rowson, 1986, 1990; Campanelli, 1963). The general age range is 7 to 16 years with an average of 11.5 years (Aplin & Rowson, 1986, 1990; Bowdler & Rogers, 1989; Campanelli, 1963). The range of hearing loss presented is wide, 35 to 75 dB, and reported averages are 40 to 60 dB (Aplin & Rowson, 1986, 1990; Campanelli, 1963; Pracy et al., 1996). The losses are predominantly sensorineural with flat configurations and are bilateral 90% of the time (Aplin & Rowson, 1986, 1990; Barr, 1963; Berger, 1965; Bowdler & Rogers, 1989; Campanelli, 1963; Lehrer, Hirschenfang, Miller, & Radpour, 1964; McCanna & DeLapa, 1981; Pracy et al., 1996).

Causes and Maintaining Factors

The most frequently named causes of childhood FEHL are school difficulties, a history of ear disease, seeking attention, and psychosocial problems. School performance tends to be low, despite generally normal or only slightly below normal intelligence (Aplin & Rowson, 1990; Barr, 1960; Berger, 1965), The presumption is that the false hearing loss is adopted as an accepted excuse (Aplin & Rowson, 1990; Barr, 1963; Berger, 1965; McCanna & DeLapa, 1981), but inferring a causal relationship seems based more on supposition than on evidence. In this author's patients, there was a rather definite time when grades declined, which coincided with both a disturbing life event and the onset of the supposed hearing loss. When one also considers reports that psychosocial problems are common among these children (discussed below), it seems equally or more likely that both the lowered school performance and the false hearing loss are cosymptoms of a third factor.

A history of middle ear problems is a common co-occurrence with FEHL (Aplin & Rowson, 1986; Barr, 1960; Lehrer et al., 1964). Many surmise that hearing loss is chosen because the history affords first-hand experience with an ear problem, but this also lacks substantiation. As otitis media is so common, it would not be unusual to find an 11-year-old child who had not had otitis media. Furthermore, the great preponderance of children with a background of otitis media do not exhibit FEHL. Besides, it also avoids the question of why a child would feel a need to present a false disorder.

Displaying a hearing loss could be seen as a way to get attention. It could well be true, but supporting empirical evidence is lacking. Children might be happy to miss school, but they might also have to miss after-school activities or risk being taken for medical care and getting a shot. Furthermore, seeking attention in this way, or learning to enjoy such attention, may well signal an underlying unmet need.

In contrast to the foregoing, there is evidence that psychological difficulties are more common than not in childhood FEHL. Aplin and Rowson (1986) found introversion and neuroticism, especially in girls, whereas boys were more likely to be aggressive and antisocial. A greater degree of false impairment suggested greater psychological problems (Aplin & Rowson, 1990). Conflict at home or school is common among children exhibiting FEHL (Barr, 1960; Berger, 1965). A number of instances of FEHL have been linked to abuse and neglect, either physical or psychological (Drake, Makielski, McDonald-Bell, & Atcheson, 1995; Lumio, Jauhiainen, & Gelhar, 1969; Riedner & Efros, 1995). Broad (1980) concluded that false hearing loss serves to protect a fragile sense of self. Lehrer et al. (1964) documented insecurity, inadequacy, hostility, tension, and anxiety. In McCanna and DeLapa's (1981) study, 62% of the children with FEHL came from broken homes, and many were living with persons who were not their parents. In several instances, parental divorce occurred just prior to the appearance of the hearing concern. The majority of children either were being seen by a psychologist or were described by their parents as being nervous, easily upset, having peer-problems, being withdrawn, or having a disorganized personality. In a clinical study (Peck, 2002), two-thirds of children with FEHL had positive scores on the Pediatric Symptom Checklist, a screening test for psychosocial disorders (Appendix 15–A).

Signs and Risk Factors

There are several signs and risk factors, before and during testing, for potential invalid responding.

Before Testing

Referral by Attorney

Almost always, this means a question of liability or compensation.

Reason for Visit

Litigation or eligibility determination, regardless of referral source, usually involves monetary benefit. This might not be evident at the outset, and the clinician may need to ask if eligibility determination is involved.

History

A report may lack credibility as to cause or onset or otherwise seem dubious. The history should cover a few important factors. A prime area is school problems, which are so prevalent in children with FEHL. Changes in the child's behavior should be checked (e.g., gloomy, acting less mature, or spending more time alone). Abuse, neglect, or a dysfunctional environment need to be considered. If the historian does not mentioned these, the clinician may need to inquire (techniques to do so are discussed later).

Observations and Behavior

The patient readily understands soft speech when speaker's face is unseen. The patient may exhibit behaviors that are out of the ordinary, such as having a flat affect, or being sullen, subdued, or argumentative.

During Testing

Behaviors

The patient understands speech softer than would be expected from test results. Other suspicious behaviors are comments about being confused, looking uncertain, concentrating strenuously, radiating cooperation, acting bored, looking around the test room, and the like (McCanna & DeLapa, 1981).

Pure-Tone Audiometry

A hallmark of FEHL is inconsistent pure-tone thresholds. Test-retest reliability should be within 5 dB, and discrepancies should not exceed 10 dB at any frequency.

As compared to true responders, pseudohypacusics have more false negative responses and especially fewer false positive responses. The manner of responding can be significant, for example, slow, elaborate, or laborious. Such behavioral observations are not available from pressing a button for a response light, which may be a drawback for this sort of behavioral audiometry.

The audiometric configurations most common in entirely false hearing loss are flat and saucer-shaped. However, if there is a coexisting organic loss with other than a flat pattern, that shape is added in to produce something other than the classic configuration. Furthermore, saucer and flat patterns are seen in purely organic hearing losses. Thus, the audiogram configuration has no diagnostic significance whatsoever.

The absence of a shadow curve in severe unilateral losses, when the good ear is not masked, is highly indicative of invalid results. Usual interaural attention is on the order of 50 to 60 dB with typical supra-aural headsets (Snyder, 2001) but can be 70 dB. Thus, there should be responses due to crossover by about 75 dB HL.

Speech Audiometry

Perhaps, the most prominent of all signs of invalid performance is the speech recognition threshold (SRT) being significantly better than the pure-tone thresholds. The pure tone average (PTA), whether the Carhart three frequency average of 500, 1000, and 2000 Hz or the Fletcher average of the two best thresholds of those frequencies, if the configuration is other than fairly flat, should agree with the SRT within about 6 dB. Differences beyond 10 dB are indicative of FEHL.

In addition to poor tone-speech threshold agreement, several telltale behaviors tend to mark FEHL and are much less often observed in true responders:

- Half-word responses during SRT (e.g., "ear" for "eardrum") are seen almost exclusively in false responders;
- Protesting, "You are too soft. I can't hear you," but otherwise responding to off-hand remarks at or below the SRT;
- Pressing the earphone to the ear;
- Claiming difficulty hearing the test signal;
- Bizarre response or error of association: "boxcar" for "railroad," "dig" for "ditch";
- Seemingly deliberate errors;
- Rising inflection, as if a question or uncertain: "sidewalk?," "pick?";
- Rhyming responses;
- Exaggerated straining to understand during the test.

Test Procedures

General Principles

With any patient, the clinician should be forming an idea during the interview of how much hearing loss a patient might have. In a real sense, testing has begun before evaluation procedures are conducted. The value of observations cannot be overstated. Pure tone and speech audiometry have practices specific to each, but many audiometric principles apply to both when it comes to testing in FEHL, as will be seen in a moment. As a rule, it is wise to begin with speech audiometry. However, it also can be worthwhile to make frequent changes in the test signal, such as type (speech/tone), frequency, intensity, interstimulus timing, and ear tested. The overarching principle is to disrupt a patient's loudness standard.

It may be helpful to think of FEHL testing as being unconventional with the conventional. The literature routinely considers the subject's behavior, but that of the tester is also critical. It might call for some guile, certainly flexibility, and definitely agility in handling the controls. There is merit in some "acting," looking confused or expectant, or telling the patient that the tester feels confused by the results. There are many adjustments that clinicians can make on the spur of the moment to normal procedures. Creativity and ingenuity are invaluable. Paradoxically, FEHL testing calls for close adherence to sound audiologic principles, and not just "winging it" or going on "gut feelings." Finally, to lend credibility to the clinician's impressions during the posttest counseling, it is valuable to have the parent observe the testing and witness the responses to very soft sounds.

Instructions

Instruct the patient face to face rather than through earphones to avoid providing a loudness standard for the patient. The person should be directed to respond to tones by a definite raising of an arm or finger, even to very faint sounds. In the case of speech, familiarize with the spondee test words prior to testing and urge the patient to repeat the word no matter how soft. During pure tone audiometry, keep the patient's hands in sight to watch for the slightest finger or hand movements that are time-related to the stimulus. If during testing discrepancies arise, offer a face-saving explanation, such as a misunderstanding, and reinstruct clearly and firmly but without putting the person on the defensive. Give the child an "out," a chance to "escape with honor." One could advise that inconsistencies might take much more time or necessitate a return session, and then invite the patient to continue. All the while, the clinician should give much encouragement and reinforce correct responses, especially those at or below the tentative threshold (Nilo & Saunders, 1976). At times, it might be appropriate to cajole and press the patient to respond, but tactfully.

Starting Levels

When there is a question of FEHL, the usual rule is to proceed with very low signal levels (0–20 dB), for both tones and speech, in ascending fashion to mitigate against the patient establishing a loudness reference. On the other hand, a good way to confirm initial results is to compare thresholds from ascending and descending intensity runs.

Ascending-Descending Threshold Comparisons

Ascending-descending (A-D) threshold comparisons can be a good screener, because false responders yield substantially lower thresholds for an ascending approach than a descending approach, whereas true responders show no difference. In pure-tone testing, a threshold difference greater than 5 dB is positive for FEHL (Harris, 1958). Testing at one frequency (1 kHz) takes about a minute and is a highly effective, simple screening tool (Woodford, Harris, Marquette, Perry, & Barnhart, 1997).

Another approach to rapid and accurate screening combines the A-D threshold gap with the effects of a pulsed tone (Martin, Martin, & Champlin, 2000). Pulsed tones tend to cause false responders to present poorer thresholds than continuous tones (Rintelmann & Harford, 1967), and pulsed tones with a longer off-time are even more likely to have a pulsed-continuous threshold difference (Hattler, 1970). Using a standard audiometer, one can obtain ascending and descending thresholds with a tone continuously on and with a pulsed tone having a lengthened off time of 700 msec. to increase the chances of finding threshold gaps > 10 dB (Martin et al., 2000).

SRTs obtained from pseudohypacusics by ascending runs have been found to be an average 9 dB lower than descending SRTs (Schlauch, Arnce, Olson, Sanchez, & Doyle, 1996). Furthermore, the gap between SRT and PTA is magnified by comparing descending pure tone thresholds and ascending SRT. For rapid, clinical screening purposes, an effective combination is an average descending threshold of only two frequencies (500 and 1000 Hz) and an ascending SRT with a criterion difference of at least 10 dB. If there is a positive outcome, subsequent pure tone threshold searches should be conducted with ascending approaches only (Schlauch et al., 1996).

Small Steps

Another variant of standard procedure is to use 2 (or 2.5) dB increments instead of the usual 5 dB, whether for tones or speech (Nilo & Saunders, 1976; Snyder, 2001). Indeed, several presentations can be made at each dB interval (Nilo & Saunders, 1976). After some presentations of small or no increments, a patient apparently feels the signals are loud enough that it is time to respond; thus, a much narrower intensity range is covered in an ascending series (Snyder, 2001). A good combination is a low starting point and small interval size (Nilo & Saunders, 1976).

Suggestibility

Clinicians can take advantage of their authority status and the element of suggestibility in various ways. Encourage the patient to be a bit bold. Give frequent prompts: "Go ahead. I think you got it," and similar ploys. Do not argue. If the child says they cannot hear it, either ignore it (i.e., do not reinforce the comment) and proceed, or deflect the comment saying something like, "sometimes they are soft, but that's OK, raise your hand/say the word anyway," or "the next ones are easier." For discrete frequency testing, the next "easier" ones could be warble tones or narrow band noises. Employ much suggestibility and expectation. There is great value in the psychological tenet that people tend to behave in the direction in which they are expected to behave.

One novel example of using suggestibility is telling the child that hearing results will be improved by a hearing aid. A behind-the-ear hearing aid is put on the ear but is not turned on and has no tubing or ear tip. In one study, 20 children showed average pure tone improvement of 26 dB and an SRT improvement of about 10 dB (the SRTs were already better than the tone thresholds; (Hosoi, Tsuta, Murata, & Levitt, 1999). Usually, such elaborate trickery will not be necessary.

Pure-Tone Audiometry

A simple way to check validity is to insert long silent intervals of 30 seconds between signals. Conscientious responders might make a few false positive responses, but invalid responders are unlikely to make any (Chaiklin & Ventry, 1965).

Pure tone audiometry can be altered in several ways. A long-standing and remarkably successful approach is the "yes-no" test (Frank, 1976; Miller, Fox, & Chan, 1968). The child is instructed to say "yes" when they hear the tone and "no" when they do not. Some children do not see the incongruity of acknowledging a supposedly inaudible signal by saying "no." The success of the test depends on responses coming within a normal time window after a signal, and also on no response when there is no signal or when the signal is below the child's true threshold. In this author's experience, some children spontaneously adopt a "no" response, which the clinician can exploit.

The variable intensity pulse count method (Ross, 1964) is presented to the child as one of counting ability. In this excellent test, the child is instructed to count how many times a tone was heard in a series of one to six pulses. Initially, a few series of tones are presented above admitted thresholds to be sure that the child can perform the task. Then, the intensity of one of the tones is given at 10 to 15 dB below the admitted threshold, and the succeeding tones are given above "threshold." A correct answer means the child most probably heard the lower tone. The intensity and number of tones are varied at random, that is, one or more tones below admitted threshold interspersed with one or more tones above admitted threshold. Intensity is varied until the lowest level of three consecutive correct responses is found. Even incorrect answers, intentional or not, can be informative, when given just after the signal. If it happens that the signal is very near the true threshold, genuine errors might be expected. Also, an error could be intentional to mislead the tester. Thus, if a child does not answer during silent control periods but answers "on time," even if wrong, it is likely that the signal was heard.

For unilateral pseudohypacusis, a quick and easy test takes advantage of the occlusion effect. While presenting a low-frequency bone-conducted signal, plugging the "good" ear would make the signal even more audible in the already admitted good ear, so there would be no reason not to respond. But occluding the "poor" (but actually normal) ear would shift the signal to that ear, and the false patient will not respond. If the loss were genuine, occluding the poor ear would have no effect, and the person would still hear the signal in the good ear and respond (Thompson & Denman, 1970). Here is an outline of the expected result in false hearing loss.

Occlude	Respond?	Reason
"good" ear	yes	signal shifted to "good" side, even more audible
"poor" ear	no	signal shifted to "poor" side where denied

Speech Audiometry

Familiarizing the patient with the spondee words prior to testing is always good practice. If a patient gives half word responses during SRT testing, there are a few options. One is to accept the response and proceed; even a correct half-word means the spondee was heard. Or, the clinician can "remind" the patient that the words had been practiced beforehand; therefore, hearing "birth" could only be "birthday." Urge the patient to say what they *think* the word might be. Or, coax the patient to say the second syllable, "birth-what?" If a patient does not respond, sometimes waiting several seconds helps lend a sense of expectancy, which can elicit a response.

If a tentative SRT has been established, obtain a speech recognition score at 10 to 15 dB SL. Alternatively, one could proceed directly to a soft conversational level (e.g., 30–40 dB HL). If hearing is actually quite good, this is a suprathreshold task, and responding to suprathreshold signals is easier than responding to very low signals. A countervailing caution is that a higher signal presentation level does help accustom the patient to greater loudness and goes against the notion of using very low signal levels. For normal hearers, word recognition scores reach 94 to 100% at about 27 dB SL re SRT (see Olsen & Matkin, 1991). In the case of FEHL, it is common to obtain a high word recognition score at only 10 dB SL, which strongly suggests that the Sensation Level is actually greater than 10 dB. The SRT could be predicted to be at least 15 to 20 dB lower than the presentation level.

Special Tests

The dividing line between special and conventional tests can be somewhat arbitrary. Here, "special" means those procedures that are not necessarily part of a basic audiologic evaluation of pure tone and speech audiometry. Also, special and conventional tests typically are separated for explanation purposes, but that should not give the idea that they are separated in practice. One might switch from a conventional to a special test and back again.

Stenger Test

The Stenger test is the most effective behavioral test for false unilateral or asymmetric hearing losses. It is applicable when there is a difference in admitted thresholds between the two ears of at least 25 dB, but accuracy rises greatly when the difference is at least 40 dB. Not only does the Stenger test identify FEHL but it can also help estimate true thresholds. The test is based on the Stenger effect: when identical signals are introduced simultaneously to each ear, the signal is perceived on the side where it is louder. The test requires a single sound source to the two ears but with independent control of the intensities. The signal can be a pure tone or speech.

The procedure is to present a signal 10 dB above threshold to the "better" ear and an identical signal simultaneously 10 dB below supposed threshold to the "poorer" ear. In contrast, if the threshold in the poorer ear is genuine, the patient will respond because of hearing the sound in the "better" ear (negative Stenger). If there truly is no hearing loss in the "poorer" ear, the patient will hear the signal only in the "poorer" ear and not respond (positive Stenger). However, a patient becoming suspicious that a stimulus is going to each ear might do some clever guessing of when and when not to respond. Thus, now and then, one should withhold the signal to the "better" ear. If the patient responds, it must be because the person hears the signal in the "poorer" ear (also sometimes considered a positive Stenger). In addition, to check the validity of a negative Stenger, now and then present the signal only to the "better" ear. Failure to respond shows that the patient is not responding validly.

This highlights the need for the procedure to be performed seamlessly. During threshold testing, the audiologist simply makes a few control changes and applies the Stenger test. To the patient, it should seem that nothing has changed. Then, the Stenger can show almost instantaneously whether the "poorer" ear threshold is valid or not. The test can be employed in an ostensibly informal manner by making offhand remarks ("Tell me again how old you are.") or asking simple questions ("Do the earphones feel OK?").

A 40 dB difference in admitted thresholds is necessary because the test gives, relatively speaking, a 10 dB lower signal to the "poorer" ear and a 10 dB greater signal to the "better" ear. Consequently, any ear difference in alleged thresholds is reduced by the test's 20 dB difference in supposed sensation levels. Therefore, the initial difference must be large enough to exceed this cancellation effect.

To estimate the true threshold of the "poorer" ear, one finds the lowest level to that ear at which the patient does respond. That lowest level at which the signal in the "poorer" ear interferes with hearing the signal in the "better" ear can be called the Minimal Contralateral Interference Level (MCIL). One can seek the MCIL either by lowering the signal to the "poorer" ear from a high starting point or raising the signal from 0 dB HL with the same result (Peck & Ross, 1970). The MCIL in the "poorer" ear roughly equals the SL in the "better" ear. For example, if the MCIL in the "poorer" ear is 40 dB HL and the signal in the "better" ear is 10 dB SL, one may infer that 40 dB HL is about 10 dB SL and that, therefore, the threshold in the "poorer" ear is about 30 dB HL. This is merely an approximation because the range at which the MCIL occurs is somewhat broad. Tone MCILs have been found to be within 14 dB of the true thresholds, permitting some degree of threshold estimate of the "poorer" ear (Peck & Ross, 1970).

Evoked Otoacoustic Emissions

As a broad guideline, the presence of evoked otoacoustic emissions (EOAEs) argues against a hearing loss greater than 40 dB, and absent EOAE are compatible with hearing loss greater than 40 dB (provided a normal tympanogram). Screening for EOAEs can be done quickly and easily and is sufficient to confirm or deny the audiometric results. However, EOAE testing provides no information about organic thresholds. Further details on the types of EOAEs and their significance are covered more fully in Chapter 19.

Acoustic Reflex Threshold

In supposed hearing losses greater than 70 dB HL, absence of the acoustic reflex (presuming normal tympanograms) lends credence to the hearing test results. However, an acoustic reflex threshold only 10 dB above a voluntary threshold makes that threshold highly suspicious, and an acoustic reflex threshold lower than the voluntary threshold clearly indicates false test results (Rintelmann & Schwan, 1999). In the 1970s, attempts were made for sensitivity prediction from the acoustic reflex (SPAR test). For various reasons, it probably is rarely used, particularly to assess FEHL.

Auditory Evoked Potentials

It is beyond the scope of this chapter to detail the various auditory evoked potentials procedures; they are covered in Chapters 20 and 21. Suffice it to say that evoked potentials can confirm FEHL and quantify true sensitivity to a large degree.

Reporting

The report of any audiologic evaluation might well have social and legal ramifications, but especially reports regarding persons with FEHL. The language used in reports should be chosen with great care. It would be wise to avoid the word "diagnosis" and, instead, give descriptions, impressions and recommendations. Audiologists should not use labels, such as "malingering," "unconscious," "hysteric", or other words that refer to state of mind (Martin, 2009; Rintelmann & Schwan, 1999; Snyder, 2001; Ventry & Chaiklin, 1962).

Protocol

Given the nature of FEHL and the need to be adaptable, it is difficult to lay out a routine test order. Flexibility is implicit in this outline.

- Consider beginning with or, as soon as suspicion arises, switching to acoustic reflex and/or OAE screening.
- Use visual signs as deterrents, for example, a picture of a tympanogram labeled "normal," pointing out deflections on the acoustic reflex meter or the indication of "present;" similarly, showing the display of normal OAEs or the indication of "pass."
- Initial instructions should be face to face whether for speech or tone audiometry.
- Begin with ascending SRT.
- Switch between speech and tones, and among frequencies and intensities from time to time.
- If validity is in question, assess ascending-descending thresholds (e.g., descending tone and ascending SRT).
- Employ the Stenger test in unilateral loss or bilateral loss with large asymmetry.
- Obtain a low level word recognition score.
- As a last resort, perform diagnostic OAE and evoked potentials testing, especially the auditory brainstem response.

Psychosocial Considerations

Nineteen percent of youth have a psychological or psychiatric problem at some time (Kashani et al., 1987), and 17% experience some depression (Sood & Sood, 2000). Many of the precipitating factors and symptoms of depression are remarkably similar to characteristics of childhood FEHL: parental divorce, family discord, and lack of emotional availability of parents (Doebelling, 2000), along with a somatic complaint, decrease in school performance, and behavioral problems (Sood & Sood, 2000; Waslick, Kandel, & Kakouros, 2002). Abuse and neglect contribute significantly to psychosocial problems, such as reduced academic achievement, poor social skills and relationships, low self-esteem, depression, and suicide risk (Erikson & Egeland, 2002; Hart, Brassard, Binggeli, & Davidson, 2002.). In 1997, 2.3 million children in the United States were reported abused or neglected (Erikson & Egeland, 2002).

The 2:1 prevalence of FEHL in favor of girls has no clear explanation. Depression might play a role in the gender difference. The onset of puberty is accompanied by a disproportionate increased risk of depressive symptoms in girls, becoming twice as common in females as in males by later adolescence (Waslick et al., 2002). Also with puberty, sexual abuse rises sharply and occurs more often against females than males (see Berliner & Elliott, 2002; Gordon & Schroeder, 1995). Twenty to 25% of women have been victimized before adulthood. Such treatment predisposes children to somatic complaints, depression, poor schoolwork, low self-esteem, and suicide.

Suicide deserves mention because it is often linked to depression and maltreatment (Waslick et al., 2002). Thoughts of suicide, suicidal gestures (Sood & Sood, 2000), and completion rise greatly during adolescence (U.S. Dept. of Commerce, 2004). In 2001, the rate of suicide among 5- to 14-year-olds was 0.7 per 100,000 whereas among 15- to 24-year-olds, the rate was 9.9 per 100,000, nearly a 14-fold increase (U.S. Dept. of Commerce, 2004)!

Given all the above, it seems most unlikely that children with FEHL are emotionally well, clever swindlers seeking some tangible benefit. In any event, one cannot know if a person is malingering because of the private nature of personal thoughts and motivations (McCann, 1998; Nemzer, 1996). Even if a person is malingering, faking at any age is a poor way to handle life situations. A nonexistent disorder may be a symptom of something serious and should not be dismissed out of hand (McCann, 1998).

Interviewing, Counseling, Referring

Should the false hearing loss resolve during the evaluation, still check for signs of psychosocial difficulty. The problem does not disappear just because the "hearing loss" disappears. Between extremes of referring no one or everyone for further evaluation, audiologists can reasonably identify those most likely in need of referral by taking a few simple measures (Peck, 2002). Talk with the child and with the parent separately. One can ask a few simple questions tactfully. Is the person "bothered about something?" One can follow up more specifically. Are there any problems with friends, school, or home? Does the child seem as well adjusted and as happy as other children? Has there been a change in behavior or mood? Also, for children 6 to 12 years of age, the caregiver can easily complete the Pediatric Symptom Checklist (see Appendix 15–A), a standardized, pass-fail screening tool for psychosocial dysfunction (Jellinek et al., 1988). Before ending, explain to the parent that the child does not deserve punishment and advise that there be little or no mention of hearing loss, so as not to reinforce the idea in the child. Leave the child with assurance that hearing is or will be getting better (taking advantage of suggestibility).

Audiologists might be concerned that they will appear to be prying or inappropriate. Yet, people usually can tell when a clinician is genuinely interested and they will not be offended. If an audiologist has reasonable suspicion of a psychosocial problem, refer to whomever can assure further evaluation and intervention. Some audiologists might hesitate to refer, fearing the harmful stigma associated with mental health care. Yet, if there are already signs of a psychosocial difficulty, it is much more likely that greater harm will be done by *not* referring. By discounting the risk, an audiologist might delay badly needed help. By recognizing it, an audiologist can take the first step toward appropriate management.

References

American Psychiatric Association. (2000). *Diagnostic and statistical manual of mental disorders (DSM-IV-TR)* (4th ed., text revision). Washington, DC: Author.

Aplin, D. Y., & Rowson, V. J. (1986). Personality and functional hearing loss in children. *British Journal of Clinical Psychology, 25,* 313–314.

Aplin, D. Y., & Rowson, V. J. (1990). Psychological characteristics of children with functional hearing loss. *British Journal of Audiology, 24,* 77–87.

Barr, B. (1960). Nonorganic hearing problems in schoolchildren. Functional deafness. *Acta oto-laryngologica, 52,* 337–346.

Barr, B. (1963). Psychogenic deafness in school-children. *International Audiology, 2,* 125–128.

Beagley, H. A., & Knight, J. J. (1968). The evaluation of suspected non-organic hearing loss. *Journal of Laryngology and Otology, 82,* 693–705.

Berger, K. (1965). Pseudohypacusis in children. *Laryngoscope, 75,* 447–457.

Berliner, L., & Elliott, D. M. (2002). Sexual abuse of children. In J. E. B. Myers, L. Berliner, J. Briere, C. T. Hendrix, C. Jenny, & T. A. Reid (Eds.), *The APSAC handbook on child maltreatment* (2nd ed., pp. 55–78). Thousand Oaks, CA: Sage.

Bowdler, D. A., & Rogers, J. (1989). The management of pseudohypacusis in school-age children. *Clinical Otolaryngology, 14*, 211–215.

Broad, R. D. (1980). Developmental and psychodynamic issues related to cases of childhood functional hearing loss. *Child Psychiatry and Human Development, 11*, 49–58.

Campanelli, P. A. (1963). Simulated hearing losses in school children following identification audiometry. *Journal of Auditory Research, 3*, 91–108.

Chaiklin, J. B., & Ventry, I. M. (1965). Patient errors during spondee and pure-tone threshold measurement. *Journal of Auditory Research, 5*, 219–230.

Doebelling, C. C. (2000). Epidemiology, risk factors, and prevention. In J. L. Levenson (Ed.), *Depression* (pp. 23–46). Philadelphia, PA: American College of Physicians.

Drake, A. F., Makielski, K., McDonald-Bell, C., & Atcheson, B. (1995). Two new otolaryngologic findings in child abuse. *Archives of Otolaryngology-Head and Neck Surgery, 121*, 1417–1420.

Erikson, M. F., & Egeland, B. (2002). Child neglect. In J. E. B. Myers, L. Berliner, J. Briere, C. T. Hendrix, C. Jenny, & T. A. Reid (Eds.), *The APSAC handbook on child maltreatment* (2nd ed., pp. 3–20). Thousand Oaks, CA: Sage.

Frank, T. (1976). Yes-no test for nonorganic hearing loss. *Archives of Otolaryngology, 102*, 162–165.

Gordon, B. N., & Schroeder, C. S. (1995). *Sexuality: A developmental approach to problems.* New York, NY: Plenum Press.

Harris, D. A. (1958). A rapid and simple technique for the detection of nonorganic hearing loss. *Archives of Otolaryngology, 68*, 758–760.

Hart, S. N., Brassard, M. R., Binggeli, N. J., & Davidson, H. A. (2002). Psychological maltreatment. In J. E. B. Myers, L. Berliner, J. Briere, C. T. Hendrix, C. Jenny, & T. A. Reid (Eds.), *The APSAC handbook on child maltreatment* (2nd ed., pp. 79–104). Thousand Oaks, CA: Sage.

Hattler, K. W. (1970). Lengthened off-time: A self-recording screening device for nonorganicity. *Journal of Speech and Hearing Disorders, 35*, 113–122.

Hosoi, H., Tsuta, Y., Murata, K., & Levitt, H. (1999). Suggestion audiometry for non-organic hearing loss (pseudohypacusis) in children. *International Journal of Pediatric Otorhinolaryngology, 47*, 11–21.

Jellinek, M. S., Murphy, J. M., Robinson, J., Feins, A., Lamb, S., & Fenton, T. (1988). Pediatric symptom checklist: Screening school-age children for psychosocial dysfunction. *Journal of Pediatrics, 112*, 201–209.

Kashani, J. H., Beck, N. C., Hoeper, E. W., Fallahi, C., Corcoran, C. M., McAllister, J. A., . . . Reid, J. C.. (1987). Psychiatric disorders in a community sample of adolescents. *American Journal of Psychiatry, 144*, 584–589.

Lehrer, N. D., Hirschenfang, S., Miller, M. H., & Radpour, S. (1964). Nonorganic hearing problems in adolescents. *Laryngoscope, 74*, 64–69.

Leshin, G. J. (1960). Childhood nonorganic hearing loss. *Journal of Speech and Hearing Disorders, 25*, 290–292.

Lumio, J. S., Jauhiainen, T., & Gelhar, K. (1969). Three cases of functional deafness in the same family. *Journal of Laryngology and Otology, 83*, 299–304.

Martin, F. N. (2009). Nonorganic hearing loss. In J. Katz (Ed.), *Handbook of clinical audiology* (6th ed.). Baltimore, MD: Lippincott Williams & Wilkins.

Martin, J. S., Martin, F. N., & Champlin, C. A. (2000). The CON-SOT-LOT Test for nonorganic hearing loss. *Journal of the American Academy of Audiology, 11*, 46–51.

McCann, J. T. (1998). *Malingering and deception in adolescents: Assessing credibility in clinical and forensic settings.* Washington, DC: American Psychological Association.

McCanna, D. L., & DeLapa, G. (1981). A clinical study of twenty-seven children exhibiting functional hearing loss. *Language, Speech, and Hearing Services in Schools, 12*, 26–33.

Mendel, L. L., Danhauer, J. L., & Singh, S. (1999). *Singular's illustrated dictionary of audiology.* San Diego, CA: Singular Publishing Group.

Miller, A. L., Fox, M. S., & Chan, G. (1968). Pure tone assessments as an aid in detecting suspected non-organic hearing disorders in children. *Laryngoscope, 78*, 2170–2176.

Nemzer, E. D. (1996). Somatoform disorders. In M. Lewis (Ed.), *Child and adolescent psychiatry: A comprehensive textbook* (2nd ed., pp. 693–702). Baltimore, MD: Williams & Wilkins.

Nilo, E. R., & Saunders, W. H. (1976). Functional hearing loss. *Laryngoscope, 86*, 501–505.

Noble, W. G. (1978). *Assessment of impaired hearing: A critique and a new method.* New York, NY: Academic Press.

Olsen, W. O. (1991). Special auditory tests: A historical perspective. In J. T. Jacobson, & J. L. Northern (Eds.), *Diagnostic audiology* (pp. 19–51). Austin, TX: Pro-Ed.

Olsen, W. W., & Matkin, N. D. (1991). Speech audiometry. In W. F. Rintelmann (Ed.), *Hearing assessment* (2nd ed., pp. 39–135). Boston, MA: Allyn & Bacon.

Peck, J. E. (2002). *Pseudophypacusis: Psychosocial issues and management.* Short course presented at the annual convention of the American Academy of Audiology, Philadelphia, PA.

Peck, J. E., & Ross, M. (1970). A comparison of the ascending and the descending modes for administration of the pure-tone Stenger test. *Journal of Auditory Research, 10*, 218–220.

Pracy, J. P., Walsh, R. M., Mepham, G. A., & Bowdler, D. A. (1996). Childhood pseudohypacusis. *International Journal of Pediatric Otorhinolaryngology, 37*,143–149.

Riedner E. D., & Efros, P. L. (1995). Nonorganic hearing loss and child abuse: Beyond the sound booth. *British Journal of Audiology, 29*, 195–197.

Rintelmann, W. F., & Harford, E. R. (1967). Type V Bekesy pattern: Interpretation and clinical utility. *Journal of Speech and Hearing Research, 10*, 733–746.

Rintelmann, W. F., & Schwan, S. A. (1999). Pseudohypacusis. In F. E. Musiek & W. F. Rintelmann (Eds.), *Contemporary perspectives in hearing assessment* (pp. 415–435). Boston, MA: Allyn & Bacon.

Roeser, R. J., Buckley, K. A., & Stickney, G. S. (2000). Pure tone tests. In R. J. Roeser, M. Valente, & H. Hosford-Dunn

(Eds.), *Audiology diagnosis* (pp. 227–251). New York, NY: Thieme.

Ross, M. (1964). The variable intensity pulse count method (VIPCM) for the detection and measurement of the pure tone threshold of children with functional hearing losses. *Journal of Speech and Hearing Disorders*, *29*, 477–482.

Schlauch, R. S., Arnce, K. D., Olson, L. M., Sanchez, S., & Doyle, T. N. (1996). Identification of pseudohypacusis using speech recognition thresholds. *Ear and Hearing*, *17*, 229–236.

Shahrokh, N. C, Hales, R. E. (Eds.). (2003). *American psychiatric glossary* (8th ed.). Washington, DC: American Psychiatric Publishing.

Snyder, J. M. (2001). Audiological evaluation for exaggerated hearing loss. In R. A. Dobie (Ed.), *Medical-legal evaluation of hearing loss* (2nd ed., pp. 49–88). San Diego, CA: Singular Thomson Learning.

Sood, A. A., & Sood, R. K. (2000). Depression in children and adolescents. In J. L. Levenson, (Ed.), *Depression* (pp. 225–250). Philadelphia, PA: American College of Physicians.

Stach, B. A. (2003). *Comprehensive dictionary of audiology: Illustrated* (2nd ed.). Clifton Park, NY: Delmar Learning.

Thompson, G., & Denman, M. (1970). The occlusion effect in unilateral functional hearing loss. *Journal of Speech and Hearing Research*, *13*, 37–40.

U.S. Department of Commerce. (2004). Statistical abstract of the United States: 2004–2005. *The national data book* (124th ed.). Washington, DC: Author.

Ventry, I. M., & Chaiklin, J. B. (1962). Functional hearing loss: A problem in terminology. *American Speech Language Association*, *4*, 251–254.

Waslick, B. D., Kandel, R., & Kakouros, A. (2002). Depression in children and adolescents: An overview. In D. Shaffer & B. D. Waslick (Eds.), *The many faces of depression in children and adolescents* (pp. 1–36). Washington, DC: American Psychiatric Publishing.

Woodford, C. M., Harris, G., Marquette, M. L., Perry, L., & Barnhart, M. (1997). A screening test for pseudohypacusis. *Hearing Review*, *11*, 23–24, 26.

APPENDIX 15–A

Pediatric Symptom Checklist

Please mark under the heading that best fits your child:

	Never	Sometimes	Often
1. Complains of aches or pains	______	______	______
2. Spends more time alone	______	______	______
3. Tires easily, little energy	______	______	______
4. Fidgety, unable to sit still	______	______	______
5. Has trouble with a teacher	______	______	______
6. Less interested in school	______	______	______
7. Acts as if driven by a motor	______	______	______
8. Daydreams too much	______	______	______
9. Distracted easily	______	______	______
10. Is afraid of new situations	______	______	______
11. Feels sad, unhappy	______	______	______
12. Is irritable, angry	______	______	______
13. Feels hopeless	______	______	______
14. Has trouble concentrating	______	______	______
15. Less interested in friends	______	______	______
16. Fights with other children	______	______	______
17. Absent from school	______	______	______
18. School grades dropping	______	______	______
19. Is down on himself or herself	______	______	______
20. Visits physician, but physician finds nothing wrong	______	______	______
21. Has trouble with sleeping	______	______	______
22. Worries a lot	______	______	______
23. Wants to be with you more than before	______	______	______
24. Feels he or she is bad	______	______	______
25. Takes unnecessary risks	______	______	______
26. Gets hurt frequently	______	______	______
27. Seems to be having less fun	______	______	______
28. Acts younger than children his or her age	______	______	______
29. Does not listen to rules	______	______	______

	Never	Sometimes	Often
30. Does not show feelings	______	______	______
31. Does not understand other people's feelings	______	______	______
32. Teases others	______	______	______
33. Blames others for his or her troubles	______	______	______
34. Takes things that do not belong to him or her	______	______	______
35. Refuses to share	______	______	______

The parent or caregiver completes the PSC by checking each statement as to "*Never*," "*Sometimes*," or "*Often*." Each "*Sometimes*" is worth one point, and each "*Often*" is worth two points. No points are scored for "*Never*." The points are totaled. A score of 28 or higher is positive for risk of psychosocial dysfunction (Jellinek et al., 1988).

IV

Early Identification of Hearing Loss

16

Principles and Methods of Population Hearing Screening in EHDI

Martyn Hyde

Introduction

This chapter examines some fundamental issues that arise in hearing screening of entire populations or large subgroups. The main context considered is that of newborn hearing screening (NHS) within an early hearing detection and intervention (EHDI) program, although many of the principles and issues discussed are relevant to almost any public health screening program. Many publications are already available on EHDI and universal newborn hearing screening (UNHS), so a basic familiarity with the area is assumed. The intent here is to consider key aspects in some depth, to examine common assumptions critically, to identify challenges, and to suggest some improvements in approach.

This chapter addresses not only the general principles of population screening but also specific hearing screening tests based on otoacoustic emissions (OAE) and the auditory brainstem response (ABR). The basic properties and applications of these phenomena have been described in a multitude of articles and review texts and are out of place here. See, for example, the excellent reviews by Burkard and Don (2007) for the ABR and by Prieve and Fitzgerald (2009) for the OAE. Here, there is some discussion on those particular aspects of the ABR and OAE that relate specifically to their validity, effectiveness, and efficiency as screening tools.

Throughout the chapter, references of special interest are cited but many excellent articles are omitted, and there is no attempt at formal evidence review of any specific area. Such reviews are necessarily exhaustive. Rather, the chapter reflects the author's experience and viewpoint and is offered as food for thought. The best judge of success in that regard is, of course, the reader herself.

A Conceptual Model of EHDI

A conceptual model is a useful starting point. Most readers will know that any EHDI program includes a newborn screening component, usually universal screening, followed by diagnostic, audiologic assessment and then various types of intervention, along with other key components such as medical management and public information. Rather than simply depict that procedural chain linearly, Figure 16–1 reflects some aspects of the *purpose* of the various stages in the EHDI process.

Figure 16–1 looks like two filter funnels joined together. The inverted funnel represents progressive filtering or selection of newborns. The baseline is some population of newborns who are then input to hearing screening through a process referred to as *coverage*. The screening may have several stages (typically two). A small proportion of the newborns will fail the screening (increasingly, use of the euphemism "refer" instead of "fail" is considered questionable) and these are then input to more definitive diagnostic audiometry. In turn, some proportion of these will have confirmed hearing loss. The lower and upper funnels are linked by key procedures grouped under the term *intervention*, which receives input from below and delivers

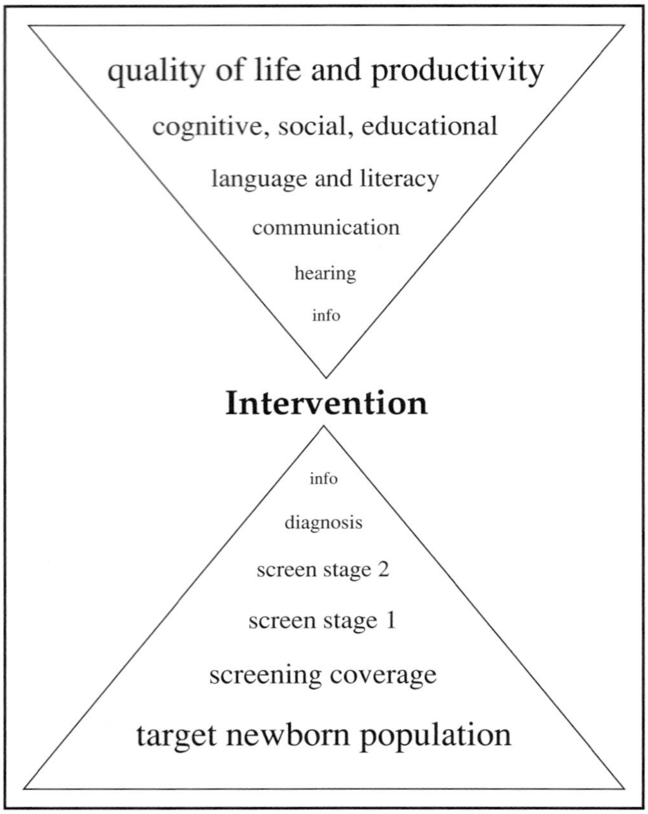

FIGURE 16–1. A simple, conceptual model of EHDI. The bottom, inverted funnel represents a progressive filtering process that extracts babies with hearing loss from the newborn population and delivers them to interventions. The upper funnel represents an expanding array of personal, familial, and societal functioning that is facilitated by the interventions.

outputs above. The upper funnel represents not individuals but their levels of functioning. The processes of intervention are intended first to enhance hearing or other communication modes. These in turn lead to an expanding array of functioning, including language, literacy, cognitive, social, and educational development, ultimately yielding a high quality of life and a full and productive participation in the family and in society at large. These are the ultimate endpoints that are the long-term purpose of the initial screening.

Consider this a little more quantitatively. Starting with the newborn population, some proportion of that population will have the *target disorder* or *target condition,* which is the set of all hearing disorders that we wish to detect and then address by interventions. That proportion (p) is the population *prevalence* of the target disorder and at baseline is often quoted to be 1 to 3 per 1,000 (0.2–0.3%) in developed countries. This is the *congenital* prevalence, that is, the prevalence of hearing loss at birth. Because we are primarily interested in permanent hearing disorders, prevalence tends to increase with age. Note the distinction between prevalence and *incidence* or *incidence rate* of hearing loss, which is the number of new cases that arise in a given period of time, often expressed as a proportion of a given population subgroup size. Technically, the proportion of newborns that have congenital hearing loss is a prevalence, not an incidence, because it refers not to a time interval but to a population cross-sectional freeze frame defined by the moment of birth. At first, we do not know who has the target disorder and who does not, so think of each newborn as having an invisible label stuck on the forehead. On each label is printed the same thing: the prevalence value 0.002, for example. That number can also be interpreted as the initial probability that any individual newborn selected at random will have the target disorder.

Newborns require levels of care ranging from routine care in the well-baby nursery through to the highest levels of care in neonatal intensive care units (NICUs). Many babies in NICUs and some in well-baby nurseries have risk indicators for hearing loss. Each risk indicator increases the number on the baby's label to some level that is often not known exactly. For some groups, the probability may be quite large and in some cases, such as total ear canal atresia, the probability achieves certainty (1.0). Typically, most babies "at risk" based on the set of known indicators are considered as a group, in which the average level of hearing loss probability (high-risk prevalence) is about 1 to 2% or about 10 times that in the newborn population as a whole. Variations in reported prevalence for entire populations and high-risk groups are due to many factors, including sampling variation, epidemiologic, demographic, and socioeconomic features of the population, risk criteria, the effectiveness of risk determination, the quality of perinatal care, and the characteristics of special-care units.

The screening itself may be *selective* or *targeted,* which is usually directed at only the at-risk group or at some limited but convenient approximation to it, such as all graduates of an extended stay in an NICU. In developed countries, about 5 to 10% of the newborn population will be found to be at risk, given current methods of assessing hearing loss risk. Alternatively, the screening may be *universal,* directed at the entire population of newborns. Whichever is the case, it is not easy to access every newborn and the coverage is always imperfect. In a good UNHS program, population coverage of at least 90% is usually achieved and sometimes (generally in geographically smaller programs) it can be as high as 99%. Those babies who are accessed successfully will receive screening and most, but not all, will have a successful screening test or tests. The imperfect coverage and success will lead to some babies with hearing loss being missed. In UNHS the proportion of babies with the disorder who will not be screened successfully typically is small. In a selective program, much larger losses will occur depending on the proportion of babies with hearing loss who are not identified as at risk. Many children with the disorder have no apparent, current risk indicator. Both the proportion of the newborn population found to be at risk and the proportion of all babies with the target disorder who are labeled as at risk are subject to many sources of variability. These include local population epidemiology and genetics, the quality of perinatal care, the risk indicator set used, the precise criteria for presence of individual indicators, the diligence with which the risk assessment is conducted, and the quality of the individual medical records. These many factors may explain why, for example, reported proportions of babies with hearing loss who are found to be at risk varies over a wide range, even though a value of about 50% is commonly quoted or assumed.

Although imperfect coverage and screening eliminate some small fraction of babies with hearing loss from consideration, the screening as a whole acts as a deliberate filter that increases the probability of the target disorder in those who pass through it. Given screening with an appropriate protocol and good quality of testing, the babies referred for diagnostic evaluation will have a much higher number on their labels than the newborn population. Suppose the baseline prevalence were 0.002 and assume for simplicity that no baby with the target disorder was missed. If 10%, say, of newborns failed a Stage 1 screen (such as by OAE), then in the referred group the number on each baby's label increases by a factor of 10, to 0.02. A subsequent Stage 2 screen (such as an automated ABR) is likely to increase the label value further, typically to about 0.1 to 0.2. This is a 50-fold to 100-fold overall enrichment of prevalence from that in the newborn population at large. The number of babies referred usually will be in the range 1 to 2% of the number of newborns screened.

Although the probability of disorder is greatly increased in babies who fail screening, a large majority of those babies *do not* have the target disorder. Therefore, it may be preferable to think of hearing screening tests not as tests that detect hearing loss, but as tests that classify babies into two groups; those with very low probability of loss and those with a much higher probability that demands follow-up action. This view is not as academic as it might seem. For example, screening personnel in EHDI programs may well fall into the trap of equating screening failure with hearing loss presence, which can result in misleading communications to families, needless levels of anxiety, and subsequent confusion when the diagnostic tests prove hearing to be normal, which they will in the majority of cases.

Certain risk indicators, such as symptomatic congenital cytomegalovirus infection (CMV), can raise the prescreen probability of hearing loss to as high as 41% (NIDCD, 2002), well above the level generally associated with conventional hearing screening test failure. Should such babies be screened at all, or should they go directly to diagnostic hearing testing? Given that screening tests are far from perfect, as will be seen shortly, beyond a certain level of risk the direct route to diagnostics is more appropriate. In fact, the presence of specific risk indicators for hearing loss, such as congenital CMV, severe hypoxia, hyperbilirubinemia, and others, can be viewed as screening "tests" in their own right, because they serve to increase the probability of hearing loss, just as do conventional screening tests.

The next step in Figure 16–1 is confirmatory and diagnostic audiometry. Although not the focus of this chapter, it should be noted that such testing is also imperfect in several respects, albeit much less so than screening. In principle, high-quality diagnostic audiometry could be thought to yield posttest probabilities of either 0 (target disorder absent) or 1 (present). In practice, due to limitations of test access and delivery (diagnostic coverage), intrinsic accuracy, test protocol, and procedural quality, real diagnostic test performance will be less than perfect. In principle, though, the bottom pyramid has filtered the newborn population down to only those babies who have the target disorder.

The entries in the upper part of Figure 16–1 are self-explanatory and the details of their performance are beyond the scope of this chapter, except in so far as the relevant intervention services either are not delivered or have limited success. That aspect will arise later, when the programmatic evaluation of EHDI is considered briefly. It is sufficient to say, at this point, that screening is not an end in itself. It is done in order to lay the groundwork to achieve the entire suite of functional outcomes outlined in Figure 16–1. Although this may seem obvious, it is worth noting that in the historical development of EHDI, attention and effort over many years was directed predominantly to screening itself, with rather less attention to the subsequent and much more complex procedures that translate screening failure into the desired short-term and long-term outcomes. The quality of diagnostic assessments and interventions has only emerged as a widespread focus of attention in the last 5 to 10 years and a great deal of further effort will be required for many years to come.

Ground Rules for Population Screening

The starting point for most discussions of the principles of screening is the seminal text written many years ago by Wilson and Jungner for the World Health Organization (WHO; Wilson & Jungner, 1968). The report was commissioned because at that time, the WHO was facing a barrage of controversy and diverse efforts to implement early detection of many chronic diseases. The key propositions put forward in that text have become widely known as "the WHO principles of screening." They have been variously adopted or adapted by many authorities and agencies in the field of health services (see, for example, the 23 criteria of the U.K. National Screening Committee, 2009), as well as by many individuals manifesting variable insight and interpretation. They are presented often enough that the reader may have met some version of them before and even be disenchanted to see them again here. However, there is no better starting point and it is hoped that the development here may include some features that are novel and informative, so the original wording is presented in Table 16–1, part A.

In 2008, again under the auspices of the WHO, Andermann, Blancquaert, Beauchamp, and Dery reviewed the history and evolution of screening principles since the original publication. In an important update of the Wilson-Jungner criteria, they synthesized

Table 16–1. Classical World Health Organization (WHO) Screening Criteria and Recent Enhancements

A. *Classical screening criteria* (Wilson & Jungner, 1968) ∞ The condition sought should be an important health problem. ∞ There should be an accepted treatment for patients with recognized disease. ∞ Facilities for diagnosis and treatment should be available. ∞ There should be a recognizable latent or early symptomatic stage. ∞ There should be a suitable test or examination. ∞ The test should be acceptable to the population. ∞ The natural history of the condition, including development from latent to declared disease, should be adequately understood. ∞ There should be an agreed policy on whom to treat as patients. ∞ The cost of case-finding (including diagnosis and treatment of patients diagnosed) should be economically balanced in relation to possible expenditure on medical care as a whole. ∞ Case-finding should be a continuing process and not a "once and for all" project.
B. *Synthesis of emerging screening criteria proposed over the past 40 years* (Andermann et al., 2008) ∞ The screening program should respond to a recognized need. The objectives of screening should be defined at the outset. ∞ There should be a defined target population. ∞ There should be scientific evidence of screening program effectiveness. ∞ The program should integrate education, testing, clinical services, and program management. ∞ There should be quality assurance, with mechanisms to minimize potential risks of screening. ∞ The program should ensure informed choice, confidentiality, and respect for autonomy. ∞ The program should promote equity and access to screening for the entire target population. ∞ Program evaluation should be planned from the outset. ∞ The overall benefits of screening should outweigh the harm.

Source: Reprinted with permission from Andermann, A., Blancquaert, I., Beauchamp, S., and Dery, V. (2008). Revisiting Wilson and Jungner in the genomic age: A review of screening criteria over the past 40 years. *WHO Bulletin*, *86*(4), 241–320. Retrieved from http://www.who.int/bulletin/volumes/86/4/07-050112/en/index.html. Copyright 2010 World Health Organization.

a list of additional or modified criteria that reflect a modern approach to health programming in the age of evidence-based practice, genuinely client-centered or family-centered care, protection of privacy and, above all, strong program accountability. These important additions are given in Table 16–1, part B. A reference of interest that addresses criteria for implementing population screening in this age of genomic medicine and of the potential to screen for not the actual presence of a disorder but the *susceptibility* to a disorder is Khoury, McCabe, and McCabe (2003). Genetic screening for hearing loss susceptibility as well as genetic testing for etiological purposes in young children with proven hearing loss are topics of great current interest that may radically affect the conduct of newborn hearing screening programs in the near future. See also Morton and Nance (2006) for an excellent, general review of newborn hearing screening with special reference to genetic causes of hearing loss.

The classical Wilson and Jungner criteria (Table 16–1, part A) have been criticized on several grounds. One issue is their susceptibility to variable interpretation and misinterpretation, using vague and subjective terms like "important," "accepted," and "suitable." Nevertheless, they have remained a cornerstone of the public health screening field. The propositions can be grouped and prioritized for the EHDI context specifically. First, there is the over-riding issue of identifying and quantifying the *important health problem* or *recognized need*. Why is it appropriate that newborns be screened for hearing loss, and what problem or deficiency of previous approaches to early identification of hearing loss is being addressed by such screening? Although the answer to this may seem obvious, there are important issues and subtleties that are often overlooked. There also is the closely related matter of the benefits that may ensue as a result of screening, which are more diverse and complex than commonly assumed. Second, the issues of latent period and natural history of hearing disorders are not really applicable and can be dispensed with easily, when considering congenital, permanent hearing disorders. Third, there must exist screening tests that are practicable, acceptable to the recipients of screening, and reasonably accurate. A substantial part of this text addresses that issue, which has many facets, wrinkles, and challenges. Fourth, the question of an effective treatment is linked not only to the array of potential benefits that can result from intervention but also to the extent to which the entire programmatic apparatus of EHDI works successfully, which raises major issues of program design and evaluation. This particular area is crucial but was not stressed in the original WHO principles, except with reference to an accepted treatment. Lastly, there is the question of costs, which will be addressed later. Before delving into these specifics, some inherent attributes and peculiarities of screening are outlined, forming the basis for much of the ensuing discussion. These attributes of screening form the rationale underlying the WHO principles.

Population Screening Is Different from Ordinary Clinical Care

One reason why the WHO saw fit to commission the Wilson-Jungner (1968) report is that screening large numbers of people for some disorder of interest differs radically in many ways from the ordinary process of delivering health care to persons who seek it. People receiving public health screening usually are not actively seeking care because they perceive a specific sign or symptom of a disorder. Rather, screening is offered to them proactively, usually at some point when the disorder is unrecognized or occult. Although any medical or related intervention is guided by a basic principle of "first, do no harm," the proactive nature of screening leads to even stronger demands in terms of its justification and the balance of benefits and possible harms that may result. As screening can become widely accepted and even sought out by the public as a perceived standard of care or as a right, the fact remains that the individuals being screened usually have no obvious expression of the disorder—if they did then not screening but diagnostic investigation would be the usual action.

Although hearing loss is perceptible by most adults, a newborn or infant will be unaware that the experience is exceptional and, above all, will be incapable of directive complaint. Similarly, the elderly individual who has an insidious decline in auditory functions may not recognize or acknowledge the extent of the dysfunction and ensuing maladaptations such as social withdrawal or dependency. It is this inability to recognize and act upon an impairment or an associated functional limitation that sets the stage for possible benefit of hearing screening. Whether such inability is intrinsic, such as for a baby, or is acquired, such as for many elderly persons, there is surely an increased onus on a productive and compassionate society to make detection and intervention services available proactively. Although such an onus does not negate the need for careful justification of screening, it can and should influence the search for a reasonable balance of benefits, harms, and resource expenditure.

A second facet of screening is that it usually seeks to identify a disorder at an early stage, usually prior to its overt expression as a significant physical or psychological deviation from the norm. This usually has several implications for the type of screening test that can be used and for the actions that normally follow a failure on such a test, that is, when the test is positive for presence of the disorder. The screening test must be sensitive to the early or unrecognized stages of the disorder and a screening failure must be followed by procedures that characterize the type, severity, impact, and probable time course of the disorder.

In the case of hearing disorders in newborns or infants, because the auditory periphery up to and including the cochlea is well developed at birth, many hearing disorders that do not immediately involve central auditory pathways are latent only in the sense that they are not accompanied by expressed symptoms, not in the sense that there is some occult precursor stage. In babies with severe or profound hearing losses, there may indeed already be signs of the disorder, such as lack of behavioral response to loud sounds. Recall that a *symptom* is something of which the subject complains, whereas a *sign* is some physical or behavioral manifestation of the disorder that may not necessarily precipitate any symptom.

A third aspect of population screening is that, by definition, it involves testing very large numbers of people, relatively few of whom may actually have the disorder of interest. This will involve major resource expenditure and organization to access the target population, explain the tests, perform the tests, document the findings, and ensure that appropriate follow-up services are delivered in a timely and effective manner. The resource expenditure itself implies that such programs should not be undertaken lightly and without a solid and well-documented expectation of sufficient benefit to the affected individuals and to society at large, especially given the major, economic constraints that exist for health care expenditures. Also, given the large numbers of individuals or families for whom the screening will prove negative, any harms or costs, even minor ones, are magnified by the large numbers involved. Typically, a large number of minor harms or inconveniences are balanced against a relatively small number of cases of major benefit from early detection.

The fourth key aspect is that no screening test is perfect at distinguishing those who do have the disorder from those who do not. Screening tests are typically cheap and relatively simple substitutes for more costly, more definitive tests that are often referred to as *gold standards*. Screening tests will make errors. They will miss (pass) some true cases of disorder (false-negative screens) and they will fail some persons who do not have the disorder (false-positive screens). For rare or infrequent disorders, it is not unusual that the majority of screening failures are false-positive. This raises important issues of credibility of screening results, labeling of persons who actually are free of disorder, as well as engagement of many persons in unnecessary diagnostic follow-up. Unnecessary interventions can also occur, if the diagnostic tests are less than perfectly accurate.

Lastly, as already noted, preoccupation with screening itself appears to have been almost endemic over the last two decades, yet the real measures of success of screening relate to subsequent delivery of valued outcomes from diagnostic testing and from various types of intervention. A consequence is the frequently stated position that all the mechanisms needed to ensure adequate levels of follow-up care for babies who fail the screen should be in place before any screening program is implemented. This follows directly from the WHO principles. Although such a view may be naïve in a political sense, it certainly expresses a necessity for overall success as well as reflecting the ethical position that one should not impose on the public a health care process (screening) that cannot, for whatever reason, offer genuine benefit to its recipients.

What Is the Real "Important Health Problem" or "Recognized Need"?

Not Only Language Delay But Also Hearing Loss Itself

Over the last 30 years or more, the majority of publications about newborn hearing screening (NHS) contained a sentence such as, "Unrecognized hearing loss in young children compromises the development of speech and language," usually leading to arguments in favor of screening. This historical focus on compromised language development in children with unmanaged hearing loss was understandable and certainly was well-intentioned, but it is not the only possible perspective. One of its consequences was that, almost without exception, the audiology and health services evaluation communities came to believe that the important health problem to be addressed was language development and, inescapably, that proof of the merit of NHS must lie in demonstration of improved long-term language outcomes. Such proof has been extremely hard to come by, as noted later, but that is not the main reason to reconsider such a view. In fact, the focus on long-term language has had the effect of unnecessarily complicating and delaying both proper evaluation and widespread acceptance of UNHS and EHDI.

A major concern with the language-based rationale is that it blatantly underestimates the importance of hearing itself. Essentially, the rationale treats hearing loss as a surrogate or proxy for delayed or deficient language development. A viewpoint that is far more appropriate in this author's opinion is that *the ability to hear is a fundamental attribute and significant deficiency of that ability is a primary health condition in itself.* Given that perspective, hearing loss is accorded much greater significance than solely as a proxy for delayed language. Rather, it is a primary, sensory impairment that, if unrecognized and unmanaged, can have a wide range of harmful effects on the affected child and family. It is also a mediator variable that, along with many other variables such as the quality of hearing health care services, various developmental disorders, parental educational level, and home language environment, can have compromised language development as one of several long-term outcomes. Using the language and conceptual framework of the WHO's International Classification of Functioning, Disability and Health (ICF, 2001), hearing loss in the young child is unequivocally an impairment and equally unequivocally it leads to disability (limitation of normal activity or functioning). It may or may not lead to significant handicap (restriction of participation in the normal range of human roles and choices) depending on the environmental demands, values, and preferences of the affected individual and family. Most informed persons would consider significant hearing impairment to confer a variety of serious functional limitations and restrictions, and the special role of hearing in facilitating oral language development is indisputable.

Although analogies are often limited in their validity, conceptualizing the problem of hearing loss as one of compromised long-term language development is akin to conceptualizing vision deficits in the newborn or young infant as a problem of reading development at school age. This seems obtuse at best, even misguided. If the underlying deficit is loss of visual acuity, surely the immediate challenge is to detect it and fix it. Translating this back to hearing, the primary, immediate purpose of hearing screening is to detect and diagnose hearing disorders, followed by efforts at their amelioration. Improvement in long-term language outcomes is a probable consequence, among many other consequences. What this means is that the "important health problem" noted in the WHO principles is not language development but hearing loss itself. A closely related and significant problem is that because the young infant is a young infant, in the absence of screening the family may be unaware of the hearing problem and will obviously fail to address it, will manifest inappropriate and ineffective communication behaviors, will experience frustration and probably misinterpretation of the child's behaviors and, when the fact of impaired hearing finally does surface, will experience guilt and anxiety. Compounding the problem, the traditional medical system was quite likely to have written off any early parental concerns as unwarranted, possibly with the common "don't worry, she'll grow out of it" response. Meanwhile, of course, the child cannot hear, has no idea that the experience is not normal, does not understand the associated pattern of abnormal family communication and response, and undergoes a period of explosive brain and behavior development without the proper range of sensory input.

None of this detracts from the unquestioned importance of long-term language development. What it does do, however, is suggest a different view of the real health problem, how it should be quantified and in terms of what outcomes the success or failure of newborn hearing screening should be measured and evaluated.

The Target Disorder and Population: What Hearing Disorders Do We Really Want to Detect?

The term *target disorder* refers to the set of all hearing disorders that the screening is intended to detect. Precise definition of this set is important but often lacking in published reports. Without such a definition it is difficult, if not impossible, to describe adequately the condition sought that is referred to in Table 16–1A. The definition also is crucial for screening test and program design and evaluation, as well as for valid comparisons of program results. Would exactly the same screening test be appropriate for bilateral, moderate, average hearing loss and for unilateral, mild, frequency-specific hearing loss? No, it would not. How can you evaluate the success of a screening program if its targets have not been defined precisely? You cannot. How can you compare in a valid manner two or more screening programs that may or may not be seeking the same set of hearing disorders? You cannot, except perhaps by sophisticated methods of meta-analysis. How can you even develop a valid rationale for screening, without declaring exactly what is to be detected and why? Not possible.

In the choice of the target disorder, there are four basic considerations that arise directly from the WHO principles of screening: all disorders within the target set must have a substantial negative impact on important hearing-related functioning, must be detectable with reasonable accuracy by available screening tests, and must be addressable by an effective intervention. Additionally, the cost of the overall endeavor must be reasonable in relation to health care costs more generally.

If detecting significant hearing loss is accepted as a rational objective of NHS and EHDI, the question is: what is meant by "significant"? With the traditional focus on long-term language as the metric of the health problem, significant hearing loss was actually a proxy target that should have been defined in terms of its quantitative relationship to long-term language itself, the question being: what hearing loss in the newborn and young infant is just sufficient to cause a meaningful decline in long-term language skills? But, the current state of knowledge was and still is unable to answer that question, so the various target levels of hearing loss adopted in various EHDI programs have emerged on some basis other than language-related evidence. Possibilities include a tendency to adopt choices made by leaders in the field, or a general sense of what is audiometrically significant in relation to speech perception in adults, or a sense of the capabilities and limitations of current hearing screening methods. If the alternative viewpoint that hearing disorders themselves are the primary issue is adopted, then "significant" must be defined in relation to hearing function directly, not to language development. Hearing sensitivity is an obvious starting point, so the target disorder could be defined in terms of the pure-tone audiogram. This generally is what has been done anyway, despite the emphasis on language and despite the additional concern that in adults, crucial functions such as speech perception have only a limited correlation with simple audiometric thresholds. Notwithstanding these limitations, hearing loss itself has the advantage of relative simplicity and broad acceptance. The challenge of target disorder definition, then, becomes to specify the least pure-tone hearing loss that belongs within the target disorder, as well as other aspects such as frequency, type, and laterality of loss. Clearly, all hearing losses greater than the least loss would also be in the target set.

As for the target population, in the context of justifying or evaluating NHS the target population is the neonate and young infant. It is desirable to be more precise with the definition of *young infant*, because the choice of appropriate screening techniques as well as their field performance may be different for older infants. Also, because the prevalence of hearing disorders increases with age (Fortnum, Summerfield, Marshall, Davis, & Bamford, 2001), difficulties will arise comparing programs with very different target population age limits. A reasonable definition might include neonates and infants under 3 months corrected age, but any upper age limit under about 6 months of age could be considered. At about 6 months of age, the possibility of behavioral screening emerges and it becomes increasingly difficult to secure an adequate behavioral state (ideally, sleep) in which to conduct automated OAE or ABR screening quickly and accurately.

It makes no sense to include in the target disorder hearing losses that have later onset than the age limits just mentioned, nor is it reasonable to criticize NHS because it will not detect hearing losses that are not present at the point of screening. Such hearing losses can only be detected by additional, programmatic means, such as longitudinal surveillance of high-risk children, later population screening (prelingually or at school entry, for example), enhanced responsiveness to family or professional concerns about hearing or about language development, or by case-finding such as in medical visits that may be unrelated to hearing. Such activities represent an extension of the target population for the EHDI program to, for example, all children from birth to school entry, but they do not relate directly to NHS itself.

The reader will be keenly aware that hearing loss categories can be characterized by common descriptors that include the following:

- Bilateral hearing loss only or unilateral plus bilateral losses
- The minimum severity (dB HL) or lower bound of the range of target losses
- Better ear or worse ear lower bounds of severity
- Average lower bound or worst case lower bound across frequencies
- Frequency range and the number of frequencies included
- Permanent losses or permanent plus long-duration losses
- Age at onset (congenital, late-onset, acquired, prelingual, preschool, etc.)
- Constancy, progression, and resolution of losses
- Type of causative pathology (conductive, cochlear OHC, cochleoneural, neural)

Many choices are available for the lower bounds of the target disorder. Is it desired to include only bilateral losses or also unilateral losses? What is the minimum severity of interest: should hearing losses of 40 dB HL or more, or down to 30 dB HL, or even less be included? Should the severity criterion chosen be applied to individual frequencies or to averages and over what range of frequencies? What types of hearing loss should be included? Should the focus be on conventional cochlear hearing loss, or should the target include auditory neuropathy spectrum disorder (ANSD) and other disorders of more central provenance in the auditory system? Should conductive disorders be included, and if so, must they be permanent or chronic, or include transient or recurrent disorders?

There are no definitive answers to many of these questions and many different choices have been made and continue to be made by program designers at various times and in various places and situations. In many current NHS programs, at least in developed countries, the target disorder is commonly assumed or stated to be permanent, unilateral, or bilateral and of 30 dB HL or more, either in terms of average hearing loss or worst-case loss at specific, key frequencies. ANSD often is included in the target, even though it may occasionally present with normal pure tone hearing sensitivity. *Permanent* is often defined to include sensorineural loss or structural conductive loss, which is mostly conductive loss that is not attributable to transient middle-ear disorders. These decisions are not etched in stone, nor are they necessarily appropriate in situations of severely limited resources, such as in developing countries. In such situations, it may be reasonable to adopt more conservative target disorder definitions, such as bilateral loss only, moderate loss or worse, or losses not including ANSD.

The choices made to date for lower bounds of the target disorder have been made in the absence of a strong evidence base about child impact and largely on the basis of informed clinical opinion, advocacy, and some limited findings about long-term educational effects attributed to minimal or mild hearing losses. A related factor is that there is little point in choosing lower bounds of hearing loss that do not match appropriately with the stimulus and recording parameters of currently available screening devices. Common choices, therefore, have taken some account of what is readily available in terms of screening technology, as well as what seems reasonable on clinical grounds with respect to early intervention.

Unfortunately, there is relatively little high-quality information available on the immediate and longitudinal functional impact of different degrees of hearing loss severity on the developing young child. The relationship between functional impact and pure-tone thresholds is likely to be highly nonlinear, with impact increasing rapidly at the low end of the moderate hearing loss range. If a reasonable, key element of the significance of the disorder is thought to be the effect of hearing loss on speech perception, then the Speech Intelligibility Index (SII; ANSI, 1997) could conceivably be a more useful impact quantifier than, say, an average pure-tone threshold.

Consider the issue of the least hearing loss severity of interest. In general, the lower the severity limit, the more cases will be defined as present in the population, that is, the prevalence of the target disorder will increase. This important effect is illustrated in Figure 16–2. Note that as the minimum target criterion hearing loss is lowered, the prevalence of the target disorder appears to increase ever more rapidly. If the limit of the standard definition of normal hearing were approached, it would increase exponentially because the number of individuals with slight hearing loss in the population is likely to be large relative to the number with mild or moderate hearing losses. Bear in mind that the definition of normal hearing is essentially arbitrary and based on a statistical distribution of hearing sensitivity.

When attempting to define these lower bounds of loss severity targets, several of the WHO criteria come into play quite forcefully: will those cases at the lower limit be detectable reliably by current screening tests? If so, given that the EHDI program resources needed to deal with the cases found will increase rapidly as

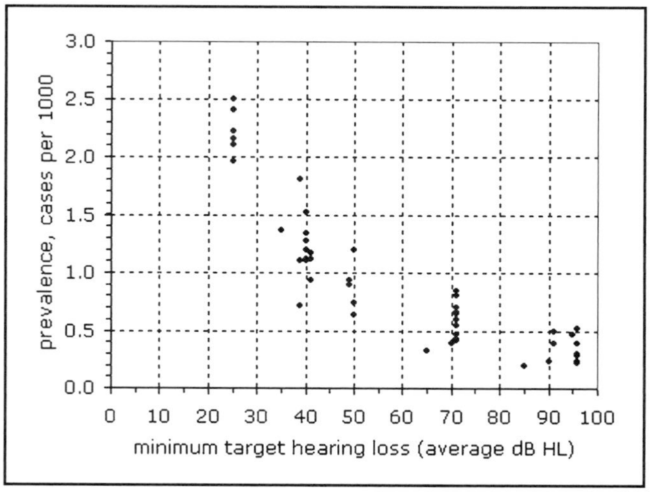

FIGURE 16–2. The prevalence of permanent hearing loss increases dramatically as the minimum (smallest) loss that is included in the target disorder definition is lowered. Note the accelerating rate of increase as the criterion is lowered. The data are extracted from studies reviewed by Fortnum (2003) and the Public Health Agency of Canada's Canadian Working Group on Childhood Hearing (CWGCH; 2005).

the lower bound of target hearing loss decreases, are there sufficient resources available? Can the diagnostic tests accurately confirm and quantify the severity and type of hearing losses at, say, the low end of the mild category? If so, what is the nature and effectiveness of the interventions required, and is there consensus on what to do? For example, should a child with a 25 dB unilateral hearing loss receive amplification? Would the child's family even believe such a loss existed or was important and, if they did not, would any such intervention be successful? Would such a child respond favorably to such aiding, given the minimal benefit that might ensue, or would the aggravation cause the device to be abandoned? Would the professional community, including family physicians, pediatricians and otolaryngologists, endorse and support such activities? If these questions do not have clear answers, is it appropriate or even ethical to detect such hearing losses? These concerns do not mean that hearing losses that are, for example, slight and bilateral or at the low end of the mild range and unilateral are unimportant and do not have deleterious effects when undetected or unmanaged. What it does mean is that very careful consideration is required as to whether such losses specifically can be addressed in a manner that comes at least close to satisfying several of the core WHO screening principles. The reader might find it interesting to search for evidence of such careful consideration in relation to the lower limits of hearing loss targeted even by current EHDI programs. An interesting review of the question was presented by Judy Gravel and her colleagues (Gravel et al., 2005). In that review, several concepts and issues covered in this chapter are addressed, mainly but not completely with conclusions similar to those given here. See also Tharpe (2008) for a broad review of unilateral and mild bilateral hearing loss in children.

Do Acceptable and Suitable Screening Tests Exist?

What Do the Words Really Mean?

Wilson and Jungner's (1968) statement that there should be a screening test that is both acceptable and suitable is a deceptively terse summary of a large topic that is profoundly relevant to whether hearing screening should be undertaken and, if so, how it should be done. The word *acceptable* relates directly to the experience of the test by its recipients. This is a matter of whether the test is unduly onerous or carries significant risk of direct harm, either in fact or as perceived by the child's family. The commonly-used screening tests such as automated OAE or ABR are not invasive by any sensible definition of the term, although reasonable care must be exercised in any skin preparation for ABR electrodes and whenever a transducer is inserted into an infant's ear canal. But these tests impose little, if any, discomfort, so the acceptability requirement is easily satisfied.

In contrast, suitability of the tests is a much more complex question. Although the word *suitable* seems vague, it covers many key aspects of any screening test, most importantly its validity and accuracy. In the original WHO document, validity was defined solely in terms of whether the test was accurate, that is, whether it made many errors. That definition of validity does not reflect modern thinking on the nature of validity. The position taken here is that validity is a deeper issue than accuracy and that the two are distinct but related: a valid test may or may not be accurate, because a valid measure could be subject to substantial random error. On the other hand, a highly accurate test is likely to be valid, because if it were not valid, the high accuracy would have to be serendipitous, which is inherently highly improbable.

Validity of OAE and ABR Screening Tests

The OAE and ABR dominate the field of screening tests for newborns and infants under about 6 months developmental age. Evoked OAEs, whether of the transient (TEOAE) or distortion-product type (DPOAE), are generated by cochlear outer hair cells (OHCs). Recording of a robust OAE by a miniature microphone in the ear canal generally is considered to reflect functioning OHCs. To evoke an OAE, there must be appropriate transmission of the stimulus through the middle ear to the cochlea and also back-transmission of the evoked emission through the middle ear. Thus, the OAE is an indicator of auditory functioning at the cochlear OHC level but its recording is mediated by the external and middle ears, causing vulnerability to minor conductive disorders. In OAE screening devices, algorithmic decisions are made about the presence or absence of OAEs from several frequency regions of the cochlea. These are made directly, in the case of DPOAEs elicited by tone pairs at specific frequencies of interest, or indirectly, by decomposition of the complex TEOAE waveform elicited by a transient stimulus such as a click.

The relationship between OAE amplitude and hearing thresholds is neither linear nor straightforward. In large groups of persons with normal hearing, there is a range of OAE amplitudes elicited by any given set of stimulus conditions. Similarly, large groups of persons with a wide range of hearing losses also show distributions of OAE amplitude. Overlap between these distributions means that perfect discrimination of normal and impaired hearing is not possible, but separation of the distributions confers useful, binary discriminative ability. See, for example, the results reported by Gorga et al. (1997) for DPOAEs.

ABRs are electrical waveforms recordable with scalp electrodes after appropriate computer processing of minute responses to many transient acoustical stimuli presented rapidly. ABRs are usually complex waveforms that are the net result of superposition of thousands of synchronized action potentials and postsynaptic potentials elicited from the auditory nerve and brainstem pathways. The relationship between cochlear activity, bilateral brainstem pathway activity, and the net ABR waveform recorded by a typical high-forehead-to-mastoid electrode derivation is extremely complex. However, there is a strong correlation between recordable ABRs and audibility of brief transient sounds. Unlike the OAE, the ABR can be used quite easily to estimate directly the threshold of hearing. In the screening context, however, specific stimulus and recording parameters are applied in order to yield a binary (yes-no) decision about ABR presence or absence. See Sininger and Hyde (2009) as well as Sininger (2007) for detailed reviews and discussions. The ABR is not appreciably affected by minor middle-ear disorders, but it *is* affected by disorders that reduce or abolish the volume or temporal synchrony of the action potential volley evoked by the stimulus. The most obvious such disorder is ANSD.

Whatever the biophysical response to be used, population hearing screening demands that the process be objective and automated, for speed, consistency, and reliability of decision-making. Although a highly skilled tester might be able to detect responses more reliably than a computer-based decision algorithm under some circumstances (such as in a diagnostic context), it is difficult if not impossible to maintain high subjective reliability over an enormous number of tests. It also is not easy to determine who is highly skilled and who is not.

With respect to the important matter of the intrinsic validity of OAE and ABR screening tests, the modern view of validity, originating in the field of psychometrics, is that it reflects the extent to which a test actually does measure what it is intended or purported to measure. The key questions are: does a detectable ABR or OAE obtained under some appropriate set of stimulus and recording conditions strongly imply normality of hearing function and conversely, does an undetectable ABR or OAE strongly imply abnormal hearing function?

In fact, neither the ABR nor the OAE are tests of hearing in the conventional sense, because there is no direct measurement of auditory perception involved. For either test, their validity is not intrinsic because in some subgroups of infants, a response (OAE or ABR) may be observed consistently in the absence of sound perception and, at least in older children and adults, perception may be observed consistently in the absence of a physiologic response. The diversity and complexity of the auditory system are such that these situations are inevitable. The obvious example of response in the absence of auditory perception occurs in situations of pathologies that lie more centrally in the auditory pathway than the site of response generation. For example, a child with ANSD may have normal OAEs but severe loss of hearing sensitivity or highly disordered temporal processing, or both. It also is possible, although rare, that a recordable ABR may occur in the presence of major central auditory disorder, such as may occur due to pathologies at thalamic or cortical levels. Conversely, infants with hearing functions grossly within normal limits may have small or absent OAEs due to natural biologic variation or to minor middle-ear conditions. It is possible to see absent or highly aberrant ABRs in the presence of normal hearing sensitivity and even normal speech perception, in some cases of ANSD, for example.

For a less obvious source of validity limitation, consider a screening test based on the click ABR. Is such an ABR a valid screening measure of the clinically important features of the pure tone audiogram that may be included in the target disorder definition? The answer is: yes, but only as long as the pure-tone audiogram is flat. Even substantial hearing losses that are low-frequency, high-frequency, notched, or U-shaped may occur despite a detectable click ABR. Similar validity concerns arise with the OAE as implemented in current screening devices, especially in relation to low-frequency losses as well as losses restricted in frequency range. Note here the importance of the target disorder definition, when discussing this aspect of validity. For example, if average hearing loss at 1, 2, and 4 kHz were the chosen parameter of the target disorder, then the click-ABR would be more valid than it would be if hearing losses at individual frequencies were included in the target, one reason being that substantial losses at single frequencies would meet the target disorder criterion (with ABR present), whereas the averaged loss would be smaller and may not meet the criterion. Furthermore, the OAE becomes less valid if ANSD is included in the target, whereas the ABR is a valid screen for ANSD, even though it is not a valid measure of hearing thresholds when ANSD is present.

These situations of invalidity are a significant concern. Although a screening test is not expected to equal the performance of any appropriate gold standard test of hearing, the existence of specific subgroups of infants for whom the target disorder will be systematically and consistently missed or for whom screening will consistently give false detection of disorder are challenging limitations of current hearing screening tests that are quite different from occasional instances of random error in screening outcomes. Taking the screened population as a whole, lack of validity in specific subgroups will cause screening errors that will contribute to the overall frequency of errors. Other errors can arise from a variety of sources, such as the level of environmental acoustical noise, physiological noise, natural biological variations across infants in OAE or ABR amplitude, variations in efficiency of response detection methods, and so on, which will be explored in more detail shortly. These other types of error are considered to be sources of inaccuracy. Thus, the overall patterns of screening error are governed by sources of both invalidity and inaccuracy. Is the distinction between the two types of error important or useful? The reader who has some familiarity with statistics may recall the difference between *bias* and *precision* when considering the overall quality of some estimator such as a sample mean. The difference between the two is that bias reflects some systematic, reproducible difference between the true value of some measure and the estimates of that measure gained from samples of observations. Precision, on the other hand, reflects some amount of random error inherent in the measurements. The practical differences in the context of screening test evaluation lie in the interpretation of observed test performance and the steps that can be taken to improve performance. Suppose, for example, two studies of OAE screening test performance came up with radically different rates of missed hearing loss. If it were found that the study with the higher rate was based on a sample with a much higher probability of ANSD, one source of bias is readily apparent. Improving the OAE detection method would have no effect whatsoever on the errors due to intrinsic invalidity, whereas they could improve the precision component substantially. This has clear implications for how screening should be done, how errors can be explained, and how test performance might be legitimately compared and improved.

It is worth noting that any limitations of screening test validity and accuracy that arise from the fact that OAE and ABR tests access different facets of auditory system activity are not in conflict with the increased ability for differential diagnosis of hearing disorders that arise from precisely those very differences. In the diagnostic context, as opposed to the screening context, the differences among the test measures are undoubtedly a source of increased insight into the location and nature of hearing disorders. An obvious example is the potential for disentanglement of a global term such as sensorineural hearing loss into more precisely defined components relating to the outer hair cells, inner hair cells, synaptic junctions with primary auditory neurons, and the auditory brainstem pathways. However, those aspects are beyond the purview of this chapter on screening.

Classical Measures of Screening Test Efficacy

This section of the chapter addresses some standard measures and approaches to quantification of screening test efficacy (how well *can* it work?). The most important aspect of efficacy has to do with the accuracy of the test, because if a test is not acceptably accurate, it matters little how quick it is, how much it costs, how easy it is to do, how much expertise is required, and so on. This section has a didactic component, and some readers already may be less than delighted to embark on yet another explanation of sensitivity, specificity, and the like. Certainly, no chapter on the fundamentals of screening could omit such issues. Two arguments to stick with it here come to mind. First, there are many ways to explain the subject so there may be something new here or a light may go on where perhaps no twilight was perceived. Second, in this chapter there are conceptual threads and a terminology that are being developed. An effort has been made not to dwell on the simplest matters and to treat the subject somewhat critically.

Sensitivity and Specificity

The *efficacy* of a screening test reflects the extent to which the test is capable of discriminating cases from noncases. A *case* is a child with the target disorder and a *noncase* is a child without such a disorder. In the simplest version of this discrimination, the screening test yields a binary (pass-fail) result. Not all screening tests are binary, but those used in the EHDI context traditionally are used in a binary manner. In any given test on any given child, the disorder may be present or absent and the test may be positive (fail) or negative (pass) for the disorder, so four outcomes are possible:

- Disorder present, test fail: a true positive (TP) event
- Disorder present, test pass: a false negative (FN) event
- Disorder absent, test fail: a false positive (FP) event, and
- Disorder absent, test pass: a true negative (TN) event.

The performance of any binary screening test is commonly summarized by two numbers: the *sensitivity*, which is the probability of a positive test when the disorder is truly present, as well as the *specificity*, which is the probability of a negative test when the disorder is truly absent. When the disorder is truly present, the outcome of a successful screening test must be either a TP or FN event, so their combined probability is 1.0. Therefore, if we know the sensitivity we can derive the false negative probability, which is its complement (1 – sensitivity). Similarly, when the disorder is truly absent either a TN or FP outcome must occur, so their combined probability is also 1.0, and if we know the specificity we can derive the false positive probability (1 – specificity). It follows that to quantify test performance in any given context of screening, *two and only two numbers are always needed*; knowing the sensitivity or the specificity alone is not enough. For example, we could adopt a ridiculous test strategy and simply call all screens positive, which would result in perfect sensitivity but useless (zero) specificity and no discrimination ability between cases and noncases. That is one of the reasons why the reader should regard skeptically any report that quotes only sensitivity or only specificity. A perfect test, which is virtually impossible except for a gold standard test itself, has unit (1.0) sensitivity and specificity. For a useless test, the sensitivity equals the false positive rate, so the false negative rate equals the specificity; in that case the result gives no information about whether the disorder is present or not, that is, the test has zero discrimination ability For a tabular illustration of test outcomes and related probabilities, test performance measures, and numerical examples, see Appendix 16–A.

Screening Test Measures and Pass-Fail Criteria

The underlying measures for common screening tests are not naturally binary (yes-no) variables. Rather, the screening result arises by applying some numerical pass-fail criterion to a measure that is inherently continuous in nature. Consider Figure 16–3A.

In generic terms, the screening device takes a measurement of some kind of biophysical function. Such measures have inherent variability, both for repeated measures within any one subject and for measurements across subjects. For a large number of such measurements there will be a statistical distribution of possible measured values, represented by the curves in Figure 16–3A. In such figures, the distributions are typically modeled as having a shape that is *normal* in the terminology of statistics and *Gaussian* in the terminology of engineering. Real measures, such as signal-to-noise ratios, may have other distributions, but the normal distribution is typically used for illustration and approximation. Moreover, the distributions are standardized, meaning that the test measure is scaled (transformed) numerically such that mean value of the disorder-absent distribution is rescaled to zero and the standard deviation is set to unity (1.0). Conventionally, the left-hand distribution is that for no disorder (D–) and the other distributions represent disorder presence (D+) for various different screening tests. The reader might imagine, for example, that the left-hand distribution represents possible blood pressure readings from a screening device in a normal population, whereas the other distributions represent such results in subjects with moderate hypertension, the tests differing in how sensitive they are to moderate hypertension. In general, for the screening measure to be useful, the distributions must be separated when the target disorder is present or absent. The more separated the distributions are, the better the test is likely to be at discriminating subjects with and without the target disorder.

The pass-fail criterion is some particular critical value of the screening measure, shown in Figure 16–3A with a numerical value of 1.64 standard deviations above the mean of the D– distribution, as an example. Any measurement value arising from a single screening act will either be above or below the criterion, and the task is to infer whether the observation came from the response-present or response-absent distributions. The usual approach is to decide that the measurement came from the D+ distribution if the observation equals or exceeds the criterion, otherwise it is deemed to have come from the D– distribution.

The reader may recall that probabilities can be represented as areas under statistical distributions. For any pair of distributions, one of which is the no-disorder distribution, the test sensitivity equals the area under the D+ distribution for all values of the test measure that are to the right of the criterion, whereas the specificity

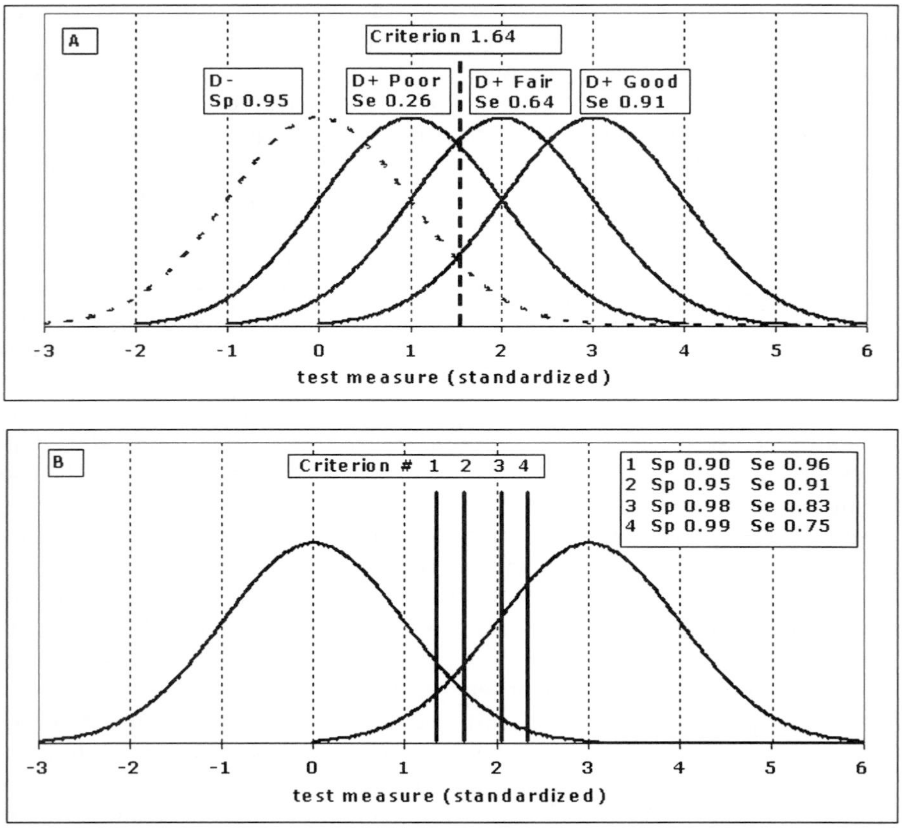

FIGURE 16–3. A. Statistical distributions of generic screening tests' underlying measures, for tests of different discrimination ability. The disorder-absent (D–) distribution stays centered on zero but the disorder-present (D+) distributions can have any position. The test measure has been "standardized" such that D– is centered at zero, both distributions have unit standard deviation (SD), and the x-axis units are in standard deviations (SDs). The greater the separation of the D– and D+ distributions, the better the test is. Three examples are shown for D+. Specificity is the area under D– left of the screening fail criterion and sensitivity is the area under D+ to the right of the criterion. A criterion value is illustrated at 1.64 SDs above the D– mean, which would yield a specificity of 95% (0.95). The differing sensitivities of the various tests are shown. The distances in SD units between the D– and D+ distribution centers are the test performance parameter d' (see text). **B.** For a given screening test and its associated, fixed pair of distributions, sensitivities and specificities for various values of the failure criterion are shown and are seen to change inversely. Note that even with three SDs of distributional separation (d' = 3), there is still substantial overlap. For a typical, desired specificity of at least 0.98 (giving a screening fail rate of no more than about 2%), the sensitivity is barely acceptable.

is the area under the D- distribution for all values to the left of the criterion. In Figure 16–3A, the three different D+ distributions shown yield sensitivities of 0.26, 0.64, and 0.91, respectively, after applying the criterion that gives a specificity of 0.9 for the fixed D– distribution. The reader should note that only the rightmost D+ distribution could represent a screening test that would be acceptable or, in other words, that substantial separation of the D– and D+ distributions is required for a good screening test.

In Figure 16–3B, two distributions are shown, one is the D– distribution and the other is the D+ distribution for a good screening test. The two things that affect the values of sensitivity and specificity are the separation of the distributions and the chosen value of the criterion itself. For any given pair of distributions, if the criterion is changed then the sensitivity and specificity will also change and *will do so inversely*—the higher the sensitivity, the lower the specificity, and vice versa. What this means is that an entire spectrum of values for sensitivity or specificity is obtainable, depending on where the criterion is set. What defines the quality of the screening test has far more to do with the distributional separation than with the criterion itself. The greater the separation, the better the test is intrinsically, regardless of which particular criterion is chosen. If two screening tests have the same distributional shape and separation on the standardized axis then they are essentially equivalent in terms of their intrinsic performance, even if they were based on different underlying measures or technologies.

In the specific case of automated OAE and ABR screening tests, the measure underlying the tests is based either directly or indirectly on a signal-to-noise ratio (SNR), either acoustic (for OAE) or electrophysiologic (for ABR). The measure might be an actual SNR calculation, a variance ratio, a correlation coefficient, a probability estimate, or any of several other possible response detector functions. Although potentially confusing, it is important here to appreciate that physiologic response detection in typical screening devices is actually a variation on the illustrative schematics shown in Figure 16–3. In an automated ABR device, for example, the outcome or scoring algorithm decides that response is absent unless a specific numerical criterion is met or exceeded. The criterion is set such that the likelihood of it being exceeded by chance in the absence of response (due to noise fluctuations alone) is very small, typically less than 1%. Response absence equates to target disorder presence and vice versa, because hearing loss is assumed to abolish response. Thus, false positive detection of a response leads to a false-negative screen and conversely, false negative response detection leads to a false positive screen. Thus, by controlling the rate of false positive response detection, the screening algorithm actually controls the false negative screening error rate, that is, it effectively controls the screening sensitivity and relates to the D+ distribution. Essentially, this amounts to a reversal of the conventional picture shown in Figure 16–3. In fact, proper performance analysis for OAE and ABR screening tests is somewhat complicated and is beyond the scope of this chapter. However, the principles discussed here and displayed in Figure 16–3 are entirely valid and useful as a basic conceptual model.

Returning to the general model of Figure 16–3, an obvious inference is that a given screening test may in effect become a different test (in terms of performance) if any change in its implementation or context of use were to alter the shape, spread or location of the underlying distributions of the test measure. The crucial aspect is the extent of distributional overlap for D– and D+. There are many possible causes of such change, but two of them will be mentioned briefly, to illustrate how easy it is to alter such distributions. One example of a contextual change is a change in the target disorder definition, such as moving the lower limit of target hearing loss severity to a lower or higher value, which will be discussed further shortly. The other example is a procedural change in how the screening device works, such as a change in stimulus type or intensity, in the amount of averaging used in OAE or ABR measurement, or in the way in which the signal-to-noise ratio is calculated. For instance, simply using more averaging sweeps or a more effective stimulus for the ABR may change the distributions and, therefore, could result in genuinely different test performance. This implies that there is not one but many substantively different versions of an ABR or an OAE screening test, even given a single, specific target disorder definition. This is important because there is a tendency to think that all OAE or all ABR screening tests have the same performance characteristics, whereas in fact, they do not.

Having clarified what is meant by two tests being equivalent or different in performance, there are three common, important questions:

1. Do the sensitivity and specificity pairs come from equivalent or different tests?
2. If they come from different tests, which test is genuinely the better or the best?
3. Whether equivalent or different, how should the optimal value for the criterion be chosen?

The Relative (Receiver) Operating Characteristic

A common method of evaluating and comparing tests makes use of the *relative operating characteristic* (also known as the receiver operating characteristic [ROC]). A definitive description of the application of ROCs to test evaluation was given by Swets (1988). An ROC is a plot of sensitivity on the *y*-axis or ordinate against the false-positive probability (1 – specificity) on the *x*-axis or abscissa, for various values of the test failure criterion. An example ROC plotted with linear probability axes is shown in Figure 16–4A. It can be seen that as the criterion is changed to make the test more liberal or lax (more likely to fail a child), both the sensitivity *and* the false-positive probability increase, which is reasonable intuitively. Figure 16–4A also shows a diagonal line, which represents the ROC for all useless tests that have no power to discriminate true positives from false positives, whatever their false-positive probability. Tossing a coin, for example, and calling the disorder present if a head came up, would give sensitivity and FP values of 0.5. Throwing a die and calling the disorder present if a six came up would make both the sensitivity and FP probability one in six (0.17). Both are tests with zero discriminant ability and both yield a point on the diagonal ROC.

ROCs are often characterized by one of two common parameters, d' (d-prime) and A. In graphical terms, d' reflects how far the ROC is shifted from the diagonal line of the useless test (which has a d' of zero), towards the upper left-hand corner (which has infinite d'). In terms of the underlying distributions of the test measure, d' is the number of standard deviations by which the means of the D– and D+ distributions are separated. If those distributions are truly normal in shape, an entire ROC (known as a binormal ROC) is specified by a single value of d'. There is, of course, an infinite number of ROCs generated as d' varies from zero to infinity. They all have the same general shape but with varying amounts of bulge toward the upper left corner of the ROC plane.

Note that an estimate of d' can be calculated easily from any sensitivity-specificity pair, simply by figuring out with statistical tables of the cumulative standard normal distribution (or using the Excel function [norminv(probability, 0, 1)]) what separation (number of standard deviations) of disorder-negative and disorder-positive distributions would give the observed values (areas to the left and right of a criterion line). For example, an FP rate of 5% (0.05), say, would require a criterion at +1.64 and if the associated sensitivity were 90%, that criterion would have to be at –1.28 relative to the mean of the disorder-positive distribution, to give the correct area under the curve. Thus, the value of d' is 2.92, based on the binormal model. Remember, a completely useless test has a d' of zero, that is, the two underlying distributions completely overlap, whereas good tests typically have d' values of about 3.0 or higher and excellent tests typically have d' greater than 4.0.

The alternative measure A is the area under the ROC curve (AUC) when it is plotted with linear probability axes. Any useless test has an A of 0.5, whereas a (nonexistent) perfect test would have an A of 1.0. The measure A has some elegant and interesting properties. For example, if many pairs of babies were presented for testing, with one baby in each pair free from disorder and the other with the disorder, the quantity A actually equals the probability of correct detection of the baby with the disorder, which is approximated by the proportion correct over a large number of selections.

If the binormal model is actually correct in any given situation, d' and A have a simple algebraic relationship. However, such a simple model is frequently a poor approximation to the truth. In such cases, the actual ROC may not have a single value of d'. Moreover, the parameter A will not be very useful because it reflects the area under the entire ROC. In screening for disorders with low prevalence we are interested only in the test performance at very low values of the FP probability (high specificity), that is, toward the left-hand end of the ROC. An alternative measure of test quality is the partial A, which may be denoted as A(max FP), for some particular acceptable maximum value of the false-positive probability. Because there is little interest in FP probabilities greater than, say, 10% or 0.1, the focus perhaps would be on A(0.1) and also on the values of the shift parameter d'. Figure 16–4B shows some ROCs with different values of d'. Only the FP range of greatest interest is shown, from 0.005 (0.5%) to 0.05 (5%).

It is worth noting that ROCs can be plotted using various different axis scales, including linear in probability (as shown here), logarithmic in probability (which is useful to zoom into interesting regions such as the region with very low FP rate) and normal deviate, which is basically linear in standard deviations of the standard normal distribution (which has mean zero and unit SD). Many real tests tend to yield ROCs that are straight lines when plotted on normal deviate axes. However, that property is less interesting if the focus is upon a small part of the ROC plane, as is the case here, because ROCs will tend to be close to linear over a small range of FP error, even when plotted with linear probability axes. There are many Web sites, some of them interactive, that explain these matters in much more detail than is appropriate in this chapter. They can be accessed, for example, simply by searching "receiver operating characteristic" or "ROC normal deviate" online.

Now consider two tests that have different sensitivity-specificity pairs such that neither test has both higher sensitivity *and* specificity. If the two points on the ROC plane corresponding to those values are

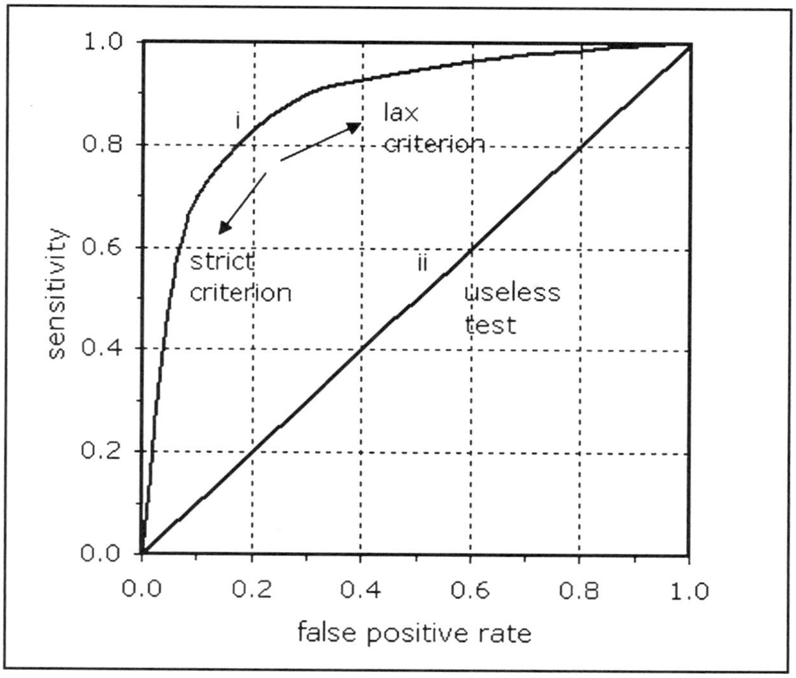

A

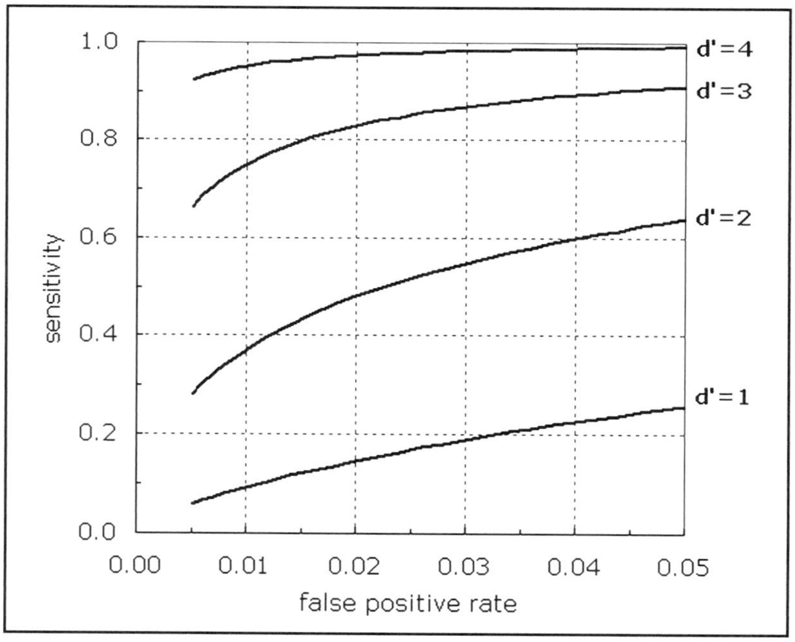

B

FIGURE 16–4. A. Relative (or receiver) operating characteristic (ROC) curves. The ordinate is the test sensitivity and the abscissa is the false positive probability (which equals 1– the specificity). As the screen fail is changed, the sensitivity and false-positive rate increase and decrease together. The upper ROC curve (i) is typical for a "good" test. The diagonal (ii) is the ROC for a useless test with no ability to discriminate persons with and without the target disorder (such as tossing a coin or throwing a die), for which the sensitivity and false-positive rate are equal for any criterion. On this type of plot, d' is the least distance from the ROC to the upper left corner. The measure A, the total area under the ROC, is 0.5 for the useless test and 1.0 for a perfect test. **B.** Segments of ROC curves for tests with different values of d'. Only the range of greatest interest for UNHS are shown, with false-positive rates less than 5% (0.05). The upper left box is the part of the ROC plane of interest for excellent test performance.

actually on the same ROC, then neither test is intrinsically superior in terms of discrimination ability. The different sensitivity and specificity pairs reflect merely different values of the pass-fail criterion and, if the binormal model were operative, they would yield the same value of the underlying d'. In contrast, if the two tests fall on different ROCs they will have different values of d' and if the differences are statistically significant, it is likely that the two tests are truly different in their discrimination ability.

A complication in this general approach occurs if the observed ROCs in the specificity range of interest do not follow the simple binormal model, which has equal SDs for the underlying distributions. In that situation, no single value of d' can be assigned as a summary parameter for the test. If this happens, it is often the case that the variability of the underlying test measure differs in the populations with and without the target disorder, or because the shapes of the underlying distributions differ substantially from normal. In such a case, the decision between two tests is still straightforward if one of the ROCs always lies above (dominates) the other, but if the ROCs cross, then the decision about which test is better requires that a single, reference value or range of desired specificity (or sensitivity) be defined.

Unfortunately, there appears as yet to be no standard approach to the description and reporting of screening test performance. Indeed, it is still not uncommon to see values of sensitivity or specificity calculated and reported singly (i.e., not in the required pairs) and not always computed in a valid manner. Evaluation or comparison of screening tests would be far easier and more informative if the clinical and technologic communities involved in NHS were to adopt a small range of specificity or a small number of key reference or index values such as the set [0.5, 1, 2, 5, and 10%]. The idea would be that screening test or screening protocol performance (estimates of sensitivity *plus* specificity) would have to be determined and reported for at least one value in such an index range or set, for any report to be taken seriously. Unfortunately, it is difficult to see how such a standardized approach would come to pass without impetus from a major funding agency or collaborative group.

Selecting the Failure Criterion

Suppose a given test with a particular ROC is chosen as the preferred test, how should the pass-fail criterion be chosen? In statistical decision theory, one way is to assign some quantitative cost to the test outcomes, usually to the FN and FP error events. The optimal criterion is the one that yields the least overall expected cost, which is the sum of error probabilities multiplied by their associated costs. However, it can be very difficult to assign valid, quantitative costs to FN and FP errors (especially FN errors), and the optimal criterion values so derived may be sensitive to changes in those numerical costs. A common viewpoint is that the cost of missing a child with hearing loss is much greater than that of a false-positive screen. In fact, it is only necessary to define the cost *ratio* for FN and FP errors in order to solve for the cost-minimizing criterion, but the ratio is no easier to define than are the costs themselves.

If it is not possible to assign meaningful error costs, then the rationale for the choice of criterion is limited to consideration of a desired sensitivity or, more commonly, a desired specificity (or its complement, the FP probability). Typically, a very high specificity in the range 0.9 to 0.99 is desired, because of the preference to limit false-positive fails in order to control the refer rate to diagnostics, among other reasons. As already noted, there are no widely accepted standards for the choice of specificity. Moreover, screening devices usually offer little or no flexibility in choice of the underlying pass-fail criterion. This renders optimization and valid comparisons of screening devices both limited and problematic.

Test Efficacy Depends on the Target Disorder Definition

The target disorder set for an NHS program clearly will include different severities and types of hearing loss, and this complicates measurement of efficacy. There is no good reason to assume that the sensitivity and specificity of any given screening test will be the same for all degrees and types of hearing loss within the target disorder set. A simple example is offered by ANSD. If it were included in the target disorder, then the sensitivity of OAE screening, for example, would immediately decrease by 5 to 10%, that is, by the prevalence of ANSD in the screened population, because almost all such cases would be missed by OAE screening. As another example, small reductions (such as 10 dB or less) in the lower severity bounds of the target disorder range could have significant adverse effects on both sensitivity and specificity. It might be expected that close to the lower severity limit, the poorer the sensitivity will be, given that most tests are based on some kind of response signal-to-noise ratio. A small hearing loss just within the target disorder range may not totally abolish the OAE or the ABR, which could in turn lead to reduced test sensitivity if the test criterion is such that small OAEs or ABRs will sometimes be detected and cause a screen pass. Conversely, the lower the hearing loss criterion, the higher is the likelihood of screen failure due to small hearing losses that may satisfy the numerical severity target but are due to transient (nontarget) conditions such as external ear debris or unresolved middle ear fluid. These will reduce the screen specificity. Although these potentially important effects are rarely described in published reports to date, they are especially relevant to the current, challenging issue of whether to screen for hearing losses at the lower end of the mild range. They also are relevant with regard to explaining some of the variability in reported accuracy of screening tests.

Interpretation of Screening Fail and Pass Results: Positive and Negative Predictive Value

The sensitivity and specificity are intrinsic measures of the test itself; together, they tell us how good it is at separating cases from noncases. But, by themselves, sensitivity and specificity tell us little about the meaning of a given screening fail or pass result, such as how much confidence we can have that a baby who fails actually has hearing loss. The level of confidence is very important in relation to the amount of effort that is justifiable in pursuing high levels of follow-up, as well as in the proper explanation of the significance of screening outcomes to affected families. The actual pattern of pass and fail results expected when screening a large number of babies depends not only on the intrinsic performance of the screening test itself, but also on the population prevalence of the disorder.

The probabilities of special interest that arise from the interaction of prevalence, sensitivity, and specificity are the *positive predictive value* (PPV) and *negative predictive value* (NPV). The PPV is the probability that any given baby who fails the screen (a positive screen) will turn out to have the disorder, whereas the NPV is the probability that any given baby who passes the screen (a negative screen) will turn out to be free of the disorder. The PPV is especially important because it governs the significance and the credibility of screening failure, and these are the babies who require strong follow-up action. A test may have very good sensitivity but still result in a low PPV if the disorder is rare, that is, if the prevalence is small. If the general population prevalence of target hearing disorders in newborns is typically about two per thousand, the vast majority of any given sample of screened babies will NOT have the disorder. Consequently, the PPV is governed strongly not by *sensitivity* (which relates to the relatively few babies who do have the disorder) but by the *specificity* of the screen (which relates to the many who do not). It is essential that good screening tests for rare disorders have very high specificity. These effects are illustrated in Table 16–2.

Table 16–2 shows PPV values for various combinations of disorder prevalence, test sensitivity and specificity. A prevalence of 0.001 (1/1000) is typical in newborns who are not at risk for hearing loss, and 0.01 (10/1000 or 1%) is typical in high-risk newborns. Compare rows 1 and 2, 3 and 4, 5 and 6, and 7 and 8, to see the effect of specificity change from 0.9 to 0.99. In every case, the effect on PPV is very large. Now compare lines 1 and 3, 2 and 4, 5 and 7, and 6 and 8, to see the effect of sensitivity change by the same amount. In every case, the change in PPV is small. To see the effects of change in prevalence, compare lines 1 and 5, 2 and 6, 3 and 7, and 4 and 8. In each case, the effect on PPV is very large. Notice an important fact that is often not appreciated. Even when test sensitivity and specificity values are excellent (and better than those usually obtained with individual OAE or ABR screening tests), namely 0.99 in this example, the PPV for a relatively rare disorder like hearing loss in the nil-risk population does not exceed 9%, meaning that 91% of all nil-risk babies who fail the screen will *not* have the disorder, even with such excellent tests. What this suggests is that further efforts to bring the real-world false-positive rate down below 1% may be very worthwhile in terms of improving the credibility of screening failure and the efficiency of referral to diagnostic assessment. Given that missing babies with genuine permanent hearing loss (PHL) usually is assigned a high cost, reduction in false positives would only be acceptable if not accompanied by a substantial loss in sensitivity. That means that a screening method with truly better performance in the ROC false-positive probability region of 0.001 to 0.01 (0.1–1%) would be a major advance. It also means that the benchmark value for the maximum acceptable false positive probability for any screening protocol would be more reasonably set at 1%, not the much larger values commonly regarded as acceptable in the literature to date. With a 3% false-positive rate (specificity 0.97), for example, the PPV for prevalence 0.001 and excellent sensitivity of 0.99 is a mere 3.2%, which many might consider unacceptably low.

The NPV, in contrast, reflects the credibility that can be placed on a screening pass. If the target disorder has low prevalence, the NPV of any reasonable

Table 16–2. Examples of the Effect of Prevalence, Sensitivity, and Specificity of the Positive Predictive Value (PPV) of a Screening Test*

	Prevalence	*Sensitivity*	*Specificity*	*PPV %*
1	0.001	0.9	0.9	0.9
2	0.001	0.9	0.99	8.3
3	0.001	0.99	0.9	1.0
4	0.001	0.99	0.99	9.0
5	0.01	0.9	0.9	8.3
6	0.01	0.9	0.99	47.6
7	0.01	0.99	0.9	9.1
8	0.01	0.99	0.99	50.0

*For the large effects of prevalence, compare Rows 1 with 5, 2 with 6, 3 with 7, and 4 with 8. For the small effects of sensitivity, compare Rows 1 with 3, 2 with 4, 5 with 7, and 6 with 8. For the large effects of specificity, compare 1 with 2, 3 with 4, 5 with 6, and 7 with 8. Given that the prevalence of hearing disorders is usually not controllable, the main strategy for enhancing PPV lies in increasing the specificity of screening, often by repeat testing or a serial protocol with different test technology. All serial screening reduces sensitivity to some degree. The challenge is to minimize such sensitivity loss.

screening test inevitably is very high (close to 1.0) and so usually is of much less interest than the PPV. However, it is important to remember and to convey to families of screened newborns that a high NPV relates strictly to the absence of hearing loss at the time of the screen; it says nothing at all about the likelihood of subsequent hearing loss.

Likelihood Ratios Are Interesting and Useful

The reader with little interest in details of test evaluation could skip this section, with the caveat that likelihood ratios could figure more prominently in the test evaluation literature in the future, as the sophistication of such evaluations develops over time.

Although the PPV reveals the probability of target disorder presence given a screen failure, because its value depends strongly on the prevalence (or, more generally, the pretest probability of the disorder) it must be recalculated for every possible pretest probability of interest. It is sometimes convenient to make use of test performance measures that are independent of pretest probability but that relate more directly and simply to the posttest probability of disorder than do sensitivity and specificity. The likelihood ratio (LR) is such a measure. It is a number associated with each screening outcome, so for a binary screen there are two LRs, one for a positive screen (fail) and one for a negative screen (pass). These are denoted as LR+ (LR positive) and LR–, respectively. LR+ is simply the ratio of sensitivity to false positive probability, whereas LR– is the ratio of specificity to false negative probability. Referring back to Figure 16–4A, note that the LR+ is simply the ratio of areas to the right of the criterion, under the disorder-present and disorder-absent distributions of the test measure. The LR– is a similar ratio of areas, but to the left of the criterion. These ratios are independent of the pretest probability.

If the LRs of a screening test pass and fail are known then it is a straightforward matter to calculate the postscreen probabilities of the target disorder (which is the PPV, given screening failure) for any specific value or range of prescreen probabilities. The latter may be either known or estimated values of the prescreen prevalence. Such estimates could be of baseline prevalence for the newborn population at large, for any given high-risk group, or even for individual babies with specific sets of risk indicators. The calculation involves not probabilities directly but odds for the disorder, which are easily converted to and from probabilities. The equation is:

Postscreen odds =
prescreen odds × likelihood ratio, where

Odds $(o) = p/(1-p)$,
conversely probability $(p) = o/(o+1)$.

For example, if the prevalence p is 0.002 or 2 per thousand, the sensitivity 0.9 and specificity 0.95, the LR+ is 0.9/0.05, which equals 18. The prescreen odds are 0.002/0.998, and it is easy to show that the post-screen probability is 0.035 or 3.5%. Referring back to the beginning of this chapter, this would mean that the number on the baby's forehead label changed from 0.2% to 3.5%. For a high-risk baby with a prescreen prevalence of 0.01, say, the result would be a probability change from 1 to 15%.

The postscreen probability can be calculated directly or by using tables that are easy to create using, for example, Excel. There are also readily available graphical tools such as nomograms that are convenient for rough estimates. See the excellent Web site of the Centre for Evidence Based Medicine in Oxford, UK, for more details on this and many other aspects of test evaluation, available at www.CEBM.net, under "EBM Tools > Critical Appraisal > Explanations and Examples > Likelihood Ratio."

A pair of Likelihood Ratios is generated by each sensitivity-specificity pair. The advantages of LRs over sensitivity-specificity pairs are that LRs are easier to conceptualize in terms of the effect of the screening result on the pretest probability. In fact, for very small values of the pretest probability, a good approximation to the posttest probability is simply the product of the pretest probability and the LR+. Thus, for the example prevalence above of 0.002 and typical LR+ of about 18, the posttest probability is crudely estimated at $0.002 \times 18 = .036$ (about 4%), whereas the exact value is 0.0348. Likelihood ratios are not commonly presented in the audiology literature, but after a little practice they are simple and intuitively useful measures of screening test impact. They are more useful, in practical terms, than sensitivity and specificity.

Yield, Refer Rate (Fail Rate), Accuracy, and Number Needed to Screen (NNS)

The *yield* of a screening test reflects the number of true cases found, usually expressed as a proportion or percentage of the number of individuals screened. It is very important not to confuse screening yield with the prevalence of the target disorder. Screening program yields are (negatively) biased estimators of prevalence, because sensitivity is never perfect and some babies will always be missed by real-world screening tests.

The refer rate reflects the number of screening tests that are positive, also usually expressed as a proportion or percentage of the number of individuals screened. It is made up of both true positive and false positive outcomes, usually with the latter dominating. It is of interest for two main reasons. First, if every screening failure must be followed up, the refer rate is related directly to the resources required to provide such follow-up, such as the number of initial diagnostic tests that will be needed. Second, the refer rate gives a sense of the number of families who will experience a screening failure, with its attendant stress and anxiety. Because for rare disorders the refer rate is usually dominated by false-positive outcomes, it also gives a sense of the number of families who experience a failure when in fact their child does not have the target hearing disorder.

Test *accuracy* is quite commonly listed in the literature on screening test measures, where the term is given a very specific meaning: the estimated proportion of all screening tests that are correct, that is, are TP or TN. Not only is use of the term *accuracy* very specific, but also the proportion so derived lumps all errors together and is uninformative when different importance is attached to FN and FP errors, which certainly is the case in NHS programs as well as in most screening programs more generally.

Finally, the reader may also meet the *number needed to screen (NNS)*, which is simply the number of screens needed to yield one additional case. The lower the NNS, the more productive is the screening, in terms of new cases found per unit of screening resource expenditure.

Real-World Challenges of Screening Performance

The Elusive Gold Standard Hearing Test for Neonates and Young Infants

In the previous discussion of efficacy measures, much reference was made to whether the screened persons did or did not have the target disorder, but nothing was said about how that truth can be determined. This is the matter of a gold standard test of a baby's hearing. How can it be determined whether a screening result is correct or not?

Comparing screening test outcomes with reliable, behavioral thresholds as soon as they can be obtained seems the only valid approach for screening test accuracy studies. However, there are two significant issues. Because the gold standard test (also referred to as a *reference* or *index test*) cannot be done at the same time as the test under investigation, there is no way of knowing whether the hearing has changed in the interval between the two tests. Also, behavioral response to sound, such as head-turning in a conditioned paradigm, is itself subject to validity and accuracy challenges. Not only might visual reinforcement audiometry (VRA) minimum response levels (MRLs) be systematically higher than true, perceptual thresholds, but what if there is a (known or unknown) disorder of vision, sensory-motor integration, motor function, attention, or even volition? Does no overt response equate to no hearing? Not in every case. Is behavioral audiometry even feasible in some groups of children? Clearly, it is not. Therefore, it can be argued that *there is no globally valid gold standard test of hearing in newborns and young infants.* Early, high quality VRA is more properly considered as a "silver" standard, by virtue of its dependency on tester expertise and its limited applicability to a significant proportion of the target population for screening, such as NICU graduates with multiple morbidities.

Automated ABR screening might be compared with the results of a comprehensive, manual diagnostic ABR. Such a comparison has the advantage that the two types of test can be done close together in time, that is, when the baby is the same age. The problem is that such a comparison does not answer the key question, "*Is the screening result correct?*" Rather, it answers the question, "*Does AABR screening agree with manual diagnostic ABR results*?" Not the same question at all, not the least because the ABR is not a direct measure of hearing but, rather, a statistical correlate and epiphenomenon (a sort of by-product) of hearing. Second, if the reference ABR is done with toneburst stimuli, there are difficulties that arise in comparing the results to those of a test with clicks. Third, the screening and reference ABR outcomes can both be right or wrong with respect to actual hearing, but they will tend to be so in tandem, which is known as a problem of correlated error. This type of positive error correlation results in overestimation of the accuracy of the screen. In fact, such test comparisons are ill-conceived as evaluations of screening test accuracy, though they may be informative with respect to other issues such as the relationship between click and tone burst ABR thresholds. Note that although comparing OAE screening outcomes to the results of diagnostic ABR remains ill-conceived as a measure of OAE screening performance with respect to auditory perception, such comparisons are less prone to correlated error and may be highly informative.

The reader may have seen or heard statements to the effect that high-quality, diagnostic ABR is a gold standard hearing test for infants under about 6 months of age. It is inappropriate to equate the best available test (the test of choice) for some population with a genuine gold standard for that population. Frequency-specific, diagnostic ABR testing conducted with a well-designed and standardized test protocol can constitute a good reference test for the follow-up of newborns who fail screening tests, but it certainly is not a gold standard in the full sense of the word. An important distinction must be made here between use of diagnostic ABR to evaluate automated ABR or OAE screening and its use as a confirmatory and diagnostic procedure in babies who fail screens. One reason for this difference is that in the evaluation of screening it is important to be able to distinguish very small percentages of error, whereas in clinical audiometric follow-up the precision demands are less stringent. Moreover, there is a substantial body of knowledge about reasonable correspondence between high-quality, frequency-specific ABR testing and conventional, behavioral measures of hearing, as well as to the factors that affect accuracy and validity in older children and adults. This is *construct validity* of the ABR, namely, a network of relationships that as a whole delimit the strengths and weaknesses of the ABR as a measure of hearing. An automated ABR screen, in contrast, is at best a limited, statistical approximation to a high-quality diagnostic ABR test. The same could be said of any automated OAE screen, in relation to its high-quality, diagnostic analog.

OAE and ABR Hearing Screening Sensitivity Are *Not* Well Understood

Values for automated OAE (AOAE) and automated ABR (AABR) screening test sensitivity are reported quite frequently, and there appears to be a tendency to believe that current screening tests detect all, or nearly all, hearing losses that are of moderate degree or greater. Unfortunately, less is known about the actual sensitivity of AOAE and AABR than the reader might imagine. There are several reasons for this. First, direct, prospective determination of sensitivity requires that ALL children screened be followed up by a definitive procedure to determine the true hearing status. It follows that sensitivity cannot be determined from a population screening program, because only screening failures are routinely followed up, usually by diagnostic ABR. To determine sensitivity it is necessary to conduct a cohort study of the entire screened group, which means simply that all group members must have a described final outcome.

It might seem an obvious approach to compare screening program yield with independent estimates of prevalence, to estimate screening test sensitivity. Although valid in principle, the main problems are the availability and reliability of such prevalence estimates. Even if estimates were obtained for specific populations, for which there are several examples, their generalizability across populations and over times is highly questionable. Prevalence is known to be subject to variation due to many facets of definition, measurement, and epidemiologic context.

Second, as noted earlier there is no definitive hearing test that can be administered concurrently with the screen. When relying on later validation, late-onset or progressive loss in the intervening period can lead to underestimation of screening sensitivity, as can positive bias in VRA minimum response levels. Also, ear canal volume increase during early growth can reduce the effective SPL of a given stimulus dial level significantly, which might also cause sensitivity to be underestimated because the actual SPL at the screen is elevated relative to that for an equivalent nominal stimulus level at the subsequent behavioral audiometry. Fluctuating sensorineural hearing loss and small levels of conductive overlay are also potential sources of bias or varibility.

Third, there is a serious problem of insufficient sample size. Suppose that in any given study the screened group were a particular birth cohort, such as all children born in some date range at some screening location. The most common estimate of sensitivity obtained from follow-up of all screened babies is simply the proportion of all screened children found to have hearing loss at follow up and who also failed the screen. There are readily available statistical tables or algorithms giving the variability of such proportions for various sample sizes (binomial confidence intervals). Examples of such confidence intervals are given in Table 16–3, derived using the *adjusted Wald* estimator calculator retrievable at www.measuringusability.com/wald. The important issues are the maximum tolerable width of confidence interval for the estimate of sensitivity and the number of babies that need to be screened and followed up in order to achieve an interval of that width or less. For example, a sample that contained only 50 babies with genuine hearing loss and 45 of these failing the screen would yield a sensitivity estimate of approximately 0.9 and would have 90% confidence limits on that estimate from about 0.81 to 0.95. Remember that the true value of sensitivity can lie anywhere in that interval. Is such an estimate useful? Probably not, in that a value of 0.81 would be considered unacceptable, whereas a value of 0.95 would be considered excellent. It can be seen from Table 16–3 that perhaps 500 babies with hearing loss are needed before the sensitivity estimate is sufficiently precise (0.88–0.92). In a natural, prospective screening sample with a prevalence of about 2 per 1,000, this would require follow-up of 250,000 babies, which is obviously prohibitive. One way around the difficulty would be to screen only NICU babies, for which the prevalence is much higher, perhaps as high as 2 per 100. This would lead to a natural sample requirement of 25,000 babies, which is still extremely demanding. Another problem with that approach is that the sensitivity in such a specialized sample may not be the same as it

Table 16–3. Point Estimates and 90% Confidence Intervals (adjusted Wald method) for True Sensitivity of About 0.9 (90%), for Different Numbers of True Cases*

Number of true cases	20	50	100	200	500	1000
Number failing screen	18	45	90	180	450	900
Sensitivity estimate (%)	86.4	88.5	89.2	89.6	89.8	89.9
Lower Confidence Limit	73.0	80.6	83.9	85.9	87.6	88.3
Upper Confidence Limit	97.5	95.3	94.0	93.0	92.0	91.5

*The precision of the sensitivity estimate is not acceptable for samples containing fewer than at least 200 babies with hearing loss and even then the range of plausible values is more than 7%. Higher, standard confidence levels such as 95% or 99% would require even larger numbers of true cases to achieve useful precision of sensitivity estimation. Note that the statistically preferred (point) estimator of sensitivity is not the simple proportion of true cases failing the screen but tends toward it as the sample size increases.

would be in the general population of all newborns. Despite the best effort to date (Norton et al., 2000), no prospective study as yet has yielded the desirable precision on sensitivity estimates for OAE or ABR screening tests. It does not matter whether a single point estimate of sensitivity is derived or an ROC curve is used: the resulting confidence intervals for feasible, prospective studies are too wide to render typical estimates of much value in test development or evaluation. The more common 95% confidence interval of course, would be wider still. Note also that these calculations take no account of any actual changes in true sensitivity for different degrees of hearing loss severity.

Fourth, there is pervasive issue of differences between sensitivity estimates obtained from controlled trials and field sensitivity that occurs in actual practice. Laxity and diversity of screening practices in actual screening programs might have unpredictable effects on actual test performance, and there is very little published information available about such effects. It can be speculated that observed variations in specificity (see later) may also occur for sensitivity. The problem is that such effects are extremely difficult to demonstrate and quantify.

In practice, perhaps the only practicable approach to large-sample estimation of sensitivity is through so-called ascertainment studies, that is, if all cases of hearing loss in a given geographical region were identifiable from, say, a retrospective review of all audiologic records, then if all those cases had been screened, a reasonably valid and precise estimate of screening sensitivity might be derived. Such an estimate however, will be affected by many challenges, including the completeness of the identification process, the quality of clinical records, the stability of the target population, the completeness of the screening and, of course, the inherent problems of longitudinal validation just mentioned. Good ascertainment studies essentially demand regionally or nationally centralized, universal hearing health care programs based on consistent protocols, such as are implemented to some extent in, for example, England and Australia.

Given all of these concerns, the apparent ease and confidence with which sensitivities of NHS tests are reported and quoted is quite remarkable. In fact, there is very little hard data on sensitivity that is valid, precise, and generalizable across studies or program populations. We may believe that the sensitivity of a well-conducted AABR screen is good, but we do not know, indeed we may never know, exactly what it is or how much it can vary across populations.

Intrinsic Sensitivity Limitations of OAE and ABR Screening

The complexity of hearing itself and of hearing screening tests raise many important issues that impinge directly on the ability to satisfy the Wilson-Jungner (1968) criteria. Although there is no doubt that AABR screening as currently implemented is vastly superior to behavioral screening methods in newborns and young infants, what are the limits of this effectiveness, particularly with reference to its ability to detect all hearing disorders within the target disorder set? There are several substantial issues.

One reason for concern, or at least for curiosity, is that in the only multicenter, prospective, comparative study of OAE and ABR screening sensitivity to date, by Susan Norton and her colleagues (2000), the ROCs for detection of average pure tone hearing loss showed that at a specificity of 0.95 the sensitivities of TEOAE, DPOAE, and ABR were in the range about 0.6 to 0.65. These are values that would be considered unacceptable for current screening programs. The main reason to doubt that such estimates apply to field performance of modern screening devices is that the yields of some screening programs (such as that in England) are broadly consistent with exceptionally well-characterized local prevalence data. However, one key to the difference may lie primarily in the fact that the hearing loss severity criterion used by Norton et al. was 30 dB HL by VRA, whereas the yield-prevalence match from the England data was based on an average loss criterion of at least 40 dB HL in the better ear. It was shown many years ago by Hyde, Riko, and Malizia (1990) that the predictive accuracy of the click ABR improves rapidly for hearing loss criteria in the 30 to 50 dB HL range, both by ROC and Likelihood Ratio measures.

Current AABR screening tests typically use click stimuli, which introduces some concerns about screening sensitivity. The click has a broad energy spectrum and potentially excites a large region of the cochlea. In principle at least, a detectable ABR could be elicited from any cochlear region in the range from about 1 to 4 kHz, even from an isolated island of hearing around a specific frequency. Therefore, there is a conceptual mismatch if a wide-band stimulus is used in an attempt to detect a target disorder that is defined to include low-, mid-, or high-frequency hearing losses or notched losses. At least one very recent screening device utilizes special types of wide-band, transient stimuli, such as chirps (Cebulla, Stürzebecher, Elberling, & Müller, 2007), which are substantially more effective at ABR elicitation than are conventional click stimuli, because they improve overall neuronal synchrony by compensating for cochlear traveling wave delay. However, any wideband, transient stimulus will suffer sensitivity limitations for frequency-specific hearing losses. To the extent that such losses are present in the screened population, the sensitivity of AABR screening will be compromised. One way of expressing this problem is to say that clicks or click-like stimuli "ask the wrong question" of the cochlea. Screening with a click basically asks "is there any frequency region in the range from about 1 to 4 kHz that has acceptable hearing sensitivity?" Perhaps a better question to ask is: "is there any frequency in the target disorder range that does *NOT* have acceptable hearing sensitivity?" This question, which is highly relevant if the target disorder definition includes losses at specific frequencies, could only be answered by some more complex screening technique that measures response from several regions along the cochlear partition.

A second concern relates to screening stimulus levels. One aspect is that ABR thresholds expressed in dB nHL do not necessarily equate directly to perceptual thresholds in dB HL, so an adjustment must be made in order to relate screening stimulus levels correctly to the desired minimum hearing loss within the target disorder range. For a detailed explanation of relationships between ABR thresholds and perceptual thresholds, see Sininger and Hyde (2009). An equally troubling concern is variation among newborns in the actual sound pressure level (SPL) of the stimulus that results from use of a constant nominal stimulus level in dB nHL. The volume and geometry of the external ear canal affect the actual intensity of the stimulus at the tympanic membrane and such effects differ over frequency (see, for example, Bagatto, Scollie, Seewald, Moodie, & Hoover, 2002). At the very least, this means that with most current AABR instruments, which do not autocalibrate stimulus levels within individual ear canals, newborns are being screened at SPLs that may differ substantially from baby to baby. Such differences may be as large as a range of 15 to 20 dB, with the highest SPLs generally occurring in those with the smallest canal volumes. Clearly, this may reduce the sensitivity of AABR screening in newborns with mild hearing losses who happen to have small canal volumes and, therefore, elevated effective stimulus SPLs. Conversely, it will increase sensitivity in newborns with unusually large volumes, because of lower effective SPLs. The size and scope of this effect on sensitivity are unknown, but it is a clear deficiency of measurement parameters that could be avoided by stimulus SPL autocalibration using a miniature microphone, as is commonly done for OAE stimuli.

As noted earlier, AABR devices all implement some statistical test for response detection. Any such test will have an implicit or explicit significance level for response detection, usually expressed as the size of the probability of false-positive response detection. This equals the algorithmic screening false-negative probability, because false-positive response detection results in a screen pass in the absence of response, namely in the presence of hearing loss. The lower the false positive response detection probability is set, the higher will be the (algorithmic) screen sensitivity and FP rate. Again, there are no standards for setting such probabilities, across screening devices.

Can the sensitivity of AABR be significantly improved without concomitant increase in FP screens? The most obvious approach is to address the issue of false-negatives due to frequency-specific hearing losses. This would require a frequency-specific, multiple-frequency method and the most obvious is to use the multifrequency 80-Hz ASSR, which basically is just a fast ABR with a simple, frequency-based detection algorithm. The big question is the choice of the number and range of test frequencies. The time taken to screen with acceptable error rates will be governed by the lowest frequency chosen (e.g., 500 Hz or 1 kHz), because EEG noise levels increase steadily at low frequencies. It remains to be seen whether such devices emerge in the near future. The pace of implementation may well be limited by problems of patent protection, a common issue in the history of newborn hearing screening.

A second approach would be to increase the separation between the case and noncase distributions, thereby increasing the value of d'. This boils down to narrowing the distributional spread of the SNR measure. Here, the main challenge is that newborns and young infants present for AABR screening with a wide range of EEG noise levels. Averaging strategies based on a fixed number of stimuli do not compensate for such a range, because they yield a fixed reduction in noise level based on the square root of the number of sweeps collected. Most screening instruments compensate by adjusting the number of sweeps in an attempt to achieve a target low level of EEG noise in the average. There are limits to the practicality and success of this method because, for example, a five-fold variation in EEG noise (probably a conservative estimate of the true range) would require a 25-fold range of sweep counts, which would lead to impractically lengthy averaging times in some babies. So, for this reason among others, the higher the EEG noise level, the greater the probability of both false-negative and false-positive response identification by the ABR detection algorithm, so the lower will be the sensitivity and specificity. The only way to avoid this effect is for the device to declare the screen void beyond a given EEG noise level; some devices do versions of this, but the methods and criteria are not standardized. The practical challenge for screening device manufacturers is that the tighter the control over required average noise levels, the higher will be the incidence of voided screens and the longer will be the maximum screening times, both of which would probably be perceived negatively by the user community.

Although there have been substantial recent advances in relation to stimulation techniques, such as the chirp methods already mentioned, current methods of ABR measurement are not very sophisticated, from a statistical perspective. There are several advanced statistical techniques that could improve SNR distributional characteristics for the ABR, but none of them is straightforward conceptually or technically. Their implementation would require an extraordinary conjunction of statistical, clinical, and technological insight and cooperation, as well as strong commercial incentive and will. Given the apparently reasonable performance of existing devices, the prospects for rapid development of better methods for ABR detection seem limited at present.

Just as is the case for the ABR, OAE screening currently only has empirical validity, based on observed correlations between OAE detectability and hearing thresholds. Leaving aside the matter of ANSD, which AOAE screening intrinsically cannot detect, current test sensitivity is limited mainly by the wide natural distribution of AOAE amplitudes in subjects with hearing losses that are at or near the lower bound of a reasonable target disorder range. It is perfectly feasible to enhance AOAE specificity by improving the power of the emission detection algorithm but improving sensitivity without concomitant increase in FP screens is very challenging. It seems indisputable that many children with hearing losses up to at least 30 dB HL will have detectable OAEs. Simply making the OAE detection criterion more conservative will increase sensitivity at the expense of already limited specificity. The prospects for accurate OAE screening for mild or minimal hearing losses seem constrained at best, because of underlying distributional overlap for the target and nontarget groups.

Current AOAE devices, whether based on transient or distortion-product emissions, effectively test OAE signal-to-noise ratio for several frequency regions. Frequencies below about 1 kHz are difficult to test accurately not because of absent OAE but because of increasing environmental and body-generated acoustical noise levels at low frequencies. In principle, sensitivity could be increased by requiring response detection at *every one* of several test frequencies, somewhat analogous to the argument made earlier for the AABR. But, there is the ever-present issue of balance between sensitivity and FP rate. To the author's knowledge, there are limited efficacy and effectiveness data addressing adequately the detailed effects of AOAE pass-fail criteria on actual test error rates in populations with diverse audiometric profiles and severities. Indeed, the scientific rationale underlying the nature and variety of current device pass-fail criteria is not readily apparent. Certainly, there is much room for evidence-driven, parametric improvement in OAE screening protocols.

OAE and ABR Screening Specificity Is Relatively Well Understood

The amount of information available about specificity values for automated OAE and ABR screens is vastly greater than that available for sensitivity. This is a fact simply because the population prevalence of hearing loss is low. Take a figure of, say, 2 per 1,000 live births. Because the vast majority of babies who fail the initial screening will *not* have hearing loss, the overall proportion of babies who fail (the refer rate) is actually an accurate estimate of the screen FP rate, given a substantial sample size that is quite easy to obtain. No follow-up at all is required for this estimation. A modest screening program sample of 50,000 babies, for example, will yield a reasonable estimate of the refer rate and the specificity estimate is simply the complement of that rate. It is important to note that using the refer rate as an estimate of the true FP rate only works when prevalence is very low, which may not be a valid assumption when considering the performance of the later stages of a multistage screening process (see later).

Specificity Limitations of OAE and ABR Screening

In newborn hearing screening, the most common questions relate to which test(s) to use and should a one-, two-, or three-stage series of screens be used. The challenge is usually to increase specificity while suffering a minimal loss in sensitivity, that is, to reduce the net rate of screening failure without missing a significant additional number of babies with hearing loss. To understand how to do this, the various causes of false positive and false negative errors must be considered.

Some possible causes of false-positive screening failure, for automated OAE and ABR screens, are as follows:

AOAE	AABR
Random algorithmic error	Random algorithmic error
High environmental noise	High electromyogenic noise
Minor or worse middle-ear conditions	Substantial transient conductive loss
Partially blocked probe	Partially blocked insert phone
Poor probe positioning	Poor earphone positioning
Naturally small OAEs	Naturally small ABRs
Suboptimal test methods	Suboptimal test methods

These sources of false-positives can be divided into categories that reflect different properties. First, there is algorithmic error. This is statistical error arising within the screening device response detection decision algorithm itself, because the pass-fail criteria are inherently statistical. Such errors are controlled in part by the choice of significance level of the response detection algorithm. The more conservative the test for response detection is the more reluctant the algorithm will be to conclude that response is present and, therefore, that the measurement comes from the disorder-absent distribution. Consequently, the higher the likelihood is of false positive screens. Note also that the lower the statistical power of the detection algorithm, the less likely the algorithm will be to detect a genuinely present response, so the higher the FP rate will be. There are no standards yet in place for the statistical performance of screening devices and their associated response detection algorithms and the algorithms themselves differ radically across devices and manufacturers. But, one important point about algorithmic error is that it is quite likely that such errors will be statistically random and independent of each other, so the probability that they will occur repeatedly declines dramatically with screen repetition.

The second group of errors that may be useful to identify could be called "transient," for lack of a better term. These errors can arise from several sources, including temporary environmental, physiologic, or physical conditions that may readily change over a short time. For example, middle ear debris or fluid may resolve within a matter of hours. A blocked probe can be unblocked, or poor position avoided. Calming a baby may improve acoustic or electromyogenic noise levels, and so on. The key point about these error sources is that they can be changed readily. If, and only if, the source of potential error is recognized and addressed, then the errors will not persist across multiple screens and, therefore, they will become independent. If the sources persist, so will the errors. Changing the test type, however, may improve independence, because different tests tend to differ in their susceptibilities to various error sources.

The third error group might be called "sustained" errors. For these, little can be done and they will tend to persist across multiple tests of the same type, although they may not persist across different test types. For example, there is a natural distribution of OAE amplitude (and ABR amplitude) in babies who do not have significant hearing loss, so inevitably some babies will fail simply because they have small responses. Repeating an OAE screen would do nothing to reduce errors from that source, so the errors would persist, whereas changing to an ABR screen, for example, could avoid that error source completely (while introducing other possible sources, but possibly independent ones). Similar remarks could be applied to screening devices that had algorithms or stimulation/recording methods that were inherently inefficient at eliciting or detecting response.

The relative magnitudes of all the different possible sources of false-positive screening error are at present poorly understood and almost certainly are very different across locations, times, test populations, and test personnel. Some sources of error, such as poor probe positioning, can be addressed by better technique; the challenge there is how to detect the deficiency and remedy it. Probe blockage can sometimes be addressed by removal, cleaning and immediate re-screening, but such rescreening will do nothing to abolish false-positives due to middle-ear debris or infection; there is no choice but to wait or to rescreen on an outpatient or community basis. Debris or fluid issues can be addressed, if practicable, by delaying the test. For example, Figure 16–5 shows the effect of age in hours on the failure rate for DPOAE screening. Clearly, the more time that elapses from birth, the lower the OAE screening failure rate will be. However, the trend towards shorter perinatal hospital stays may limit options, if predischarge screening is the chosen mode. Movement noise, whether acoustical (AOAE) or electrophysiologic (AABR), is addressed by screening when the baby is in as quiet a state as possible but, again, this may or may not be achievable practically under the constraints of predischarge test scheduling. Moreover,

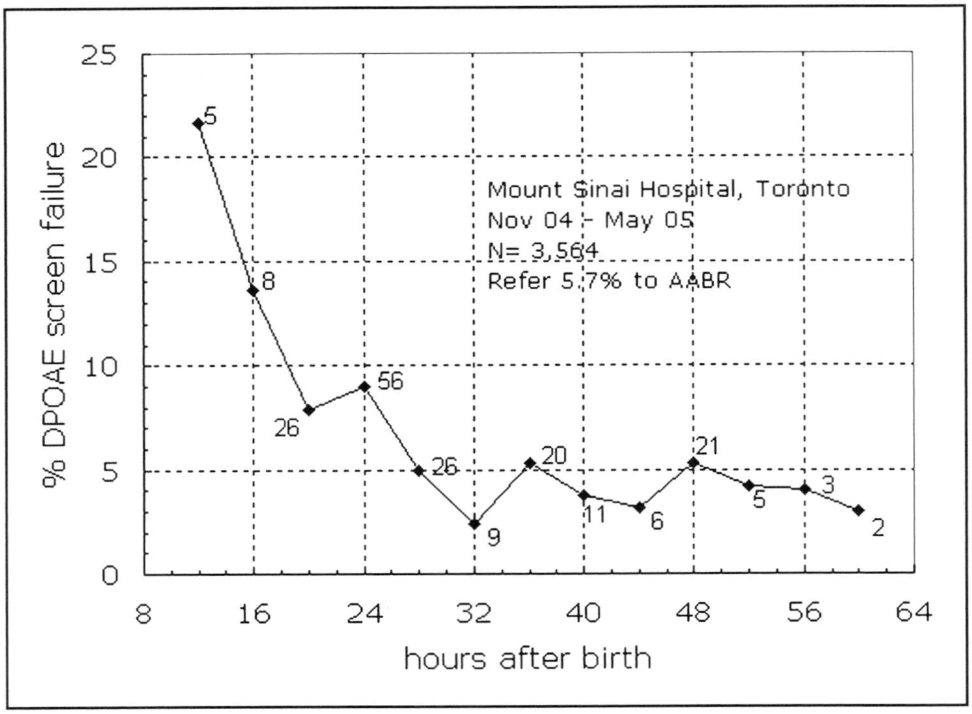

FIGURE 16–5. The fail rate from Stage 1 DPOAE screening declines rapidly with age of vaginal-birth babies in hours, with an asymptotic value achieved at about 24 hours of age. The interval between birth and OAE screening is a strong source of variability in screening fail (refer) rates.

high levels of such noise are not always readily apparent and accompanied by gross movement of the baby. In many ways, the predischarge hospital stay is not necessarily the most favorable situation with respect to false positives, but outpatient or community screening presents a common challenge of reduced access to the child, so the choice may be between high access and high FP rate versus poorer access and lower FP rate.

Refer Rate Variation: Does a Single Specificity Value Actually Exist?

While test efficacy measures such as sensitivity and specificity reflect the extent to which the test *can* discriminate cases from noncases, *effectiveness* reflects the extent to which it *does* discriminate in actual, field practice. Effectiveness is rarely, if ever, as good as efficacy studies lead us to expect. The reasons for this are many; some are obvious and some are more subtle. Test efficacy is typically established by controlled studies. Such studies are usually undertaken with very careful optimization and standardization of procedures, instrumentation, and criteria. They are usually designed and implemented by experts in the specific area of interest, with training and oversight of practices. Moreover, studies almost always target specific populations of subjects that are filtered by clear inclusion and exclusion criteria.

In actual field practice, very few of these factors may operate. In contrast to the controlled study context, the populations are unfiltered and reflect the full range of natural variation in subject characteristics and behaviors. Instrumentation, protocols, and procedures may vary from place to place, tester to tester, subject to subject and over time. The levels of understanding and expertise may vary substantially among testers and over time, perhaps improving with practice and perhaps deteriorating with carelessness or the development of idiosyncratic variations of practice. Each and every one of these factors will increase the variability of outcomes and will also tend to reduce test performance.

In the light of all of these concerns and sources of false-positive screens, it should be no surprise to the reader that reported screening refer rates for any given screening technology or specific device vary widely.

What is remarkable is the large amount of variation in refer rates, not only across screening studies or service programs, but across regions, centers and even across screening personnel within centers. Figure 16–6 shows an example of such variation. Although there are few published reports of variation analysis, the author is aware of similar ranges of refer rate variation in several state or national programs.

What does screening refer rate variation, which is attributable primarily to variation in false-positive rates, really mean at a deeper level, with respect to program quality? First, it means that there is a loss of screening *equity*, in the sense that children may have radically different likelihoods of false-positive screening, depending on where they go for screening and who screens them. Second, there will be widely variable demand for follow-up services, such as diagnostic testing. These are important issues that have received little attention in published reports on EHDI programs.

Perhaps the most interesting implication of refer rate variation is that reports of screen test performance must be viewed with great caution. Of course, there is the basic matter of sampling error, which is more important than commonly believed and are discussed shortly. But, more fundamentally, there is the question of whether it is actually meaningful to attribute a single, specific false-positive rate to a specific screening test technology or device. The reason is that FP rates are intimately dependent on a host of practical variables that have to do with technique, environment and the precise characteristics of the screened population. For example, if two programs have different practices or constraints with respect to scheduling of initial screening tests, their FP rates will differ, perhaps substantially. Also, it is commonly reported that refer rates of screening programs decrease substantially over a period of years from program initiation. None of these reported rates is correct. In fact, it can be argued that there is no correct rate for any given screening test technology or device. There is a typical rate, a best rate, a median rate, and a range of rates, but it is the detailed procedures and factors that lead to the lowest rates that are of greatest interest in terms of screening program quality.

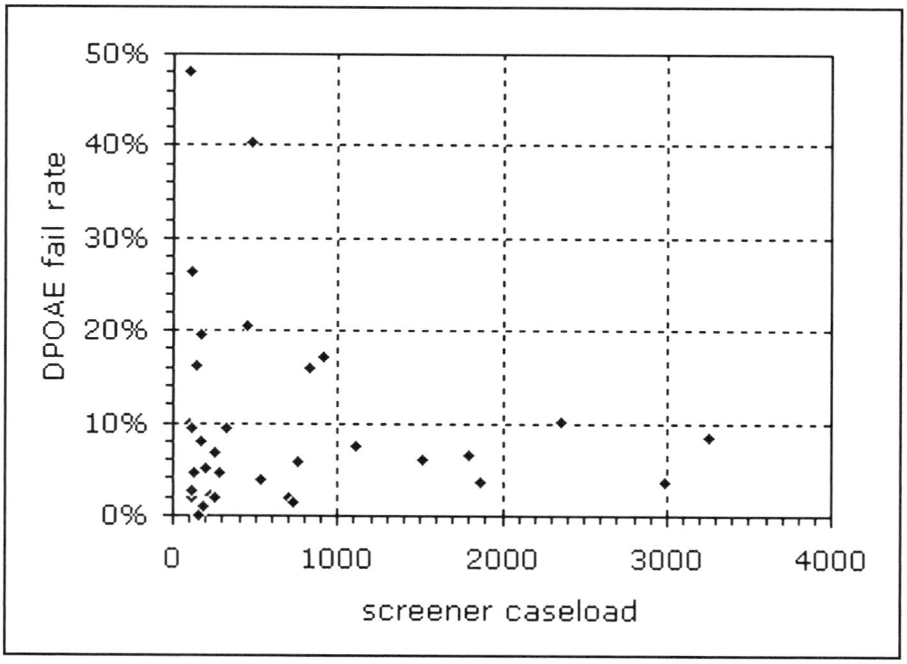

FIGURE 16–6. DPOAE Stage 1 screening fail (refer) rates for individual screening personnel can differ dramatically. The more babies an individual screens, the lower the failure rates tend to be, but substantial differences can occur even with very experienced screeners. These effects are dominated by false-positive screens. They raise the issue of whether it is meaningful to think of a single fail rate as valid for any screening test.

In summary, the challenge with specificity is not so much to obtain accurate estimates of it, but rather to make any valid use of those estimates, in light of the many sources of local variability in refer rates and, by implication, FP rates, which were discussed earlier. Note that *it is the variation of observed FP rates across individual screeners, locations, and time, as well as the lowest observed rates, that are of most interest in relation to screening program quality.*

AOAE and AABR Combinations and Screening Protocol Performance

A *screening protocol* is defined here as a set of screening tests and decision rules that determine how the outcomes of individual screening tests are combined into an overall, pass-fail outcome for the whole protocol. Many screening programs make use of more than one screening test. The tests may be repetitions of a single test technology or mixtures of different test technologies, or both. Decision rules for combining test results into a pass or fail for the overall protocol may be *serial* or *parallel*. A common serial rule involves only those who fail a first (Stage 1) screen going on to another (Stage 2) screen, so an overall fail is a fail on both tests. An example of this is the use of AOAE as an initial screen, followed by AABR in AOAE failures. For a parallel rule, two (or more) tests are done on all subjects and an overall fail is a fail on any one of the tests. Such parallel protocols are less common, except for programs in which the nature of the screening follow-up differs depending on the pattern of failure. For example, newborns who fail an OAE and pass an AABR might be simply monitored by developmental questionnaire or interview, whereas those who fail AABR would go on to immediate diagnostic tests. Alternatively, those who pass OAE and fail AABR might be referred directly to a special follow-up for possible ANSD candidates. Finally, a *mixture* protocol may include different protocols for subgroups of the screening population. For example, babies who are not at risk might receive serial OAE/AABR, whereas babies at risk might receive only AABR. One rationale for that approach is that at-risk newborns will include the majority of ANSD cases, which is speculated but not yet proven and which may depend, as do so many aspects of screening, on local population epidemiology. A more traditional rationale is that the much higher prevalence of hearing loss in the at-risk group justifies the use of a more expensive test with higher intrinsic efficacy.

The purpose of using tests in combination is usually to control overall errors. Most commonly, it is to increase specificity, that is, to lower the net FP rate. What exactly is the effect of combining tests on the overall sensitivity and specificity? In the simplest case, the errors for each test are assumed to be statistically unrelated (independent), in which case probabilities can be calculated easily. For example, suppose we have two screens (S1 and S2) with sensitivities and specificities denoted as (se1, sp1) and (se2, sp2).

For S1 and S2 both with se and sp of 0.9 for simplicity, and with a serial decision rule:

$$\text{se (overall)} = \text{se1} \times \text{se2} = 0.9 \times 0.9 = 0.81, \text{ and}$$

$$\text{sp (overall)} = 1-[(1-\text{sp1}) \times (1-\text{sp2})], = 1-[0.1 \times 0.1] = 1 - 0.01 = 0.99,$$

so the sensitivity is reduced by 10% but the specificity increases dramatically, with a 90% reduction in false positives (from 0.1 to 0.01). This is a typical result-serial protocols usually improve specificity dramatically and reduce sensitivity slightly.

In contrast, for S1 and S2 with a parallel decision rule:

$$\text{se (overall)} = 1-[(1-\text{se1}) \times (1-\text{se2})] = 0.99, \text{ and}$$

$$\text{sp (overall)} = \text{sp1} \times \text{sp2} = 0.81,$$

so the sensitivity increases to 0.99 and the specificity is reduced to 0.81. Parallel protocols usually increase sensitivity dramatically and reduce specificity slightly. One reason why they are less common is the high FP rates and the large workload involved if all protocol failures were to be followed up diagnostically. It is not possible to enhance sensitivity dramatically without FP cost.

In actual practice, the effects of multiple screens are not as dramatic as those just calculated, because the errors in the two screens are usually *not* completely independent. Suppose, for example, we took the extreme case of complete correspondence between the errors for S1 and S2. In the serial model, doing S2 will have no effect at all on the outcomes of S1, because all the FPs from S1 will also fail S2 and none of the FNs from S1 make it to S2. The overall performance equals that of S1 alone. In the parallel model, precisely the same subjects will be FP or FN so again the addition of S2 changes nothing. In the real world, neither the full independence or full dependence assumptions is true. There will be some degree of correlation between the errors for the two tests, and the amount of correlation will dictate the impact of adding the second screen.

Consider a situation in which about half of the false-positive screening errors arising in S1 were identical in S2. What that means is that the actual specificity of S2 in those subjects who fail S1 is very much lower (sp2 = 0.5) than when S2 is used alone as a first screen (sp2 = 0.9) because half of all the false-positive errors from S1 were propagated by S2. Another way of putting this is that the *conditional specificity* of S2 given S1 failure is much lower than the unconditional (ordinary) specificity of S2. Redoing the above calculation example for the serial protocol now gives an overall specificity of 0.95, not 0.99. This is, however, still a 50% reduction in false-positives, which is a big improvement.

Other Limitations of Current OAE and ABR Screening Instruments

Although test efficacy and effectiveness have been discussed in some detail, the actual performance of current screening tests is constrained not only by the intrinsic nature of such tests but also by limited flexibility that is granted the user by the manufacturers of screening instruments. There is limited ability to adjust screening tests to reflect different desired levels of performance. Furthermore, it is of limited interest and somewhat moot to define, for example, a 20dB HL hearing loss at a specific frequency as within the target disorder range, if the available screening devices cannot be configured and tuned to have acceptable performance for such hearing losses. Certainly, one cannot and should not rely on device manufacturers to be in a position to conduct large-sample efficacy optimization studies. In a sense, the situation that has emerged is one of the "tail (manufacturers) wagging the dog" (the screening community), albeit doubtless with the best of intentions.

What flexibility might be desired in current OAE screening tests? Despite the inherent limitation that statistical distributions of OAE amplitude overlap substantially when such hearing losses are present and absent, could test performance be improved by more flexibility? Take DPOAE screens, for example. What quantitative, evidence-driven rationale underlies the choice of test frequencies in range and number, the amount of averaging for each stimulus frequency pair, the SNR criterion value(s) and the nature of the pass-fail decision rule? What is the practical relevance of DPOAE measurements above 4 kHz? Why should failure to detect an OAE at any single F2 frequency not lead to overall failure, especially if such rules as "2 out of 3" or "3 out of 4" frequency passes could lead to a child with no hearing below 2 kHz passing the screen? The amount of information available on these issues is really quite limited, especially in relation to newborn screening for diverse hearing losses under a wide range of measurement conditions. Certainly, there is evidence that more sophisticated approaches to decision rules, such as the use of multivariate statistical tests, could improve performance (see, for example, Gorga et al., 2005). It seems fair to say that despite the considerable body of work that has led to viable and valuable screening tools to date, the surface of OAE screen optimization has barely been scratched. However, all of this is not about flexibility so much as it is about optimization.

In click-AABR screens, improvement such as autocalibration is also an optimization issue. However, unlike the situation for OAE, wherein optimal stimulus intensity parameters are understood quite well, stimulus levels for AABR screening could be selectable in order to accommodate different program criteria and target disorder choices. Notwithstanding the issues of actual ear canal SPL, if it were desired to detect only hearing losses of at least moderate degree, current nominal click levels of about 30 dB nHL are too low. Conversely, if it were desired to detect the full range of mild losses, 30 dB nHL is probably too high to achieve good sensitivity at the lower limits of loss. Currently, the willingness of device manufacturers to permit such adjustment is limited at best.

These limitations of flexibility are not without benefit. Imagine a world in which every program designer were able to chose a different screening stimulus intensity. Would this flexibility be beneficial, or would it increase an already problematic situation in terms of performance variability and the ability to evaluate or compare results across programs? A challenge sometimes expressed by device designers and manufacturers is that device users vary hugely in their level of knowledge and sophistication, so granting more flexibility would be appropriate for some but not all. One approach to this problem is to embed limited flexibility but to require a certain level of rationale in order to be able to access it. Although this smacks uncomfortably of policing, the downside of not doing it is that many reasonable program decisions, as well as many much-needed investigations of performance, are difficult if not impossible.

The fundamental point is that at present, *screening instruments do what they are configured to do and what individual screening program designers may want them to do is somewhat moot*, at least in the absence of evidence-based professional consensus of sufficient strength to influence equipment designers and manufacturers. Therefore, appropriate definitions of the target disorder, especially in terms of lower severity bounds, are substantially constrained by the capability and flexibility of available instruments and technologies.

Despite such restrictions, there remain important decisions that can be made about target disorder definition, and there are indeed important options for the design of screening programs. For the target disorder, the most important decisions to be made about screening with current instruments are whether it is desired to detect unilateral hearing loss and whether ANSD should be included in the target disorder set. With respect to screening efficacy, there are also program decision options that involve using combinations of screening tests.

The Impact of Hearing Screening

Having explored the WHO-inspired questions of the "significant health problem" and the "acceptable screening test" in some detail, we turn now to the issue of the effects of implementing a population hearing screening program.

The effect or impact of any new program of care must be predicted as part of the rationale for introducing the program. Impact must also be evaluated after the program is introduced, both to verify the performance projections and to provide the basis for correction of mistakes, fine-tuning, and overall quality improvement. Program impact can be evaluated in absolute or comparative terms. The absolute terms usually reflect the values and mores of society. For example, an absolute, value-driven position might be that every child has a basic right to services that will maximize the potential for a full and productive life. More specifically, this could be expressed in terms of the right to develop and realize the best possible communication, social, and educational potential, areas that are known to be compromised significantly by sustained hearing loss that goes undiagnosed for a substantial period. In contrast, comparative evaluation might address the question of whether a proposed program has improved the achievement of a valued outcome relative to current or historical performance, namely, the projected value added of the new program. Alternatively, it may address the relative performance of more than one alternative program model. The quantification of the important health problem, discussed at some length earlier, is crucial and is inextricably tied to the question of screening program impact, because impact can only be measured meaningfully in terms of a change in the state of the important health problem.

The possible effects of NHS programs in the EHDI context are far more diverse than is commonly considered. Impacts can be identified at least at three levels: the individual child, the individual family unit and the society at large. Table 16–4 presents some of the facets of program impact that should be considered. A full dis-

Table 16–4. Some Possible Components of Hearing Screening Impact

Child level
Earlier, improved hearing function
Enhanced family communication
Improved medical/developmental care
Improved language development
Improved cognitive and social development
Improved early literacy and educational readiness
Improved quality of life
Improved socioeconomic opportunity
Consequences of false-positive screening
Consequences of diagnostic error
Consequences of intervention failure
Family level
Exercise of the right to know the child's hearing status
Exercise of the right to make informed decisions
Avoidance of guilt due to ignorance or inaction
Avoidance of inappropriate or maladaptive behaviors
Improved family communication
Reduced long-term anxiety, uncertainty and stress
Reduced long-term costs
Long-term benefit from child's improved socioeconomic capacity
Short-term anxiety
Effects of false-positive screening
Immediate inconvenience and costs
Dissatisfaction with program deficiencies or failures
Societal level
Fulfillment of societal values and responsibilities
Reduced late-diagnosis and management costs
Reduced long-term special education costs
Reduced drop-out and delinquency costs
Increased individual productivity
Increased taxation revenue
Immediate program costs
Resource wastage due to program deficiencies

cussion of each of these factors is beyond the scope of this chapter, but several of them are touched upon briefly.

In the present author's view, three areas or clusters of these facets of impact merit particular emphasis as primary outcomes of screening. They are: (1) the acquisition of knowledge about the child's hearing status by the family and by relevant professionals, (2) the improvement in the child's hearing function, and (3) the child's development of language, with its broad array of consequences and correlates. The family knowledge outcomes occur through the process of audiologic diagnosis, as well as the subsequent, effective communication of its nature and meaning to the affected family. The latter is an area that is commonly overlooked despite its potential importance with respect to family understanding and behavior. The hearing improvement outcomes are contingent upon delivery of verified and valid technology-based intervention, typically through amplification or cochlear implants. These outcomes generally occur rapidly upon fitting of an appropriate device. The language outcomes, in contrast, are highly longitudinal, developing over an extended period of time and mediated by many factors such as family choices, language intervention services access, style, content and quality, service uptake and engagement by the family, translation of language development techniques into the home language environment and many other factors, such as the effects and management of concurrent sensory, cognitive, and developmental disorders.

Measurement of Screening Program Effectiveness

We now consider some of the approaches that have been taken to measuring the impact or effectiveness of a newborn hearing screening program. The evaluation of program effectiveness is an essential component of program improvement as well as a key facet of the justification for program continuation. Relatively few reports have addressed the matter of benefits of early knowledge for the family and for professionals involved with the child's health and developmental status. In contrast, many reports have focused upon screening coverage, age at screening, diagnosis and intervention, as well as the yield and characteristics of cases identified. Other important facets of program impact include costs, cost-effectiveness, and cost benefit. Lastly, we touch on issues of societal ethics, in relation to program rationale and impact.

Age at Hearing Loss Diagnosis and Intervention

Despite the traditional emphasis on language development, reports about age at diagnosis and age at hearing aid or cochlear implant fitting are perhaps the most common expressions of screening program impact. This is curious, because if language development was actually the primary health problem, then language performance should be the primary measure in terms of which system performance and change in performance due to screening are quantified. The child's age at diagnosis and at amplification are remote and very poor proxies for language status, albeit much easier to measure. The shift in viewpoint to include hearing itself as a primary dimension of the problem and of program impact renders the ages at diagnosis and amplification much more relevant and valid as measures of program success.

If it is accepted that family ignorance of the child's hearing status is an important part of the significance of the primary health problem, then the associated primary outcome measure is the child's age at which the family becomes fully informed, which is at least closely related to the age at diagnosis. It is also curious that with so much focus on age at diagnosis, the importance of the immediate knowledge outcomes has received relatively little attention in the literature to date.

If hearing function also is accepted as a primary measure of *health state* in itself, then the time a child spends in the state of hearing deficiency is an important measure of the *burden* of the disorder. It follows that the population distribution of ages at *effective provision* of improved hearing becomes the key quantifier not only of the important health problem but also of program impact.

The most common routes to improved hearing are amplification or a cochlear implant. Age at diagnosis is a credible proxy for age at device fitting, because it represents the least age at which fitting could occur. It is not a perfect proxy, because many factors can cause substantial delay between diagnosis and fitting, especially for an implant. Another complication in figuring out the actual age at onset of meaningful hearing improvement, especially for mild hearing loss, is that if diagnosis leads to knowledge and knowledge in turn leads to better communication strategies in the family, then some hearing benefit may ensue before the actual fitting of amplification.

One of the largest North American retrospective studies to date of age at diagnosis and age at hearing aid fitting was reported by Durieux-Smith and Whittingham (2000). Unfortunately, the study has not received the audience it deserves, probably because it was published in a Canadian journal. A re-analysis of some results of the study is illustrated in Figure 16–7.

Figure 16–7 shows that the average age at diagnosis in unscreened groups depended strongly on hearing loss severity; the less the severity, the greater the mean age at diagnosis. This is true whether or not the children had a risk indicator for hearing loss, the mean ages being somewhat lower for children with risk indicators. This is a very important observation, as will be made clear shortly. In addition, both unscreened groups have mean ages at diagnosis far greater than those for a screened group, for which severity had no effect on the mean age. This is all very reasonable intuitively.

Limitations of the Mean Age at Diagnosis or at Intervention

It is common in the audiology literature to see large values (such as 2–3 years) of the mean age at diagnosis as a quantifier of the problem prior to introduction of a screening program and much lower values (such as 3–6 months) as a measure of the effectiveness of screening. Such an approach is useful but can be improved. First, despite its popularity, the mean or average is notoriously unstable relative to the median when sample sizes of babies with hearing loss are not large and when statistical distributions of age at any given event are contaminated by extreme values or are systematically different from the normal (Gaussian) distribution. Both of these conditions are very probable. Second, the mean tells us something about the middle of a symmetric distribution but nothing at all about the spread or the upper end of the distribution, which are of much interest because they inform about the range of values and the cases of greatest concern. In general, it can be asserted that averages or mean values of variables obscure interesting properties and behaviors, rather than reveal and illuminate them. Third, use of the overall mean age at diagnosis contains an implicit

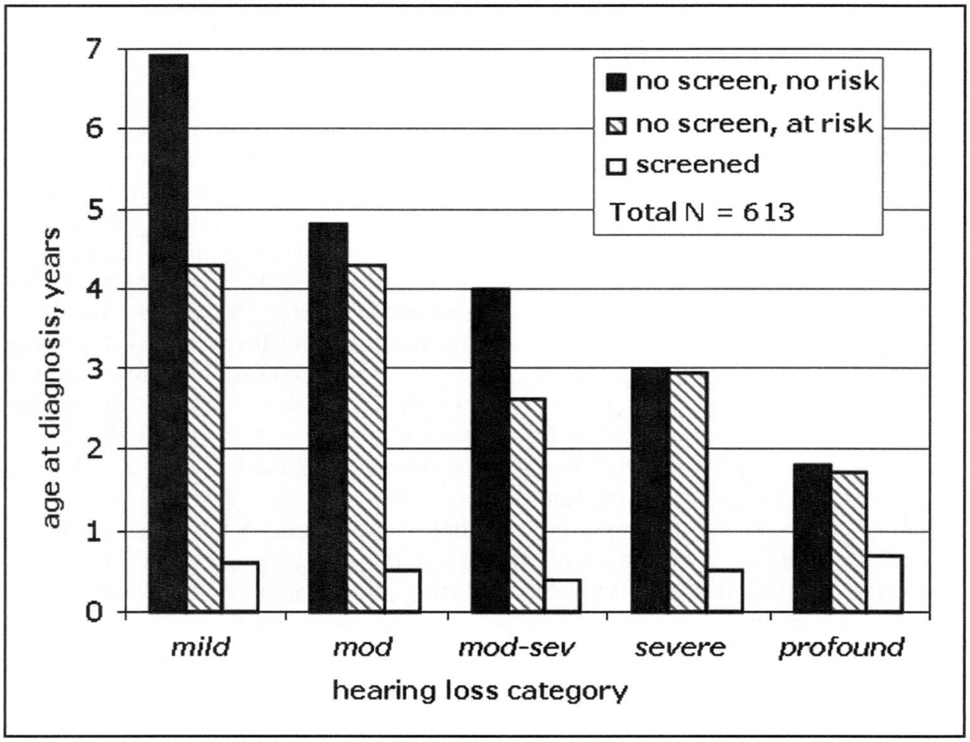

FIGURE 16–7. Some results from a retrospective chart analysis of age at diagnosis of hearing loss in 613 infants and young children fitted with hearing aids, from Durieux-Smith and Whittingham (2000). Three groups are shown: screened, unscreened with high-risk indicators, and unscreened without high-risk indicators. Note the very strong effect of increasing hearing loss severity on mean age at diagnosis in unscreened cases, as well as the differences across groups at each severity level.

assumption of equal importance for all severities of hearing loss, whereas it is manifestly false that a six-month delay in diagnosis of a mild and a severe hearing loss are equally important. Fourth, as the data in Figure 16–7 show, the absolute ages at diagnosis (and the effects of screening on age at diagnosis) are different for different degrees of loss, so the baseline (pre-screening) problem of late diagnosis is very different in magnitude across hearing loss severities. Fifth, the overall mean takes no explicit account of the prevalence of different hearing loss severities in any given sample, so it does not permit generalization of inferences to different populations with different patterns of severity prevalence.

Part of the problem is the natural desire for a very simple way to quantify the state of affairs but, as Albert Einstein once said, "everything should be made as simple as possible, *but not simpler*." The median (50th percentile) is often a more stable and useful index of the center of a distribution than is the mean. Other percentiles of the distribution of ages, such as the 90th or the 95th percentile, are also of interest. The measure that is most relevant for any given enquiry depends on the precise question being asked, and many questions of interest have little to do with the mean. An elegant approach is to use the entire cumulative distribution of ages, as shown in Figure 16–8. From such a plot, any required percentile of the distribution is immediately available. The cumulative distribution curve is *much* more informative than any single distributional parameter.

Improving the statistical description of age at diagnosis does not overcome the problem of grouping all hearing loss severities together. Therefore, in quantifying the state of affairs or the effectiveness of a program, the degree of hearing loss should be stratified; that is, the descriptive statistics should be given for subject groups with different ranges of hearing loss. While there are many possible measures of hearing loss severity, a rational choice might be the conventional audiometric

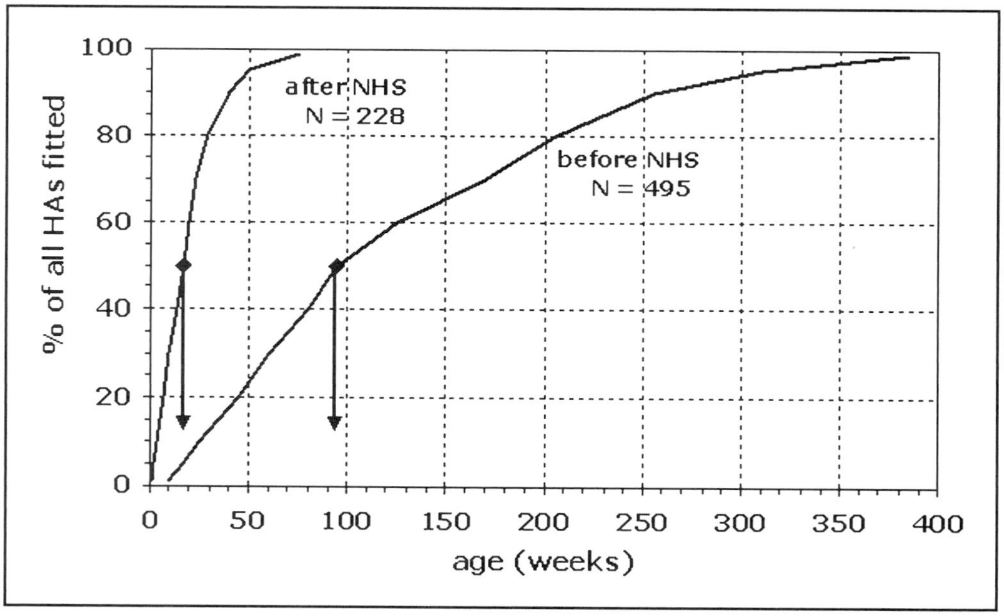

FIGURE 16–8. Sample cumulative distributions (CDs) of age at hearing aid fitting before and shortly after introduction of newborn hearing screening in England, showing a dramatic reduction in the median (50th percentile) age at device provision. The CD is a powerful and elegant summary of program performance, more robust and informative than the mean age at fitting or the percentage fitted by a single, specific age, because all such percentages are readily apparent. Such CDs are strongly recommended as an obligatory, standard component of all program performance reports involving age at occurrence of key events in UNHS and EHDI and of the intervals between such events. These data were provided to the author by kind permission of Dr. Adrian Davis.

severity category of the average loss at 0.5 to 4 kHz in the better ear.

Even without using the cumulative distribution approach, a much better quantification of both the important health problem and the effectiveness of any screening program can be obtained, for example, by using a minimum of five numbers, such as the medians for each severity group. This gives a *median age profile by severity*. If a single absolute target maximum age at diagnosis has been set, such as the Joint Committee on Infant Hearing (JCIH, 2007) recommendation of 3 months of age, then the median age minus three months for each severity group summarizes the shortfall from that target and the cumulative distributions of age minus three months give all the information available about the distribution of ages and shortfalls. One could, of course, set different targets for different severities. The overall burden of late diagnosis of hearing loss depends on the numbers of children affected as well as the amount of shortfall for each child in each severity group.

It is certainly possible, even desirable, to go further than this in quantifying both the problem and program impact. This would involve allocating some numerical value to each hearing loss severity that described the actual impact of a given severity of loss on the child. How could a meaningful magnitude of impact be expressed? One could assign a zero to normal hearing, unity or 100% to a profound hearing loss and intermediate values to intermediate severities. But, the effect of a given hearing impairment is not captured well simply by the average hearing threshold. A more natural measure might relate to the unaided speech intelligibility index. This is an area that has not received much attention, from the standpoint of quantifying the true burden of late detection of hearing loss or the effect of screening programs.

The Question of Program Costs

The importance of screening program cost is obvious, especially so in this era of accountability and economic concern. Cost can be viewed in several ways. In a *logic model* approach to program evaluation, cost is often treated as an input variable, expressed as required funding. In at least one classical approach to program evaluation, cost is treated as an element of program structure, just as are people, equipment, and buildings. In other models, cost may be treated as an outcome variable, so a program delivers both desired outcomes and costs. Whatever model is applied, cost basically is a negative attribute or parameter of any health services system and the associated health state of the population. Even to have no NHS program at all is one particular system choice, with an array of associated costs, such as the direct costs of the old medical referral system and the costs of special schooling to address compromised language development, for example.

Inevitably, the achievement of screening program objectives and desired clinical outcomes are constrained in the real world by consideration of the resources required. This necessarily invokes the methods of *cost-effectiveness* and *cost-benefit* analysis. In cost-effectiveness analysis (CEA), different programs or systems of care are compared in terms of the resources required to produce a given unit of desired outcome. For example, one might examine the communication skills of children at school entry in relation to three programs: a default program such as that historically based on medical referral for hearing services as and when suspicion of hearing loss arises, a system that includes targeted screening of newborns at high risk for hearing loss, and a system that includes universal screening of all newborns. Some of the outputs of each system may be desired and these are positive benefits. Others may be undesirable, and these are negative benefits, more commonly referred to as *harms*. These benefits and harms may relate directly to the intended program goals, or they may be unanticipated side-effects. The essence of CEA is computation of the costs of a given amount of net product or outcome of any given activity. Various methods are available for exploring quantitatively the values (positive or negative) that people assign to different outcomes or health states, broadly referred to as *health state utility analysis*.

Cost-benefit analysis (CBA) is a specific variant of CEA in which *all* of the inputs (resources) and outcomes are expressed in the same units, usually monetary and usually discounted for change in the value of money over time. The latter is especially important when calculating cost-benefit over periods of many years. A major challenge in applying CBA to NHS outcomes is to assign meaningful and valid monetary values to the variety of outcomes, be they benefits or harms. What is the monetary value, for example, of an earlier diagnosis or of an improved education readiness of a child? What is the cost of failure to achieve a valued societal goal for an individual child? Frequently, the cost values assigned are incomplete, approximate or even speculative. This can render the conclusions of CBA very unstable, and at the very least, it is essential to explore how those conclusions may vary with changes in the monetary values assigned. This is known as *sensitivity analysis*, an unfortunate term that the reader should not confuse with the very specific meaning of the word *sensitivity*, discussed earlier.

The reader interested in cost analysis of newborn hearing screening is encouraged to review carefully a report by Keren, Helfand, Homer, McPhillips, and Lieu (2002), which includes a substantial bibliography of relevant references. This detailed and sophisticated study used well-founded estimates of program performance parameters, costs and cost-savings to build a quantitative, comparative model of UNHS, selective screening and no screening. They included much sensitivity analysis, to test stability of the model's implications for ranges of assumed parameters. The bottom line was that UNHS is likely to result in long-term cost savings relative to selective screening or no screening, but that more evidence is required to substantiate the impact of EHDI on long-term language development, educational and occupational performance, and quality of life.

A significant, further limitation of many cost-oriented analyses of UNHS and EHDI to date has been a lack of separation of both absolute costs and changes in costs that can arise for different levels of hearing loss severity. Some cost analyses appeal to estimates of lifetime earnings with and without hearing loss, or special education costs with and without early interventions to improve hearing and language, but it cannot be valid to apply the same cost values to all children detected by screening and diagnosis. Different degrees of hearing loss cause different patterns not only of disadvantage and associated educational costs, but also of timing and delay in identification and intervention, both with and without screening programs. There may even be an unintended bias toward lines of argument that amplify the costs of undetected hearing loss as well as the cost saving attributable to UNHS programs. See, for example, an important report by Schroeder and her colleagues in 2006 and a commentary on it by Grosse and Ross (2006). Notwithstanding these benefit-inflationary concerns, it can also be said that most cost analyses to date have not taken into account the full array of potential benefits of EHDI to individuals, families and society, both ethical and functional. It is hoped that higher standards of economic analysis such as those illustrated and recommended by Schroeder and colleagues will come to pass.

Universal Versus Selective Newborn Hearing Screening

Although universal screening has emerged as almost a standard of care in many economically developed countries, the current rationale for it should not be considered as etched in stone or necessarily valid under all circumstances. It is instructive to review some of the underlying considerations for *any* NHS program, which can become quite complicated if all the pertinent factors are taken into account.

Hearing screening of newborns and infants identified as at risk for hearing loss (such as those with low birth weight, severe hypoxia, certain perinatal infections or a family history of childhood hearing loss) was widely advocated for many years prior to the more recent interest in universal screening. Part of the rationale is that selective screening concentrates effort and resources upon the children more likely to have the disorder. This remains to some extent true and especially relevant in situations of severe economic constraint, such as in developing countries with major resource limitations and serious health care challenges, often involving high mortality. Selective screening, as a minimum necessary practice, seems intuitively defensible, subject to the caveat that any screening at all can only be justified by the delivery of prompt and effective diagnosis and intervention.

Selective screening requires identification of the population at risk. As noted earlier, comprehensive determination of risk can be time-consuming and variable in quality. However, there are several approaches to efficient risk determination. If the purpose is solely to establish whether the infant is at risk or not, for the purpose of deciding whether or not to screen, then it is a matter of going through a list of indicators, preferably ordered by decreasing prevalence (of each indicator) and stopping as soon as any single indicator is positive. The indicator list for the well-baby nursery is very short (family history and craniofacial anomalies), while that for NICU babies is quite lengthy. Note that in this approach the purpose is not to develop a complete risk profile and establish whether each and every risk indicator is present, only to establish whether at least one of them is present.

One way of simplifying risk determination further is to consider only those infants who attend an NICU for some minimum duration (such as 5 days or more) as automatically at risk and all others to be not at risk. This avoids exploration of individual risk indicators. Limitations of that approach are that many NICU graduates may not actually be at risk, although some babies who do not attend an NICU certainly will be at risk. The latter is a more serious concern, because missing children at risk carries an elevated probability of missing true cases and, of all babies ultimately found to have the target disorder, a substantial proportion will not have attended an NICU.

Another problem with short-circuiting determination of the complete risk profile relates to an issue that goes beyond newborn hearing screening. It is now well-recognized that a significant (but currently unknown) proportion of all children who have hearing loss at school entry, say, do not have it at the neonatal stage and so they will be missed by newborn screening. Some, but not all, of those children who develop late-onset or progressive hearing loss (as distinct from hearing loss acquired in early childhood due to adventitious causes) will have perinatal risk indicators, even some specific indicators for late-onset or progressive hearing loss. If these children are to be monitored over time in some way, as is done in some comprehensive EHDI programs, then a perinatal risk review is required for that purpose alone, that is, to establish candidacy for monitoring or surveillance, not for newborn screening in itself. What this implies is that risk review of all babies is required whether the screening is selective or universal.

A further issue that must be accounted for, especially in the NICU population, is that some children will be very sick for a long time, or recurrently, which can cause substantial and justifiable delays in hearing screening. A significant proportion of NICU graduates with hearing loss, perhaps one-third, will have disorders additional to those of hearing that may include visual, motor and neurodevelopmental disorders, which can complicate diagnosis and intervention greatly.

With respect to the impact of hearing screening, it must be remembered that many NICU graduates attend high-risk follow-up clinics as a matter of course and assessing their hearing may have been a natural part of developmental evaluations, even in the absence of any formal hearing screening program. These factors reduce the value added of a systematic screening program, whether selective or universal, because some of these children would already have been identified early anyway, as part of a high-quality, traditional system of care.

The conventional argument used against selective screening has been that it is unacceptable to miss the substantial proportion of newborns and infants who have the disorder but no apparent risk indicator. This position essentially takes selective screening of at-risk newborns as a baseline and weighs the incremental benefits and costs of expansion to universal screening. Let us consider a simple, quantitative model. The reader with little interest in program costing can skip the next two paragraphs.

Because only 5 to 10% of newborns are typically determined to be at risk, screening all newborns increases the screening workload by a factor of 10 to 20 times. With perfect coverage, this could capture most of the affected infants not at risk, which may be anything from 20 to 50% of the total number with the target disorder. Because the majority of infants who fail screening do not have the disorder, many infants without the disorder will end up having diagnostic tests following UNHS and the number of such tests may also increase by a factor of 5 to 10 in a universal program.

Modern UNHS programs typically can achieve overall screening failure rates of about 1%, that is, the group referred to diagnostic tests is two orders of magnitude smaller than the screened population. Although a diagnostic test may be up to one order of magnitude (i.e., 10×) more costly than a screen, it follows that screening costs typically dominate diagnostic costs by an order of magnitude. For simplicity, let us consider only the direct costs of screening itself. In a large program, the capital costs of instrumentation are usually insignificant relative to personnel costs, because the life span of a single screening device will service thousands of babies. Supplies costs may be nontrivial for some screening systems but are ignored here. Assume perfect coverage and that any true case will fail the screen. Then, the four parameters that really matter are the screening personnel cost per screen (c), the prevalence of the disorder (p), the population proportion that are at risk (r) and the proportion of all true cases that are at risk (a). The outcome measure of most interest is the so-called *marginal cost per additional case identified*, that is, the cost per case for those cases identified by UNHS but missed by selective NHS. It turns out that the cost per case for UNHS is simply the personnel cost per case divided by the prevalence, namely, c/p. This is a simple, approximate but useful guide; for example, at $20 per screen and with a prevalence of 2 per 1,000 births, the cost per case is 20 per 0.002 or $10,000. It is easily shown that the selective NHS cost per case is the UNHS cost c/p times the ratio r/a and the marginal cost per additional case from UNHS is c/p times an inflation factor (1–r)/(1–a). For the values $c = 20$, $p = 0.002$, $r = 0.08$, and $a = 0.5$, for example, the UNHS, selective NHS and marginal costs per additional case are $10,000, $1,600, and $18,400. Note in particular that the inflation factor is very sensitive to the proportion of true cases that are at risk (a). The marginal cost of $18,400 was obtained using a proportion of 50%, whereas if the proportion were actually 80%, then the marginal cost would be $46,000. Note also that because determination of risk is always imperfect, actual proportions at risk that are reported are likely to be underestimates of true proportions, resulting in underestimates of marginal cost per additional case.

Suppose in a birth cohort of 100,000 we would find 200 babies with UNHS, versus 100 with selective screening. The 100 additional babies have a total marginal cost for screening of $1.8 million using the most favorable (lowest) estimate of the true case proportion at risk. The obvious question is whether it is worth the expense to discover the additional cases. But, introduced earlier, how do you put a meaningful dollar value on improving a child's hearing or giving a family vital knowledge? The cost-benefit argument traditionally is focused upon long-term returns on the investment, especially in terms of mainstreaming at school. Such figures are not only quite speculative and variable but also fail to capture many of the benefit components addressed earlier.

These types of cost-effectiveness and cost-benefit analyses are all very well, but it is not entirely clear whether absolute resource costs or cost per case identified are actually what dominate decisions about whether to implement UNHS or targeted screening. Moving away from the quantitative numbers game, it might strike the reader that missing a few children due to selective screening rather than UNHS could be tolerated but not missing half of them. On that line of argument it is not so much the cost per additional case but the major shortfall in proportion identified that drives the decision about what type of screening should be implemented. The key questions would then become: what is the actual proportion of true cases that are at risk and what value (if any) of that proportion would be acceptable to justify only selective screening . . . 80%, 90%, 95%? It is possible, though, that there is no fixed value of the proportion, and it will differ according to the demographic, epidemiologic, and health care quality characteristics of individual populations and societies.

Questions of Policy, Values, and Ethics

Although costs are often raised as a key aspect of health policy, they are by no means the only driving force. One viewpoint is that ethical considerations that reflect underlying societal values are the fundamental initiator of change in practice. The ensuing debate invokes considerations of the quality of evidence for benefit. Given ethical drive and reasonable evidence, cost is then invoked as a qualifier, to a greater or lesser extent, depending on the general economic environment and the strength of the ethical and evidential positions. Societal ethics actually have had an important, but somewhat covert, contributory role in many decisions about large-scale implementation of screening programs, with cost-based arguments taking a secondary role. There are many interesting ethical questions raised by population hearing screening, for example:

- Does a family have a fundamental right to know if their baby can hear?
- Does a child have a fundamental right to the best possible hearing ability?
- Does a child have a right to choose whether to be able to hear?
- Does a family have the right to choose not to maximize their child's hearing options?
- Does society have an obligation to detect hearing loss proactively, given absence of overt symptoms?
- Is it discriminatory to deny by inaction the child's right to care equivalent to that given an adult with the same disorder?

These are large questions that the reader may note have little to do directly with long-term language ability. They actually transcend and to some extent preempt or qualify the interpretation of the basic WHO principles of screening. Any of these questions could occupy this entire book and some of them are quite controversial. They embrace not only issues of rights, values, fairness, equity, and discrimination, but also the contention between family-centered and child-centered care. The reader who has a clinical background may answer some, if not all, of these questions with "of course," although an ethicist might have a harder time of it. What is surprising, however, is that most such questions have not been thoroughly debated in the specific context of justifying newborn hearing screening. If, for example, the answer about the rights of the child is a resounding "yes," then the interpretation of the WHO screening principles changes considerably, in essence because society would then consider undetected hearing loss to be virtually unacceptable in itself. Moreover, if a child has a basic right to hear or to equity of care in relation to that routinely provided for adults, then what does that mean for decisions about screening program design and what is the relevance of somewhat speculative cost-benefit arguments? What it probably means is that the acceptable proportion of true cases that could be missed by design is very small and that the virtually pandemic enthusiasm for UNHS actually reflects qualitative societal values (perhaps covertly) more than it does any dollar-based rationale. Of course, this is not to say that EHDI programs can be fiscally irresponsible. They must be implemented as efficiently as possible. One position is simply that a child's hearing and all that flows from it are worth a lot more than $20,000 or even $50,000 per case detected. However, many cases of hearing loss would be detected eventually anyway, without systematic screening, so the real issue is more about early detection than detection itself. Moreover, the cost issue has as much to do with *opportunity cost* rather than absolute cost or cost-benefit. Opportunity cost is basically the cost of not being able to implement alternative programs in some other deserving areas of care, as a result of having depleted the finite pool of health care resources.

For a thought-provoking approach to some of these ethical issues just raised, the reader might search the Internet for the terms "open future" and "respect for autonomy." The main question raised therein is one of balancing the rights of the child to make future decisions about matters that will affect his or her life against the rights of the family to pursue their own preferences, where such pursuit may restrict or abrogate the choices the child eventually may be able to make. To go directly to the source of the open future concept, see Feinberg (1994).

The Question of Evidence

In an era of increased attention to the quality of scientific evidence underlying health care in general and large public health programs in particular, it is beyond question that some kind of evidence base for effectiveness of NHS is necessary. What is more debatable, however, is what constitutes acceptable evidence. Indeed, the history of evidence review in relation to NHS is fascinating and has been characterized by dissent and variability of standards and conclusions. The reader may be familiar with some of the evidence reviews that have occurred for NHS, such as those carried out at the behest of the U.S. Agency for Healthcare Research and Quality (AHRQ) via the U.S. Preventive Services Task Force (USPSTF). See, for example, the systematic review by Thompson, McPhillips, Davis, Lieu, Homer, and Helfand (2001) and the most recent USPSTF recommendation on newborn hearing screening (U.S. Preventive Services Task Force, 2008). Publications such as the National Institutes of Health (NIH) Consensus Statement on newborn hearing screening (National Institutes of Health, 1993) are influential but do not constitute formal evidence reviews. Rather, they are basically statements grounded in expert opinion, as are the Position Statements typically put forward by professional organizations. The methodological standards applied by the USPSTF and other agencies internationally are more stringent than those that are typical in recommendations by clinically driven bodies. See Harris et al. (2001) for a description of the evaluative methods used by the third USPSTF.

Proper systematic reviews follow well-defined approaches that incorporate established hierarchies of study quality, careful attention to elements such as population sampling and sample size, details of screening methods and protocols, outcome variables, analytical methods and validity of study inferences. This is all entirely appropriate, given the generally questionable methodological quality of many published reports despite the current peer-review system. Moreover, proper evaluations of screening programs take account not only of whether procedures such as individual screening tests can in principle work well, which is a question of efficacy, but whether they actually do work well in the field, in terms of their ability to deliver the desired program outcomes, which is a question of field effectiveness. The distinction between efficacy and effectiveness is important, because efficacy is necessary but by no means sufficient for effectiveness. For example, efficacy studies are often reported by expert groups in specific contexts using rigorous methodological control and restrictive subject eligibility criteria. In the field, however, programs may be delivered by persons with variable expertise, exercising variable attention to details of protocol and with application to highly diverse and variable populations of subjects. It should be no surprise that efficacy results frequently are far better than those found in widespread practice. Thus, a focus on actual, delivered outcome is completely justifiable.

Unfortunately, the major evidence reviews of NHS focused on long-term language outcomes. Some limitations of such a focus were noted earlier. The combination of specific methodology and language focus led the USPSTF, for example, to conclude in 2000 that the available evidence was insufficient to recommend UNHS. Well-known studies such as those by Yoshinaga-Itano and her colleagues (Yoshinaga-Itano, Sedey, Coulter, & Mehl, 1998) and by Moeller (2000), despite the acclaim they deservedly received in the clinical community were, rightly or wrongly, considered insufficient to establish the case for UNHS. It is instructive to read Yoshinaga-Itano's response to the USPSTF, available on Audiology Online. The USPSTF cautiously modified their recommendation in 2008, it appears to the present author mainly as a result of a high-quality clinical trial with long-term language outcomes, reported by Kennedy et al. (2006), which is the only report to date addressing long-term language outcomes from a controlled, large-sample clinical trial (Wessex Universal Neonatal Hearing Screening Trial Group, 1998).

If not language but hearing dysfunction is the primary health problem, then systematic reviews of evidence of effectiveness of UNHS should be focused on the questions of whether or not amplification and cochlear implants actually improve the ability to hear. A formal review of that evidence is beyond the scope of this chapter, but the important point is that the key question is completely different from that addressed in past reviews and consensus statements. One obvious point is that it does not require a lengthy clinical trial to determine that hearing aids and cochlear implants *can* improve the audibility of sounds, when fitted appropriately (efficacy). The real, effectiveness question then becomes: to what extent are amplification and cochlear implants actually fitted appropriately and with valid and reliable outcome measures addressing primarily the audibility of sounds? The question is not as simple as it may appear, because there are many challenges involved in prompt, consistent, high-quality fitting of devices to very young children, but it is by no means the traditional question in terms of which the justification of NHS has been framed.

Two other points are worth mentioning in relation to evidence. First, what if the child is not a candidate for amplification or for a cochlear implant? Examples include children with profound hearing loss who have no cochlear nerves or for whom the family chooses to embrace Deaf culture. The key question then becomes: does early determination of deafness still confer substantive benefit, even in the absence of device candidacy? This leads back to the issue of early family knowledge as a primary outcome, the possible benefit being earlier engagement in communication development services based on visual languages. Second, although the evaluation community focusing exclusively on speculative harms such as anxiety and bonding disruption allegedly associated with false-positive screens, it is an extraordinary omission that equal consideration was not given to avoidance of the spectrum of anxieties and frustrations typically encountered by families of children who actually were deaf or hard of hearing but were mislabeled as delayed or as having behavioral disorders, often until school entry and often despite enduring parental concern. Indeed, it is tempting to conclude more generally that the history of evidence evaluation of newborn hearing screening has been characterized more by idiosyncratic, even ideologic position-taking than by deep insight and balanced consideration of the broad range of issues and factors involved.

The Programmatic Approach to Screening and EHDI

The reader may have noticed that early in this chapter the word *test* was very common, but that it morphed into the word *program* in more recent sections. This was a reflection of the fact that there is much more to delivering high-quality screening than just the screening test itself as well as of the shift of focus from the somewhat idealized flavor of test efficacy to the larger, more practical questions of real-world effectiveness in field use. Now, this shift will be taken one step further, to the macroscopic view of the role of screening in the overall EHDI context. The reader may look back and see that in Table 16–1B, five of the 10 recent additions to the original Wilson-Jungner screening criteria include the word *program*. This reflects the emergence of a distinct, programmatic approach to health services delivery over the last two decades. That approach incorporates a strong focus on the quality of services and, concomitantly, an emphasis on program performance evaluation (PE) and continuous quality improvement (CQI). Indeed, health services research and program evaluation have emerged as major disciplines in their own right. What have driven this evolution are fundamentally the burgeoning cost of public services and health care in particular, the emergence of an evidence-based mindset, a transition toward patient-centered or client-centered care and, perhaps, a fuller recognition of the complexity, frailty and vulnerability of large systems of human services. For a comprehensive text on many aspects of program evaluation, see the *Handbook of Practical Program Evaluation* edited by Wholey, Hatry, and Newcomer (2004).

A key to the programmatic approach lies in the concept of quality, as distinct from simple, service activity. Does a new health service actually deliver what it seeks to deliver? Do we even know and define precisely what is sought? What structures, which include funding, personnel and physical facilities (buildings, instruments, supplies, client transport services, etc.), are necessary? What processes are essential, including accessing target populations, clinical procedures such as screening, diagnostics and interventions, tracking and reporting, training and monitoring of personnel, connections delivering people between procedures, public and professional education, and information? What outcomes must be measured, including "simple" activities such as screening, recording and databasing of procedural results and, most critically, measurement of actual effects and impacts on service recipients? Quality, in relation to all of these aspects, is comprised fundamentally of three core ingredients: effectiveness, equity, and efficiency. Effectiveness, which term we have already met, relates to whether procedures or processes actually do what they are intended to do, in real-world practice, as distinct from the laboratory or the controlled clinical trial. Equity, also briefly introduced earlier, reflects the extent to which process effectiveness is fairly and equally accessible to all intended service recipients. Efficiency reflects the extent to which given levels of effectiveness and equity are achieved in relation to the quantity of resource expenditure (ultimately, dollar costs) required. The remainder of this chapter addresses these issues briefly.

An example of a procedures and linkages between them for a simple UNHS process is shown in Figure 16–9A. An expanded model of an EHDI program is shown in Figure 16–9B. It is clear that UNHS is embedded within a larger structure that serves the ultimate purposes of the screening. Such a structure is obligatory in order to comply with the expanded WHO principles. EHDI programs usually include UNHS as a key component, although there is no reason why they could not include selective or targeted screening (TNHS) in situations of very limited resources. The NHS itself is a subprogram of EHDI and is the primary source of subjects who should receive confirmatory, diagnostic audiologic assessments, but it is not the only source. A comprehensive EHDI program also includes other intake routes such as surveillance of children at high-risk for progressive or late-onset disorders, as well

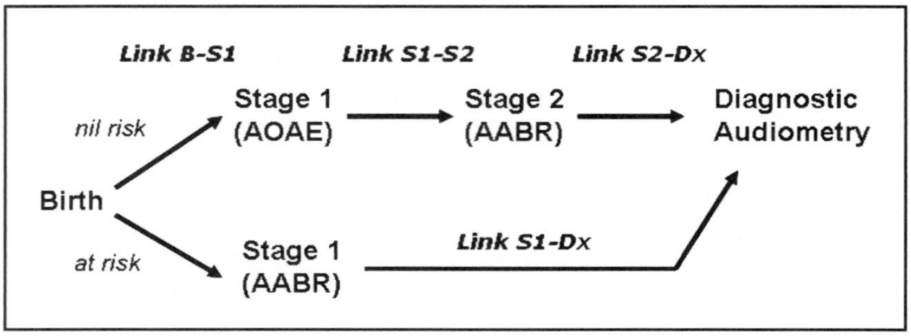

A

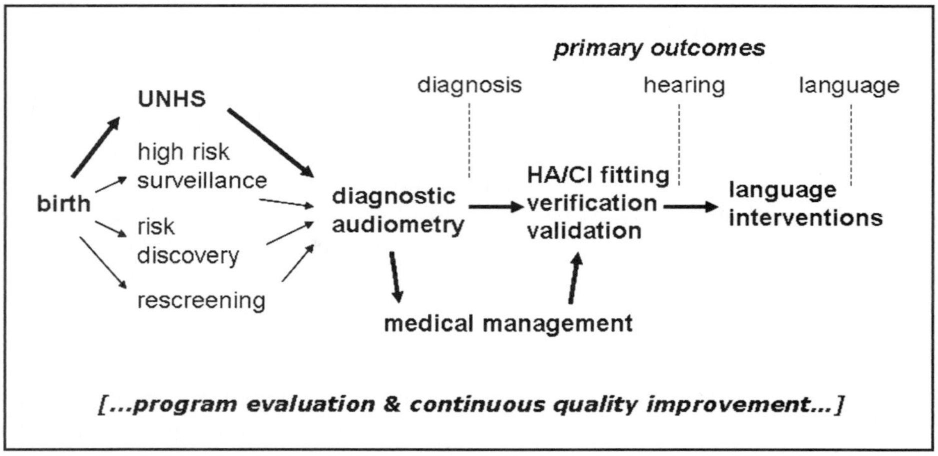

B

FIGURE 16–9. A. A simplified process diagram of UNHS procedures and links between them, for a mixed protocol involving two-stage, sequential automated OAE and automated ABR screening for newborns with no known risk indicator for hearing loss, and a single-stage AABR screen for newborns at risk. The links are points of potential failure of the care pathway and are at least as important as the clinical procedures themselves; for evaluation and quality improvement purposes the links should be viewed simply as a different kind of key "procedure." **B.** A simplified process diagram for an EHDI program. Note the several sources of babies. The major links from the UNHS path are the heavy arrows. Three different primary outcomes are shown (see text). The subprogram for program evaluation and quality improvement operates on all major stages of EHDI.

as referral-in routes such as for case-finding from medical visits unrelated to hearing loss, or for self-referral in case of family concern about response to sound or about speech and language development. There may even be included subsequent population or subgroup screening at some age prior to, or at, school entry. Each major component of EHDI can be and should be conceptualized as a subprogram in itself, the whole being an integrated matrix of linked subprograms.

What Makes a Program a Program?

Most readers may be directly involved in the provision or supervision of clinical services, including many of the major elements of EHDI. Some services are delivered more or less programmatically, especially in a large hospital or agency context, but there is more to a program worthy of the name than simply providing a service. Some important attributes of the programmatic approach, some of which are made explicit in the expanded WHO criteria, are presented in Table 16–5.

Goals and Core Values

Although services may or may not have explicitly defined and documented goals, a program *must* have them and, moreover, such goals must be carefully crafted. Statements of program missions or goals are usually large in scope and somewhat fuzzy but, nevertheless, they are important in that they reflect a large and generally accepted societal need. Furthermore, a well-stated goal can help to bind program personnel who may come from various professions or backgrounds to a common overall reason for their particular roles and activities. In large programs, it is not uncommon for those working on various parts of the program to lose sight of their overall purpose and as a result, to diverge into variable and even misguided beliefs and practices. An example of this from the author's experience is variability in screening practices and communication of results and their meaning to families. Screeners may screen repeatedly out of a desire to avoid alarming a family, or may overly minimize the significance of a screening failure, for the same reason. Both of these are inappropriate and may compromise goal achievement. Goals must be compelling, insightful, and frequently reinforced in order to enhance understanding, consistency, and commonality of purpose. Not only that, but goals should reflect the core values of the program. For example, it might be stated that all components of a program will be designed and delivered in a manner or style that is evidence-based and family-centered. Provided that such terms are executed faithfully and not merely given lip-service, they can have profound effects on the effectiveness and overall quality of services. Family-centered practice, for example, includes informed choice, confidentiality of personal information and respect for autonomy as key attributes. Autonomy basically is the right of a family to determine the services they wish to receive as well as the desired outcomes of those services, according to the dictates of their individual values and culture. What is critical is that the family be given full, timely, unbiased information about the implications of test results and the options available to them, in order to be in a position to exercise their autonomy in a proper manner. Moreover, the information must be presented in a way that is comprehensible and acceptable, bearing in mind that incomprehensible or unacceptable information is actually no information at all, or worse. It is the service recipients' understanding that matters, over and above that of the service provider.

Table 16–5. Key Attributes of the Programmatic Approach to Service Delivery

Program goal definition
Program core values definition
Explicit, specific overall and component objectives
Evaluability of defined objectives
Program process and outcome measurement
Continuous evaluation and quality improvement
Collateral effect measurement
Size, scope, and diversity of components
Effective linkage, integration, and cohesion of program components
Strong mechanisms of program oversight and consistency control

Objectives and Program Evaluability

Although goals are a centripetal (binding) force across a program, precisely because they are large and fuzzy, it is usually difficult to evaluate their achievement in quantitative terms. Therefore, the goals must be translated into a set of very specific objectives. These objectives must be defined for the EHDI program as a whole as well as for each and every subprogram, including NHS, diagnostics, amplification and cochlear implants, and language intervention subprograms. The importance of objectives is specifically stated in the expanded WHO guidelines.

An objective is a concrete, explicit, and precise statement of a desired outcome, for any program or subprogram. *An objective is worthless if its achievement or nonachievement cannot be measured.* That is what is meant by the term *evaluability*, which is the ability of a program to be evaluated in a valid and quantitative, as well as qualitative, manner. Table 16–6 shows examples for a screening (sub)program of a goal statement, a related objective and some challenges of definition and measurement that can arise, even with a seemingly precise statement of objective.

For every objective that can be formulated, for whatever part of the EHDI program is considered, these kinds of issues of definition, criteria and limitations of measurement will arise. To be genuinely useful in program evaluation, all such questions and more must be answered. It is difficult to overemphasize the attention to detail that is required when planning program data collection and analysis in order to effect genuine quality improvement. Moreover, to contribute to public knowledge, the precise definitions involved must be clearly stated. If they are not, which is frequently the case, then comparison of results across programs may be invalid or, worse, misleading. There are no sufficient procedural or definitional standards for these many factors that can affect the quantitative outcomes of EHDI programs and subprograms. There is an urgent need for such standards but the process of developing them will be challenging, largely because it requires drive, insight, and consensus across diverse groups.

Process and Outcome Measures

Any well-formulated, specific program objective must possess closely associated *outcome measures* or *endpoints* that are valid, accurate, and reliable measures of the achievement or nonachievement of that objective. In the parlance of program evaluation, these are often referred to as *indicators*. Usually, any indicator variable will have associated *benchmarks* and *targets*. A benchmark is usually taken to be a best-practice level of performance, whereas a target is a plausible value of range

Table 16–6. Examples of a Goal, Objective, and Issues of Definition and Measurement

Goal
To screen all newborns for significant, permanent hearing loss
Objective
In the 2010 birth cohort, to screen successfully at least 95% of all newborns by 1 month of age for permanent hearing loss of 30 dB or more at one or more frequencies in the range 500 Hz to 4000 Hz.
Issues
What types, degrees, frequencies, and laterality of hearing loss should be targeted and why?
What if there is significant hearing dysfunction but little, if any, loss of hearing sensitivity?
What exactly is meant by the term "permanent"? For example, would it embrace chronic or recurrent middle-ear pathology?
Is age to be chronologic or gestation-corrected? Until what age should gestation correction be applied?
Does screening at 5 weeks represent success or not? Is by one day better than by one month?
What if prompt access to the baby were impossible due to prolonged illness at home?
What constitutes a "screen"? Is an offer to screen important in itself? A consent to screen? Accessing a baby? A failed attempt to screen?
What is a successful screen? A pass or fail result in one ear? In both ears? Can screening stop if the first ear fails?
How many attempts are reasonable? How many repetitions in cases of questionable baby state? How many immediate rescreens of those who fail?

of performance that represents practical and reasonable progress towards the benchmark. These are expressed as values or ranges of key indicators, which represents program success. An example is the percentage of an annual live birth cohort screened successfully by 1 month corrected age, perhaps with a benchmark of 90% in Program Year 1, 95% in Year 2, and with targets within 5% of the benchmark values.

Common indicators of program performance are the percentage of newborns screened by one month, diagnosed by 3 months and entering intervention by 6 months of age, the so-called "1-3-6" model. A merit of such straightforward indicators is that they are easy to understand and they focus widespread attention on specific, numerical targets, which is vastly better than having no targets. There are concerns about the specific ages used, because they are not apparently evidence-based but arose through influential, consensus opinion. There is a related question of validity. There is no known sense in which a child diagnosed by 4 months, say, as opposed to by 3 months, is unsuccessful. Nor is it apparent whether a program should expend even more resources in order to diagnose newborns by one month of age or enter children into intervention by 4 months of age, not 6.

Part of the issue here is the natural urge for clarity and simplicity of targets, which carries an attendant risk of being uninformative or misleading. For example, Figure 16–10 shows hypothetical data for two programs that have precisely the same performance by age 3 months, but for which the pattern of shortfall from that target and the ensuing steps that would be required to improve the programs would be very different. More generally, a strong argument can be made

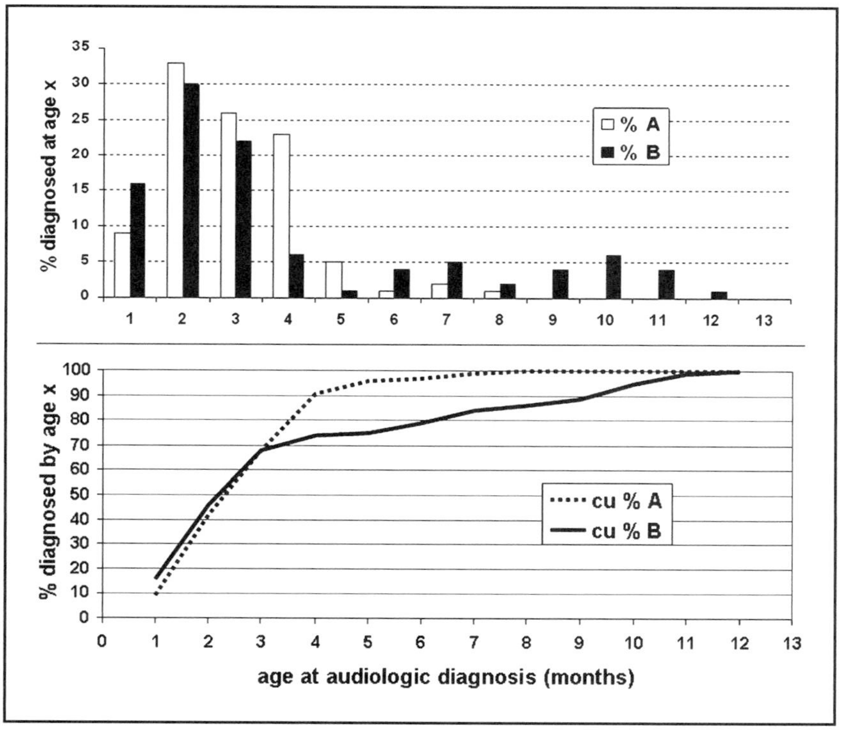

FIGURE 16–10. Distributions of ages at successful screening are shown for two hypothetical programs. The upper part shows age histograms and the lower part shows sample cumulative distributions CDs. The CDs show diverging program performance more clearly than the histograms. The programs have identical screening delivery performance at 3 months (a common benchmark) but the severities of shortfall for the two programs are different, as would be any remedial action for program improvement. This illustrates a weakness of simplistic performance targets based on a count at a single, specific age.

for retaining the 1-3-6 targets but augmenting them with an analysis that is more complete and informative than simply a binary count of "done" or "not done." In fact, as introduced earlier in Figure 16–8, whenever there is an indicator that is based on an event in time or an interval of time, the cumulative distribution of event times or intervals achieved is an elegant tool that offers much more information than the "success" counts that are commonly reported. It would be overly cynical to suggest that one reason why cumulative distributions are not more commonly reported might be precisely the large amount of information that they reveal. See Uus and Bamford (2006) for a good example of a program effectiveness report, including use of cumulative distributions and their benchmark percentiles.

The reader may have noticed that indicators such as the proportion of newborns screened by some particular corrected age or similar indicators for diagnostics and various interventions vary in the directness of their relationship to the actual, desired outcomes of EHDI. Reflecting the early discussion, suppose the focus is upon three major outcomes: determination of hearing loss presence and a well-informed and empowered family, improvement in actual hearing function and optimized language development over time. Successful screening is necessary but not sufficient for any of these primary child outcomes. Successful screening is a real outcome from the limited perspective of a screening subprogram, but it does not equate to an EHDI objective in the big-picture sense. In contrast, early, successful diagnostic audiometry leading to hearing loss confirmation is a real, primary outcome, because one EHDI objective is to detect children with a target hearing loss. It is wise to include the informational and counseling process for affected families as a component of a complete diagnostic test, because failure to achieve belief, acceptance, and empowerment for the family could result in major loss to follow-up. What is the ultimate value of a diagnosis that is denied or ignored? In a sense, a successful diagnostic assessment is a proxy outcome for an affected but empowered family.

The second, primary EHDI outcome is early, improved hearing and for that, there must be an appropriate fitting of either amplification or a cochlear implant. Successful diagnostics are necessary but not sufficient for such fitting, so diagnosis is a proxy for improved hearing. The real outcome indicators are the age at which a verified and validated device fitting is achieved and the amount of hearing function that results. With respect to language interventions, the percentage of enrolment in early intervention and the age at such enrollment are *not* primary outcomes, but are merely *process proxies* for real language outcomes, and poor proxies at that. Again, enrolment is a necessary but not sufficient condition for achievement of the actual desired outcome, which is optimized language development. In that regard, the entire language development trajectory is relevant as a primary outcome measure, for which standardized, norm-based, age-referenced language assessment tools are obligatory as components of an array of indicators.

The proper analysis of program performance is based on what is referred to as *cohort* analysis, a term that was introduced earlier. A cohort is simply a group of individuals who share some common, defining set of characteristics, such as birth between dates x and y, diagnosis of the target disorder between dates x and y, and so on. Cohort analysis requires that the outcome for each and every individual in the cohort be determined and included. This is usually expressed using tree diagrams that cover all major results at different steps of the program.

Another common type of performance analysis is the *period* report, which is a count of different program activities in a given period of time such as a calendar quarter or year. Period reports are tools to assess the amount of activity or workload in a period of time, but they cannot and must not be interpreted as cohort analyses, because individual subjects outcomes are not tracked through the program. For example, the subjects who are identified with hearing loss in a given period will not necessarily all arise from the subjects who are screened in that same period, because some screened subjects will not yet have had the opportunity to be diagnosed. Of course, it would be folly to interpret the ratio of positive diagnoses to successful screens in a period report as any kind of prevalence estimate or even as a meaningful program yield measure. Yield can only be determined properly from a specific birth cohort and even then it will not reveal the true prevalence of the disorder, because of unknown, missed cases.

The Program Evaluation and Quality Improvement Subprogram

Quality Assurance and Program Evaluation are explicitly mandated in the expanded WHO criteria. Given the emphasis here on program evaluability, precise objectives, associated indicators and benchmarks, it should come as no surprise that program evaluation

(PE) and quality improvement (QI) are virtually obligatory components of any well-designed program. PE addresses the extent to which objectives are achieved. QI is a process that takes the results of the PE and, where deficiencies are identified, implements changes and evaluates their success. This last step is critical and is sometimes overlooked. "Cosmetic" PE and QI simply measure things, with or without making improvements. Real QI absolutely must close the loop and prove whether any program changes have improved performance, have had no effect, or even have degraded performance. The endless, iterative nature of a well-designed PE and QI subprogram has led to such activities sometimes being referred to as continuous quality improvement (CQI).

The importance of a PE and QI program as a component of EHDI cannot be overstated. How well the program is working and whether it can be done better or more efficiently are fundamental questions. Few programs for which such question cannot be answered will have much prospect of long-term survival in a health care world replete with competing priorities for funding. The overarching message here is that it is one thing to start an EHDI program and quite another for it to survive and flourish. Constant attention to outcome evaluation and quality improvement is a crucial program survival tool, as well as being necessary ethically and clinically.

Three Key Facets of Program Quality: Effectiveness, Equity, and Efficiency

The simple examples of indicators just given focus on program effectiveness, which reflects the achievement of desired quantities and timeliness of key program events, but effectiveness is only part of the story and the simplest part, at that. Comprehensive program evaluation also addresses equity and efficiency of program deliverables. Equity is a very important construct that addresses the variability or distribution of effectiveness across different segments of the target population for the program. Put another way, equity reflects the degree to which all recipients of program services experience equivalent quality of service. For example, suppose a screening coverage benchmark of 95% was achieved in an overall birth cohort for a particular state or region, but that newborns of a particular ethnicity or newborns born in a particular county or at a particular hospital fell far short of the benchmark when broken out from the whole cohort. Despite the overall success, these particular groups are not being served equally by the program. This is a failure of program equity. Such failures are hidden by gross benchmarks—the basket of fruit looks good, but the oranges at the bottom are rotten. Lack of equity, therefore, is as important a target for PE and QI as is global program performance. An important concept related to equity is "area variation" in any aspect of program performance. The area in area variation may be a geographic unit, such as a county or a provider hospital or community center, but it also may be nongeographic, such as a cultural group, a socioeconomic group, or even the individual providers of services. Thus, the analysis of and elimination of area variations are an important component of deep program evaluation. It may even reveal the reason for limitations of overall program effectiveness.

Collateral Effect Measurement

The term *collateral effects* is sometimes used in reference to outcomes of a program that are unintended or are deemed undesirable. In the latter case, the effect may be called a harm, negative benefit, or even a cost, depending on the context and viewpoint. For example, consider the family anxiety that may arise from a screening failure. Anxiety, while seemingly undesirable in and of itself, can have both adaptive and maladaptive connotations. Is it not perfectly normal, even appropriate, for a certain amount of anxiety to accompany realization of a significant risk of hearing loss? One outcome of anxiety may be a tendency to comply with requests to attend for follow-up procedures and, in that sense, the anxiety can be beneficial. If, however, the anxiety is excessive or inappropriate, it might lead to denial and thereby undermine attendance for diagnostic assessment. What seems reasonable is to control the amount of anxiety by reducing excessive false-positive screens and by careful, culturally and individually appropriate conveyance to the family of screening failure implications and essential next steps. Note that early in the history of EHDI, concerns about bonding disruption were expressed, but now no concrete evidence has yet arisen to support such speculations.

An example of a beneficial collateral effect would be an increase in public and professional awareness of the importance and feasibility of early detection and management of hearing loss in newborns and infants. Another would be any spinoff benefit from the increasing prominence of evidence-based and programmatic practices on the general quality of pediatric audiology in a given region or locale.

Size, Scope, and Diversity

Clinical services may cater to any size of patient intake, but population-level services with very large intake demand a substantial organizing structure and processes that promote economies of scale, efficient tracking and scheduling mechanisms, commonality of goals and style as well as consistency of practices. In the absence of such constraints, there is a natural tendency for the beliefs and practices of individual providers to diverge and become somewhat idiosyncratic, even inappropriate. This may occur even when service providers are obliged to conform to typical practice standards associated with professional, regulatory oversight. At some ill-defined point, depending on the strength of the organizing forces, the large service may acquire a programmatic flavor. For example, a group of audiologists providing diagnostic audiometry services for a group of otolaryngologists may well deliver services of high quality but it is not programmatic unless there are mechanisms that promote goal-directedness, consistency of practice and serious efforts at performance evaluation and improvement.

Diversity of service components increases further the requirement for an organized and controlled approach. Although audiometry services alone could possess a programmatic flavor, effective linkage to, say, amplification and rehabilitation services clearly increases the potential benefit of well-defined overall structure and effective integration processes. The greater the range and diversity of activities, the greater the tendency towards service inconsistency and fragmentation in the absence of strong oversight.

Linkage and Integration

Close attention to linkage and integration are crucial to overall effectiveness of diverse activities. Clues to the truth of this are found readily in the literature on EHDI, wherein the importance of patient tracking and inter-service communications is widely recognized and almost universally found to be challenging. For example, screening effectiveness is readily undermined by poor performance of the linkage to definitive audiologic assessment. Because an immediate objective of screening is to detect the target disorder, the linkage between screening and diagnostic is fundamental to achievement of the program objective. The linkage typically consists of screening outcome documentation, databasing, timely transmission of or access to the fail outcome, family contact, diagnostic appointment scheduling and attendance promotion. This set of events is sufficiently complex to require a programmatic approach in itself. Then same can be said for all linked activities that are necessary for a given program outcome. This viewpoint is discussed in more detail shortly.

Program Oversight and Control

Adequate oversight and control are crucial to high, sustained program quality. Oversight refers to a mechanism by which overall program effectiveness, equity, and efficiency are monitored, with accompanying programmatic intervention if deficiencies in performance are detected. Thus, the oversight should embrace all aspects of quality as well as cost-effectiveness and cost-efficiency. Local or regional program management typically will not have the expertise or big-picture information necessary to detect or address quality shortfalls. Of course, oversight without teeth is somewhat pointless, and the most effective teeth are likely to be budgetary. Therefore, an effective oversight mechanism should include some measure of budgetary and cost-control capability. The detailed mechanisms of oversight are beyond the scope of this chapter, but may include statistical review of program activities, processes, and real outcomes at the state, regional or local level, even at the level of individual provider performance. Area variations analysis and cost-workload analysis are important tools. Some programs internationally also include adverse-event-driven or random performance audit of institutions', agencies', or individuals' performance. If done in a constructive manner, such audits can be accepted as beneficial, even necessary, for providers and recipients alike.

The word *control* applies not only to budget but to service practices. For the latter, control is not meant to be taken as meaning some kind of dictatorial restriction of freedom of professional practice. Rather, it refers to mechanisms that promote commonality of goals and practice styles, adoption of well-defined procedural protocols and methods of ensuring and verifying achievement of desired clinical outcomes in an efficient and consistent manner. The best practice control mechanisms are those that are driven by professional integrity, consensus and drive for quality, putting quality of service above personal opinions and idiosyncrasy of viewpoints. The tendency toward adoption of evidence-based practices can be very helpful in this regard, provided that it is taken seriously and does not descend into a waving around of decision-makers' favorite, often discordant, pieces of published evidence.

In the author's experience, it is not unusual to encounter professional resistance to detailed, mandatory practice protocols. Investment in one's own clinical opinion and perceived expertise is perfectly understandable. However, there is good reason why even expert clinical opinion is the lowest level of scientific evidence. In fact, rigorous, evidence-driven protocols are an important tool for enhancing program quality, provided it is realized that such protocols do not threaten freedom of practice. Rather, they can encourage easier achievement of minimum practice standards and focus professional skills on the unique characteristics and needs of individual patients or clients. Another objection often voiced is that protocols do not accommodate the diversity and individuality of children and families. Given a well-designed protocol, that is a misconception. People like their coffee in various ways, but boiling the water is a universally valid component, and attention can be directed at what blend, how strong and how much sugar. Similarly, it is not rocket science that common errors in judgment of ABR presence or absence in diagnostic assessment recordings can be reduced by rational attention to measures of signal-to-noise ratio and EEG quality. Nor is it unreasonable to propose that language interventions should be organized around longitudinal, repeated measurement using standardized norm-based and criterion-based tools, with structured intervention changes contingent on individual progress criteria.

EHDI Program Performance Analysis: A Chain Model

A comprehensive EHDI program is viewed properly as a complex, integrated network of subprograms. However, at its core lies a series or chain of key procedures and critical linkages between those procedures. At several points in the chain from birth through screening, diagnostics, devices, and interventions, the valued, primary program outcomes emerge. Here, we retain the focus on diagnosis and family information, improved hearing and language development. These are delivered by procedural chains of different length, and at every point in the chains there may arise sources of shortfall or performance deficiency. An inherent property of serial chains is that the shortfalls at various points cumulate as the series progresses. The more elements involved, the greater the cumulative deficiency.

For any core procedure such as screening or diagnostics, three areas of performance limitation can be defined: the input or capture of candidates for the given procedure, the inherent properties of the procedure itself and its delivery in the field, and the output of candidates for the next procedure in the chain. The initial procedure that starts the chain is of course the live birth. The linkages between procedures can be defined to include all aspects of the transfer of individuals from the output from one procedure to the input for the next. Table 16–7 illustrates some possible sources of program performance deficiency in this chain process.

One might find the information presented in Table 16–7 discouraging. Certainly, there are many challenges to achievement of high quality in each major program area and in the linkages between areas. However, explicit recognition of those challenges is an important step toward their solution. There are obvious themes underlying many of the entries in Table 16–7. These include the critical importance of provider training and skills maintenance, procedure information management and subject tracking, valid and comprehensive procedural protocols and protocol compliance, as well as very judicious and appropriately individualized informing and counseling of families throughout the entire process.

Acknowledging that there are various sources of shortfall, now consider the core chain of EHDI as separated into clinical procedures and output-input linkages. The overall chain is:

> Birth, birth link to screen, screen, screen link to diagnostics, diagnostics, diagnostics link to devices, devices, devices link to intervention, intervention

This chain can be expressed in shorthand as:

> B, L(B-S), S, L(S-Dx), Dx, (O1), L(Dx-D), D, (O2), L(D-I), I,(O3),

where O1, O2, and O3 represent the delivery points of the diagnosis and information, improved hearing and language development primary outcomes, respectively. Now, for each procedure and linkage, let the deficiencies arising from each associated source be lumped together and expressed as a percentage yield of success. For example, suppose all the above table elements for Screen Input resulted in a net input shortfall of 7% from the total target newborn population, then the link L(B-S) would have a performance value of 93%. Put more simply, the birth cohort would have a 93% net access performance. Similarly, the Screen Procedure elements might yield a net success rate of 95%. If screening coverage were defined to include not just

Table 16–7. Some Sources of Program Chain Performance Deficiency

Chain Stage	*Input*	*Procedural*	*Output*
Screening	Unknown birth Family not accessed Consent denied Child not accessed Lost between screen stages Chronic illness	Validity limitation Sensitivity limitation Poor screen technique Poor screen environment Poor child state Inappropriate info to family	Unsuccessful screen Erroneous result Documentation error/failure Database entry error/failure Inappropriate anxiety Lack of commitment to diagnostics
Diagnostics and Information	Follow-up tracking failure (Screen fail unrecognized, family untraceable or not contactable) Declined or deferred Chronic child illness Recurrent no-show	Inadequate test protocol Noncompliance with protocol Poor test technique Poor test environment Poor child state Comorbidity challenges Test interpretation error Fluctuating/progressive disorder Lost during diagnostic process Inappropriate info/counseling	Unsuccessful test Erroneous test results Documentation error/failure Database entry error/failure Inadequate info to family Family denial of loss Family confusion/indecision
Amplification/ Cochlear Implant	Follow-up tracking failure (Case not recognized or family lost) Declined or deferred Cultural or socioeconomic barriers to amplification/CI Recurrent middle-ear disease	Device contraindication Inappropriate fitting Failure to verify and validate Inappropriate device use Inadequate device maintenance Inappropriate info/counseling	Limited device effectiveness Documentation error/failure Database entry error/failure Family denial of intervention need Family confusion/indecision
Language Intervention	Follow-up tracking failure (Case not recognized, Family lost) Declined or deferred Cultural or socioeconomic barriers to intervention	Inappropriate mode choice Limited provider skills Suboptimal therapy Family incapacity Family challenges and priorities	Limited intervention effectiveness Documentation error/failure Database entry error/failure Family nonengagement Family disillusionment

access to the newborn but also the actual delivery of timely and successful screens, then the coverage performance value is the product of 93% and 95% or just over 88%. From the standpoint of the screening subprogram alone, the key subprogram outcome is timely and successful screens, so the performance analysis can stop at that point. Note that if the screening comprised multiple stages in series, the screening procedure-linkage chain would increase in length.

Viewing this process from the standpoint of the EHDI program as a whole, a successful screen is not in itself sufficient as a primary outcome. Because we have chosen to define a successful diagnostic test as the first of the three primary outcomes (disregarding, for simplicity, the related act of delivering information about the diagnosis to the affected families), the performance values for the L(S-Dx) link and the Dx procedure itself must be added into the chain for successful diagnosis of the target disorder. If we denote the performance of each step as P(step), because each performance value can be understood as a probability of step success, then for the three primary outcomes of EHDI chosen here the chain success probabilities are:

for successful target disorder diagnosis (O1):

$$P(O1)=P[L(B\text{-}S)]\times P(S)\times P[L(S\text{-}Dx)]\times P(Dx),$$

for successful improved hearing (O2):
P(O2)=P(O1)×P[L(Dx-D)]×P(D), and

for successful language development (O3):
P(O3)=P(O2)xP[L(D-I)]xP(I).

Several important inferences follow from this viewpoint. First, the chain performance can be no better than that of the lowest step performance. Therefore, any efforts at improving the chain should be directed at the weakest step, which is quite obvious. Second, what is less obvious is that the cumulative performance of the outcome chains deteriorates quite rapidly, even if each step performs very well. Of course, the more steps to the outcome, the greater the cumulative effect. As a simple example, let each step have a success rate of 95%. The cumulative performance values are then:

For successful target disorder diagnosis:
$(0.95)^4 = 0.81$ or 81%,

For successful improved hearing:
$(0.95)^6 = 0.74$ or 74%, and

For successful language development:
$(0.95)^8 = 0.66$ or 66%.

What this simple model makes painfully clear is that serial processes are inherently vulnerable, perhaps alarmingly so, given that what might be considered as excellent performance from the standpoint of each individual step (95%, in this example) cumulates such that only two thirds of children with the target disorder actual achieve the desired primary language outcome. Couple this with the fact that some of the steps may not achieve anything close to 95% performance and the cumulative performance picture deteriorates much further. The reader is left to contemplate the implications of a cumulative performance value of 50% or less, which is entirely plausible.

Toward Better Program Evaluation and Reporting

The chain performance analysis suggests an obvious approach to quantitative summary of subprogram and overall program effectiveness: *for a given birth cohort, develop a complete cohort outcome analysis tree, plus a serial listing of % successful performance values for each major step (both procedures and links), together with a serial listing of the cumulative performance values up to and including each successive step. This should be done for each and every defined, primary program outcome.* These step and cumulative numeric series could easily be graphed and would comprise a highly informative tool to direct quality improvement efforts as well as to characterize and report program results in substantially more depth and detail than is the norm in published reports to date. Most program reports focus on only one or two procedures, especially screening and diagnosis, yet loss to follow-up is known to be a major challenge to overall program success. Genuine loss to follow-up (as distinct from mere loss to documentation) is primarily an issue of multiple linkage deficiency. Moreover, many program reports appear to routinely overlook many of the sources of deficiency in field practice for both linkages and current clinical procedures themselves. Although the type of analysis just suggested is not rocket science, the author has not yet seen any such analysis, despite the large number of program reports published to date. Test and protocol sensitivity for screening tests were discussed earlier. Program sensitivity simply generalizes that idea to incorporate cumulative shortfall in the ensuing steps required to deliver the desired overall program outcome. The development given here is merely an elaboration of that concept as a program evaluation tool. This type of comprehensive approach to program performance analysis approach is essential, not only to satisfy fully the expanded WHO criteria but also to fulfill the ultimate promise of EHDI of the highest possible quality. It can be argued that the more complete and revelatory the program performance analysis is, the closer we have come to clear identification of the areas of deficiency and the necessary efforts at improvements.

Conclusions

It is hoped sincerely that this chapter has helped to convince the reader that the real challenges of EHDI have only just begun to be realized and addressed. Far from being a done deal, it is actually an area of enormous potential and opportunity for advance. The major points discussed in this chapter are as follows:

1. WHO screening principles originally defined by Wilson and Jungner (1968) and updated by Andermann et al. (2008) continue to provide a solid basis for screening program development and evaluation.
2. Population screening is a public health endeavor that differs radically from response to symptomatic disorders. Although many, minor harms must be balanced against relatively few, major benefits, the predicament of the young child imposes an onus of proactivity on society.

3. Fundamental societal values and ethical principles of equality of care can influence strongly the rationale for early detection of hearing loss, as well as program design.
4. Screening is not an end in itself but a vehicle for delivery of beneficial outcomes. It must be conceptualized, justified, and evaluated in the larger context of the entire EHDI program.
5. Compromised language development is only one facet of the problem to be addressed by screening. Disorder of hearing is the primary health deficit and improved hearing function is a primary health benefit in itself, not only a proxy for language development.
6. Explicit, quantitative definition of the set of hearing disorders targeted by screening is important and affects almost every aspect of program design, performance, and evaluation.
7. We know less than is commonly believed about the prevalence of hearing disorders in early childhood. Prevalence is difficult to determine and is strongly affected by the target disorder criteria, age at determination and population epidemiology. Screening programs do not provide good estimates of prevalence, but only of yield.
8. Sensitivity and specificity estimates are key measures of screening test efficacy. They tend to vary inversely and both are necessary to characterize test performance. Isolated estimates of one or the other are of limited value.
9. ROC methods are a useful tool to summarize, optimize, evaluate, and compare screening tests, but only a small part of any ROC is relevant in screening for hearing disorders.
10. The predictive value of a positive screen is very important practically and is strongly affected by prevalence and specificity. Most infants who fail a screen will not have significant hearing loss. Likelihood ratios are a useful tool for deriving post-screen probabilities of hearing loss.
11. Much less is known than is commonly believed about the actual sensitivity of automated OAE and ABR screens. Direct determination of sensitivity requires that all babies screened be followed up. In contrast, a great deal is known about screening test specificity.
12. In the estimation of both prevalence and sensitivity, there are formidable challenges of study sample size, precision of estimates, validity, and generalizability of results.
13. Screening test effectiveness in field practice can be very different from that determined by controlled studies and may vary dramatically across testers and locations.
14. The click-ABR and the OAE have substantial limitations of validity, accuracy, flexibility, and consistency. Improvements are necessary and feasible but may be a coherent driving force.
15. Proper evaluation of the field effectiveness of single screening tests or test combinations requires extraordinary attention to detail, matters of definition and data quality.
16. Most, but not all analyses to date of EHDI cost-effectiveness and cost-benefit are simplistic in health-economic terms. A common deficiency is failure to account for major differences in both the burden of unidentified hearing loss and the overall effectiveness of EHDI for young children with different degrees of permanent hearing loss severity.
17. A programmatic approach to EHDI as a whole and to its major components is obligatory and has many distinct and important defining characteristics.
18. Without explicit objectives, the achievement of which can be evaluated quantitatively, a program cannot be rationally designed, evaluated, and improved. You cannot verify achievement of anything that is not defined or not able to be measured.
19. Lack of practice consistency across all key components of an EHDI program is a serious threat to program quality, including the ability to evaluate and improve the program, effectiveness of services, equity, or fairness of service delivery, and program efficiency. Centralized governance and strong, evidence-based, well-accepted procedural protocols are virtually mandatory for high program quality.
20. An EHDI subprogram that is not cosmetic but that actually delivers program evaluation and demonstrable continuous quality improvement is essential.
21. Popular, age-based performance benchmarks have significant limitations and better methods are available, especially those based on cumulative distributions of age at key events and intervals between events.
22. Programs such as EHDI that involve serial chains of key activities are highly vulnerable to cumulative deficits in overall performance. The linkages that transfer children between the key program stages are just as important as the clinical procedures themselves.
23. More comprehensive methods of program performance analysis and reporting are necessary and feasible. A birth cohort approach with cumulative chain performance display for all primary outcomes is strongly recommended.

24. The real challenge of achieving the true promise of EHDI has only just begun.

References

American National Standards Institute (ANSI). (1997). *Methods for calculation of the Speech Intelligibility Index, ANSI S3.5-1997*. New York, NY: Acoustical Society of America.

Andermann, A., Blancquaert, I., Beauchamp, S., & Dery, V. (2008). Revisiting Wilson and Jungner in the genomic age: A review of screening criteria over the past 40 years. *WHO Bulletin*, *86*(4), 241–320. Retrieved June 24, 2010, from http://www.who.int/bulletin/volumes/86/4/07-050112/en/index.html

Bagatto, M. P., Scollie, S. D., Seewald, R. C., Moodie, S., & Hoover, B. M. (2002). Real-ear-to-coupler difference predictions as a function of age for two coupling procedures. *Journal of the American Academy of Audiology*, *13*(8), 407–415.

Burkard, R. F., & Don, M. (2007). The Auditory brainstem response. In R. F. Burkard, M. Don, & J. Eggermont (Eds.), *Auditory evoked potentials—Basic principles and clinical application* (pp. 229–253). Baltimore, MD: Lippincott Williams & Wilkins.

Canadian Working Group on Childhood Hearing (CWGCH). (2005). *Resource document: Early hearing and communication development* (Chap. 3, Burden of the target disorder). Retrieved June 24, 2010, from http://www.phac-aspc.gc.ca/publicat/eh-dp/index-eng.php

Cebulla, M., Stürzebecher, E., Elberling, C., & Müller, J. (2007). New clicklike stimuli for hearing testing. *Journal of the American Academy of Audiology*, *18*(9), 725–738.

Durieux-Smith, A., & Whittingham, J. (2000). The rationale for neonatal hearing screening. *Journal of Speech-Language Pathology and Audiology*, *24*(2), 59–67.

Feinberg, J. (1994). The child's right to an open future. In *Freedom and fulfillment: Philosophical essays* (pp 76–97). Princeton, NJ: Princeton University Press.

Fortnum, H. M. (2003). Epidemiology of permanent childhood hearing impairment. *Journal of Audiological Medicine*, *1*, 155–164.

Fortnum, H. M., Summerfield, A. Q., Marshall, D. H., Davis, A. C., & Bamford, J. M. (2001). Prevalence of permanent childhood hearing impairment in the United Kingdom and implications for Universal Neonatal Hearing Screening: Questionnaire based ascertainment study. *British Medical Journal*, *323*, 536–539.

Gorga, M. P., Dierking, D. M., Johnson, T. A., Beauchaine, K. L., Garner, C. A., & Neely, S. T. (2005). A valid and potential clinical application of multivariate analysis of distortion-product otoacoustic emission data. *Ear and Hearing*, *26*(6), 593–607.

Gorga, M. P., Neely, S. T., Ohlrich, B., Hoover, B., Redner, J., & Peter, J. (1997). From laboratory to clinic: A large scale study of distortion product otoacoustic emissions in ears with normal hearing and ears with hearing loss. *Ear and Hearing*, *18*(6), 440–455.

Gravel, J. S., White, K. R., Johnson, J. L., Widen, J. E., Vohr, B. R., James, M., . . . Meyer, S. (2005). A multisite study to examine the efficacy of the otoacoustic emission/automated auditory brainstem response newborn hearing screening protocol: Recommendations for policy, practice, and research. *American Journal of Audiology*, *14*, S217–S228.

Grosse, S. D., & Ross, D. S. (2006). Cost savings from universal newborn hearing screening. *Pediatrics*, *118*(2), 844a–845a.

Harris, R. P., Helfand, M., Woolf, S. H., Lohr, K. N., Mulrow, C. D., Teutsch, S. M., & Atkins, D., (2001). For the Methods Work Group, third U.S. Preventive Services Task Force. Current methods of the U.S. Preventive Services Task Force: A review of the process. *American Journal of Preventive Medicine*, *20*(3S), 21–35.

Hyde, M. L., Riko, K., & Malizia, K. (1990). Audiometric accuracy of the click ABR in infants at risk for hearing loss. *Journal of the American Academy of Audiology*, *1*(2), 59–66.

International Classification of Functioning, Disability and Health (ICF). (2001). Geneva, World Health Organization (WHO). Retrieved from the WHO Library Database June 24, 2010, from http://www.who.int/publications/en/

Joint Committee on Infant Hearing (JCIH). (2007). Year 2007 position statement: Principles and guidelines for early hearing detection and intervention programs. *Pediatrics*, *120*, 898–921.

Kennedy, C. R., McCann, D. C., Campbell, M. J., Law, C. M., Mullee, M., Petrou, S., . . . Stevenson, J. (2006). Language ability after early detection of permanent childhood hearing impairment. *New England Journal of Medicine*, *354*, 2131–2141.

Keren, R., Helfand, M., Homer, C., McPhillips, H., & Lieu, T. A. (2002). Projected cost-effectiveness of statewide universal newborn hearing screening. *Pediatrics*, *110*(5), 855–864.

Khoury, M. J., McCabe, L. L., & McCabe, E. R.B. (2003). Population screening in the age of genomic medicine. *New England Journal of Medicine*, *348*, 50–58.

Moeller, M. P. (2000). Early intervention and language development in children who are deaf and hard of hearing. *Pediatrics*, *106*(3), e43.

Morton, C. C., & Nance, W. E. (2006). Newborn hearing screening—a silent revolution. *New England Journal of Medicine*, *354*, 2151–2164.

NIDCD: National Institute on Deafness and other Communication Disorders. (2002). *Report and recommendations: NIDCD workshop on congenital cytomegalovirus infection and hearing loss*. Retrieved June 24, 2010, from www.nidcd.nih.gov/funding/programs/hb/cmvwrkshop.asp

National Institutes of Health. (1993). Early identification of hearing impairment in infants and young children. *NIH Consensus Statement*, *11*(1),1–24. Retrieved June 24, 2010, from http://www.ncbi.nlm.nih.gov/books/bv.fcgi?rid=hstat4.chapter.11796

Norton, S. J., Gorga, M. P., Widen, J. E., Folsom, R. C., Sininger, Y., Cone-Wesson, B., . . . Fletcher, K. (2000). Identification of neonatal hearing impairment: Evaluation of transient evoked otoacoustic emission, distortion product otoacoustic emission, and auditory brain stem response test performance. *Ear and Hearing*, *21*(5), 508–528.

Prieve, B., & Fitzgerald, T. (2009). Otoacoustic emissions. In J. Katz, L. Medwetsky, R. Burkard, & L. Hood (Eds.), *Handbook of clinical audiology* (6th ed., pp. 293–321). Baltimore, MD: Lippincott Williams & Wilkins.

Schroeder, L., Petrou, S., Kennedy, C., McCann, D., Law, C., Watkin, P., . . . Ho, M. Y. (2006). The economic costs of congenital bilateral permanent childhood hearing impairment. *Pediatrics*, *117*(4), 1101–1112.

Sininger, Y. S. (2007). The use of auditory brainstem response in screening for hearing loss and audiometric threshold prediction. In R. F. Burkard, M. Don, & J. Eggermont (Eds.), *Auditory evoked potentials—basic principles and clinical application* (pp. 254–274). Baltimore, MD: Lippincott Williams & Wilkins.

Sininger, Y. S., & Hyde, M. L. (2009). Auditory brainstem response in audiometric threshold prediction. In J. Katz, L. Medwetsky, R. Burkard, & L. Hood (Eds.), *Handbook of clinical audiology* (6th ed., pp. 293–321). Baltimore, MD: Lippincott Williams & Wilkins.

Swets, J. (1988). Measuring the accuracy of diagnostic systems. *Science*, *240*, 1285–1293.

Tharpe, A. (2008). Unilateral and mild bilateral hearing loss in children: Past and current perspectives. *Trends in Amplification*, *12*, 7–15.

Thompson, D. C., McPhillips, H., Davis, R. L., Lieu, T. L., Homer, C. J., & Helfand, M. (2001). Universal newborn hearing screening: Summary of evidence. *Journal of the American Medical Association*, *286*(16), 2000–2010.

U.K. National Screening Committee. (2009). *Criteria for appraising the viability, effectiveness and appropriateness of a screening programme* (updated June 2009). Retrieved June 24, 2010, from http://www.screening.nhs.uk/criteria

U.S. Preventive Services Task Force. (2008, July). *Universal screening for hearing loss in newborns*, topic page. Agency for Health care Research and Quality, Rockville, MD. Retrieved June 23, 2010, from http://www.ahrq.gov/clinic/uspstf/uspsnbhr.htm

Uus, K., & Bamford, J. (2006). Effectiveness of population-based newborn hearing screening in England: Ages at identification and profile of cases. *Pediatrics*, *117*(5), e887–e893.

Wessex Universal Neonatal Hearing Screening Trial Group. (1998). Controlled trial of universal neonatal screening for early identification of permanent childhood hearing impairment. *Lancet*, *352*, 1957–1964.

Wholey, J. S., Hatry, H. P., & Newcomer, K. S. (Eds.). (2004). *Handbook of practical program evaluation* (2nd ed., p. 720). San Francisco, CA: Jossey-Bass.

Wilson, J. M. G., & Jungner, G. (1968). *Principles and practice of screening for disease.* Geneva: World Health Organization. Public Health Paper # 34. Retrieved June 24, 2010, from http://whqlibdoc.who.int/php/WHO_PHP_34.pdf

Yoshinaga-Itano, C., Sedey, A. L., Coulter, K., & Mehl, A. L. (1998). Language of early- and later-identified children with hearing loss. *Pediatrics*, *102*(5), 1161–1171.

APPENDIX 16–A

Conventional Probability Table

A conventional probability table relating target disorder presence (D+) and absence (D–) to screening test outcomes of Fail (T+) and Pass (T–).

	D+	D–	sum
T+	p.se	(1–p).(1–sp)	P(fail)
T–	p.(1–se)	(1–p).sp	P(pass)
sum	p	(1–p)	1

Sensitivity = P(T+ *given* D+) = p.se/p = se

Specificity = P(T– *given* D–) = (1–p).sp/(1–p) = sp

P(fail) = p.se + (1–p).(1–sp)

Fail (refer) rate (%) = 100. P(fail)

P(pass) = p.(1–se) + (1–p).sp

Pass rate (%) = 100. P(pass)

Positive predictive value (PPV) = p.se/ P(fail)

Negative predictive value (NPV) = (1–p).sp / P(pass)

Likelihood Ratio LR+ = se/(1–sp)

LR– = (1–se) /sp

A conventional table showing expected counts of the four possible combinations of screening outcome and disorder status (True Positive (TP), False Negative (FP), False Positive (FP), and True Negative (TN)) for a hypothetical sample of 100,000 babies with prevalence 2/1000 (0.2%), sensitivity 0.95 (95%), and specificity 0.90 (90%). Results for actual samples from this population would usually differ from these expected values because of statistical sampling variation. The resulting summary statistics would then be estimates of their true values shown below.

	D+	D–	sum
T+	190 TP	FP 9,980	10,170
T–	10 FN	TN 89,820	89,830
sum	200	99,800	100,000

Sensitivity = 190/200 = 0.95

Specificity = 89,820/99,800 = 0.9

P(pass) = 89,830/100,000 = 0.898

P(fail) = 10,170/100,000 = 0.102

PPV = 190/10,170 = 0.019 (1.9%)

NPV = 89,820/89,830 = 0.999

LR+ = 0.95/0.1 = 9.5

LR– = 0.1/0.95 = 0.11

17

Screening for Hearing Loss and Middle Ear Disorders: Beyond the Newborn Period

Jackson Roush and Robert J. Nozza

Introduction

Screening for hearing loss in children was among the first public health initiatives undertaken in the United States over 70 years ago. Schools, clinics, and health departments have employed a variety of hearing screening methods to identify children needing referral for comprehensive assessment. Methods have also been developed for detection of middle ear disorders. Considering the long history of screening for hearing loss and middle ear disorders one would expect to find consistent and well-standardized protocols and procedures. Instead there remains considerable variability in screening procedures and, in many cases, limited evidence to support current practices. Indeed, some screening protocols appear to be guided more by history than by evidence. This chapter examines behavioral and physiologic screening for hearing loss and middle ear disorders in the months and years that follow the newborn period, with emphasis on older infants and children from preschool to school age. The chapter provides an evidence-based review of methodology and screening protocols as well as a review of instrumentation, personnel, follow-up, and other factors that must be considered in the design, implementation, and evaluation of a screening program. Where evidence is lacking we highlight areas of need for future research.

Purpose of Screening

The purpose of screening is to identify children most likely to have a targeted disease or disorder in need of treatment. It is important to differentiate screening from diagnostic procedures. Screening is applied to populations with no apparent signs or symptoms of the target disorder. Diagnostic procedures, which are more expensive and time consuming, are applied only to a subset of individuals who are more likely to have the disorder. Thus, screening may be defined as an activity that separates individuals with high and low probability of a disease or disorder, from the general population (Feightner, 1992; Roush, 2001). Decisions regarding whether to screen for a disease or disorder are guided by several considerations:

- *Importance to Society.* Each disease or disorder has a cost to society. The greater the societal cost, the greater the justification for screening.
- *Diagnostic Criteria.* There must be a clear and measurable definition of the disease or disorder and a gold standard diagnostic test.
- *Availability of Treatment.* For those identified by screening there must be treatment available that is known to be effective.
- *Access to Those Who Will Benefit.* The target population must be available and accessible.
- *Resources and Compliance.* Resources needed for diagnosis and treatment must be available, and those referred must be willing to comply with recommendations for follow-up.
- *Feasibility of the Screening Test.* In order to be accepted by the public, by program administrators, and by those responsible for screening, the test must be rapid, inexpensive, easy to administer, and acceptable to the person screened.
- *Program Evaluation.* The screening program must have a monitoring and evaluation process to determine its efficacy and to allow for modifications based on experience and accumulated evidence.

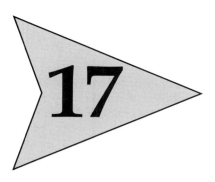

- *Costs and Benefits.* For each screening outcome there are costs and benefits. Costs are determined by the number of individuals who actually have the condition in proportion to the total number screened and the expenses associated with the screening process; costs are also influenced by the number of incorrect screening outcomes. Benefits generally are associated with correct screening outcomes.

Screening Test Characteristics

A screening *test* result may be positive, suggesting increased risk for the target disorder, or negative, suggesting no risk or reduced risk. However, a screening *outcome* can only be determined based on the results of a subsequent "gold-standard" diagnostic test. A positive screening test that results in a positive diagnostic test would be a *true positive;* that is, it occurs when the target condition is correctly identified. This outcome is beneficial because treatment that otherwise might have been denied or delayed can be provided. Screening can also result in a *true negative;* that is, a negative screening test is confirmed with a negative diagnostic test in an individual who is truly free of the condition. A true negative is beneficial because the patient or the parents are assured of the condition's absence. A *false positive* occurs when the screening results indicate the need for referral but subsequent diagnostic tests indicate absence of the condition. This outcome is costly from a financial standpoint because it entails an unnecessary diagnostic procedure. It is also costly in human terms if individuals or their families are needlessly concerned or inconvenienced. Finally, a *false negative* occurs when the screening procedure indicates a pass even though the disorder is, in fact, present. This is considered the most serious error because the screening procedure fails to uncover an existing disorder. The costs associated with a false negative may be harm to the patient (exacerbation of the condition, delayed and/or inappropriate intervention or educational placement) and/or misinformation conveyed to the family.

To determine the performance of a screening protocol it is necessary to calculate its *validity*. Several terms developed in the field of clinical epidemiology are useful in this regard. The first is *prevalence*, which is defined as the number of cases of a disease existing in the population during a specified time period. A related term sometimes mistakenly used interchangeably is *incidence*. Incidence is defined as the number of new cases identified over a given period of time, usually one year.

In addition to the incidence or prevalence of a disorder, determining the validity of a screening procedure requires calculation of *sensitivity* and *specificity*. Sensitivity refers to the number of people with a given disorder who test positive; that is, the rate of correct classification for affected individuals. It is calculated by dividing the number of true positives by all those in the screened group with the disorder (the sum of the true positives and false negatives), or:

$$Sensitivity = \frac{TruePositives}{TruePositives + FalseNegatives} \times 100$$

Thus, if 100 infants have a hearing loss and the test is able to identify 90 of them, the test has a sensitivity of 90%.

In contrast, specificity refers to the test's accuracy in correctly identifying persons who *do not* have the condition; that is, the rate of correct classification for unaffected individuals. It is calculated by dividing the number of true negatives by all those in the screened group without the disorder (the sum of the true negatives and false positives), or:

$$Specificity = \frac{TrueNegatives}{TrueNegatives + FalsePositives} \times 100$$

Thus, if 100 infants have normal hearing and the screen is able to classify 90 of them as normal, the test has a specificity of 90%.

The ideal screening test would have high sensitivity and high specificity, meaning that false-negatives (misses) as well as false-positives (unnecessary referrals) are few. There is an important tradeoff, however, between sensitivity and specificity, the extent of which is determined by the pass-fail criteria; that is, the rules that define a pass or a fail on a given screening test. The relationship between sensitivity and specificity is illustrated in Figure 17–1.

Figure 17–1 shows two hypothetical distributions, one representing individuals without the disorder of interest (nondiseased curve) and the other representing those with the disorder (diseased curve). In this example, the two groups have very different screening outcomes. As is typical of most screening scenarios, there are many more people without the disorder in comparison to those who have it. Also, affected individuals show greater variability in their test results. In Figure 17–1, the nondiseased population, with no disorder, exhibits hypothetical screening results with test values ranging from approximately 0 to 9. The population with disease (diseased curve) exhibits hypothetical screening results with test values ranging from approximately 3 to 13. Note that the two distributions overlap from about 3 to 9, meaning that there are a few

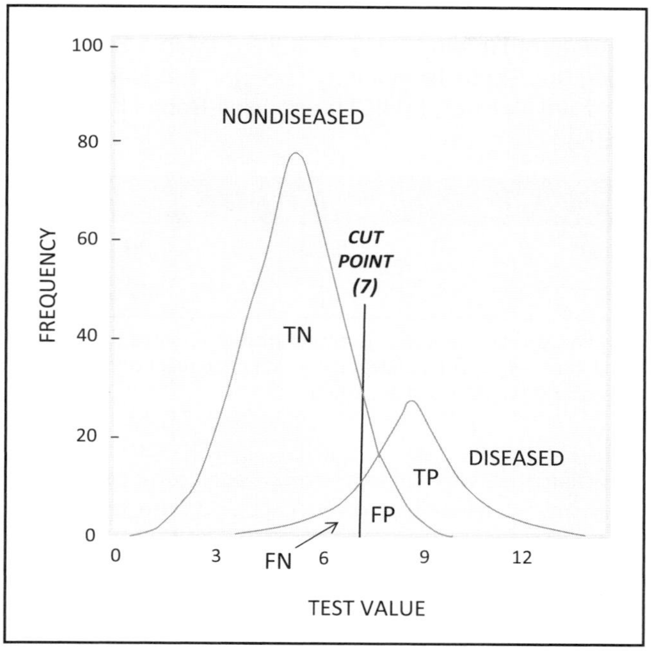

FIGURE 17–1. Hypothetical screening distributions showing the overlap of diseased and nondiseased populations. TN = true negative; TP = true positive; FP = false positive; FN = false negative.

individuals without the disorder whose screening outcome measures were unusually high, and a few with the disorder whose measures were unusually low. This is the case for all screening tests. There is always overlap of the distributions of those with and those without the disease along the screening test score continuum. If the two distributions were totally separated along that continuum, one could pick a test score that perfectly separates the two groups, in which case there would be a perfect gold standard diagnostic test. The area of overlap is where the screening test cannot differentiate normal from abnormal. In this example, the clinician must choose a cut-point (vertical black line) above which the screening is considered positive and below which the screening is said to be negative. The cut-point will determine the number of true positives (TP; area under the disease curve, to the right of the cut point), false positives (FP; area under the nondisease curve to the right of the cut point), true negatives (TN; area under the nondisease curve to the left of the cut point), and false negatives (FN; area under the nondisease curve to the left of the cut point). Moving the cut-point (vertical bar) to the left would increase the sensitivity, but the tradeoff would be lower specificity as more nondisordered individuals would be referred. Conversely, moving the cut-point to the right would increase the specificity at the expense of lower sensitivity. The cut-point may be adjusted differently depending on the purpose of the screening and the implications of an incorrect outcome.

In assessing a screening procedure, it is also important to consider the *predictive value. Positive predictive value* (PPV) refers to the percentage of cases with positive screening outcomes that are found, by diagnostic evaluation, to actually have the disorder. Stated differently, PPV indicates the likelihood of the target condition being present when the screening test is positive. In contrast, *negative predictive value* (NPV) refers to the percentage of cases with negative screening outcomes that are found, by diagnostic evaluation, to be free of the disorder. A test's predictive value is especially important to clinicians since the goal of the practitioner is to apply a screening test to determine whether *an individual child* has the disorder (PPV) or does not have the disorder (NPV). The PPV is calculated by dividing the number of true positives by all positives, or:

$$PPV = \frac{TruePositives}{TruePositives + FalsePositives} \times 100$$

The NPV is determined by dividing the number of true negatives by all negatives, or:

$$NPV = \frac{TrueNegatives}{TrueNegatives + FalseNegatives} \times 100$$

Unlike sensitivity and specificity, which remain the same regardless of disease prevalence, predictive value is heavily influenced by the prevalence of the disorder being screened. This is illustrated in Figure 17–2, which includes calculation of sensitivity, specificity, and predictive value. Note that prevalence has no effect on sensitivity or specificity, whereas predictive values are greatly affected by prevalence. This is because in the computing of predictive values the denominator represents the total number screened with a positive test (PPV) or negative test (NPV), which will vary with prevalence even when sensitivity and specificity remain the same.

The affect of prevalence on PPV is also illustrated in a study by Prieve et al. (2000) that compared hearing screening outcomes in the well-baby nursery (WBN) to those observed in the neonatal intensive care unit (NICU), where the prevalence of permanent hearing loss was known to be approximately ten times higher (Prieve & Stevens, 2000). Infants who did not pass a screening auditory brainstem response (ABR) were referred for diagnostic ABR assessment. As expected, the PPV for permanent hearing loss was significantly

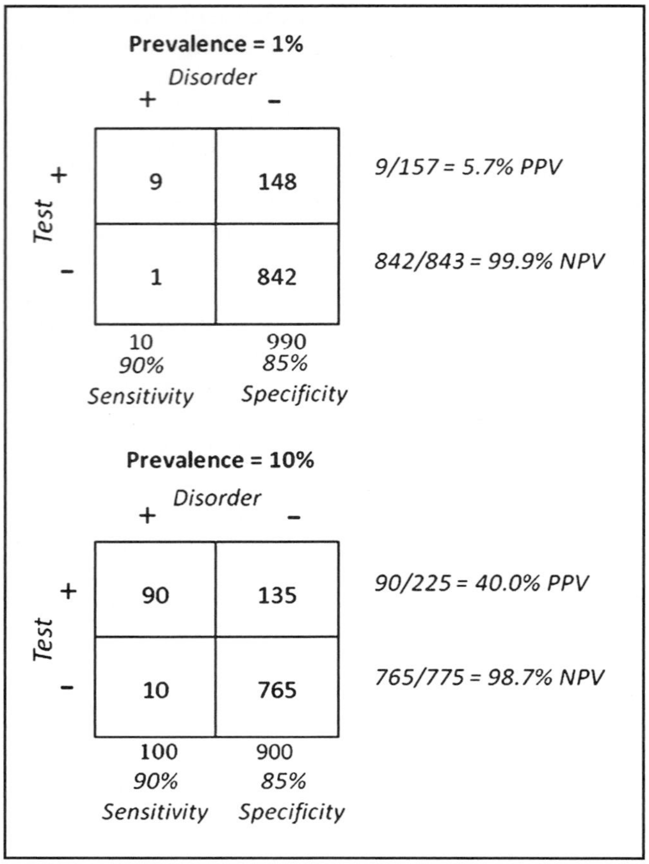

FIGURE 17–2. Two-by-two matrices of hypothetical data illustrating the effects of disease prevalence on test performance. In both cases, the test has sensitivity of 90% and specificity of 85%; however, positive predictive value (PPV) changes considerably with increase in disease prevalence. NPV = negative predictive value.

Table 17–1. Positive Predictive Value (PPV) for Permanent Hearing Loss (PHL), for Infants Screened Using the Same Technology (ABR) in the Neonatal Intensive Care Unit (NICU) and Well-Baby Nursery (WBN)

PPV for PHL	Inpatient Fail	Outpatient Fail
NICU	12.5%	25.9%
WBN	2.2%	17.9%

Note how prevalence, which is approximately 10 times higher in the NICU than in the WBN, affects the PPV for inpatient and outpatient screening (from Prieve et al., 2000).

higher in the NICU than in the WBN for both inpatient and outpatient screening (Table 17–1).

Disorders with low prevalence are likely to have lower PPVs and higher NPVs. Thus, the less prevalent the disease, the lower the PPV because the proportion of true positives is smaller. Similarly, the less prevalent the disease, the higher the NPV because of the larger proportion of true negatives. As the true status of each individual is unknown at the time of screening, knowledge of the predictive values for each screening procedure is critically important. Despite their importance, predictive values are for many clinicians the least understood screening principles. Without them, however, a screening protocol cannot be properly evaluated. Moreover, consideration only of sensitivity and specificity without regard to predictive values can result in a distorted view of how well a screening protocol is performing. Measures of predictive value require an understanding of their relationship to sensitivity and specificity, and what can be done to improve them. In particular, it is important to remember that the vast majority of individuals screened in any program will *not* have the target condition. Thus, the false positives are derived from this relatively large pool of individuals. Consequently, problems with low PPV are usually caused not only by the low prevalence of the disorder, but by low specificity as well. Even a small reduction in specificity can result in a large decline in PPV because the proportion of individuals without the disorder is so great. Thus, the goal is to increase sensitivity with minimal effect on specificity. There are at least two ways this might be accomplished. One way is to limit screening to those individuals already known to be at increased risk. The disadvantage, in the context of infant hearing screening, is that no more than half of the infants with congenital hearing loss have high risk factors. Thus, improving PPV would occur at the expense of lower sensitivity and a reduction in early detection of hearing loss. A more favorable approach is to do repeated measures or a multiple-stage screening procedure. A rescreening or a two-stage approach, used in many screening programs, may involve rescreening with the same technology or a different technology. In a two-stage protocol, the patient who fails the first screen is rescreened using the second technology and must also fail that test before being referred. If the number of referrals can be lowered by rescreening, the rate of false positives and the corresponding specificity and PPV will improve. It should be remembered, however, that multiple screening procedures increase the amount of clinician time and, in some cases, the instrumentation and space required, thus adding to the overall cost of the program. Multiple rescreenings can also increase the possibility of a false negative outcome. Each of these factors must be considered based on the goals of the screening program, the costs and benefits derived, and individual circumstances unique to each setting.

A key point here is that sensitivity and specificity of the test and prevalence of the disorder can only be determined through diagnostic testing applied to a large number of cases in the target population. Sensitivity and specificity must be known prior to implementing the screening program and can only be determined by comparing screening test data with diagnostic test results in a controlled study of cases representative of the population to be screened. Likewise, the diagnostic data will only provide an *estimate* of the disorder's prevalence in that population. Data on sensitivity and specificity must be monitored within the screening program over time and adjustments made to pass-fail criteria and/or definition of the disorder, as appropriate. Specificity is especially hard to monitor because those who pass the screening are typically not followed diagnostically. Those who pass are typically a much larger group than those referred, so following all of them to determine specificity is not practical within a screening program and, in fact, would defeat the purpose of screening. However, it is possible to periodically check a small sample of those who pass to ensure that the false negative rate is in line with screening program objectives.

Screening for Hearing Loss

Prevalence of Permanent Hearing Loss

Sensorineural hearing loss is the most common abnormality affecting newborn infants in the United States and in most developed countries. Population-based estimates of the prevalence for moderate to profound permanent hearing loss in one or both ears range from 1 to 3 per 1,000 (0.1 to 0.3%; Finitzo, Albright, & O'Neal, 1998; Mauk & Behrens, 1993; Vohr, Carty, Moore, & Letourneau, 1998) whereas milder degrees of permanent hearing loss in infants account for a prevalence of approximately 0.55/1000 (0.06%; Gravel et al., 2005).

The prevalence of permanent hearing loss is at least 10 times higher for infants whose birth history required admission to the NICU with a prevalence ranging from 8 to 20 per 1,000 or 0.8 to 2.0% (Gerber, 1990; Mauk, White, Mortensen, & Behrens, 1991; Prieve et al., 2000; Stein, 1999). Most permanent hearing losses detected in the NICU are cochlear in origin; however, NICU history is also an important risk factor for auditory neuropathy (Berg, Spitzer, Towers, Bartosiewicz, & Diamond, 2005), a condition characterized by absent or abnormal ABR in the presence of intact cochlear hair cell function (Starr, Sininger, & Pratt, 2000). The condition has also been called auditory neuropathy/dys-synchrony (JCIH, 2007) and more recently, auditory neuropathy spectrum disorder (ANSD) to account for its variable nature and etiology (Guidelines Development Conference on the Identification and Management of Infants with Auditory Neuropathy, 2008). ANSD is more prevalent than once thought and is now believed to affect 7 to 10% of all children with sensorineural hearing loss (Madden, Rutter, Hilbert, Greinwald, & Choo, 2002; Rance, 2005).

Children with congenital *conductive* hearing loss comprise another special population of permanent hearing loss. Some of the congenital conditions associated with permanent conductive hearing loss, such as aural atresia, are apparent at birth. Others, due to ossicular fixation or other middle ear anomalies, may be more insidious and difficult to detect.

The overall prevalence of permanent hearing loss in children appears to increase during the preschool years. Bamford et al. (2007), in the United Kingdom, examined the prevalence of sensorineural hearing loss at school entry, noting that among approximately 3.5 per 1,000 children known to have permanent hearing loss at school entry, nearly 1.9 in 1,000 required identification *after* the newborn screen. There is evidence of further increase in permanent hearing loss during the school years. Estimates vary based on methodological differences; however, two investigations published in 1998 (Bess, Dodd-Murphy, & Parker, 1998; Niskar et al., 1998) found a prevalence of sensorineural loss ranging from 11 to 15% in school-age children when all types and degrees of hearing loss were included. Both studies reported a variety of audiometric configurations with more unilateral than bilateral losses. For hearing losses greater than 20 dB HL in the "speech frequencies," Mehra, Eavey, and Keamy (2009) estimated a prevalence of 3.1% for all children and youth; the prevalence was relatively higher for Hispanic-American children and those from low-income households.

The reasons for the increasing occurrence of permanent hearing loss from birth to school age are not fully understood but several contributing factors are evident. Some infants with congenital hearing loss are missed at newborn screening; others are unreported or lost to follow-up. Still others have progressive or acquired sensorineural hearing loss due to genetic disorders, infectious diseases, noise exposure and other environmental hazards, or exposure to ototoxic medications. Of particular concern is the number of children with mild hearing loss who appear to be missed by newborn screening. In the study by Bess et al. (1998) cited earlier, the prevalence of mild permanent unilateral and bilateral hearing loss was estimated to be 54 per 1,000 (5.4%). These findings suggest that current screening outcomes do not account for the number of children who present with mild bilateral or unilateral hearing loss in later childhood (Gravel et al., 2005).

In the following section, we review physiologic and behavioral methods of screening for hearing impairment. We also examine controversies associated with screening for middle ear disorders and the application of pass-refer criteria when tympanometric screening is justified.

Justification for Hearing Screening Beyond the Newborn Period

The detrimental effects of hearing loss on speech, language, and educational development are well established (e.g., Moeller, Osberger, & Eccarius, 1986). Even mild hearing loss has been associated with educational and psychosocial delays (Bess et al., 1998). Moreover, there is the intrinsic right of children to hear and for families to be informed when their child's access to sound is compromised. Fortunately, there is growing evidence that early identification and intervention for young children with congenital hearing loss results in favorable developmental outcomes (Moeller, 2000; Yoshinaga-Itano, Sedey, Coulter, & Mehl, 1998). Consequently, neonatal hearing screening is now considered a standard of care across the United States, and over 94% of newborns are screened for hearing loss prior to hospital discharge (Centers for Disease Control and Prevention [CDC], 2007a). It is important to emphasize, however, that even well-managed programs are unlikely to screen 100% of their newborns prior to hospital discharge. Furthermore, among those who are successfully screened but do not pass, an alarming number are lost to follow-up. In some states, the proportion of infants unreported or lost to follow-up exceeds 50% (CDC, 2007). Also, as noted earlier, there is the potential for missed screenings, loss to follow-up, missing documentation, late onset or progressive cochlear impairment, and undetected auditory neuropathy. In addition, a substantial number of children experience chronic conductive hearing loss secondary to otitis media. For all of these reasons ongoing surveillance of hearing status in children is essential.

Does this mean every child should undergo multiple hearing screenings after the newborn period, even if there are no hearing concerns or risk factors? This is an important question and one that has been answered differently by various professional organizations and public health agencies. Recommendations for hearing screening have been published by the American Speech-Language-Hearing Association (ASHA, 1997, 1997), the American Academy of Audiology (AAA, 1997), and most recently, by the American Academy of Pediatrics (AAP; Harlor & Bower, 2009). It is important to emphasize, however, that policies regarding implementation and management of hearing screening programs are determined at the state and local levels. All 50 states in the United States currently provide *newborn* hearing screening, but there is considerable variability in policies and procedures for screening that occurs after the newborn period. Some states have both legislative mandates and detailed protocols for hearing screening. Others have neither a legislative requirement nor statewide policies for screening beyond the newborn period, leaving decisions to individual health departments, school districts, and local educational agencies. Federal guidelines require that children in the United States receiving healthcare through the Medicaid program be monitored according to the guidelines established for Medicaid's Early and Periodic, Screening, Diagnosis and Treatment (EPSDT) well-child examination program. In 2004, the EPSDT screening guidelines committee recommended that hearing screenings be performed according to the methodology and periodicity guidelines established by the AAP. AAP recently updated its guidelines for "Hearing Assessment in Infants and Children: Recommendations Beyond Neonatal Screening" (Harlor & Bower, 2009). Key points from this document call for periodic "objective screening" (e.g., otoacoustic emissions [OAEs]) in the medical home of all children and surveillance of those with one or more risk indicators. The document also calls for careful attention to parental concern regarding a child's hearing status; application of pneumatic otoscopy and tympanometry; referral to a pediatric audiologist for children who do not pass the screening; and comprehensive audiologic and otologic assessment for children with developmental abnormalities or behavioral conditions that preclude routine screening. The AAP recommendations emphasize the importance of interdisciplinary management an appropriate intervention for children with confirmed hearing loss.

In summary, there is strong evidence to support screening after the newborn period whenever there are caregiver concerns or risk indicators for late onset hearing loss. It is also recognized that hearing screening should be provided periodically for all children, even in the absence of concerns or risk indicators. States and municipalities vary substantially with regard to how and where screenings are performed and in the methodology employed. The recently updated recommendations of the AAP (Harlor & Bower, 2009) provide an important commitment from the medical community and a useful framework for physicians willing to conduct hearing screening in the medical home; however, implementation of these recommendations and evaluation of their efficacy will take time and additional research. In the meantime, programs for early hearing detection and intervention (EHDI), state health departments, and school-based hearing screening programs, must work together to achieve functional, well-coordinated policies, procedures, and referral criteria. The process must consider the advantages and limitations of each screening method and the considerations relevant to various special populations of infants and children.

Methods of Screening for Hearing Loss

Behavioral Hearing Screening Procedures

It is well established that behavioral hearing screening cannot be reliably conducted in the newborn period (JCIH, 1971). Once infants reach a developmental age of 5 to 6 months, however, behavioral assessment is possible using visual reinforcement audiometry (VRA; Widen et al., 2000). For typically developing infants, VRA can be used for behavioral hearing screening or to estimate hearing threshold levels. Because the VRA technique requires specialized instrumentation and the expertise of a pediatric audiologist, however, it cannot be routinely applied as a tool for behavioral hearing screening outside the pediatric audiology clinic.

Screening children in the age range of 2 to 4 years can be challenging even for pediatric audiologists. The experienced clinician is often able to adapt behavioral methods to combine VRA with conditioned play procedures using a method known as visual reinforced operant condition audiometry (VROCA). As with VRA, however, the procedure cannot be used outside the pediatric audiology clinic because it requires specialized instrumentation and expertise. For these reasons, physiologic methods, described below, are often preferred for routine screening of children in this age group.

Once a child reaches the age of 3 to 4 years, pure-tone audiometry can be performed using developmentally-appropriate assessment procedures. Behavioral pure-tone screening has been employed for many years by a variety of health care professionals. It is typically conducted at a fixed intensity of 20 dB HL at the frequencies 1000, 2000, and 4000 Hz; a pass requires repeatable responses in each ear to all stimuli (AAA, 1997; ASHA, 1997). Depending on the goals of the screening program and the target population, other frequencies may be included (Holmes, Niskar, Kieszak, Rubin, & Brody, 2004). Pure-tone screening has several advantages. Portable audiometers are relatively inexpensive and uncomplicated, and because behavioral pure-tone screening involves the auditory system at all levels, it may be considered a true hearing test. There are, however, a number of limitations. First, behavioral screening requires an experienced examiner with the qualifications needed to select and apply developmentally-appropriate methods and materials. It also requires a child capable of attending and responding appropriately to the test stimuli. Additionally, pure-tone screening necessitates an acoustic environment that is quiet enough to meet published standards for allowable levels of ambient noise (ANSI S3.1, 1999, 2008).

Considering the many prerequisites and pitfalls associated with behavioral pure-tone screening, it is not surprising the procedure has had mixed success. In a study of approximately 3,500 kindergarten and first grade children using well-prepared examiners in a controlled acoustic environment, FitzZaland and Zink (1984) reported sensitivity and specificity of 93% and 99%, respectively. A far less favorable outcome was reported by Halloran, Hardin, and Wall (2009) when pure-tone screening was conducted in a primary care medical setting. In the study by Halloran and colleagues, which involved approximately 1,000 preschool and school-age children screened in eight pediatric offices using conventional pure-tone screening procedures, sensitivity and specificity was only 50 and 78%, respectively. Thus, it is evident that pure-tone screening can be applied successfully for identification of hearing loss in preschool and school-age children, but only under relatively ideal conditions. Because of the difficulties associated with behavioral pure-tone screening there is growing interest in the use of physiologic measures, not only for newborns, but for screening older infants and preschool-age children.

Physiologic Screening Procedures

The physiologic procedures most commonly used to screen for sensorineural hearing loss are based on the recording of ABR and OAE, including transient evoked otoacoustic emissions (TEOAE) and distortion product otoacoustic emissions (DPOAE). As both technologies are objective in nature they can be applied to a variety of pediatric populations including those too young or too developmentally delayed to be screened behaviorally. There are important differences between the two technologies, however, and it is important to consider the advantages and limitations of each.

OAEs are cochlear responses generated by the outer hair cells in response to acoustic stimuli. As such they provide useful information regarding the *preneural* status of the auditory system. In contrast, ABRs, recorded from surface electrodes attached to the head, reflect neural activity in the auditory nerve and brainstem. Thus, OAEs provide an assessment of cochlear function while ABRs include activity generated by the cochlea, as well as a measure of neural integrity and synchrony beyond the level of the cochlea, in the auditory brainstem. OAE screening provides a more broadband test of the cochlea (multiple frequencies) whereas ABR screening, using only clicks, is dominated by a more restricted range of frequencies. Although neither method is considered a true test of hearing in the perceptual sense, both ABRs and OAEs are sensitive to abnormalities at different levels of the auditory system making them useful for both screening and diagnostic purposes.

OAEs can be applied to awake children at any age using a variety of screening personnel. In contrast, ABR screening can be performed in natural sleep for the first few months of life, but after 4 to 6 months requires sedation or anesthesia, and thus can only be carried out in a medical setting by an audiologist. The two technologies also differ with regard to the nature of the physiologic recording. Because OAEs require the conductive pathway for both delivery of the acoustic stimulus and for reverse transmission of low amplitude cochlear emissions, middle ear status affects OAEs to a greater extent than ABR. Emissions are generally absent in the presence of middle ear effusion (Lonsbury-Martin, Martin, McCoy, & Whitehead, 1995; Margolis & Trine, 1997; Owens, McCoy, Lonsbury-Martin, & Martin, 1993) and even negative middle ear pressure can obscure their measurement (Marshall, Heller, & Westhusin, 1997; Prieve, Calandruccio, Fitzgerald, Mazevski, & Georgantas, 2008; Trine, Hirsch & Margolis, 1993). Thus, a child with a normal cochlea may fail an OAE screening because of middle ear abnormalities. ABR and OAE, when used for hearing screening, are also limited in their ability to detect milder degrees of hearing loss (e.g., < 25 to 35 dB HL). A large multicenter study funded by the National Institutes of Health compared the relative sensitivity of TEOAEs with ABR (Gorga et al., 2000; Norton et al., 2000; Sininger et al., 2000). Each method performed well in the identification of moderate, severe, and profound hearing loss. The study also found pass rates similar for ABRs, TEOAEs, and DPOAEs. However, mild hearing loss was detected at a rate of only about 50% (Prieve, 2008). Finally, the two technologies differ in their ability to detect disorders of the auditory pathway beyond the level of the cochlea. As OAEs are generated by the cochlear hair cells they may be unaffected by disorders of the auditory nerve or brainstem pathway. Since most permanent hearing loss in children is cochlear in origin, OAEs provide a viable screening tool for all but the mildest hearing losses. However, if the goals of the screening program include detection of ANSD, ABR is the screening procedure of choice (JCIH, 2007).

There are many studies of OAEs applied to newborn screening but far fewer that have investigated OAE screening in toddlers, preschoolers, and school-age children. The studies that have employed OAEs with older age groups reveal generally good test characteristics, comparable to other methods. But the studies are difficult to compare because of differences in degree of hearing loss targeted; the population of interest; stimulus and recording variables; pass-fail criteria and test environment (Dille, Glattke, & Earl, 2007; Driscoll, Kei, & McPherson, 2001; Eiserman et al., 2008; Glattke, Pafitis, & Cummiskey, 1995; Lyons, Kei, & Driscoll, 2004; Nozza, Sabo, & Mandel, 1997; Shi et al., 2000; Sideris & Glattke, 2006). There is also evidence of differences in performance for TEOAEs and DPOAEs when applied to screening (Dille et al., 2007; Shi et al., 2000). Clinicians must determine the appropriate application of OAEs based on the target population and the goals of their screening program, taking into account each of the variables noted above.

Although the focus of this chapter is on screening after the newborn period, a discussion of newborn hearing screening is relevant because the outcome at initial screening will influence sensitivity and specificity, and thus the number of children requiring later identification and follow-up. In general, OAE screening takes less time than ABR and is less costly with regard to consumable supplies needed for each screen (electrodes and ear couplers). Consequently, many newborn hearing screening programs employ both OAE and ABR using a two-step protocol that uses OAE for the initial screen followed by automated ABR for infants who do not pass the OAE. The two-step protocol, whereby the child must fail both stages to be referred, is designed to reduce loss to follow-up by decreasing the number of false-positive screening results. Johnson et al. (2005) evaluated the sensitivity of a two-stage protocol in a study that included VRA at 9 months as a gold standard for assessing the accuracy of OAE and ABR screening for infants who failed the initial screen. Their findings indicated that combining the two technologies resulted in a lower refer rate but at the expense of lower sensitivity. Specifically, nearly one-fourth of the infants with confirmed hearing loss would have passed the ABR screening. Not surprisingly, most of those infants had mild cochlear hearing losses. Johnson and colleagues note that this finding is due, in part, to the fact that most ABR screening instruments are designed to identify infants with moderate or greater degrees of hearing loss. One of the fundamental principles of screening, that of defining the target disease or disorder, is relevant here. Audiologists responsible for screening programs who rely on automated ABR or OAE screening, neither of which is highly sensitive to mild cochlear hearing loss, must consider the feasibility of targeting mild hearing loss (Gravel et al., 2005). There are trade-offs in screening that require balancing many factors including the nature of the disorder, the performance of the screening test, costs associated with screening/referral, and the implications of delayed identification and intervention. Most would agree, however, that missing over 20% of infants with congenital and early onset hearing loss in infancy (White et al., 2005) is an unacceptable scenario that places an even greater burden on screening after the newborn period (Gravel et al., 2005).

Screening for Middle Ear Disorders

Prevalence of Middle Ear Disease

Otitis media is a highly prevalent disease that affects nearly all children at least once during early childhood. In fact, middle ear disease is cited as the most frequently diagnosed pediatric disease (Daly & Giebink, 2000). The incidence is affected by seasonal variation and other factors; however, it is estimated that over one-third of preschool-age children experience recurrent otitis media and concomitant conductive hearing loss. Otitis media has its highest incidence before 2 years of age although some pediatric populations are at risk throughout childhood (Daly et al., 2010). Those at highest risk include children in group daycare and those exposed to passive cigarette smoke. Others at risk include indigenous groups (e.g., American Indian) and children with predisposing conditions (e.g., Down syndrome, craniofacial anomalies).

Screening for Middle Ear Disorders: Is There Justification?

In contrast to hearing screening, which is widely accepted as necessary and appropriate, screening for middle ear disorders has been the subject of considerable discussion and debate for many years (Bluestone et al., 1986; Northern, 1992). From its inception as a clinical tool in the 1970s, tympanometric screening for asymptomatic otitis media with effusion (OME) has been questioned by the medical community and by some audiologists. Although tympanometry has good sensitivity and specificity for detection of middle ear effusion (MEE), the natural history of otitis media and lack of consensus regarding its sequelae have caused many to question its appropriateness for mass screening. Much of the controversy has been due to high false-positive rates when tympanometry is applied to large numbers of preschool or school-age children. Early immittance screening protocols recommended medical referral based on abnormality of a single tympanometric screen (ASHA, 1979). This resulted in dissatisfaction from both pediatricians and parents when, by the time the child was seen for medical examination, many of the middle ear disorders had resolved (Bess, 1980; Bluestone et al., 1986; Roush & Tait, 1985).

It is now recognized that OME is a transient condition that resolves without treatment in over 50% of cases within 6 months (Rosenfeld & Kay, 2003). It may or may not cause significant hearing loss and its prevalence varies with age, time of year, and a variety of environmental factors (Bluestone & Klein, 2007; Daly & Giebink, 2000). If the decision is made to include screening for middle ear disorders it must be applied judiciously as part of a comprehensive program designed to identify children with chronic or recurrent middle ear disorders, while minimizing false-positive medical referrals. Recently, clinical practice guidelines for OME were revised by a subcommittee of the American Academy of Family Physicians, the American Academy of Otolaryngology-Head and Neck Surgery, and the American Academy of Pediatrics (2004). The guidelines discourage mass tympanometric screening and recommend that population-based screening programs for OME not be performed in healthy, asymptomatic children. Screening for middle ear disorders is clearly justified, however, for children who are at high risk for otitis media. This would include children with predisposing conditions such as cleft palate or Down syndrome. Tympanometric screening also is justified for children likely to suffer adverse consequences from even a mild conductive hearing loss. Included in this group are children already experiencing developmental delays and those with concomitant sensorineural hearing loss. Monitoring of middle ear status is especially important for children who use amplification since the benefits of hearing aid use are seriously compromised by a transient conductive component.

Decisions regarding inclusion of tympanometric screening in a preschool or school setting are often made by school administrators based on the advice of a consulting audiologist. It is incumbent upon audiologists responsible for these programs to consider the advantages and controversies associated with screening for middle ear disorders, as well as the epidemiological principles of screening in general. They should be familiar with local and state regulations pertinent to screening, and willing to consider the recommendations of the medical community as reflected in various practice guidelines and position statements. Where inconsistencies exist it is important to communicate directly with health care providers in the community to achieve consensus on screening and referral criteria.

Methods of Screening for Middle Ear Disorders

Tympanometry

If the decision is made to include tympanometric screening it should be preceded by visual inspection of the external ear to detect observable signs of disease or malformation. The outer ear examination is followed by otoscopic inspection. Visual inspection is essential to identify conditions requiring immediate medical attention and to ensure that the ear canal is free of obstructions that might cause injury or affect screening results. Immittance screening criteria, protocols, and procedures have been outlined by several professional organizations. Although some of these recommendations were published over a decade ago, most are still applicable. AAA published a position statement in 1997 entitled: Identification and Diagnosis of Hearing Loss and Middle-Ear Dysfunction in Preschool and School-Age Children; a similar document was issued by ASHA, Guidelines for Audiologic Screening (1997). The recommendations contained in both the AAA (1997) and ASHA (1997) screening documents are guided by two general tenets: (1) referral for medical examination should not be based on a single tympanometric screening; a follow-up test should occur at some later point in time, for example, in four to six weeks, to determine if there is evidence of persistent MEE, and (2) tympanometric data should be interpreted based on quantitative values rather than gross pattern detection. The latter recommendation is based on the fact that the A, B, C pattern-identification method of classification originated with tympanograms from impedance meters that used arbitrary units of measurement. In 1987, standards for acoustic immittance instruments were developed (ANSI, 1987) that required direct measurement of acoustical admittance or impedance. The resulting tympanometric patterns are not consistent with those from early impedance meters and now provide absolute physical values. Although many clinicians have developed their own criteria for classifying tympanograms according to A, B, and C patterns, there is no standard for such a classification, and consequently, considerable variability exists among clinics and screening programs. In addition, the pattern classification system gives weight to tympanometric peak pressure, a measure shown to be ineffective in the detection of MEE (Nozza, 1994; Smith et al., 2006). Furthermore, the ABC classification system does not incorporate measures of tympanometric shape or gradient. In particular, tympanometric width (TW) has been shown to have good performance in identifying MEE. With current instruments, peak admittance and TW values are consistent across instruments and there are data available relating these values to identification of MEE (Margolis & Heller, 1987; Nozza, Bluestone, Kardatzke, & Bachman, 1994; Nozza, 1998; Roush, Drake, & Sexton, 1992; Smith et al., 2006).

The tympanogram is quantified using four measures: equivalent volume (ml), tympanometric peak pressure (daPa), peak acoustic admittance (Peak Y in mmho) and TW (daPa). The pass-fail criteria recommended by AAA (1997) and ASHA (1997) are similar and are based on research designed to estimate sensitivity and specificity (Nozza, Bluestone, Kardatzke, & Bachman, 1992; Nozza et al., 1994; Roush & Tait, 1985; Roush, 1990; Silman, Silverman, & Arick, 1992). For example, the AAA position statement suggests referral for children ages 3 to 7 years if peak $Y < 0.2$ mmho or $TW > 250$ daPa. ASHA guidelines recommend a referral from an initial screening be made for children age 1 year through school age if peak Y is < 0.3 mmho or $TW > 200$ daPa. ASHA Guidelines recommend slightly different criteria for infants 6 to 12 months of age: peak $Y < 0.2$ or $TW > 235$ daPa (Roush et al, 1995). Chapter 18 in this volume provides a useful summary of several studies that have reported normative data for various age groups.

The guidelines published by AAA (1997) and the ASHA (1997) do not differentiate between the general population and high-risk groups in their recommended pass/refer criteria for MEE. However, it is important to remember that the prevalence of the disorder in the population being tested will affect predictive values. Therefore, it is advisable to consider different criteria for different populations. Having good prevalence data for the target population is essential for estimating predictive values (Nozza et al., 1994). Current technology for immittance screening relies almost exclusively on measurement of acoustic admittance. A low frequency (226 Hz) probe tone is commonly used for tympanometric screening in children over the age of 4 to 6 months.[1]

Clearly there are many issues that need to be taken into account when tympanometry is used to screen for MEE. Decisions regarding pass/refer criteria must consider normative data and research findings on sensitivity and specificity, but they must also consider instrumentation variables, the population screened (especially age and prevalence of MEE), available resources for re-screening and follow-up and most importantly, agreement between the screening refer criteria and the definition of the disorder according to the diagnostician. Referrals from a screening program that result in too many false positives according to the diagnostic practitioner will result in failure of the screening program.

When planning a program to screen for middle ear disorders, audiologists must determine if the goal is to detect *any* middle ear disorder or only MEE, and whether the program seeks to identify children with MEE at a single point in time or the subset of children with chronic conditions. Those responsible for the supervision of screening programs should monitor outcomes associated with screening, and communicate with local health care providers to determine if changes in referral criteria are needed. Achieving an acceptable balance between sensitivity and specificity requires thoughtful consideration of the issues noted above and careful evaluation of screening outcomes.

Is There a Dual Role for OAE in Screening for Middle Ear Disorders and Cochlear Hearing Loss?

The impact of middle ear disorders on the recording of OAEs is often cited as a limiting factor for OAE; however, some investigators have suggested that a combined protocol consisting of OAEs followed by tympanometry could be useful in the detection of both middle ear disorders and cochlear hearing loss (Koivunen et al., 2000; Lyons et al., 2004; Nozza et al., 1997). Because OAEs typically are abnormal in ears with hearing loss and/or middle ear disorders, a group of children screened with OAEs could produce referrals that include cochlear hearing loss, middle ear disorders with or without concomitant conductive hearing impairment, or a combination of these conditions. A few false positives would likely be included as well. Ears that pass the OAE screen would be assumed to have hearing threshold levels ≤ 25 to 35 dB HL and normal middle ear function. Those not passing the OAE screen would undergo tympanometry. This would be a small subset of the target population making the number of children requiring both tests significantly reduced in comparison to a protocol requiring a hearing test (e.g., pure-tone screening or OAE) and tympanometry on all children. For example, even if 20 to 30% failed the initial OAE screening, 70 to 80% of the children would likely have passed and would not need a second screening test. Those who fail the initial OAE screening and who demonstrate abnormal tympanometry would follow the protocol for immittance screening and return at a later date (e.g., 4 to 6 weeks) for tympanometric re-screening. When the child passes the tympanometric rescreening and/or is found by medical examination to be free of middle ear disease, a repeat OAE or behavioral hearing screening could be provided to rule out permanent hearing loss. A child referred from an OAE screening who passes the tympanometric screening would be referred to a pediatric audiologist for comprehensive assessment.

The suggestion that OAE might be useful for both hearing screening and detection of MEE was initially made in the context of school-age children (Nozza et al., 1997). Since then, the combined protocol has been explored with younger children (Hunter, Davey, Kohtz, & Daly, 2007). It is important to remember that this approach will be influenced by the age and demographics of the target population as well as the setting where screening is performed and the skill of the examiners. Also, young children (< 4 years old) have a higher prevalence of MEE than school-age children so a higher proportion will fail OAE screening. In nearly all cases the OAE fail will be due to a middle ear disorder rather than cochlear hearing loss. This raises an important philosophical question regarding the use of OAE for detection of MEE. When normal cochlear function cannot be demonstrated there is heightened concern regarding the possibility of permanent hearing loss, even if the failed screen is likely due to a middle ear disorder. Thus, it is important to consider the potential for over-referring children for comprehensive audiologic assessment when the underlying cause

[1]If tympanometry is used before 6 months of age it is necessary to employ a high-frequency probe tone (e.g. 1000 Hz) and apply normative data for young infants (Kei, Mazlan, Hickson, Gavranich, & Linning, 2007; Margolis, Bass-Ringdahl, Hanks, Holte, & Zapala, 2003).

is MEE. This issue comes down to the goals of the screening program as illustrated by Ho, Daly, Hunter, and Davey (2002). Ho and colleagues performed OAE and tympanometry in a group of children ranging in age from birth to 5 years, in a study designed to evaluate the concordance of tympanometry and TEOAE and how these measures compared to physician findings. Their results suggest that TEOAE screening is a useful complement to tympanometry screening and that the combination is more effective than either technique alone because both conductive and sensorineural hearing loss, as well as middle ear effusion, can be detected with a combination of screening measures. Ho and colleagues concluded that if the goal of a screening program is to detect sensorineural and conductive hearing loss, then TEOAE screening alone would be effective in accomplishing that goal. However, if the goal is to detect OME, then both tympanometry and TEOAE screening are recommended.

It is important to emphasize that OAE screening is susceptible to environmental noise and noise generated by the child. When measuring OAEs in a clinical setting with a parent or caretaker present, movement and noise can often be controlled. In contrast, when OAEs are used in a pediatrician's office or preschool setting, noise and other distractions can produce an excessive number of unsuccessful or false positive results, thus diminishing the overall performance of the screening protocol (Nozza, 2001). This, in fact, was the outcome reported by Hunter et al. (2007) in a cohort of approximately 400 American Indian children followed prospectively from birth to 2 years of age. Hunter and colleagues found OAE screening to be challenging with these young children, even when using well-trained examiners. A more favorable experience was reported by Eiserman et al. (2008) in a study that employed "lay screeners" to assess 4,500 preschoolers in multiple child care settings. In any setting, the outcome of an OAE screening program will be influenced by several factors including the examiner's level of skill and experience with OAEs, the state of the child, noise levels, and the screening environment. Problems with any one of these factors can lead to an excessive number of unsuccessful tests. For many years the authors have observed these problems, anecdotally, particularly in primary care offices and preschool settings.

Future Technologies: Acoustic Reflectance

An alternative method for identification of MEE relies on acoustic reflectivity or wideband acoustic reflectance. Sound introduced into the ear canal is reflected off the tympanic membrane based on the admittance characteristics of the middle ear. If the middle ear has normal admittance characteristics, sound will pass through easily and little will be reflected. Conversely, if the middle ear has low admittance as with MEE, more sound will be reflected back into the ear canal. Different technologies use different means of quantifying the reflectance; some measure the amplitude of the response whereas others consider the broadband frequency response. A potential advantage of reflectance over traditional immittance testing is that it uses a wideband stimulus (e.g., a chirp) and therefore measures transfer of sound through the tympanic membrane across the frequency spectrum, not just at a single probe frequency (e.g., 226 Hz). See Chapter 18 in this volume for details.

There has been considerable research on the potential role of acoustic reflectance for identification of MEE (Babb, Hilsinger, Korol, & Wilcox, 2004; Hunter, Tubaugh, Jackson, & Propes, 2008; Lampe & Schwartz, 1989; Lampe, Weir, Spier, & Rhodes, 1985; Teele & Teele, 1984; Vander Werff et al., 2007). A commercially available device, the EarCheck™ Middle Ear Monitor, is currently marketed to pediatricians and consumers for quick and easy screening for MEE; however, it has met with mixed results. Data are limited on the sensitivity and specificity of the device and it has reportedly lacked acceptance in the medical community because of difficulty setting standards and establishing pass-fail criteria (Waseem & Aslam, 2008). A recent study in Finland by Teppo and Revonta (2009) examined the diagnostic accuracy of the EarCheck™ Monitor in a prospective study of preschool-age children that compared the results of acoustic reflectometry performed by parents, to otomicroscopic myringotomy conducted immediately following reflectometry. Their findings indicated good performance in identifying MEE. The authors emphasize, however, that parents performed the reflectance measures in the hospital shortly after being instructed in the use of the instrument and that all children in the study had chronic MEE or "glue ear." Thus, their findings may not easily be generalized to screening at home in the general population where various degrees of middle ear disease would be encountered. It also should be noted that the EarCheck™ instrument is not recommended for use with young infants or with children who have craniofacial abnormalities.

Instruments that employ "wideband acoustic reflectance" measures have been studied with neonates for use in conjunction with newborn hearing screening programs (Keefe et al., 2000; Keefe, Gorga, Neely, Zhao, & Vohr, 2003; Keefe, Zhao, Neely, Gorga & Vohr, 2003). Some studies have included older children, but there is a paucity of data from which to determine sensitivity and specificity (Hunter et al., 2008; Waseem & Aslam, 2008). Also, much of the recent work has been done in research laboratories using computer-based instrumentation that would be impractical in a typical screening environment. Audiologists responsible for or in any way involved with screening for middle ear disorders should be familiar with wideband acoustic reflectance and aware of future development. Advances may lead to improved methods of screening for middle ear disorders in young children. Further study is needed, however, before this technology can be recommended for general implementation as a screening tool.

Special Populations and Settings

The issues outlined in the foregoing discussion apply to most settings where screening is conducted. There are additional considerations, however, that pertain to special populations of children based on age, risk factors, and setting. These include infants in the neonatal intensive care unit; older children with risk factors; and routine screening of preschool and school-age children.

Infants in the Special Care Nursery

The NICU provides specialized treatment in a hospital setting for infants with prematurity or serious illness. Special care facilities for infants are classified by the AAP as Level I Nurseries, which provide basic care to well-infants; Level II Nurseries, which provide specialty care for infants at moderate risk of serious complications; and Level III Nurseries where infants receive specialty and subspecialty care including mechanical ventilation (Stark, 2004). There are approximately 120 Level-II NICUs and 760 Level-III NICUs in the United States (AAP, 2004). NICU infants represent approximately 10% of the newborn population or about 400,000 infants per year (JCIH, 2007).

Several reports have shown that infants whose birth history includes hospitalization in the NICU are at increased risk for both cochlear hearing loss and ANSD (Berg et al., 2005; D'Agostino & Austin, 2004). As noted earlier, the prevalence of sensorineural hearing loss is at least 10 times higher than it is in the well-infant population, and recent studies have shown that NICU history is a significant risk factor for ANSD (Xoinis et al., 2007). Consequently, the JCIH now recommends separate protocols for the NICU and well-infant nurseries (JCIH, 2007). Specifically, for NICU infants at greatest risk for auditory impairment (defined as those admitted to the NICU for more than five days) ABR screening is recommended to avoid missing ANSD. The JCIH further recommends that infants who do not pass an initial ABR screen in the NICU be referred directly to an audiologist for rescreening. The JCIH 2007 Position Statement also recommends that infants requiring readmission in the first month of life (NICU or well infant) for conditions associated with potential hearing loss (e.g., hyperbilirubinemia requiring exchange transfusion or culture-positive sepsis), undergo a repeat hearing screening with ABR prior to discharge.

Table 17–2 provides a summary of risk indicators for hearing loss in children including conditions that require surveillance for late onset/progressive hearing loss. Many of these conditions occur more frequently in infants with a NICU history. Indeed, of all pediatric settings where screening is conducted, the NICU is likely to yield the highest number with previously undetected sensorineural hearing loss. Thus, it is vitally important that screening in the NICU be conducted with careful attention to optimal test protocols, and that infants who do not pass the ABR screening receive immediate referral to a pediatric audiologist.

Older Infants/Toddlers with Risk Factors

Although most permanent hearing loss in children can be detected at birth, some infants are at risk for later onset sensorineural hearing impairment. Those infants pose a significant challenge for audiologists and EHDI personnel because once they are discharged from the hospital, access for rescreening becomes more difficult. In an earlier JCIH position statement (JCIH, 2000) it was recommended that infants at risk for postnatal hearing impairment be rescreened at intervals of approximately six months, until 3 years of age. This recommendation proved to be impractical because of the burden it placed on audiologists and referral sources, especially in regions where pediatric audiology services were limited. It was also recognized that there are infants with unknown risk factors who develop late onset hearing loss. Thus, in the most recent position statement (JCIH, 2007; Clarification, 2007) responsibility for "surveillance" is shifted to the pediatrician or family physician as part of the child's ongoing care within the "medical home" (AAP, 2002). According to this recommendation, surveillance does not occur through actual hearing screening but in conjunction with the use of a "global developmental screening tool" to be administered at 9, 18, 24, and 30 months to all infants or whenever there is parental concern. It is assumed

Table 17–2. Risk Indicators Associated With Permanent Congenital, Delayed-Onset, or Progressive Hearing Loss in Childhood. The Risk Indicators Underlined Are of Greatest Concern for Delayed-Onset Hearing Loss (JCIH, 2007)

1. Caregiver concern regarding hearing, speech, language, or developmental delay.
2. Family history of permanent childhood hearing loss.
3. Neonatal intensive care of more than 5 days or any of the following regardless of length of stay: ECMO, assisted ventilation, exposure to ototoxic medications (gentimycin and tobramycin) or loop diuretics (furosemide/Lasix), and hyperbilirubinemia that requires exchange transfusion.
4. In utero infections, such as CMV, herpes, rubella, syphilis, and toxoplasmosis.
5. Craniofacial anomalies, including those that involve the pinna, ear canal, ear tags, ear pits, and temporal bone anomalies.
6. Physical findings, such as white forelock, that are associated with a syndrome known to include a sensorineural or permanent conductive hearing loss.
7. Syndromes associated with hearing loss or progressive or late-onset hearing loss, such as neurofibromatosis, osteopetrosis, and Usher syndrome; other frequently identified syndromes include Waardenburg, Alport, Pendred, and Jervell and Lange-Nielson.
8. Neurodegenerative disorders, such as Hunter syndrome, or sensory motor neuropathies, such as Friedreich ataxia and Charcot-Marie-Tooth disease.
9. Culture-positive postnatal infections associated with sensorineural hearing loss, including confirmed bacterial and viral (especially herpes viruses and varicella) meningitis.
10. Head trauma, especially basal skull/temporal bone fracture that requires hospitalization.
11. Chemotherapy.

that physicians will refer children with suspected hearing impairment to an audiologist. The JCIH (2007) Position Statement further advises that the timing and number of hearing re-evaluations for children with risk factors be "customized and individualized" based on the likelihood of a subsequent, delayed-onset hearing loss. Furthermore, according to JCIH (2007), infants who pass the neonatal screening but have a risk factor should undergo at least one diagnostic audiology assessment by 24 to 30 months of age, even in the absence of hearing concerns (this recommendation was also included in the AAP 2009 recommendations for screening after the newborn period). The JCIH (2007) position statement notes that early and more frequent assessment may be indicated for children with a history of cytomegalovirus infection, syndromes associated with progressive hearing loss, neurodegenerative disorders, trauma, or culture-positive postnatal infections associated with sensorineural hearing loss. Closer surveillance is also justified for children who have received extracorporeal membrane oxygenation (ECMO) or chemotherapy, and whenever there are caregiver concerns or a family history of hearing loss (see Table 17–2).

The efficacy of a program that places responsibility for early detection of hearing loss in the medical home is yet to be determined; however, it has been shown that many primary care physicians, although concerned about hearing in children, have significant gaps in their knowledge (Moeller, White, & Shisler, 2006). Efforts to educate pediatricians and primary care physicians about risk factors and signs of hearing loss are ongoing but few studies have prospectively investigated the efficacy of hearing screening in the primary care setting, especially for children under the age of 3 years. Now that most infants undergo hospital-based newborn hearing screening, detection of later onset sensorineural hearing loss in the medical home is an important priority for future investigation. Permanent hearing loss in children is of primary concern but it is also important to identify chronic or recurrent *conductive* hearing loss associated with otitis media. Otitis media remains the most common cause of hearing loss in this age group. In order for detection of hearing loss to occur in the medical home, primary care physicians must have the instrumentation and personnel needed for valid screening. They must also be willing to take the time needed to administer the global developmental screening tools described earlier. These are not trivial expectations in a busy practice but when successful can lead to earlier identification and treatment.

Preschool Children and School-Age Children

Children over 3 years of age present a different set of challenges. Typically they are not seen as frequently in the primary care setting as younger children, but many are in daycare settings or preschools where hearing screening, and in some cases, screening for middle ear disorders, is provided. Most typically developing children 3 years of age and older can be screened using developmentally-appropriate pure-tone procedures, but behavioral screening is susceptible to the challenges and limitations described earlier (Allen, Stuart, Everett, & Elangovan, 2004). If personnel from the daycare facility or preschool are involved in screenings, they should be carefully trained by an audiologist who also provides oversight and program evaluation. Children who are difficult to screen because of behavioral challenges or those already suspected of having a hearing impairment, developmental delays, or risk indicators for sensorineural hearing loss, should be referred directly to a pediatric audiologist for comprehensive assessment.

Among the greatest challenges to identification of hearing loss beyond the newborn period is access to children who are economically disadvantaged. Those at greatest risk for communication disorders are often from impoverished home environments. They may or may not attend child care programs or preschool, and if they do it may be provided in homes or other locations difficult to access for screening purposes. Furthermore, children from low income families may not be receiving regular examinations by a primary care physician because they lack financial resources, health insurance, or documentation of citizenship. These vulnerable children are in particular need of early identification and intervention aimed at building the foundations necessary for optimal developmental and academic success. The challenges are many but when successful outcomes are achieved there are important benefits for the child and for the community.

Once children enter school they are more accessible for screening purposes, but even then significant challenges remain. Hearing screening of school-age children has been conducted in the United States for decades, but despite the long history of school-based hearing screening programs there is considerable variability in policies, procedures, and protocols. Some states have comprehensive and well-defined policies and procedures; some have even enacted legislation regarding school-age hearing screening. For example, one Midwestern state has a law that requires children to be screened for hearing loss once before school entry, between 3 to 5 years. Upon reaching school age they are screened in kindergarten and grades 1, 2, 3, 5, 8, and 11. Annual hearing screening is also recommended for children with known hearing losses, those in special education classes, or those with one or more risk factors. In contrast to this state, which has both a legislative mandate and detailed protocols for implementation, many states have neither a legislative requirement nor statewide policies for screening beyond the newborn period, leaving decisions to individual health departments and local educational agencies. Furthermore, even among school districts that conduct hearing screening through adolescence, fewer than one-fourth employ protocols that will detect noise-induced hearing loss (Meinke & Dice, 2007).

Regardless of whether preschool and school-age screening is provided by legislative mandate or according to policies determined at the local or regional level, many programmatic elements must be considered in addition to the methodological issues reviewed earlier. These components, compiled from several sources (AAA, 1997; ASHA, 1997; Harlor & Bower, 2009; Roush, 1990, 2001) include screening personnel, when to screen, the screening environment, instrument calibration and maintenance, documention, and follow-up.

Screening Personnel

United States licensure laws and regulations must be consulted regarding screening personnel. In most states a variety of health care providers, support personnel, and even volunteers are permitted to engage in screening. It is essential, however, that institutional screening programs be conducted under the general supervision of an audiologist. Although most instrumentation designed for screening is relatively uncomplicated, personnel must undergo comprehensive orientation and training. It is recommended that instruction be provided by an audiologist and that screening personnel be required to demonstrate proficiency in the administration of screening procedures and the accurate recording of screening results.

When to Screen

Recommendations vary with regard to age and screening intervals, but it is generally agreed that asymptomatic children without risk factors who passed newborn hearing screening should be screened for hearing loss at least once in the preschool years and at school entry.

Most guidelines recommend screening at several different early elementary grade levels. For example, the AAP, in its Recommendations for Preventive Pediatric Health Care (AAP, 2008) recommends that hearing screening be performed beyond the newborn period at the age of 4, 5, 6, 8, and 10 years, with yearly "risk assessment" for children who may require screening on a more frequent basis. With regard to time of year, hearing screening can be conducted any time; however, for institutional programs there are advantages to screening in the fall of the year. It is desirable to identify hearing problems early in the school year so appropriate intervention can be initiated. In addition, fall and winter months are associated with a higher incidence of otitis media. Although prevalence rates vary, more children with transient hearing loss due to middle ear disorders are likely to be identified during the fall and winter months. The time of day is also important. Young children usually perform best from mid to late morning. Time of day is less critical for older children and likely will be dictated by instructional schedules.

The Screening Environment

Pure-tone screening requires a quiet environment, free of visual distractions and competing background noise. Table 17–3 provides a summary of permissible noise levels according to the American National Standards Institute (ANSI S3.1, 1999, 2008) for screening at 20 dB HL using supra-aural earphones and insert receivers.

The values shown are sound pressure levels for octave bands. Ambient noise levels must be at or below the levels indicated. It is important to note that ANSI S3.1 requires the measurement of octave or one-third octave bands within the inclusive range of 125 to 8000 Hz, regardless of the test condition or frequency range to be employed (Frank, 2000). It may be necessary for sound level measures to be made by an audiologist or acoustic engineer; however, screening personnel, if properly trained and equipped, can often perform these measures. It is essential that the screening environment meet ANSI specifications for acceptable noise levels. Unfortunately, two practical problems often arise. First, the equipment and personnel needed to accomplish sound level measurements may be unavailable. Second, even if the measurements are made, ambient levels may vary over time. Screening personnel must exercise good judgment at all times in evaluating the adequacy of the acoustic environment. When sound level measures are not available or if conditions vary, ANSI S3.1 includes a provision for applying a psychoacoustic check of ambient noise levels, using two listeners known to have normal hearing.

In any screening environment the supervising audiologist must ensure that screening personnel are

Table 17–3. Octave Band Maximum Permissible Ambient Noise Levels With Ears Covered for Pure Tone Screening at 20 dB HL Using Supra-Aural and Insert Earphones as Specified in ANSI/ASA S3.1-1999 (R 2008).

	Supra-Aural Earphone			*Insert Earphone*		
Octave Band Intervals	***125–8000 Hz***	***Screening Level***	***Maximum Allowable Ambient Level***	***125–8000 Hz***	***Screening Level***	***Maximum Allowable Ambient Level***
125	35	20	55	59	20	79
250	25	20	45	53	20	73
500	21	20	41	50	20	70
1000	26	20	46	47	20	67
2000	34	20	54	49	20	69
4000	37	20	57	50	20	70
8000	37	20	57	56	20	76

Note: The ANSI Standard requires measurement of octave (or one-third octave) bands within the inclusive range of 125 to 8000 Hz, regardless of the test condition or frequency range employed. For pure-tone screening at a fixed intensity the screening level is added to the maximum permissible noise level at each octave band, as illustrated here for screening at a fixed intensity of 20 dB HL. Values are in dB re: 20 Pa to the nearest 0.5 dB (ANSI, 1999, 2008).

not tempted to increase the presentation level when screening is performed in a less than ideal environment. Attempts to "compensate" for a poor acoustic environment could result in failure to identify a child with a hearing loss whose thresholds are below the screening level. School administrators must understand the importance of an adequate acoustic environment and recognize that time and financial resources will be wasted if children are referred unnecessarily for diagnostic assessment.

Instrument Calibration and Maintenance

Audiometers and tympanometers require calibration checks by a qualified technician at least once each year according to ANSI (1999, 2008) specifications. In addition to formal calibration measures, daily visual inspection and listening checks are essential. It is also important to insure that equipment is carefully transported to and from screening sites and well-maintained when not in use. Time spent on proper maintenance and handling of equipment will be compensated by fewer repairs and less down time.

Documentation and Follow-Up

Screening itself does not improve the wellness of children; it is the action taken as a result of screening that leads to improved outcomes. A detailed examination of data management, reporting, and follow-up is beyond the scope of this chapter; however, it is essential that findings be accurately documented and promptly disclosed to parents and caretakers. It also is important to obtain parental consent, when required, and to inform the child's pediatrician or family practice physician of screening results. For permanent conditions or those likely to be chronic or recurrent it is important to notify school personnel and to make recommendations for environmental modifications when indicated. See DeConde Johnson, Benson, and Seaton (1997) for additional information on screening and follow-up in the educational setting.

Screening Beyond the Newborn Period: Current Challenges and Future Needs

Hearing screening after the newborn period has existed in one form or another for decades, yet few large-scale prospective studies have addressed the efficacy of preschool and school-based hearing screening programs. Research is needed to better understand the validity of traditional screening practices as well as the advantages and disadvantages of replacing conventional methods, such as pure-tone hearing screening, with OAEs or other methods. Research is needed not only to validate hearing screening methods, but also to better understand the causes of hearing loss in young children and the reasons for the increasing prevalence of permanent hearing loss after the newborn period. It is important to determine the proportion of children with hearing losses missed at the time of newborn hearing screening versus those added because of late onset or progressive conditions. In addition to traditional analyses based on sensitivity and specificity it is important to consider costs, benefits, and societal implications. A recent article by Porter, Neely, and Gorga (2009) provides a useful framework for calculating benefit-cost ratios for evaluation of hearing screening protocols.

Improved detection of mild cochlear losses could be achieved by increasing the sensitivity of ABR or OAE screening protocols, but this would occur at the expense of increasing the number of false positive referrals (Gravel et al., 2005; White et al., 2005; Widen et al., 2005). Research is needed to determine pass-refer rates associated with various OAE and ABR protocols alone and in combination, the impact of multilevel screens, the role of screening middle ear function, and the relative costs associated with each (Gravel et al., 2005). There is also a need for continued efforts to decrease the number of infants unreported or lost to follow-up. Data management systems that provide on-going tracking and surveillance are vital components of EHDI programs. Unfortunately, they often are compromised by inaccurate recording or incomplete data entry (Allen et al., 2004).

There is a particular need for standards that pertain to the stimulus and recording parameters used in OAE and ABR screening instruments as well as a need for more complete and uniform technical specifications (Durrant, Sabo, & Delgado, 2007). As noted by Gravel and Kurman (2006) the lack of ANSI standards for calibration of OAE and ABR devices has led to variability among commercially available screening instruments. Specifically, variation in acoustic stimuli and sound pressure levels at the tympanic membrane can result in different pass-refer criteria among devices. This is a particular issue with instruments designed for screening purposes, many of which are designed to restrict users from altering test parameters to meet recommended criteria. For example, among DPOAE screeners there are differences in the tonal pairs used, and among automated ABR screeners there are differences in stimulus levels (e.g., 35 dB nHL versus 40 dB nHL). These issues, according to Gravel and Kurman, not only affect calibration but create obstacles to the implementation of uniform pass-refer criteria. They also make it difficult to compare data across programs and settings, and they limit the ability to conduct prevalence estimates for various populations and geographic regions. This is a critical area of need, with important implications for EHDI programs at the time of initial screening and for screening conducted after the newborn period. Fortunately, there is now progress on the development of an ANSI standard for calibration of acoustic transients and it is likely that standards will be forthcoming the near future (Burkard, 2010).

Finally, and perhaps most pressing, is a need for improved coordination of screening efforts and better communication among agencies and service providers. As new and updated guidelines and position statements emerge from various organizations, it is important to seek consensus at the state and local levels to achieve well-coordinated policies and procedures. Newborn hearing screening is mandated in most states and the procedures employed are similar among hospitals. But screening *after* the newborn period involves a multitude of settings, service providers, public policies, and screening methods. Successful programs require evidence-based protocols and the concurrence of numerous stakeholders including those in health departments, hospitals, community clinics, and educational settings, working in partnership with clinicians and service providers in the public and private sectors. Without effective coordination and communication, screening may be insufficient or excessive. Responsibility will vary among states and municipalities based on legislative requirements, public policies, and local history, but the active engagement of pediatric and educational audiologists is needed at each level to achieve effective policies and procedures.

Summary and Conclusions

Hearing screening beyond the newborn period is supported by a substantial body of evidence that confirms the detrimental sequelae associated with undetected hearing loss. This includes speech, language, social development, and psychoeducational outcomes. Moreover, it is supported by the intrinsic right of all children to hear and for families to be informed if there is uncertainty regarding their child's access to sound. The role and efficacy of tympanometric screening is less clear but it too remains vital for children at risk for middle ear disorders and those with concomitant sensorineural hearing loss. The key points in this chapter are summarized as follows:

- Permanent hearing loss is the most common abnormality affecting newborn infants. Moreover, the prevalence appears to increase dramatically during the preschool and school years due to a variety of factors including: failure to detect mild losses at the time of newborn screening, late onset or progressive sensorineural hearing loss, and an alarming number of young children lost to follow-up whose diagnosis inevitably will be delayed.
- The prevalence of permanent hearing loss is especially high among infants whose birth histories include special care in the NICU. In addition to higher prevalence of cochlear hearing loss, many infants with NICU histories are at increased risk for ANSD or delayed onset/progressive cochlear hearing loss. ABR is the only technology appropriate for detection of sensorineural hearing loss in the NICU because of its sensitivity to ANSD. Because of the relatively high incidence of sensorineural hearing loss in this population, JCIH 2007 recommends that NICU infants who do not pass an initial ABR screening be referred to an audiologist for assessment and follow-up. Infants *readmitted* to the hospital after the newborn period for a condition that increases the risk of sensorineural hearing loss should be rescreened with ABR prior to discharge.
- Routine behavioral hearing screening from birth to 3 years cannot be reliably conducted by nonaudiologists. Once a child reaches the age of 3 to 4 years, behavioral pure-tone screening is feasible, but it requires a capable and experienced examiner and a cooperative child with the motivation and developmental maturity necessary to provide reliable responses. Behavioral pure-tone screening also requires a suitable acoustic environment, free of visual distractions and excessive noise.
- Physiologic measures based on ABR and OAE are essential screening tools, but as typically applied in newborn screening (e.g., a two-step screening OAE/ABR protocol) they are likely to miss a substantial number of newborns with milder degrees of permanent hearing loss in one or both ears. This unfortunate reality increases the burden of accurately detecting hearing loss after the newborn period. Unfortunately, ABR screening without sedation is difficult in older infants. OAEs can be used with children at any age but may miss mild cochlear hearing loss and auditory neuropathy. OAE screen-

ing is also prone to error or over-referral in the hands of an inexperienced user.

- The use of tympanometry to screen for middle ear disorders in young children is widely practiced in the United States even though current recommendations from the medical community discourage mass tympanometric screening in healthy, asymptomatic children. Middle ear monitoring is clearly justified, however, for children with histories of recurrent otitis media or for those with concomitant sensorineural hearing loss.
- OAEs are sensitive to otitis media *and* cochlear hearing loss. Applied judiciously in combination with tympanometry they can be used to screen for both conditions; however, because OAEs may miss mild cochlear hearing loss and auditory neuropathy, a combined approach is best suited for routine screening of asymptomatic children who do not have risk factors for sensorineural hearing loss.
- There is an urgent need for standards that define calibration of OAE and ABR screening devices and that set forth stimulus and recording parameters that make it possible to establish uniform pass-refer criteria among commercially available screening instruments.
- The AAP 2009 recommendations for screening after the newborn period represent an important commitment from the medical community and a useful conceptual framework. Effective screening in the medical home would facilitate earlier detection of hearing loss, especially among children who require surveillance because of a risk factor for late onset or progressive hearing loss. However, the efficacy of hearing screening in the primary care setting has not been clearly established and further research is needed.
- There is considerable variability among, and even within, states with regard to screening policies and procedures employed with older infants, preschoolers, and school-age children. Inconsistencies exist in technology, personnel, pass-fail criteria, and surveillance of children with risk indicators for late onset-progressive hearing loss. Within most states and local communities there is a need for better coordination of screening and follow-up, and improved communication with families and primary care providers. This requires the endorsement of many stakeholders, public and private, with the aim of achieving an effective continuum of screening, referral, and follow-up, balanced with a reasonable expenditure of public health resources.
- Because of limitations inherent in each of the screening methods currently available, children with known or suspected developmental delays, caregiver concerns, educational concerns, risk indicators for sensorineural hearing loss, or characteristics that make them "difficult to test" by conventional means, should be referred to a pediatric audiologist for comprehensive assessment.

The nationwide implementation of hospital-based, newborn hearing screening programs is a remarkable achievement. But many challenges remain, among them the screening and follow-up needed in the months and years that follow the newborn period. The same level of commitment and advocacy that led to the successful implementation of neonatal hearing screening is needed on behalf of the infants and children who require screening and surveillance beyond the newborn period.

References

Allen, R. L., Stuart, A., Everett, D., & Elangovan, S. (2004). Preschool hearing screening: Pass/refer rates for children enrolled in a head start program in eastern North Carolina. *American Journal of Audiology, 13*(1), 29–38.

American Academy of Audiology (AAA). (1997). *Identification of hearing loss and middle ear dysfunction in preschool and school-age children*. Reston, VA: Author.

American Academy of Family Physicians (AAP), American Academy of Otolaryngology-Head and Neck Surgery, & American Academy of Pediatrics (AAP) Subcommittee on Otitis Media With Effusion. (2004). Otitis media with effusion. *Pediatrics, 113*(5), 1412–1429.

American Academy of Pediatrics (AAP). (2002). Medical Home Initiatives for Children with Special Needs, Project Advisory Committee. The medical home. *Pediatrics, 110*, 184–186.

American Academy of Pediatrics (AAP). (2008). *Recommendations for preventive pediatric health care (periodicity schedule)*. Retrieved January 23, 2010, from http://practice.aap.org/content.aspx?aid=1599

American National Standards Institute (ANSI). (1987). *Specifications for instruments to measure aural acoustic impedance and admittance (aural acoustic immittance)*. ANSI S3.39-1987. New York, NY: Acoustical Society of America.

American National Standards Institute (ANSI). (1999, 2008). *American National Standard maximum permissible ambient noise levels for audiometric test rooms* (ANSI/ASA 3.1-1999, R 2008). Melville, NY: Acoustical Society of America.

American Speech-Language-Hearing Association (ASHA). (1979). *Guidelines for acoustic immittance screening of middle ear function*. Rockville, MD: American Speech-Language-Hearing Association.

American Speech-Language-Hearing Association (ASHA). (1997). Panel on audiologic assessment. *Guidelines for audiologic screening*. Rockville, MD: Author.

Babb, M. J., Hilsinger, R. L. Jr., Korol, H. W., & Wilcox, R. D. (2004). Modern acoustic reflectometry: Accuracy in diagnosing otitis media with effusion. *Ear, Nose, and Throat Journal, 83*(9), 622–624.

Bamford, J., Fortnum, H., Bristow, K., Smith, J., Vamvakas, G., Davies, L., . . . Hind, S. (2007). Current practice, accuracy, effectiveness and cost-effectiveness of the school entry hearing screen. *Health Technology Assessment (Winchester, England), 11*(32), 1–168, iii–iv.

Berg, A. L., Spitzer, J. B., Towers, H. M., Bartosiewicz, C., & Diamond, B. E. (2005). Newborn hearing screening in the NICU: Profile of failed auditory brainstem response/passed otoacoustic emission. *Pediatrics, 116*(4), 933–938.

Bess, F. H. (1980). Impedance screening for children. A need for more research. *Annals of Otology, Rhinology and Laryngology Suppl., 89*(3 Pt 2), 228–232.

Bess, F. H., Dodd-Murphy, J., & Parker, R. A. (1998). Children with minimal sensorineural hearing loss: Prevalence, educational performance, and functional status. *Ear and Hearing, 19*(5), 339–354.

Bluestone, C. D., Fria, T. J., Arjona, S. K., Casselbrant, M. L., Schwartz, D. M., Ruben, R. J., . . . Rogers, K. D. (1986). Controversies in screening for middle ear disease and hearing loss in children. *Pediatrics, 77*(1), 57–70.

Bluestone, C. D., & Klein, J. O. (2007). *Otitis media in infants and children* (4th ed.). Philadelphia, PA: B.C. Decker.

Burkard, R. (2010). Update on a standard for the calibration of acoustic transients. *ASHA Audiology Connections, 15.* Retrieved August 16, 2010, from http://www.asha.org/uploadedFiles/10AudConn.pdf

Centers for Disease Control and Prevention (CDC). (2007a). *Annual EHDI data, 2007.* Retrieved January 23, 2010, from http://www.cdc.gov/ncbddd/ehdi/data.htm

Centers for Disease Control and Prevention (CDC). (2007b). *Summary of 2007 national CDC EHDI data.* Retrieved January 23, 2010, from http://www.cdc.gov/ncbddd/ehdi/documents/DataSource2007.pdf

D'Agostino, J. A., & Austin, L. (2004). Auditory neuropathy: A potentially under-recognized neonatal intensive care unit sequela. *Advances in Neonatal Care: Official Journal of the National Association of Neonatal Nurses, 4*(6), 344–353.

Daly, K. A., & Giebink, G. S. (2000). Clinical epidemiology of otitis media. *Pediatric Infectious Disease Journal, 19*(5 Suppl), S31–S36.

Daly, K. A., Hoffman, H. J., Kvaerner, K. J., Kvestad, E., Casselbrant, M. L., Homoe, P., & Rovers, M. M. (2010). Epidemiology, natural history, and risk factors: Panel report from the Ninth International Research Conference on Otitis Media. *International Journal of Pediatric Otorhinolaryngology, 74*(3), 231–240.

Deconde Johnson, C., Benson, P. V., & Seaton, J. B. (1997). *Educational audiology handbook.* San Diego, CA: Singular.

Dille, M., Glattke, T. J., & Earl, B. R. (2007). Comparison of transient evoked otoacoustic emissions and distortion product otoacoustic emissions when screening hearing in preschool children in a community setting. *International Journal of Pediatric Otorhinolaryngology, 71*(11), 1789–1795.

Driscoll, C., Kei, J., & McPherson, B. (2001). Outcomes of transient evoked otoacoustic emission testing in 6-year-old school children: A comparison with pure-tone screening and tympanometry. *International Journal of Pediatric Otorhinolaryngology, 57*(1), 67–76.

Durrant, J. D., Sabo, D. L., & Delgado, R. E. (2007). Call for calibration standard for newborn screening using auditory brainstem responses. *International Journal of Audiology, 46*(11), 686–691.

Eiserman, W. D., Hartel, D. M., Shisler, L., Buhrmann, J., White, K. R., & Foust, T. (2008). Using otoacoustic emissions to screen for hearing loss in early childhood care settings. *International Journal of Pediatric Otorhinolaryngology, 72*(4), 475–482.

Feightner, J. W. (1992) Screening in the 1990's: Some principles and guidelines. In F. H. Bess & J. W. Hall (Eds.), *Screening children for auditory function* (pp. 1–16). Nashville, TN: Bill Wilkerson Center Press.

Finitzo, T., Albright, K., & O'Neal, J. (1998). The newborn with hearing loss: Detection in the nursery. *Pediatrics, 102*(6), 1452–1460.

FitzZaland, R. E., & Zink, G. D. (1984). A comparative study of hearing screening procedures. *Ear and Hearing, 5*(4), 205–210.

Frank, T. (2000). ANSI update: Maximum permissible ambient noise levels for audiometric test rooms. *American Journal of Audiology, 9*(1), 3–8.

Gerber, S. E. (1990). Review of a high risk register for congenital or early-onset deafness. *British Journal of Audiology, 24*(5), 347–356.

Glattke, T., Pafitis, I. A., & Cummiskey, C. (1995). Identification of hearing loss in children and young adults using measures of transient evoked otoacoustic emission reproducibility. *American Journal of Audiology, 4*, 71–86.

Gorga, M. P., Norton, S. J., Sininger, Y. S., Cone-Wesson, B., Folsom, R. C., Vohr, B. R., . . . Neely, S. T. (2000). Identification of neonatal hearing impairment: Distortion product otoacoustic emissions during the perinatal period. *Ear and Hearing, 21*(5), 400–424.

Gravel, J., & Kurman, B. (2006). *Standards for newborn hearing screening equipment: What are we measuring in newborn hearing screening programs?* National Conference on Early Hearing Detection and Intervention, February, 2006, Washington, DC.

Gravel, J. S., White, K. R., Johnson, J. L., Widen, J. E., Vohr, B. R., James, M., . . . Meyer, S. (2005). A multisite study to examine the efficacy of the otoacoustic emission/automated auditory brainstem response newborn hearing screening protocol: Recommendations for policy, practice, and research. *American Journal of Audiology, 14*(2), S217–S228.

Guidelines Development Conference on the Identification and Management of Infants with Auditory Neuropathy. (2008). International Newborn Hearing Screening Conference, June 19–21, Como, Italy. Available at http://www.thechildrenshospital.org/conditions/speech/danielscenter/ANSD-Guidelines.aspx

Halloran, D. R., Hardin, J. M., & Wall, T. C. (2009). Validity of pure-tone hearing screening at well-child visits. *Archives of Pediatrics and Adolescent Medicine, 163*(2), 158–163.

Harlor, A. D. Jr., Bower, C., Committee on Practice and Ambulatory Medicine, & Section on Otolaryngology-Head and Neck Surgery. (2009). Hearing assessment in infants and children: Recommendations beyond neonatal screening. *Pediatrics, 124*(4), 1252–1263.

Ho, V., Daly, K. A., Hunter, L. L., & Davey, C. (2002). Otoacoustic emissions and tympanometry screening among 0–5 year olds. *Laryngoscope, 112*(3), 513–519.

Holmes, A. E., Niskar, A. S., Kieszak, S. M., Rubin, C., & Brody, D. J. (2004). Mean and median hearing thresholds among children 6 to 19 years of age: The third national health and nutrition examination survey, 1988 to 1994, United States. *Ear and Hearing, 25*(4), 397–402.

Hunter, L. L., Davey, C. S., Kohtz, A., & Daly, K. A. (2007). Hearing screening and middle ear measures in American Indian infants and toddlers. *International Journal of Pediatric Otorhinolaryngology, 71*(9), 1429–1438.

Hunter, L. L., Tubaugh, L., Jackson, A., & Propes, S. (2008). Wideband middle ear power measurement in infants and children. *Journal of the American Academy of Audiology, 19*(4), 309–324.

Johnson, J. L., White, K. R., Widen, J. E., Gravel, J. S., James, M., Kennalley, T., . . . Holstrum, J. (2005). A multicenter evaluation of how many infants with permanent hearing loss pass a two-stage otoacoustic emissions/automated auditory brainstem response newborn hearing screening protocol. *Pediatrics, 116*(3), 663–672.

Joint Committee on Infant Hearing (JCIH). (1971). *Joint Statement on Neonatal Screening for Hearing Impairment.* Retrieved January 23, 2010, from http://jcih.org/posstatemts.htm

Joint Committee on Infant Hearing (JCIH). (2000). Year 2000 position statement: Principles and guidelines for early hearing detection and intervention programs. *Pediatrics, 106*(4), 798–817.

Joint Committee on Infant Hearing (JCIH). (2007). Year 2007 position statement: Principles and guidelines for early hearing detection and intervention programs. *Pediatrics, 120*(4), 898–921.

Joint Committee on Infant Hearing. *Clarification, year 2007 statement.* Retrieved January 23, 2010, from: http://jcih.org/Clarification%20Year%202007%20statement.pdf

Keefe, D. H., Folsom, R. C., Gorga, M. P., Vohr, B. R., Bulen, J. C., & Norton, S. J. (2000). Identification of neonatal hearing impairment: Ear-canal measurements of acoustic admittance and reflectance in neonates. *Ear and Hearing, 21*(5), 443–461.

Keefe, D. H., Gorga, M. P., Neely, S. T., Zhao, F., & Vohr, B. R. (2003). Ear-canal acoustic admittance and reflectance measurements in human neonates. II. predictions of middle-ear in dysfunction and sensorineural hearing loss. *Journal of the Acoustical Society of America, 113*(1), 407–422.

Keefe, D. H., Zhao, F., Neely, S. T., Gorga, M. P., & Vohr, B. R. (2003). Ear-canal acoustic admittance and reflectance effects in human neonates. I. Predictions of otoacoustic emission and auditory brainstem responses. *Journal of the Acoustical Society of America, 113*(1), 389–406.

Kei, J., Mazlan, R., Hickson, L., Gavranich, J., & Linning, R. (2007). Measuring middle ear admittance in newborns using 1000 Hz tympanometry: A comparison of methodologies. *Journal of the American Academy of Audiology, 18*(9), 739–748.

Koivunen, P., Uhari, M., Laitakari, K., Alho, O. P., & Luotonen, J. (2000). Otoacoustic emissions and tympanometry in children with otitis media. *Ear and Hearing, 21*(3), 212–217.

Lampe, R. M., & Schwartz, R. H. (1989). Diagnostic value of acoustic reflectometry in children with acute otitis media. *Pediatric Infectious Disease Journal, 8*(1), 59–61.

Lampe, R. M., Weir, M. R., Spier, J., & Rhodes, M. F. (1985). Acoustic reflectometry in the detection of middle ear effusion. *Pediatrics, 76*(1), 75–78.

Lonsbury-Martin, B. L., Martin, G. K., McCoy, M. J., & Whitehead, M. L. (1995). New approaches to the evaluation of the auditory system and a current analysis of otoacoustic emissions. *Otolaryngology-Head and Neck Surgery: Official Journal of American Academy of Otolaryngology-Head and Neck Surgery, 112*(1), 50–63.

Lyons, A., Kei, J., & Driscoll, C. (2004). Distortion product otoacoustic emissions in children at school entry: A comparison with pure-tone screening and tympanometry results. *Journal of the American Academy of Audiology, 15*(10), 702–715.

Madden, C., Rutter, M., Hilbert, L., Greinwald, J. H., Jr., & Choo, D. I. (2002). Clinical and audiological features in auditory neuropathy. *Archives of Otolaryngology-Head and Neck Surgery, 128*(9), 1026–1030.

Margolis, R. H., Bass-Ringdahl, S., Hanks, W. D., Holte, L., & Zapala, D. A. (2003). Tympanometry in newborn infants —1 kHz norms. *Journal of the American Academy of Audiology, 14*(7), 383–392.

Margolis, R. H., & Heller, J. W. (1987). Screening tympanometry: Criteria for medical referral. *Audiology: Official Organ of the International Society of Audiology, 26*(4), 197–208.

Margolis, R. H., & Trine, M. B. (1997). Effects of middle ear disease on otoacoustic emissions. In M. S. Robinette, & T. Glattke (Eds.), *Otoacoustic emissions: Clinical applications* (pp. 130–150). New York, NY: Thieme.

Marshall, L., Heller, L. M., & Westhusin, L. J. (1997). Effect of negative middle-ear pressure on transient-evoked otoacoustic emissions. *Ear and Hearing, 18*(3), 218–226.

Mauk, G. W., & Behrens, T. R. (1993). Historical, political, and technological context associated with early identification of hearing loss. *Seminars in Hearing, 14*(1), 1–17.

Mauk, G. W., White, K. R., Mortensen, L. B., & Behrens, T. R. (1991). The effectiveness of screening programs based on high-risk characteristics in early identification of hearing impairment. *Ear and Hearing, 12*(5), 312–319.

Mehra, S., Eavey, R. D., & Keamy, D. G., Jr. (2009). The epidemiology of hearing impairment in the United States: Newborns, children, and adolescents. *Otolaryngology-Head and Neck Surgery: Official Journal of American Academy of Otolaryngology-Head and Neck Surgery, 140*(4), 461–472.

Meinke, D. K., & Dice, N. (2007). Comparison of audiometric screening criteria for the identification of noise-induced hearing loss in adolescents. *American Journal of Audiology, 16*(2), S190–202.

Moeller, M. P. (2000). Early intervention and language development in children who are deaf and hard of hearing. *Pediatrics, 106*(3), E43.

Moeller, M. P., Osberger, M. J., & Eccarius, M. (1986). Language and learning skills of hearing-impaired students. receptive language skills. *ASHA Monographs, 23*, 41–53.

Moeller, M. P., White, K. R., & Shisler, L. (2006). Primary care physicians' knowledge, attitudes, and practices related to newborn hearing screening. *Pediatrics, 118*(4), 1357–1370.

Niskar, A. S., Kieszak, S. M., Holmes, A., Esteban, E., Rubin, C., & Brody, D. J. (1998). Prevalence of hearing loss among children 6 to 19 years of age: The third national health and nutrition examination survey. *Journal of the American Medical Association, 279*(14), 1071–1075.

Northern, J. L. (1992) Special issues concerned with screening for middle ear disease in children. In F. H. Bess & J. W. Hall (Eds.), *Screening children for auditory function.* Nashville, TN: Bill Wilkerson Center Press.

Norton, S. J., Gorga, M. P., Widen, J. E., Folsom, R. C., Sininger, Y., Cone-Wesson, B., . . . Fletcher, K. (2000). Identification of neonatal hearing impairment: Evaluation of transient evoked otoacoustic emission, distortion product otoacoustic emission, and auditory brain stem response test performance. *Ear and Hearing, 21*(5), 508–528.

Nozza, R. J. (1996). Pediatric hearing screening. In F. N. Martin & J. G. Clark (Eds.), *Hearing care in children* (pp. 95–114). Needham Heights, MA: Allyn and Bacon.

Nozza, R. J. (1998). Identification of otitis media. *Proceedings of the Fourth International Symposium on Childhood Deafness* (pp. 207–214). Kiawah Island, South Carolina, October, 1996, Nashville, TN: Wilkerson Center Press.

Nozza, R. J. (2001). Screening with otoacoustic emissions beyond the newborn period. In J. Durrant (Ed.), *Special topics in bases and applications of measurements of otoacoustic emissions. Seminars in Hearing, 22*(4), 415–425.

Nozza, R. J., Bluestone, C. D., Kardatzke, D., & Bachman, R. (1992). Towards the validation of aural acoustic immittance measures for diagnosis of middle ear effusion in children. *Ear and Hearing, 13*(6), 442–453.

Nozza, R. J., Bluestone, C. D., Kardatzke, D., & Bachman, R. (1994). Identification of middle ear effusion by aural acoustic admittance and otoscopy. *Ear and Hearing, 15*(4), 310–323.

Nozza, R. J., Sabo, D. L., & Mandel, E. M. (1997). A role for otoacoustic emissions in screening for hearing impairment and middle ear disorders in school-age children. *Ear and Hearing, 18*(3), 227–239.

Owens, J. J., McCoy, M. J., Lonsbury-Martin, B. L., & Martin, G. K. (1993). Otoacoustic emissions in children with normal ears, middle ear dysfunction, and ventilating tubes. *American Journal of Otology, 14*(1), 34–40.

Porter, H. L., Neely, S. T., & Gorga, G. (2009). Using benefit-cost ratio to select universal newborn hearing test criteria. *Ear and Hearing, 30*, 447–457.

Prieve, B. (2008). Otoacoustic emissions in infants and children. In J. Madell & C. Flexer (Eds.), *Pediatric audiology: Diagnosis, technology, and management.* New York, NY: Thieme Medical.

Prieve, B. A., Calandruccio, L., Fitzgerald, T., Mazevski, A., & Georgantas, L. M. (2008). Changes in transient-evoked otoacoustic emission levels with negative tympanometric peak pressure in infants and toddlers. *Ear and Hearing, 29*(4), 533–542.

Prieve, B., Dalzell, L., Berg, A., Bradley, M., Cacace, A., Campbell, D., . . . Stevens, F. (2000). The New York state universal newborn hearing screening demonstration project: Outpatient outcome measures. *Ear and Hearing, 21*(2), 104–117.

Prieve, B. A., & Stevens, F. (2000). The New York state universal newborn hearing screening demonstration project: Introduction and overview. *Ear and Hearing, 21*(2), 85–91.

Rance, G. (2005). Auditory neuropathy/dys-synchrony and its perceptual consequences. *Trends in Amplification, 9*(1), 1–43.

Rosenfeld, R. M., & Kay, D. (2003). Natural history of untreated otitis media. *Laryngoscope, 113*(10), 1645–1657.

Roush, J. (1990). Identification of hearing loss and middle ear disease in preschool and school-age children. *Seminars in Hearing, 11*(4), 357–371.

Roush, J. (Ed.). (2001). *Screening for hearing loss and otitis media in children.* San Diego, CA: Singular/Thomson Learning.

Roush, J., Bryant, K., Mundy, M., Zeisel, S., & Roberts, J. (1995). Developmental changes in static admittance and tympanometric width in infants and toddlers. *Journal of the American Academy of Audiology, 6*(4), 334–338.

Roush, J., Drake, A., & Sexton, J. E. (1992). Identification of middle ear dysfunction in young children: A comparison of tympanometric screening procedures. *Ear and Hearing, 13*(2), 63–69.

Roush, J., & Tait, C. A. (1985). Pure-tone and acoustic immittance screening of preschool-aged children: An examination of referral criteria. *Ear and Hearing, 6*(5), 245–250.

Shi, S., Kei, J., Murdoch, B., McPherson, B., Smyth, V., Latham, S., & Loscher, J. (2000). Paediatric hearing screening in the community: A comparison of outcomes from transient evoked and distortion product otoacoustic emission measures. *Scandinavian Audiology, 29*(2), 83–92.

Sideris, I., & Glattke, T. J. (2006). A comparison of two methods of hearing screening in the preschool population. *Journal of Communication Disorders, 39*(6), 391–401.

Silman, S., Silverman, C. A., & Arick, D. S. (1992). Acoustic-immittance screening for detection of middle-ear effusion in children. *Journal of the American Academy of Audiology, 3*(4), 262–268.

Sininger, Y. S., Cone-Wesson, B., Folsom, R. C., Gorga, M. P., Vohr, B. R., Widen, J. E.,. . . Norton, S. J. (2000). Identification of neonatal hearing impairment: Auditory brain stem responses in the perinatal period. *Ear and Hearing, 21*(5), 383–399.

Smith, C. G., Paradise, J. L., Sabo, D. L., Rockette, H. E., Kurs-Lasky, M., Bernard, B. S., . . . Colborn, D. K. (2006). Tympanometric findings and the probability of middle-ear effusion in 3686 infants and young children. *Pediatrics, 118*(1), 1–13.

Stark, A. R., & American Academy of Pediatrics Committee on Fetus and Newborn. (2004). Levels of neonatal care. *Pediatrics, 114*(5), 1341–1347. doi:10.1542/peds.2004-1697

Starr, A., Sininger, Y. S., & Pratt, H. (2000). The varieties of auditory neuropathy. *Journal of Basic and Clinical Physiology and Pharmacology, 11*(3), 215–230.

Stein, L. K. (1999). Factors influencing the efficacy of universal newborn hearing screening. *Pediatric Clinics of North America, 46*(1), 95–105.

Teele, D. W., & Teele, J. (1984). Detection of middle ear effusion by acoustic reflectometry. *Journal of Pediatrics, 104*(6), 832–838.

Teppo, H., & Revonta, M. (2009). Consumer acoustic reflectometry by parents in detecting middle-ear fluid among children undergoing tympanostomy. *Scandinavian Journal of Primary Health Care, 27*(3), 167–171.

Trine, M. B., Hirsch, J. E., & Margolis, R. H. (1993). The effect of middle ear pressure on transient evoked otoacoustic emissions. *Ear and Hearing, 14*(6), 401–407.

Vander Werff, K. R., Prieve, B. A., & Georgantas, L. M. (2007). Test-retest reliability of wideband reflectance measures in infants under screening and diagnostic test conditions. *Ear and Hearing, 28*(5), 669–681.

Vohr, B. R., Carty, L. M., Moore, P. E., & Letourneau, K. (1998). The Rhode Island hearing assessment program: Experience with statewide hearing screening (1993–1996). *Journal of Pediatrics, 133*(3), 353–357.

Waseem, M., & Aslam, M., (2008). Otitis media: Differential diagnosis and work-up. *eMedicine, 2008.* Retrieved January 16, 2010, from: http://emedicine.medscape.com/article/994656-overview

White, K. R., Vohr, B. R., Meyer, S., Widen, J. E., Johnson, J. L., Gravel, J. S., . . . Weirather, Y. (2005). A multisite study to examine the efficacy of the otoacoustic emission/automated auditory brainstem response newborn hearing screening protocol: Research design and results of the study. *American Journal of Audiology, 14*(2), S186–S199.

Widen, J. E., Folsom, R. C., Cone-Wesson, B., Carty, L., Dunnell, J. J., Koebsell, K., . . . Norton, S. J. (2000). Identification of neonatal hearing impairment: Hearing status at 8 to 12 months corrected age using a visual reinforcement audiometry protocol. *Ear and Hearing, 21*(5), 471–487.

Widen, J. E., Johnson, J. L., White, K. R., Gravel, J. S., Vohr, B. R., James, M., . . . Meyer, S. (2005). A multisite study to examine the efficacy of the otoacoustic emission/automated auditory brainstem response newborn hearing screening protocol: Results of visual reinforcement audiometry. *American Journal of Audiology, 14*(2), S200–S216.

Xoinis, K., Weirather, Y., Mavoori, H., Shaha, S. H., & Iwamoto, L. M. (2007). Extremely low birth weight infants are at high risk for auditory neuropathy. *Journal of Perinatology: Official Journal of the California Perinatal Association, 27*(11), 718–723.

Yoshinaga-Itano, C., Sedey, A. L., Coulter, D. K., & Mehl, A. L. (1998). Language of early- and later-identified children with hearing loss. *Pediatrics, 102*(5), 1161–1171.

V

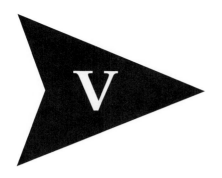

Approaches to Assessment

18

Middle Ear Measurement

Lisa L. Hunter and Robert H. Margolis

Overview

Middle ear measurement is a cornerstone of the basic audiologic test battery, and a physiologic measure that should be a part of all comprehensive audiologic assessments, particularly in infants and children. Middle ear measures provide a cross-check for other physiologic and behavioral measures, do not require behavioral response, are low cost and require minimal time. Also known generically as acoustic immittance measures, these tests are simple to perform, yet complex to interpret in relation to the physical properties of the ear. The immittance battery contains three main components: single frequency tympanometry, acoustic stapedial reflexes, and broadband or multifrequency immittance measures. The immittance battery is able to provide important diagnostic information about middle ear, cochlear, and neural functioning. Combined with other physiologic measures such as otoacoustic emissions and auditory brainstem response, useful diagnostic information may be gleaned even when behavioral tests are not possible. Although single-frequency tympanometry and acoustic reflexes have comprised the standard immittance battery for the past 30 years, newer procedures using broadband stimuli have been developed recently, including broadband tympanometry and acoustic reflex measures. To fully realize the diagnostic potential of these broadband measures, an understanding of the physical bases of aural acoustic immittance is useful. A brief overview is provided in this chapter, but for a more complete discussion, the reader is referred to Keefe and Feeney (2008), Margolis and Hunter (2000), and Wiley and Fowler (1997).

Middle ear measurement is particularly important in infants and children, since the highest incidence of middle ear problems occurs in the first few years of life. In addition, as infants and young children are not able to provide their own perspectives about ear symptoms, and they are less able to provide us with behavioral test results, it is vitally important that sensitive and specific physiologic measures be available to provide information about functioning of the middle ear.

Middle Ear Characteristics and Postnatal Development

Although the cochlea is mature and adult in size at birth, the ear canal and middle ear are immature and undergo continued development, especially during the first six months after birth. Major changes that occur postnatally are:

1. An increase in diameter, length and orientation of the ear canal, especially in the first two years of life.
2. An increase in the rigidity of the ear canal. Initially, the neonate ear canal is relatively flaccid and prolapsed, making visualization of the tympanic membrane difficult. The inner half of the infant ear canal begins ossifying prenatally and continues through the first year; thus, before this time, the ear canal is highly compliant (Holte, Margolis, & Cavanaugh, 1991). Stiffness of the ear canal increases as the medial bony portion ossifies and lengthens.
3. As depicted in Figure 18–1, a change in orientation and thickness of the tympanic membrane (TM) occurs after birth. The TM is oriented horizontally with respect to the ear canal at birth, and gradually becomes more perpendicular to the long axis of

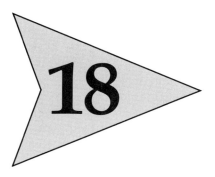

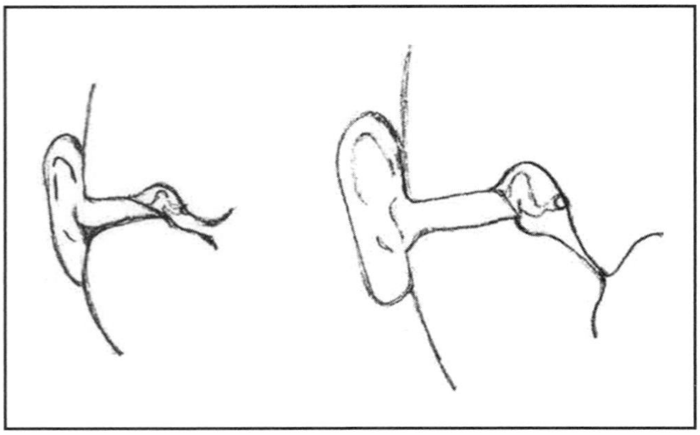

FIGURE 18–1. Newborn (*left panel*) and adult (*right panel*) ear canal, tympanic membrane, middle ear cavity, and eustachian tube showing changes in diameter, length, size, and orientation with development.

the ear canal, allowing better visualization. The appearance of the TM is normally dull, white and thickened at birth. Over time, it thins due to loss of mesenchymal tissue (Ruah, Schachern, Zelterman, Paparella, & Yoon, 1991).

4. An increase in aeration and size of the middle ear cavity, including pneumatization of the mastoid air cells. At birth, the middle ear may not be completely aerated. Based on temporal bone studies of deceased neonates, which likely are not reflective of normal newborns, contaminates in the middle ear space may be present including amniotic fluid, exudates, blood, desquamated epithelial cells and hair, keratinized cells, inflammatory cells, mucosal infiltrate and reactive polyps (Palva, Northrup, & Ramsay, 1999). Estimates of the physical size of the middle ear and mastoid vary considerably among studies. A recent careful review of large consecutive planimetric studies by Cinamon (2009) revealed a development pattern of growth. There are three distinct phases of mastoid pneumatization from birth to adult size. The mastoid bone and air cell compartments share a similar growth pattern and bone expansion lags behind aeration. The mastoid antrum is well developed at birth with a volume of 1 to 1.5 cm^3. The mastoid cells are 3.5 to 4 cm^3 at age 1 year and grow linearly until the age of 6 years at a rate of 1 to 1.2 cm^3 per year. Thereafter, growth slowly continues, reaching adult size at puberty (approximately 12 cm^3). The mastoid bone expansion is about 0.6 to 0.9 cm per year in length and width and 0.4 cm per year in depth in the first year, followed by half that rate until the age of 6 to 7 years. At puberty, there is a slower growth trajectory to adult size. Different ethnic groups share similar mastoid aeration and bone growth patterns. Interestingly, there were no differences between mastoid aeration measured in the preantibiotic era and after its widespread use (Cinamon, 2009).

   Physiologic studies of normal newborns using auditory brainstem response, otoacoustic emissions, videorecorded otoscopy, and multifrequency tympanometry are also consistent with the presence of fluid or other material in the middle ear space causing conductive hearing loss during the first few days after birth. Aeration normally occurs during the first 48 hours, but fluid and other materials may persist longer in some newborn ears. Infants born with meconium-stained amniotic fluid have a higher prevalence of material in the middle ear space (Piza, Gonzalez, Northrop, & Eavey, 1989). By the end of the first 24 hours after birth, approximately 50% of ears retain middle ear fluid, decreasing to 27% after 48 hours and 13% after 2 weeks (Roberts et al., 1992). In addition, the middle ear space is much smaller than that of an older child or adult. The length of the middle ear cavity increases in the first six months, from the tympanic membrane to the stapes footplate.
5. Finally, the ossicles become less dense over the first six months as they resorb mesenchyme and ossify (Eby & Nadol, 1986), and the ossicular joints stiffen as well (Saunders, Kaltenbach, & Relkin, 1983).

Physiologically, these anatomic changes mean that at birth, the infant middle ear is more mass-loaded and less compliant than the adult ear. These developmental effects translate into lower static admittance, broader tympanometric width, appearance of notching at low frequencies (such as 226 Hz), transmission of low-frequency energy into the flaccid ear canal walls, and less energy transmission in middle to high frequencies into the middle ear due to the smaller and less aerated middle ear cavity and mastoid air cells. Thus, age-related normative values are important for middle ear measures.

Immittance Instrumentation

Most commercially available immittance instruments use a single probe tone frequency (Figure 18–2 shows a diagram of immittance instrumentation), usually 226 Hz,

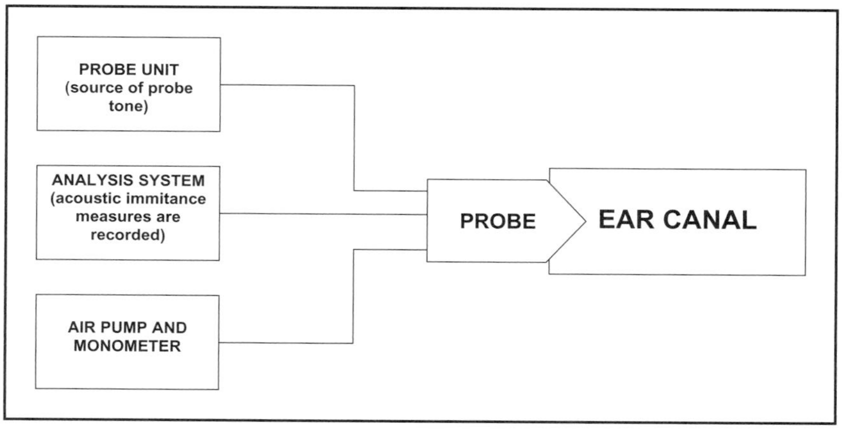

FIGURE 18–2. Block diagram of an electroacoustic immittance system showing the necessary hardware components.

and measure the voltage delivered to the probe tone transducer that produces a constant sound pressure level in the sealed ear canal. That voltage is proportional to the acoustic admittance at the probe tip. As the ear canal is pressurized it takes less voltage to produce the desired sound pressure level because some of the energy is reflected from the stiffened TM. Thus, when air pressure is high in the sealed ear canal, and the voltage to the probe tone transducer is low, the admittance is correspondingly low. This is indicated by the mimimal admittance at the positive (a) and the negative (b) tails of the tympanogram (Figure 18–3). As air pressure in the sealed ear canal approaches ambient pressure (0 daPa), the admittance of the middle ear increases as the tympanic membrane assumes its normal flexibility and the voltage needed to maintain constant SPL in the ear canal increases. The peak of the tympanogram corresponds to maximum admittance of the middle ear, which occurs at the ear-canal air pressure that is approximate to the middle-ear pressure (Figure 18–3[c]). This same principle holds for other probe tone frequencies, except that the physical volume relationship (in cm^3) to admittance (in mmho) is not 1:1 as it is at 226 Hz. For this reason, estimates of the volume of the tympanogram should be made when using a probe tone at 226 Hz.

The American National Standards Institute (ANSI) published the first standard for immittance instruments in 1987. Manufacturers generally adhere to this standard for design and calibration. The standard provides uniform terminology and plotting formats as well as calibration standards.

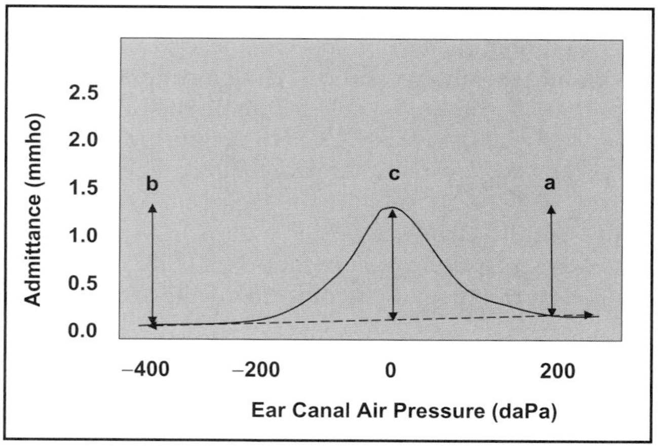

FIGURE 18–3. A single frequency tympanogram (226-Hz), showing measurement of static compensated acoustic admittance, compensated using: (a) positive, (b) negative, and (c) average of two-tail compensation.

Single-Frequency (226 Hz) Tympanometry

Tympanometric Shapes

Two approaches have been used in the interpretation of 226-Hz tympanograms—qualitative and quantitative. Many of the early instruments that were used for tympanometry were uncalibrated and presented tympanometric results as "arbitrary compliance units." Because it was not appropriate to make quantitative measurements using uncalibrated instruments, qualitative measurements were based on the shapes of tympanograms. The most popular of these was the classification scheme originally described by Lidén (1969), Jerger (1970), and Lidén, Harford, and Hallen (1974). As shown in Figure 18–4, tympanograms using the Lidén-Jerger classification scheme are typed according to the height and location of the tympanogram peak. Type A tympanograms have normal peak height and location on the pressure axis. Type B tympanograms are flat with no discernable peak. A type C tympanogram has a peak that occurs at negative middle-ear pressure. Lidén also described a type D tympanogram characterized by a double peak. Later, subtypes A_D and A_S were added (Feldman, 1976), indicating a high-peaked and shallow-peaked pattern, respectively. Although this qualitative approach is useful for identifying abnormal tympanometric features, and simplifies interpretation, its lack of precision leads to occasional errors and misinterpretations. For example, without quantitative criteria, no rule for distinguishing among types A, A_D, and A_S exists. Even distinguishing between types B and A is sometimes problematic when small or broad peaks occur, or shifts in the positive compared to the negative tails occur.

After the publication of the ANSI (1987) standard, manufacturers began to conform to the requirement that immittance instruments provide calibrated physical units of measurement rather than arbitrary compliance units. Virtually all immittance instruments produced since then have been admittance meters. Quantitative analysis of tympanograms is preferable, especially when assessing infants and children, for which different normative values based on age are needed and the cut-points used for distinguishing normal and abnormal middle ear function require precise measurement of admittance and width. Four tympanometric features are used to quantify tympanograms. Table 18–1 provides age-related normative values for these measures.

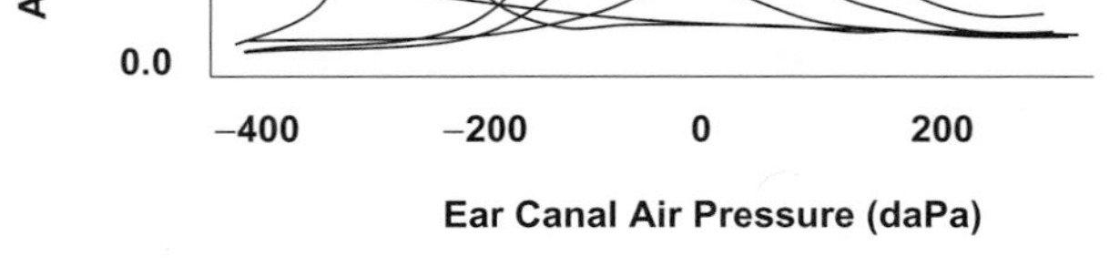

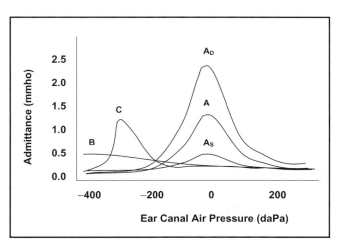

FIGURE 18–4. Lidén-Jerger classification scheme for tympanometric shapes, based on qualitative analysis of the height and location of the primary peak (Jerger, 1970; Lidén, 1969).

Peak Compensated Static Admittance (Ytm)

The peak compensated static acoustic admittance, or Ytm, is the most often used measurement of the 226 Hz tympanogram. The peak of the tympanogram includes the admittance due to the middle ear (Ytm) and admittance of the ear canal. Compensation, or subtraction of the admittance of the ear canal, is necessary to determine Ytm. There are three primary methods to compensate the tympanogram as shown in Figure 18–3: positive tail, negative tail, and the two-tails method. The positive tail method uses the value at +200 daPa to estimate the admittance of the ear canal, which is then subtracted from the peak admittance, as shown in Figure 18–3. The negative tail method uses the minimum tail value at –400 daPa, and the two-tails method uses the interpolated value of the positive and negative tail values, obtained by drawing a line between the two tails and measuring the value corresponding to the peak of the tympanogram (Baldwin, 2006).

There are advantages and disadvantages for the three methods of compensation. The negative tail of the tympanogram presents some disadvantages for compensation. First, artifactual spikes are more common with extremes in negative pressure, which can affect measurements at the negative tail. Second, in newborns and infants, the ear canal may collapse with negative pressure, which complicates measurement of the minimum tail value.

Static admittance is specific to many middle-ear conditions, such as distinguishing otitis media with effusion (OME) and ossicular discontinuity from normal middle-ear function. Sensitivity of Ytm is poorer for conditions such as ossicular fixation or cholesteatoma that do not restrict mobility of the tympanic membrane. Conversely, Ytm is sensitive to unimportant

Table 18–1. Normative Data by Age for Single-Frequency Tympanometry

Study	*Age*	*Probe Frequency Hz*	*Peak Compensated Static Admittance 5 to 95% tiles mmho*	*Tympanometric Width daPa*	*Pump Speed/ Direction daPa*
Margolis et al. (2003)	Birth to 4 weeks CA	1 k Hz	.60 to 4.3 –400 tail to peak	NA	+200 to –400 (600 daPa/sec @ tails, 200 daPa/sec @ peaks)
Kei et al. (2003)	1 to 6 days	1 k Hz	Right ears +200 tail to peak .39 to 2.28	Right ears 56.6 to 154	+200 to –200 @ 50 daPa/sec
	1 to 6 days	1 k Hz	Left ears +200 tail to peak .39 to 1.95	Left ears 46.1 to 144.2	+200 to –200 @ 50 daPa/sec
Roush et al. (1995)	6–12 mo	226 Hz	.20 to .50 +200 tail to peak	102 to 234 Ytm ≥ .3mmho	+200 to –300
	12–18 mo	226 Hz	.20 to .60 +200 tail to peak	102 to 204 Ytm ≥ .3mmho	+200 to –300
	18–24 mo	226 Hz	.30 to .70 +200 tail to peak	102 to 204 Ytm ≥ .3mmho	+200 to –300
	24–30 mo	226 Hz	.30 to .80 +200 tail to peak	96 to 192 Ytm ≥ .3mmho	+200 to –300
Marchant et al. (1986)	< 5 mo	660 Hz	Peak Compensated Static Susceptance Baseline to peak .18 mmho lower limit	NA	+300 to –400 @ 50 daPa/sec
Holte et al. (1991)	≥ 4 mo	Up to 900 Hz	Vanhuyse Model 1B1G up to 900 Hz, 3B1G @ 900 Hz	NA	

conditions such as tympanic-membrane scarring because tympanometry is more affected by conditions that have close proximity to the measurement probe. Thus, other measurements have been suggested to complement Ytm, specifically tympanometric width.

Tympanometric Width (TW)

A number of studies have demonstrated that the sharpness of the tympanometric peak is an indicator of middle ear pathology (Fiellau-Nikolajsen, 1983; Nozza, Bluestone, Kardatze, & Bachman, 1992, 1994). Brooks (1968) introduced the term *gradient* for this measurement. Methods for quantifying gradient were first proposed by Brooks (1968), Paradise, Smith, and Bluestone (1976), and Lidén (1969). Two studies have compared gradient measures obtained with the various techniques in normal children and adults (de Jonge, 1986; Koebsell & Margolis, 1986). These studies concluded that the preferred technique is the tympanometric width (TW). Figure 18–5 illustrates the measurement of TW. Diagnostically, only broad TW is important in children for diagnosis of otitis media.

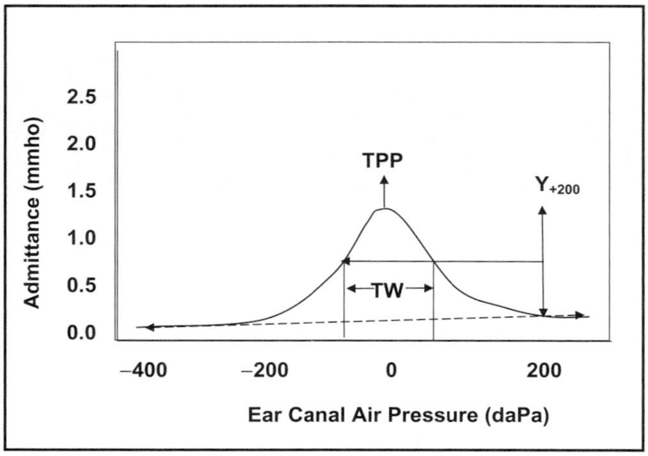

FIGURE 18–5. A single frequency tympanogram (226-Hz), showing measurement of tympanometric width (TW), compensated using +200 tail. A horizontal line is drawn at 1/2 of the Y + 200 value, and the points where this line intersects the tympanogram are measured on the pressure axis in daPa.

Tympanometric Peak Pressure (TPP)

The ear-canal air pressure at which the peak of the tympanogram occurs is the tympanometric peak pressure (TPP), as shown in Figure 18–5. TPP is an indicator of the pressure in the middle-ear space. Although TPP overestimates the actual middle-ear pressure, sometimes by as much as 100% (Elner, Ingelstedt, & Ivarsson, 1971; Renvall & Holmquist, 1976), it is a general indicator of the status of middle-ear pressure. A TPP of -300 daPa, for example, could occur with actual middle-ear pressure of only −150 daPa. Negative TPP has not been shown to provide reliable diagnostic specificity or sensitivity to otitis media in children (Fiellau-Nikolajsen, 1983; Nozza et al., 1994; Paradise et al., 1976), and thus is not currently recommended as a reason to refer children for treatment (American Speech-Language-Hearing Association [ASHA], 2004).

Measurement of TPP may be useful for equilibrating ear-canal air pressure to enhance acoustic-reflex and otoacoustic-emission responses (Trine, Hirsch, & Margolis, 1993). Hof, Anteunis, Chenault, and van Dijk (2005) compensated middle-ear pressure while measuring transient evoked otoacoustic emissions (TEOAEs) in 59 children and reported a mean amplitude increase of 1.9 dB between 1 to 2 kHz. Self-induced negative TPP has been shown to affect distortion product otoacoustic emission (DPOAE) responses below 1000 Hz by about 4 to 6 dB (Sun & Shaver, 2009). However, Prieve, Calandruccio, Fitzgerald, Mazevski, and Georgantis (2008) measured TEOAE and noise levels in 18 children under two conditions: on a day when the tympanogram TPP was normal and on a day when the tympanogram TPP was negative. They reported that average TEOAE level was about 4 dB lower for all frequency bands from 1000 to 4000 when TPP was negative, but noise levels did not change between the two conditions. Importantly, the presence of negative TPP affected the pass rate in only 5 to 6% of cases.

Equivalent Ear Canal Volume (Veq)

Acoustic immittance measures using a 226 Hz probe tone are useful for estimating the volume of air in front of the probe (Lindeman & Holmquist, 1982; Shanks, Stelmachowicz, Beauchaine, & Schulte, 1992). In the presence of a flat tympanogram, an estimate of the volume of air in front of the probe can be useful for detecting eardrum perforations and evaluating the patency of tympanostomy tubes. Although a normal Veq does not rule out a perforation, a flat tympanogram with a large Veq is evidence of tympanic membrane perforation or a patent tympanostomy tube. In normal ears, the admittance at high positive or negative pressure is primarily determined by the ear canal volume. This measurement is the same as the tail value used to compensate the tympanogram, as shown in Figure 18–5. However, because the eardrum and ear-canal walls are not perfectly rigid when the ear is pressurized, the admittance at 226 Hz, expressed as Veq, overestimates the actual ear-canal volume by about 25% in adults, partly due to distension of the ear-canal wall (Shanks & Lilly, 1981). For this reason, the negative tail value is a more accurate estimate of Veq than the positive tail.

The average tympanometrically measured Veq is about 0.3 cm^3 in 4-month-old infants (Holte et al., 1991), 0.75 cm^3 in preschool children (Margolis & Heller, 1987), and 1.0 to 1.4 cm^3 in adults (Margolis & Heller, 1987; Wiley et al., 1996). An opening in the TM adds the volume of the middle-ear space and contiguous mastoid air cells to the volume of the ear canal. On the basis of these tympanometric measurements, it should be possible to distinguish between ears with intact eardrums and those with perforations without difficulty. However, ears with perforations may have past or present middle-ear disease that causes volumes to be decreased for several reasons. An ear with active middle-ear disease may contain inflammation, fluid, granulation tissue, fibrosis, polyps, or cholesteatoma in the middle-ear space. Mastoid air cells may be blocked by tissue or underdeveloped with poor pneumatization due to inflammation. Shanks et al. (1992) recommended an abnormal criterion of 1.0 $cm^3$for children for equivalent volume. Another useful clinical application for equivalent volume is to monitor the course of middle-ear disease after placement of tympanostomy tubes. It has been shown that equivalent volume correlates with disease severity (Hunter, Margolis, Daly, & Giebink, 1992) and with recurrence of otitis media (Takasaka et al., 1996). Progressively larger equivalent volume after tube insertion is an indication of recovery from otitis media. When equivalent volume remains small, it is an indicator of continued disease. In a prospective study of 157 children aged 6 months to 8 years, treated with tubes for OME, equivalent volume of less than 1.5 cc was associated with greater OME recurrence (Hunter & Margolis, 1992). A large recent study by the MRC Multicentre Otitis Media Study Group (2003) provides equivalent volume measurements in 3- to 7-year-old children randomized to one of three interventions (tube insertion with or without adenoidectomy and nonsurgical observation). The study reported otoscopy for 336 ears with functioning tubes and 205 nonsurgery ears compared to equivalent ear-canal volume (Veq) before and after tube insertion. Cutoff Veq were evaluated in terms of classification accuracy against otoscopy after intervention. Age range did not influence Veq, or the optimum Veq cutoff, but boys had significantly larger Veq (by 0.09 cm^3) than girls. The recommended mean cutoff for tube patency is greater than or equal to 1.13 cm^3, slightly higher than the 1.00 cm^3 recommended by Shanks et al. (1992).

Sensitivity and Specificity of Tympanometry

To gauge the clinical usefulness of any diagnostic test, a complete understanding must be developed of the test's performance in various populations at high and low risk for the disease of interest. Tympanometry is one of the most highly utilized diagnostic tests for diagnosing a specific condition in audiology. In most studies before 1990, tympanometry was measured with arbitrary units and therefore qualitative types were compared with pneumatic otoscopy or with surgery. More recent studies have used quantitative analysis of tympanometry. Silman, Silverman, and Arick (1992) investigated several protocols for sensitivity and specificity of detection of OME in children. Children were identified with OME on the basis of pneumatic otoscopy. Combinations of static admittance, width, peak pressure and ipsilateral acoustic reflex resulted in sensitivity varying from 76 to 95%.

Performance of two screening measures was also assessed by Roush, Drake, and Sexton (1992) in 374 ears of 3- to 4-year-old children in a preschool program. A "traditional" procedure, based on TPP less than −200 daPa or absent acoustic reflexes was compared with interim norms (ASHA, 1990) both against the gold standard of pneumatic otoscopy by an experienced, validated otoscopist. The traditional procedure had high sensitivity (95%), but low specificity (65%). The ASHA interim norms had high sensitivity (84%) and specificity (95%), with a positive predictive value of 69% and a negative predictive value of 98%. The interim 1990 ASHA screening guidelines have since been updated (ASHA, 1997), and are described in Chapter 17 in this volume.

Nozza and colleagues (1992, 1994) have made important contributions in their studies of acoustic immittance in various populations of children. In the first study (1992), two groups of children were evaluated. One group (n = 61, aged 1 to 8 years) received tympanostomy tubes and thus was at high risk for OME. Tympanometry was performed no more than 30 minutes before surgery. The surgeon was unaware of the results of tympanometry. Six different protocols were evaluated; three of these included ipsilateral acoustic reflex thresholds. Sensitivity, specificity, positive predictive values, and negative predictive values were reported. Positive and negative predictive values are affected by the prevalence of the disease, which was high in this population (73%). Sensitivity (90%) and specificity (86%) were highest for gradient combined with acoustic reflexes. Gradient combined with static admittance also produced relatively high sensitivity (83%) and specificity (87%). A second group of children who attended an allergy clinic (n = 77, aged 3 to 16 years) were unselected with regard to otitis media history and were reported in the same study with the same six protocols and gold standard. In that group, sensitivity was 78% for all protocols except ipsilateral acoustic reflex alone (sensitivity = 88%) and gradient or static admittance < 0.1 mmho (sensitivity = 67%). Gradient + ipsilateral reflex and gradient + static admittance performed equally well for specificity (99%). Positive predictive value was higher for gradient + static admittance (88%) than it was for gradient + ipsilateral reflex (78%).

In a subsequent study (Nozza et al., 1994), a group of children (n = 171, aged 1 to 12 years) with recurrent or chronic OME, who were scheduled for myringotomy and tubes, received otoscopy by a validated otoscopist and tympanometry by a certified audiologist. The prevalence of OME in this group was 55%. Eleven criteria, with various cut-points for each criterion, were evaluated. As expected, there was a tradeoff between sensitivity and specificity. Best overall performance was found for TW or Ytm combined with pneumatic otoscopy (sensitivity and specificity = 80%), or for TW alone greater than 275 daPa (sensitivity = 78%, specificity = 82%). Interim norms (ASHA, 1990) showed high sensitivity (95%), but poor specificity (24%).

These studies demonstrate that the choice of cutoff criteria affects test performance greatly. It appears that combinations of criteria, such as otoscopy and TW, perform better than single criteria. Static admittance (Y) alone has poor sensitivity but good specificity, but this depends on the cutoff criteria selected. Use of either ipsilateral reflex or TW combined with Y provides good test performance, as does otoscopy combined with TW. If Y is used diagnostically, it should be combined with pneumatic otoscopy, width, gradient or ipsilateral acoustic reflexes.

It is important to note that all studies examining test performance of pneumatic otoscopy have used experienced otoscopists who have received specific training and have been validated, or compared to other expert otoscopists. Most OM is diagnosed by primary care physicians. In many cases, clinicians who use otoscopy to diagnose OME do not use pneumatic otoscopy, and have not been validated against experienced otoscopists. In order for otoscopy to reach high levels of sensitivity and specificity, pneumatic otoscopy must be performed after ear canal cleaning by a highly experienced clinician. Due to these practical considerations, tympanometry is very useful as an alternative, especially when pneumatic otoscopy is unsuccessful or an experienced otoscopist is not available.

Screening Tympanometry

Tympanometry has been widely used in screening programs primarily for identifying middle ear disease in pediatric populations. Roush and Nozza discuss the principles underlying screening for hearing loss and middle ear disease in children after the neonatal period in Chapter 17. The value of mass screening programs in children has been controversial (American Academy of Audiology [AAA], 1997, Bluestone et al., 1986). Although various conferences, organizations, and agencies have been hesitant to recommend large-scale screening programs, many programs for preschool and school age children have incorporated tympanometric screening into the protocol. Most programs combine audiometric screening with tympanometric screening to detect both sensorineural hearing loss and middle ear disorders (AAA, 1997; ASHA, 1990).

Universal newborn hearing screening (UNHS) programs do not usually include middle-ear assessment in either well baby nurseries (WBNs) or neonatal intensive care units (NICUs) for several reasons (Joint Committee on Infant Hearing [JCIH], 2007). Pneumatic otoscopy and bone-conducted ABR are impractical in UNHS due to the use of untrained personnel in many settings. Low-frequency tympanometry (e.g., 226 Hz) is insensitive to middle ear dysfunction in newborns (Hunter & Margolis, 1992; Paradise et al., 1976; Sprague, Wiley, & Goldstein, 1985), as described in more detail below.

Tympanometry in Newborns and Infants

226-Hz Tympanometry

Tympanograms recorded from normal ears of newborn infants are very different from those obtained from older infants, children, and adults. The earliest tympanometric recordings from neonate ears were made with single-component instruments that used a 220 Hz probe tone and expressed the results as "arbitrary compliance units" (Bennett, 1975; Keith, 1973, 1975; Poulsen & Tos, 1978). These studies reported a frequent occurrence of double-peaked tympanograms. Later studies recorded two-component tympanograms at two probe frequencies, 220 and 660 Hz (Himelfarb, Popelka, & Shanon, 1979; Sprague et al., 1985). These two-component recordings permit an analysis of the reactance and resistance of the infant ear. These studies indicated that at low frequencies, the newborn ear is highly resistive and has low negative reactance, suggesting a significant mass effect that offsets the stiffness of the middle-ear system. These effects are probably related to developmental differences between infant middle ears and those of older children and adults. The reasons for differences in admittance characteristics between adults and newborns are not fully known. However, anatomical differences in the infant ear, such as a more compliant ear-canal wall (Holte et al., 1991), smaller ear canal and middle-ear space, tympanic-membrane thickening, middle-ear fluid and mesenchyme, and a more horizontal orientation of the tympanic membrane with respect to the axis of the ear canal, are the most likely contributors (Eavey, 1993; Ikui, Sando, & Fujita, 1997; Ruah et al., 1991; Saunders et al., 1983).

In neonate ears with confirmed middle-ear disease, 226-Hz tympanograms are not reliably different from those obtained from normal ears. In addition, the variability of 226-Hz probe-tone admittance tympanometry characteristics in young infants has led to conflicting interpretation of what tympanometric criteria define a normal infant middle ear, which casts doubt on the clinical utility of these measures for newborns. (Hunter & Margolis, 1992; Keith, 1975; Paradise, et al., 1976; Sprague et al., 1985). Infants with diagnosed middle-ear fluid have been demonstrated to have normal 226-Hz tympanograms (Hunter & Margolis, 1992; Paradise et al., 1976). For these reasons, 226-Hz tympanometry is not an effective test for middle-ear measurement in newborns.

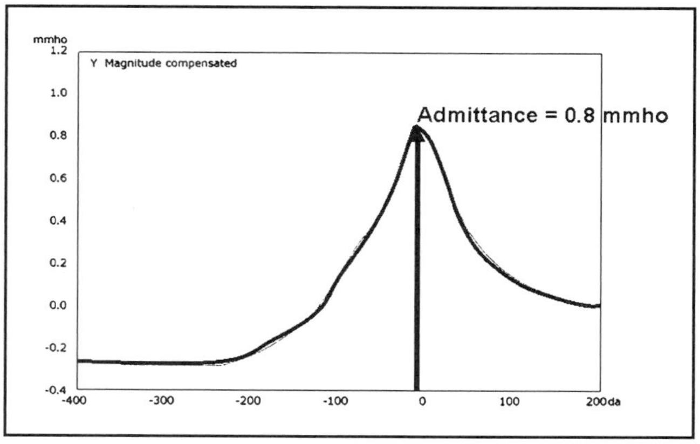

FIGURE 18–6. Example of a 1000-Hz tympanogram measured in a 1-day-old infant who passed newborn hearing screening with DPOAE. Normal admittance magnitude, tymoanometric width and peak pressure are present. The tympanogram is asymmetric due to volume changes with positive versus negative pressure, characteristic of the newborn ear canal.

660- and 1000-Hz Tympanometry

Evidence has accumulated that tympanometry using higher probe-tone frequencies (up to and including 1000 Hz) is more sensitive to changes in middle-ear status in infants less than 4 months old compared to 226-Hz tympanometry (Alaerts, Lutz, & Woulters, 2007; Calandruccio, Fitzgerald, & Prieve, 2006; Hunter & Margolis, 1992; Marchant et al., 1986; Rhodes, Margolis, Hirsch, & Napp, 1999; Swanepoel et al., 2007). Some studies have reported normative data for a variety of young ages, and some have investigated test performance of specific 1000-Hz admittance criteria in predicting otoacoustic emission (OAE) screening results. A tympanogram measured at 1000 Hz in a normal newborn is shown in Figure 18–6. A normally shaped single peak is typical even in newborns if the middle ear is aerated and the ear canal is not prolapsed. An example of a tympanogram measured in a newborn with a prolapsed ear canal is shown in Figure 18–7. To complicate matters, the tympanogram is also notched at the peak, which frequently occurs in newborns. Despite these considerations, Margolis, Bass-Ringdahl, Hanks, Holte, and Zapala (2003) recommend use of negative tail compensation because the tympanogram is often so asymmetric that the peak to positive tail difference is very small and therefore insensitive to fluid. The two-tail compensation method recommended by Baldwin (2006) averages or interpolates across the positive and negative tail, so offers a reasonable compromise over the use of one tail value alone.

Margolis et al. (2003) assessed 1000-Hz tympanometric test performance in predicting whether a newborn infant passed or failed a DPOAE test. The 1000-Hz tympanometry criterion had a specificity of 91% in predicting which ears passed the DPOAE test, but a sensitivity of only 50% in predicting which ears failed the DPOAE test. Kei et al. (2003) reported 1000 Hz tympanometric data that was obtained from both ears of 106 infants (1 to 6 days old) who passed a click-evoked OAE hearing screening and presented with "single peaked" tympanograms. Kei et al. suggested that a tympanogram representing normal middle-ear function should include a single peak (which was the case in 92.3% of their sample) and that its tympanometric variables (six were identified) should lie within the 90% range of a population of normal-hearing infants (which would exclude at least 10% of their sample with single-peaked tympanograms). With their proposed six tympanometric variables, some normal-hearing infants would be within the 90% range on some variables and outside for others, but no procedure for choosing among these various criteria was described. Baldwin (2006) compared admittance tympanometry results at 226, 678, and 1000 Hz between groups of infants (mean age of 10 weeks) classified as having either normal or disordered middle-ear function. Baldwin classified the infant tympanograms using a traditional visual classification scheme (Jerger, 1970; Lidén, 1969), and a classification scheme proposed by Marchant et al. (1986). Comparisons of sensitivity and specificity values for the method after Marchant et al. revealed the best results for 1000-Hz tympanometry (sensitivity of 0.99 and specificity of 0.89). Baldwin cautioned that these

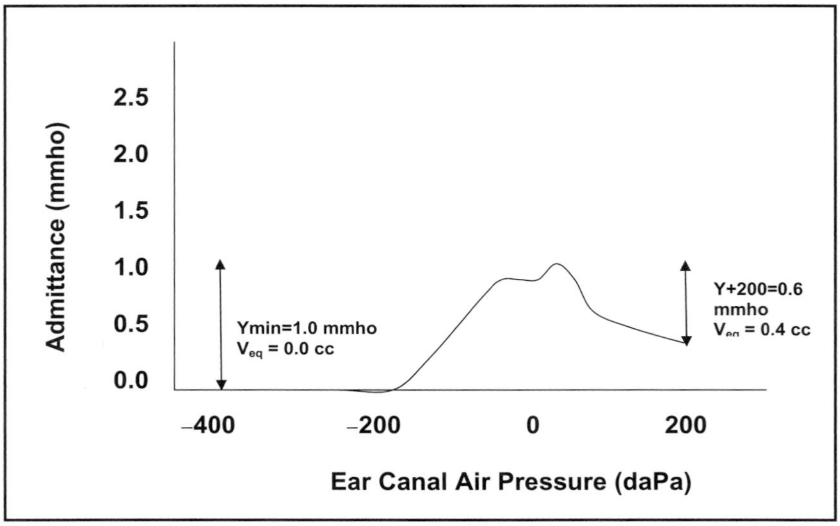

FIGURE 18–7. Example of a tympanogram measured in a newborn with collapsing ear canal, indicated by a sudden decrease to a volume of 0 cc with negative pressure. The collapsing volume measurement is reflected in the minimum tail value, and the notched peak of the tympanogram complicates measurement of peak admittance. The first peak was used to calculate static admittance. Note the differences in static admittance measured using the positive, minimum and interpolated tail values, as well as the differences in equivalent ear canal volume.

findings may not apply to neonates, as the youngest infant tested in her study was 2 weeks old. Swanepoel et al. (2007) reported sensitivity of 57% and specificity of 95% for 1000-Hz tympanometry, 57% and 90% for acoustic reflex presence, and 58% and 87% for combined tympanometry and acoustic reflex results, respectively. The Joint Committee on Infant Hearing (JCIH, 2007) has recommended 1000-Hz tympanometry for assessment of babies younger than 6 months on the basis of these studies.

Multifrequency Tympanometry

Earlier studies of multifrequency tympanometry give some clues as to why higher frequency regions provide different results in neonates than in adults. For example, Holte et al. (1991) recorded multifrequency tympanometry (226 to 900 Hz) from newborns and followed them to 4 months of age. Tympanometric shapes were classified according to the model described by Vanhuyse and colleagues (Vanhuyse, Creten, & Van Camp, 1975). For newborns, (1–7 days), at 226 Hz, all tympanograms conformed to the Vanhuyse model classifications. At higher frequencies, more tympanograms were classified as "other," meaning they did not adhere to the Vanhuyse classification model. At 900 Hz, none of the shapes conformed to the classification. With increasing age, more of the tympanograms became adult-like, following the Vanhuyse model. By 4 months of age, tympanometric patterns adhered to the Vanhuyse model, indicating that significant development had occurred. Reasons for the disorganized pattern of tympanograms in newborns are not entirely clear. Because the osseous portion of the ear canal of the newborn is not rigid, it has been suggested that ear canal wall motion influences the shape of the tympanogram (Paradise et al., 1976). There is evidence for and against this hypothesis. Holte, Margolis, and Cavanaugh (1990) found no relationship between canal wall movement of neonates measured with video otomicroscopy and their tympanometric patterns. Hsu, Margolis, and Schachern (2000) found similarly complex tympanometric patterns in newborn chinchillas despite the fact that their canal walls appeared to be fully ossified on histologic analysis. On the other hand, Keefe, Bulen, Arehart, and Burns (1993) measured complex impedance in infants at various ages and found a mass effect that was similar to the acoustic properties of soft tissue elsewhere in the body. Because this effect dominates at frequencies below 1000 Hz, they argued that low frequencies are a poor choice for evaluating middle-ear function in newborns. In addition to the flaccidity of the ear-canal walls, the fluid and material that is found in newborn middle ears likely contributes to greater mass loading, which results in more complex, notched patterns at lower frequencies, consistent with the Vanhuyse model predictions. Thus, as a result of these studies, it has become apparent that higher frequency probe tones are needed to adequately assess middle ear status in newborns, and that 226-Hz tympanometry becomes more adult-like by 4 months of age.

Wideband Immittance Measures

Single-frequency admittance tympanometry contrasts with other tests of auditory function such as behavioral audiometry, OAE and ABR tests. These tests all use stimuli over multiple octaves of the frequency range of human hearing. Techniques to classify such multi-frequency admittance tympanometric patterns have been used to measure responses up to approximately 2000 Hz (Colletti, 1977; Vanhuyse, Creten, & Van Camp, 1975; Wada, Koike, & Kobayashi, 1998) to measure the middle-ear resonance frequency. Nevertheless, use of multifrequency tympanometry is not widely accepted in clinical settings, largely due to the complexity of the responses. Thus, middle-ear function may not be adequately assessed at the higher frequencies important for audition. Single-frequency tympanometry and acoustic reflexes perform reasonably well for detection of middle-ear effusion, but there are some ways these tests fall short:

- In babies under 6 months, 226-Hz tympanometry has very poor sensitivity to middle ear effusion and the jury is still out on sensitivity of 1000 Hz in newborns;
- Tympanometry does not accurately predict conductive hearing loss;
- Tympanometry does not accurately detect otosclerosis;
- Acoustic reflexes have poor sensitivity to acoustic neuroma and carry some risk of causing noise-induced hearing loss;
- Single-frequency tympanometry cannot be realistically compared to broadband tests such as otoacoustic emissions.

A new method known variously as: wideband energy reflectance (ER), wideband impedance or admittance (generically, wideband acoustic immittance) makes possible measurements at any frequency up to approximately 10 kHz through advances in calibration and measurement techniques that are relatively unaffected by standing waves in the ear canal. These newer wideband acoustic-immittance tests have the potential to improve clinical diagnosis of auditory pathology in infants, children and adults with various types of middle-ear disease. Two wideband immittance instruments are commercially available: The Hear-ID ambient pressure system from Mimosa Acoustics, which is approved by the Food and Drug Administration (FDA) in the United States and can be combined with TEOAE and DPOAE in the same system, and an experimental (non-FDA approved) system from Interacoustics, which includes tympanometry and acoustic reflexes elicited and monitored by broadband stimuli. This technique was first developed to measure acoustic impedance in cats (Allen,1986) and was later adapted for noninvasive clinical use in humans (Keefe, Ling, & Bulen,1992). These wideband tests (ambient and pressurized reflectance and absorbance, admittance, impedance, and acoustic reflexes) have been shown to enhance newborn hearing screening (NHS) programs for early identification of infants with sensorineural hearing loss, and to detect middle ear dysfunction and conductive hearing loss in children and adults. These tests use a wideband "chirp" stimulus that allows measurements over the range 200 to 10,000 Hz in a few seconds, are noninvasive, use a standard soft immittance probe tip, and provide a comprehensive set of measurements to assess the middle ear over the entire range of sound frequencies important to speech perception. Figure 18–8 shows a laptop based system produced by Mimosa Acoustics, Inc. (Hear-ID, Champaign, IL). The system is calibrated with probes inserted into each of four cavities of varying volumes (Figure 18–9).

As shown in Figure 18–10, the calibrated chirp stimulus is presented to the ear canal from a speaker housed inside a probe, which is seated in the ear with a soft probe tip, just as in tympanometry or OAE tests. The test can be done with ambient ear-canal air pressure or with varying pressure as in tympanometry. The SPL and phase of the sound in calibration cavities is compared to that of the sound recorded in the ear canal. The difference is energy that is absorbed by the middle ear structures. Energy reflectance (ER) is the ratio of the incident sound (input to the ear canal) and the reflected sound and varies between 0 and 1. The normal range for ambient pressure ER in infants and children reported by Hunter, Tubaugh, Jackson, and Propes (2008a) and Hunter, Feeney, Lapsley Miller, Jeng, and

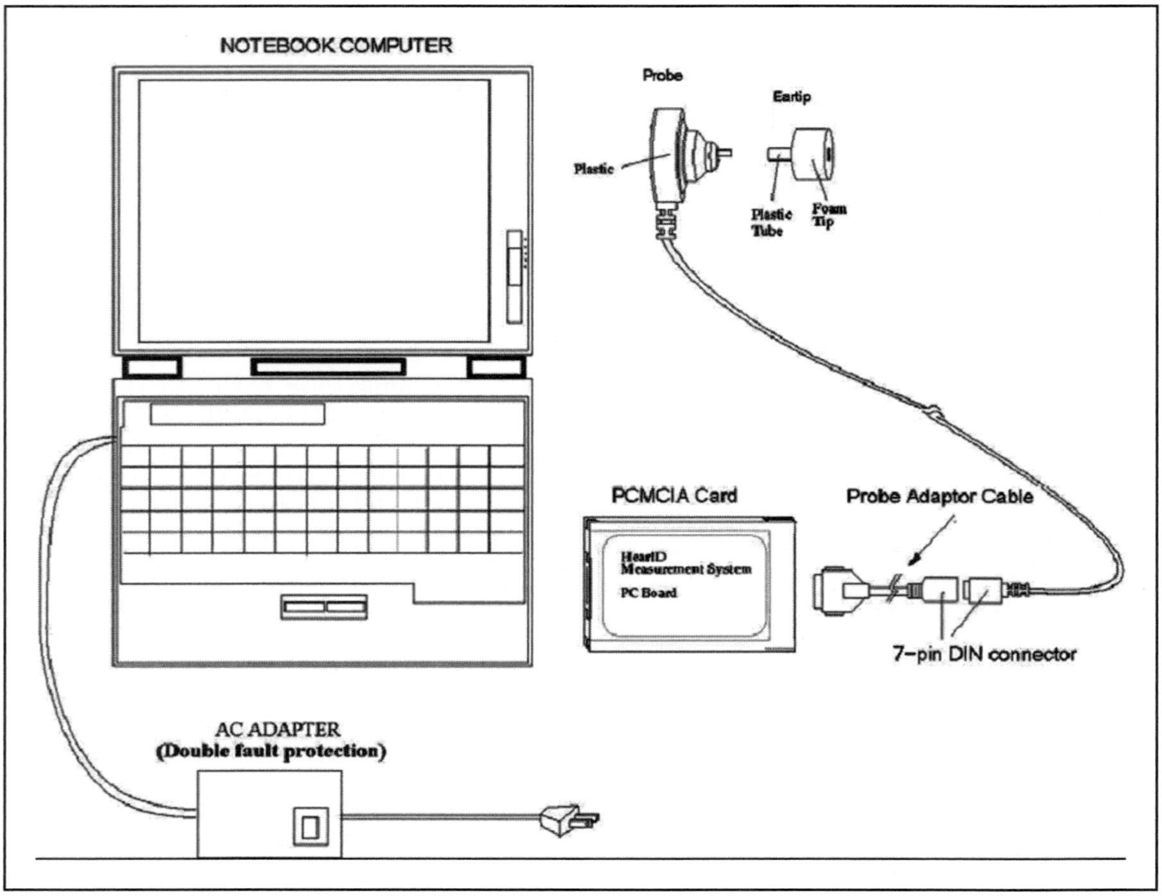

FIGURE 18–8. Diagram of instrumentation used to measure wideband middle ear power. A broadband chirp stimulus was produced and played through the probe into the ear canal. The sound energy travels down the ear canal and is either reflected or absorbed by the tympanic membrane.

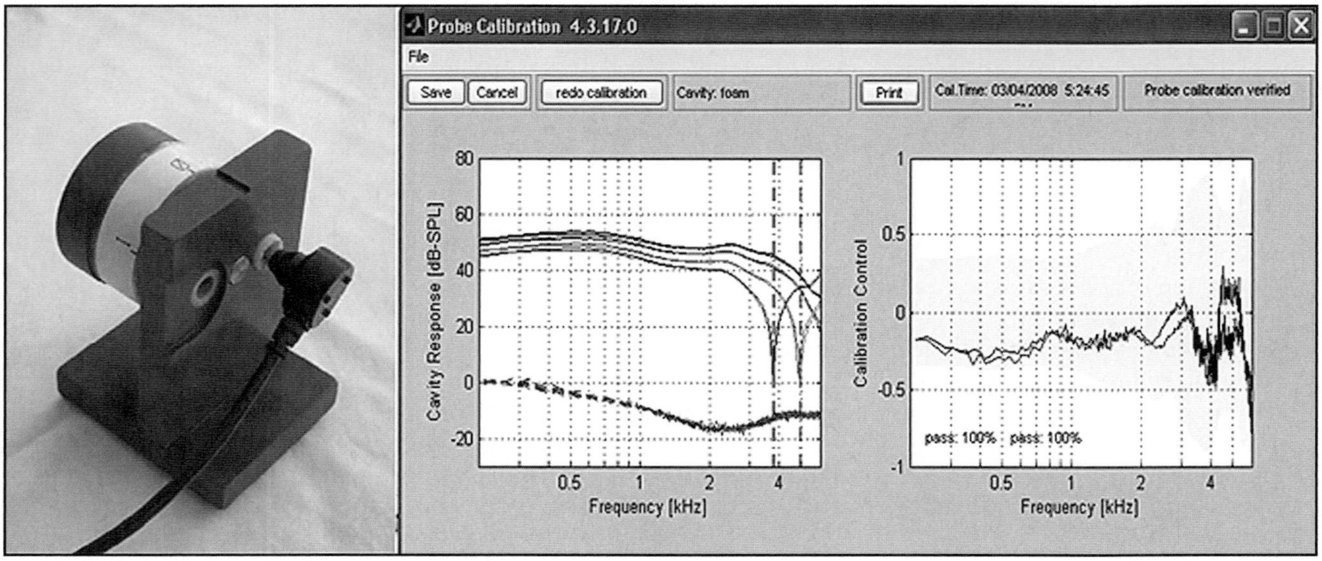

FIGURE 18–9. CC-4 calibration cavity set along with the Thevenin equivalent measurements representing a passing calibration.

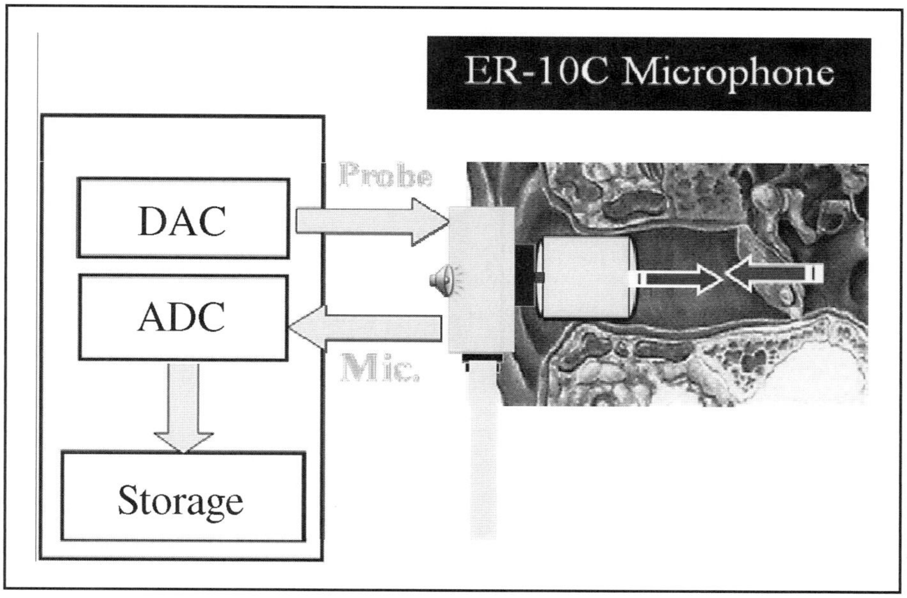

FIGURE 18–10. Wideband reflectance data collection and storage system. The right-facing arrow represents the chirp stimulus directed toward the tympanic membrane, whereas the left-facing arrow represents the energy that is reflected back into the ear canal (Feeney & Hunter, 2008).

Bohning, 2010 is shown in Figure 18–11. Computer algorithms for noise and artifact reduction, and calculation of impedance and admittance quantities such as admittance, impedance and their subcomponents provides a rapid, quantitative analysis of the acoustical response of the middle ear into the ear-canal walls.

Wideband ambient-pressure ER and related measurements have been reported in normal children and infants (Keefe et al., 1993; Prieve & Georgantis, 2007; Sanford & Feeney, 2008; Vander Werff, Prieve, & Georgantas, 2007), and newborn infants (Abdala, Keefe, & Oba, 2007; Keefe et al., 2000; Keefe & Abdala, 2007). The first developmental study of ER was reported by Keefe et al. (1993), who investigated middle-ear maturation on wideband immittance measures in adults and in five groups of infants and children (1, 3, 6, 12, and 24 months of age). This study reported that age-related variations in ER over a frequency range of 0.125 to 10 kHz were most significant between 1 and 6 months of age. The greatest changes in ER occurred at frequencies below 0.5 kHz where ER increased by up to 30% between 1 and 6 months of age. Keefe et al. (1993) concluded that greater energy transfer due to ear-canal flaccidity was responsible for lower ER in young infants and that these effects may account for the variability of 226-Hz admittance tympanograms and poor test sensitivity for detecting middle-ear effusion in infants. Conversely, Hunter et al. (2008a) did not find significant low-frequency effects from 1 month to 4 years of age using a different ER measurement system and probe type, but did find high-frequency development changes (specifically at 6000 Hz), which may be due to mass effects at high frequencies. Another recent study (Sanford & Feeney, 2008) reported wideband tympanometry in infants, with 20 infants tested in each of three age groups (4, 12, and 24 weeks). Sanford and Feeney found developmental changes in wideband ER measurements varied as a function of frequency. For frequencies from 0.25 to 0.75 kHz there was as much as a 30% increase in mean ER with changes in static ear-canal pressure between 4 and 24 weeks of age. This change was hypothesized to be due to corresponding increases in stiffness of the external ear canal. The frequency region from 0.75 to 2 kHz was reported to be a developmentally stable frequency range with few age-related changes. Between 2 and 6 kHz, there were differential effects of pressure for the youngest infants; negative pressures caused increased ER and Y, and positive pressures caused decreased ER and Y, and the magnitude of this effect decreased with age. The authors hypothesized that the differential effects could be due to ossicular decoupling for negative pressure and

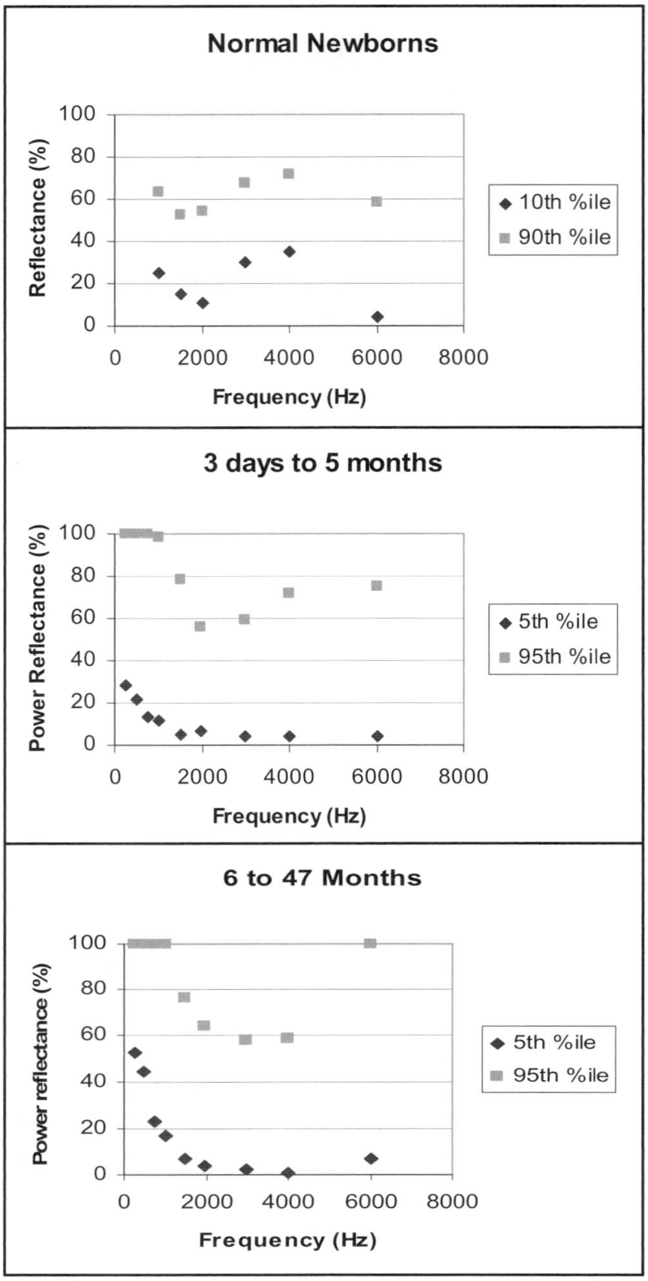

FIGURE 18–11. The normal range for ambient pressure reflectance in infants and children. Modified from Hunter et al. (2008a, 2010).

increased coupling for positive pressure. Additionally, high-frequency ER due to changes in mass, possibly related to mesenchyme absorption was also hypothesized.

Two recent studies of ER normal and abnormal characteristics have recently been reported. Hunter, Feeney, Lapsley Miller, Jeng, and Bohning (2010) reported normative data for wideband middle-ear power reflectance using the Mimosa Acoustics HEAR-ID System in a newborn hearing screening population in comparison to 1-kHz tympanometry for prediction of DPOAE-screening outcome in 324 infants. Normative frequency regions were reported, and receiver-operator characteristic (ROC) curve analyses showed that reflectance provides the best prediction of DPOAE status in the frequency ranges around 2 kHz. Power reflectance produced much better prediction of DPOAE status than 1-kHz tympanometry. Reflectance decreased with age over the first 3 days of age. Birth type and birth weight did not contribute to differences in reflectance. This study concluded that referrals in OAE-based infant hearing screening can be evaluated by simultaneously measuring wideband power reflectance. The study recommended that newborns obtaining high reflectance scores be rescreened within a few hours to a few days, as most middle-ear problems are transient, whereas newborns with normal reflectance and a refer result for the OAE screen should be referred for immediate diagnostic testing with threshold ABR.

Another recent study by Sanford et al. (2009) compared sensitivity and specificity of 1-kHz tympanometry to wideband reflectance tests in 455 newborn ears (375 passed and 80 referred), and found excellent prediction of DPOAE screening results by ER, while 1000-Hz tympanometry was shown to produce poorer results. Of the 80 infants referred on day one, 67 infants were evaluated again after a second UNHS DPOAE test the next day (day 2). Clinical decision theory analysis was used to assess the test performance of wideband and 1-kHz tests in terms of their ability to classify ears that passed or were referred, using DPOAE UNHS test outcomes as the "gold standard." This study found that the highest area under the ROC curve was 0.87 for an ambient WB test predictor, whereas the highest area under the ROC curve among several variables derived from 1-kHz tympanometry was 0.75. In general, ears that passed the DPOAE UNHS test had higher energy absorbance compared with those that were referred, indicating that infants who passed DPOAE had a more acoustically efficient conductive pathway. The authors concluded that wideband immittance results in newborns ears that refer from UNHS are related to transient conditions affecting the sound conduction pathway; that wideband data reveal changes in sound conduction during the first 2 two days of life; and that wideband measurements are objective, quick, and feasible to consider implementing in conjunction with UNHS programs.

ER measurements have also been reported in middle-ear disorders including infants and children with otitis media with effusion (Hunter et al., 2008a), otosclerosis, ossicular discontinuity and perforation of the tympanic membrane (Feeney, Keefe, & Marryott, 2003; Piskorski et al., 1999). Figures 18–12, 18–13, and 18–14 illustrate examples of ER in normal ears, in negative pressure and tympanic membrane perforation, respectively.

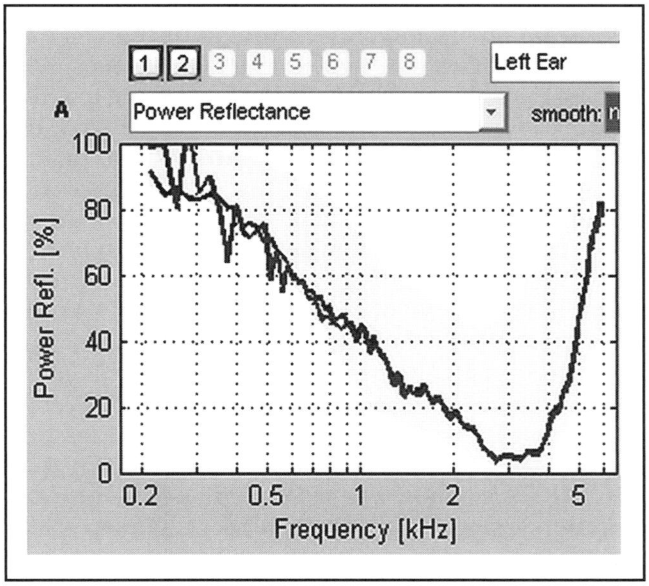

FIGURE 18–12. Normal WBR responses from children 6 years; 0 month to 6 years; 11 months.

Because ER provides reliable information of middle-ear function in young infants, it could potentially be a useful tool in UNHS and EHDI programs. For example, Keefe et al. (2003a, 2003b) analyzed a subset of data obtained from two-stage hearing screening protocols (TEOAE/ABR and DPOAE/ABR) that had a 5% false positive rate. They reported significant correlations between two ambient-pressure ER variables and CEOAE responses, suggesting that ER measures could be useful in interpreting TEOAE responses. Applying ER factors identified in Keefe et al. (2003a) to a predictive test of middle-ear dysfunction in infants, Keefe et al. (2003b) showed that inclusion of the ambient-pressure ER test decreased the false positive rate from 5% to 1%. Thus, ER is able to detect transient middle-ear dysfunction in newborns.

Test-retest reliability has been reported in infants (Hunter et al., 2008a; Vander Werff et al., 2007) and children (Hunter et al., 2008a). In the study by Vander Werff et al., test-retest reliability and differences between ER measures in an infant group receiving outpatient hearing screenings (mean age 7.6 weeks, SD = 5.3 weeks) was compared to an infant group receiving outpatient diagnostic hearing assessments (mean age 12.4 weeks, SD = 8.5 weeks). Lower (better) test-retest variability was reported for the diagnostic than the screening group, and the difference was attributed to

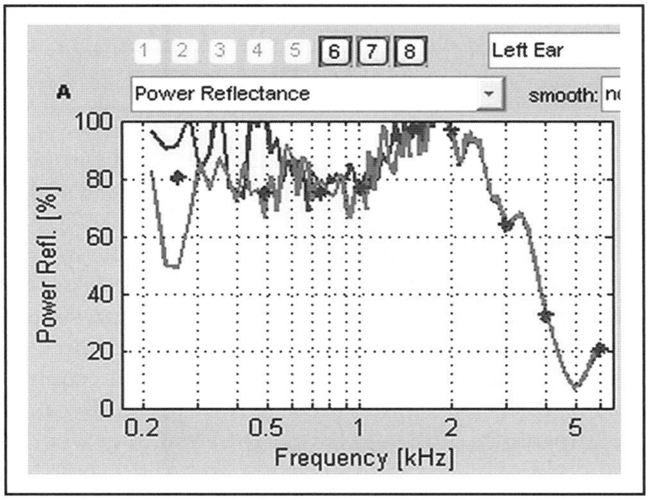

FIGURE 18–13. Abnormal WBR response from a 6-year-old with negative middle ear pressure. The shaded region shows previously collected normative data from adults. Note the increase in reflectance between 1 and 3.5 kHz for both ears.

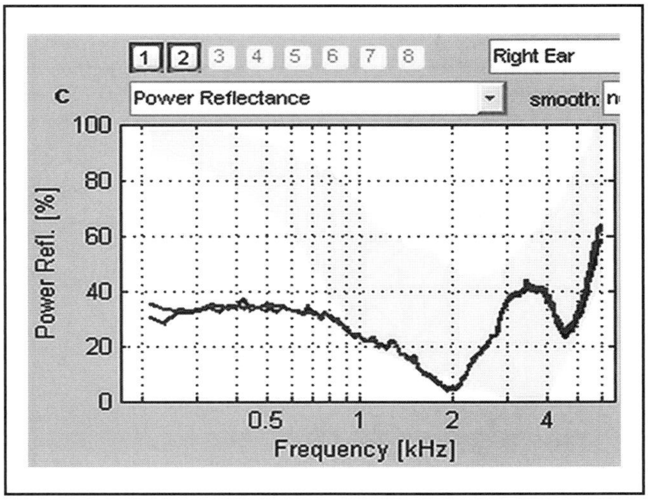

FIGURE 18–14. WBR measures showing a perforation of the eardrum in comparison to the normative region. Notice that frequency responses below 1 kHz are outside the shaded normative area.

decreased noise in the testing environment of the diagnostic group. Infants who failed the OAE screening had significantly higher ER values (exceeding test-retest variability) for frequencies ranging from 630 to 2000 Hz compared to infants who passed, suggesting the presence of a middle-ear conductive component in infants who failed the OAE screening. In the Hunter et al. (2008a) study, ER showed high test-retest reliability in the same test session after removal and replacement of the probe tip. ER was significantly higher in infants and children who failed a combination of otoscopy, OAE and single-frequency tympanometry. A study of infants with unrepaired cleft lip and palate (Hunter et al., 2008a) also demonstrated agreement between wideband reflectance and DPOAE that was higher than between otoscopy, 226-Hz, or 1000-Hz tympanometry and DPOAE (Hunter, Bagger-Sjöbäck, & Lundberg, 2008b). However, variability in ER measurements can occur if the probe fit is loose. As shown in Figure 18–15, the low frequencies are significantly lower when the probe fit is inadequate, similar to ER effects seen in eardrum perforation.

WB energy reflectance can be considered an alternative middle-ear assessment technique to single-frequency admittance tympanometry. Wideband measurements of ER tympanograms were first reported by Keefe and Levi (1996), and found in other studies to reveal more information than does an ER test at ambient pressure (Margolis, Saly, & Keefe, 1999; Sanford & Feeney, 2008). Studies of tympanograms measured with a wideband stimulus predicted the presence of a conductive hearing loss more accurately than did an wideband immittance measured at ambient pressure, indicating that pressurization may be important even if a wideband stimulus is employed (Keefe & Simmons, 2003). That study investigated the test performance of 226-Hz admittance tympanometry, ambient-pressure ER, and WB tympanometry as predictors of conductive hearing loss in children 10 years of age or older. Data were obtained from 42 normal-functioning ears and 18 ears with conductive hearing loss. The sensitivity of these measures to detect conductive hearing loss was only 28% for static acoustic admittance (226-Hz), but was higher (72%) for ambient-pressure ER, and highest (94%) for WB tympanometry. Thus, available research demonstrates that WB tympanometry is a useful diagnostic tool for detection of conductive hearing loss.

Wideband immittance measurements can also be presented in terms of energy absorbance (EA), the inverse of ER. To the extent that the ear-canal walls absorb no sound energy, EA is the fraction of incident energy absorbed by the middle ear (Keefe & Feeney, 2008); both EA and ER vary between 0 and 1 (assuming no OAE contribution). EA can also be converted into a dB scale known as transmittance. Use of EA is worthwhile since it is easily relatable to admittance, as measured in tympanometry. EA is largest at frequencies for which the middle ear is efficient in collecting sound energy (1000-3000 Hz). An EA tympanogram in a healthy adult middle ear, like a 226-Hz admittance-magnitude tympanogram, has a single peak in its response across air pressure.

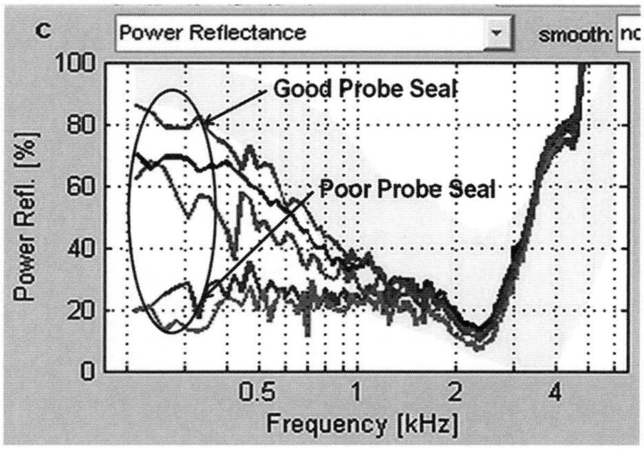

FIGURE 18–15. WBR measurement is made by placing the probe in the canal. Results can vary depending on probe seal; this figure shows the difference between a good and a poor probe seal.

Acoustic Stapedial Reflex Measures

Historically, several methods have been used for measurement of the acoustic stapedial reflex (ASR), also known as the middle ear muscle reflex (MEMR), but the method used in all commercially available instruments is monitoring of admittance changes evoked by a brief, loud pure tone or broadband noise presented to the ear in which the admittance measurement is made (ipsilateral ASR) or to the opposite ear (contralateral ASR). The ASR is present at birth, but because the impedance of the ear is very different in newborns as discussed earlier in this chapter, the ASR is not reliably detected using low probe frequencies. Higher frequency probe tones, at 660 Hz or higher, do evoke the ASR reliably in newborns (McMillan, Bennett, Marchant, & Shurin, 1985; Weatherby & Bennett, 1980).

As in adults, the ASR is useful in pediatric assessment to define middle ear problems, cochlear hearing loss, and problems beyond the outer hair cells, such as auditory neuropathy spectrum disorders (ANSD), retrocochlear disorders, central auditory processing disorder, and facial nerve disorders. For a detailed review of the history of ASR measurement, and anatomy and physiology of the ASR pathway, refer to Margolis and Hunter (2000) or Wiley and Fowler (1997).

Studies of the acoustic reflex in the pediatric populations have focused on two fundamental issues: normative studies in various age groups and studies in middle ear disease. Studies of the ASR in ANSD and auditory processing disorders consist primarily of cases or case series.

ASR Normative Studies

A summary of normative studies of ASR thresholds for infants and children for various probe and stimulus frequencies is shown in Table 18–2 for studies that included probe tone frequency information. In newborns, three studies examined the effect of probe tone frequency. Weatherby and Bennett (1980) studied broadband reflex thresholds with a series of probe tone frequencies in 49 newborns from 10 to 169 hours old, and found that probe tones between 800 and 1800 Hz provided the lowest ASR thresholds. In a study of 95 well babies, McMillan and colleagues (1985a, b) found that ipsilateral and contralateral acoustic reflexes were detected three times more frequently with a 660-Hz probe tone than with 220 Hz. Acoustic reflex thresholds were similar to adult values for activator stimuli at 500, 1000, and 4000 Hz and were 8 dB higher than adult values for a 2000-Hz activator stimulus (660 Hz probe tone). Ipsilateral thresholds were lower than contralateral thresholds, and were similar to adult thresholds for a 660-Hz probe tone. Sprague and colleagues (1985) studied 53 newborns who were 24 to 105 hours old, using probe tones of 220 and 660 Hz and evoked by 1000-Hz pure tones and broadband noise presented both ipsilaterally and contralaterally. They reported that 80% of the newborns had observable ASR for 660-Hz probe tones whereas only 50% had observable ASR with a 220-Hz probe tone. ASR thresholds for broadband noise were significantly lower than for the 1000-Hz pure tone. Ipsilateral presentation produced lower thresholds than contralateral presentation. They also reported that flat 660-Hz tympanograms were associated with absent ASR. Thus, these studies taken together can be summarized as follows: The ASR is measurable in a high proportion of newborns when a probe tone of 660 Hz or higher is used, the measured thresholds are similar to adults, and broadband stimuli provide lower ASR thresholds than pure-tone stimuli. Limited information indicates a correlation between flat tympanometry at 1000 Hz and absent ASR at the same frequency. Important data on test-retest reliability of the ASR in neonates was recently reported by Mazlan, Kei, and Hickson (2009). In this study, 194 healthy neonates aged between 24 and 192 hours passed an automated ABR screening test and were assessed with TEOAE, 1000-Hz tympanometry and ASR using a 1000-Hz probe tone with 2 kHz and broadband ipsilateral activators. The Madsen Otoflex diagnostic immittance system was used. Ipsilateral ASRs were present in 91% of neonates,

Table 18–2. Summary of Acoustic Reflex Studies in Infants and Children

Study	*Ages*	*Probe Frequency*	*Test Frequencies*	*Presentation Levels*	*Normative Values*
Kankkunen & Lidén (1984)		660 Hz	500, 1000, 2000, 4000 Hz and broadband noise—all with Ipsilateral presentation	Up to limits of equipment, 90 dB HL at 500 and 4000 Hz, 100 dB HL at 2000 Hz, and 110 dB HL at 1000 Hz.	Upper normal ART limits 500 = 95, 1000 = 101, 2000 = 102, 4000 = 96 dB HL
Gerber, Gong, & Mendel (1984)	12 to 36 weeks	Unknown	500, 1000, 2000, 4000 Hz, broadband noise	70 to 110 dB HL Contralateral presentation	12 wks: 500 = 81 ± 7.8, 1000 = 82 ± 9.3, 2000 = 83 ± 8.5, 4000 = 84 ± 8.8 dB HL.

continues

Table 18–2. *continued*

Study	*Ages*	*Probe Frequency*	*Test Frequencies*	*Presentation Levels*	*Normative Values*
Abahazi & Greenberg (1977)	1 to 12 months	unknown	500, 1000, 2000 Hz and low-pass, high-pass, and white noise.	70 dB ascending in 5 dB steps until AR elicited	Mean values in dB SPL: 500 = 105.3, 100 = 97.9, 2000 = 98.9, low pass = 90.7, high pass = 88.3, white noise = 84.2
Nozza, Bluestone, Kardatzke, & Bachman (1992)	1 to 8 years for group 1. 3 to 16 years old for group 2.	unknown	1000 Hz	100 dB HL screening ipsilateral presentation at peak pressure or atmospheric pressure Group 1. Group 2 was presented at 85, 95, and 105 dB HL.	N/A
Freyss, Narcy, Manac'h, & Toupet (1980)	6 mos to 8 yrs	unknown	1000 Hz contralateral presentation	Up to 115 dB	N/A
McMillan et al. (1985b)	2 wks to 12 mos	220 and 660 Hz	500, 1000, and 2000, 4000 Hz ipsilateral presentation	70 dB HL raised in 5 dB steps to the limits of the equipment. A deflection 0.11 mmhos for 660 Hz and 0.036 mmhos for 220 Hz signified a reflex.	N/A
Schwartz & Schwartz (1980)	4 mos to 17 yrs	unknown	1000 and 2000 Hz contralateral presentation	unknown	N/A
McMillan, Bennett, Marchant, & Shurin (1985a)	0 to 2 days	220 and 660 Hz	500, 1000, 200, 4000 Hz at peak pressure from 660-Hz tymp or ambient pressure if no peak present.	70 dB HL raised in 5 dB steps until the limits of the equipment.	N/A
Casselbrant et al. (1985)	2 to 6 years	unknown	1000 Hz	105 dB SPL	N/A
Marchant et al. (1986)	0 to 4 months	660 Hz	1000 Hz	80 to 110 dB HL Ipsilateral presentation	N/A
Weatherby & Bennett (1980)	10 to 169 hours old	220 to 2000 Hz	broadband noise	95 dB SPL decreased in 10 dB steps until response extinguished.	N/A
Sprague, Wiley, & Goldstein (1985)	24 to 105 hours old	220 and 660 Hz	1000 Hz and broadband noise	40 dB HL ascending in 10 dB steps Ipsilateral and contralateral presentation	N/A
Mazlan, Kei, & Hickson (2009)	24 to 192 hours	1000 Hz	2000 Hz and broadband noise	Madsen otoflex system	2000 Hz Mean = 76 dB HL; BBN Mean = 65 dB HL

whereas 9% showed flat tympanograms and absent ASR as well as a "refer" result for the TEOAE test. The mean ASR threshold was 76 dB HL for the 2-kHz activator and was 65 dB HL for the broadband noise (BBN) activator. ASR thresholds did not differ significantly for the first test and second tests for either ASR activator, and showed high intracorrelation coefficients (0.83). This study shows that 1000-Hz probe tone ASRs are consistently elicited from healthy neonates who pass automated ABR and TEOAE screening and 1000-Hz tympanometry, thus ASR test holds promise as a useful diagnostic/screening instrument in ascertaining the hearing status in neonates.

Caution should be exercised when introducing high-level stimuli to the ear canal in infants and children for ASR testing, due to the potential risk of permanent threshold shift and because SPL developed in a smaller ear canal can be at least 10 dB higher than in an adult ear (Hunter, Ries, Schlauch, Levine, & Ward, 1999). McMillan, Bennett, Marchant, and Shurin (1985a) measured ear canal SPL with a probe microphone compared to the level indicated on the immittance instrument. At maximum HL presentation permitted (generally 110 dB HL), the measured SPL in infant ears reached 126 dB and 130 dB SPL at 1000 and 2000 Hz, respectively. These levels are clearly a hazard, and despite this, levels on acoustic immittance instruments are not limited, and the audiologist must be aware of these potential hazards when testing infants and children. In general, acoustic reflex thresholds for infants and children are similar to those of adults, and an upper limit of 90 dB HL is considered the normal range for pure tone stimuli (Kankkunen & Lidén, 1984; McMillan, Marchant, & Shurin, 1985b). The study indicated that the mean acoustic reflex threshold averaged for 500-Hz, 1000-Hz, 2000-Hz, and 4000-Hz pure tones was 85 dB HL. Results demonstrated that the acoustic reflex threshold increased with age from 1 month to 5 years of age. Gerber, Gong, and Mendel (1984) measured acoustic reflex thresholds for contralateral stimulation in 45 infants, ages 12 to 36 weeks, and found average thresholds between 81 and 84 dB HL for pure tone stimuli at 500, 1000, 2000, and 4000 Hz. Maximum presentation levels should be limited to no greater than 105 dB SPL (Hunter et al., 1999), but unfortunately this limits interpretation of the ASR, as the upper limit of the ASR in infants can exceed 105 dB SPL (see Table 18–2). Broadband noise is recommended as an alternative stimulus to pure tones, as thresholds will be lower, and the risk of iatrogenic hearing loss is lower since the energy is distributed across the basilar membrane, rather than concentrated as for pure tones.

ASR in Otitis Media and Middle Ear Effusion

Other studies have examined the usefulness of the acoustic reflex test in children as an indicator of middle ear effusion. Studies suggest the presence of the acoustic reflex at normal levels can indicate an effusion-free middle ear. Freyss, Narcy, Manac'h, and Toupet (1980) used a 1000-Hz stimulus to elicit the acoustic reflex in 99 ears for infants and children 6 months to 8 years of age immediately prior to myringotomy. They found that ears with an acoustic reflex threshold of 115 dB or lower were effusion-free at the time of surgery. Conversely, those ears with an absent reflex above 115 dB were ears positive for MEE. This study did not specify if presentation levels were measured in dB SPL or dB HL. Nozza and colleagues (1992) used myringotomy as a standard determination for middle ear effusion in a study of 264 ears for children 1 to 16 years of age. This study reported that up to 85% of ears without middle ear effusion had the acoustic reflex present at 1000 Hz with a 100 dB HL presentation tone. Only 12% of ears with effusion had a measurable reflex. Marchant et al. (1986) found that an acoustic reflex at 100 dB HL or less for 1000 Hz in infants was strongly associated with the absence of middle ear effusion and with a normal tympanometric peak.

The acoustic reflex is most reliable as a predictor of middle ear status when coupled with tympanometric measurements including static admittance (Casselbrant et al., 1985; Marchant et al., 1986) and gradient (Nozza et al., 1992). The acoustic reflex alone may not be the best predictor of middle ear effusion. Nozza et al. (1992) found 76% of ears without effusion had a measurable acoustic reflex. They concluded the absence of the acoustic reflex alone was not a sufficient predictor of middle ear effusion in children because 28% of ears had no reflex present and were also effusion-free. However, coupled with tympanometric gradient of less than 0.1 mmhos, the absence of the acoustic reflex was a powerful indicator. The test parameters used in the above research are summarized in Table 18–2.

The suggested protocol for acoustic reflex measurement in infants less than 6 months of age includes ipsilateral presentation of a broadband noise or pure tones at 1000 Hz and 2000 Hz at levels that do not exceed 105 dB SPL and the use of a 660 or 1000-Hz probe tone. At ages greater than 6 months, a standard 226-Hz probe tone is adequate for detection of the ASR. These parameters should serve to elicit the acoustic reflex at the lowest possible sound pressure levels and provide reliable information regarding middle-ear status complimentary to tympanometric data for the detection of middle ear effusion.

ASR in Auditory Neuropathy Spectrum Disorder (ANSD)

ANSD (previously known as auditory neuropathy/auditory dyssynchrony disorder or AN/AD) has been identified and described over the past 15 years but is still elusive in terms of etiology. It appears that multiple etiologies may be present, and there is a wide range of severity and clinical presentations, thus a recent consensus conference at the International Newborn Hearing Screening Conference in 2008 recommended the addition of the qualifier "spectrum" to the disorder. Newborns may present with referral from ABR screening procedures, as ABR waveforms are markedly abnormal or absent by definition. Detailed descriptions of ANSD are beyond the scope of this chapter and are covered elsewhere in this text (see Chapters 13 and 37). However, it is important to recognize the value of ASR measurements in infants and children suspected of having ANSD. ASR is an effective low-cost test that can be employed in the newborn nursery or the outpatient clinic to assess the possibility of ANSD, in combination with behavioral audiometry and otoacoustic emissions. Berlin et al. (2005) examined a subpopulation of 136 patients (from their database of 257 subjects with ANSD) in whom middle ear muscle reflexes had been measured. They found *that none of the patients had normal acoustic reflexes* for both 1000 and 2000 Hz, whether ipsilaterally or contralaterally elicited. Berlin and colleagues urged use of the ipsilateral ASR at least at 1 kHz and 2 kHz in any perinatal hearing screening that depends solely on otoacoustic emissions. If the emissions are present and the reflexes are absent or elevated, an ABR is recommended to determine whether ANSD may be present.

Wideband Acoustic Reflex Measures

As in tympanometry, ASRs can be measured using wideband stimuli and reflectance measurements. For example, Keefe, Fitzpatrick, Liu, Sanford, and Gorga (2009) studied a wideband aural acoustical test battery of middle-ear status, including acoustic-reflex thresholds and acoustic-transfer functions (ATFs, i.e., absorbance and admittance). Ipsilateral acoustic-reflex thresholds were assessed with a stimulus including four broadband-noise or tonal activator pulses alternating with five clicks presented before, between and after the pulses. Acoustic reflex thresholds were measured using maximum likelihood both at low frequencies (0.8-2.88 kHz) and high (2.8-8 kHz). The median low-frequency acoustic reflex threshold was elevated by 24 dB in NHS refers compared to passes. ATF and acoustic reflex threshold tests performed better than either test alone in predicting NHS outcomes, and WB tests performed better than 1-kHz tympanometry.

Summary

Acoustic immittance tests have long been a critical component of physiologic assessment for newborns, infants, and children. With significant advancements in the past few years that have brought multifrequency and now broadband measures into clinical use, it is now possible to more effectively diagnose newborns with middle ear problems, and to more directly compare middle ear measures to cochlear measures in the same frequency range.

Acknowledgment. The assistance of Erin Davis, AuD, in preparation of figures is gratefully acknowledged.

References

Abahazi, D. A., & Greenberg, H. J. (1977). Clinical acoustic reflex threshold measurements in infants. *Journal of Speech and Hearing Disorders*, *42*, 514–519.

Abdala, C., Keefe, D. H., & Oba, S. I. (2007). Distortion product otoacoustic emission suppression tuning and acoustic admittance in human infants: Birth through 6 months. *Journal of the Acoustical Society of America*, *121*, 3617–3627.

Alaerts, J., Lutz, H., & Woulters, J. (2007). Evaluation of middle ear function in young children: Clinical guidelines for the use of 226- and 1,000-Hz tympanometry. *Otology and Neurotology*, *28*, 727–732.

Allen, J. B. (1986). Measurement of eardrum acoustic impedance. In J. B. Allen, J. L. Hall, A. E. Hubbard, S. T. Neely, & A. Tubis (Eds.), *Peripheral auditory mechanisms* (pp. 44–51). New York, NY: Springer-Verlag.

American Academy of Audiology (AAA). (1997). Identification of hearing loss & middle-ear dysfunction in preschool and school-age children. *Audiology Today*, *9*, 3.

American National Standards Institute (ANSI). (1987). *American National Standard specifications for instruments to mea-*

sure aural acoustic impedance and admittance (aural acoustic immittance). ANSI S3.39-1987. New York, NY: Author.

American Speech-Language -Hearing Association (ASHA). (1990). Guidelines for audiologic screening for hearing impairment and middle-ear disorders. *American Speech-Language-Hearing Association, 32* (Suppl. 2), 17–24.

American Speech-Language-Hearing Association (ASHA). (2004). *Guidelines for the audiologic assessment of children from birth to 5 years of age.* Available from http://www.asha.org/policy

Baldwin, M. (2006). Choice of probe tone and classification of trace patterns in tympanometry undertaken in early infancy. *International Journal of Audiology, 45,* 417–427.

Bennett, M. (1975). Acoustic impedance bridge measurements with the neonate. *British Journal of Audiology, 9,* 117–124.

Berlin C. I., Hood L. J., Morlet T., Wilensky D., St John, P., Montgomery, E., & Thibodaux M. (2005). Absent or elevated middle ear muscle reflexes in the presence of normal otoacoustic emissions: A universal finding in 136 cases of auditory neuropathy/dys-synchrony. *Journal of the American Academy of Audiology, 16,* 546–553.

Bluestone, C. D., Fria, T. J., Arjona, S. K., Casselbrandt, M. L., Schwartz, D. M., Ruben, R. J., . . . Jerger, J. F. (1986). Controversies in screening for middle ear disease and hearing loss in children. *Pediatrics, 77,* 57–70.

Brooks, D. N. (1968). An objective method of determining fluid in the middle ear. *International Journal of Audiology, 7,* 280–286.

Calandruccio, L., Fitzgerald, T. S., & Prieve, B. A. (2006). Normative multifrequency tympanometry in infants and toddlers. *Journal of the American Academy of Audiology, 17,* 470–480.

Casselbrant, M. L., Brostoff, L. M., Cantekin, E. I., Flaherty, M. R., Doyle, W. J., & Bluestone, C. D. (1985). Otitis media with effusion in preschool children. *Laryngoscope, 95,* 428–436.

Cinamon, U. (2009). The growth rate and size of the mastoid air cell system and mastoid bone: A review and reference. *European Archives of Otorhinolaryngology, 266,* 781–786.

Colletti, V. (1977). Multifrequency tympanometry. *Audiology, 16,* 278–287.

de Jonge, R. R. (1986). Normal tympanometric gradient: A comparison of three methods. *Audiology, 25,* 299–308.

Eavey, R. D. (1993). Abnormalities of the neonatal ear: Otoscopic observations, histologic observations, and a model for contamination of the middle ear by cellular contents of amniotic fluid. *Laryngoscope, 103,* 1–31.

Eby, T. L., & Nadol, J. B. (1986). Postnatal growth of the human temporal bone. Implications for cochlear implants in children. *Annals of Otology, Rhinology and Laryngology, 95,* 356–364.

Elner, A., Ingelstedt, S., & Ivarsson, A. (1971). The elastic properties of the tympanic membrane. *Acta Otolaryngologica, 72,* 397–403.

Feeney, M. P., & Hunter, L. L. (2008). *May the Force be with you: Wideband middle ear power measures.* Presentation at the annual convention of the American Academy of Audiology. Charlotte, North Carolina.

Feeney, M. P., Keefe, D. H., & Marryott, L. P. (2003). Contralateral acoustic reflex threshold for tonal activators using wideband reflectance and admittance. *Journal of Speech, Language, and Hearing Research, 46,* 128–136.

Feldman, A. S. (1976). Tympanometry—Procedures, interpretations and variables. In A. S. Feldman & L. A. Wilber (Eds.), *Acoustic impedance and admittance—The measurement of middle ear function* (pp. 103–155). Baltimore, MD: Williams and Wilkins.

Fiellau-Nikolajsen, M. (1983). Tympanometry and secretory otitis media. Observations on diagnosis, epidemiology, treatment, and prevention in prospective cohort studies of three-year-old children. *Acta Otolaryngolica, 394*(Suppl.), 1–73.

Freyss, G. E., Narcy, P. P., Manac'h, Y., & Toupet, M. G. (1980). Acoustic reflex as a predictor of middle ear effusion. *Annals of Otology, Rhinology and Laryngology, 89*(Suppl.), 196–199.

Gerber, S. E., Gong, E. L., & Mendel, M. I. (1984). Developmental norms for the acoustic reflex. *Audiology, 23,* 1–8.

Himelfarb, M. Z., Popelka, G. R., & Shanon, E. (1979). Tympanometry in normal neonates. *Journal of Speech and Hearing Research, 22,* 179–191.

Hof, J. R., Anteunis, L. J., Chenault, M. N., & van Dijk, P. (2005). Otoacoustic emissions at compensated middle ear pressure in children. *International Journal of Audiology, 44,* 317–320.

Holte, L., Cavanaugh, R. M., Jr., & Margolis, R. H. (1990). Ear canal wall mobility and tympanometric shape in young infants. *Journal of Pediatrics, 117,* 77–80.

Holte, L., Margolis, R. H., & Cavanaugh, R. M. (1991). Developmental changes in multifrequency tympanograms. *Audiology, 30,* 1–24.

Hsu, G. S., Margolis, R. H., & Schachern P. A. (2000). Development of the middle ear in neonatal chinchillas. I. Birth to 14 days. *Acta Otolaryngologica, 120,* 922–932.

Hunter, L. L., Bagger-Sjöbäck, D., & Lundberg, M. (2008b). Wideband reflectance associated with otitis media in infants and children with cleft palate. *International Journal of Audiology, 47,* 57–61.

Hunter, L. L., Feeney, M. P., Lapsley Miller, J. A., Jeng, P. S., & Bohning, S. (2010). Wideband reflectance in newborns: Normative regions and relationship to hearing screening results. *Ear and Hearing,* May 29 (Epub ahead of print).

Hunter, L. L., & Margolis, R. H. (1992). Multifrequency tympanometry, current clinical application. *American Journal of Audiology, 1,* 33–43.

Hunter, L. L., Margolis, R. H., Daly, K. A., & Giebink, G. S. (1992). Relationship of tympanometric estimates of middle ear volume to middle ear status at surgery. In *Abstracts of the midwinter research meeting of the association for research in otolaryngology.* St. Petersburg Beach, FL.

Hunter, L. L., Ries, D. T., Schlauch, R. S., Levine, S. C., & Ward, W. D. (1999). Safety and clinical performance of acoustic reflex tests. *Ear and Hearing, 20,* 506–514.

Hunter, L. L., Tubaugh, L., Jackson, A., & Propes, S. (2008a). Wideband middle ear power measurement in infants and children. *Journal of the American Academy of Audiology, 19*, 309–324.

Ikui, A., Sando, I., & Fujita, S. (1997). Postnatal change in angle between the tympanic annulus and surrounding structures: Computer-aided three-dimensional reconstruction study. *Annals of Otolaryngology Rhinology and Laryngology, 106*, 33–36.

Joint Committee on Infant Hearing. (JCIH). (2007). Year 2007 position statement: Principles and guidelines for early hearing detection and intervention programs. *Pediatrics, 120*, 898–921.

Jerger, J. (1970). Clinical experience with impedance audiometry. *Archives of Otolaryngology, 92*, 311–324.

Kankkunen, A., & Lidén, G. (1984). Ipsilateral acoustic reflex thresholds in neonates and in normal-hearing and hearing-impaired pre-school children. *Scandinavian Audiology, 13*, 139–144.

Keefe, D. H., & Abdala, C. (2007). Theory of forward and reverse middle-ear transmission applied to otoacoustic emissions in infant and adult ears. *Journal of the Acoustical Society of America, 121*, 978–993.

Keefe, D. H., Bulen, J. C., Arehart, K. H. & Burns, E. M. (1993). Ear-canal impedance and reflection coefficient in human infants and adults. *Journal of the Acoustical Society of America, 94*, 2617–2638.

Keefe, D. H., & Feeney, M. P. (2008). Principles of acoustic immittance and acoustic transfer functions. In J. Katz, R. F. Burkhard, L. Medwetsky & L. J. Hood (Eds.), *Handbook of clinical audiology*. New York, NY: Lippincott, Williams & Wilkins.

Keefe, D. H., Fitzpatrick, D., Liu, Y. W., Sanford, C. A., & Gorga, M. P. (2009). Wideband acoustic-reflex test in a test battery to predict middle-ear dysfunction. *Hearing Research, 263*(1–2), 52–65.

Keefe, D. H., Folsom, R., Gorga, M. P., Vohr, B. R., Bulen, J. C., & Norton, S. (2000). Identification of neonatal hearing impairment: Ear-canal measurements of acoustic admittance and reflectance in neonates. *Ear and Hearing, 21*, 443–461.

Keefe, D. H., Gorga, M. P., Neely, S. T., Zhao, F., & Vohr, B. R. (2003b). Ear-canal acoustic admittance and reflectance measurements in human neonates. II. Predictions of middle-ear in dysfunction and sensorineural hearing loss. *Journal of the Acoustical Society of America, 113*, 407–422.

Keefe, D. H, & Levi, E. (1996). Maturation of the middle and external ears: Acoustic power-based responses and reflectance tympanometry. *Ear and Hearing, 17*, 361–373.

Keefe, D. H., Ling, R., & Bulen, J. C. (1992). Method to measure acoustic impedance and reflection coefficient. *Journal of the Acoustical Society of America, 91*, 470–85.

Keefe, D. H., & Simmons, J. L. (2003c). Energy transmittance predicts conductive hearing loss in older children and adults. *Journal of the Acoustical Society of America, 114*, 3217–3238.

Keefe, D. H., Zhao, F., Neely, S. T., Gorga, M. P., & Vohr, B. R. (2003a). Ear-canal acoustic admittance and reflectance effects in human neonates. I. Predictions of otoacoustic emission and auditory brainstem responses. *Journal of the Acoustical Society of America, 113*, 389–406.

Kei, J., Allison-Levick, J., Dockray, J., Harrys, R., Kirkegard, C., Wong, J., . . . Tudehope, D. (2003). High-frequency (1000 Hz) tympanometry in normal neonates. *Journal of the American Academy of Audiology, 14*, 20–28.

Keith, R. W. (1973). Impedance audiometry with neonates. *Archives of Otolaryngology, 97*, 465–476.

Keith, R. W. (1975). Middle ear function in neonates. *Archives of Otolaryngology, 101*, 376–379.

Koebsell, K. A., & Margolis, R. W. (1986). Tympanometric gradient measured from normal preschool children. *Audiology, 25*, 149–157.

Lidén, G. (1969). The scope and application of of current audiometric tests. *Journal of Laryngology and Otology, 83*, 507–520.

Lidén, G., Harford, E., & Hallén, O. (1974). Tympanometry for the diagnosis of ossicular disruption. *Archives of Otolaryngology, 99*, 23–29.

Lindeman, P., & Holmquist, J. (1982). Volume measurement of middle ear and mastoid air cell system with impedance audiometry on patients with eardrum perforation. *Acta Otolaryngologica, 386* (Suppl.), 70–73.

MRC Multicentre Otitis Media Study Group. (2003). The role of ventilation tube status in the hearing levels in children managed for bilateral persistent otitis media with effusion. *Clinics in Otolaryngology and Allied Sciences. 28*, 146–153.

Marchant, C. D., McMillan, P. M., Shurin, P. A., Johnson, C. E., Turczyk, V. A., & Feinstein, J. C. (1986). Objective diagnosis of otitis media in early infancy by tympanometry and ipsilateral acoustic reflex thresholds. *Journal of Pediatrics, 109*, 590–595.

Margolis, R. H. (1993). Detection of hearing impairment with the acoustic stapedius reflex. *Ear and Hearing, 14*, 3–10.

Margolis, R. H., Bass-Ringdahl, S., Hanks, W. D., Holte, L., & Zapala, D. A. (2003). Tympanometry in newborn infants —1 kHz norms. *Journal of the American Academy of Audiology, 14*, 383–392.

Margolis, R. H., & Heller, J. W. (1987). Screening tympanometry: Criteria for medical referral. *Audiology, 26*, 197–208.

Margolis, R. H., & Hunter, L. L. (2000). Acoustic immitance measurement. In R. J. Roeser, M. Valente. & H. Hosford-Dunn (Eds.), *Audiology: Diagnosis*. New York, NY: Thieme Medical.

Margolis, R. H., Saly, G. L., & Keefe, D. H. (1999). Wideband reflectance tympanometry in normal adults. *Journal of the Acoustical Society of America, 106*, 265–280.

Mazlan, R., Kei, J., & Hickson, L. (2009). Test-retest reliability of the acoustic stapedial reflex test in healthy neonates. *Ear and Hearing, 30*, 295–301.

McMillan, P. M., Bennett, M. J., Marchant, C. D., & Shurin, P. A. (1985a). Ipsilateral and contralateral acoustic reflexes in neonates. *Ear and Hearing, 6*, 320–324.

McMillan, P. M., Marchant, C. D., & Shurin, P. A. (1985b). Ipsilateral acoustic reflexes in infants. *Annals of Otology, Rhinology, and Laryngology, 94*, 145–148.

Nozza, R. J., Bluestone, C. D., Kardatzke, D., & Bachman, R. (1992). Towards the validation of aural acoustic immittance measures for diagnosis of middle ear effusion in children. *Ear and Hearing, 13*, 442–453.

Nozza, R. J., Bluestone, C. D., Kardatzke, D., & Bachman, R. (1994). Identification of middle ear effusion by aural acoustic admittance and otoscopy. *Ear and Hearing, 15*, 310–323.

Palva, T., Northrop, C., & Ramsay, H. (1999). Spread of amniotic fluid cellular content within the neonate middle ear. *International Journal of Pediatric Otorhinolaryngology, 48*, 143–153.

Paradise, J. L., Smith, C. G., & Bluestone, C. D. (1976). Tympanometric detection of middle ear effusion in infants and young children. *Pediatrics, 58*, 198–210.

Piskorski, P., Keefe, D. H., Simmons, J., & Gorga, M. P. (1999). Prediction of conductive hearing loss based on acoustic ear-canal response using a multivariate clinical decision theory. *Journal of the Acoustical Society of America, 105*, 1749–1764.

Piza, J., Gonzalez, M., Northrop, C. C., & Eavey, R. D. (1989). Meconium contamination of the neonatal middle ear. *Journal of Pediatrics, 115*, 910–914.

Poulsen, G., & Tos, M. (1978). Screening tympanometry in newborn infants and during the first six months of life. *Scandinavian Audiology, 7*, 159–166.

Prieve, B. A., Calandruccio, L., Fitzgerald, T., Mazevski, A., & Georgantas, L. M. (2008). Changes in transient-evoked otoacoustic emission levels with negative tympanometric peak pressure in infants and toddlers. *Ear and Hearing, 29*, 533–542.

Renvall, U., & Holmquist, J. (1976). Tympanometry revealing middle ear pathology. *Annals of Otology, Rhinology and Laryngology, 85* (Suppl. 25), 209–215.

Rhodes, M. C., Margolis, R. H., Hirsch, J. E, & Napp, A. P. (1999). Hearing screening in the newborn nursery: A comparison of methods. *Otolaryngology-Head and Neck Surgery, 120*, 799–808.

Roberts, D. G., Johnson, C. E., Carlin, S. A., Turczyk, V., Karnuta, M. A., & Yaffee, K. (1992). Resolution of middle ear effusion in newborns. *Archives of Pediatric Adolescent Medicine, 149*, 873–877.

Roush, J., Bryant, K., Mundy, M., Zeisel, S., & Roberts, J. (1995). Developmental changes in static admittance and tympanometric width in infants and toddlers. *Journal of the American Academy of Audiology, 6*, 334–338.

Roush, J., Drake, A., & Sexton, J. E. (1992). Identification of middle ear dysfunction in young children: A comparison of tympanometric screening procedures. *Ear and Hearing, 13*, 63–69.

Ruah, C. B., Schachern, P. A., Zelterman, D., Paparella, M. M., & Yoon, T. H. (1991). Age-related morphologic changes in the human tympanic membrane. A light and electron microscopic study. *Archives of Otolaryngology-Head and Neck Surgery, 117*, 627–634.

Sanford, C. A., & Feeney, M. P. (2008). Effects of maturation on tympanometric wideband acoustic transfer function in human infants. *Journal of the Acoustical Society of America, 124*, 2106–2122.

Sanford, C. A., Keefe, D. H., Liu, Y. W., Fitzpatrick, D., McCreery, R. W., Lewis, D. E., & Gorga, M. P. (2009). Sound-conduction effects on distortion-product otoacoustic emission screening outcomes in newborn infants: Test performance of wideband acoustic transfer functions and 1-kHz tympanometry. *Ear and Hearing, 30*, 635–652.

Saunders, J. C., Kaltenback, J. A., & Relkin, E. M. (1983). The structural and functional development of the outer and middle ear. In R. Romand & M. R. Romand (Eds.), *Development of auditory and vestibular systems* (pp. 3–25). New York, NY: Academic Press.

Schwartz, D. M., & Schwartz, R. H. (1980). Acoustic immittance findings in acute otitis media. *Annals of Otology Rhinology and Laryngology, 89*(Suppl.), 211–213.

Shanks, J. E., & Lilly, D. J. (1981). An evaluation of tympanometric estimates of ear canal volume. *Journal of Speech and Hearing Research, 24*, 557–566.

Shanks, J. E., Stelmachowicz, P. G., Beauchaine, K. L., & Schulte, L. (1992). Equivalent ear canal volumes in children pre- and post-tympanostomy tube insertion. *Journal of Speech and Hearing Research, 35*, 936–941.

Silman, S., Silverman, C. A., & Arick, D. S. (1992). Acoustic immittance screening for detection of middle-ear effusion in children. *Journal of the American Academy of Audiology, 3*, 262–268.

Sprague, B. H., Wiley, T. L., & Goldstein, R. (1985). Tympanometric and acoustic-reflex studies in neonates. *Journal of Speech and Hearing Research, 28*, 265–272.

Sun, X. M., & Shaver, M. D. (2009) Effects of negative middle ear pressure on distortion product otoacoustic emissions and application of a compensation procedure in humans. *Ear and Hearing, 30*(2), 191–202.

Swanepoel, D. W., Werner, S., Hugo, R., Louw, B., Owen, R., & Swanepoel, A. (2007). High frequency immittance for neonates: A normative study. *Acta Otolaryngologica, 127*, 49–56.

Takasaka, T., Hozawa, K., Shoji, F., Takahashi, Y., Jingu, K., Adachi, M., & Kobayashi, T. (1996). Tympanostomy tube treatment in recurrent otitis media with effusion. In D. J. Lim, C. D. Bluestone, M. Casselbrandt, J. O. Klein, & P. L. Ogra (Eds.), *Recent advances in otitis media* (pp. 197–199). Hamilton, Ontario: B. C. Decker, Inc.

Trine, M. B., Hirsch, J. E., & Margolis, R. H. (1993). The effect of middle ear pressure on transient evoked otoacoustic emissions. *Ear and Hearing, 14*, 401–407.

Vander Werff, K. R., Prieve, B. A., & Georgantas, L. M. (2007). Test-retest reliability of wideband reflectance measures in infants under screening and diagnostic test conditions. *Ear and Hearing, 28*, 669–681.

Vanhuyse, V. J., Creten, W. L., & Van Camp, K. J. (1975). On the W-notching of tympanograms. *Scandinavian Audiology, 4*, 45–50.

Wada, H., Koike, T., & Kobayashi, T. (1998). Clinical applicability of the sweep frequency measuring apparatus for diagnosis of middle ear diseases. *Ear and Hearing, 19*, 240–249.

Weatherby, L. A., & Bennett, M. J. (1980). The neonatal acoustic reflex. *Scandinavian Audiology*, *9*, 103–110.

Wiley, T. L., Cruikshanks, K. J., Nondahl, D. M., Tweed, T. S., Klein, R., & Klein, B. E. K. (1996). Tympanometric measures in older adults. *Journal of the American Academy of Audiology*, *7*, 260–268.

Wiley, T. L., & Fowler, C. G. (1997). *Acoustic immittance measures in clinical audiology: A primer.* San Diego, CA: Singular.

19

Otoacoustic Emissions

Beth A. Prieve and Laura Dreisbach

Introduction

Simply stated, otoacoustic emissions (OAEs) are sounds that are generated in the inner ear, travel through the middle ear and into the ear canal where they can be measured by a miniature microphone. David Kemp is credited with first reporting and describing OAEs (Kemp, 1978). Since the time of their first description, considerable research has been conducted on OAEs, and they now play an essential role in the pediatric test battery. The goal of this chapter is to provide information about OAEs in infants and children so that they can be used in the most effective manner for the diagnosis of hearing loss. First, the cochlear physiology underlying OAE generation is briefly reviewed.[1] Second, types of OAEs are described. Next, clinical considerations for identifying hearing loss in infants and children are given. Finally, possible future uses of OAEs are discussed.

Physiology of OAEs

Motion of the middle ear ossicles moves the stapes footplate in and out of the oval window, delivering vibrations to the cochlear fluids with reciprocal movement at the round window. The vibrations are transmitted throughout the cochlea simultaneously because the cochlea is small and cochlear fluids are incompressible. The pressure variations produce a traveling wave on the basilar membrane, which is the "floor" of the cochlear duct. The traveling wave is created due to the properties of the basilar membrane, which is stiffer and narrower at the base than it is at the apex. The basal end of the basilar membrane moves sooner than the apex because there is less inertia to overcome. The magnitudes of the vibrations are relatively small at the base and progressively increase to a maximum in a confined area corresponding to the incoming frequency. Just apical to this region, the magnitude decreases rapidly. Said another way, different parts of the basilar membrane respond to incoming sounds based on their frequencies, with high frequencies processed at the base and low frequencies processed at the apex. This tonotopic organization of the cochlea was first described by Békèsy (1960). The contribution of mechanical energy from outer hair cells to low and moderate intensity stimuli is known to amplify basilar membrane motion, allowing inner hair cells to transduce vibratory signals to electrochemical signals, which are eventually processed at the cortex.

The cochlear origin of OAE generation is well documented (e.g., Gaskill & Brown, 1990; Harris, Lonsbury-Martin, Stagner, Coats, & Martin, 1989; Probst, Lonsbury-Martin, & Martin, 1991; Wilson, 1980). It is hypothesized that all types of evoked OAEs (EOAEs) in response to low-to-moderate intensity stimuli depend on normal cochlear function and are a by-product of the cochlear amplifier. Specifically, OAEs are tied with normal outer hair cell (OHC) function; however, the specific site and action of production are yet to be determined. Some have proposed that somatic motility, the rapid change in OHC shape and length with electrical stimulation is involved in OAE production

[1]For a more thorough description of OAE generation, see Ryan (2007).

(Brownell, 1990; Liberman et al., 2002) while others have proposed the nonlinearity of the OHC stereocilia bundle (Manley, Kirk, Koppl, & Yates, 2001; Ricci, 2003). It is possible that both of these mechanisms contribute to the generation of mammalian OAEs, but their contributions could differ depending on stimulus levels (Liberman, Zuo, & Guinan, 2004).

OAEs are vulnerable to cochlear disruptions known to affect OHC function, including ototoxic drugs, hypoxia, and intense noise exposure (Norton, Mott, & Champlin, 1989). Additionally, observable emissions are related to the amount of hearing loss present in an individual. Thus, damage to the cochlea in specific regions can reduce or eliminate OAEs in that region while sparing emissions in other regions that are healthy (Probst et al., 1991; Stover, Gorga, & Neely, 1996; Stover, Neely, & Gorga, 1999).

Studies examining the suppression phenomenon, in which the level of an OAE is reduced by stimulation with additional tones, support the cochlear origin theory of emissions (Probst et al., 1991). Using suppression, it has been suggested that OAEs originate from a highly tuned, frequency selective mechanism within the cochlea, which is believed to be a part of the biomechanical process that also results in sharp tuning and enhancement of basilar membrane motion (Harris & Glattke, 1992). The majority of studies reporting results from suppression of distortion-product otoacoustic emissions (DPOAEs) conclude that the major generation site is near the region of the primary frequencies (f_1 and f_2; Harris, Probst, & Xu, 1992; Kemp & Brown, 1983). However, it has been shown that the distortion-product frequency place also is involved in the generation of DPOAEs (Heitmann, Waldmann, Schnitzler, Plinkert, & Zenner, 1998; Kemp & Brown, 1983; Konrad-Martin et al., 2002; Kummer, Janssen, & Arnold, 1995; Wilson, 1980).

In order for clinicians to use OAEs effectively with children in the clinic, it is important for them to have an appreciation for how different parts of the auditory system affect OAEs. First, OAEs are dependent on metabolic processes, as they are reduced or abolished under hypoxic conditions. OAEs are not generated in the middle ear but can be affected or altered by the status of the external and middle ears, as will be discussed later in this chapter. OAEs are generated pre-neurally in the cochlea, as their properties are inconsistent with responses of neural origin. For example, there is absence of adaptation with increasing stimulus rates, complete response polarity reversal with changes in stimulus polarity, and the routine finding that OAE detection thresholds are lower than corresponding psychoacoustical thresholds (Probst et al., 1991). OAE generation is independent of afferent synaptic transmission. In a study using channel blockers that inhibit synaptic transmission, it was demonstrated that OAEs were independent of neural activity whereas, the auditory brainstem response (ABR) was essentially abolished. Similarly, when the eighth nerve is severed, DPOAE measurements are not altered. In summary, OAE generation appear to be peripheral to the eighth nerve and independent of afferent innervation. However, OAE results can be influenced, in a reversible manner, by activation of medial olivocochlear reflex, which includes both afferent and efferent auditory pathways (Harris & Glattke, 1992). It is believed that the medial olivocochlear pathway exerts control over the amplification provided by outer hair cells. When the medial olivocochlear system is activated, OAEs can be influenced in subtle ways using either ipsilateral or contralateral simultaneous stimuli. Because changes in OAEs due to the medial olivocochlear reflex are not routinely used in diagnosis of hearing loss at this time, readers are referred to Guinan (2006) and Hood (2007) for detailed information.

In summary, OAEs are generated in the cochlea. In mammalian species, OHCs are involved in OAE generation, but the exact mechanism(s) contributing to their generation is(are) still under investigation. Although the condition of the external and middle ears can influence OAE measures, the middle ear is not generating OAEs. Additionally, OAEs are not generated by neurons and are unaffected by neural disruption. Knowledge of the physiology underlying the generation of OAEs makes them a powerful tool in the diagnostic test battery for pediatric patients. Because they are indicative of mechanical, preneural activity, clinicians have an idea whether there is a "sensory" component to a more commonly described "sensorineural" hearing loss. If the middle ear is normal and OAEs are reduced or absent along with the finding of elevated auditory brainstem response (ABR) or behavioral thresholds, there is evidence that OHCs are damaged and hearing aids are a reasonable rehabilitative choice.

General Equipment and Recording Considerations

Most clinical measurement devices have some basic, common features. Digital-to-analog and analog-to-digital conversions are used to deliver signals to the ear and sample output from the microphone, respectively. Because OAEs are low-level phenomena, averaging of recordings and procedures to extract the low-level OAEs from the input stimuli are necessary. Artifact rejection of external (e.g., room noise) and internal (e.g., heavy breathing, swallowing) noise is needed, especially for infants and children. Most importantly, a good coupling of the probe to the ear is essential to reduce external noise from getting into the ear canal and ensure the OAE level remains high. There currently are no industry standards for OAE equipment, so hardware, software, and peripherals vary across clinical instruments. Probes can be different in many ways, such as frequency response, impedance, and calibration. In addition, there are differences in how responses are averaged and how "noise" is calculated.

Types of OAEs

Two distinct classes of emissions exist according to the type of eliciting stimulus. The first class of OAEs is spontaneously present without external stimulation, and the second class is evoked by different types of acoustic stimulation. EOAEs can be divided into subclassifications according to the eliciting stimulation used: transient-evoked OAEs (TEOAEs), distortion-product OAEs (DPOAEs), and stimulus-frequency OAEs (SFOAEs). Even though TEOAEs and DPOAEs are the only types of OAEs typically used clinically, a review of each type follows as unique applications of each may be useful.

Spontaneous Otoacoustic Emissions

Spontaneous otoacoustic emissions (SOAEs) are narrow-band signals that can be measured without any eliciting acoustic stimuli. They are relatively stable signals and have been studied in some individuals as long as 19.5 years (Burns, 2009). SOAEs can be recorded in premature infants (Brienesse, Maertzdorf, Anteunis, Manni Blanco, 1998; Smurzynski, 1994), newborns (Bonfils, Uziel, & Narcy, 1989; Burns, Arehart, & Campbell, 1992; Kok, van Zanten, & Brocaar, 1993) and children (Bonfils et al., 1989; Lambrecht-Dinnison et al., 1998). SOAEs measured in infants generally are higher in level and frequency than those measured from adults. The majority of SOAEs in infants occur between 3 to 4 kHz (Kok et al., 1993), whereas the majority of adult SOAEs occur between 1 to 2 kHz. Although adults can have SOAEs at frequencies above 2 kHz, the possibility of measuring higher frequency SOAEs decreases with age. In fact, there is a general decline in SOAE frequency across time on average of 0.25% per year (Burns, 2009). The exception to this finding is for preterm infants, whose SOAE frequencies increase with post conceptional age (PCA; Brienesse et al., 1998; Smurzynski, 1994). In newborns, SOAE amplitudes range from −12 to 42 dB SPL (Burns et al., 1992; Burns, Campbell, & Arehart, 1994; Kok et al., 1993) with a mean amplitude of 10 dB SPL as compared to a mean of −3 to 0 dB SPL for adults. Average SOAE levels in children and adults decrease across time; however, within an individual, they may decrease, increase or stay relatively stable (Burns, 2009). Nevertheless, it can be stated that the largest decreases in amplitude with age are found for higher frequency SOAEs (Burns et al., 1994). There is a decrease in SOAE amplitude with development, with decreases from 1 to 24 months of age (Burns et al., 1992) and continued decreases until 6 years of age (Lamprecht-Dinneson et al., 1998). SOAEs occur in 30 to 40% of normally hearing adults (Bilger, Matthies, Hammel, & Demorest, 1990; Bonfils, 1989; Lamprecht-Dinneson et al., 1998), but prevalence as high as 72% has been recorded using noise reduction techniques (Talmadge, Long, Murphy, & Tubis, 1993) and as high as 83% in a select population of females (Penner & Zhang, 1997). Kuroda (2007) reports that the majority of SOAEs are measured in subjects 20 years of age or less, with an overall prevalence of 30 to 40% in subjects 49 years of age or less. Most reports of newborn SOAEs suggest a higher prevalence, 64 to 78% (Bonfils et al., 1989; Kok et al., 1993). Some researchers report that SOAEs occur more in females than males and in right ears than left ears (Bilger et al., 1990; Kuroda, 2007). The presence of a SOAE in one ear increases the likelihood of SOAEs in the other ear. The explanation provided for these observations assumed that the tendency to exhibit emissions is inherited, perhaps a sex-linked trait. Also, ears are asymmetric with respect to anatomic anomalies of the apical portion of the organ of Corti, which also may be linked with SOAEs (Bilger et al., 1990). SOAEs are never found in frequency regions where cochlear hearing loss exceeds 40 dB HL. Thus, SOAE presence suggests near normal cochlear sensitivity near the frequency of the SOAE.

Transient-Evoked Otoacoustic Emissions

Transient-evoked otoacoustic emissions (TEOAEs) are evoked by brief (transient) acoustic stimuli such as rectangular or Gaussian-shaped clicks, single-cycle sinusoids, half-cycle sinusoids, or tone bursts (Probst et al., 1991). Transient stimuli have brief durations that result in a broad frequency spectrum that excites a wide portion of the basilar membrane. The TEOAE occurs in the time period following stimulation, and in clinical instruments, is monitored for approximately 20 msec. TEOAEs evoked by clicks exhibit what has been referred to as "frequency dispersion"; that is, high frequencies appear earlier in time after the stimulus, with lower frequency energy returning with successively longer delays. A similar property is found for TEOAEs evoked by tonebursts, with longer latencies for lower frequency tonebursts (e.g., DeVries & Decker, 1992; Prieve, Gorga, & Neely, 1996). The waveform pattern of TEOAEs evoked by clicks is quite variable among individuals, but very repeatable within an individual.

The top panel in Figure 19–1 is an example of a TEOAE from an infant with normal ABR toneburst thresholds and was obtained using Otodynamics ILO96 software and accompanying hardware. The "nonlinear" mode of stimulus recording and processing was used[2] and the first 2.5 ms of the averaged response was eliminated to reduce stimulus artifact. The output has many details about the response and the recording. The waveform of the click stimulus in the ear canal and the TEOAE are shown in the upper left-hand and large, middle portions of the plot, respectively. For the TEOAE, there are two responses plotted, noted as "A" and "B," which were recordings from the ear canal that were directed in tandem into two different buffers. Comparison of the waveforms stored in the two buffers allows calculations to quantify the reproducibility between waveforms, the emission-to-noise ratio (ENR), and overall TEOAE level. The ENR is a ratio of the level of the TEOAE (the "signal") to the level of the noise expressed in dB. The ENR is calculated for the overall TEOAE trace or in a given frequency band, in this case, half-octave bands. The difference between waveforms "A" and "B" was calculated and reported as noise level in dB SPL, displayed next to "A-B" in the right-hand column (4.9 dB SPL). The cross power spectrum of the two waveforms was calculated and displayed in the upper, middle portion of the display under the heading "Response FFT" (response fast fourier transform). TEOAE levels are indicated by the dark gray regions and noise levels are indicated by the light gray area.

The third box on the right-hand column with the word "Response" presents many of the quantitative results for the OAE. The heading "Response" indicates the TEOAE level in dB SPL for responses higher than the noise floor across all frequencies. Under the heading "Band Repro% SNR dB," the first row of numbers indicates the percentage reproducibility of the cross-power spectrum from both traces (A and B) of the TEOAE in half-octave bands centered at 1, 1.5, 2, 3, and 4 kHz and below that, the ENR (SNR in Figure 19–1) in dB.

The remaining boxes on the right-hand column of the display indicate information about noise levels, the number of noisy traces, the stimulus level and reproducibility and the file name. The bottom of the display prints the TEOAE level in half-octave bands (function denoted by circles) and the noise levels (gray shaded area), along with TEOAE and noise levels in each half-octave band in the right column.

The bottom panel in Figure 19–1 shows TEOAE results from an infant with severe sensorineural hearing loss as measured by air- and bone- toneburst ABR thresholds at the time of TEOAE testing and later, by behavioral threshold measurements at 10 months of age. The response is different from that of the infant with normal hearing in regard to response level, percent reproducibility, and ENR. Notable is that there were sufficient averages to obtain a response, and the stimulus stability was acceptable.

Distortion-Product Otoacoustic Emissions

Distortion-product otoacoustic emissions (DPOAEs) represent evoked responses at frequencies not present in the eliciting stimuli. The frequencies of the two primary stimuli, f_1 and f_2 ($f_2 > f_1$), are related to the frequency of the distortion product. In humans, the largest DPOAE occurs at the frequency expressed as $2f_1–f_2$, or cubic difference tone (Probst et al., 1991). DPOAEs can be elicited at any frequency throughout the range of human hearing (Dreisbach & Siegel, 2001). Current commercially available equipment produces signals to approximately 8 kHz, but with modified speakers signals can be generated at the highest frequencies of human hearing.

DPOAEs are generated in the frequency region of the basilar membrane corresponding to the interaction or overlap of the primary tones (f_1 and f_2). The DPOAE that is measured in the ear canal is, minimally, a combination of the $2f_1–f_2$ generated from the primary frequency region (f_1 and f_2) and the component generated from the traveling wave causing the basilar membrane (BM) to move at the characteristic frequency (CF) of $2f_1–f_2$. In contrast to TEOAEs, DPOAEs are measured

[2]For detailed information about the "nonlinear" stimulation and recording paradigm and details on the Otodynamics equipment, please refer to Bray (1989).

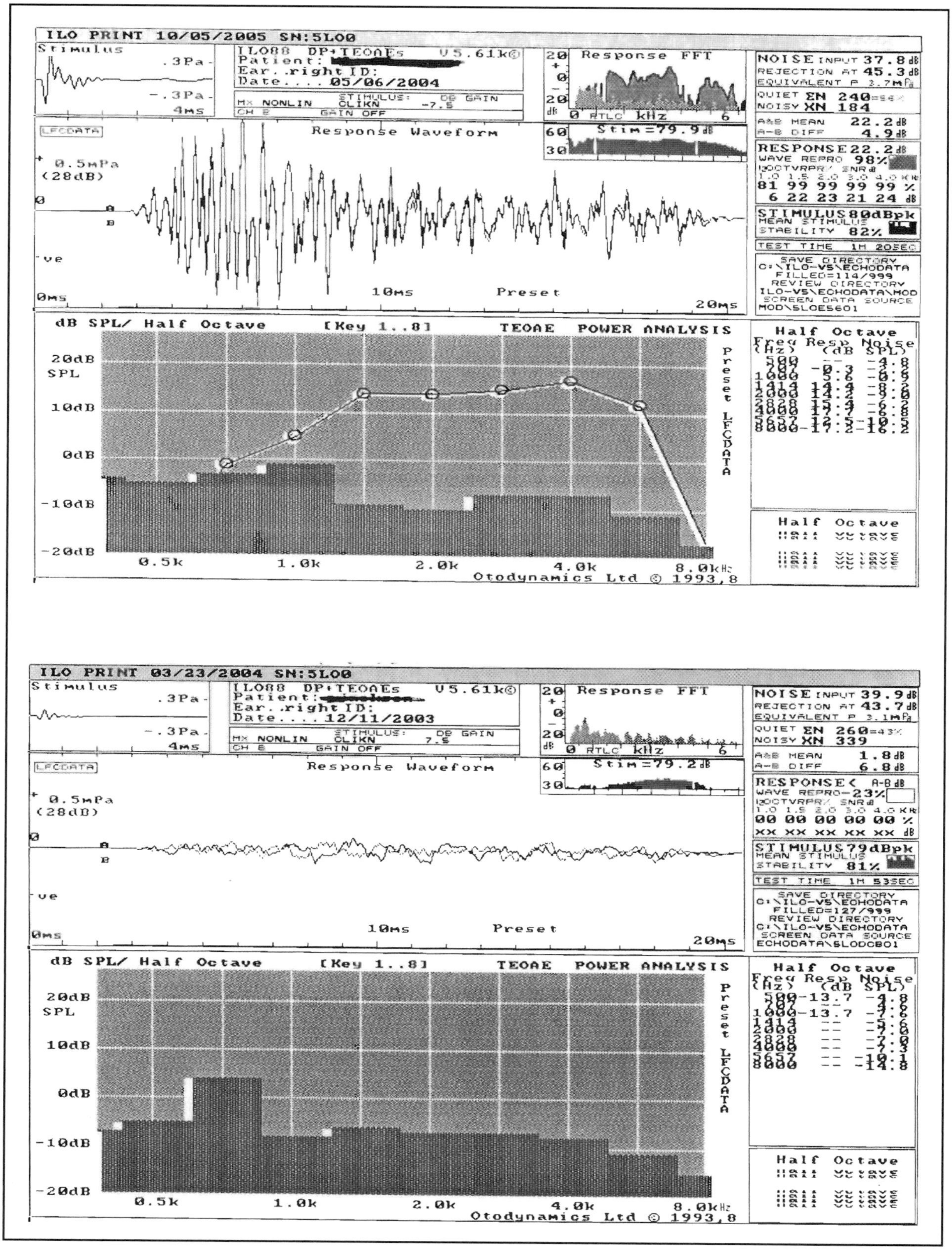

FIGURE 19–1. TEOAEs measured using clinical equipment from one manufacturer. The top panel illustrates TEOAEs from an infant with normal hearing measured by ABR tone burst thresholds. The bottom panel illustrates recordings from an infant with severe-to-profound hearing loss.

in the presence of the stimulating tones and are detected using narrowband filtering. The DPOAE level measured in the ear canal is dependent on the primary frequency ratio (f_2/f_1) of the stimulus tones, their levels (L_1 and L_2), and level difference (e.g., $L_1 > L_2$). When only f_2/f_1 was varied for a particular frequency region, it was determined that on average across frequency, an f_2/f_1 of 1.21 produced the largest DPOAE levels in normally hearing ears. However, narrower and wider ratios produced larger DPOAE amplitudes at higher and lower frequencies, respectively (Dreisbach & Siegel, 2001; Gaskill & Brown, 1990). It has also been determined that unequal stimulus levels generate the highest DPOAE levels for stimulus levels less than 70 dB SPL, regardless of frequency (Dreisbach & Siegel, 2005; Gaskill & Brown, 1990; Whitehead, Stagner, Lonsbury-Martin, & Martin, 1995). The DPOAE level is more dependent on L_1 than L_2, so for low and moderate stimulus levels L_1 should be greater than L_2 (e.g., L_1 = 65 and L_2 = 50 dB SPL; Whitehead et al., 1995).

Figure 19–2 illustrates the most common clinical method for measuring DPOAEs, referred to as a "DP-gram." The f_2/f_1 is usually fixed at approximately 1.2 and L_1 and L_2 are in the range of 65 and 55 dB SPL, respectively. The f_2 and f_1 sample a range of fixed frequencies, with f_2 ranging between 0.7 and 6 kHz. The DPOAE levels at $2f_1$-f_2 in dB SPL for each f_2 frequency are plotted as a function of f_2 frequency in an infant. The top panel illustrates data from an infant with normal DPOAEs and the bottom panel illustrates responses from an infant with severe sensorineural hearing loss. With current clinical equipment, DPOAEs can be recorded in patients with greater hearing loss and at higher test frequencies than TEOAEs (DeVries & Decker, 1992; Dreisbach & Siegel, 2001). Typical clinical measures of DPOAEs include their level (in dB SPL) and the ENR for a given frequency. It is typical for the noise floor to be averaged across adjacent frequency bins higher and lower than the DPOAE frequency.

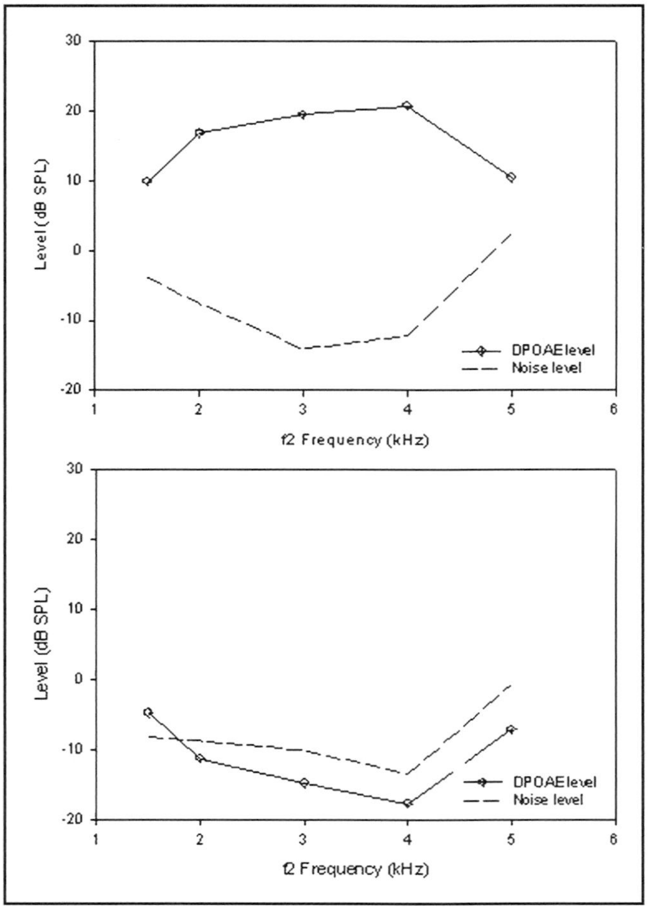

FIGURE 19–2. DPOAEs measured using clinical equipment. The top panel illustrates DPOAEs from an infant with normal hearing measured by ABR tone-burst thresholds. The bottom panel illustrates recordings from an infant with severe-to-profound hearing loss. The solid lines depict DPOAE levels and the dashed lines depict the noise floor.

Stimulus-Frequency Otoacoustic Emissions

A stimulus-frequency otoacoustic emission (SFOAE) is evoked with a single, pure tone. When measuring SFOAEs the evoking probe tone must be differentiated from the emission. One way to differentiate between the emission and the probe tone is based on the cochlear phenomenon of suppression. This is accomplished by subtracting two recordings of the sound measured in the ear canal; one when the probe tone is presented alone and another when the probe tone is presented along with a suppressor tone. The assumption is that the suppressor tone will reduce the emission in response to the evoking stimulus (Brass & Kemp, 1991, 1993; Dreisbach, 1999; Souter, 1995), so that the subtracted waveform (after the stimuli are removed) is the SFOAE evoked by the probe tone. SFOAEs using this methodology are shown in Figure 19–3. Other ways to measure SFOAEs is to vary the level of the stimulus from a high intensity stimulus to a low intensity stimulus (Kemp & Chum, 1980; Probst et al., 1991) or use three equal-duration, equal-frequency, equal-level stimuli as described by Keefe (1998). SFOAEs are the most frequency specific OAE as they are evoked with a single probe tone and they occur in approximately 94% of

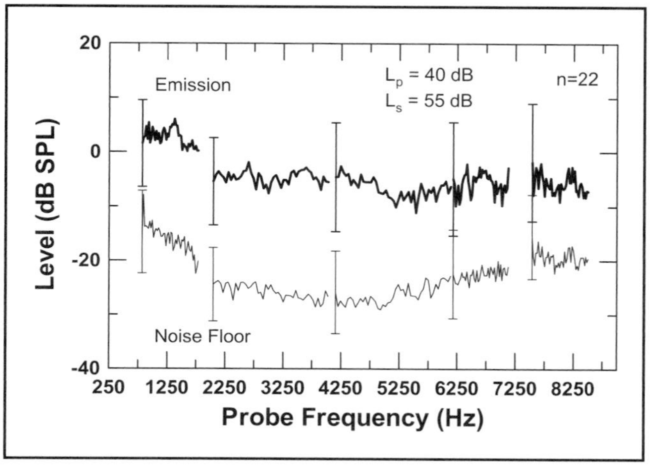

FIGURE 19–3. Average SFOAE responses from 22 adults are shown for varying frequency regions from approximately 750 to 8750 Hz with a probe tone of 40 dB SPL (L_p) and a suppressor tone 43 Hz less than the probe tone frequency and a level of 55 dB SPL (L_s). The SFOAE is indicated by heavy solid lines and the average noise floor is shown with thin solid lines. Standard errors are shown for each frequency region for both the SFOAE and noise floor.

examined normal hearing humans (Probst et al., 1991). SFOAEs currently are not measured in clinical settings. However, their utility to detect hearing loss has been explored in a laboratory study in 85 ears with normal hearing and hearing loss (Ellison & Keefe, 2005). Additional studies measuring SFOAEs in clinical settings are necessary before determining whether they may be useful in the diagnostic test battery.

Developmental Changes in OAEs

TEOAEs and DPOAEs in normal-hearing ears change over the life span, with the most rapid changes occurring during the early childhood years. The changes with development are frequency dependent, meaning that they are greater for some frequencies than others. In general, TEOAEs and DPOAEs increase in level from preterm through term birth, from birth to 1 month of age, then decrease in childhood. Thus, both TEOAEs and DPOAEs have higher levels in infants and young children than in older children and adults.

OAEs have been recorded from preterm newborns less than 25 weeks gestational age (Gorga et al., 2000; Norton et al., 2000a). Cross-sectional (Abdala Oba & Ramanathan, 2008; Gorga et al., 2000; Norton et al., 2000a) and longitudinal (Abdala et al., 2008; Smurzynski, 1994) data from infants cared for in the NICU suggest that DPOAEs and TEOAEs can be measured over broad frequency ranges from 1.0 to 5.6 kHz and that OAE levels increase for most frequencies with increasing postconceptional age (PCA). Between birth and 1 month of age (newborns), TEAOEs increase in level across half-octave bands centered from 1.5 to 4 kHz by an average of 4 to 7 dB, with levels in the 3 and 4 kHz bands increasing more than those centered at 1.5 and 2 kHz (Prieve, Hancur-Bucci, & Preston, 2009). DPOAE levels do not appear to change in babies 40 weeks PCA through 6 months of age (Abdala et al., 2008; Gorga et al., 2000; Zang & Jiang, 2007), although slight decreases have been noted at 12 months of age (Zang & Jiang, 2007).

OAE levels decrease significantly during childhood for frequencies higher than 1 kHz. Cross-sectional data indicate that DPOAE and TEOAE levels are higher in infants than toddlers, preschoolers and adults. Children aged 1 to 5 years have significantly higher OAE levels than do school-age children and adults (Groh et al., 2006; Kon, Inagaki, & Kaga, 2000; Prieve, Fitzgerald, & Schulte, 1997a; Prieve, Fitzgerald, Schulte, & Kemp, 1997b). These developmental changes occur whether or not an infant or child has SOAEs (Prieve et al., 1997a, 1997b).

Contributors to Developmental Changes in OAEs

The most obvious reasons for developmental changes in OAEs are growth of the outer and middle ears, which go through significant anatomic changes with development. At birth, the human ear canal wall is composed mostly of soft tissue (McLellan & Webb, 1957). Unlike older children and adults, who have a bony portion of their ear canals, infants have only a thick layer of cartilage (Anson & Donaldson, 1981). The tympanic membrane relative to the ear-canal wall is almost horizontal in newborns, and the angle increases with maturation (Ikui, Sando, Sudo, & Fujita, 1997; Northern & Downs, 2002). Not surprisingly, the transmission of sound through the ear canal changes with development. Acoustic estimates of the ear-canal area (Keefe & Abdala, 2007; Keefe, Bulen, Arehart, & Burns, 1993) and length (Keefe et al., 1993) increase through infancy until 2 years of age (the oldest participants that were studied). Because of the smaller cross-sectional areas of infant ears, a model predicts that the level of sound in the newborn ear canal is greater by 18 dB than it is in the adult ear canal (Keefe & Abdala, 2007).

The tympanic cavity also enlarges with development (Anson & Donaldson, 1981). Model estimates of tympanic cavity volume are 454 mm^3 in infants and 640 mm^3 in adults (Ikui, Sando, Haginomori, & Sudo, 2000). In the first 6 months of life the distance between the tympanic membrane and footplate of the stapes increases (Eby & Nadol, 1986). Developmental changes have also been noted in middle ear measures. Middle-ear admittance (Holte, Margolis, & Cavanaugh, 1991) increases in the first 2 years of life, with greater increases for frequencies around 1 kHz than for lower frequencies (Holte et al., 1991; Prieve, Chasmawala, & Jackson, 2005). Conductance (Keefe et al., 2000) increases with development. There is some disagreement on whether energy reflectance through the ear canal and middle ear system change with development, however, these differences may be due to calibration and estimation of the ear-canal area (Hunter, Tubaugh, Jackson, & Propes, 2008b; Keefe et al., 1993; Keefe & Abdala, 2007). Based on a model of ear canal and middle ear transmission based on energy reflectance and DPOAEs, Keefe and Abdala (2007) determined that the forward flow of energy into the cochlea is lower in infants than it is in adults, but because of the smaller ear-canal area, the reverse flow of power into the ear canal is seven times greater than that of adults. The general trend for decreasing DPOAE level with development is explained mostly by the rapid increase in ear-canal area. The model described by Keefe and Abdala (2007) accounts for all but 4 dB of DPOAE level differences between infants and adults.

OAEs as Part of the Audiologic Test Battery in Pediatric Populations

OAEs are a standard part of pediatric diagnostic protocols. It has long been observed that OAEs are absent or reduced in people with cochlear hearing loss (e.g., Kemp, 1978; Probst et al., 1991). However, as pediatric clinicians, we need to know the best criteria that will separate normal from impaired ears and the accuracy with which the criteria predict hearing loss. In addition, it must be taken into account if developmental changes influence clinical decisions. The studies referred to in this chapter review only those that included some children under the age of 10 years in their data sets.

Both TEOAEs and DPOAEs are excellent predictors of hearing loss in children (Glattke, Pafitis, Cummisky, & Herer, 1995; Harrison & Norton, 1999), mixed populations of children and adults (Gorga et al., 1997, 2005; Hussain, Gorga, Neely, Keefe, & Peters, 1998; Prieve et al., 1993), newborns (Norton et al., 2000b) and infants (Prieve et al., 2009). Based on relative operating curve (ROC) characteristics, the accuracy of identification of hearing loss is best from 2 to 4 kHz, with identification of hearing loss poorer at 0.75, 1, 6, and 8 kHz (Gorga et al., 1997, 2000, 2005; Hussain et al., 1998; Nicholson, 2003; Norton et al., 2000b; Prieve et al., 1993). When several different OAE parameters (such as OAE level and the surrounding noise for various frequencies) are included in a multiple variable analysis, identification of hearing loss at low frequencies improves dramatically (Gorga, Neely, & Dorn, 1999; Gorga et al., 2005; Hussain et al., 1998). Although ROC analysis is an excellent technique for describing the "goodness" of a clinical test for identifying hearing loss, it is difficult to ascertain what response criteria result in a particular hit/false alarm rate. Currently, two methods are in use clinically: templates and ENR.

Templates

Templates include the distribution of OAE levels from normal and impaired ears. OAE templates were first introduced for DPOAEs by Gorga and his colleagues (1997). DPOAEs and hearing thresholds were measured in 806 patients ranging in age from 1.3 to 96.5 years, resulting in a total of 1,267 ears. The levels of f_2 and f_1 were 55 and 65 dB SPL, respectively and the f_2/f_1 was 1.22. Cumulative distributions were plotted as a function of DPOAE level in ears with normal hearing and hearing loss, so that any combination of "hit," "true positive," "true negative," and "correct rejections" could be found for any DPOAE criterion. Based on these distributions, templates were constructed, a replica of which is shown on the left side of Figure 19–4. This DP-gram has four solid lines plotted on it, two representing levels from normally-hearing ears and two representing levels from ears with hearing loss. The lowest line represents the fifth percentile of DPOAE level for normally hearing ears (≤ 20 dB HL). The line just above it represents the 10th percentile of DPOAE levels from normally hearing ears. The top two lines represent the 90th and 95th percentiles, respectively, of DPOAE levels in ears with hearing loss. If a clinician is testing a patient, and the DPOAEs from that ear fall below the fifth percentile from ears with normal hearing, there is reasonable confidence that the ear has a hearing loss. If the DPOAE level falls above the 95th percentile for ears with hearing loss, we are reasonably confident that the ear is normally hearing. If the DPOAEs fall above the 10th percentile from normally hearing ears and below the 90th percentile for ears

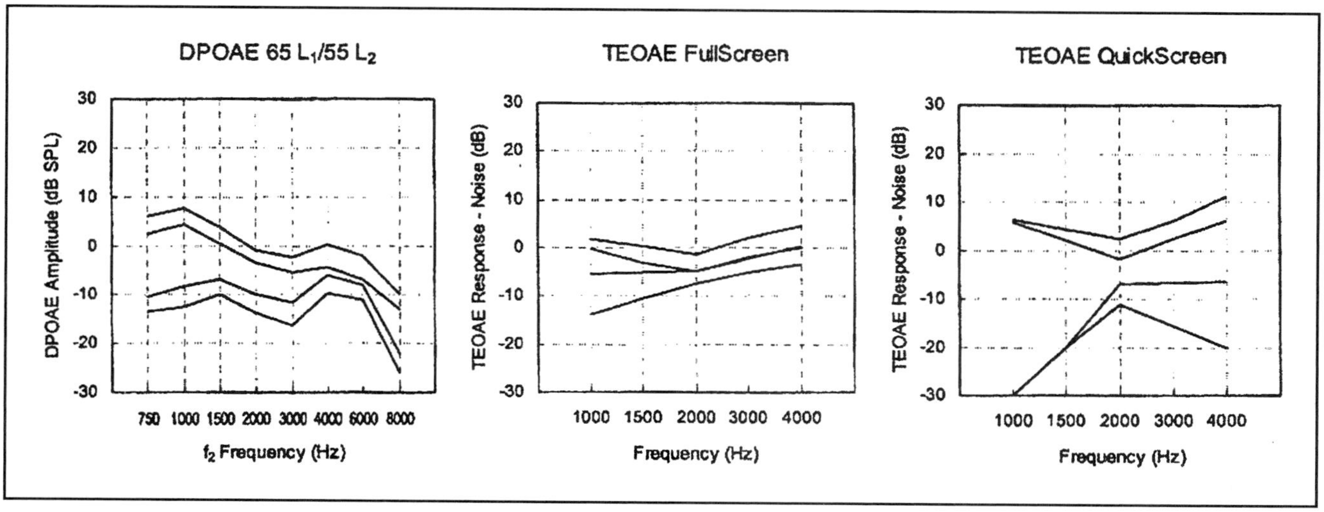

FIGURE 19–4. Illustrations of DPOAE (*left panel*), TEOAE Full-Screen (*middle panel*), and TEOAE Quickscreen (*right panel*) templates. Reprinted with permission from Nicholson, N., and Widen, J. (2007). "Evoked Otoacoustic Emissions in the Evaluation of Children. " In M. Robinette and T. Glattke (Eds.), *Otoacoustic Emissions: Clinical Application* (3rd ed., p. 379), Thieme, Copyright 2007.

with hearing loss, then it is uncertain whether the ear is normally hearing or has hearing loss because these OAE levels are within the overlapping ranges from these two populations. However, there is some evidence that OAE responses in this range may come from ears with mild hearing loss (Gorga et al., 2005; Nicholson & Widen, 2007).

Nicholson (2003) and Nicholson and Widen (2004) applied this template technique for TEAOEs measured with the ILO88 equipment using the FullScreen and QuickScreen modes (see Robinette & Glattke, 2007 for detailed information on these two types of stimulus/recording paradigms). Nicholson and Widen measured TEOAEs using the FullScreen mode on 240 ears of 135 participants aged 3.1 to 29.1 years and the QuickScreen mode in 84 ears of 49 participants aged 1.0 to 17.5 years. For both of these studies, the TEOAEs were analyzed into half-octave bands and the click stimulus was presented at 80 dB ±3 dB pSPL. A minimum of 50 averages contributing to the final OAE was required. The resulting template for TEOAE level using the FullScreen is shown in the middle panel and that for the QuickScreen mode is shown in the right panel of Figure 19–4. Templates such as these can be used in clinical decision-making to determine whether a particular ear has normal hearing or hearing loss. Nicholson and Widen (2007) present individual case studies in children using these templates.

Gorga and colleagues have developed another template for DPOAEs. Instead of DPOAE level or ENR, the template uses the probability that an ear has normal hearing. They used the Logit function (LF) coefficient constants generated by their earlier work (Dorn et al., 1999), and applied them to a new data set. In the new data set, DPOAEs were collected using the Biologic Scout system (version 3.45) from 345 ears of 187 participants ranging in age from 2 to 86 years (median = 29.7 years) with the same collection parameters used in their earlier work (Gorga et al., 1997). ROC curves and the area underneath them using the new data were similar to their former results, confirming that the equations could be generalized to new data sets. Similar to their previous work, they found that using the LF scores rather than DPOAE levels or ENR alone resulted in larger areas under ROC curves, especially for lower frequency primaries. Also similar to their previous work, many participants with mild hearing loss in the new data set met "passing" DPOAE criteria. Most interesting in this study was the way they transformed LF scores to the probability that an ear was normal, denoted as P(N). This conversion allowed for data from individual patients to be converted to a probability that the results were from a normal ear. Although there is no commercial equipment that currently makes the conversion automatically, clinicians could use the information in this manuscript to compute it themselves.

Before using a published template in the clinic, audiologists will want to ensure that their equipment and recording parameters are similar to those used to construct the template. In addition, the patients seen by the clinician should be similar to, or at least included in the population tested and used to construct the template. For example, Figure 19–5 compares cumulative distributions of DPOAE levels for two groups of patients that were different in age ranges and tested with different DPOAE systems. The black lines illustrate data collected from over 1200 normally hearing ears aged 1 to 96 years using the laboratory precurser of the Bio-Logic Scout® (Gorga et al., 1997). The gray lines illustrate DPOAE levels collected from 45 ears of infants aged 3 to 35 weeks (median is approximately 10 weeks) using the Otodynamics system. All infants had hearing within normal limits based on air- and tone-burst ABR thresholds (Vander Werff, Prieve, & Georgantas, 2009). Each line type represents DPOAE level by a different f_2 frequency. The graph illustrates that DPOAE levels from young infants tested with the Otodynamics system are higher than those from a mixed population of children and adults tested with a different system. The higher level DPOAEs measured from the infants would move the lower two lines on the DPOAE template shown in the left panel of Figure 19–4 to a higher position on the template. These data suggest that clinicians may want to validate that the templates they are using in their clinics are appropriate for their data collection system and the patient population.

ENR Criteria

Many clinicians use a priori ENR criteria to assess DPOAEs. Gorga, Neely, and Dorn (1999) performed an analysis on the a priori DPOAE criteria of 3, 6, and 9 dB DPOAE/noise ratios for various combinations of audiometric behavioral thresholds. There are many significant findings reported in this article and only a few are mentioned here. First, they found that using their most stringent criteria, 9 dB, the accuracy with which DPOAEs identified hearing loss was never more than 90%. Most errors were made when hearing loss ranged between 21 and 40 dB HL, with sensitivity approaching 100% for hearing loss greater than 40 dB HL (Gorga et al., 1999). A second important finding is that using an a priori criterion of 6 dB ENR to diagnose hearing loss using four f_2 frequencies (2, 3, 4, and 6 kHz),

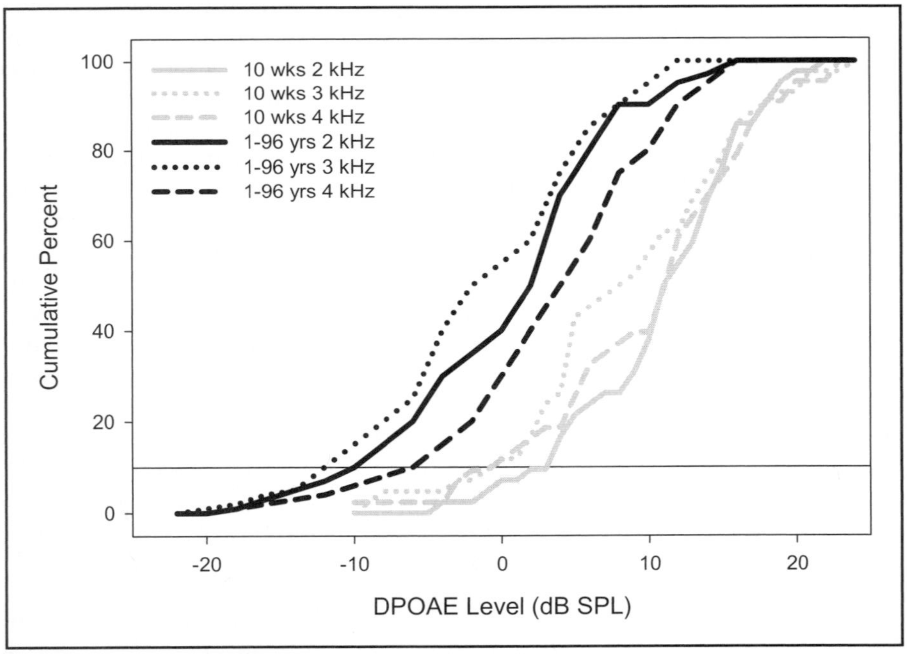

FIGURE 19–5. Cumulative distributions for normally hearing ears from Gorga et al., 1997 and a group of infants tested with the Otodynamics equipment. Reprinted with permission from Prieve, B. A. (2007). "Otoacoustic Emissions in Infants and Children." In J. R. Madell and C. Flexer (Eds.), *Pediatric Audiology: Diagnosis, Technology and Management* (p. 128), Thieme, Copyright 2007.

identified severe and profound hearing loss at approximately 100% and moderate hearing loss close to 100%. The ability to identify hearing loss using three f_2 frequencies was slightly lower. The results suggest that using either three, four, or five frequencies improves identification of hearing loss in an ear instead of using just one frequency. Although not addressed in this study, clinicians should be aware of default protocols on equipment for a "passing" OAE may be set at meeting an ENR criterion at 3/3, 3/4, or 4/5 f_2 frequencies without specifying at which frequencies the criteria were met. Often in infants and young children, acceptable ENR at lower frequencies (i.e., 1.5 kHz) may not be possible because of high noise levels. However, sometimes a child will meet ENR criteria at 1.5, 2, and 3 kHz, but not 4 kHz, meeting 3 out of 4 criteria to pass a screen. If a baby does not have OAEs at high frequencies, this may truly indicate hearing loss, as noise in this frequency band is usually quite low. It is important to note *why* a child doesn't meet ENR criteria at a particular frequency: whether the noise level is high, or whether the noise level is low and it is likely an OAE is not present. A final, critical note is that audiologists should not be performing the same ENR screen on pediatric diagnostic patients as they do for newborn hearing screening. Diagnostic tests are meant to capture a higher number of people with hearing loss because the prevalence of hearing loss in a diagnostic population is higher than that in a general, newborn population. Stricter criteria or broader frequency regions may be used to determine whether low-frequency or high-frequency areas of the cochlea may be functioning. In summary, the results from OAE studies in infants and children in clinical populations establish their use in a pediatric test protocol, although clear OAE criteria in infants are still emerging.

Effect of Middle Ear Status on OAEs

OAEs are affected by even slight changes in the middle ear. Although the cochlea produces OAEs, the evoking stimulus must pass through the external and middle ears to the cochlea to evoke the OAEs. The OAEs travel back through the middle ear into the ear canal, so minor changes can alter their levels. TEOAE and DPOAE levels are reduced in infants and children having negative tympanometric peak pressure (TPP) as measured from tympanograms (Choi, Pafitis, & Zalzal, 1999; Hof, Anteunis, Chenault, & van Dijk, 2005a; Hof, van Dijk, Chenault, & Anteunis, 2005b; Koike & Wetmore, 1999; Koivunen, Uhari, Laitakari, Alho, & Luotonen, et al., 2000; Lonsbury-Martin, Martin, McCoy, & Whitehead, 1994; Owens et al., 1993; Prieve, Calandruccio, Fitzgerald, Georgantas, & Mazevski, 2008). The reduction of OAE level is not correlated with the severity of the negative pressure (Koike & Wetmore, 1999; Prieve et al., 2008; Trine, Hirsch, & Margolis, 1993). Prieve and colleagues (2008) measured TEOAEs in infants and toddlers when their TPP was normal and again when it was negative. They found an approximately 4 dB reduction in TEOAE level for frequency bands from 1 to 4 kHz. The mean change in TPP between the two measurements was −169 daPa. The mean level reduction in TEOAE level between the two sessions was statistically significant, however, when using a 6 dB ENR criterion as a "passing" OAE, there was not a significant change in "pass" rate. In children, small changes in "pass" rates using a priori criteria have been reported (Hof et al., 2005b; Koike & Wetmore, 1999). Taken together, research results suggest that although negative TPP reduces OAE level, it may not be a major problem for infants and children undergoing a diagnostic test battery.

The situation is quite different when tympanograms have no measurable peak ("flat"). OAEs are dramatically reduced in level and often are not measurable in children having "flat" tympanograms (Choi et al., 1999; Koike & Wetmore, 1999; Koivunen et al., 2000; Lonsbury-Martin et al., 1994; Owens et al., 1993). Absent TEOAEs is a common finding in children with confirmed otitis media, most often when middle ear fluid is viscous (Amedee, 1995) or when there is a large quantity of effusion (Koivunen et al., 2000). Absence of OAEs have also been compared to elevated energy reflectance through the external/middle ear (Hunter, Bagger-Sjöbäck, & Lundberg, 2008a; Keefe, Gorga, Neely, & Zhao, 2003). Audiologists should be aware that OAEs are measurable in a portion of cases in infants and children with otitis media, flat tympanograms, or elevated energy reflectance (Prieve, 2009). Infants and children with negative TPP often have measurable, but reduced-level OAEs. Because the importance of obtaining some idea of whether there is sensory loss is critical, clinicians should still include OAEs in the test battery even in infants and children whose tympanograms are flat or have negative TPP.

Future Directions

As we have learned more about how otoacoustic emissions are generated, the way we classify OAEs has evolved. Additionally, different methodologies have been employed that may be more sensitive to cochlear change in comparison to traditional, clinical methodologies. A few of these topics are discussed in this section.

Measurement Versus Mechanism Based OAEs

OAEs can be classified as measurement or mechanism based. Measurement based OAEs, meaning they are described based on the stimuli (or lack thereof) used to evoke them, were previously discussed. Mechanism based OAEs relate to how an emission is generated in the cochlea. It has been theorized that emissions can arise by linear reflection, known as reflection emissions, or they can arise by nonlinear distortion, known as distortion emissions. Reflection emissions are hypothesized to be due to random impedance perturbations or irregularities along the cochlear partition that cause a reflection of energy. The types of irregularities that actually cause the reflection in the cochlea are unknown and Kemp (2002) has recommended that reflection emissions can be further differentiated between potentially passive mechanisms, such as an irregularity in hair cell number, and active mechanisms, such as variation in cochlear amplifier gain. Distortion emissions are thought to arise from nonlinearities associated with the injection of energy into basilar membrane motion by the action of the cochlear amplifier, which in turn, produces cochlear traveling waves. SOAEs measured in the absence of deliberate, acoustic stimulation are an example of linear reflection. All evoked emissions are a combination of linear reflection and nonlinear distortion mechanisms. SFOAEs and TEOAEs are reflection emissions at low levels and distortion emissions at high levels, whereas DPOAEs are always initiated by nonlinear distortion and may have additional reflection components (Shera, 2004; Shera & Guinan, 1999). Thus, using the mechanism based classification of OAEs, at low levels SOAEs, SFOAEs, and TEOAEs are generated similarly, whereas DPOAEs differ. The details of the mechanism(s) responsible for these theories are still under investigation and continue to refine the theories (He, Fridberger, Porsov, Grosh, & Ren, 2008; Siegel et al., 2005). It is uncertain how this information will be used clinically. One recent report failed to show an improvement in identification of hearing loss using only the DPOAE distortion component in adult ears (Johnson et al., 2007). However, further investigation into using a combination of both distortion and reflection emissions is still under investigation, especially in infants and children.

DPOAE Input/Output and Group Delay

In addition to the DP-gram, other characteristics of DPOAEs that may provide the clinician with information regarding cochlear function in a specified frequency region are input/output (I/O) functions and group delay. To create a DPOAE I/O function, the stimulus frequencies (f_1 and f_2) and ratio (f_2/f_1) are fixed and both stimulus levels (L_1 and L_2) can be varied together, with or without a level difference between them, or one stimulus level can be varied (L_1) as the other stimulus level (L_2) is fixed. In the later scenario, the response at low stimulus levels grows linearly and becomes compressive with increasing levels (e.g., Dorn et al., 2001). Figure 19–6A represents results for 12 kHz using this later scenario. From the resultant DPOAE I/O function, the slope of the function can be evaluated and a threshold can be determined. Typically, threshold is defined as the lowest stimulus level producing a DPOAE that is 3 dB above the noise floor with subsequent growth in level for successively higher stimulus levels. DPOAE I/O functions in cochlear impaired human ears reveal elevated thresholds, reduced compression, and a steeper slope of the I/O function in comparison to normal ears (Dorn et al., 2001; Janssen, Boege, Oestreicher & Arnold, 2000; Janssen, Kummer, & Arnold, 1998; Kummer, Janssen, & Arnold, 1998).

DPOAE group delay, the slope of the phase versus frequency curve, can be determined by varying the f_2/f_1 (e.g., 1.1 to 1.3) for a particular frequency region (e.g., $f_2 = 4$ kHz), keeping the stimulus levels constant. The group delay estimate is thought to be related to the region of origin of the DPOAE in the cochlea. The pattern of wave motion in the cochlea predicts a longer group delay as frequency decreases, corresponding to excitation of more apical locations. Studies of DPOAEs elicited throughout the range of human hearing show that the group delay estimate increases for $2f_1–f_2$ as the frequencies of the primary stimuli are lowered (Dreisbach & Siegel, 2001; Kimberley, Brown, & Eggermont, 1993; Moulin & Kemp, 1996; O'Mahoney & Kemp, 1995; Whitehead, Stagner, Martin, & Lonsbury-Martin, 1996). Figure 19–6B illustrates DPOAE group delay values for frequencies from 2 to 13 kHz. DPOAE group delay estimates involve travel times of the primary frequencies and the return trip of the DPOAE, as well as the delays associated with the response time of the cochlear filter. Therefore, DPOAE group delay estimate measurements may reflect changes in cochlear frequency selectivity that may be associated with a variety of sensorineural hearing losses (Whitehead et al., 1996). Significant differences between males and

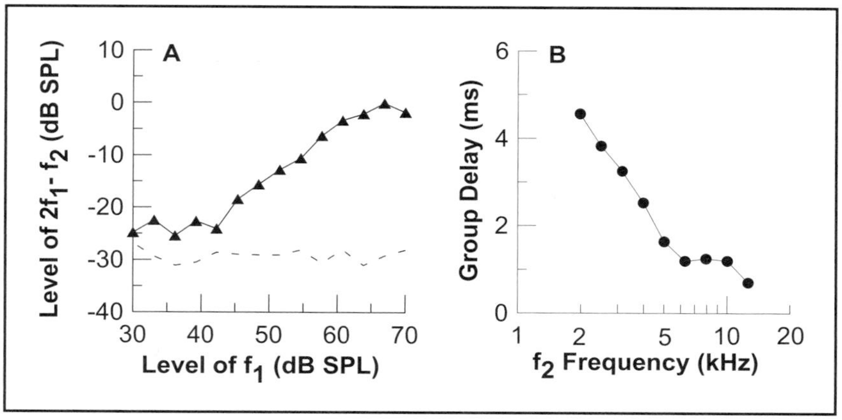

FIGURE 19–6. DPOAE I/O function for an f_2 of 12 kHz with L_2 fixed at 50 dB SPL and L_1 varied from 30 to 70 dB SPL in 3 dB steps with f_2/f_1 of 1. 2 **(A)**. DPOAE group delay **(B)** for f_2 from 2 to 13 kHz for one individual.

females have been reported for DPOAE group delay values in the lower frequencies (Bowman, Brown, & Kimberely, 2000; Dunckley & Dreisbach, 2004; Kimberley et al., 1993; Moulin & Kemp, 1996). These differences have been attributed to cochlear length according to gender.

Applications of DPOAE I/O functions and group delay calculations include ototoxic monitoring (drugs, noise) and determination of artifactual results. If the results from a DP-gram seem suspicious (e.g., large amplitude DPOAE(s) with a poor audiogram when cochlear damage is suspected), a DPOAE I/O function or group delay measurement can be made to determine if the results obtained in the DP-gram are of cochlear origin.

Monitoring Change due to Ototoxicity

Ill infants and children can be given drugs that cause ototoxicity. It has been shown that there is a higher incidence of hearing loss due to ototoxic medications in children than in adults who are exposed to ototoxic medications (e.g., Li, Womer, & Silber, 2004). Children less than 5 years of age at the time of treatment were 21 times more likely to acquire moderate-severe high-frequency hearing loss compared to those 15 to 20 years of age (Li et al., 2004). Because children are more susceptible to certain ototoxic agents than are adults it is critical for audiologists to monitor them for hearing loss.

Studies have shown that otoacoustic emission measures identify damage due to ototoxicity (drugs, noise) prior to threshold measures in both humans and animals (Biro, Baki, Buki, Noszekand, & Jokuti, 1997; Hall & Lutman, 1999; Katbamna, Homnick, & Marks, 1999; Littman, Magruder, & Strother, 1998; Mulheran & Degg, 1997; Plinkert & Krober, 1991; Ress et al., 1999; Sie & Norton, 1997; Stavroulaki, Nikolopoulos, Psarommatis, & Apostolopoulos, 2001b; Stavroulaki et al., 2002; Zorowka, Schmitt, & Gutjahr, 1993). Stavroulaki et al. (2001b) found that hearing loss predominantly occurred at high frequencies (HF), especially 12 kHz, for young patients with chronic renal failure having hemodialysis and that DPOAE levels were decreased whether patients did or did not have hearing loss up to 4 kHz versus age-matched controls. These authors suggested that DPOAE measures might possibly be more predictive in the case of substantial threshold shifts for a given frequency prior to a measurable sensitivity loss. Ress et al. (1999) reported that DPOAEs were as sensitive as HF audiometry for detecting changes in hearing due to cis-platinum ototoxicity, but that DPOAEs were superior to HF audiometry as an ototoxic screening tool. Measuring I/O functions to determine DPOAE detection thresholds, Mulheran and Degg (1997) found a significant elevation in the stimulus levels that generated a DPOAE at 4 kHz in young patients with cystic fibrosis (CF) receiving frequent aminoglycoside treatments with normal hearing from 0.25 to 8 kHz in comparison to control volunteers. The authors suggested that the elevation could represent an early change in OHC function caused by the treatment, or it could be a result of the CF condition. To differentiate the cause of reduced DPOAEs in patients with CF, Stavroulaki and colleagues (2002) compared behavioral audiometry and DPOAE measures in audiologically normal children with CF receiving and not receiving aminoglycosides and age-matched healthy volunteers. They found that the CF group receiving aminoglycosides had significantly lower DPOAE levels at 5 kHz compared to the children with CF not receiving aminoglycosides and the healthy volunteers. Thus, the reduction in DPOAE levels was attributed to the aminoglycoside treatments, not the CF condition. At the end of the treatments, the children with CF still had normal behavioral thresholds but exhibited further decreases in DPOAE levels at frequencies higher than 3 kHz. Based on their results when examining children who received a first cisplatin-infusion, Stavroulaki, Apostolopoulos, Segas, Tsakanikos, and Adamopoulos (2001a) concluded that DPOAE levels were sensitive indicators of cochlear damage and were superior to behavioral audiometry for identifying cochlear changes due to aminoglycosides (up to 8 kHz). In a case report by Littman et al. (1998), they found that DPOAE levels that were present at baseline testing were in the noise floor following treatment radiation, cisplatin, and etoposide when behavioral thresholds at the same frequency were unchanged. Thus, these authors suggested that DPOAE testing has the possibility of being predictive of the earliest stages of progressive hearing loss before changes are noted behaviorally.

When comparing different DPOAE paradigms, Katbamna et al. (1999) found that DPOAE group delay and detection threshold values, determined from I/O functions, were earlier indicators of cochlear ototoxicity compared to conventional and HF behavioral hearing thresholds and the more common DPOAE level measures obtained from DP-grams in a group of children and young adults with CF receiving tobramycin. Group delay values were reduced or prolonged, dependent on cumulative doses of tobramycin, and some of the subjects demonstrated significant elevations in DPOAE detection thresholds compared to controls. These results suggest that assessment of DPOAE group delay and detection thresholds may be more effective tools for monitoring cochlear ototoxicity than the more traditional DP-gram.

In addition to cochlear changes due to ototoxicity, TEOAE and DPOAE amplitude measures, as well as DPOAE group delay calculations, have been monitored to evaluate temporary and permanent effects of noise on hearing. Noise exposure is a public health issue in children, with reports that 5.2 million children aged 6 to 19 years have hearing loss directly related to excessive levels of noise (Niskar et al., 2001). Furthermore, studies in animals suggest that exposure to noise early in life produces neural, but undetected peripheral changes as the individual ages (Kujawa & Liberman, 2006). For an extensive review of the effects of noise on OAE levels, the reader is referred to Lapsley, Miller, and Marshall (2007). Similar to ototoxicity, group delay may be important for evaluating the effects of noise on hearing. DPOAEs have a shorter group delay in individuals after noise exposure, producing temporary effects (Engdahl & Kemp, 1996; Kramer et al., 2006). However, longer group delays have been found in miners with long-term histories (8–15 years) of exposure to occupational noise than for healthy young adults (Namyslowski, Morawski, Trybalska, & Urbaniec, 2004). These results suggest that group delay might be a way to measure noise exposure with expectations being that group delay may depend on the duration of exposure and/or underlying physiologic consequences of noise exposure. Telischi, Stagner, Widick, Balkany, and Lonsbury-Martin (1998) found that changes in group delay occurred much sooner (1–5 seconds) than DPOAE amplitude changes (15–30 seconds) following interruption of cochlear blood flow.

In the discussions above, OAEs were used for monitoring cochlear change because DPOAE testing has been found to be repeatable over short and long periods of time (Beattie & Bleech, 2000; Beattie, Kenworthy, & Luna, 2003; Cacace, McClelland, Weiner, & McFarland, 1996; Franklin, McCoy, Martin, & Lonsbury-Martin, 1992; Roede, Harris, Probst, & Xu, 1993; Shehata-Dieler, Dieler, Teichert, & Moser, 1999; Zhao & Stephens, 1999) allowing for the possibility that a patient's inner ear function can be monitored during prolonged noise exposure and the administration of ototoxic medications. When testing during the same trial (test-retest) or across 5 to 10 days, DPOAE levels differing by more than 6 to 7 dB can be determined to be significantly different (Beatie & Bleech, 2000; Beattie et al., 2003). DPOAEs are also stable over longer periods of time. Franklin et al. (1992) reported that DPOAE levels were repeatable in normally hearing adults over consecutive days and weeks using equal level primary tones over the $2f_1$-f_2 frequency range of 1 to 8 kHz. Some individuals demonstrated greater variability, especially at 1 and 8 kHz, but it was concluded that DPOAE testing can be used to monitor hearing with the expectation that only 5 percent of the population will have greater than a 4 dB change in DPOAE level during monitoring. Using a similar paradigm, Roede et al. (1993) concluded that a change of more than 6 to 9 dB in DPOAE level would constitute a significant change in cochlear status based on monitoring over a 6-week period. The greatest variability was noted at frequencies greater than 6 kHz. Dreisbach, Long, and Lees (2006) examined the repeatability of DPOAEs measured with HF stimuli (f_2 of 2-16 kHz) in normally hearing adult subjects across 4 trials. At each trial, DP-grams and ratio sweeps were used to measure DPOAE levels and calculate DPOAE group delay values, respectively. For DP-grams, greater variability was found in DPOAE levels for the higher frequencies. The average DPOAE level differences-between-trials for the higher (> 8 kHz) and lower (< 8 kHz) frequencies were 5.15 (SD = 4.40 dB) and 2.80 (SD = 2.70 dB) dB, respectively. For DPOAE group delay calculations, greater variability was noted at lower frequencies and at 10 kHz. The average difference-between-trials for the higher and lower frequencies was 0.22 (SD = 0.20 ms) and 0.28 (SD = 0.24 ms) ms, respectively. Even though the data obtained at frequencies greater than 8 kHz were more variable than at low frequencies, the responses at higher frequencies were not significantly different between trials for either paradigm tested. Thus, it seems that DPOAEs have excellent repeatability, even over time, so that changes greater than approximately 9 dB constitute a cochlear change. Future research is needed to determine if HF DPOAE shifts are capable of detecting initial changes due to ototoxicity, especially in children where behavioral measures may be difficult to obtain reliably.

Summary

In conclusion, OAEs are an essential part of the pediatric test battery because of their strong ties to cochlear health and ease of administration. In the future, it is possible that we may use them for monitoring ototoxicity and noise exposure, two significant causes of hearing loss in children.

References

Abdala, C., Oba, S., & Ramanathan, R. (2008). Changes in the DP-gram during the preterm and early postnatal period. *Ear and Hearing*, *29*, 512–523.

Amadee, R.G. (1995). The effects of chronic otitis media with effusion on the measurement of transiently evoked otoacoustic emissions. *Laryngoscope*, *105*, 589–595.

Anson, B. J., & Donaldson, J. A. (1981). *Surgical anatomy of the human temporal bone*. Philadelphia, PA: W. B. Saunders.

Beattie, R. C., & Bleech, J. (2000). Effects of sample size on the reliability of noise floor and DPOAE. *British Journal of Audiology*, *34*, 305–309.

Beattie, R. C., Kenworthy, O. T., & Luna, C. A. (2003). Immediate and short-term reliability of distortion-product otoacoustic emissions. *International Journal of Audiology*, *42*, 348–354.

Békèsy, G. von. (1960). *Experiments in hearing* (transl. and ed. by E. G. Wever). New York, NY: McGraw-Hill.

Bilger, R.C., Matthies, M. L., Hammel, D. R., & Demorest, M. E. (1990). Genetic implications of gender differences in the prevalence of spontaneous otoacoustic emissions. *Journal of Speech and Hearing Research*, *33*, 418–432.

Biro, K., Baki, M., Buki, B., Noszek, L., & Jokuti, L. (1997). Detection of early ototoxic effect in testicular-cancer patients treated with cisplatin by transiently evoked otoacoustic emission: A pilot study. *Oncology*, *54*, 387–390.

Bonfils, P. (1989). Spontaneous otoacoustic emissions: Clinical interest. *Laryngoscope*, *99*, 752–756.

Bonfils, P., Uziel, A., & Narcy, P. (1989). The properties of spontaneous and evoked acoustic emissions in neonates and children: A preliminary report. *Archives of Otorhinolaryngology*, *246*, 249–251.

Bowman, D. M., Brown, D. K., & Kimberley, B. P. (2000). An examination of gender differences in DPOAE phase delay measurements in normal-hearing human adults. *Hearing Research*, *142*, 1–11.

Brass, D., & Kemp, D. T. (1991). Time-domain observation of otoacoustic emissions during constant tone stimulation. *Journal of the Acoustical Society of America*, *90*, 2415–2427.

Brass, D., & Kemp, D. T. (1993). Suppression of stimulus frequency otoacoustic emissions. *Journal of the Acoustical Society of America*, *93*, 920–939.

Bray, P. J. (1989) *Click evoked otoacoustic emissions and the development of a clinical otoacoustic hearing test instrument*. Doctoral dissertation, University of London, UK.

Brienesse, P., Maertzdorf, W., Anteunis, L., Manni, J., & Blanco, C. (1998). Long-term and short-term variations in amplitude and frequency of spontaneous otoacoustic emissions in pre-term infants. *Audiology*, *37*, 278–284.

Brownell, W. E. (1990). Outer hair cell electromotility and otoacoustic emissions. *Ear and Hearing*, *11*, 82–92.

Burns, E. M. (2009). Long-term stability of spontaneous otoacoustic emissions. *Journal of the Acoustical Society of America*, *125*, 3166–3176.

Burns, E. M., Arehart, K. H., & Campbell, S. L. (1992). Prevalence of spontaneous otoacoustic emissions in neonates. *Journal of the Acoustical Society of America*, *91*, 1571–1575.

Burns, E. M., Campbell, S. L., & Arehart, K. H. (1994). Longitudinal measurements of spontaneous otoacoustic emissions in infants. *Journal of the Acoustical Society of America*, *95*, 385–394.

Cacace, A. T., McClelland, W. A., Weiner, J., & McFarland, D. J. (1996). Individual differences and the reliability of 2F1-F2 distortion-product otoacoustic emissions: Effects of time-of-day, stimulus variables, and gender. *Journal of Speech and Hearing Research*, *39*, 1138–1148.

Choi, S. S., Pafitis, I. A., & Zalzal, G. H. (1999). Clinical applications of the transiently evoked acoustic emissions in the pediatric population. *Annals of Otology, Rhinology, and Laryngology*, *108*, 132–138.

DeVries, S. M., & Decker, T. N. (1992). Otoacoustic emissions: Overview of measurement methodologies. *Seminars in Hearing, 13,* 15–22.

Dorn, P. A., Konrad-Martin, D., Neely, S. T., Keefe, D. H., Cyr, E., & Gorga, M. P. (2001). Distortion product otoacoustic emission input/output functions in normal-hearing and hearing-impaired human ears. *Journal of the Acoustical Society of America, 110,* 3119–3131.

Dorn, P. A., Piskorski, P., Gorga, M. P., Neely, S. T., & Keefe, D. H. (1999). Predicting audiometric status from distortion product otoacoustic emissions using multivariate analyses. *Ear and Hearing, 20,* 149–163.

Dreisbach, L. E. (1999). *Characterizing the $2f_1$-$2f_2$ distortion-product otoacoustic emission and its generators measured from 2 to 20 kHz in humans.* Ph.D. thesis, Northwestern University, Evanston, IL.

Dreisbach, L. E., Long, K. M., & Lees, S. E. (2006). Repeatability of high-frequency distortion-product otoacoustic emissions (DPOAEs) in normally hearing adults. *Ear and Hearing, 27,* 466–479.

Dreisbach, L. E., & Siegel, J. H. (2001). Distortion-product otoacoustic emissions measured at high frequencies in humans. *Journal of the Acoustical Society of America, 110,* 2456–2469.

Dreisbach, L. E., & Siegel, J. H. (2005). Level dependence of distortion-product otoacoustic emissions measured at high frequencies in humans. *Journal of the Acoustical Society of America, 117,* 2980–2988.

Dunckley, K. T., & Dreisbach, L. E. (2004). Gender effects on high frequency distortion product otoacoustic emissions in humans. *Ear and Hearing, 25,* 554–564.

Eby, T. L., & Nadol, Jr. J. B. (1986). Postnatal growth of the human temporal bone: Implications for cochlear implants in children. *Annals of Otoogy Rhinology and Laryngology, 95,* 356–364.

Ellison, J. C., & Keefe, D. H. (2005) Audiometric predictions using SFOAE and middle-ear measurements. *Ear and Hearing, 26,* 487–503.

Engdahl, B., & Kemp, D. T. (1996). The effect of noise exposure on the details of distortion product otoacoustic emissions in humans. *Journal of the Acoustical Society of America, 99,* 1573–1587.

Franklin, D. J., McCoy, M. J., Martin, G. K., & Lonsbury-Martin, B. L. (1992). Test/retest reliability of distortion product and transiently evoked otoacoustic emissions. *Ear and Hearing, 13,* 417–429.

Gaskill, S. A., & Brown, A. M. (1990). The behavior of the acoustic distortion product, 2f1-f2, from the human ear and its relation to auditory sensitivity. *Journal of the Acoustical Society of America, 88,* 821–839.

Glattke, T. J., Pafitis, I. A., Cummiskey, C., & Herer, G. R. (1995). Identification of hearing loss in children and young adults using measures of transient otoacoustic emission reproducibility. *America Journal of Audiology, 4,* 71–86.

Gorga, M. P., Dierking, D. M., Johnson, T. A., Beauchaine, K. L., Garner, C. A., & Neely, S. T. (2005). A validation and potential clinical application of multivariate analyses of distortion-product otoacoustic emission data. *Ear and Hearing, 26,* 593–607.

Gorga, M. P., Neely, S. T., & Dorn, P. A. (1999). DPOAE test performance for a priori criteria and for multifrequency audiometric standards. *Ear and Hearing, 20,* 345–362.

Gorga, M. P., Neely, S. T., Ohlrich, B., Hoover, B., Redner, J., & Peters, J. (1997). From laboratory to clinic: A large scale study of distortion product otoacoustic emissions in ears with normal hearing and ears with hearing loss. *Ear and Hearing, 18,* 440–455.

Gorga, M. P., Norton, S. J., Sininger, Y. S., Cone-Wesson, B., Folsom, R. C., Vohr, B. R., Widen, J. E., & Neely, S. T. (2000). Identification of neonatal hearing impairment: Distortion product otoacoustic emissions during the perinatal period. *Ear and Hearing, 21,* 400–424.

Groh, D., Pelanova, J., Jilek, M., Popelar, J., Kabelka, Z., & Syka, J. (2006). Changes in otoacoustic emissions and high-frequency hearing thresholds in children and adolescents. *Hearing Research, 212,* 90–98.

Guinan, J. (2006). Olivocochlear efferents: Anatomy, physiology, function and measurement of efferent effects in humans. *Ear and Hearing, 27,* 589–607.

Hall, A. J., & Lutman, M. E. (1999). Methods for early identification of noise-induced hearing loss. *Audiology, 38,* 277–280.

Harris, F. P., & Glattke, T. J. (1992). The use of suppression to determine the characteristics of otoacoustic emissions. *Seminars in Hearing, 13,* 67–80.

Harris, F. P., Lonsbury-Martin, B. L., Stagner, B. B., Coats, A. C., & Martin, G. K. (1989). Acoustic distortion products in humans: Systematic changes in amplitudes as a function of f2/f1 ratio. *Journal of the Acoustical Society of America, 85,* 220–229.

Harris, F. P., Probst, R., & Xu, L. (1992). Suppression of the 2f1-f2 otoacoustic emission in humans [published erratum appears in Hear Res, 1993; 66(1):121]. *Hearing Research, 64,* 133–141.

Harrison, W., & Norton, S. J. (1999). Characteristics of transient evoked otoacoustic emissions in normal-hearing and hearing-impaired children. *Ear and Hearing, 20,* 75–86.

He, W., Fridberger, A., Porsov, E., Grosh, K., & Ren, T. (2008). Reverse wave propagation in the cochlea. *Proceedings of the National Academy of Sciences, 105,* 2729–2733.

Heitmann, J., Waldmann, B., Schnitzler, H. U., Plinkert, P. K., & Zenner, H. P. (1998). Suppression growth functions of DPOAE with a suppressor near f1-f2 depends on DP fine structure—evidence for two generations sites of DPOAE. *Journal of the Acoustical Society of America, 103,* 1527–1531.

Hof, J. R., Anteunis, L. J. C., Chenault, M. N., & Van Dijk, P. (2005a). Otoacoustic emissions at compensated middle ear pressure in children. *International Journal of Audiology, 44,* 317–320.

Hof, J. R., van Dijk, P., Chenault, M. N., & Anteunis, L. J. C. (2005b). A two-step scenario for hearing assessment with otoacoustic emissions at compensated middle ear pressure (in children 1–7 years old). *International Journal of Pediatric Otorhinolaryngology, 69,* 649–655.

Holte, L., Margolis, R. H., & Cavanaugh, R. M. Jr. (1991). Developmental changes in multifrequency tympanograms. *Audiology, 30*, 1–24.

Hood, L. (2007). Suppression of otoacoustic emissions in normal individuals and in patients with auditory disorders. In M. Robinette and T. Glattke (Eds.), *Otoacoustic emissions: Clinical applications* (3rd ed., pp. 297–319). New York, NY: Thieme.

Hunter, L., Bagger-Sjöbäck, D., & Lundberg, M. (2008a). Wideband reflectance associated with otitis media in infants and children with cleft palate. *International Journal of Audiology, 47*(Suppl. 1), 57–61.

Hunter, L., Tubaugh, L., Jackson, A., & Propes, S. (2008b). Wideband middle ear power measurement in infants and children. *Journal of the American Academy of Audiology, 19*, 309–324.

Hussain, D. M., Gorga, M. P., Neely, S. T., Keefe, D. H., & Peters, J. (1998) Transient evoked otoacoustic emissions in patients with normal hearing and in patients with hearing loss. *Ear and Hearing, 19*, 434–449.

Ikui, A., Sando, I., Haginomori, S. -I, & Sudo, M. (2000). Postnatal development of the tympanic cavity: A computer-aided reconstruction and measurement study. *Acta Oto-Laryngologica, 120*, 375–379.

Ikui, A., Sando, I., Sudo, M., & Fujita, S. (1997). Postnatal changes in angle between the tympanic annulus and surrounding structures. *Annals of Otology Rhinology and Laryngology, 106*, 33–36.

Janssen, T., Boege, P., Oestreicher, E., & Arnold, W. (2000). Tinnitus and 2f1–f2 distortion product otoacoustic emissions following salicylate overdose. *Journal of the Acoustical Society of America, 107*, 1790–1792.

Janssen, T., Kummer, P., & Arnold, W. (1998). Growth behavior of the 2f1–f2 distortion product otoacoustic emission in tinnitus. *Journal of the Acoustical Society of America, 103*, 3418–3430.

Johnson, T. A., Neely, S. T., Kopun, J. G., Dierking, D. M., Tan, H., Converse, C., . . . Gorga, M. P. (2007). Distortion product otoacoustic emissions: Cochlear-source contributions and clinical test performance. *Journal of the Acoustical Society of America, 122*, 3539–3553.

Katbamna, B., Homnick, D. N., & Marks, J. H. (1999). Effects of chronic tobramycin treatment on distortion product otoacoustic emissions. *Ear and Hearing, 20*, 393–402.

Keefe, D. (1998). Double-evoked otoacoustic emissions. I. Measurement theory and nonlinear coherence. *Journal of the Acoustical Society of America, 103*, 3489–3498.

Keefe, D. H., & Abdala, C. (2007). Theory of forward and reverse middle-ear transmission applied to otoacoustic emissions in infant and adult ears. *Journal of the Acoustical Society of America, 121*, 978–993.

Keefe, D. H., Bulen, J. C., Arehart, K. H., & Burns, E. M. (1993). Ear-canal impedance and reflection coefficient in human infants and adults. *Journal of the Acoustical Society of America, 94*, 2617–2638.

Keefe, D. H., Folson, R. C., Gorga, M. P., Vohr, B. R., Bulen, J. C., & Norton, S. J. (2000). Identification of neonatal hearing impairment: Ear canal measurements of acoustic admittance and reflectance in neonates. *Ear and Hearing, 21*, 443–461.

Keefe, D. H., Gorga, M. P., Neely, S. T., & Zhao, F. (2003). Ear-canal acoustic admittance and reflectance measurements in human neonates. II. Predictions of middle-ear dysfunction and sensorineural hearing loss. *Journal of the Acoustical Society of America, 113*, 407–422.

Kemp, D. T. (1978). Stimulated acoustic emissions from the human auditory system. *Journal of the Acoustical Society of America, 64*, 3566–3576.

Kemp, D. T. (2002). Exploring cochlear status with otoacoustic emissions: The potential for new clinical applications. In M. S. Robinette & T. J. Glattke (Eds.), *Otoacoustic emissions: Clinical applications* (2nd ed., pp. 1–47). New York, NY: Thieme.

Kemp, D. T., & Brown, A. M. (1983). An integrated view of cochlear mechanical nonlinearities observable from the ear canal. In E. de Boer & M. A. Viergever (Eds.), *Mechanics of hearing* (pp. 75–82). Delft, Netherlands: Delft University Press.

Kemp, D. T., & Chum, R. A. (1980). Observations on the generation mechanism of stimulus frequency acoustic emissions—two tone suppression. In G. van den Brink, & F. A. Bilsen (Eds.), *Psychophysical, physiological and behavioral studies in hearing* (pp. 35–42). Delft, Netherlands: Delft University Press.

Kimberley, B. P., Brown, D. K., & Eggermont, J. J. (1993). Measuring human cochlear traveling wave delay using distortion product emission phase responses. *Journal of the Acoustical Society of America, 94*, 1343–1350.

Koike, K. J., & Wetmore, S. J. (1999). Interactive effects of the middle ear pathology and the associated hearing loss on transient-evoked otoacoustic emission measures. *Otolaryngology–Head and Neck Surgery, 121*, 238–244.

Koivunen, P., Uhari, M., Laitakari, K., Alho, O. -P., & Luotonen, J. (2000). Otoacoustic emissions and tympanometry in children with otitis media. *Ear and Hearing, 21*, 212–217.

Kok, M. R., van Zanten, G. A., & Brocaar, M. P. (1993). Aspects of spontaneous otoacoustic emissions in healthy newborns. *Hearing Research, 69*, 115–123.

Kon, K., Inagaki, M., & Kaga M. (2000). Developmental changes of distortion product and transient evoked otoacoustic emissions in different age groups. *Brain Development, 22*, 41–46.

Konrad-Martin, D., Neely, S. T., Keefe, D. H., Dorn, P. A., Cyr, E., & Gorga, M. P. (2002). Sources of DPOAEs revealed by suppression experiments, inverse fast Fourier transforms, and SFOAEs in impaired ears. *Journal of the Acoustical Society of America, 111*, 1800–1809.

Kramer, S., Dreisbach, L., Lockwood, J., Baldwin, K., Kopke, R., Scranton, S., & O'Leary, M., (2006). Efficacy of the antioxidant N-acetylcysteine (NAC) in protecting ears exposed to loud music. *Journal of the American Academy of Audiology, 17*, 265–278.

Kujawa, S. G., & Liberman, M. C. (2006). Acceleration of age-related hearing loss by early noise exposure: Evidence of a misspent youth. *Journal of Neuroscience, 26*, 2115–2123.

Kummer, P., Janssen, T., & Arnold, W. (1995). Suppression tuning characteristics of the 2f1-f2 distortion-product otoacoustic emission in humans. *Journal of the Acoustical Society of America, 98*(1), 197–210.

Kummer, P., Janssen, T., & Arnold, W. (1998). The level and growth behavior of the 2f1–f2 distortion product otoacoustic emission and its relationship to auditory sensitivity in normal hearing and cochlear hearing loss. *Journal of the Acoustical Society of America, 103*, 3431–3444.

Kuroda, T. (2007). Clinical investigation on spontaneous otoacoustic emission (SOAE) in 447 ears. *Auris Nasus Larynx, 34*, 29–38.

Lamprecht-Dinneson, A., Pohl, M., Hartmann, S., Heinecke, A., Ahrens, S., Muller, E., & Riebandt, M. (1998). Effects of age, gender, and ear side on SOAE parameters in infancy and childhood. *Audiology and Neuro-Otology, 3*, 386–401.

Lapsley Miller, J. A., & Marshall, L. (2007). Otoacoustic emissions as a preclinical measure of noise-induced hearing loss and susceptibility to noise-induced hearing loss. In M. S. Robinette & T. J. Glattke (Eds.), *Otoacoustic emissions: Clinical applications* (3rd ed., pp. 321–341). New York, NY: Thieme.

Li, Y., Womer, R. B., & Silber, J. H. (2004). Predicting cisplatin ototoxicity in children: The influence of age and the cumulative dose. *European Journal of Cancer, 40*, 2445–2451.

Liberman, M. C., Gao, J., He, D. Z., Wu, X., Jia, S., & Zuo, J. (2002). Prestin is required for electromotility of the outer hair cell and for the cochlear amplifier. *Nature, 419*, 300–304.

Liberman, M. C., Zuo, J., & Guinan, J. J., Jr. (2004). Otoacoustic emissions without somatic motility: Can stereocilia mechanics drive the mammalian cochlea? *Journal of the Acoustical Society of America, 116*, 1649–1655.

Littman, T. A., Magruder, A., & Strother, D. R. (1998). Monitoring and predicting ototoxic damage using distortion-product otoacoustic emissions: Pediatric case study. *Journal of the American Academy of Audiology, 9*, 257–262.

Lonsbury-Martin, B. L., Martin, G. K., McCoy, M. J., & Whitehead, M. L. (1994) Otoacoustic emissions testing in young children: Middle-ear influences. *American Journal of Otology, 15*(Suppl. 1), 13–20.

Manley, G. A., Kirk, D. L., Koppl, C., & Yates, G. K. (2001). In vivo evidence for a cochlear amplifier in the hair-cell bundle of lizards. *Proceedings of the National Academy of Sciences, USA, 98*, 2826–2831.

McLellan, M. S., & Webb, C. H. (1957). Ear studies in the newborn infant. *Journal of Pediatrics. 51*, 672–677.

Moulin, A., & Kemp, D. T. (1996). Multicomponent acoustic distortion product otoacoustic emission phase in humans. I. General characteristics. *Journal of the Acoustical Society of America, 100*, 1617–1639.

Mulheran, M., & Degg, C. (1997). Comparison of distortion product OAE generation between a patient group requiring frequent gentamicin therapy and control subjects. *British Journal of Audiology, 31*, 5–9.

Namyslowski, G., Morawski, K., Trybalska, G., & Urbaniec, P. (2004). The latencies of the 2f1–f2 DPOAE measured using phase gradient method in young adults and workers chronically exposed to noise. *Polish Otolaryngology, 58*, 131–138.

Nicholson, N. (2003). Transient evoked otoacoustic emissions in relation to hearing loss: Univariate and multivariate analyses. *Dissertation Abstracts International, 64*, 5432.

Nicholson, N., & Widen, J. E. (2004). *Templates for diagnostic interpretation of TEOAEs*. Poster presented at the 16th Annual American Academy of Audiology convention, Salt Lake City, UT.

Nicholson, N., & Widen, J. E. (2007). Evoked otoacoustic emissions in the evaluation of children. In: M. Robinette, & T. Glattke (Eds.), *Otoacoustic emissions: Clinical application* (3rd ed., pp. 365–399). New York, NY: Thieme.

Niskar, A. S., Kieszak, S. M., Holmes, A. E., Esteban, E., Rubin, C., & Brody, D. J. (2001). Estimated prevalence of noise-induced hearing threshold shifts among children 6 to 19 years of age: The Third National Health and Nutrition Examination Survey, 1988–1994, United States. *Pediatrics, 108*, 40–43.

Northern, J. L., & Downs, M. P. (2002). *Hearing in children* (5th ed.). Baltimore, MD: Lippincott Williams & Wilkins.

Norton, S. J., Gorga, M. P., Widen, J. E., Folsom, R. C., Sininger, Y., Cone-Wesson, B., . . . Fletcher, K. A. (2000b). Identification of neonatal hearing impairment: Evaluation of transient evoked otoacoustic emission, distortion product otoacoustic emission, and auditory brainstem response test performance. *Ear and Hearing, 21*, 508–528.

Norton, S. J., Gorga, M. P., Widen, J. E., Vohr, B. R., Folsom, R. C., Sininger, Y. S., . . . Fletcher, K. A. (2000a). Identification of neonatal hearing impairment: Transient evoked otoacoustic emissions during the perinatal period. *Ear and Hearing, 2*, 425–442.

Norton, S. J., Mott, J. B., & Champlin, C. A. (1989). Behavior of spontaneous otoacoustic emissions following intense ipsilateral acoustic stimulation. *Hearing Research, 38*, 243–258.

O Mahoney, C. F., & Kemp, D. T. (1995). Distortion product otoacoustic emission delay measurement in human ears. *Journal of the Acoustical Society of America, 97*, 3721–3735.

Owens, J. J., McCoy, M. J, Lonsbury-Martin, B. L., & Martin, G. K. (1993). Otoacoustic emissions in children with normal ears, middle ear dysfunction, and ventilating tubes. *American Journal of Otology, 14*(1), 34–40.

Penner, M. J., & Zhang, T. (1997). Prevalence of spontaneous otoacoustic emissions in adults revisited. *Hearing Research, 103*, 28–34.

Plinkert, P. K., & Krober, S. (1991). Early detection of cisplatin-induced ototoxicity using evoked otoacoustic emissions. *Laryngorhinootologie, 70*, 457–462.

Prieve, B. A. (2009). *Big sounds from little ears: OAEs in children*. Presentation at Academy Research Conference held in conjunction with the American Academy of Audiology, Dallas, TX. April, 2009.

Prieve, B. A., Calandruccio, L., Fitzgerald, T., Georgantas, L., & Mazevski, A. (2008). Changes in transient-evoked otoacoustic emission levels with negative tympanometric peak pressure in infants and toddlers. *Ear and Hearing*, *29*, 533–542.

Prieve, B., Chasmawala, S., & Jackson, M. (2005). *Development of middle-ear admittance in humans.* Abstracts of the Midwinter Meeting of the Association for research in Otolaryngology. New Orleans, Louisiana.

Prieve, B. A., Fitzgerald, T. S., & Schulte, L. E. (1997a). Basic characteristics of COAEs in infants and children. *Journal of the Acoustical Society of America*, *102*, 2860–2870.

Prieve, B. A., Fitzgerald, T. S., Schulte, L. E., & Kemp, D. (1997b). Basic characteristics of DPOAEs in infants and children. *Journal of the Acoustical Society of America*, *102*, 2871–2879.

Prieve, B. A., Gorga, M. P., & Neely, S. T. (1996). Click- and toneburst-evoked otoacoustic emissions in normal-hearing and hearing-impaired ears. *Journal of the Acoustical Society of America*, *99*, 3077–3086.

Prieve, B. A., Gorga, M. P., Schmidt A. L., Neely, S. T., Peters, J., Schulte, L., & Jesteadt, W. (1993). Analysis of transient-evoked otoacoustic emissions in normal-hearing and hearing-impaired ears. *Journal of the Acoustical Society of America*, *93*, 3308–3319.

Prieve, B. A., Hancur-Bucco, C., & Preston, J. (2009). Transient-evoked otoacoustic emissions in the first month of life: Frequency changes and debris. *Ear and Hearing*, *30*, 330–339.

Probst, R., Lonsbury-Martin, B. L., & Martin, G. K. (1991). A review of otoacoustic emissions. *Journal of the Acoustical Society of America*, *89*, 2027–2067.

Ress, B. D., Sridhar, K. S., Balkany, T. J., Waxman, G. M., Stagner, B. B., & Lonsbury-Martin, B. L. (1999). Effects of cisplatinum chemotherapy on otoacoustic emissions: The development of an objective screening protocol. *Otolaryngology-Head and Neck Surgery*, *121*, 693–701.

Ricci, A. (2003). Active hair bundle movements and the cochlear amplifier. *Journal of the American Academy of Audiology*, *14*, 325–338.

Robinette, M., & Glattke, T. (Eds.) (2007). *Otoacoustic emissions: Clinical application* (3rd ed.). New York, NY: Thieme.

Roede, J., Harris, F. P., Probst, R., & Xu, L. (1993). Repeatability of distortion product otoacoustic emissions in normally hearing humans. *Audiology*, *32*, 273–281.

Ryan, A. F. (2007). The anatomic, physiologic, and molecular basis of cochlear function. In M. S. Robinette & T. J. Glattke (Eds.), *Otoacoustic emissions: Clinical applications* (3rd ed., pp. 43–66). New York, NY: Thieme.

Shehata-Dieler, W. E., Dieler, R., Teichert, K., & Moser, L. M. (1999). Intra- and intersubject variability of acoustically evoked otoacoustic emissions. II. Distortion product otoacoustic emissions. *Laryngo-Rhinootologie*, *78*, 345–350.

Shera, C. A. (2004). Mechanisms of mammalian otoacoustic emission and their implications for the clinical utility of otoacoustic emissions. *Ear and Hearing*, *25*, 86–97.

Shera, C. A., & Guinan, J. J. (1999). Evoked otoacoustic emissions arise by two fundamentally different mechanisms: A taxonomy for mammalian OAEs. *Journal of the Acoustical Society of America*, *105*, 782–798.

Sie, K. Y., & Norton, S. J. (1997). Changes in otoacoustic emissions and auditory brainstem response after cisplatinum exposure in gerbils. *Otolaryngology-Head and Neck Surgery*, *116*, 585–592.

Siegel, J. H., Cerka, A. J., Recio-Spinoso, A., Temchin, A. N., van Dijk, P., & Ruggero, M. A. (2005). *Journal of the Acoustical Society of America*, *118*, 2434–2443.

Smurzynski, J. (1994). Longitudinal measurements of distortion-product and click-evoked otoacoustic emissions of preterm infants: Preliminary results. *Ear and Hearing*, *15*, 210–223.

Souter, M. (1995). Stimulus frequency otoacoustic emissions from guinea pig and human subjects. *Hearing Research*, *90*, 1–11.

Stavroulaki, P., Apostolopoulos, N., Segas, J., Tsakanikos, M., & Adamopoulos, G. (2001a). Evoked otoacoustic emissions—An approach for monitoring cisplatin induced ototoxicity in children. *International Journal of Pediatric Otorhinolaryngology*, *59*, 47–57.

Stavroulaki, P., Nikolopoulos, T. P., Psarommatis, I., & Apostolopoulos, N. (2001b). Hearing evaluation with distortion-product otoacoustic emissions in young patients undergoing haemodialysis. *Clinical Otolaryngology*, *26*, 235–242.

Stavroulaki, P., Vossinakis, I. C., Dinopoulou, D., Doudounakis, S., Adamopoulos, G., & Apostolopoulos, N. (2002). Otoacoustic emissions for monitoring aminoglycoside-induced ototoxicity in children with cystic fibrosis. *Archives of Otolaryngology-Head and Neck Surgery*, *128*, 150–155.

Stover, L., Gorga, M. P., Neely, S. T. (1996). Toward optimizing the clinical utility of distortion product otoacoustic emission measurements. *Journal of the Acoustical Society of America*, *100*, 956–967.

Stover, L. J., Neely, S. T., & Gorga, M. P. (1999). Cochlear generation of intermodulation distortion revealed by DPOAE frequency functions in normal and impaired ears. *Journal of the Acoustical Society of America*, *106*, 2669–2678.

Talmadge, C. L., Long, G. R., Murphy, W. J., & Tubis, A. (1993). New off-line method for detecting spontaneous otoacoustic emissions in human subjects. *Hearing Research*, *71*, 170–182.

Telischi, F., Stagner, B., Widick, M., Balkany, T., & Lonsbury-Martin, B. (1998). Distortion-product otoacoustic emission monitoring of cochlear blood flow. *Laryngoscope*, *108*, 837–842.

Trine, M., Hirsch, J., & Margolis, R. (1993). The effect of middle ear pressure on transient evoked otoacooustic emissions. *Ear and Hearing*, *14*, 401–407.

Vander Werff, K., Prieve, B., & Georgantas, L. (2009). Infant air and bone conduction tone burst auditory brain stem responses for classification of hearing loss and the relationship to behavioral thresholds. *Ear and Hearing*, *30*, 350–368.

Whitehead, M. L., Stagner, B. B., Lonsbury-Martin, B. L., & Martin, G. K. (1995). Effects of ear-canal standing waves on measurements of distortion-product otoacoustic emissions. *Journal of the Acoustical Society of America*, *98*, 3200–3214.

Whitehead, M. L., Stagner, B. B., Martin, G. K., & Lonsbury-Martin, B. L. (1996). Visualization of the onset of distortion-product otoacoustic emissions, and measurement of their latency. *Journal of the Acoustical Society of America, 100*, 1663–1679.

Wilson, J. P. (1980). The combination tone, 2f1-f2, in psychophysics and ear-canal recording. In G. van den Brink, & F. A. Bilsen (Eds.), *Psychophysical, physiological and behavioral studies in hearing* (pp. 43–52). Delft, The Netherlands: Delft University Press.

Zang, Z., & Jiang, Z. D. (2007). Distortion product otoacoustic emissions during the first year in term infants: A longitudinal study. *Brain Development*, *29*, 346–351.

Zhao, F., & Stephens, D. (1999). Test-retest variability of distortion-product otoacoustic emissions in human ears with normal hearing. *Scandinavian Audiology*, *28*, 171–178.

Zorowka, P. G., Schmitt, H. J., & Gutjahr, P. (1993). Evoked otoacoustic emissions and pure tone threshold audiometry in patients receiving cisplatinum therapy. *International Journal of Pediatric Otorhinolaryngology*, *25*, 73–80.

20

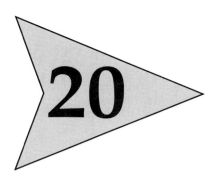

Frequency-Specific Threshold Assessment in Young Infants Using the Transient ABR and the Brainstem ASSR

David R. Stapells

Introduction

The importance of early identification and habilitation of hearing loss for improved access to auditory stimuli and for positive prognosis of speech and language is well established in the literature (ASHA, 2004; Hyde, 2005; JCIH, 2007; Kennedy, McCann, Campbell, Kimm, & Thornton, 2005; Yoshinaga-Itano & Gravel, 2001; Yoshinaga-Itano, Sedey, Coulter, & Mehl, 1998). As a result of the importance of early identification of hearing loss, many countries have established newborn hearing screening programs. Diagnostic audiologic assessment is required for follow-up for infants who do not pass newborn hearing screening, with the goal for most newborn hearing screening, follow-up and intervention programs, including the British Columbia Early Hearing Program (BCEHP), of confirmation and characterization of hearing loss (of a mild degree or worse) by age 3 months, and amplification by the age of 6 months (JCIH, 2007). An auditory evoked potential (AEP) with high correlation to behavioral threshold is essential for the young infant population and for those older infants and children where accurate behavioral thresholds cannot be obtained. This chapter describes the two frequency-specific AEP methods currently considered appropriate for infant threshold measures: the tone-evoked auditory brainstem response (ABR), the current gold-standard measure, and the relatively new brainstem auditory steady-state response (ASSR).

Transient Versus Steady-State Responses

Auditory evoked potentials such as wave V of the ABR or N1 of the slow cortical potential are considered "transient" responses, where the response to one stimulus ends before the next stimulus occurs. An ASSR is a repetitive evoked potential, which is best considered in terms of its constituent frequency components rather than in terms of its waveform (Regan, 1989, p. 35). If stimulus rates are high enough, the resulting response often resembles a sinusoidal waveform whose fundamental frequency is the same as the stimulation rate, although it may be more complex (Regan, 1989, p. 35). In evoking an auditory steady-state response, stimulus rates are sufficiently rapid such that the transient response to one stimulus overlaps with responses to succeeding stimuli (Picton, John, Dimitrijevic, & Purcell, 2003).

With transient responses, longer latency responses tend to originate from sources higher in the auditory system; for example, wave V, which occurs approximately 6 to 15 ms following a brief stimulus, originates in the brainstem, whereas N1 occurs 80 to 150 ms following a stimulus and has its main sources within the auditory cortex. Latencies and intracranial origins of ASSRs are more complicated. Whereas with transient responses it is relatively straightforward to relate stimulus timing with evoked potential measures (i.e., amplitude and latency), with the overlapped nature of ASSRs, this relationship is quite complex (Picton et al., 2003). Different stimulus rates result in ASSRs with different neural origins; ASSRs to faster rates tend to reflect earlier/lower processing. For example, the ASSR to a stimulus with an 80-Hz modulation rate has its main sources in the brainstem (and has thus been termed the "brainstem ASSR"), whereas the 40-Hz ASSR has its main source in the auditory cortex, but also has brainstem contributions (Herdman, Lins, et al., 2002).

There also exist, in practice, differences between transient and steady-state responses in how they are detected (presence versus absence) and measured (timing and amplitude). As the ASSR typically resembles a sinusoidal waveform whose fundamental frequency is same as the stimulation rate, it is best (and easily) measured using frequency-domain analyses, such as fast Fourier transforms (FFT). Well-tested procedures exist to provide objective (computer-determined) measures of ASSR presence/absence as well as the amplitude and phase (timing) of the ASSR. In contrast, transient responses such as the ABR typically involve more subjective visual detection (e.g., is a peak replicable?) and measurement of peak latencies/amplitudes. The use of objective measures for the ASSR has been touted as an "advantage" of the ASSR over the transient ABR; however, this advantage may be less than commonly believed, as expert clinicians well-trained in ABR measures can be very accurate; also, objective statistical measures of the ABR are increasingly becoming available (see below).

What Information Is Required?

Many of the goals of AEP audiometry in infants are (or should be) the same as those of behavioral threshold estimation in older children and adults. Thus, as is routinely done in behavioral audiometry, AEP thresholds must be obtained for *frequency-specific* (i.e., tonal) stimuli, and to distinguish between sensorineural, conductive and mixed hearing losses, AEP techniques must provide results for both air- and bone-conduction stimuli (Gravel, 2002; JCIH, 2007). Frequency-specific thresholds and identification of the type of hearing loss are necessary to make decisions regarding medical intervention and planning aural (re)habilitation. Uncertainty with regards to hearing loss type leads to large delays in medical treatment and audiologic intervention (Gravel, 2002).

This chapter therefore assumes, as indicated by the 2007 Joint Committee on Infant Hearing Position Statement (JCIH, 2007), that clinicians will use frequency-specific stimuli and, when thresholds are elevated, bone-conduction stimuli. Although frequency-specific (e.g., tone-evoked ABR) testing has been proven reliable for many years, surprisingly many clinicians today persist in using broadband click stimuli for ABR thresholds, even though the inadequacy of click-ABR threshold has been known and documented for many years (e.g., Eggermont, 1982; Picton, 1978; Picton & Stapells, 1985; Stapells, 1989; Stapells & Oates, 1997). As a single "point" estimate, it is impossible for the click threshold to provide estimates for thresholds at each octave frequency of the audiogram. More importantly, as a broadband stimulus, the click stimulates most of the cochlea and one cannot say with certainty which frequency the click-ABR threshold represents—at best it represents the "best" hearing in the 500 to 8000 Hz range. Thus, click-ABR should not be routinely used for *threshold* determinations. Interestingly, the use of broadband stimuli has never been an issue with the brainstem ASSR; ASSR threshold testing has always utilized frequency-specific stimuli.[1] However, ASSR and ABR share another problem in their use by many clinicians: although bone-conduction testing is known to be essential, many clinicians still continue to use only air-conduction stimuli when estimating thresholds in infants using the ABR (or ASSR).

A key difference between behavioral assessments in older children and adults and electrophysiologic threshold assessments in infants concerns practical limits on the level of precision one seeks to attain. In behavioral testing of adults, one normally continues a threshold search until actual threshold is obtained, even when well within normal limits (e.g., 0 or −10 dB HL). Furthermore, one normally ends the search using a 5-dB step size. Electrophysiologic testing of infants does not have the luxury of time for such precision: infants must be tested while sleeping and thus test time is limited. Modern, efficient protocols therefore limit the lowest level tested to those which will indicate the threshold is within normal limits. Most programs consider behavioral thresholds of 25 dB HL or better to be normal, thus minimum ABR intensities are chosen to test no lower than required to indicate if thresholds are

[1]That ASSRs from the beginning have utilized tonal stimuli is interesting in itself, as it demonstrates how a new measure avoids the pitfalls of long-held beliefs and practice, even though the brainstem ASSR is quite likely equivalent to ABR wave V.

25 dB HL or better. Thus, ABR minimum normal levels for air conducted (AC) stimuli are currently 25 to 35 dB nHL. Similarly, threshold searches normally end with a minimum stepsize of 10 dB, with the exception of hearing loss greater than 70 dB where 5-dB may be important given the much reduced dynamic range of hearing (BCEHP, 2008; OIHP, 2008).

"Response Present," "No Response," and "Could Not Assess"

As the above paragraph suggests, problems persist with the current practice of AEP audiometry. In addition to the above, one also sees misinterpretation of results, especially that of indicating a response is "present" or "absent" when the data are not of sufficient quality to make such a statement. Thus, one may get an inaccurate threshold because an ABR wave V was identified as "present" even though it was not significantly greater than the background noise (typically determined through replicability and/or flatness of tracings). As interpretation of the ABR usually relies on visual observation, ASSR thresholds based on statistical measures are thought by some to be more objective and thus better. However, even the ASSR is not immune to misinterpretation, as current clinical use of ASSR measures routinely violates statistical assumptions, and thus even "significant" ASSRs may sometimes be random noise (John & Purcell, 2008; Luts, Van Dun, Alaerts, & Wouters, 2008). Moreover, both ABR and ASSR current clinical practices are plagued by the common mistake of indicating a "no response" when the data are too noisy to say so (i.e., the amplitude of the residual EEG noise is larger than the amplitude of a typical threshold response, and thus a response might have been missed). Fortunately, for both ABR and ASSR, solutions to the above problems are relatively straightforward, and are covered in the sections below.

Clinical Implementation of New Techniques

Widescale clinical implementation of a procedure requires evidence of reasonable quality in a sizeable subject group that is similar to the population requiring the clinical testing. A history of successful clinical use over many patients and over a long enough time to indicate any problems also provides evidence of a procedure's usefulness. Preferably, these data have been published in peer-reviewed journals and by different research groups. In addition to numerous publications by many different investigators, the ABR to air- and bone-conducted brief tones has had a long history of successful clinical use (BCEHP, 2008; OIHP, 2008). In comparison, the brainstem ASSR has had a more limited history of clinical use. More importantly, there is much diversity in ASSR stimulus and analysis procedures/parameters, thus reducing both the clinical history and the clinical data. As we shall see, this limits the current clinical use of the ASSR.

Estimating Behavioral Thresholds Using AEPs

The primary goal of frequency-specific ABR or ASSR audiometry is to estimate behavioral thresholds. Brief-tone ABR thresholds (typically in dB nHL) and ASSR thresholds (typically in dB HL) are not directly equivalent to perceptual thresholds in dB HL, and there is no reason one should expect them to be. Therefore, offset adjustments for bias of ABR or ASSR thresholds are required. There are several methods of obtaining this estimated behavioral hearing level (EHL; Bagatto, 2008; BCEHP, 2008; OIHP, 2008), with the most common methods being: (i) application of a regression formula (e.g., Rance et al., 2005; Stapells, Gravel, & Martin, 1995) or (ii) subtraction of a correction factor (BCEHP, 2008; OIHP, 2008). Recording variables, such as averaging time and residual EEG noise (Picton, Dimitrijevic, Perez-Abalo, & van Roon, 2005) and subject factors, such as maturation, affect the accuracy of these methods. For example, because of the effects of ear-canal maturation, the observed relationships between ABR/ASSR and behavioral thresholds will incorporate the effects of maturational SPL changes in the developing ear. Due to the effects of changing size/properties of the ear canal with age, less intensity is required to generate a given dB SPL at the eardrum in a neonate as would be required in an older child. The actual SPLs in early infancy will be greater than those for the same stimulus at the time of later behavioral threshold measurement, especially at higher frequencies, so the results may give an impression of progressive impairment (Bagatto, 2008). Cognitive maturation also affects thresholds, such that behavioral VRA thresholds in a 7-month-old are typically higher than a behavioral threshold obtained when the child is 3 years of age. ABR/ASSR threshold accuracy (and thus the estimated behavioral hearing level accuracy) is affected by procedural factors, including recording time (longer recording times per intensity typically equal less noisy recordings and thus more accurate thresholds) and final intensity stepsize (a 10-dB final step-size could easily miss true threshold by 5–10 dB).[2] Finally, differences between AEP and behavioral thresholds typically show standard deviations of about 10 dB; thus, in about one in 20 subjects, behavioral thresholds are under- or overestimated by 20 dB (Picton et al., 2005). When using any thresholds obtained in infancy, and especially AEP thresholds, one must keep in mind that the estimated behavioral threshold is an estimate, and is often off by 10 dB and occasionally by 15 to 20 dB. Thus, EHL correction factors must take this possibility into account, as must any subsequent fitting of amplification.

Auditory neuropathy spectrum disorder (ANSD) or any significant neurologic dysfunction within the VIIIth nerve and/or brainstem will reduce or eliminate both the transient and steady-state brainstem responses. Thus, whenever no clear response is present at highest intensities (and for transient ABR, no clear wave V), one must investigate the possibility that the elevated ASSR/ABR threshold is due to ANSD (e.g., no neural components) or neurologic (e.g., present early waves but absent wave V) disorder. This is accomplished by recording the transient ABR to high-intensity mono-polarity clicks as well as evoked otoacoustic emissions (EOAEs; see Chapter 13 in this volume on ANSD). When ANSD or neurologic disorder is present that significantly degrades (or eliminates) ABR wave V, neither the transient ABR nor the brainstem ASSR may provide accurate measures of hearing thresholds.

The Transient Tone-Evoked ABR

The ABR to brief tones has been used successfully for threshold assessment for more than 30 years, since the first publications in the 1970s. Nevertheless, despite early and subsequent success, there existed much misinformation about the tone-evoked ABR. Many clinicians erroneously believed that tone-ABR thresholds lacked frequency specificity especially at low frequencies (i.e., they did not reflect the nominal frequency of the tone), that they did not provide accurate estimates of the behavioral audiogram and, finally, that they were too difficult and too time-consuming to obtain. In fact, there were relatively few research articles noting problems with tone-ABR, and most of these articles had significant technical problems and/or presented results from only a few cases. In contrast, our meta-analysis of the tone-ABR literature in 2000 (Stapells, 2000b) demonstrated that the great majority of research papers considering the tone-ABR for threshold estimation showed reasonably accurate results. More recent studies have confirmed the utility and accuracy of the tone ABR and have expanded the results to even younger infants (Lee, Hsieh, Pan, & Hsu, 2007; Lee, Jaw, Pan, Hsieh, & Hsu, 2008; Rance, Tomlin, & Rickards, 2006; Ribeiro & Carvallo, 2008; Vander Werff, Prieve, & Georgantas, 2009). Importantly, clinical programs have effectively used the ABR to air- (and bone-) conducted tones for many years. Experience with provincewide universal early hearing programs in Ontario and British Columbia indicates that with appropriate training and use of efficient parameters and test sequences, a substantial amount of information is typically obtained within one test session, thus the tone-ABR is neither too difficult nor too time consuming (Janssen, Usher, & Stapells, 2010). Figure 20–1 shows typical tone-ABR recordings from a young infant in response to brief tones presented at "normal" levels (25–35 dB nHL, see below).

How well the air-conduction tone-ABR threshold estimates threshold in infants with normal hearing or hearing loss is presented in Tables 20–1 and 20–2, which show results from the previous meta-analysis, as well as results from several more recent studies, and compares these to adults. As shown in Table 20–1, normal infants show mean thresholds of about 15 to 20 dB nHL for 500 through 4000 Hz, similar to adult thresholds. However, not all normal-hearing infants show responses at 20 dB nHL, and for clinical purposes programs are rarely interested in determining normal thresholds better than 25 to 30 dB EHL, thus criteria for "normal" are higher than the mean thresholds. Typically, these normal levels are in the range of 30 to 40 dB nHL for 500 Hz, 25 to 35 dB nHL for 1000 Hz, 20 to 30 dB nHL for 2000 Hz, and 20 to 25 dB nHL for 4000 Hz. Currently, the BCEHP specifies normal levels of 35 dB nHL for 500 Hz, 30 dB nHL for 1000 and 2000 Hz, and 25 dB nHL for 4000 Hz (BCEHP, 2008). If a response is present at the normal level, the EHLs at that frequency are within the normal range.

The scatterplots presented in Figure 20–2 plot tone-ABR (in dB nHL) and follow-up behavioral thresholds (in dB HL) for a relatively large group of infants

[2]However, due to test-time constraints imposed by the requirement that infants must sleep during ABR/ASSR testing, normally one uses a final step-size of 10 dB for ABR/ASSR testing.

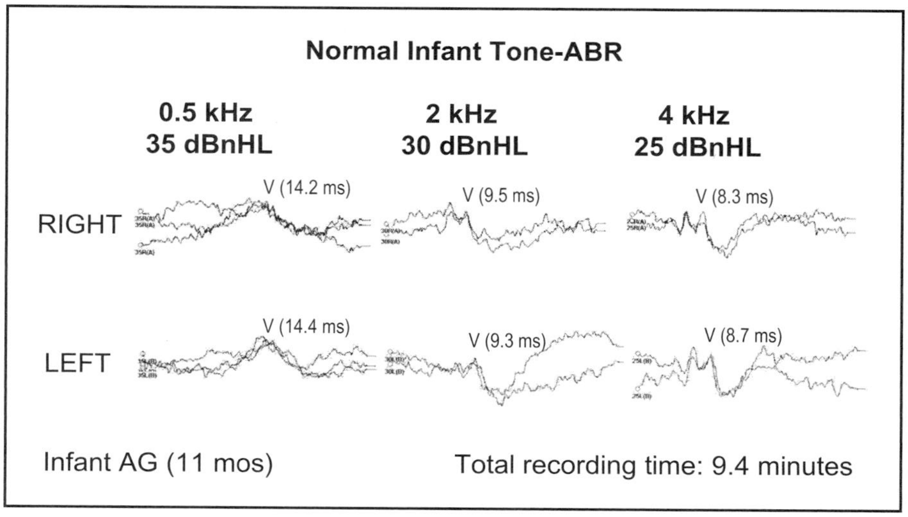

FIGURE 20–1. Tone-evoked ABR waveforms obtained from an infant (aged 11 months) with normal hearing. Brief-tone stimuli were presented at the "normal" intensity levels for each frequency. Replicable responses are clearly present for each waveform set, with wave V location and latency indicated. Total time required to obtain these results was 9.4 minutes. Timebase for waveforms is 25.6 ms. Results obtained in collaboration with Renée Janssen.

Table 20–1. Air-Conduction Tone-ABR Thresholds (in dB nHL) in Infants and Young Children With Normal Hearing

AC TONE-ABR STUDY	*500 Hz*	*1000 Hz*	*2000 Hz*	*4000 Hz*
Meta-analysis of adult data (1977–1999; 22 studies; Stapells, 2000b)	*20 ± 13 (271)*	*16 ± 10 (271)*	*13 ± 8 (216)*	*12 ± 8 (258)*
Meta-analysis of infant data (1977–1999; 9 studies; Stapells, 2000b)	20 ± 9 (369)	17 ± 6 (78)	14 ± 7 (65)	15 ± 10 (209)
Rance et al., 2006 (age 6 weeks data; thresholds converted using nHL calibrations in Table 20–5)	30 ± 7 (17)			15 ± 6 (17)
Lee et al., 2007	18 ± 8 (88)	17 ± 7 (75)	13 ± 7 (69)	11 ± 6 (56)
Vander Werff et al., 2009	27 ± 8 (40)		14 ± 6 (40)	12 ± 6 (30)

Note: Adult results from Stapells (2000b) meta-analysis are shown for comparison. Mean (dB nHL) ± standard deviation; Results rounded off to closest decibels; Number of subjects in parentheses.

with normal hearing and hearing loss (Stapells et al., 1995). Typical of the literature, correlations between infant tone-ABR and behavioral thresholds in this study were high: $r = .94$, $r = .95$ and $r = .97$ for 500, 2000, and 4000 Hz, respectively. Table 20–2 presents difference scores (i.e., tone-ABR threshold in dB nHL minus pure-tone behavioral threshold in dB HL) from many studies for infants and young children with hearing loss, and compares these to those from adults. Typically, tone-ABR thresholds are within 5 to 10 dB of the behavioral thresholds. Across most studies, standard deviations are typically on the order of 9 to 12 dB

Table 20–2. Air-Conduction Tone-ABR Minus Behavioral Threshold Difference Scores in Infants and Young Children with Hearing Loss

AC TONE-ABR STUDY	HL type	500	1000	2000	4000
Meta-analysis of adult data (1977–1999; 8 studies; Stapells, 2000b)	*ADULT SNHL*	*+13 ± 11 (85)*	*+10 ± 12 (167)*	*+8 ± 10 (100)*	*+5 ± 13 (84)*
Meta-analysis of infant data (1977–1999; 6 studies; Stapells, 2000b)	SNHL	+6 ± 14 (125)	+5 ± 14 (118)	+1 ± 11 (110)	–8 ± 12 (35)
Lee et al., 2008 † (Group with behavioral thresholds >40 dB HL)	SNHL	+5 ± 5 (135)	0 ± 5 (119)	–5 ± 8 (112)	–5 ± 8 (91)
Vander Werff et al., 2009	SNHL	+13 ± 12 (3)		0 ± 9 (7)	–3 ± 14 (6)
Stapells & Gravel, unpublished (ABR and behavioral obtained on same day)	Otitis Media	+10 ± 19 (30)		+1 ± 18 (26)	–11 ± 15 (11)

Note: Adult results from Stapells (2000b) meta-analysis are shown for comparison. Difference score (dB) = tone-ABR threshold (in dB nHL) minus pure-tone behavioral threshold (in dB HL); Mean (dB) ± standard deviation († Lee et al. results are median difference scores ± 1 quartile) Results rounded off to closest decibels; Number of subjects in parentheses.

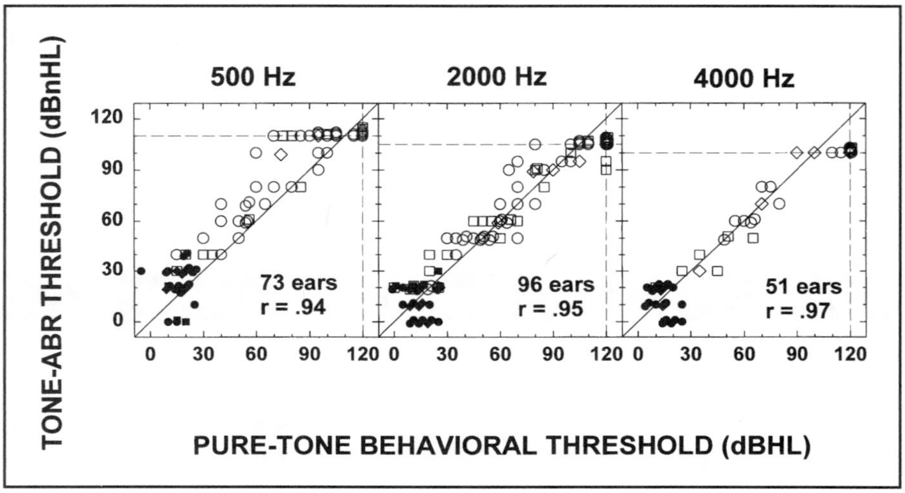

FIGURE 20–2. Threshold estimation using the ABR to 500 Hz (*left*), 2000 Hz (*middle*), and 4000 Hz (*right*) tones presented in notched noise. Results for normal-hearing (*filled symbols*) and sensorineural-impaired (*open symbols*) ears are plotted with three age ranges (at time of ABR) identified: 0 to 6 months (*diamonds*); 7 to 48 months (*circles*); 49 months or greater (*squares*). Shown also are the correlation coefficients for each frequency across all subjects and the number of ears involved. Dashed lines (- - - - -) indicate the no-response range for each frequency and test, equivalent to the equipment maximum output plus 10 dB. Points plotted ≥ the dashed line indicate no-response for the measure. Points with multiple subjects have symbols offset (± 1 dB per subject) to show clearly the overlapping data. Diagonals (*solid lines*) represent perfect ABR-behavioral threshold correspondence and are not regression lines. Reproduced with permission from Stapells, D. R., Gravel, J. A., and Martin, B. A. (1995). Thresholds for auditory brain stem responses to tones in notched noise from infants and young children with normal hearing or sensorineural hearing loss. *Ear and Hearing*, *16*(4), 361-371. Copyright 1995 Lippincott Williams & Wilkins.

(Stapells, 2000b), and differences of 20 dB are occasionally found, although most (≥ 65%) thresholds are within 10 dB. Figure 20–3 shows ABR-predicted and behavioral audiograms for several infants. Table 20–2 also suggests there may be somewhat greater variability in tone-ABR minus-behavioral threshold differences scores for infants with otitis media, highlighting the importance of obtaining bone-conduction results for these infants (Gravel, 2002; Stapells, 1989).

Although it is widely held that difference scores decrease (i.e., tone-ABR threshold is closer to behavioral threshold) as hearing loss increases, the existing data do not clearly support this (Sininger & Hyde, 2009). Slope of ABR versus behavioral threshold regression lines are typically close to unity, indicating thresholds are not closer with severe loss. However, the issue is complicated by the fact that: (i) most ABR measures in the normal range do not seek true thresholds and (ii) the presence of no-response results for ABR occur at a lower intensity (in dB nHL) than for pure-tone behavioral (in dB HL), due in part to transducer limitations. It does appear that it is difficult to

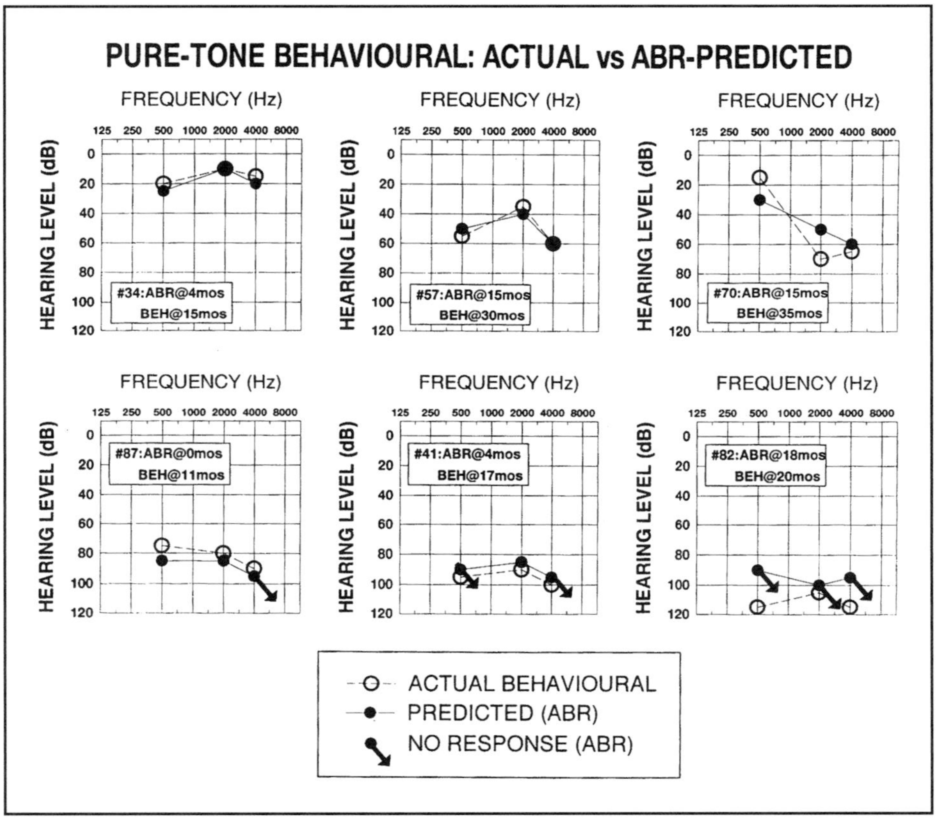

FIGURE 20–3. Comparison of ABR-predicted audiograms with actual behavioral audiograms obtained on follow-up testing for six infants. Results for individuals with normal hearing (*upper left corner*) to profound sensorineural hearing loss (*lower right corner*) are shown. ABR-predicted thresholds were determined using the linear regression equations presented in Stapells, Gravel, and Martin (1995). Predicted thresholds with arrows were ABR "no response" results—note the ABR's inability to differentiate between 90 and 110 dB HL. Otherwise, most ABR-predicted thresholds are quite close to actual behavioral thresholds. BEH = behavioral. Reproduced with permission from Stapells, D. R. (2000a). Frequency-specific evoked potential audiometry in infants. In R. C. Seewald (Ed.), *A sound foundation through early amplification: Proceedings of an international conference* (pp. 13–31). Stäfa, Switzerland: Phonak AG. Copyright 2000 Phonak.

get close to true normal threshold (e.g., –5 to 10 dB nHL) in individuals with normal hearing, but this is complicated by acoustic noise (ambient noise in room) and electrical noise (room and subject) issues. Given near-unity slopes, estimation of behavioral thresholds (EHL) using either regression functions or correction factors should yield equivalent results. Importantly, as Table 20–2 shows, difference scores for infants and young children are clearly different from those of adults; it is therefore important that we use infant data to determine appropriate correction factors. The British Columbia and Ontario provincial programs currently use conservative correction factors of –15, –10, –5, and 0 dB for estimating 500-, 1000-, 2000-, and 4000-Hz pure-tone behavioral thresholds (in dB HL) from tone-ABR thresholds (in dB nHL; BCEHP, 2008; OIHP, 2008; Sininger & Hyde, 2009).

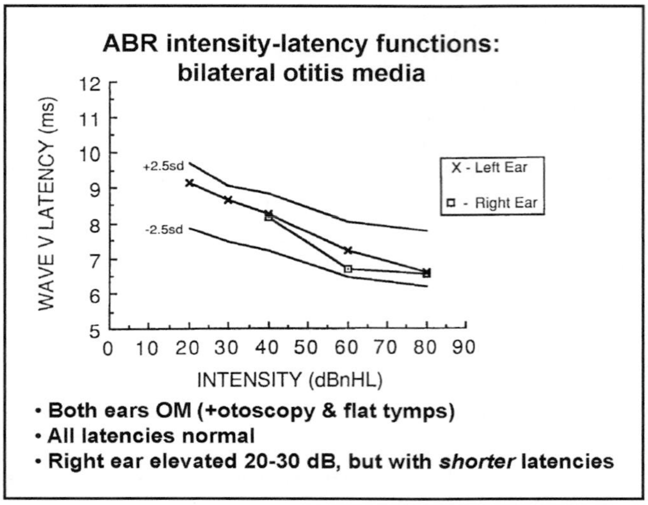

FIGURE 20–4. Click-evoked air-conduction ABR wave V intensity-latency functions in an infant with bilateral otitis media (and normal bone-conduction hearing). Otitis media indicated by pneumatic otoscopy (i.e., presence of fluid) and flat tympanograms bilaterally. Despite bilateral otitis media and a 20 to 30 dB elevation for the right-ear ABR, all latencies are well within normal limits, with latencies for right-ear stimulation slightly shorter than for the left ear. Follow-up testing indicated normal ABR and behavioral thresholds, and normal middle-ear function, indicating sensorineural loss was not present and the elevation was conductive in nature. Thus, reliance on air-conduction ABR intensity-latency functions could have erroneously suggested no conductive loss, with the right-ear elevation being sensorineural in nature. Results obtained in collaboration with Judy Gravel.

ABR Assessment of Conductive Loss

The most common cause of elevated ABR (or ASSR) thresholds in young infants is conductive loss (Canadian Working Group on Childhood Hearing, 2005; Gravel, 2002). This is especially so for young infants referred for diagnostic ABR/ASSR testing after failing one or more newborn hearing screenings. Protocols, therefore, must be able to determine whether a significant conductive component is present. When testing older children and adults, this assessment is primarily achieved through comparison of air- versus bone-conduction thresholds. Additional information may be gained from immittance and EOAE measures; however, these latter measures are unable to quantify the degree of conductive loss. In the presence of conductive pathology, they are typically abnormal whether the conductive component is relatively minor (e.g., only 5 dB) or substantial (e.g., 30 dB). Others have suggested that analysis of ABR wave V or wave I latencies in response to air-conducted clicks can differentiate conductive from sensorineural losses, and perhaps can even quantify the conductive component (e.g., Fria & Sabo, 1979; McGee & Clemis, 1982; Yamada, Yagi, Yamane, & Suzuki, 1975). Our research, using click-ABR wave I latencies, has indicated that although air-conducted latencies are indeed prolonged *on average* in infants with conductive hearing loss, latency-based measures of the conductive component are not reliable. Some infants with conductive loss showed normal latencies (Figure 20–4), whereas some infants with either sensorineural hearing loss or normal thresholds showed prolonged latencies (Mackersie & Stapells, 1994). The overlap between groups is even greater for wave V latencies (Vander Werff et al., 2009). Given these overlaps, it should not be surprising that attempts to quantify the amount of conductive component using AC click-ABR wave V or wave I latency shifts have not proven reliable, with large errors in many infants (Eggermont, 1982; Mackersie & Stapells, 1994) and relatively low correlations between latency and the size of the air-bone gap (Vander Werff et al., 2009). Furthermore, latency-based measures typically require responses to air-conducted clicks (especially for wave I measures); as discussed above, no frequency-specific information can be reliably obtained using clicks; given the large amount of information required from sleeping infants, modern ABR protocols thus rarely use clicks, except when assessing infants suspected of ANSD or other neurologic problem that may disrupt the ABR.

The problems with latency-based measures are demonstrated in Figure 20–4, which presents results from an infant whose air-conducted click-ABR wave V thresholds were normal (20 dB nHL or better) for the left ear but mildly elevated (40 dB nHL) for the right ear; wave V latencies for both ears were both well within normal limits; indeed, latencies for the right ear with elevated thresholds were shorter in latency. Relying on latency shifts, one might interpret no conductive component was present in either ear and the right-ear threshold elevation was a sensorineural loss. This infant, however, had normal thresholds for bone-conduction stimuli and otoscopic examination revealed bilateral otitis media; air-conduction thresholds returned to normal at a subsequent visit.

It is therefore not possible to reliably determine the presence or degree of a conductive component using air-conduction ABR latency information. With the exception of ABR assessment of ANSD and/or neurologic involvement, we do not use any ABR latency results when determining *threshold*.[3] Rather, we rely on the combination of air- (AC) and bone- (BC conduction tone-ABR results. An elevated tone-ABR (or ASSR) threshold to air-conduction stimuli with tone-ABR responses to bone-conduction stimuli at normal levels clearly indicates the presence and degree of a conductive loss; if ABR thresholds to bone-conduction stimuli are elevated, a sensorineural component is present. Current comprehensive diagnostic protocols for infants emphasize the importance of obtaining bone-conduction information early in the process (i.e., as soon as an elevation in air-conduction thresholds is indicated)—this information is needed to determine the next test step and is important both for appropriate follow-up and for parent counseling. Indeed, when bone-conduction thresholds turn out to be within normal limits, indicating a conductive loss, the thresholds for air-conduction stimuli in many cases are of less importance because, when resulting from fluctuating conditions such as otitis media, they may be quite different in days following the assessment. Unfortunately, currently many clinicians routinely fail to obtain ABR results for bone-conduction stimuli after finding elevated air-conduction threshold(s), relying instead on immittance results. Tone-ABR (and to a much lesser extent, ASSR) protocols, test parameters, and results are currently available for the assessment of conductive loss.

Bone-Conduction Tone-ABR

Bone-conduction tone-ABR has a history of over two decades of regular use in the clinic (Gravel, Kurtzberg, Stapells, Vaughan, & Wallace, 1989; Stapells, 1989; Stapells & Ruben, 1989), and protocols using bone-conduction tonal stimuli are currently routinely employed in large programs such as BCEHP (2008) and OIHP (2008).[4] Despite their history of clinical use and importance for clinical assessment, it is somewhat surprising that relatively few bone-conduction tone-ABR data in infants have been published in the peer-reviewed literature (Cone- Wesson, 1995; Cone-Wesson & Ramirez, 1997; Foxe & Stapells, 1993; Nousak & Stapells, 1992; Stapells & Ruben, 1989; Vander Werff et al., 2009), with most published for data in infants having normal hearing or conductive hearing loss.

Young infants' thresholds for bone-conduction stimuli differ significantly from adults (Foxe & Stapells, 1993; Small & Stapells, 2006, 2008c; Stapells & Ruben, 1989; Stuart, Yang, & Green, 1994; Stuart et al., 1993; Vander Werff et al., 2009; Yang et al., 1987), likely due primarily to the immaturity of the infant skull (Anson & Donaldson, 1981; Small & Stapells, 2008c; Yang et al., 1987). Table 20–3 shows normal infant BC tone-ABR thresholds obtained by several studies. There is some variability in the literature, but all show mean thresholds that are: (i) better for low versus high frequencies, and (ii) better than expected compared to those for adults. Thus adult "normal" levels for bone-conduction stimuli do not apply to infants; criteria for infants must be determined directly from infant BC ABR results. We have found that to be considered "normal" (for bone-conduction hearing), infants should show ABRs to bone-conducted tones presented at 20 dB nHL for 500 Hz and at 30 dB nHL for 2000 Hz (Stapells,

---

[3]We do not evaluate whether a tone-ABR wave V latency is "normal" or "prolonged," as this typically provides no extra (or reliable) information over AC versus BC tone-ABR results. We do use latency differences when considering differences between wave V recorded in ipsilateral and contralateral EEG channels (see below). Also, if a "wave V" latency appears to be too early to be wave V, we will be concerned the thresholds are unreliable (e.g., neurologic or ANSD concerns). Of course, for neurologic/ANSD assessment, we do consider normality of click-ABR latency measures.

[4]The ABR to bone-conduction clicks has also been used clinically, preceding the use of bone-conducted tones (e.g., Cone-Wesson, 1995; Cornacchia, Martini, & Morra, 1983; Hooks & Weber, 1984; Kavanagh & Beardsley, 1979; Mauldin & Jerger, 1979; Muchnik, Neeman, & Hildesheimer, 1995; Stuart, Yang, Stenstrom, & Reindorp, 1993; Yang, Rupert, & Moushegian, 1987; Yang & Stuart, 1990). However, as with air-conducted clicks, bone-conducted clicks lack frequency specificity (Kramer, 1992); also, due to maturational issues, the "effective" spectra for air- and bone-conducted clicks differ (Small & Stapells, 2008c), making comparison between the two difficult in infants.

Table 20–3. Bone-Conduction Tone-ABR Thresholds (in dB nHL) in Infants and Young Children With Normal Bone-Conduction Hearing

BC TONE-ABR STUDY	500	1000	2000	4000
Stapells & Ruben, 1989 (normal group)	2* (24)		6* (24)	
Stapells & Ruben, 1989 (all infants)	−2* (66)		4* (66)	
Foxe & Stapells, 1993	3 ± 10 (9)		14 ± 7 (8)	
Cone-Wesson & Ramirez, 1997 (age: 1–2 days)	−15 ± 10† (24)			7 ± 7† (20)
Vander Werff et al., 2009	11 ± 8 (40)		17 ± 7 (40)	

Mean (dB nHL) ± standard deviation (where available); Results rounded off to closest decibels.
Number of subjects in parentheses; * Threshold = 50% point on cumulative response-presence distribution for "normal" and "all" infants; † Thresholds converted to dB nHL using calibrations in Table 20–5 standard deviations estimated from graph in original study.

1989; Stapells & Ruben, 1989). Currently, there are too few infant ABR data for 1000- and 4000-Hz bone-conduction tones (see Table 20–3), so these frequencies are not routinely tested using bone-conducted stimuli. Because the upper limits (before distortion) of the most commonly used bone oscillator (B71) for brief tones is 51 dB nHL at 500 Hz and 63 dB nHL at 2000 Hz (Small & Stapells, 2003), a range of only 30 dB above these normal levels can be tested. Due to several reasons (limited dynamic range; 10-dB step-size; lack of published data for AC-BC differences in infants), the "air-bone gap" is usually not calculated. Rather, the BC results are primarily used to indicate whether bone thresholds are "normal" or "elevated" and thus whether or not there is a sensorineural component (i.e., BC elevated) to an elevated AC threshold. The approximately 30-dB dynamic range essentially only allows one to classify bone thresholds as "normal," "mildly elevated" or "at least moderate." Figure 20–5 shows bone-conduction tone-ABR results from young children with conductive and sensorineural hearing loss.

Bone-Conduction ABR: Isolating the Responding Cochlea

Masking of the contralateral ear, typically required with bone-conduction testing in adults, currently is not feasible and likely not necessary for ABR audiometry in young infants. Masking is not feasible because: (i) effective masking levels for bone-conduction brief-tone stimuli in infants are not known and (ii) time is too limited to record using several masking levels, such as one might when attempting plateau masking (Stapells, 2000a). However, because of their immature skulls, young infants show substantial interaural attenuation of bone-conducted stimuli, as much as 25 dB (Small & Stapells, 2008b; Yang et al., 1987). Thus stimuli presented to the temporal bone at the low stimulus levels (20–30 dB nHL) required to demonstrate normal versus impaired cochlear function will stimulate primarily the cochlea ipsilateral to the oscillator placement, and masking may not be required. Furthermore, the laterality of ABR origin (i.e., which cochlea is resulting in the recorded ABR) can be determined using 2-channel EEG recordings, and observing the large ipsilateral/contralateral wave V latency and amplitude asymmetries present in infants and young children (but not in older children or adults). As shown in Figure 20–5, in the infant with a normal ABR to BC tones, wave V is larger and earlier in the EEG channel ipsilateral to the stimulated cochlea (Edwards, Durieux-Smith, & Picton, 1985; Foxe & Stapells, 1993; Stapells, 1989; Stapells & Mosseri, 1991); thus, if one sees this pattern in the channel on the same side as the bone oscillator, one can infer that stimulation of the cochlea on the same side has resulted in the ABR. However, if one sees the opposite pattern, as shown in the child with sensorineural hearing loss (SNHL) in Figure 20–5, then the opposite cochlea has produced the response, and a sensorineural impairment is pres-

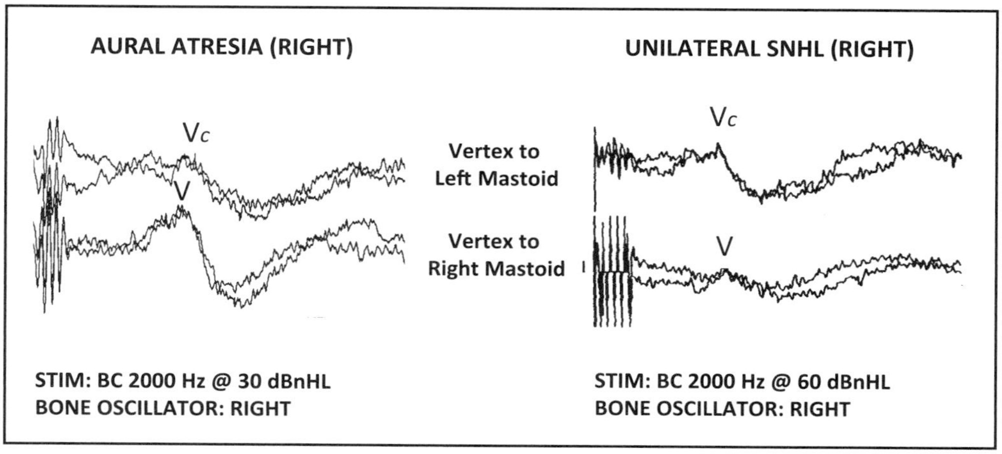

FIGURE 20–5. ABR to 2000-Hz bone-conducted tones in two children, one with conductive hearing loss (*right panel*) and one with unilateral sensorineural hearing loss (*left panel*). Shown are the results for the left ("Vertex to Left Mastoid") and right ("Vertex to Right Mastoid") EEG channels, obtained simultaneously, with the bone oscillator placed on the right temporal bone. In the infant with conductive loss due to right-ear atresia, wave V in the right EEG channel (i.e., ipsilateral to bone oscillator placement) is both earlier and larger than the wave V in the left (contralateral) EEG channel. This is a *normal asymmetry* and indicates the right cochlea is the primary contributor to the response to these bone-conduction tones at the normal (30 dB nHL) intensity. This indicates a normal 2000-Hz bone-conduction response for this ear. In the child with a unilateral (right-ear) sensorineural loss, 60 dB nHL 2000-Hz bone-conduction tones presented to the right temporal bone resulted a wave V in the right EEG channel (i.e., ipsilateral to bone oscillator placement) that is much smaller and later than the wave V seen in left (contralateral) EEG channel. This is an *abnormal asymmetry*, indicating the left ear is the primary contributor to the response, and thus indicating the presence of a sensorineural hearing loss. Further ABR and behavioral testing indicated a severe unilateral sensorineural hearing loss in the right ear. Vc: wave V in contralateral EEG channel. Waveform timebase: 25 ms.

ent (Sininger & Hyde, 2009; Stapells, 1989). Although reasonably well-tested in infants with conductive loss (Stapells, 1989; Stapells & Ruben, 1989), the ipsi/contra technique requires further assessment in infants with sensorineural or mixed loss; the author's clinical experience as well as that of larger programs (e.g., BCEHP, OIHP) indicates reasonable results in these latter groups.[5]

Tone-ABR Technical Details

Tables 20–4 and 20–5 present specific recording and stimulus parameters we recommend for tone-ABR, based on more than 30 years of research and 20 years of clinical application. The data supporting each choice are discussed in detail elsewhere (BCEHP, 2008; Stapells, 2000a; Stapells & Oates, 1997) and thus are not elaborated on here. Test sequences for tone-ABR are provided below in a later section concerning clinical ABR/ASSR protocols.

Most clinical AEP equipment is reasonably capable of basic tone-evoked ABR measures. However, not all systems are optimal and some are not up to the task. Optimally, a very wide and flexible range of stimulus and recording settings should be available. Currently, we consider the following to be *minimum* requirements for tone-ABR systems (additional capabilities are required for other AEPs such as slow-cortical responses).

[5]The normal infant ABR wave V ipsi/contra asymmetries are also useful when recording responses to high-intensity for air-conduction stimuli when one suspects a significant interaural difference in the degree of hearing loss.

Table 20–4. Recommended Recording Parameters for Tone-ABR

	Air Conduction	*Bone Conduction*
EEG channels	Minimum: 1 channel Cz- Mastoid-ipsi Preferred: 2 channels † Cz- Mastoid-ipsi Cz- Mastoid-contra	Minimum: 2 channels † Cz- Mastoid-ipsi Cz- Mastoid-contra
EEG filters (12 dB/octave slope)	30 Hz (high pass) to 1500–3000 Hz (low pass)	
Gain	50,000–100,000	
Artifact rejection	Trials exceeding ±25 V(±15 Vis acceptable if there are < 10% rejections). Set artifact region to start *after* end of stimulus so that stimulus artifact does not trigger artifact rejection (if available)	
Number of accepted trials per replication	Typically, 2,000 per replication; additional trials may be required to reduce noise (achieved either by increasing the number of trials per replication or by averaging together replications)* Minimum 1000 per replication *After 1,000 trials, if online residual noise measure available, may stop when waveform noise reduced to ≤ criterion (e.g., IHS RN ≤ .08 V)	
Number of replications	At least two (often three, sometimes four)	
Recording (time) window and stimulus rate	Typically 25 ms which usually allows a rate up to about 39.1/s ‡ Some systems are slower so either a slightly shorter window (e.g., 23–24 ms) or a slightly slower rate (e.g., 37.1/s) must be used. Clinicians must check that their system *averages* at 39.1/s and does not skip stimuli. 2000 trials should take about 51 seconds; if it requires substantially longer, it is skipping stimuli and either a slower rate or a shorter recording window is required.	
Visual Display Scale	Waveforms must be displayed with a sufficient display gain such that very small responses would not be missed. A rule of thumb is to "blow-up" waves such that peak-to-peak height of largest wave is *at least* 1/4 the length of the recording window (i.e., if ABR waveform displayed is 10 cm in length then the display should be increased such that the peak-to-peak amplitude of wave V-V' is *at least* 2.5 cm in height)	

† Laterality (cochlear origin) of BC-ABR determined from wave V ipsi/contra asymmetries (infants/young children only). Consider this also for air conduction if a large difference in thresholds between ears exists. ‡ Although a 25-ms window works for all frequencies, infant responses to 2000- and 4000-Hz stimuli are shorter in latency and thus a shorter time window (18-20 ms) and a faster rate (49.1/s) could be used.

Recording

Two EEG channels allowing for simultaneous ipsilateral/contralateral recordings (with artifact reject locked/chained across channels); EEG filters allowing for 30- to 3000-Hz and 30- to 1500-Hz settings; Flexible stimulus artifact setting (allowing for ± 10 μV to ± 25 μV), which can be set to exclude rejection due to voltages within the region of stimulus artifact; Flexible recording sweep time, with at least a 24- to 25-ms sweep time allowed; An online calculation and visual presentation of residual noise (RN) in the waveform (e.g.,"RN" from "±" average: Özdamar & Delgado, 1996; Picton, Linden, Hamel, & Maru, 1983; or "single-point variance": Don & Elberling, 1996), to indicate whether the waveform is quiet enough to conclude

Table 20–5. Stimuli for Tone-ABR: Rise/Fall Times, Durations, Acoustic Calibrations for 0 dB nHL, and Signal-to-Noise (SNR) Regions

	Linear window	Blackman window	Acoustic calibration for 0 dB nHL			SNR region†† (begin to end, in ms)	
Frequency (Hz)	**Rise/Fall (r/f) & Plateau (2-1-2 cycles)**	**Total Duration (5 cycles total)**	**Insert (AC) ER-3A dB ppe SPL†**	**Supra (AC) TDH-49 dB ppe SPL**	**Bone (BC) B-71 dB ppe re: 1 µN RMS**	**Air (AC)**	**Bone (BC)**
500	4-ms r/f 2-ms plateau	10-ms total	22	25	67	10.5–20.5	20dB: 10.5–20.5 ≥ 30dB: 14–24‡
1000	2-ms r/f 1-ms plateau	5-ms total	25	23	54	7.5–17.5	
2000	1-ms r/f 0.5-ms plateau	2.5-ms total	20	26	49	6.5–16.5	6.5-16.5
4000*	AC: 0.5-ms r/f 0.25-ms plateau	AC: 1.25-ms total	26	29	46	5–15	
	BC: 1-ms r/f 0.25-ms plateau	BC: 2.25-ms total					

Rate: 37.1-39.1/s (assuming 23- to 25-ms averaging window); Polarity: alternating; ppe: peak-to-peak equivalent dB ("peak" = ppe + 3 dB for brief tones). † Insert earphones calibrated using a DB0138 2-cc coupler. †† SNR region (for waveform noise and response presence measures) must not include stimulus artifact. May be a problem for high-intensity 500-Hz stimuli. ‡ Window later to exclude stimulus artifact but also excludes much of response. Valid for residual noise measures only (i.e., not CCR, SNR or Fsp). *BC stimuli at 4000 Hz must be extended in total duration to reduce ringing by bone oscillator.

"no-response," with flexible parameters such the duration and location of the window over which the noise is calculated; A signal-to-noise measure (preferably calculated automatically while recording data) to assist clinicians in concluding a response is present (e.g., standard deviation ratio [SDR]; Picton et al., 1983; or signal-to-noise ratio [SNR; Özdamar & Delgado, 1996]; F-test using single-point variance [Fsp; Don, Elberling, & Waring, 1984]; or correlation between waveforms [CCR; Hyde, Sininger, & Don, 1998; Picton et al., 1983]), again, all with flexible parameters; Ability to add or subtract waveforms offline (e.g., to increase the number of trials; to calculate "alternating" from rarefaction and condensation click results, etc.); and Standard measures of latency and amplitude.

Stimuli

Possibility of air- (insert and supra-aural earphones) and bone-conduction transducers; Acoustic calibrations specific to each stimulus and transducer (with the possibility of the user adjusting the calibrations); Octave frequencies from 500 through 8000 Hz; Linear and/or Blackman (or exact-Blackman) windowing functions, with flexible rise/fall times, and plateau times (or total durations) allowing for stimuli with total durations of 5 cycles (e.g., linear windows with 2 cycles rise, 1 cycle plateau, and 2 cycles fall times, or Blackman-windowed tones with 5-cycle total duration and no plateau); Stimulus rates of at least 37 per second when using a 24- to 25-ms sweep time (i.e., without skipping stimuli); Ability to use rarefaction, condensation and alternating onset polarity.

Preferably, tone-ABR systems will provide the above *plus* wider ranges of settings and additional features; better systems are those with maximum flexibility and allow for speedy changing of stimulus parameters, addition of waves, marking/measuring of waveforms and subsequent printouts. Because some infants will have neurologic dysfunction or ANSD, all systems must also allow for switching to click-ABR or slow-cortical potential parameters.

Interpretation of Tone-ABR Waveforms

Although the tone-ABR has the capability to provide reasonably accurate estimates of threshold, a continuing major problem with the clinical use of the ABR today lies largely with the clinicians who carry out the testing and/or interpret the waveforms, rather than with the ABR itself. Currently, clinicians typically determine response presence/absence and waveform noisiness "subjectively" by visually assessing the repeatability and noisiness of multiple "replicate" waveforms. Most clinicians become reasonably proficient in this; some become so good as to be considered "experts"; however, some clinicians seem never to gain the skill. The differences are likely due to training, experience (e.g., number and diversity of cases) and inherent abilities. Fortunately, with modern systems, clinicians need not base their interpretation solely on their visualization of the responses (although for very experienced observers, this may currently be the best method). Objective measures of response replicability/signal-to-noise ratio and, importantly, response noisiness, are available and should be used.

Too often, clinicians indicate a response is "present" or "absent" when they do not have the data of sufficient quality to make such a statement. As noted above, to conclude a response is present, the clinician must have evidence of a significant signal-to-noise ratio. When assessed visually, a "present" response must contain a replicable waveform, one which is repeatable over its total duration, usually at least 3 to 4 ms for wave V. To be sure it has a significant signal-to-noise ratio, the waveform's peak-to-peak amplitude (the average of all replications) must be at least three times the average difference between the replications (Don & Elberling, 1996; Picton et al., 1983; Picton & Maru, 1984). On the other hand, a decision that a wave is "absent" can only be made if replications are essentially flat and show little or no difference between them (i.e., repeatably flat over at least the 3- to 4-ms duration in the region of wave V). If the waveform peak in question is not repeatable or if the replications are not flat (i.e., noisy), the clinician must obtain more replications. Otherwise, the result should be interpreted only as "could not interpret" or "data incomplete" (Sininger & Hyde, 2009; Stapells, 2000a). Figure 20–6 shows examples of waveforms in each of these three categories. Much of the variability of ABR thresholds and the inconsistency with subsequent behavioral thresholds are the result of basing waveform interpretation on insufficiently replicable responses and waveform tracings too noisy to be called "no response." Fortunately, the solutions to this problem are quite simple: obtain additional replications when needed (this assumes one has made every attempt to ensure the infant is quietly asleep), average together replications to increase the number of trials in an average and thus reduce residual noise in waveform, and do not interpret conditions with insufficient replications and/or noisy data.

As noted above, statistical measures of ABR signal-to-noise ratio and waveform noisiness are currently available. Currently, of the two, an online measure of waveform noisiness is the most important and must be considered a requirement when considering any new clinical ABR system.[6] It is important that any system implementing these statistical measures must allow for flexibility in their parameters, as they differ depending upon stimulus and response characteristics (e.g., settings are different for 500 versus 2000 Hz tones; as well as wave V versus later responses). Table 20–5 includes recommendations for latency windows ("SNR Regions," each 10 ms in duration) over which these measures are calculated. Exact parameters and especially criteria are not easily available; some information is provided below (further details are provided in BCEHP, 2008; HAPLAB, 2009). Statistical measures of waveform noisiness or response presence/absence (signal-to-noise) include the following.

Waveform Noisiness (Residual Noise)

Single-point (sp) variance (waveform noise; Don & Elberling, 1996; Don et al., 1984): This measure, available on only a couple of systems, measures the trial (stimulus) by trial variance in amplitude of a single time point in the evoked potential waveform, usually in the region of the expected response and always beyond any stimulus artifact. As the number of trials averaged increases, the variance goes down. The location of the single point is typically placed in the middle of the signal to noise ratio (SNR) region. For threshold measures, in order to conclude "no response," one usually must have the final sp variance down to 10 to 20 nV, a level smaller than a typical threshold wave V response. *Residual noise* (RN; i.e., waveform noise; Özdamar & Delgado, 1996; Picton et al., 1983) as with sp variance, is available on only one or two systems. The standard

[6] At the time of writing this chapter, appropriate statistical measures, especially waveform noise, were available on only a few clinical systems. However, several other manufacturers were in the process of implementing these measures.

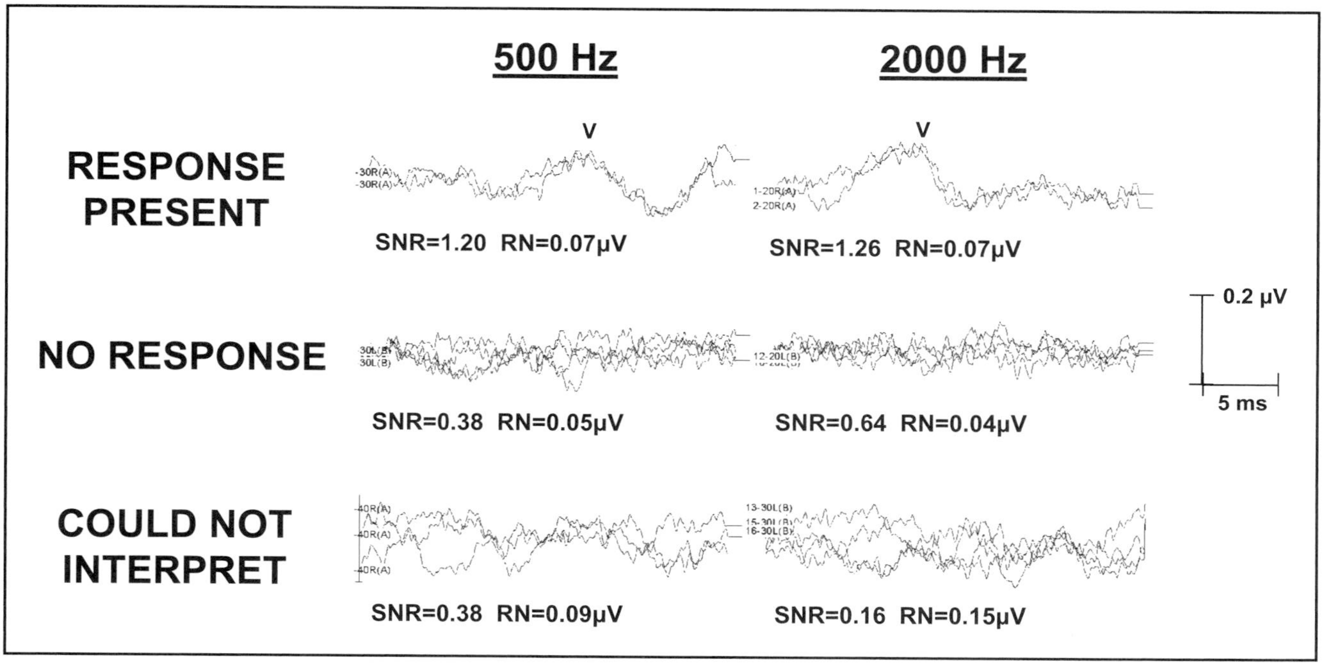

FIGURE 20–6. Interpretation of ABR waveforms. Infant ABR waveforms in response to 500- and 2000-Hz brief tones typical of "response present" (*top row*), "no response" (*middle row*), and "could not interpret" (*bottom row*) results. Shown also are the IHS Smart-EP "SNR" and "RN" measures calculated over a 10-ms window (see Table 20–5) on the average of all replications for a given set. The "response present" waveforms show a clear repeatable wave V, the peak-to-peak amplitude of which is at least three times the average difference between the replications in the 3- to 4-ms region surrounding wave V. The SNR measures are above 1.0, also consistent with response presence. Although not required for a present response, the RN values of 0.07 μV indicate reasonably quiet results. The "no response" waveforms do not show a repeatable waveform that is larger than the background noise (i.e., difference between replications is at least as large as any peak), and the waveforms are essentially flat. SNR values are well below 1.0 and thus consistent with no response. Most importantly, the waves are acceptably quiet (indicated both visually and by the low RN values which are less than the 0.08-μV criterion). The "could not interpret" waveforms do not show any repeatable peak and SNR values are well below 1.0; hence, they do not show any response. However, one cannot be sure a small, threshold-level response was not missed as these recordings are noisy. Thus, because the waves are too noisy (indicated by large differences between replications and nonflat waveforms and RN values that are above the 0.08-μV criterion) one must interpret these waves as "could not interpret." SNR: IHS Smart-EP "signal-to-noise ratio"; RN: IHS Smart-EP "residual noise level." Waveform timebase: 25.6 ms.

deviation of the plus-minus average is similar to that used on transient EOAE systems ("A-B" in dB). RN (from average of all replications) must be lower than a set value to conclude a "no response." Currently, BCEHP ABR protocols require the RN over all replications to be 0.8 μV or less before a "no response" is concluded.[7] Details are available in the BCEHP protocols (BCEHP, 2008), as well as on the HAPLAB Web site (HAPLAB, 2009). Figure 20–6 shows RN values (calculated for the average of all replications) for results showing "response present," "no response," and "could not interpret" (i.e., too noisy to conclude no response).

[7] The Intelligent Hearing Systems (IHS) SmartEP calculation of "RN" does not divide the A-B difference wave by 2 (required to calculate the plus-minus average), thus this measure over-estimates the residual noise in the waveforms by a factor of 2. The BCEHP RN criterion of 0.08 μV is thus equivalent to 0.04 μV (i.e., 40 nanovolts). Others have recommended lower noise levels (e.g., Don & Elberling, 1996).

Response Presence/Absence (Waveform Signal-to-Noise Ratio)

Correlation coefficient between replications (CCR; Hyde et al., 1998; Picton et al., 1983): Most current clinical ABR machines have the capability to calculate the correlation coefficient between two replications (Picton, Durieux-Smith, & Moran, 1994; Picton et al., 1983), a measure similar to the "reproducibility" measure used in transient EOAEs (Kemp, 1988; Picton et al., 1994). However, few systems calculate and update the correlation online as trials are averaged. Normally calculated using a 10-ms window centered on the typical response (see Table 20–5), a correlation of 0.5 and higher provides clinicians with an indication that a response is present—the higher the correlation, the more likely a response is present. Although it is not a perfect measure, individual clinicians can determine their own criterion correlation (over many sets of waves) and use this objective measure to aid in their response determination. *F-test using single-point variance* (Fsp; Don et al., 1984; Elberling & Don, 1984; Hyde et al., 1998): A somewhat better measure than correlation, the "Fsp," also provides an online/ongoing indication of response presence/absence. Unfortunately, Fsp is implemented on only a few clinical machines and few data are available. Also, typically calculated over a 10-ms window, "significant" Fsp values are typically in the range of 2.9 to 3.1 (Sininger & Hyde, 2009). *Signal-to-noise ratio (SNR) or standard deviation ratio (SDR)*; Özdamar & Delgado, 1996; Picton et al., 1994; Picton et al., 1983).[8] Also, calculated over a 10-ms window (see Table 20–5), the SNR (or SDR) provides an online/ongoing calculation but is implemented on only a few clinical machines. SNR is nearly identical to the transient EOAE signal-to-noise measures. After a study of SNRs of tone-ABRs in nearly 100 infants with normal or impaired hearing (Haboosheh, 2007), the BCEHP has recently implemented the use of SNR for determination of response presence in tone-ABR waves (BCEHP, 2008). Typically, SNR values of 1.0 or greater (or SDR ≥ 2) suggest a likely response (occasionally, "present" responses show SNR values < 1.0). Figure 20–6 shows SNR values (calculated for the average of all replications) for results showing "response present," "no response," and "could not interpret" (i.e., too noisy to conclude no response).

None of the measures above are perfect, and occasionally suggest "no response" when visual examination by experts conclude otherwise. Moreover, these measures are quite sensitive to the presence of stimulus artifact or 60-Hz (50-Hz in Europe) line noise, thus care must be taken to ensure these are excluded from the SNR region. As noted above, measures of waveform noise (RN or sp-variance) are currently most important and essential. Statistical measures described above may be particularly helpful in training new clinicians and in ensuring consistency among clinicians within a facility or across multiple facilities within a larger program (such as the BCEHP).

Current Issues and Questions Concerning the Tone-ABR

Frequency Specificity of the Tone-ABR

In order to evoke ABRs of reasonable amplitude, brief tones with relatively short rise/fall times and durations must be used (Beattie & Torre, 1997; Brinkmann & Scherg, 1979; Kodera, Yamane, Yamada, & Suzuki, 1977; Stapells & Picton, 1981; Suzuki & Horiuchi, 1981). As shown in Table 20–5, we (as well as others) recommend brief tones with total durations of 5 cycles and rise/fall times of 2 to 2.5 cycles. Such brief tones demonstrate reasonable frequency specificity (Klein, 1983; Nousak & Stapells, 1992; Oates & Stapells, 1997a, 1997b; Purdy & Abbas, 2002; Stapells & Oates, 1997; Stapells, Picton, & Durieux-Smith, 1994), and many studies have shown these brief stimuli provide adequate estimates of the audiogram for all but very steep (≥ 50 dB/octave slope) hearing losses. When hearing losses are very steep, the tone-ABR threshold will indicate an elevated threshold, but may underestimate the amount of hearing loss; this occurs as a result of the acoustic splatter to the better hearing at adjacent frequencies (Purdy & Abbas, 2002). Fortunately hearing losses with such steep slopes (≥ 50 dB/octave) are relatively uncommon, especially in infants, thus the ABR threshold to brief (5-cycle) tones provides a good estimate of the audiogram for the large majority of infants.

It has been claimed that the frequency-specificity of the tone-ABR threshold estimate can be improved by using more complex nonlinear stimulus windowing functions, such as Blackman or exact-Blackman windows (Gorga, 2002; Gorga & Thornton, 1989). Although the acoustics based on the total duration of the stimuli might lead one to conclude these nonlinear windows would be better, such a claim assumes the

[8] Due to overestimation of the residual noise by RN (see preceding footnote), the IHS SmartEP system's SNR measure is equivalent to SDR/2. Both SNR and SDR measures use a measure of the "signal" that contains both response and noise. One can estimate the true signal-to-noise ratio by $[(SNR * 2)^2 - 1]$ or $[SDR^2 - 1]$ (Picton et al., 1983).

ABR reflects the whole stimulus, whereas the "effective" portion of the stimulus is almost certainly less than the whole stimulus. The ABR appears not to be sensitive to the small differences in the temporal waveforms of the linear versus Blackman stimuli. Results published to date do not support the claim for superiority of these nonlinear windows, with at least five studies showing equivalent ABR results between linear and nonlinear (Blackman or exact-Blackman) windows (Beattie, Kenworthy, & Vanides, 2005; Johnson & Brown, 2005; Oates & Stapells, 1997a, 1997b; Purdy & Abbas, 2002). Thus, either linear- or Blackman-windowed stimuli may be used with equal accuracy.

Another technique proposed to improve the frequency specificity of the ABR to brief tones, especially in the presence of very steep losses, is that of band-reject ("notched") noise masking (Picton, Ouellette, Hamel, & Smith, 1979; Stapells & Picton, 1981; Stapells et al., 1994). The notched noise restricts the region of the basilar membrane that is capable of contributing to the response to the frequencies within the notch. The noise has a 1-octave-wide notch centered on the tone's nominal frequency; slopes of the noise filters must be quite steep (at least 48 dB/octave slope) and the intensity of the noise (before filtering) set 20 dB below the peak-to-peak equivalent SPL of the brief-tone stimulus. In recent years, we have de-emphasized the need for notched noise, as it adds complexity to equipment setup and test protocol, few clinical machines provide the capability for notched noise, and more importantly, results have shown the need for notched noise is limited to only very steep losses. Thus, ABR threshold results with and without notched noise masking are similar for more typical groups of individuals with hearing loss (Johnson & Brown, 2005; Stapells, 2000b).

It is important to remind readers that without special noise masking procedures, *no measure* is cochlear place-specific when using moderate-to-high stimulus levels; not even a behavioral response to long-duration pure-tone stimuli. That is, when presented at 60 to 80 dB HL (and higher), even pure-tone stimuli result in fairly wide cochlear excitation (Moore, 2004). Thus, elevated thresholds obtained using behavioral pure-tone audiometry are affected by this broad cochlear excitation, and it is unreasonable to expect the ABR (or ASSR) at these intensities to exhibit any better frequency specificity (Picton et al., 2003).

Stimulus Onset Polarity: Alternating or Single Polarity?

Concern has often been expressed about the use of alternating onset polarity. Specifically, it has been suggested that response amplitudes with alternating polarity will be reduced due to phase cancellation, and thus thresholds elevated (e.g., Gorga et al., 2006; Gorga, Kaminski, & Beauchaine, 1991). However, there is no evidence for this concern, especially concerning thresholds in infants. Indeed, in an unpublished study in our lab, in nine normal infants, we found no difference between single polarity (rarefaction or condensation onset polarity) and alternating polarity for wave V amplitudes and thresholds for clicks, 500-Hz brief tones, or 2000-Hz brief tones (Wu & Stapells, unpublished). This is consistent with the fact that the majority of tone-ABR threshold studies have utilized alternating onset polarity and, as noted above, threshold estimates have been quite accurate (see Tables 20–1 through 20–3). In fact, there are good reasons for employing alternating polarity tones: (i) at high intensities, electromagnetic stimulus artifact can significantly contaminate responses, especially at 500 and 1000 Hz. This artifact can make it difficult to recognize the physiologic response; if objective response detection measures are employed, the artifact can render these measures useless. Alternating polarity largely removes the artifact (though not completely at highest intensities); and (ii) especially for moderate and higher stimulus intensities, there may be steady-state responses to each cycle of the tone's carrier frequency, such as the cochlear microphonic and/or the frequency following response, which often make it more difficult to recognize or measure the transient (e.g., wave V-V') response. Alternating the polarity, for the most part, removes these unwanted responses. Although we recommend routine use of alternating polarity for all brief-tone intensities, at lower stimulus intensities there is likely no difference and little concern about polarity, and either single polarity or alternating polarity are fine. It is important to note, however, that due to the very large electromagnetic stimulus artifact occurring with bone-conduction transducers, alternating polarity should always be used for bone-conduction stimuli.

Maximum Stimulus Intensities for ABR

For several reasons, there are limits to the maximum intensities of stimuli for the ABR. First, current transducers have limitations, beyond which significant distortion occurs. Insert earphones (ER-3A) typically are limited to a maximum of about 120 dB SPL. This limits 500- to 4000-Hz pure-tone stimuli to about 110 dB HL. Because behavioral and ABR thresholds for the brief stimuli used to elicit the ABR are in the 20 to 30 dB SPL range (see Table 20–5), maximum intensities are thus limited to about 90 to 100 dB nHL. This is not necessarily the maximum possible output for ABR stimuli, as other air-conduction transducers, including sound-field speakers, do have higher output. The maximum outputs (before distortion) are even more limited for the B-71 bone oscillator: about 70 dB HL for pure-tone stimuli, and 50 to 60 dB nHL for brief-tone stimuli (Small & Stapells, 2003).[9] A second reason there are maximum output limitations is the contamination of responses by large stimulus artifact at very high intensities. For the most part, the presence of stimulus artifact does not preclude interpretable recordings, as ABR wave V-V′ usually occurs later than the artifact. Furthermore, stimulus polarity may be alternated to at least partially cancel stimulus artifact, and in extreme cases special shielding can reduce artifact. High-amplitude stimulus artifact has been shown to result in artifactual ASSRs (Gorga et al., 2004; Jeng, Brown, Johnson, & Vander Werff, 2004; Small & Stapells, 2004), although appropriate processing of the EEG largely removes these nonphysiologic spurious responses (Brooke, Brennan, & Stevens, 2009; Picton & John, 2004; Small & Stapells, 2004). A third cause of output limitation is the possibility of high stimulus levels producing non-auditory responses. Vibrotactile responses, especially to bone-conduction stimuli, place well-known limits for behavioral audiometry (Boothroyd & Cawkwell, 1970). Although vibrotactile responses are not likely to produce an ABR or brainstem ASSR, there is evidence that stimulation of the vestibular system can produce responses in the ABR and brainstem-ASSR time frame. Vestibular responses are especially problematic for interpretation of ASSRs to high-intensity stimuli in individuals with severe-profound hearing loss. This issue is discussed in the ASSR section below. Finally, a fourth cause of output limits is the real concern that maximum output stimuli may cause cochlear damage. This is of greatest concern for the ASSR where at least 10 minutes of averaging may be required to reduce the residual EEG noise to a level below that of the amplitude of a near-threshold response. As ASSR stimuli are continuous, stimulation at levels such as 90 to 110 dB HL must be regularly interrupted in order to rest the cochlea and protect it from damage. This is less of a concern for the transient ABR, as stimuli are already presented with a less than 50% duty cycle (a 500-Hz brief tone present using a 39 per second rate has at least a 15 ms quiet blank between each 10-ms stimulus). Similarly, damage from high-intensity stimuli is much less of a concern for behavioral testing, as stimuli are presented for only very brief durations.

How to Couple the Bone Oscillator to an Infant's Head

In our early research, we had an assistant hand-hold the bone oscillator to the infant's head during bone-conduction ABR testing, and found little difficulty with this procedure (Gravel et al., 1989; Stapells, 1989; Stapells & Ruben, 1989). However, other researchers expressed concern with this practice, so our subsequent bone-conduction research (Foxe & Stapells, 1993; Ishida, Cuthbert, & Stapells, submitted; Nousak & Stapells, 1992; Small & Stapells, 2003, 2004, 2005, 2006, 2008b, 2008c) utilized the technique described by Yang and colleagues (Yang, 1991; Yang, Stuart, Mencher, Mencher, & Vincer, 1993), which uses a wide elastic band with Velcro. However, we find this technique often awkward clinically, sometimes waking an infant and always requiring a longer time. Subsequently, we carried-out research comparing the elastic-band and hand-held procedures, and found the hand-held procedure was at least as reliable (indeed, it was less variable) and accurate as the elastic band procedure, provided assistants were appropriately trained (Small, Hatton, & Stapells, 2007). For clinical use, we currently recommend hand-holding the bone oscillator, given the relative ease and, importantly, speed and non-intrusiveness, of hand-holding.[10]

Establishing Normative Data

Many popular textbooks instruct clinicians to obtain (i) normal hearing levels (nHL) for their ABR stimuli, and (ii) their own normative latency data. Both of these practices have significant problems. Obtaining nHLs for click and brief-tone stimuli requires appropriate quiet sound booths, careful psychoacoustic procedures, and appropriate subjects (e.g., large number of normal young adults)—error in any of these can make a clinic's results uninterpretable, especially if no acoustic calibration of the obtained 0-dB nHL is made. Unless using a radically different stimulus for which no research exists, clinicians should use the acoustic calibrations of published research—in the same fashion (but with different calibration values) as how they calibrate their equipment for behavioral audiometry. Although official "standards" for ABR stimuli are not yet available, there are several publications providing well-researched acoustic levels of normal thresholds for

[9] As with air conduction, there are other bone-conduction transducers with a higher maximum output (e.g., MAICO KLH96), but for which there are no published ABR (or ASSR) data.

[10] The elastic-band technique is preferable when it is difficult to hand-hold the bone oscillator due to equipment setup or lack of a trained assistant.

these stimuli. Table 20–5 presents our recommended 0-dB nHL values for three transducers.

Clinicians often ask for tone-ABR latency normative data. As noted above, we do not assess whether latencies are normal or prolonged when evaluating ABR thresholds. Thus, tone-ABR latency "norms" are not that helpful, other than to give an idea of where wave V typically occurs. This information is available from the waveforms in Figures 20–1 and 20–5 (as well as other publications) and quickly comes after testing a few infants. On the more-general question of clinicians obtaining their own latency norms (e.g., for click-ABRs), we strongly believe that the literature already contains excellent normative data, obtained for a greater number of subjects than is typically possible for most clinicians (good latency norms require large samples of subjects—sample sizes of 10–20 are too small). The most important click-ABR latency measures—the I-V interpeak interval and wave V interaural latency difference—are quite consistent across most studies and little affected by stimulus and recording factors (except for rates > 20 per second), making it quite acceptable to use published norms. Thus, we do not recommend that clinicians determine their own norms; rather, we suggest they use published norms from a larger study for reasonably similar parameters and subject population (for a listing of many normative samples, see textbook by Hall, 1992). To ensure their results are similar, clinicians may test a small group (e.g., 10 subjects) and then compare statistically their results with the larger study. If no practically significant differences exist, clinicians can feel comfortable using the larger sample published norms for their clinical testing.

The Brainstem Auditory Steady-State Response

The auditory steady-state responses to stimuli presented using repetition (or modulation) rates in the 70- to 110-Hz range (the "80-Hz" or "brainstem" ASSR) have recently gained considerable attention and some excitement by audiologists, especially by those involved in the assessment and subsequent hearing-aid fitting of very young infants identified as having a hearing loss. Equipment manufacturers are marketing their new ASSR systems for such testing. Readers will find the recent text edited by G. Rance contains many excellent up-to-date chapters describing in detail the brainstem ASSR (Rance, 2008b).

What Is the Auditory Steady-State Response?

First recorded in 1960 from the scalp of humans by Geisler (1960), ASSRs were subsequently recorded in response to clicks, to sinusoidally modulated tones, and to square-wave modulated tones by Campbell and colleagues (Campbell, Atkinson, Francis, & Green, 1977). Major audiologic interest in the ASSRs came with the publication by Galambos et al. in 1981 concerning the "40-Hz ASSR" (Galambos, Makeig, & Talmachoff, 1981). Subsequent studies indicated frequency-based (Fourier) analyses could be used to accurately measure the ASSRs (e.g., Rickards & Clark, 1984; Stapells, Linden, Suffield, Hamel, & Picton, 1984). From 1981 through to the mid-1990s, the clinical audiology community went through its first phase of excitement concerning this new evoked potential threshold measure, with one manufacturer developing and marketing "the first objective infant audiometer" utilizing the ASSR to stimuli presented with a 40-Hz repetition rate. Unfortunately, subsequent research showed the 40-Hz ASSR was decreased in sleeping subjects (e.g., Cohen, Rickards, & Clark, 1991; Linden, Campbell, Hamel, & Picton, 1985) and, more importantly, it is very difficult to record in infants (e.g., Stapells, Galambos, Costello, & Makeig, 1988; Suzuki & Kobayashi, 1984). Interest and use of ASSRs by clinicians thus quickly disappeared. However, some researchers persevered and demonstrated that ASSRs to near-threshold stimuli presented with rates of 70- to 110-Hz—the brainstem ASSR—are easily recordable in sleeping infants (e.g., Lins & Picton, 1995; Lins, Picton, Picton, Champagne, & Durieux-Smith, 1995; Lins et al., 1996; Rance, Rickards, Cohen, De Vidi, & Clark, 1995), and today there is a growing body of data as well as availability of clinical systems that automatically stimulate and analyze these responses.

Discussion concerning the generators of the ASSR has thus far primarily focused on the ASSRs evoked by stimulus rates in the 30- to 50-Hz range. Studies investigating the neural sources of the 40-Hz response have concluded the response has both brainstem and cortical generators (e.g., Herdman, Lins, et al., 2002; Mauer & Döring, 1999). Recent studies investigating the neural sources of the 80-Hz ASSRs in humans and animals indicate they originate primarily from brainstem structures (Herdman, Lins, et al., 2002; Kuwada et al., 2002; Mauer & Döring, 1999). Although not yet confirmed, it is quite likely that the 80-Hz ASSRs are actually ABR waves V to rapidly presented stimuli. The ASSR stimulation and analysis techniques may differ, but the underlying physiology and interpretation of these brainstem ASSRs are likely very similar to those for ABR wave V.

ASSR Analysis Techniques

As noted above, an important feature of the ASSR is that frequency-domain analyses, such as the fast Fourier transform (FFT), provide excellent measures of the response, and there are clear procedures to determine response presence and absence. For example, similar to procedures for distortion-product otoacoustic emissions (DPOAEs), an FFT of the response provides the amplitude at exactly the stimulus modulation rate, which is compared to the amplitudes of "noise" frequencies immediately surrounding the modulation rate ("sidebins"; Figure 20–7). Thus, the amplitude and phase of the response at the rate of stimulation, as well as measures of response noise, are measured entirely objectively and automatically by a computer. In contrast to DPOAE measures, however, ASSR systems go a step further, and determine the statistical probability of a response being present. A number of statistical tests have been employed, with most studies employing either a measure of phase variability ("phase coherence") or comparison of the amplitude at the stimulus rate (or modulation frequency) to amplitudes of surrounding noise frequencies ("F-test"; for detailed reviews, see John & Purcell, 2008; Picton et al., 2003). Thus, with current ASSR systems, response determination is entirely objective; a human interpreter does not view waveforms or determine the replicability and location of peaks. This objectivity of response determination

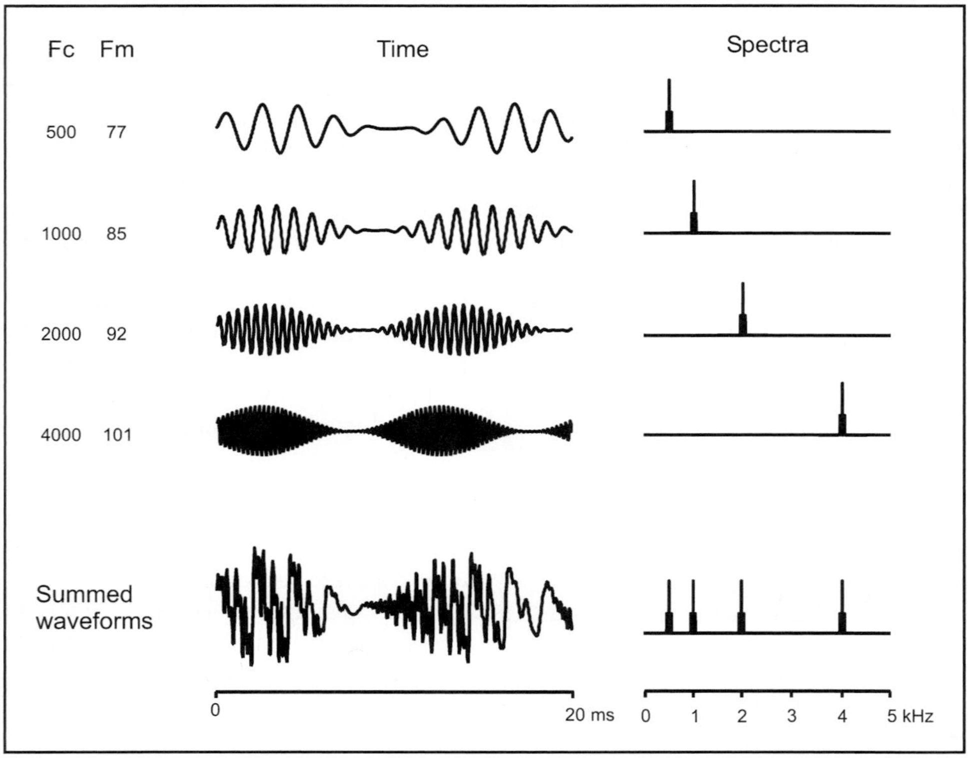

FIGURE 20–7. A. ASSR stimuli: Time and frequency spectra of multiple auditory steady-state stimuli. Four individual amplitude-modulated stimuli with carrier frequencies (Fc) ranging from 500 to 4000 Hz and modulation frequencies (Fm) ranging from 77 to 101 Hz are shown. Time waveforms spanning 2 cycles are shown (*left panel*). The corresponding spectra are shown in the right panel. The summed time and frequency spectra are shown at the bottom left and right panels, respectively. *continues*

is a major advantage of the ASSR over the transient ABR, although as noted above, objective techniques are also available for the ABR.

As when interpreting the ABR, the "response noise" estimate is also an essential measure for ASSR interpretation. When concluding a "no-response" result, it is important that a clinician continues recording until the level of response noise is below the typical amplitude of a threshold-level response. That is, ensure that a small-amplitude response was not missed because of a noisy recording. Unfortunately, not all ASSR systems provide this noise measure and, importantly, not all research studies (or clinicians) have employed such noise measures. Furthermore, there remains some uncertainty concerning what is the appropriate noise criteria (e.g., what is an acceptably low level of noise?). Because near-threshold 80-Hz ASSRs have amplitudes of about 20 to 30 nV, mean noise levels (e.g., side-bin noise) of 10 nV or lower are typically required before one can conclude that no response is present, although this level appears to differ somewhat for different analysis methods (van Maanen & Stapells, 2009). The above notwithstanding, an appropriate noise criterion must be reached before concluding "no response."

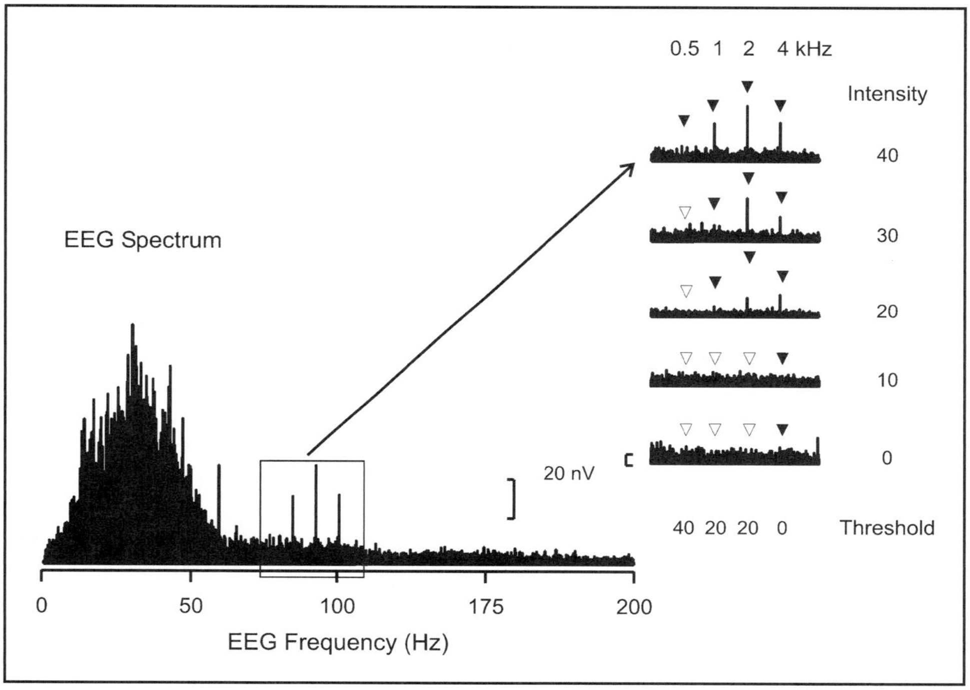

A

FIGURE 20–7. *continued* **B.** Response analyses: Threshold intensity series of multiple auditory steady-state responses recorded from an 11-week-old infant with normal hearing. Intensities are in dB nHL (Herdman & Stapells, 2001, 2003). Responses were elicited using the stimuli shown in Figure 20–7A. Bottom right shows the entire EEG frequency spectra. Right panel shows the spectra over the frequency range near the modulation frequency. Carrier frequencies corresponding to the four signals are shown on the top. Filled triangles indicate responses that reached significance ($p < .05$); open triangles indicate no-response ($p \geq .05$ *and* EEG noise < 11nV). Thresholds of 40, 20, 20, and 0 dB nHL at 500, 1000, 2000, and 4000 Hz are equivalent to 46, 29, 24, and 2 dB HL. Reproduced with permission from Stapells, D. R., Herdman, A., Small, S. A., Dimitrijevic, A., and Hatton, J. (2005). Current status of the auditory steady-state responses for estimating an infant's audiogram. In R. Seewald and J. Bamford (Eds.), *A sound foundation through early amplification 2004: Proceedings of the Third International Conference* (pp. 43–59). Stäfa, Switzerland: Phonak AG. Copyright 2005 Phonak.

As indicated above, there is considerable research demonstrating the effectiveness of phase coherence and F-test response statistics, and some ASSR systems employ these well-tested measures (for review: John & Purcell, 2008). Some recent ASSR systems, however, use modifications of these measures, or altogether entirely different algorithms. Few studies, however, have assessed these new or modified measures—it may be premature for individuals to consider purchase of these new and relatively untested systems.

ASSR Stimulus Paradigms

Although the earliest studies of the ASSRs tended to use brief tonal stimuli, similar to those used to evoke the ABR, most recent research has focused on continuous sinusoidally amplitude-modulated (AM) tonal stimuli, sometimes with 10 to 25% frequency modulation. Most current ASSR systems use such stimuli, as have most research studies. The acoustics of continuous sinusoidal AM stimuli are very frequency specific: their spectra show energy at the carrier frequency plus two sidelobes at frequencies equal to the carrier frequency plus/minus the modulation frequency. Thus, as shown in Figure 20–7A, a 1000-Hz tone modulated at 85 Hz would contain energy at 915, 1000, and 1085 Hz. Because no energy is present at the modulation rate, interpretation of response presence/absence by the computer is less susceptible to stimulus artifact (assuming linear stimulus systems and appropriate EEG digitization; see below). Adding 10 to 25% frequency modulation results in somewhat larger ASSR amplitudes, but also complicates the stimulus spectra (Purcell & Dajani, 2008). One possible reason most researchers studying the brainstem ASSR have used continuous stimuli (sine AM or AM/FM) may lie in a belief that these ASSRs are inherently different from the transient ABR. However, as discussed above, the 80-Hz ASSRs are brainstem responses and thus may show similar stimulus-response limitations as ABR wave V. For example, the transient ABR shows larger responses to stimuli with faster rise times (e.g., Stapells & Picton, 1981); similarly, larger amplitude ASSRs are obtained using AM tones with more-rapid envelopes, such as brief-duration tones (Mo & Stapells, 2008) or exponential envelopes (John, Dimitrijevic, & Picton, 2002). Indeed, one recently introduced clinical ASSR system's default stimuli are brief tones (4–8 ms duration), which may result in larger-amplitude ASSRs. However, to obtain a significant improvement in ASSR amplitude (compared to longer stimuli), durations must be reduced to quite brief (< 4 cycles); such durations result in reduced frequency specificity as well as increased interactions (amplitude reductions) between responses to multiple simultaneous stimuli (Mo & Stapells, 2008). As noted above, stimuli with broader frequency spectra lead to larger amplitude ASSRs. AM/FM stimuli do show broader frequency spectra and result in larger amplitudes, and the small loss in frequency specificity has generally been considered acceptable. Some studies have investigated the use of stimuli with much broader frequency spectra (e.g., clicks or modulated noise), specifically for the purpose of newborn hearing screening (Cebulla, Sturzebecher, Elberling, & Muller, 2007; John, Brown, Muir, & Picton, 2004). The broad frequency spectra result in large-amplitude ASSRs, making response detection (and thus screening) much faster. However, as with the click-ABR, there is no frequency specificity to this screening. Research into the use of more frequency-specific stimuli for newborn screening is also underway (Cone-Wesson, Parker, Swiderski, & Rickards, 2002; John et al., 2004; Savio, Perez-Abalo, Gaya, Hernandez, & Mijares, 2006; Sturzebecher, Cebulla, Elberling, & Berger, 2006;).

The Multiple ASSR Technique

A unique feature of the ASSR is that responses to multiple stimuli can be separated and independently assessed, all simultaneously. Because the ASSR to a stimulus presented at a specific modulation rate has its major response energy at exactly the stimulus modulation rate, it is possible to present several stimuli each with different carrier frequencies and, importantly, different modulation rates (Figure 20–7). Responses to each stimulus can then be evaluated by examining the response energy at each stimulus' exact modulation rate. First demonstrated by Lins and Picton in 1995, this multiple-stimulus ASSR technique has subsequently been developed to allow assessment of responses from both ears and four carrier frequencies (i.e., eight different modulation rates) simultaneously. Research to date suggests that: (i) amplitudes are not reduced using the multiple-ASSR technique (compared to single stimuli) provided stimulus carrier frequencies (within an ear) are at least an octave apart in frequency and 60 dB SPL or less (Herdman & Stapells, 2001; John, Lins, Boucher, & Picton, 1998); (ii) presenting multiple AM stimuli does not appear to reduce the frequency specificity of the stimulus-response pairing (Herdman, Picton & Stapells, 2002; Herdman & Stapells, 2003); (iii) at higher intensities (> 60 dB SPL), amplitudes decrease due interactions between responses to the multiple stimuli (John et al., 1998; Picton, van Roon, & John,

2009; Wood, 2009); and (iv) the multiple stimulus technique is more efficient (faster) than the single-stimulus technique, although not as much as initially expected. Especially for high intensities, the multiple-ASSR technique may be less efficient than the ASSR to single stimuli. Issues such as sloping audiograms, smaller amplitudes at some frequencies compared to others, and amplitude reductions due to interactions decrease the efficiency of the multiple stimulus technique such that it is, at best, only 1.5 to 3 times faster than the single-stimulus technique (Herdman & Stapells, 2001, 2003; John, Purcell, Dimitrijevic, & Picton, 2002).

Although many clinical systems employing the multiple-ASSR are currently being marketed to clinicians, there are surprisingly few studies that have investigated the efficiency of the single versus multiple ASSR techniques. Our recent studies indicate that (i) normal infants show significant interactions with the multiple-ASSR, even at 60 dB SPL, but their thresholds are not affected and the multiple technique remains more efficient (Hatton & Stapells, submitted), and (ii) stimuli with broader spectra, such as AM/FM, show significantly greater interactions, even at 60 dB SPL in adults, significantly reducing the efficiency of the multiple-ASSR technique (Mo & Stapells, 2008; Wood, 2009).[11]

Frequency Specificity of the Brainstem ASSR

The *acoustic frequency specificity* of sinusoidally amplitude-modulated tones, even when combined with 10 to 25% frequency modulation (AM/FM), is reasonably narrow, a fact that is often touted as one advantage of the ASSR over the tone-evoked ABR. However, the *cochlear place specificity* and the *neuronal specificity* of the stimulus-response pairing must also be considered (Herdman, Picton, et al., 2002; Picton, Dimitrijevic, & John, 2002). Use of acoustically specific stimuli does not always translate into responses that are more frequency specific, for example, as noted above, although Blackman-windowed tones show better acoustic specificity, the brainstem responses to these stimuli have the same frequency specificity as do those to brief tones shaped by linear windows (Oates & Stapells, 1997a, 1997b; Purdy & Abbas, 2002). Research into the frequency specificity of the brainstem ASSR is quite limited. Nevertheless, using two distinct methods: (i) high-pass noise masking/derived response analyses in subjects with normal hearing (Herdman, Picton, et al., 2002) and (ii) assessment of thresholds in individuals with steeply sloping SNHL (Herdman & Stapells, 2003; Johnson & Brown, 2005), results indicate the ASSR has reasonably good frequency specificity. However, ASSR frequency specificity was not as good as would be expected from the acoustic specificity of the AM stimuli, with the ASSR frequency specificity being very similar to that previously shown for the tone-evoked ABR (Herdman, Picton, et al., 2002), a finding consistent with the view that ABR wave V underlies the 80-Hz ASSR. Importantly, no difference in ASSR frequency specificity was seen for responses to multiple versus single stimuli (Herdman, Picton, et al., 2002; Herdman & Stapells, 2003). It must be noted, however, that we currently know little of the frequency specificity of the brainstem ASSR to newer, more complex (compared to sinusoidal AM) stimuli, with no studies of the frequency specificity of brainstem ASSRs to exponential or brief-tone stimuli and only one such study for AM/FM stimuli (Johnson & Brown, 2005).

Calibration of Stimuli for the Brainstem ASSR

Similar to the long-duration pure-tone stimuli used for behavioral audiometry, the continuous nature of most ASSR stimuli makes them easy to measure using a sound-level meter set to "normal" (dB RMS) sound pressure level. Behavioral thresholds for continuous AM and AM/FM ASSR stimuli are close to those for long-duration pure tones, thus most studies (and ASSR systems) have calibrated these stimuli in dB HL (ANSI, 1996). This is in contrast to the transient brief-tone stimuli used for the ABR, where calibrations are in dB "peak" or "peak-to-peak equivalent" SPL as well in dB "normal hearing level" (nHL). The nHL is employed because behavioral and ABR thresholds are elevated due to their brief duration (e.g., Stapells & Oates, 1997). However, as shown below, ASSR thresholds (in dB HL) are also significantly elevated compared to normal behavioral thresholds, especially in young infants. Interestingly, when expressed in dB peak-to-peak equivalent SPL, air-conduction ASSR thresholds in normal infants are within about 5 dB of those for the tone-evoked ABR (e.g., Rance et al., 2006). Thus, similar to the situation for the ABR, brainstem ASSR

[11]Spectra for 100% AM/25% FM tones are about 3× wider (at –20 dB) than sine-AM and 2× wider than AM^2 stimuli (Wood, 2009).

thresholds likely reflect a brief portion of the stimulus rather than the long-term RMS SPL of the whole stimulus. Another problem for the use of dB HL is that there remain large gaps in our understanding of the relationship between ASSR thresholds (in dB HL) and pure-tone behavioral thresholds (in dB HL), especially in infants with hearing loss. Caution is thus required when interpreting infant ASSR thresholds in "dB HL."

The Problem of New ASSR Technology and Methodology

ASSR technology is quickly evolving and expanding. Fifteen years ago, there were no commercial clinical ASSR systems; 10 years ago, there were only two systems: the single-stimulus Viasys/GSI "Audera" (based on the Australian "ERA" system) and the multiple-stimulus Neuronic "Audix." Today, there are many commercial ASSR systems available.[12] A looming concern is the lack of standardization among the different systems. Some of these systems are fairly closely based on the equipment (and thus techniques) used in much of the foundational ASSR research. However, many of the new systems employ new stimulation and analysis techniques that are quite different from published research. There are few published studies to support these changes or, when available, the research has only been carried out in adults with normal hearing. With differing methodologies, new systems and few published data (especially for infants with hearing loss), the current situation is one of "buyer beware" and caution must be advised. Individuals considering purchase of a particular ASSR system should ensure evidence (including clinical data) exists for that system's methodology. Preferably, such data would be available in the peer-reviewed scientific literature, be obtained in the target population (infants, especially hearing-impaired infants) and (at least some) be at arms-length from manufacturers and patent holders.

Artifactual ASSRs and Nonauditory Responses

One clear example of the pitfalls of using of a "new" response or technique (in this case, the 80-Hz ASSR), new system, or new technology, is demonstrated by the recent findings in our laboratory as well as others of spurious or artifactual ASSRs to high-intensity air- and bone-conduction stimuli (Gorga et al., 2004; Jeng et al., 2004; Narne, Nambi, & Vanaja, 2006; Picton & John, 2004; Small & Stapells, 2004).[13] In these studies, clear "responses" were shown to be present for individuals who were deaf and could not hear the stimuli. Some of these artifactual ASSRs are now known to be due to high-amplitude stimulus artifact contaminating the recorded EEG, and aliasing to mimic physiologic responses (Picton & John, 2004; Small & Stapells, 2004). By changing the analog-to-digital (AD) rate, filtering the EEG, and alternating the stimuli, thus removing any aliased energy, we showed that *most* of these artifactual ASSRs disappeared (Small & Stapells, 2004). This finding prompted an immediate change in at least one clinical ASSR system, but not until after many clinicians had reported ASSR responses to high-intensity stimuli for infants, some of which must have been due to technical error. Although the artifactual ASSRs as a result of aliased stimulus artifact appear to have been solved through stimulus and analysis modifications—this has not been formally evaluated for many, if not most, clinical systems—nevertheless, there are also physiologic but nonauditory ASSRs in individuals with severe or profound hearing loss (Narne et al., 2006; Small & Stapells, 2004). In our 2004 study, we found that even when using an appropriate AD rate, anti-aliasing filter, and alternated-polarity stimuli, many of the deaf subjects still showed responses to 500- and 1000-Hz stimuli (no responses were seen at 2000 or 4000 Hz; Small & Stapells, 2004). We suggested these responses might be vestibular in origin, as suggested by other studies using transient-evoked potentials (e.g., Cheng, Huang, & Young, 2003; Kato et al., 1998; Murofushi, Iwasaki, Takai, & Takegoshi, 2005; Papathanasiou et al., 2004; Sheykholeslami, Kermany, & Kaga, 2000; Welgampola & Colebatch, 2001). At this time, we do not have a method to differentiate the auditory and nonauditory (vestibular) responses in an ASSR recording, nor do we know how this finding will impact audiologic decisions. The responses occur in response to high-intensity stimuli, usually low-frequency, for air-conduction stimuli (at least 100 dB HL; Gorga et al., 2004; Narne et al., 2006) and for bone-conduction stimuli (50 dB HL or higher; Narne et al., 2006; Small & Stapells, 2004).

---

[12]ASSR systems change and new systems appear regularly. A commentary on several available ASSR systems is presented at: http://www.audiospeech.ubc.ca/partners/resources-for-practioners

[13]Another clear example was the development and marketing of a 40-Hz ASSR "objective infant audiometer" before infant studies demonstrated the 40-Hz ASSR was not easily recorded in infants.

One drawback with ASSRs compared to transient-evoked ABRs is that ASSRs do not provide sensible time-domain waveforms to review when unexpected or questionable results are obtained. Sometimes, the time-domain waveforms can help differentiate auditory from nonauditory responses. Figure 20–8 shows ABR and ASSR results from an infant with profound hearing loss whose brainstem ASSR shows significant ($p < .05$) responses to 110 dB HL 500 to 4000 Hz air-conducted tones. However, his ABR waveforms to high-intensity air-conducted clicks and 2000-Hz brief tones are clearly abnormal, showing a clear early negative wave (3–4 ms poststimulus) with no wave V following. Present even with alternating stimuli (i.e., not cochlear microphonic), this "N3" wave has been suggested to originate from stimulation of the vestibular system (Colebatch, 2001; Kato et al., 1998; Murofushi et al., 2005; Papathanasiou et al., 2004), and is likely the cause of the low-amplitude but significantly present ASSRs. Current ASSR methodologies typically do not provide the ability to view resulting waveforms in the time domain, and the use of rapid multiple stimuli (and thus overlapping responses) make determination of response latency very complicated. This highlights the importance of the transient ABR when thresholds are elevated.

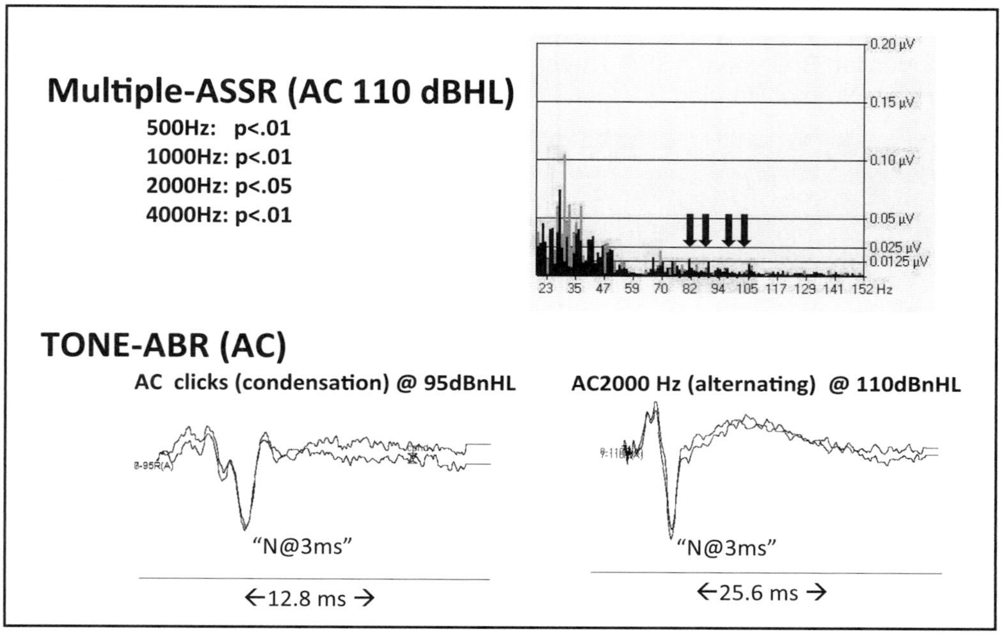

FIGURE 20–8. Air-conduction ASSR (*top panel*) and ABR (*bottom panel*) results in a 19-month-old infant with severe-profound bilateral sensorineural hearing loss. The multiple-ASSR showed small-amplitude statistically significant responses (*arrows*) in response to all four frequencies presented at the system's maximum intensity. The click-evoked (*bottom left*) and tone-evoked (*bottom right*) ABR waveforms show a large negative wave at approximately 3 to 4 ms following stimulus onset, with no clear waves V present. This "N3" wave is neural (i.e., not cochlear microphonic), as it remains present with the alternating-polarity tonal stimuli. N3 has been suggested to reflect a brainstem response originating from stimulation of the vestibular system. The presence of the significant ASSRs is likely due to repetition of the N3 to each stimulus modulation cycle—amplitudes are likely reduced due to a combination of: (i) response refractoriness due to high modulation rates and multiple simultaneous stimuli, and (ii) ASSR analysis focusses on energy at the modulation rate, which is lower than this short-latency response. These abnormal, vestibular, results are clearly evident in the time-domain waveforms of the ABR. It is much more difficult to differentiate vestibular from near-threshold auditory responses using current ASSR methodology (i.e., using frequency-domain analyses and/or multiple stimuli). Results obtained in collaboration with Renée Janssen.

Brainstem ASSR Thresholds to Air-Conduction Stimuli

Adults With Hearing Loss

There are now many studies of 80-Hz air-conduction ASSRs in adults and older children with sensorineural hearing loss. Detailed review of these studies can be found in the recent chapter by Vander Werff and colleagues (Vander Werff, Johnson, & Brown, 2008) as well as the 2007 meta-analyses by Tlumak and colleagues (Tlumak, Rubinstein, & Durrant, 2007). For most studies, the ASSR threshold provided a good-to-excellent prediction of pure-tone behavioral threshold, with correlations between ASSR and behavioral thresholds typically in the .8 to .95 range for 1000 to 4000 Hz, and .7 to .85 range for 500 Hz. The slightly poorer correlation at 500 Hz has been suggested to be due to reduced neural synchrony for responses to 500-Hz stimuli (e.g., Lins et al., 1996), although the lower correlations could also be due to some studies having relatively few 500-Hz thresholds in the severe/profound range (i.e., a restriction of range problem). Nevertheless, 500-Hz ASSR thresholds do appear to be 5 to 10 dB worse than other frequencies, similar to those for the ABR (Stapells, 2000b; Vander Werff et al., 2008). As shown on the top of Table 20–6, Tlumak and colleagues' recent meta-analysis of nine studies showed mean difference

Table 20–6. Air-Conduction Brainstem ASSR Thresholds and Maximum "Normal" Levels (in dB HL) in Infants and Young Children With Normal Hearing

			500		1000		2000		4000	
AC ASSR study	***STIM***	***Age***	***Mean ± SD***	***Norm MAX***	***Mean ± SD***	***Norm MAX***	***Mean ± SD***	***Norm MAX***	***Mean ± SD***	***Norm MAX***
Tlumak et al., 2007 (Meta-analyses of adult data)	*M*	*ADULT*	*17 ± 12*		*13 ± 12*		*11 ± 10*		*15 ± 10*	
Lins et al., 1996 (Ottawa data)	M	1–10 mos	45 ± 13	48	29 ± 10	43	26 ± 8	41	29 ± 10	40
Cone-Wesson, Parker, et al., 2002	S	<4 mos		>71		>72		50		54
John, Brown, et al., 2004 (older group)	M	3–15 wks		>46		>50		>50		40
Rance et al., 2005 †	S	1–3 mos	32 ± 8	52	33 ± 7	47	24 ± 6	40	28 ± 8	43
Swanepoel & Steyn, 2005	M	3–8 wks	37 ± 8	50	34 ± 10	>50	34 ± 11	>50	30 ± 11	40
Luts et al., 2006	M	<3 mos	42 ± 10	>44	35 ± 10	>50	32 ± 10	42	36 ± 9	44
Rance & Tomlin, 2006	S	6 wks	40 ± 7	50					33 ± 8	40
van Maanen & Stapells, 2009	M	≤6 mos	39 ± 7	49	33 ± 5	45	29 ± 7	36	24 ± 10	32
van Maanen & Stapells, 2009	M	6.1–66 mos	41 ± 7	49	37 ± 11	45	31 ± 8	36	22 ± 10	32

Note: Adult results from Tlumak et al. (2007) meta-analysis are shown for comparison. STIM: S = single-stimulus ASSR; M = multiple-stimulus ASSR; Norm MAX: Maximum intensity (in dB HL) to be considered "normal" (i.e., level required for 90-95% response presence). Mean ± SD Mean threshold in dB HL and standard deviation. Results rounded off to closest decibels. † calculated from Figure 1 of Rance et al., 2005.

scores (ASSR threshold minus behavioral threshold) for hearing-impaired adults ranging from 8 to14 dB, with individual studies showing standard deviations ranged from 7 to 18 dB (Tlumak et al., 2007). Some data suggest greater error (larger standard deviations) in estimating mild compared to more-significant hearing loss, especially at 500 Hz (D'Haenens et al., 2009; Rance et al., 2005). Studies using longer recording times (i.e., more averaging and thus lower residual EEG noise) tend to report better accuracy (Luts & Wouters, 2004; Picton et al., 2005; Vander Werff et al., 2008). In addition to estimating thresholds for individual frequencies reasonably accurately in adults, the brainstem ASSR also appears to accurately estimate audiometric shape/configuration, as demonstrated by presentation of individual audiograms (e.g., Aoyagi et al., 1994; Herdman & Stapells, 2003) and through formal statistical analyses (Herdman & Stapells, 2003; Perez-Abalo et al., 2001). Thus, at least for adults with sensorineural hearing loss, the 80-Hz ASSR provides a reasonably good estimate of behavioral threshold. Interestingly, these ASSR difference scores are very similar to those shown in Table 20–2 for the tone-ABR (Stapells, 2000b).

Given that, as noted above, conductive loss is very common in young infants, it is surprising that there appears to be only one published study of the AC ASSR in adults with true conductive loss (D'Haenens et al., 2009) and none studying individuals with mixed loss. An additional two studies have recorded ASSRs in adults with *simulated* conductive loss (produced by blocking the tubes of insert earphones; Dimitrijevic et al., 2002; Jeng et al., 2004). Overall, results suggest that difference scores (AC-ASSR minus behavioral thresholds) are somewhat larger in conductive loss than in SNHL. However, given that the results include only seven adults with true conductive loss (D'Haenens et al., 2009), more research is clearly required.

A number of studies have suggested that, compared to the ABR, the ASSR provides a better indication of residual sensitivity in individuals with profound hearing loss (Rance & Briggs, 2002; Rance, Dowell, Rickards, Beer, & Clark, 1998; Rance & Rickards, 2002; Rance, Rickards, Cohen, Burton, & Clark, 1993; Stueve & O'Rourke, 2003; Swanepoel & Hugo, 2004; Swanepoel, Hugo, & Roode, 2004). That is, ASSRs are present (especially for lower frequencies) when the ABR is absent. Although this may indeed be a real phenomenon, there are a number of issues with this suggestion: (i) Most studies used clicks to evoke the ABR. Clicks spread their energy over a wide frequency range (e.g., 100–8000 Hz), rather than concentrating their energy into a specific frequency region as do AM tones. The click-evoked ABR is well-known not to provide an accurate assessment for specific frequencies, especially for low frequencies. This is even worse when high-pass EEG filter settings of 100 Hz or higher are used (e.g., Stapells & Oates, 1997), which is the case of many of the above studies. Another problem is that the maximum click intensity of most studies was only about 90 dB nHL compared to 120 dB HL for the ASSR. Thus, for these two reasons (frequency spread and maximum intensity), the ASSR and ABR data have not been compared when the stimuli have equivalent energy at the frequency of interest. (ii) The studies that compared 500-Hz tone-evoked ABR and the ASSR also had issues, such as: lower maximum intensities for the ABR tones (in dB nHL) than the ASSR stimuli (in dB HL), incorrect (100 Hz) high-pass EEG filters, and waveform interpretation concerns (e.g., figures show clear ABR to 500 Hz but were indicated as "absent"). (iii) Finally, and importantly, at least some of the ASSRs to high-intensity stimuli may have been artifactual, either due to stimulus artifact contamination or to a nonauditory physiologic response as previously discussed and shown in Figure 20–8 (Gorga et al., 2004; Jeng et al., 2004; Narne et al., 2006; Picton & John, 2004; Small & Stapells, 2004).

In summary, although the ability to assess profound hearing losses is stated as a feature of the ASSR and an advantage over the ABR, there has yet to be an appropriate comparison which controls stimulus energy or artifactual (or nonauditory) responses. Further research and careful thought is required. Finally, it must be reiterated that presentation of high-intensity continuous tones for prolonged periods (at least 5 to 10 minutes may be required to reduce response noise below that required to state "no response") may result in noise-induced trauma to hair cells. Rest time for the cochlea must be provided by interrupting the stimuli.

Young Infants with Normal Hearing

As discussed above and shown in Table 20–1, there is a fairly reasonable database for the ABR to air-conducted brief tones thresholds in normal infants, as well as consensus as to what should be the criteria for "normal" in clinical testing (Stapells, 2000a, 2000b). The normative database for infant brainstem-ASSR thresholds is less well understood, and more recent. As noted above, the issue for ASSR is complicated further because studies have used differing stimulus (e.g., single versus multiple) and analysis (e.g., signal-to-noise and noise criteria, and thus recording time) techniques. Nevertheless, there are now many studies providing normative thresholds for infants. Figure 20–7B presents air-conduction results for a normal 11-week-old infant, showing multiple ASSR thresholds of 46, 29, 24, and 2 dB HL at 500, 1000, 2000, and 4000 Hz, thresholds which are quite different from those of adults (see Table 20–6, top line). Table 20–6 presents a detailed summary of normal infant thresholds from eight studies: mean infant thresholds (in dB HL) across studies range from 32 to 45, 29 to 37, 26 to 34, and 22 to 36 dB HL for 500, 1000, 2000, and 4000 Hz, respectively, most (85%) with standard deviations ≤ 10 dB. Importantly, infant air-conduction ASSR thresholds (uncorrected for ear-canal differences) are elevated relative to those of adults by about 20 dB for 500 to 2000 Hz, and by 10 to 15 dB for 4000 Hz. Thresholds appear to be even more elevated in very young infants (especially less than age 3–6 weeks; John et al., 2004; Rance & Tomlin, 2006; Rance et al., 2006; Savio, Cardenas, Perez Abalo, Gonzales, & Valdes, 2001); in our recent study, however, we did not find a difference in thresholds between younger (≤ 6 months) and older (6.1–66 months) infants (van Maanen & Stapells, 2009).[14] Interestingly, the higher ASSR threshold in infants compared to adults contrasts with the similar tone-ABR thresholds (in dB nHL) for the two age groups (see Table 20–1). Rance and colleagues recently compared tone-ABR and ASSR thresholds in very young infants and showed elevated ASSR thresholds in 1-week-old infants that improved over at least six weeks; tone-ABR thresholds, however, were better (lower) than the ASSR thresholds and did not change over the first six weeks of life (Rance et al., 2006). The reasons for these differences are not clear; one possible explanation is that very young auditory systems have reduced abilities to process the very rapid modulation rates (80-110 Hz) used for the brainstem ASSR, whereas the relatively slower rates (30-50/s) for the tone-ABR pose no problem (Burkard, Shi, & Hecox, 1990; Lasky, 1991; Rance, 2008a). Until recently, there has been little discussion in the literature concerning what constitutes a "normal" ASSR threshold in infants (i.e., above what intensity should an infant's thresholds be considered "elevated"). Given that mean AC-ASSR thresholds in normal infants are significantly elevated relative to adults (Table 20–7), clearly one cannot use the "normal" levels typically used for adults (i.e., one cannot use 20 to 25 dB HL as criterion for normal). To establish the criterion for "normal" for clinical testing, one does not use the mean or median thresholds (at which only ~50% of normal infants will demonstrate a response). Rather, the "normal" crite-

Table 20–7. Air-Conduction Brainstem ASSR Minus Behavioral Threshold Difference Scores (in dB) in Infants and Young Children (< 7 yrs) with Hearing Loss

AC ASSR STUDY	*STIM*	*Age*	*500*	*1000*	*2000*	*4000*
Tlumak et al., 2007 (Meta-analyses of adult data)	*M*	*Adults*	*14 ± 13 (327)*	*10 ± 13 (330)*	*9 ± 12 (328)*	*8 ± 13 (329)*
Rance & Briggs, 2002†	S	1–8 mos	6 ± 9 (160)	6 ± 7 (232)	4 ± 8 (125)	3 ± 11 (131)
Han et al., 2006	M	6–60 mos	15 ± 9 (46)	9 ± 8 (45)	8 ± 8 (42)	11 ± 9 (27)
Luts et al., 2006	M	0–50 mos	8 ± 13 (12)	6 ± 15 (25)	7 ± 13 (25)	9 ± 12 (20)
Van Maanen & Stapells, in press‡	M	1–79 mos	14 ± 9 (50)	13 ± 9 (52)	9 ± 9 (54)	−2 ± 10 (56)

Note: Adult results from Tlumak et al. (2007) meta-analysis are shown for comparison. Difference score (dB) = air-conduction ASSR threshold minus pure-tone behavioral threshold. Mean (dB) ± standard deviation. Results rounded off to closest decibels. Number of ears in parentheses. † Rance and colleagues (2005) updated their 2002 results with additional infants; however, no difference scores were provided. ‡ Behavioral threshold estimated from tone-ABR threshold using Stapells (2000b) meta-analysis difference scores (see Table 20–2).

[14]The thresholds reported above are in dB HL re: ANSI, 1996, and are not levels measured in the ear-canal, which change due to maturation of the ear canal (Bagatto, Seewald, Scollie, & Tharpe, 2006; Rance & Tomlin, 2006; Seewald, Moodie, Scollie, & Bagatto, 2005; Sininger, Abdala, & Cone-Wesson, 1997).

rion must be a level where at least 90 to 95% of infants should show a response at that level. Table 20–6 thus also presents "normal" levels for infant AC-ASSRs from eight studies. Considering these published results as well as our recent data, we recently recommended infant normal AC-ASSR levels of 50, 45, 40, and 40 dB HL for 500, 1000, 2000, and 4000 Hz, respectively, provided low-noise ASSR recordings are obtained in a quiet sound booth (Table 20–8; van Maanen & Stapells, 2009).[15]

Young Infants with Hearing Loss

Perhaps the greatest concern for clinical implementation of ASSRs is that there are very few studies of ASSR thresholds in infants with hearing loss where ASSR thresholds have been compared with gold-standard frequency-specific measures of their actual thresholds (i.e., behavioral audiometry or tone-ABR). Although several studies of ASSR thresholds in children exist, the majority of these either compare ASSR only to click-ABR thresholds; some study older children (e.g., 13 years old); and others have technical problems, especially with their tone-ABR methodology (for review see Stapells, Herdman, Small, Dimitrijevic, & Hatton, 2005). Table 20–7 lists those studies that have published difference scores (AC-ASSR thresholds minus frequency-specific behavioral or tone-ABR thresholds) in infants and young children with hearing loss. The studies by Rance and colleagues, using the single-stimulus ASSR technique, have provided the largest sample size (285 with normal hearing and 271 with sensorineural hearing loss; Rance et al., 2005). Three other studies used the multiple-ASSR technique and have a total sample size of approximately 120 ears (Han, Mo, Liu, Chen, & Huang, 2006; Luts, Desloovere, & Wouters, 2006; van Maanen & Stapells, in press). Han and colleagues' study is one of the first hearing-impaired infant threshold studies to record ASSRs to multiple brief-tone stimuli (in contrast to the more common AM or AM/FM stimuli).

As is the case with adult ASSR data, assessment of infants and children with conductive loss has received little attention. There appears to be only one study of AC-ASSR thresholds in children with conductive loss (Swanepoel, Ebrahim, Friedland, Swanepoel, & Pottas, 2008), and none for children with hearing loss of mixed origin. Although the results are promising, in Swanepoel and colleague's study (using the single-stimulus ASSR), the "conductive loss" group had no confirmation of the conductive component by frequency-specific air- and bone-conduction behavioral or tone-ABR

Table 20–8. Normal Maximum Levels and Threshold Correction Factors for Infant Tone-ABR and ASSR Thresholds

		500 Hz		1000 Hz		2000 Hz		4000 Hz	
		AC	BC	AC	BC	AC	BC	AC	BC
ABR	NORMAL MAX (dB nHL)	35	20	30	na	30	30	25	na
	Mid-Range EHL correction in dB (from Table 20–2)	10	na	5	na	0	na	–5	na
	Conservative EHL correction in dB	15	na	10	na	5	na	0	na
ASSR	NORMAL MAX (dB HL)	50	30	45	20	40	40	40	30
	EHL correction in dB † *(preliminary, conservative)*	10–20	na	10–15	na	10–15	na	5–15	na

NORMAL MAX = response must be present at this level to be considered normal.
EHL correction: ABR (dB nHL) or ASSR threshold (dB HL) minus correction = estimated behavioral hearing threshold (in dB HL).
"Conservative" ABR corrections used by BCEHP (2008) and OIHP (2008).
na: not available or not applicable.
† EHL correction factors for ASSR are preliminary. Further research is required.

[15]Interestingly, considered in ppe SPL, these normal ASSR levels are close, within 10, to those recommended for the tone ABR.

thresholds, relying, instead, on air-conducted click-ABR, EOAE, tympanograms, and otoscopy, none of which can provide an estimate of the amount of a conductive component.

Although the data to date are somewhat limited, especially for the multiple-ASSR, the results in Table 20–7 provide preliminary difference scores (i.e., corrections) to convert ASSR thresholds to EHL. Conservative AC-ASSR to EHL corrections (i.e., corrections less likely to over- estimate the amount of hearing loss) appear to be about 10 to 15 dB (see Table 20–8). These corrections apply to young children with SNHL and will require elaboration and confirmation through further research.[16]

Brainstem ASSRs to Bone-Conduction Stimuli

ASSRs to bone-conduction stimuli have not been thoroughly investigated. Several studies have reported bone-conduction ASSR thresholds in adults with normal hearing (Dimitrijevic et al., 2002; Jeng et al., 2004; Lins et al., 1996; Small & Stapells, 2005, 2008b, 2008c). Four studies have assessed the presence of spurious ASSRs in adults with severe/profound SNHL (Gorga et al., 2004; Jeng et al., 2004; Narne et al., 2006; Small & Stapells, 2004). One study has assessed bone-conduction ASSRs in adults with simulated conductive loss (Jeng et al., 2004). Recently, we studied the multiple-ASSR in adults with bone-conduction thresholds elevated either by masking noise or by SNHL. We found reasonably high correlations (.8–.9) between BC-ASSR and BC behavioral thresholds at 1000, 2000, and 4000 Hz, and somewhat poorer (.7–.8) correlations at 500 Hz. We concluded that, at least for 1000 to 4000 Hz, the BC-ASSR should provide reasonable estimates of bone-conduction thresholds (Ishida et al., submitted). However, results from infants with hearing loss are still required to confirm appropriate normal levels and determine corrections.

Our recent research has investigated the maturation of BC-ASSR thresholds in groups of premature infants, young infants, older infants as well as adults (Small et al., 2007; Small & Stapells, 2005, 2006, 2008b, 2008c). A detailed summary of our infant BC-ASSR research can be found in Small and Stapells (2008a). As shown earlier by ABR research, infant thresholds to bone-conduction stimuli are significantly different from those of adults, especially in the low frequencies. Young infants' low-frequency BC-ASSR thresholds are better (i.e., lower dB HL) than those of older infants; similarly, older infants' low-frequency BC-ASSR thresholds are better than those of adults. Thus, BC stimuli in infants are effectively more intense than the same stimuli in adults, likely due to infant skull maturation and other issues (reviewed in Small & Stapells, 2008c). Overall, low-frequency BC thresholds increase (become worse) by about 15 to 20 dB from infancy to adulthood. ASSR thresholds to 2000- and 4000-Hz BC stimuli show little or no change (Small & Stapells, 2008c). Additionally, young infant ASSR thresholds to 500- and 1000-Hz BC stimuli are better than those to 2000- and 4000-Hz BC stimuli (Small & Stapells, 2008b, 2008c) These patterns are clearly different than those for air-conduction stimuli, and indicate that "normal levels" and BC-ASSR-to-behavioral correction factors must be determined from infant data. The existing infant data are currently limited to research in our lab; based on this research, we have recommended normal BC-ASSR levels of 30, 20, 40 and 30 dB HL for infants aged 0 to 11 months, and 40, 20, 40, and 30 dB HL for infants aged 12 to 24 months (see Table 20–8; Small & Stapells, 2008a).[17]

We have also investigated methodological issues such as: (i) bone oscillator placement (mastoid versus upper temporal bone versus forehead), (ii) bone oscillator coupling technique (handheld versus elastic band), and (iii) the occlusion effect (Small et al., 2007). These infant studies indicate that: (i) forehead placement should be avoided as thresholds are elevated; upper temporal bone and mastoid results are similar although upper temporal bone may be easier to accomplish; (ii) either hand-held or elastic band may be used, provided individuals are adequately trained, and (iii) as infants do not demonstrate an occlusion effect, insert earphones may be left an infant's ear canal during testing with no correction required.

[16] In reviewing the AC-ASSR normal levels (see Table 20–6) and the difference scores with hearing loss (see Table 20–7), it becomes clear that current information makes separation of normal hearing and mild hearing loss difficult, especially at 500 Hz. For example, even a 20–dB correction factor applied to the normal level of 50 dB HL at 500 Hz results in a predicted behavioral threshold of 30 dB HL, a result still in the elevated range.

[17] We have also recommended normal levels of: (i) 30, 30, 50+, and 50 dB HL for premature infants (Small & Stapells, 2006), and (ii) 40–50, 40, 30 and 30 for adults (Small & Stapells, 2008c). We have recently suggested normal levels for adults should be reduced to 40, 30, 30, and 20 dBHL for adults (Ishida et al., submitted).

Similar to the ABR, two-channel EEG recordings of infants' brainstem ASSRs also show significant ipsilateral/contralateral asymmetries, with the responses larger and earlier (in latency) in the EEG channel ipsilateral to the stimulated ear (Small & Stapells, 2008b). Our preliminary research suggests these asymmetries may be useful in determining which cochlea is responding to bone-conduction stimuli, as is currently possible with two-channel recordings of the ABR. However, further research is required, especially in infants with hearing loss, before these ASSR ipsilateral/contralateral asymmetries can be used clinically. Currently, there are no bone-conduction ASSR studies in young infants with hearing loss. Swanepoel and colleagues recently published the first study to assess bone-conduction ASSRs in young children (mean age: 3.6 years) with elevated air-conduction click-ABR thresholds (Swanepoel et al., 2008). They also reported possible "spurious" responses using the single stimulus system, with results suggesting more spurious responses than studies using the multiple-ASSR technique (Jeng et al., 2004; Small & Stapells, 2004). Unfortunately, as noted above, Swanepoel and colleagues did not confirm the hearing status or levels of their subjects. Additional research comparing BC-ASSR thresholds in infants with hearing loss confirmed by behavioral (or tone-ABR) thresholds to air- and bone-conduction stimuli is required.

Current Status of the ABR and ASSR for Frequency-Specific Threshold Assessment in Infants and Young Children

As the preceding review indicates, using the 80-Hz ASSR to estimate hearing threshold in infants is very promising; however a number of important concerns remain. These concerns include: (i) New stimulus parameters and/or new analysis methods as well as new clinical systems have received little assessment, with few peer-reviewed data supporting their use clinically, especially for infants with hearing loss. (ii) Data for ASSR estimation of threshold in infants with hearing loss are limited to air-conduction thresholds in infants with sensorineural hearing loss. No data exist for infants with conductive or mixed hearing loss where ASSR thresholds have been compared with gold-standard behavioral and/or tone-evoked ABR thresholds. (iii) Very limited data of the bone-conduction ASSR, especially for infants with hearing loss. (iv) The relationship of ASSR thresholds in individuals with profound hearing loss is not adequately studied. The impact of nonphysiologic (artifactual) or nonauditory physiologic (e.g., vestibular) "spurious" responses on results, especially in those with profound loss remains unclear.

Without resolution of these issues, it remains premature to recommend the use of ASSRs as the primary electrophysiologic measure for threshold estimation in infants. Given the current rapid pace of ASSR research, the much-needed results *may* be available within a few years—when considering the results of future ASSR studies, clinicians must critically appraise them to ensure they involved infants with hearing loss confirmed using frequency-specific gold-standard methods (i.e., behavioral or tone-ABR thresholds using air- and bone-conduction stimuli). Until then, only the tone-evoked ABR has the sufficient research, clinical database, and clinical history to recommend it as the *primary* technique for threshold estimation in young infants. Only the tone-evoked ABR can provide both the air- and bone-conduction results required for early intervention for children with conductive, mixed, and sensorineural hearing loss. Except when air-conduction thresholds are normal, the ASSR thus is only appropriate if used *in conjunction with* the tone-evoked ABR.

Currently, there are two ways the ASSR may be used in conjunction with the tone-ABR. First, the ASSR can be very fast as the first step in the diagnostic "ABR/ASSR" protocol, quickly determining whether elevated or normal thresholds are present, by recording responses to air-conduction stimuli at "normal" levels. We have found the dichotic (two-ear) multiple stimulus ASSR to be very fast, requiring only about 4 to 6 minutes total in infants with normal hearing (Janssen & Stapells, 2009; van Maanen & Stapells, 2009). In normal infants, this is about 50 to 70% of the time required for the tone-ABR; in infants with elevated thresholds, we found the multiple-ASSR in this first step indicated "elevated" only slightly faster, requiring about 80 to 90% of the tone-ABR time (Janssen & Stapells, 2009). If the AC-ASSR is absent at the normal levels (i.e., elevated thresholds are present), testing is then quickly switched to the tone-ABR using both bone-conduction and air-conduction stimuli. The second use of the ASSR involves threshold searches *after* required tone-ABR thresholds have been obtained; these ASSR thresholds can provide an important cross-check for the tone-ABR thresholds. The following section outlines our current recommended test sequence and the rationale behind it.

Protocols and the Sequence of Testing using the ABR/ASSR

It is essential to use a test sequence that is fast and efficient, and provides the greatest increase in clinical information with each successive step.[18] Several principles guide the general strategy of stimulus conditions: (i) Test time is limited—the infant may wake-up at any moment—so the most important question must be assessed first; (ii) The choice of stimulus condition should be based on what is the most probable outcome: for example, most infants coming to the diagnostic ABR stage after referral during the newborn period have normal hearing. This is usually due to a middle-ear disorder that has resolved since the screening referral, although screening errors also occur. Thus, starting at a low intensity (i.e., at the "normal" levels discussed above) will quickly obtain the necessary results for most infants; (iii) Choice of stimulus condition should be based on provision of results that make a difference in management as well as information to the parents: for example, when no response is present at the air-conduction "normal" intensity, spending time collecting precise air-conduction threshold information is less useful than obtaining bone-conduction results, because air-conduction threshold in most infants with conductive hearing loss is a "moving target" (i.e., it changes over time). Having information about the type of impairment directs subsequent management (including medical management) and provides more certain information for the family; (iv) Efficient strategies require clinicians to frequently switch ears and mode (AC versus BC) of stimulation—insert earphones should be placed in both ears at the beginning of testing, and the bone oscillator ready for application: for example, after obtaining a "no response" at the air-conduction screening intensity in the first ear, one should switch to the other ear rather than seek threshold. Otherwise, one may have spent time determining threshold for one ear, only to have the infant wake-up before determining that the other ear was normal (determined on a second ABR appointment). Obviously, it would have been better, both for management and for the family, to know that at least one ear was normal.

For most infants, therefore, the diagnostic ABR/ASSR assessment should aim to answer the following three questions, in order of priority: (1) Is an ear's AC threshold normal or elevated? Is the other ear's AC threshold normal or elevated? (2) If elevated, is the elevation conductive in nature or is there a sensorineural component? (3) If elevated, what are the specific thresholds (AC and/or BC)? The first question is answered by testing *each ear* at the "normal" AC level; that is, the minimum level required to conclude normal thresholds for that ear. Results for 2000 Hz are typically obtained first, and this step does not normally involve a threshold search. If the baby wakes up at the end of this, the clinician is still able to state whether one or both ears' thresholds are normal/elevated. If one has multiple-ASSR available, one can answer this question quite quickly by recording the ASSR to 500, 1000, 2000, and 4000 Hz air-conducted stimuli presented at the normal levels to both ears. Table 20–8 summarizes the normal levels currently recommended for AC (and BC) stimuli for tone-ABR and ASSR.

The second question is answered by BC testing (at the minimum "normal" BC level) of the ear(s) with AC elevation(s). This question currently can only be answered by the tone-ABR, given the current lack of BC-ASSR data. This step should occur as soon as both ears have been tested in step one at 2000 Hz and one or both ears show no-response (at the normal level). If the infant wakes up at the end of this bone-conduction stage, the clinician is able to state that the elevation in AC threshold is either conductive in nature or has a sensorineural, and thus permanent, component. As the majority of infants referred from universal newborn hearing screening (UNHS) with elevated AC thresholds will turn out to have conductive losses, this procedure will most often quickly identify an infant's elevation as conductive in nature, providing important information for subsequent management and for the parents.

The third question is answered by detailed determination of AC (and BC) thresholds. AC thresholds for each required frequency are required for subsequent interventions, including amplification (when chosen by the family) when sensorineural hearing loss is present. Currently, this information must be provided by the tone-ABR. Given the relatively few ASSR data for infants with hearing loss, and uncertainties concerning appropriate ASSR-behavioral corrections, any threshold information obtained using the ASSR should come after completing the tone-ABR.

The above does not clearly indicate the priority sequence of testing for stimulus frequencies. In general, greatest priority is given to 2000 Hz, and results

[18]Greater detail of our protocols and their rationale are provided in the BCEHP and OIHP protocol documents (BCEHP, 2008; OIHP, 2008), as well as in the excellent chapter by Sininger and Hyde (2009).

for this frequency are normally obtained first. Next in priority is 500 Hz, then 4000 Hz following, and, if required, 1000 Hz following.[19] Prior information (excluding hearing screening results), history (e.g., ototoxic medications) and actual results obtained during the assessment may alter the relative priority of frequencies, but the above sequence should be appropriate for the majority infants requiring diagnostic ABR/ASSR assessment. Selecting the frequency test order is less of an issue for threshold searches carried out using the multiple-ASSR, as results are obtained for four frequencies simultaneously.

Generally, regularly using intensity stepsizes smaller than 20 dB are inefficient; however, thresholds should be established using a *final* step-size of 10 dB (except, as noted above, when thresholds are greater than 70 dB nHL, where a 5-dB final stepsize may be helpful). It is inefficient to routinely use a 5-dB stepsize or test at levels below the 25 to 35 dB nHL normal levels (with perhaps the exception of ototoxic monitoring, the management of a "threshold" at the 25 to 35 dB nHL levels is unlikely to be different from a 10 to 20 dB nHL threshold; Sininger & Hyde, 2009). Intensities tested should bracket threshold: for example, if no response is seen at 30 dB nHL (2000 Hz), choosing the next level to be 40 dB nHL will give little information if there is no response at 40 dB nHL. A better compromise is 60 dB nHL. If both 30 and 60 dB nHL at 2000 Hz have been tested (as well as BC 2000 Hz at 30 dB) before the infant wakes up, then we know the following: (i) an impairment exists for one or both ears, (ii) whether a sensorineural component exists, and (iii) whether the loss is mild/moderate (if 60 dB nHL response is present) or more severe (if 60 dB nHL is absent). Unfortunately, all too often, clinicians use smaller stepsizes, and follow a sequence which does not switch ears (and AC/BC mode), with the end result that the infant wakes up before a clear picture of the status of *both* ears, as well as the type and severity of loss, has been obtained (BCEHP, 2008; OIHP, 2008).

ABR (and ASSR) assessment of young infants can be seriously compromised by auditory neuropathy spectrum disorder and/or neurologic involvement (in such cases, especially in ANSD, ABR and ASSR thresholds typically do not reflect cochlear or behavioral sensitivity; BCEHP, 2008; OIHP, 2008; Rance, 2005). As a rule, if a clinician sees a distinct wave that is *clearly* ABR wave V (to a brief tone of any frequency, whether AC or BC), then they can be reasonably confident that an elevated ABR threshold is *not* due to ANSD or neurologic dysfunction (Providing wave V is clear and the V/I amplitude ratio is normal, the finding of a prolonged wave I-V interpeak latency should not be interpreted as suggesting any threshold elevation is due to neurologic dysfunction). On the other hand, the lack of a *clear* ABR wave V in any waveform, even at the highest intensity, may be the result of profound peripheral (conductive and cochlear) impairment *or* ANSD/neurologic dysfunction. In such a situation (no tone-ABR response with a clear wave V), the clinician must obtain recordings to high-intensity clicks (90–100 dB nHL, mono-polarity, ~19 per second rate). Unfortunately, with ASSR one does not have interpretable time-domain waveforms, thus for any elevated ASSR threshold, one requires confirmation by tone-ABR, and, if no clear wave V is present to the brief tones, by click-ABR.[20]

The question is often asked: "How much time will this tone-ABR testing require?" It definitely takes longer than a simple air-conducted click-evoked ABR; after all, far more information is being sought. Because of this, clinicians must be skilled in carrying out and interpreting tone-ABR results, and they now must use appropriate and efficient test protocols. We recently reviewed 188 tone-ABR assessments (184 infants) carried out over a 20–month period in one of our clinical facilities utilizing tone-ABR protocols (BCEHP, 2008) similar to the sequence outlined above, and found that on average, we had 58 minutes of test time for sedated infants, during which we obtained about eight "measures" (e.g., four thresholds in each ear). Nonsedated infants, all aged under 6 months, had an average of 49 minutes of test time, with six "measures" obtained. Importantly, we obtained at least six measures (e.g., three frequencies per ear) for most infants (> 80%), thus providing the required information in one session for most infants (Janssen et al., 2010). Nevertheless, even with efficient protocols, there will be infants for whom complete information is not obtained within one test session, and a second test session will be required. Although sedation provides, on average, about nine additional minutes of test time, our experience is that nonsedated appointments are much easier and flexible

---

[19]Often, there is little gained in testing 1000 Hz if thresholds for 500 and 2000 Hz are within 20 dB of each other. Thus, testing at 1000 Hz should only be carried out: (i) if 500 to 2000 Hz thresholds differ by more than 20 dB, or (ii) all other required testing has been completed (BCEHP, 2008; OIHP, 2008).

[20]It also is important to obtain other measures of auditory responsivity to cross-check the ABR/ASSR results, especially evoked otoacoustic emissions and behavioral responses.

to schedule (no evaluation or monitoring by medical personnel need be arranged), and are typically more accepted by families. Importantly, with today's very early identification, many infants are now seen at a very young age when they sleep naturally, and sedation is rarely necessary or appropriate. There should be no hesitation in scheduling a second diagnostic ABR session.

What is the minimum information required from ABR/ASSR threshold assessment? Assuming results are deemed reliable and no neurologic/ANSD component to the threshold elevation is suspected (i.e., a clear wave V is present), then, at a minimum, a "complete" tone-ABR evaluation should provide AC thresholds for 500 and 2000 Hz (or, responses at the normal levels) and, if thresholds are elevated, BC tested at least for 2000 Hz and AC thresholds for 4000 Hz (BCEHP, 2008; OIHP, 2008). Normally, additional information (EOAE, immittance) is also obtained (Janssen et al., 2010), but these additional measures are usually obtained *after* the tone-ABR testing is completed (i.e., they should not take up ABR test/sleep time; BCEHP, 2008). With this information, appropriate management can be initiated early, to be modified later as further information, especially behavioral thresholds, becomes available (Gravel, 2002; JCIH, 2007; Sininger, 2003).

Acknowledgments. This chapter is dedicated to my friend, colleague, and audiology mentor, Judith S. Gravel. I thank the many individuals with whom I have collaborated in this area, in particular: Judy Gravel, Anthony Herdman, Martyn Hyde, Sasha John, Peggy Korczak (Oates), Terence Picton, and Susan Small, and my colleagues at British Columbia's Children's Hospital Audiology Department/ BCEHP, especially Renée Janssen, Laurie Usher, and Anna van Maanen. In many cases, the "we" referred to in this chapter includes these individuals. The research and preparation of this chapter were supported by funds from the Canadian Institutes of Health Research and the Natural Sciences and Engineering Research Council of Canada.

References

American Speech-Language-Hearing Association (ASHA). (2004). *Guidelines for the audiologic assessment of children from birth to 5 years of age*. American Speech-Language-Hearing Association. Retrieved September 3, 2009, from http://www.asha.org/NR/rdonlyres/0BB7C840-27D2-4DC6-861B-1709ADD78BAF/0/v2GLAudAssessChild.pdf

ANSI. (1996). *American National Standard specifications for audiometers (ANSI S3.6-1996)*. New York, NY: Author.

Anson, B. J., & Donaldson, J. A. (1981). The ear: Developmental anatomy. In B. J. Anson & J.A. Donaldson (Eds.), *Surgical anatomy of the temporal bone*. Philadelphia, PA: W. B. Saunders.

Aoyagi, M., Kiren, T., Furuse, H., Fuse, T., Suzuki, Y., Yokota, M., & Koike, Y. (1994). Pure tone threshold prediction by 80-Hz amplitude-modulation following response. *Acta Otolaryngologica, Supplemental, 511*, 7–14.

Bagatto, M. (2008). Baby waves and hearing aids: Using ABR to fit hearing aids to infants. *Hearing Journal, 61*(2), 10–16.

Bagatto, M. P., Seewald, R. C., Scollie, S. D., & Tharpe, A. M. (2006). Evaluation of a probe tube insertion technique for measuring the real-ear-to-coupler difference (RECD) in young infants. *Journal of the American Academy of Audiology, 17*(8), 573–581.

Beattie, R. C., Kenworthy, O. T., & Vanides, E. L. (2005). Comparison of ABR thresholds using linear versus blackman gating functions for predicting pure tone thresholds in hearing impaired subjects. *Australian and New Zealand Journal of Audiology, 27*(1), 1–9.

Beattie, R. C., & Torre, P. (1997). Effects of rise-fall time and repetition rate on the auditory brainstem response to 0.5 and 1 kHz tone bursts using normal-hearing and hearing impaired subjects. *Scandinavian Audiology, 26*, 23–32.

Boothroyd, A., & Cawkwell, S. (1970). Vibrotactile thresholds in pure tone audiometry. *Acta Otolaryngologica, 69*(6), 381–387.

Brinkmann, R. D., & Scherg, M. (1979). Human auditory on- and off-potentials of the brainstem. *Scandinavian Audiology, 8*, 27–32.

British Columbia Early Hearing Program (BCEHP). (2008). *Diagnostic audiology protocol* [pdf document]. Retrieved September 1, 2009, from http://www.phsa.ca/NR/rdonlyres/EAD072EA-0C0E-40C6-830A-557357C14DA5/32441/DAAGProtocols1.pdf

Brooke, R. E., Brennan, S. K., & Stevens, J. C. (2009). Bone conduction auditory steady state response: investigations into reducing artifact. *Ear and Hearing, 30*(1), 23–30.

Burkard, R., Shi, Y., & Hecox, K. E. (1990). A comparison of maximum length and Legendre sequences for the derivation of brain-stem auditory-evoked responses at rapid rates of stimulation. *Journal of the Acoustical Society of America, 87*, 1656–1664.

Campbell, F. W., Atkinson, J., Francis, M. R., & Green, D. M. (1977). Estimation of auditory thresholds using evoked potentials. A clinical screening test. *Progress in Clinical Neurophysiology, 2*, 68–78.

Canadian Working Group on Childhood Hearing. (2005). *Early Hearing and Communication Development: Canadian Working Group on Childhood Hearing (CWGCH) Resource document*. Ottawa: Minister of Public Works and Government Services Canada. Retrieved September 20, 2009, from http://www.phacaspc.gc.ca/publicat/eh-dp/index-eng.php

Cebulla, M., Sturzebecher, E., Elberling, C., & Muller, J. (2007). New clicklike stimuli for hearing testing. *Journal of American Academy of Audiology, 18*(9), 725–738.

Cheng, P.-W., Huang, T.-W., & Young, Y.-H. (2003). The influence of clicks versus short tone bursts on the vestibular evoked myogenic potential. *Ear and Hearing, 24*, 195–197.

Cohen, L. T., Rickards, F. W., & Clark, G. M. (1991). A comparison of steady-state evoked potentials to modulated tones in awake and sleeping humans. *Journal of the Acoustical Society of America, 90*, 2467–2479.

Colebatch, J. G. (2001). Vestibular evoked potentials. *Current Opinion in Neurology, 14*(1), 21–26.

Cone-Wesson, B. (1995). Bone-conduction ABR tests. *American Journal of Audiology, 4*, 14–19.

Cone-Wesson, B., Parker, J., Swiderski, N., & Rickards, F. (2002). The auditory steady-state response: Full-term and premature neonates. *Journal of the American Academy of Audiology, 13*(5), 260–269.

Cone-Wesson, B., & Ramirez, G. M. (1997). Hearing sensitivity in newborns estimated from ABRs to bone-conducted sounds. *Journal of the American Academy of Audiology, 8*, 299–307.

Cornacchia, L., Martini, A., & Morra, B. (1983). Air and bone conduction brain stem responses in adults and infants. *Audiology, 22*, 430–437.

D'Haenens, W., Dhooge, I., Maes, L., Bockstael, A., Keppler, H., Philips, B., . . . Vinck, B. M. (2009). The clinical value of the multiple-frequency 80–Hz auditory steady state response in adults with normal hearing and hearing loss. *Archives in Otolaryngology–Head and Neck Surgery, 135*(5), 496–506.

Dimitrijevic, A., John, M. S., van Roon, P., Purcell, D. W., Adamonis, J., Ostroff, J., . . . Picton, T. W. (2002). Estimating the audiogram using multiple auditory steady state responses. *Journal of the American Academy of Audiology, 13*(4), 205–224.

Don, M., & Elberling, C. (1996). Use of quantitative measures of auditory brain-stem response peak amplitude and residual background noise in the decision to stop averaging. *Journal of Acoustical Society of America, 99*, 491–499.

Don, M., Elberling, C., & Waring, M. (1984). Objective detection of averaged auditory brainstem responses. *Scandinavian Audiology, 13*, 219–228.

Edwards, C. G., Durieux-Smith, A., & Picton, T. W. (1985). Neonatal auditory brainstem responses from ipsilateral and contralateral recording montages. *Ear and Hearing, 6*, 175–178.

Eggermont, J. J. (1982). The inadequacy of click-evoked auditory brainstem responses in audiological applications. *Annals of the New York Academy of Sciences, 388*, 707–709.

Elberling, C., & Don, M. (1984). Quality estimation of averaged auditory brainstem responses. *Scandinavian Audiology, 13*, 187–197.

Foxe, J. J., & Stapells, D. R. (1993). Normal infant and adult auditory brainstem responses to bone conducted tones. *Audiology, 32*, 95–109.

Fria, T. J., & Sabo, D. L. (1979). Auditory brainstem responses in children with otitis media with effusion. *Annals of Otology, Rhinology and Laryngology, 89*, 200–206.

Galambos, R., Makeig, S., & Talmachoff, P. (1981). A 40-Hz auditory potential recorded from the human scalp. *Proceedings of the National Academy of Sciences (USA), 78*(4), 2643– 2647.

Geisler, C. D. (1960). Average response to clicks in man recorded by scalp electrodes. *M.I.T. Technical Report, 380*, 1–158.

Gorga, M. P. (2002). Some factors that may influence the accuracy of auditory brainstem response estimates of hearing loss. In R. C. Seewald & J. S. Gravel (Eds.), *A sound foundation through early amplification 2001. Proceedings of the second international conference* (pp. 49–61). Stäfa, Switzerland: Phonak AG.

Gorga, M. P., Johnson, T. A., Kaminski, J. R., Beauchaine, K. L., Garner, C. A., & Neely, S. T. (2006). Using a combination of click- and tone burst-evoked auditory brain stem response measurements to estimate pure-tone thresholds. *Ear and Hearing, 27*(1), 60–74.

Gorga, M. P., Kaminski, J. R., & Beauchaine, K. L. (1991). Effects of stimulus phase on the latency of the auditory brainstem response. *Journal of the American Academy of Audiology, 2*, 1–6.

Gorga, M. P., Neely, S. T., Hoover, B. M., Dierking, D. M., Beauchaine, K. L., & Manning, C. (2004). Determining the upper limits of stimulation for auditory steady-state response measurements. *Ear and Hearing, 25*(3), 302–307.

Gorga, M. P., & Thornton, A. R. (1989). The choice of stimuli for ABR measurement. *Ear and Hearing, 10*, 217–230.

Gravel, J. S. (2002). Potential pitfalls in the audiological assessment of infants and young children. In R. C. Seewald & J. S. Gravel (Eds.), *A sound foundation through early amplification 2001. Proceedings of the second international conference* (pp. 85–101). Stäfa, Switzerland: Phonak AG.

Gravel, J. S., Kurtzberg, D., Stapells, D. R., Vaughan, H. G. J., & Wallace, I. F. (1989). Case studies. *Seminars in Hearing, 10*, 272–287.

Haboosheh, R. (2007). *Diagnostic auditory brainstem response analysis: Evaluation of signal- to-noise ratio criteria using signal detection theory.* Unpublished M.Sc. thesis, University of British Columbia, Vancouver, B.C.

Hall, J. W. (1992). *Handbook of auditory evoked responses.* Needham Heights, MA: Allyn & Bacon.

Han, D., Mo, M., Liu, H., Chen, J., & Huang, L. (2006). Threshold estimation in children using auditory steady-state responses to multiple simultaneous stimuli. *ORL, 68*, 64–68.

HAPLAB. (2009). *Evoked potential audiometry: Tips for clinicians.* Retrieved September 20, 2009 from http://www.audiospeech.ubc.ca/partners/resources-for-practioners

Hatton, J. L., & Stapells, D. R. (manuscript submitted for publication). *Efficiency of single- vs. multiple-stimulus auditory steady-state responses in infants.*

Herdman, A., Lins, O., van Roon, P., Stapells, D., Scherg, M., & Picton, T. (2002). Intracerebral sources of human auditory steady-state responses. *Brain Topography, 15*, 69–86.

Herdman, A. T., Picton, T. W., & Stapells, D. R. (2002). Place specificity of multiple auditory steady-state responses. *Journal of the Acoustical Society of America, 112*, 1569–1582.

Herdman, A. T., & Stapells, D. R. (2001). Thresholds determined using the monotic and dichotic multiple auditory

steady-state response technique in normal-hearing subjects. *Scandinavian Audiology, 30*, 41–49.
Herdman, A. T., & Stapells, D. R. (2003). Auditory steady-state response thresholds of adults with sensorineural hearing impairments. *International Journal of Audiology, 42*(5), 237–248.
Hooks, R. G., & Weber, B. A. (1984). Auditory brain stem response of premature infants to bone-conducted stimuli: A feasibility study. *Ear and Hearing, 5*, 42–46.
Hyde, M., Sininger, Y. S., & Don, M. (1998). Objective detection and analysis of auditory brainstem response: An historical perspective. *Seminars in Hearing, 19*(1), 97.
Hyde, M. L. (2005). Newborn hearing screening programs: Overview. *Journal of Otolaryngology, 34*(Suppl. 2), S70–S78.
Ishida, I. M., Cuthbert, B. P., & Stapells, D. R. (manuscript submitted for publication). *Multiple-ASSR thresholds to bone conduction stimuli in adults with elevated thresholds*.
Janssen, R. M., & Stapells, D. R. (2009). *Which is faster to establish "normal" versus "elevated" thresholds in infants and young children: Tone-evoked ABR or multiple-ASSR?* Paper presented at the XXI Biennial Symposium of the International Evoked Response Audiometry Study Group, June 8–11. Rio de Janeiro, Brazil.
Janssen, R. M., Usher, L., & Stapells, D. R. (2010). The British Columbia's Children's Hospital tone-evoked ABR protocol: How long do infants sleep, and how much information can be obtained in one appointment? *Ear and Hearing, 31*, 722–724.
Jeng, F. C., Brown, C. J., Johnson, T. A., & Vander Werff, K. R. (2004). Estimating air-bone gaps using auditory steady-state responses. *Journal of the American Academy of Audiology, 15*(1), 67–78.
John, M. S., Brown, D. K., Muir, P. J., & Picton, T. W. (2004). Recording auditory steady-state responses in young infants. *Ear and Hearing, 25*(6), 539–553.
John, M. S., Dimitrijevic, A., & Picton, T. W. (2002). Auditory steady-state responses to exponential modulation envelopes. *Ear and Hearing, 23*(2), 106–117.
John, M. S., Lins, O. G., Boucher, B. L., & Picton, T. W. (1998). Multiple auditory steady-state responses (MASTER): Stimulus and recording parameters. *Audiology, 37*, 59–82.
John, M. S., & Purcell, D. W. (2008). Introduction to technical principles of auditory steady-state response testing. In G. Rance (Ed.), *The auditory steady-state response. Generation, recording, and clinical application* (pp. 11–53). San Diego, CA: Plural.
John, M. S., Purcell, D. W., Dimitrijevic, A., & Picton, T. W. (2002). Advantages and caveats when recording steady-state responses to multiple simultaneous stimuli. *Journal of the American Academy of Audiology, 13*, 246–259.
Johnson, T. A., & Brown, T. A. (2005). Threshold prediction using the auditory steady-state response and the tone burst auditory brain stem response: A within-subject comparison. *Ear and Hearing, 26*, 559–576.
Joint Committee on Infant Hearing (JCIH). (2007). Year 2007 position statement: Principles and guidelines for early hearing detection and intervention programs. *Pediatrics, 120*(4), 898–921.
Kato, T., Shiraishi, K., Eura, Y., Shibata, K., Sakata, T., Morizono, T., & Soda, T. (1998). A "neural" response with 3-ms latency evoked by loud sound in profoundly deaf patients. *Audiology and Neurotology, 3*(4), 253–264.
Kavanagh, K. T., & Beardsley, J. V. (1979). Brain stem auditory evoked response. Clinical uses of bone conduction in the evaluation of otologic disease. *Annals of Otology, Rhinology, and Laryngology, 88*, 22–28.
Kemp, D. T. (1988). Developments in cochlear mechanics and techniques for noninvasive evaluation. *Advances in Audiology, 5*, 27–45.
Kennedy, C., McCann, D., Campbell, M. J., Kimm, L., & Thornton, R. (2005). Universal newborn screening for permanent childhood hearing impairment: An 8–year follow-up of a controlled trial. *Lancet, 366*(9486), 660–662.
Klein, A. J. (1983). Properties of the brain-stem response slow-wave component. II. Frequency specificity. *Archives of Otolaryngology, 109*, 74–78.
Kodera, H., Yamane, H., Yamada, O., & Suzuki, J.-I. (1977). The effects of onset, offset and rise-decay times of tone bursts on brain stem responses. *Scandinavian Audiology, 6*, 205–210.
Kramer, S. J. (1992). Frequency specific auditory brainstem responses to bone-conducted stimuli. *Audiology, 31*, 61–71.
Kuwada, S., Anderson, J. S., Batra, R., Fitzpatrick, D. C., Teissier, N., & D'Angelo, W. R. (2002). Sources of the scalp-recorded amplitude-modulation following response. *Journal of the American Academy of Audiology, 13*, 188–204.
Lasky, R. E. (1991). The effects of rate and forward masking on human adult and newborn auditory evoked brainstem response thresholds. *Devevelopmental Psychobiology, 24*, 51–64.
Lee, C. Y., Hsieh, T. H., Pan, S. L., & Hsu, C. J. (2007). Thresholds of tone burst auditory brainstem responses for infants and young children with normal hearing in Taiwan. *Journal of the Formosan Medical Association, 106*(10), 847–853.
Lee, C. Y., Jaw, F. S., Pan, S. L., Hsieh, T. H., & Hsu, C. J. (2008). Effects of age and degree of hearing loss on the agreement and correlation between sound field audiometric thresholds and tone burst auditory brainstem response thresholds in infants and young children. *Journal of the Formosan Medical Association, 107*(11), 869–875.
Linden, R. D., Campbell, K. B., Hamel, G., & Picton, T. W. (1985). Human auditory steady-state evoked potentials during sleep. *Ear and Hearing, 6*(3), 167–174.
Lins, O. G., Picton, P. E., Picton, T. W., Champagne, S. C., & Durieux-Smith, A. (1995). Auditory steady-state responses to tones amplitude-modulated at 80–110 Hz. *Journal of the Acoustical Society of America, 97*, 3051–3063.
Lins, O. G., & Picton, T. W. (1995). Auditory steady-state responses to multiple simultaneous stimuli. *Electroencephalography and Clinical Neurophysiology, 96*, 420–432.
Lins, O. G., Picton, T. W., Boucher, B. L., Durieux-Smith, A., Champagne, S. C., Moran, L. M., . . . Savio, G. (1996). Frequency-specific audiometry using steady-state responses. *Ear and Hearing, 17*, 81–96.

Luts, H., Desloovere, C., & Wouters, J. (2006). Clinical application of dichotic multiple-stimulus auditory steady-state responses in high-risk newborns and children. *Audiology and Neurotology, 11*, 24–37.

Luts, H., Van Dun, B., Alaerts, J., & Wouters, J. (2008). The influence of the detection paradigm in recording auditory steady-state responses. *Ear and Hearing, 29*(4), 638–650.

Luts, H., & Wouters, J. (2004). Hearing assessment by recording multiple auditory steady-state responses: the influence of test duration. *International Journal of Audiology, 43*(8), 471–478.

Mackersie, C. L., & Stapells, D. R. (1994). Auditory brainstem response wave I prediction of conductive component in infants and young children. *American Journal of Audiology, 3*, 52–58.

Mauer, G., & Döring, W. H. (1999). *Generators of amplitude modulation following response (AMFR)*. Paper presented at the XVI Biennial Meeting of the International Evoked Response Audiometry Study Group. Tromso, Norway.

Mauldin, L., & Jerger, J. (1979). Auditory brainstem evoked responses to bone-conducted signals. *Archives of Otolaryngology, 105*, 656–661.

McGee, T. J., & Clemis, J. D. (1982). Effects of conductive hearing loss on auditory brainstem response. *Annals of Otology, Rhinology and Laryngology, 91*, 304–309.

Mo, L., & Stapells, D. R. (2008). The effect of brief-tone stimulus duration on the brain stem auditory steady-state response. *Ear and Hearing, 29*(1), 121–133.

Moore, B. C. J. (2004). *An introduction to the psychology of hearing* (5th ed.). San Diego, CA: Elsevier Academic Press.

Muchnik, C., Neeman, R. K., & Hildesheimer, M. (1995). Auditory brainstem response to bone-conducted clicks in adults and infants with normal hearing and conductive hearing loss. *Scandinavian Audiology, 24*, 185–191.

Murofushi, T., Iwasaki, S., Takai, Y., & Takegoshi, H. (2005). Sound-evoked neurogenic responses with short latency of vestibular origin. *Clinical Neurophysiology, 116*(2), 401–405.

Narne, V. K., Nambi, P. A., & Vanaja, C. S. (2006). *Artifactual responses in auditory steady state responses recorded using phase coherence method*. Retrieved September 21, 2009, from http://www.aiish.ac.in/pdf/Microsoft%20Word%20–%20Article%2017.pdf

Nousak, J. K., & Stapells, D. R. (1992). Frequency specificity of the auditory brain stem response to bone-conducted tones in infants and adults. *Ear and Hearing, 13*, 87–95.

Oates, P., & Stapells, D. R. (1997a). Frequency specificity of the human auditory brainstem and middle latency responses to brief tones. I. High pass noise masking. *Journal of the Acoustical Society of America, 102*, 3597–3608.

Oates, P., & Stapells, D. R. (1997b). Frequency specificity of the human auditory brainstem and middle latency responses to brief tones. II. Derived response analyses. *Journal of the Acoustical Society of America, 102*, 3609–3619.

OIHP. (2008). Ontario Infant Hearing Program, *Audiologic assessment protocol* [pdf document]. Retrieved January 1, 2009, from http://www.mountsinai.on.ca/care/infant-hearingprogram/resolveUid/b84c6bf5acbf70c86347eecd6be66b1f

Özdamar, Ö., & Delgado, R. E. (1996). Measurement of signal and noise characteristics in ongoing auditory brainstem response averaging. *Annals of Biomedical Engineering, 24*(6), 702–715.

Papathanasiou, E. S., Zamba-Papanicolaou, E., Pantziaris, M., Kleopas, K., Kyriakides, T., Papacostas, S., . . . Piperidou, C. (2004). Neurogenic vestibular evoked potentials using a tone pip auditory stimulus. *Electromyography and Clinical Neurophysiology, 44*(3), 167–173.

Perez-Abalo, M. C., Savio, G., Torres, A., Martin, V., Rodríguez, E., & Galán, L. (2001). Steady state responses to multiple amplitude-modulated tones: An optimized method to test frequency-specific thresholds in hearing-impaired children and normal-hearing subjects. *Ear and Hearing, 22*, 200–211.

Picton, T. W. (1978). The strategy of evoked potential audiometry. In S. E. Gerber & G. T. Mencher (Eds.), *Early diagnosis of hearing loss* (pp. 297–307). New York, NY: Grune & Stratton.

Picton, T. W., Dimitrijevic, A., & John, M. S. (2002). Multiple auditory steady-state responses. *Annals of Otology, Rhinology and Laryngology Suppl., 189*, 16–21.

Picton, T. W., Dimitrijevic, A., Perez-Abalo, M. C., & Van Roon, P. (2005). Estimating audiometric thresholds using auditory steady-state responses. *Journal of the American Academy of Audiology, 16*(3), 140–156.

Picton, T. W., Durieux-Smith, A., & Moran, L. M. (1994). Recording auditory brainstem responses from infants. *International Journal of Pediatric Otorhinolaryngology, 28*, 93–110.

Picton, T. W., John, M., Dimitrijevic, A., & Purcell, D. (2003). Human auditory steady-state responses. *International Journal of Audiology, 42*, 177–219.

Picton, T. W., & John, M. S. (2004). Avoiding electromagnetic artifacts when recording auditory steady-state responses. *Journal of the American Academy of Audiology, 15*(8), 541–554.

Picton, T. W., Linden, R. D., Hamel, G., & Maru, J. T. (1983). Aspects of averaging. *Seminars in Hearing, 4*, 327–341.

Picton, T. W., & Maru, J. T. (1984). Comments on obtaining signals from noise. In A. Starr, C. Rosenberg, M. Don, & H. Davis (Eds.), *Sensory evoked potentials: An international conference on standards for auditory brainstem response (ABR)* (pp. 147–151). Milan, Italy: Amplifon.

Picton, T. W., Ouellette, J., Hamel, G., & Smith, A. D. (1979). Brainstem evoked potentials to tonepips in notched noise. *Journal of Otolaryngology, 8*, 289–314.

Picton, T. W., & Stapells, D. R. (1985). A "Frank's Run" latency-intensity function. In J. T. Jacobson (Ed.), *The auditory brainstem response* (pp. 410–413). San Diego, CA: College-Hill Press.

Picton, T. W., van Roon, P., & John, M. S. (2009). Multiple auditory steady state responses (80–101 Hz): effects of ear, gender, handedness, intensity and modulation rate. *Ear and Hearing, 30*(1), 100–109.

Purcell, D. W., & Dajani, H. R. (2008). The stimulus-response relationship in auditory steady state response testing. In G. Rance (Ed.), *The auditory steady-state response. Generation, recording, and clinical application* (pp. 55–82). San Diego, CA: Plural.

Purdy, S. C., & Abbas, P. J. (2002). ABR thresholds to tonebursts gated with Blackman and linear windows in adults with high frequency sensorineural hearing loss. *Ear and Hearing, 23*(4), 358–368.

Rance, G. (2005). Auditory neuropathy/dys-synchrony and its perceptual consequences. *Trends in Amplification, 9*(1), 1–43.

Rance, G. (2008a). Auditory steady-state responses in neonates and infants. In G. Rance (Ed.), *The auditory steady-state response. Generation, recording, and clinical application* (pp. 161–184). San Diego, CA: Plural.

Rance, G. (Ed.). (2008b). *The auditory steady-state response. Generation, recording, and clinical application*. San Diego, CA: Plural.

Rance, G., & Briggs, R. S. J. (2002). Assessment of hearing in infants with moderate to profound impairment: The Melbourne experience with auditory steady-state evoked potential testing. *Annals of Otology Rhinology and Laryngology, 111*(Suppl.189), 22–28.

Rance, G., Dowell, R. C., Rickards, F. W., Beer, D. E., & Clark, G. M. (1998). Steady-state evoked potential and behavioral hearing thresholds in a group of children with absent click-evoked auditory brain stem response. *Ear and Hearing, 19*(1), 48–61.

Rance, G., & Rickards, F. (2002). Prediction of hearing threshold in infants using auditory steady-state evoked potentials. *Journal of the American Academy of Audiology, 13*(5), 236–245.

Rance, G., Rickards, F. W., Cohen, L. T., Burton, M. J., & Clark, G. M. (1993). Steady state evoked potentials: A new tool for the accurate assessment of hearing in cochlear implant candidates. *Advances in Otorhinolaryngology, 48*, 44–48.

Rance, G., Rickards, F. W., Cohen, L. T., De Vidi, S., & Clark, G. M. (1995). The automated prediction of hearing thresholds in sleeping subjects using auditory steady-state evoked potentials. *Ear and Hearing, 16*(5), 499–507.

Rance, G., Roper, R., Symons, L., Moody, L.-J., Poulis, C., Dourlay, M., & Kelly, T. (2005). Hearing threshold estimation in infants using auditory steady-state responses. *Journal of the American Academy of Audiology, 16*, 291–300.

Rance, G., & Tomlin, D. (2006). Maturation of auditory steady-state responses in normal babies. *Ear and Hearing, 27*(1), 20–29.

Rance, G., Tomlin, D., & Rickards, F. (2006). Comparison of auditory steady-state responses and tone-burst auditory brainstem responses in normal babies. *Ear and Hearing, 27*, 751–762.

Regan, D. (1989). *Human brain electrophysiology: Evoked potentials and evoked magnetic fields in science and medicine*. New York, NY: Elsevier.

Ribeiro, F. M., & Carvallo, R. M. (2008). Tone-evoked ABR in full-term and preterm neonates with normal hearing. *International Journal of Audiology, 47*(1), 21–29.

Rickards, F. W., & Clark, G. M. (1984). Steady-state evoked potentials to amplitude-modulated tones. In R. H. Nodar & C. Barber (Eds.), *Evoked potentials II* (pp. 163–168). Boston, MA: Butterworth.

Savio, G., Cardenas, J., Perez Abalo, M., Gonzales, A., & Valdes, J. (2001). The low and high frequency auditory steady-state responses mature at different rates. *Audiology and Neurotology, 6*, 279–287.

Savio, G., Perez-Abalo, M. C., Gaya, J., Hernandez, O., & Mijares, E. (2006). Test accuracy and prognostic validity of multiple auditory steady state responses for targeted hearing screening. *International Journal of Audiology, 45*(2), 109–120.

Seewald, R., Moodie, S., Scollie, S., & Bagatto, M. (2005). The DSL method for pediatric hearing instrument fitting: Historical perspective and current issues. *Trends in Amplification, 9*(4), 145–157.

Sheykholeslami, K., Kermany, M. H., & Kaga, K. (2000). Bone-conducted vestibular-evoked myogenic potentials in patients with congenital atresia of the external auditory canal. *International Journal of Pediatric Otorhinolaryngology, 57*, 25–29.

Sininger, Y. S. (2003). Audiologic assessment in infants. *Current Opinions in Otolaryngology-Head and Neck Surgery, 11*(5), 378–382.

Sininger, Y. S., Abdala, C., & Cone-Wesson, B. (1997). Auditory threshold sensitivity of the human neonate as measured by the auditory brainstem response. *Hearing Research, 104*, 27–38.

Sininger, Y. S., & Hyde, M. L. (2009). Auditory brainstem response in audiometric threshold prediction. In J. Katz, L. Medwetsky , R. Burkard, & L. Hood (Eds.), *Handbook of clinical audiology* (6th ed., pp. 293–321). Baltimore, MD: Lippingcott, Williams & Wilkins.

Small, S. A., Hatton, J. L., & Stapells, D. R. (2007). Effects of bone oscillator coupling method, placement location, and occlusion on bone-conduction auditory steady-state responses in infants. *Ear and Hearing, 28*(1), 83–98.

Small, S. A., & Stapells, D. R. (2003). Normal brief-tone bone-conduction behavioral thresholds using the B-71 transducer: Three occlusion conditions. *Journal of the American Academy of Audiology, 14*(10), 556–562.

Small, S. A., & Stapells, D. R. (2004). Artifactual responses when recording auditory steady-state responses. *Ear and Hearing, 25*(6), 611–623.

Small, S. A., & Stapells, D. R. (2005). Multiple auditory steady-state response thresholds to bone-conduction stimuli in adults with normal hearing. *Journal of the American Academy of Audiology, 16*, 172–183.

Small, S. A., & Stapells, D. R. (2006). Multiple auditory steady-state response thresholds to bone-conduction stimuli in young infants with normal hearing. *Ear and Hearing, 27*, 219–228.

Small, S. A., & Stapells, D. R. (2008a). Bone conduction auditory steady-state responses. In G. Rance (Ed.), *The auditory steady-state response. Generation, recording, and clinical application* (pp. 201–228). San Diego, CA: Plural.

Small, S. A., & Stapells, D. R. (2008b). Normal ipsilateral/contralateral asymmetries in infant multiple auditory steady-state responses to air- and bone-conduction stimuli. *Ear and Hearing, 29*(2), 185–198.

Small, S. A., & Stapells, D. R. (2008c). Maturation of bone conduction multiple auditory steady state responses. *International Journal of Audiology, 47*(8), 476–488.

Stapells, D. R. (1989). Auditory brainstem response assessment of infants and children. *Seminars in Hearing, 10*, 229–251.

Stapells, D. R. (2000a). Frequency-specific evoked potential audiometry in infants. In R. C. Seewald (Ed.), *A sound foundation through early amplification: Proceedings of an international conference* (pp. 13–31). Stäfa, Switzerland: Phonak AG.

Stapells, D. R. (2000b). Threshold estimation by the tone-evoked auditory brainstem response: A literature meta-analysis. *Journal of Speech-Language Pathology and Audiology, 24*(2), 74–83.

Stapells, D. R., Galambos, R., Costello, J. A., & Makeig, S. (1988). Inconsistency of auditory middle latency and steady-state responses in infants. *Electroencephalography and Clinical Neurophysiology, 71*, 289–295.

Stapells, D. R., Gravel, J. A., & Martin, B. A. (1995). Thresholds for auditory brain stem responses to tones in notched noise from infants and young children with normal hearing or sensorineural hearing loss. *Ear and Hearing, 16*, 361–371.

Stapells, D. R., Herdman, A., Small, S. A., Dimitrijevic, A., & Hatton, J. (2005). Current status of the auditory steady-state responses for estimating an infant's audiogram. In R. Seewald & J. Bamford (Eds.), *A sound foundation through early amplification 2004: Proceedings of the third international conference* (pp. 43–59). Stäfa, Switzerland: Phonak AG.

Stapells, D. R., Linden, D., Suffield, J. B., Hamel, G., & Picton, T. W. (1984). Human auditory steady state potentials. *Ear and Hearing, 5*(2), 105–113.

Stapells, D. R., & Mosseri, M. (1991). Maturation of the contralaterally recorded auditory brainstem response. *Ear and Hearing, 12*, 167–173.

Stapells, D. R., & Oates, P. (1997). Estimation of the pure-tone audiogram by the auditory brainstem response: A review. *Audiology and Neurotology, 2*, 257–280.

Stapells, D. R., & Picton, T. W. (1981). Technical aspects of brainstem evoked potential audiometry using tones. *Ear and Hearing, 2*, 20–29.

Stapells, D. R., Picton, T. W., & Durieux-Smith, A. (1994). Electrophysiologic measures of frequency-specific auditory function. In J. T. Jacobson (Ed.), *Principles and applications in auditory evoked potentials* (pp. 251–283). Needham Hill, MA: Allyn and Bacon.

Stapells, D. R., & Ruben, R. J. (1989). Auditory brain stem responses to bone-conducted tones in infants. *Annals of Otology, Rhinology and Laryngology, 98*, 941–949.

Stuart, A., Yang, E. Y., & Green, W. B. (1994). Neonatal auditory brainstem response thresholds to air- and bone-conducted clicks: 0 to 96 hours postpartum. *Journal of the American Academy of Audiology, 5*, 163–172.

Stuart, A., Yang, E. Y., Stenstrom, R., & Reindorp, A. G. (1993). Auditory brainstem response thresholds to air and bone conducted clicks in neonates and adults. *American Journal of Otology, 14*, 176–182.

Stueve, M. P., & O'Rourke, C. (2003). Estimation of hearing loss in children: Comparison of auditory steady-state response, auditory brainstem response, and behavioral test methods. *American Journal of Audiology, 12*(2), 125–136.

Sturzebecher, E., Cebulla, M., Elberling, C., & Berger, T. (2006). New efficient stimuli for evoking frequency-specific auditory steady-state responses. *Journal of the American Academy of Audiology, 17*(6), 448–461.

Suzuki, T., & Horiuchi, K. (1981). Rise time pure tone stimuli in brain stem response audiometry. *Audiology, 20*, 101–112.

Suzuki, T., & Kobayashi, K. (1984). An evaluation of 40-Hz event-related potentials in young children. *Audiology, 23*, 599–604.

Swanepoel, D., & Hugo, R. (2004). Estimations of auditory sensitivity for young cochlear implant candidates using the ASSR: Preliminary results. *International Journal of Audiology, 43*(7), 377–382.

Swanepoel, D., Hugo, R., & Roode, R. (2004). Auditory steady-state responses for children with severe to profound hearing loss. *Archives of Otolaryngology-Head and Neck Surgery, 130*(5), 531–535.

Swanepoel, D. W., Ebrahim, S., Friedland, P., Swanepoel, A., & Pottas, L. (2008). Auditory steady-state responses to bone conduction stimuli in children with hearing loss. *International Journal of Pediatric Otorhinolaryngology, 72*(12), 1861–1871.

Swanepoel, D. W., & Steyn, K. (2005). Short report: Establishing normal hearing for infants with the auditory steady-state response. *South African Journal of Communication Disorders, 52*, 36–39.

Tlumak, A. I., Rubinstein, E., & Durrant, J. D. (2007). Meta-analysis of variables that affect accuracy of threshold estimation via measurement of the auditory steady-state response (ASSR). *International Journal of Audiology, 46*(11), 692–710.

van Maanen, A., & Stapells, D. R. (2009). Normal multiple auditory steady-state response thresholds to air-conducted stimuli in infants. *Journal of the American Academy of Audiology, 20*(3), 196–207.

van Maanen, A., & Stapells, D. R. (in press). Multiple-ASSR thresholds in infants and young children with hearing loss. *Journal of the American Academy of Audiology.*

Vander Werff, K. R., Johnson, T. A., & Brown, C. J. (2008). Behavioral threshold estimation for auditory steady-state response. In G. Rance (Ed.), *The auditory steady-state response. Generation, recording, and clinical application* (pp. 125–147). San Diego, CA: Plural.

Vander Werff, K. R., Prieve, B. A., & Georgantas, L. M. (2009). Infant air and bone conduction tone burst auditory brain stem responses for classification of hearing loss and the relationship to behavioral thresholds. *Ear and Hearing, 30*(3), 350–368.

Welgampola, M. S., & Colebatch, J. G. (2001). Characteristics of tone burst-evoked myogenic potentials in the sternocleidomastoid muscles. *Otology and Neurotology, 22*, 796–802.

Wood, L. L. (2009). *Multiple brainstem auditory steady-state response interactions for different stimuli.* Unpublished M.Sc. thesis, The University of British Columbia, Vancouver, B.C.

Yamada, O., Yagi, T., Yamane, H., & Suzuki, J.-I. (1975). Clinical evaluation of the auditory evoked brain stem response. *Aurix-Nasus-Larynx, 2*, 97–105.

Yang, E. Y., Rupert, A. L., & Moushegian, G. (1987). A developmental study of bone conduction auditory brainstem responses in infants. *Ear and Hearing, 8*, 244–251.

Yang, E. Y., & Stuart, A. (1990). A method of auditory brainstem response testing of infants using bone-conducted clicks. *Journal of Speech Language Pathology and Audiology, 14*, 69–76.

Yang, E. Y., Stuart, A., Mencher, G. T., Mencher, L. S., & Vincer, M. J. (1993). Auditory brain stem responses to air- and bone- conducted clicks in the audiological assessment of at-risk infants. *Ear and Hearing, 14*, 175–182.

Yoshinaga-Itano, C., & Gravel, J. S. (2001). The evidence for universal newborn hearing screening. *American Journal of Audiology, 10*(2), 62–64.

Yoshinaga-Itano, C., Sedey, A. L., Coulter, D. K., & Mehl, A. L. (1998). Language of early- and later-identified children with hearing loss. *Pediatrics, 102*, 1161–1171.

21

Electrophysiologic Assessment of Hearing With Auditory Middle Latency and Auditory Late Responses

James W. Hall III, Anuradha R. Bantwal, Vidya Ramkumar, and Neha Chhabria

Introduction

Historical Perspective on Cortical Auditory Evoked Responses

Cortical auditory evoked responses were first reported 70 years ago. The auditory late response (ALR) was described by P. Davis in 1939. Throughout the 1960s, the ALR was explored, and even relied on clinically, as an electrophysiologic index of auditory function, especially for objectively determining auditory thresholds in young children (for details see Hall, 1992, 2007). About 20 years later, the auditory middle latency response (AMLR) was discovered by Geisler (Geisler, Frishkopf, & Rosenblith, 1958) and almost immediately applied by Robert Goldstein and colleagues at the University of Wisconsin (Goldstein, 1967) in the assessment of auditory thresholds in young children, including newborn infants. With the emergence in the mid-1970s of the auditory brainstem response (ABR) as a clinical tool for pediatric auditory assessment, clinical use of the AMLR and ALR quickly diminished. However, within 10 years clinical audiologists and researchers (e.g., Hall, Huangfu, & Gennarrelli, 1982; Kraus, Özdamar, Hier, & Stein, 1982; Musiek, Guerkink, Weider, & Donnelly, 1984) began to recognize the need for an electrophysiological measure (or measures) of higher level auditory function. Although the auditory brainstem response (ABR) clearly was valuable in the estimation of auditory threshold, and to document overt brainstem auditory dysfunction, it provided no information on suprabrainstem (e.g., thalamic and cortical) auditory dysfunction.

Within the past 20 years, reports of clinical application of cortical auditory evoked responses, many of them case reports, periodically have appeared in the literature. However, neither the AMLR nor the ALR, or any other cortical auditory evoked responses (e.g., the P300 response), are consistently included within the test battery for assessment of central auditory nervous system function. To date, cortical auditory evoked responses have mostly been employed by investigators in the laboratory setting or in clinical research rather than in the clinical setting by practicing audiologists. We predict that cortical auditory evoked responses in the near future will play a more important, and regular, role in the assessment of central auditory function and processing. An increasing number of publications describe findings for cortical auditory evoked responses in various pediatric patient populations, including the application of the responses as objective indexes of central nervous system changes with intervention strategies. Also, we are now witnessing the first attempts to incorporate technologic features of laboratory instrumentation, including sophisticated algorithms for stimulus generation, response detection, and statistical analysis of responses, into clinical evoked response systems.

Rationale for the Application of AMLR and ALR in Children

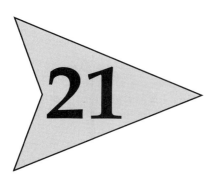

There are multiple compelling clinical reasons for measurement of cortical auditory evoked responses in

the assessment of auditory function and processing of children. General and well-appreciated advantages of electrophysiologic measures argue for inclusion of the AMLR and the ALR in the diagnostic test battery for selected patient populations. That is, electrophysiologic measures are not influenced by the quality, validity, or feasibility of behavioral responses to sound. Thus, valid and clinically useful AMLRs and ALRs can be recorded independent of listener (patient) variables that may confound traditional behavioral audiometry, such as motivation, fatigue, cognition, attention, motor function, and language. In addition, auditory evoked responses offer a degree of site specificity not available from most behavioral auditory procedures. In other words, some information on the site of dysfunction within the auditory system is gained from close analysis of auditory evoked responses. Of course, some of these advantages apply also to electroacoustic auditory measures (e.g., acoustic reflexes and otoacoustic emissions). Specific clinical advantages and disadvantages for recording the AMLR and ALR in the assessment of children are summarized in Table 21–1.

The following review focuses on clinical applications of the AMLR and the ALR in children. A complete review of the basic principles of the cortical auditory evoked response, including anatomic and physiologic underpinnings, and measurement techniques and procedures is far beyond the scope of this chapter. For more information and in-depth and current coverage of the topic, the reader is referred to recent textbooks devoted exclusively to auditory evoked responses (e.g., Hall, 2007; Burkard, Don & Eggermont, 2007).

Auditory Middle Latency Response (AMLR)

Measurement and Analysis

A protocol for clinical measurement of the AMLR, including major components Na, Pa, and Pb, is summarized in Table 21–2. For selected parameters in Table 21–2, changing the specific value or type of the

Table 21–1. Clinical Advantages and Disadvantages of Auditory Middle Latency (AMLR) and Auditory Late Response (ALR) in the Assessment of Children

Advantages	*Disadvantages*
AMLR	
• Accepted test protocols and procedures • Primary auditory cortex origins are known • Measurable in infants and young children • Analyses strategies are defined • Can be recorded with a clinical ABR system	• Influenced by sleep and sedatives • Requires hemispheric electrodes for neurodiagnostic information • Equipment must have $\geq$ 3 channels for simultaneous AMLR measurement with hemispheric and midline electrodes • Complex interaction among age, stimulus rate and duration • Influenced by state of arousal and some medications • Few data available on relation between AMLR and behavioral findings (e.g., in APD)
ALR	
• Generally accepted test protocols and procedures • Can be recorded with a clinical ABR system • Measureable in infants and young children • Analyses strategies are defined • Can be elicited with speech stimuli • Provides information on integrity of secondary auditory cortical regions • Clinical findings for various clinical populations	• Influenced by sleep and sedatives • Influenced by state of arousal and some medications • Some confusion about appropriate test parameters

Note: Electrophysiologic assessment for auditory processing disorders (APD) represents an example of a clinical application of these cortical auditory evoked responses.

Table 21–2. Guidelines for Auditory Middle Latency Response (AMLR) Test Protocol

Parameter	*Suggestion*	*Rationale/Comment*
Stimulus Parameters		
Transducer	ER-3A	Supra-aural earphones are acceptable for AMLR, but insert earphones are more comfortable and, because the insert cushions are disposable, contribute to infection control.
Type	Click	For neurodiagnosis only. However, a more robust AMLR is usually recorded with longer duration tone burst signals.
	Tone-Burst	For neurodiagnosis or frequency-specific estimation of auditory sensitivity Detection of the Pb component of the AMLR is enhanced for lower frequency tone-burst signals.
Duration		
Click Signal	0.1 ms	Click signals are less effective than tone bursts in evoking the AMLR.
Tone-Burst Signal Rise/Fall	2 cycles	Rather abrupt tone burst onset is important for AMLR as it is for the ABR.
Plateau	Multiple Cycles	Plateau durations of 10 ms or longer are appropriate for evoking the AMLR, and especially for detection of the Pb component.
Rate	≤ 7.1/second	A slower rate of signal presentation is indicated for younger children, or for patients with cortical pathology. Signal presentation rates as low as 1 per second, or 0.5/second (one signal every two seconds) are required to consistently record the Pb component.
Polarity	Rarefaction	An AMLR can also be recorded for condensation or alternating polarity signals.
Intensity	≤ 70 dB nHL	For neurodiagnosis, a moderate signal intensity level is appropriate. Signal intensity is decreased, of course, for estimation of thresholds. High signal intensity levels should be avoided. Tone-burst signals should be biologically calibrated to dB nHL in the space where clinical AMLRs are recorded.
Number	≤ 1,000	Signal repetitions vary depending on size of response and background electrical noise. Remember the signal-to-noise ratio is the key. Averaging may require as few as 50 to 100 signals at high-intensity levels for a very quiet and normal hearing patient.
Presentation ear	Monaural	For estimation of auditory sensitivity and neurodiagnosis. There is no apparent clinical indication for binaural AMLR measurement.
Masking	50 dB	Rarely required with insert earphones, and not needed for stimulus intensity levels of ≤ 70 dB nHL.
Acquisition Parameters		
Amplification	75,000	Less amplification is required for larger responses such as the AMLR.
Sensitivity	50 volts	Lower sensitivity values are equivalent to higher amplification.
Analysis time	100 ms	Long enough to encompass the Pa and Pb components.
Prestimulus time	10 ms	Provides a convenient estimate of background noise and a baseline for calculation of the amplitudes for waveform components (Na, Pa, Nb, and Pb).
Data points	512	
Sweeps	1,000	See comments above for signal number.

continues

Table 21–2. *continued*

Parameter	Suggestion	Rationale/Comment
Filters		
Band-pass	10 to 1500 Hz	For recording an ABR, and AMLR with an Na and Pa component.
	10 to 200 Hz	For recording an AMLR with an Na and Pa component. Do not overfilter (e.g., high-pass setting of 30 Hz and low pass setting of 100 Hz) as it may remove important spectral energy from the response, and it may produce a misleading filter artifact.
	0.1 to about 200 Hz	Decrease high-pass filter to 1 Hz or less to detect the Pb (P50) component.
Notch	None	A notch filter (removing spectral energy in the region of 60 Hz) is never indicated with AMLR measurement because important frequencies in the response (around 40 Hz or below for young children) may also be removed.
Electrodes		
Type	Disk	Disk electrodes applied with paste (versus gel) secure the noninverting electrodes on the scalp. It is helpful to use red and blue colored electrode leads for the right and left hemisphere locations, respectively. Ear clip electrodes are recommended when an earlobe inverting electrode site is used.
Sites		
Channel 1	C3 to Ai/Ac or C3 to NC	Hemisphere electrode locations are required for neurodiagnosis. A linked earlobe inverting electrode arrangement (Ai = ipsilateral ear; Ac = contralateral ear) or a noncephalic (NC) inverting electrode (on the nape of the neck) is appropriate, and reduces likelihood of PAM artifact.
Channel 2	C4 to Ai/Ac or NC	C3 = left hemisphere site; C4 = right hemisphere site.
Channel 3	Fz to Ai/Ac or NC	A third channel (3) is optional for neurodiagnosis. Only the midline noninverting electrode channel is needed for the estimation of hearing sensitivity.
Channel 4	Outer canthi of eye	Optional for detection of eye blinks, and rejection of averages contaminated by eye blinks.
Ground	Fpz	

Note the modifications in the test protocol that are required for consistent detection of the Pb component. Adapted from Hall (2007).

parameter does not affect consistent detection of the AMLR, for example, the stimulus transducer (e.g., supra-aural versus insert earphone) or stimulus polarity (e.g., rarefaction, condensation, or alternating). Other measurement parameters, however, are critical to ensure that an AMLR will be recorded and/or to minimize the likelihood of contamination of the waveform with artifact.

Although calculation of both latency and amplitude of wave components is routinely included in analysis of the AMLR, most clinical information is derived from amplitude values. Specifically, AMLR analysis relies on a comparison of the magnitude or amplitude of the three major wave components (Na, Pa, and Pb) among two or more channels of AMLR recordings. The most commonly reported and simplest analysis strategy calls for calculation of the amplitude of the Pa wave recorded simultaneously with a 3-channel arrangement with noninverting electrodes located over the right hemisphere (C4 location), the left hemisphere (C3 location), and the midline (Fz location). The emphasis in AMLR analysis therefore, is on the size of the response produced by the auditory cortex in the left hemisphere versus the right hemisphere versus subcortical (e.g., thalamic or thalamocortical pathways) regions. A secondary concern is analysis of the amplitude of components of an AMLR elicited with right versus left ear stimulation, or with stimulation of the ear ipsilateral versus contralateral to the noninverting recording electrode.

AMLR analysis in a hypothetical patient with dysfunction within the right primary auditory cortex is illustrated in Figure 21–1. The AMLR was recorded with a 3-channel electrode array, as just described, with tone-burst stimuli presented separately to the right and then the left ears. Each replicated waveform was

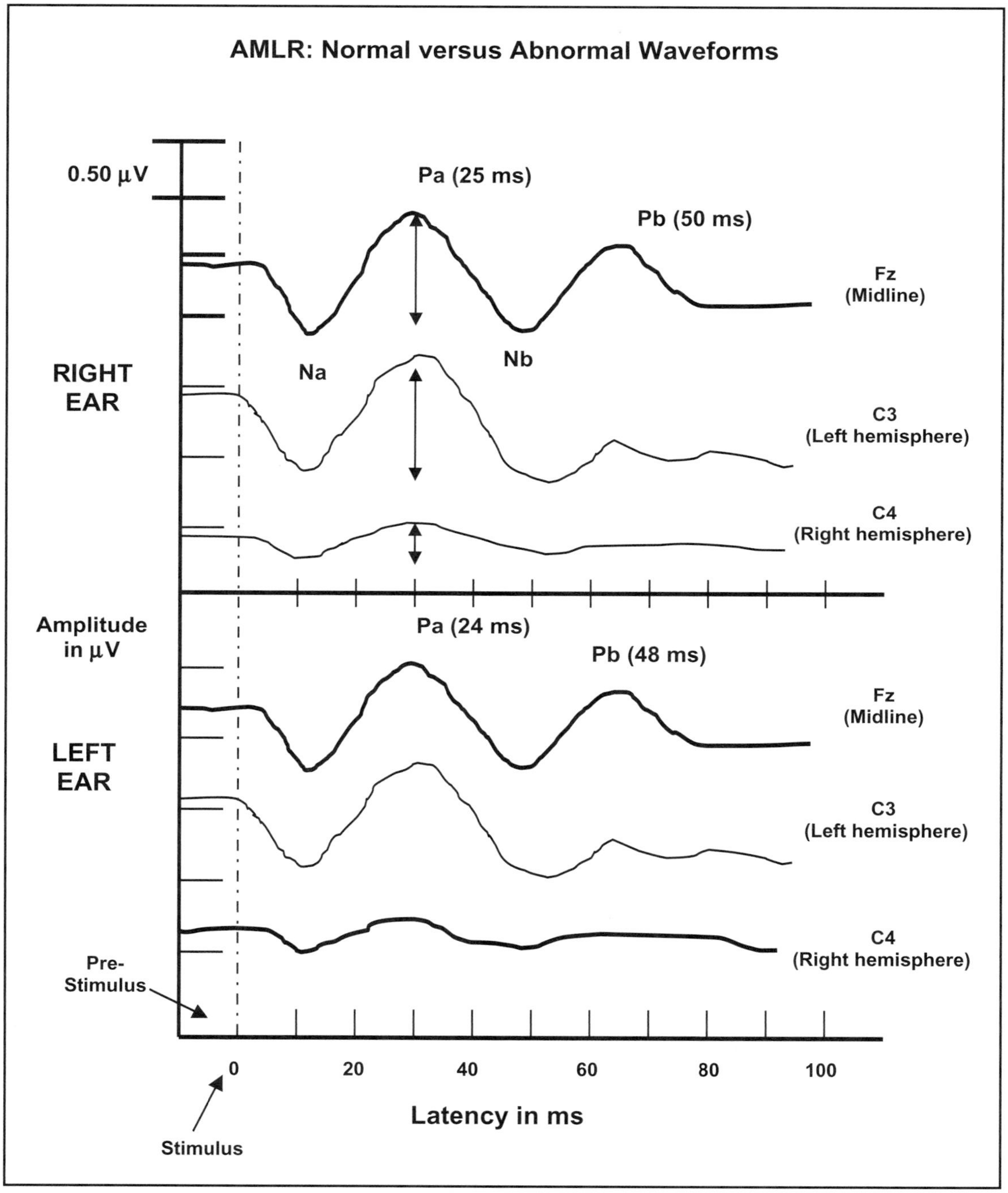

FIGURE 21–1. Auditory middle latency response (AMLR) waveforms elicited with tone burst stimuli presented monaurally to the right and left ears and recorded with three noninverting electrode arrays from the left hemisphere (C3), right hemisphere (C4), and midline (Fz). The illustrative patient is a young adult with right-sided dysfunction within the primary auditory cortex. Note the abnormality of Pa and Pb amplitude as recorded with the C4 electrode, regardless of the side of stimulation.

recorded (averaged) minimally with 500 stimuli. Notice that for right and left ear stimulation, the amplitudes of the Pa and Pb components are normal (about 1.0 μvolt) when recorded with a non-noninverting electrode located over the left hemisphere and the midline site. Importantly, amplitude of these AMLR components is about two times the amplitude of the ABR wave V under the same stimulus conditions. Whenever the AMLR is recorded with a noninverting electrode located over the right hemisphere (the site of dysfunction), amplitudes of the Pa and Pb components are markedly reduced in comparison to the AMLR detected over the opposite (left) hemisphere and midline. In fact, for the right hemisphere electrode condition, amplitude of the Pa and Pb components is smaller than even the amplitude for ABR wave V (0.5 μvolt). For this case, localization of the AMLR amplitude abnormalities to the right hemisphere is compatible with auditory dysfunction within the thalamocortical pathways on the right side and, most likely, the right primary auditory cortex. This conclusion is unaffected by various patient characteristics that would interfere with analysis of behavioral measures of central auditory functioning (e.g., attention, motivation, cognitive variables, language level, or native language, etc.).

Table 21–3. Major Nonpathologic Factors Influencing Measurement, Analysis, and Interpretation of the Auditory Middle Latency Response (AMLR)

Test Parameters

- Filtering: Avoid restricted high-pass filter setting (e.g., 30 Hz) and use HP setting of ≤ 1 Hz to detect the Pb component
- Stimulus intensity level: Avoid very high (> 75 dB nHL) levels (PAM artifact)
- Stimulus duration: Longer (> 10 ms) is better (avoid clicks)
- Stimulus rate: Slower rates for children and in pathology, with very slow rate (< 1/sec) to detect the Pb component

Subject Factors

- Age: Age is a factor for children under 10 years, and interacts with stimulus rate
- Sleep: AMLR is more variable during sleep
- Postauricular muscle (PAM) artifact: Avoid if possible
- Sedation: Amplitude is reduced and variable
- Anesthesia: Typically suppresses AMLR activity (reticular formation generators)

Nonpathologic Factors

Major nonpathologic factors influencing the AMLR, including measurement and subject variables, are summarized in Table 21–3. For children under the age of 10 years, age must be considered in AMLR measurement and analysis. This is not to say that the AMLR cannot be recorded from young children but, rather, that adjustments must be made in the test protocol, and expectations are altered for response parameters. In general, slower stimulus presentation rates are required for younger children. The use of relatively slow stimulus presentation rates (e.g., < 5 stimuli per second) is advised for children under the age of 10 years, and ≤ 1 per second for infants and very young children). Otherwise, AMLR measurement in children differs little from the approach taken with older children and adults. Given the well-documented influence of sleep on the AMLR, especially on amplitude, every attempt should be made to maintain a consistent state of arousal throughout the recording session. The challenge during pediatric AMLR recording is to prevent the child from falling asleep while keeping the child physically inactive. The most effective technique for accomplishing this goal is to encourage the child to view an engaging and age-appropriate DVD or videotape (preferably one chosen by the child or parents).

AMLR in Pediatric Populations

Introduction

The term middle latency response (MLR) was coined following the discovery of ABR because the response follows the ABR in time and precedes the ALR. The term auditory middle latency response (abbreviated AMLR) is more accurate, and preferred, as it distinguishes the response from somatosensory, visual, and vestibular evoked response components within the same time frame. AMLR components occur between approximately 10 ms and 50 ms after the presentation of a stimulus (Cacace & McFarland, 2002; Hall, 1992, 2007; Kraus, Kileny, & McGee, 1994; Picton, Hillyard, Krausz, & Galambos, 1974).

AMLR in Children with Normal Hearing

Typical of other auditory evoked responses, the human AMLR was first recorded in adults and the initial reported recommendations on recording parameters and waveform descriptions were in the context of adult data. In the late 1970s, there were attempts to record AMLRs in infants and to apply them clinically as objective measures for threshold estimation. For example, Wolf and Goldstein (1978) described findings in five newborn infants in an attempt to validate the AMLR for threshold estimation. The authors did record responses and concluded that wave components were obtained at intensity levels "approaching voluntary adult behavioral thresholds" (Wolf & Goldstein, 1978, p. 513). Subsequent studies of AMLR in children were also conducted mostly to validate the response as a tool for threshold estimation. Although initial work on optimization of AMLR recording procedures and parameters was completed with healthy adults, the same parameters were then applied to pediatric auditory assessment. It is now known, however, that AMLR measurement in infants and children requires modification of stimulus and recording parameters from those used in adults (Hall, 1992, 2007). In order to optimize the test parameters for pediatric application of AMLR, one must understand the developmental changes in the response from infancy through adulthood. This in turn mandates knowledge of the anatomic generators of the AMLR because neurophysiologic development and neuromaturational status directly affect the morphology and characteristics of the response.

Developmental Changes in the AMLR and Anatomic Correlates

The AMLR in adult humans consists of scalp or vertex negative and positive peaks, including the Na, Pa, and Pb (also referred to as the P50) components. The Pb component of the AMLR is probably the same as the P1 of the ALR, but this point is debated in the literature. The AMLR components are widely distributed over the frontocentral scalp region and can be recorded using the same electrode montage (i.e., array) used for ABR (Kraus et al., 1994). The anatomic generators of the AMLR have been debated over the years, but it is now generally accepted that the Pa component is a reflection of activity in the central nervous system within pathways leading from, and including, the thalamus and the primary auditory cortex (specifically Heschl's gyrus). For a detailed review of literature on the anatomic generators of the AMLR, the reader is directed to Hall (2007). According to McGee and Kraus (1996) the AMLR seems to have a relatively long developmental time course and continues to develop through the first decade of life. AMLR components show developmental changes not only with respect to waveform morphology, but also with respect to response reliability. The likelihood of recording an AMLR consistently increases with age up to the age of 10 years (Hall, 2007).

In a review of literature on the development of the auditory system from the gestational period to adulthood, Moore and Linthicum (2007) report original findings and correlate various research findings on histologic examination with information on the development of AMLR components. These authors describe changes that take place during the prenatal, perinatal, and postnatal period. During the perinatal period, myelination is observed in the axons that project through the brachium of the inferior colliculus to the medial geniculate body. These axons probably contribute to the AMLR component most easily detectible in infants, the Po-Na complex. This complex is barely detectible between the 25th and 27th fetal weeks but generally is present by the 33rd week and even more pronounced in full-term neonates. The rate of detection of the Pa and Na components reaches 80 to 90% at about 30 weeks conceptional age (Rotteveel, Stegeman, de Graaf, Colon, & Visco, 1987). The latency of Na decreases from approximately 28 ms at the 30th fetal week to approximately 20 ms at term (Pasman, Rotteveel, de Graaf, Maassen, & Notermans, 1991; Rotteveel et al., 1987). Po and Na are the most consistent components in the AMLR wave sequence in 3-month-old babies (Rotteveel et al., 1986). The latency of Na decreases to 18 ms by the age of 3 months and remains unchanged into adulthood (Kraus, Smith, Reed, Stein, & Cartee, 1985). According to Moore and Linthicum (2007), this early maturation follows that of the ABR closely and, hence, it seems likely that the Po-Na components reflect transmission in the brachial pathway from the inferior colliculus to the thalamus.

There is an increasing prominence of the Na component of the AMLR across early childhood. This may be reflective of the newly maturing system of thalamocortical connections (Moore & Linthicum, 2007). The Pa component increases in detectability in early childhood with a latency of approximately 25 to 30 ms (Kraus et al., 1985). This increased likelihood of detecting Pa with age occurs regardless of whether the subject is a normally developing child or a child with any of a wide range of neurologic, cognitive, or speech and language disorders (Kraus et al., 1985).

According to McGee and Kraus (1996), the Pa component has a major dipole source in the temporal region. Moore and Linthicum (2007) add that as the Pa wave matures by early childhood, and closely follows the Na wave, it probably reflects activity in the pathway running from the medial geniculate body to the cortex. The Pb component of the AMLR has a much longer course of development and reaches its adult value later than the Na component. The results of studies of AMLR maturation vary depending on whether the Pb (P1) component is considered part of the AMLR or the ALR. Other major factors that seem to determine the age of maturation are the stimulus rate and state of consciousness. The detectability of wave Pa increases monotonically, from 20% at birth to 90% at 12 years of age (Kraus et al., 1985), assuming the effect of sleep is ruled out. Other researchers (e.g., Tucker & Ruth, 1996) also have reported that the variables of age, signal level, and site of recording significantly affect the peak amplitude and absolute latency of the Pa component.

Little information exists relating AMLR findings to those for behavioral measures of central auditory function. In a study conducted on 150 participants with normal hearing ranging from 7 to 16 years of age, Schochat and Musiek (2006) described relations between data on the duration and pitch pattern tests (behavioral) and AMLR. Their results showed increased performance with age on both the behavioral tests up to age 12 years. These authors, however, did not find significant changes across this age range for either latency or amplitude measures on the AMLR. This finding seems to agree with the observation of Moore and Linthicum (2007) that the Pa component of the AMLR reflects activity in the pathways from the medial geniculate body to the cortex rather than solely in the cortical areas and, therefore, develops relatively early.

In another recent study, Frizzo, Funayama, Isaac, and Colafêmina (2007) examined the components of AMLRs using tone-burst stimuli at 50, 60, and 70 dB HL in healthy children aged 10 to 13 years. They found that the mean latencies of the Na, Pa, Nb, and Pb components at 70 dB HL were 20.8 ms, 35.3 ms, 43.3 ms, and 53.4 ms, respectively. The Na-Pa amplitude in their subjects ranged from 0.2 to 1.9 μV with a mean of 1.0 μV. Predictably, as the stimulus intensity increased, the amplitude of the wave components increased and latency decreased. These findings indicate that within the age range of 10 to 13 years, AMLR patterns resemble those of adults.

Developmental Changes and Recording Parameters

Age and the Effect of Filter Settings. Although some early researchers did not observe the Pa component consistently in neonates and young children with normal hearing (Davis, 1976), other studies showed that the Pa could be recorded reliably in newborns and young children (e.g., McRandle, Smith, & Goldstein, 1974; Mendel, Adkinson, & Harker, 1977; Mendelson & Salamy, 1981; Wolf & Goldstein, 1980). Surprisingly, as noted by Hall (2007), the latency of Pa reported in the studies did not change as a function of age and, in some cases, was even shorter in infants than in adults. It is probable that the Pa reported by some of the studies was in fact an artifact caused by excessive band pass filtering. Removing the low frequencies, by raising the high pass filter setting from 10 or 15 Hz to 100 Hz usually results in a loss of the actual Pa component and creates a positivity that mimics the Pa. Hence, an apparent (artifactual) Pa may be recorded when there is no true response. Artifacts of this nature would obviously not show any change in latency across age groups.

Age and Stimulus Rate. Stimulus rate is another factor that probably contributed to differences in findings across developmental AMLR studies. Early studies on infants and children used stimulus rates of 10 per second or slightly faster rates in the interest of saving test time. Recent literature indicates that this rate of stimulation is much too fast to elicit an AMLR from children (Fifer, 1985; Hall, 1992; Kraus, Reed, Smith, Stein, & Cartee, 1987). One principle of auditory evoked response measurement bears repeating at this juncture. Slower stimulus rates are required for longer latency responses. A stimulus rate as slow as 1 per second may be required to elicit the AMLR in infants and young children. When stimulus rates approach 11 stimuli per second, the proportion of children yielding a detectable AMLR reduces directly with a decrease in age (Hall, 2007).

Developmental Changes and State of Arousal

The AMLR can be recorded from adult subjects in sleep and even during sedation, but in infants and children, sleep, sedation, and attention are important variables that must be considered when interpreting the response (Hall, 2007). In general, there is an interaction between the AMLR response and all stages of sleep, but the response is more likely to be detected as stimulus rate is decreased (Hall, 2007). Kraus, McGee, and Comperatore (1989) recorded the AMLR in six normal-hearing children between the ages of 4 and 9 years in waking state and natural sleep. Sleep state was monitored during AMLR recordings that lasted for an average of about 2.1 hours per subject. The Pa component was consistently detected during wakefulness, alpha, stage 1, and REM sleep. AMLR was inconsistently detected in sleep stages 2 and 3, and rarely detected during stage 4 sleep especially in younger children (within the tested age range). The probability of obtaining the Pa component during stage 4 sleep increases steadily with age. The authors suggested that the differences in the effect of sleep on the adult versus child AMLR response could be arising from the difference in the neural generators at different developmental stages. The AMLR in children seems to be dominated by activity from the reticular formation and, thus, is more susceptible to sleep whereas in adults, thalamocortical activity dominates the response, minimizing sleep effects.

Other studies reported similar findings. Collet, Duclaux, Challamel, and Revol (1988) recorded AMLR, with two click-rates (1.3 stimuli/s and 8.9 stimuli/s) in 6- or 7-week-old infants in an attempt to define the effect of sleep on the amplitude of AMLR. The Na-Pa complex was always greater during waking states than sleep states regardless of stimulus rate. Okitsu (1984) reported that in young children, the Na component was only 10% lower in sleep, but the presence of Pa decreased considerably during sleep. Later waves such as Nb and Pb were rarely observed in both waking and sleep conditions. Contrary to these findings, Rogers, Edwards, Henderson-Smart, and Pettigrew (1989) found no change in wave latency or reproducibility of AMLRs recorded during different sleep states in infants between the ages of 3 to 5 days and 1 year. In summary, the majority of studies confirm an effect of the state of consciousness on the pediatric AMLR. Indeed, there is a recent literature devoted to the application of the AMLR in documenting depth of anesthesia.

Clinical Applications of AMLR in Pediatric Populations

Threshold Estimation

The AMLR can be used objectively to estimate hearing threshold. AMLR offers several advantages for this clinical application. The amplitude of the major component (Pa) is about twice the size of the ABR wave V. In theory, then, the AMLR can be identified at lower signal levels and with less averaging. Another advantage is that the AMLR can easily be elicited using highly frequency-specific longer duration tone bursts. In contrast, the ABR waves are not as robust when elicited with tone bursts, and stimulus duration must be shorter (with corresponding increase in spectral splatter). A third advantage is that AMLR measurement does not require specialized instrumentation, and typically can be recorded with ABR instrumentation using (for threshold estimation) a simple one-channel electrode montage. Despite these apparent advantages, there are compelling reasons why the AMLR is not as popular as the ABR for estimation of hearing threshold. AMLR is markedly affected by muscle and movement artifact, a major problem in pediatric populations. Sedation and anesthesia, the solution to the problem of movement interference for ABR measurement, greatly affects the AMLR and is, therefore, not an option. For this reason, AMLR has given way to ABR for electrophysiological auditory threshold estimation in children. As ABR measurement with tone-burst stimulation, and more recently the auditory steady-state response (ASSR), are the techniques of choice for frequency-specific estimation of auditory thresholds in infants and young children and are recommended for this purpose (e.g., Joint Committee on Infant Hearing-JCIH, 2007), we do not review here the literature on this application of the AMLR.

AMLR as an Index of Depth of Anesthesia

The sensitivity of the AMLR to changes in sleep state has been exploited clinically to document and quantify level of consciousness (see Hall, 2007 for detailed review). In an early study, Prosser and Arslan (1985) evaluated the AMLR and ABR in persons under general anesthesia. The authors found that ABR components remained normal under the effects of anesthesia, but AMLR was grossly abnormal, as reflected by poor stability of the components and abnormalities in the latencies of any peaks that could be detected. The study confirmed the role of the auditory cortex, and perhaps the reticular formation, in the generation of the AMLR response and the effect of drugs on these structures. More recently, Lamas et al. (2006) evaluated the utility of the AMLR in monitoring the level of sedation in six critically ill children. The level of sedation was measured using the COMFORT scale and the Bispectral Index (BIS). AMLR showed a good correlation with the COMFORT scale and BIS in light and deep sedation and, in one patient, was effective in the early detection of brain death. In another patient who was chemically paralyzed, AMLR detected inadequate (under-) sedation.

Documentation of Cochlear Implant and Hearing Aid Performance

The AMLR offers two distinct advantages for objective assessment of cochlear implant and hearing aid performance. Because it is generated by suprabrainstem (thalamocortical) pathways, AMLR provides information on higher regions of the auditory system, more closely related to "hearing," than the ABR. In addition, the AMLR with latency values far beyond the ABR is easy to record electrically without the problem of electrical or measurement artifacts. For these reasons, beginning with the investigation by Kileny, Kemink, and Miller (1989), the AMLR has been applied clinically in the evaluation of cochlear implant users. Gordon, Papsin, and Harrison (2004, 2005) more recently recorded electrically evoked AMLRs (EMLRs) in a series of 81 children with pre- or perilingual deafness. Fifty of these children were studied longitudinally with repeated measures obtained first at the time of implantation, then at the initial device stimulation, and then again after 2, 6, and 12 months of implant use. EMLRs were measured only once in the remaining 31 children who had an average of 5.3 years (± 2.9 years) of experience with their implant. These investigators found that EMLRs were rarely detected at the time of implantation under anesthesia or sedation and were detected only in 35% of awake children on the day of device activation. The percentage of detection improved significantly with consistent implant use, reaching a detectability of 100% after at least one year after implantation. They reported that older children had a greater likelihood of showing detectable EMLRs in the initial period of device use compared to younger children. However, with consistent use of the device, the younger children showed more rapid rates of increase in detectability of the evoked response compared to the older children. This observation might reflect the developmental plasticity of the thalamocortical pathways. Developmental plasticity and the deprivation effects of hearing loss on the central auditory system are discussed in detail in the following section on ALRs. In a sample of 12 postlingually deaf and 4 prelingually deaf subjects, Groenen, Snik, and van den Broek (1997) found that the electrical auditory middle latency responses (EAMLR) of both groups were remarkable similar though their speech perception skills were different. The researchers pointed out that the difference in speech perception ability between congenitally deaf and postlingually deaf cochlear implant users did not seem to be reflected in the EAMLR. Within the postlingually deaf subjects there was more diversity in the amplitude of the EAMLR component peaks and a more diffuse EAMLR peak latency organization across the electrodes in individuals with poorer speech perception performance than those with better performance.

Auditory Processing Disorders (APD) and Language/Learning Disabilities

Hall (2007), in a review of studies of the AMLR in children with auditory processing disorders, noted that many of the early studies used recording parameters that have more recently proved to be inappropriate for children. A general finding across studies was latency prolongation and amplitude reduction for the Na and Pa components in children with APDs. Among auditory evoked responses, the AMLR and P300 most often show abnormalities in patients referred for APD assessment (Hall & Mueller, 1997). Purdy, Kelly, and Davies (2002) studied ABR, AMLR, and ALR in a small sample of 10 children in the age range of 7 to 11 years with "learning disability (LD)" and a control group of 10 age-matched children. They reported delayed Na latency and smaller amplitude of the Nb component in the LD group. Based on close review of the behavioral findings for the LD group, it is difficult to verify whether the children would meet current diagnostic criteria for auditory processing disorder (e.g., American Speech-Language and Hearing Association [ASHA], 2005). Arehole, Augustine, and Simhadri (1995) reported that for certain recording conditions, the latencies of AMLR for pediatric subjects with LD were significantly different from the group of normal hearing children. Again, criteria for definition of LD were neither well defined, nor consistent with current criteria for APD.

AMLR was used by Cone-Wesson, Kurtzberg, and Vaughan (1987) as one of the tests to study auditory system integrity in a group of 59 infants at risk for subsequent hearing and language disorders due to low birth weight and/or perinatal asphyxia. In addition to the AMLR these researchers recorded the ABR. Cone-Wesson et al. (1987) reported that 63% of the subjects had findings consistent with either normal peripheral hearing or slight unilateral impairment; 84% showed test findings reflecting normal auditory system functioning up to the level of the brainstem; 82% had normal AMLRs; and 81% showed normal ALRs. Some infants showed diverse patterns of peripheral, brainstem, and cortical abnormalities. The topography of the ABR, AMLR, and "cortical evoked responses (ACR)" was investigated by Mason and Mellor (1984) in children with normal speech and language development and those with either a language or motor speech disorder. They reported that AMLR amplitude in the group with motor speech disorders was significantly larger at the mastoid and temporal electrode sites than in either the control group or the group with language disorders. The authors interpreted that this pattern could be indicative of a larger myogenic response similar to brainstem reflexes, which are known to be often more intense in individuals with congenital suprabulbar paresis. The ACRs showed significantly larger amplitudes in the motor speech group at the Cz site. This phenomenon was attributed to a possibility of less than normal levels of activity in the cortical inhibitory system. In the language disordered children, the cortical responses showed an abnormal hemispheric dominance in the left temporal region and a more inverted or "dissimilar" wave form at the site of the T3 electrode. Mason and Mellor (1984) concluded that the AMLR findings suggested impaired functioning of the left temporal cortex in children who failed to develop language normally. Formal investigation of the AMLR in a series of children with APD as diagnosed with current criteria is certainly warranted. The findings would probably contribute to the inclusion of AMLR into the clinical APD test battery.

Brain Injury

In contrast to the plentiful studies of AMLR in adults with brain injuries (e.g., Drake, Weate & Newell, 1996; Gaetz & Weinberg, 2000; Hall, 1992), there are relatively few in children. A possible explanation for the limited neurodiagnostic application of AMLR in children is the concern that absence of an AMLR may not always be a manifestation of an auditory pathway dysfunction (Kraus et al., 1985). Hall, Brown, and Mackey-Hargadine (1985) made serial auditory brainstem (ABR) and middle-latency (AMLR) response measurements in 12 children ranging in age from 2 weeks to 10 years. Of these five had acute, severe head injury, two had hydrocephalus, two had meningomyelocele, one was a case of hyperbilirubinemia, one had ototoxic drug overdose, and one had severe developmental delay. In most cases, AMLR findings were related to neurologic status and outcome.

Other Pediatric Populations

In a large sample study, Kraus et al. (1985) studied AMLRs as a function of age in 217 subjects aged 6 days to 20 years. All the subjects had normal auditory brainstem responses (ABRs). They grouped the subjects into the following diagnostic categories: normal, communicative disorders (language delay, learning disability), mentally retarded, multiply handicapped, and post-meningitis. The authors examined age effects, and effects of diagnostic category, and also compared the AMLRs of males versus females and right versus left ears. Consistent with other studies, detectability of both Na and Pa components increased significantly as a function of age. There were no significant differences among diagnostic categories, nor any gender and ear differences. Kraus et al. (1985) made the important point that every clinician using the AMLR must keep in mind that "when responses are present, they may be useful indicators of hearing sensitivity, but the absence of [A] MLRs in children cannot be taken as an indication of hearing loss" (p. 343). Kraus and colleagues (1985) also concluded that if AMLRs are absent or abnormal one cannot infer a dysfunction of the auditory pathway beyond doubt as there does not seem to be much difference between the AMLRs of normal subjects and those of patients with a "wide range of neurologic, cognitive, and speech and language disorders" (p. 343).

Studies on the AMLR in individuals with Down syndrome showed abnormal findings. Diaz and Zuron (1995) reported longer Na latency in Down syndrome subjects compared to normal subjects, whereas the Pa latency was not significantly different from normals. Poblano et al. (1991) studied the AMLR in 11 children with Down syndrome between the ages of 6 and 9 years. They reported a significant reduction in AMLR amplitude, and often absence of the Pa component. The authors hypothesized that the abnormalities of AMLR amplitude could be linked to the presence of fewer neurons in the brains of patients with Down syndrome. They also opined that microcephaly might account for reduced central transmission time and higher rates of action potential depolarization, and repolarization as well as decreased spike duration. The authors pointed out that the Pa component might have been absent in their subjects due to microgyria in the Heschl's gyrus, a finding that has been reported in earlier studies on individuals with Down syndrome.

Cottrell and Gans (1995) found that the amplitude of AMLR in children with disabilities was depressed, and that waveform morphology varied substantially and differed from normal children or infants. Vandana and Tandon (2006) reported for a group of malnourished children prolonged overall ABR peak latencies, whereas AMLRs were not significantly different from normal subjects. The authors postulated that malnutrition seems to have a negative impact on the development of auditory pathways in the brainstem while a similar impact is not seen in the central and thalamocortical connections related to these pathways. Rodríguez Holguín, Corral, and Cadaveira (2001) observed differences in AMLR among children of alcoholics with a multigenerational family history of alcoholism and controls. The children of alcoholics showed prolonged latency of Pa and Pb and, reduced Pa amplitude.

Children with autism spectrum disorders are known to be selective to certain auditory stimuli while ignoring others that are not of their interest. Kemner, Oranje, Verbaten, and van Engeland (2002) measured sensory filtering in children with autism using the P50 (Pb) gating paradigm in 12 nonmentally retarded children with autism and 11 healthy controls. They did not find any differences in absolute P50 amplitude and P50 (Pb) suppression between the children with autism and the control children. Naveen and colleagues (1998) reported that the peak latency of the AMLR P50 (Pb) component was significantly shorter for congenitally blind children than for normally sighted children. They inferred that perhaps information processing at the levels of the ascending reticular activating system or the primary auditory cortex occurs more efficiently in blind individuals.

Based on the hypothesis that the auditory afferent control is an important feedback mechanism in speech generation and that a different organization of auditory afferent pathways in children with speech alterations exists, Milicic et al. (1998) recorded ABR and AMLR elicited with monoaural and binaural click stimulation in a group of 17 children with normal speech and in 16 children with dyslalia (eight with systematic and eight with nonsystematic errors of speech). All subjects were approximately 7 years old. A successive latency prolongation (average of 2.97 ms) of AMLR wave Na was registered between the two groups. A difference between groups in the binaural interaction of AMLR of the Na component was also reported suggesting that children with dyslalia may have an atypical (different) organization in their auditory afferent pathway.

Cone-Wesson, Ma, and Fowler (1997) reported that binaural interaction (BI) responses in ABR and AMLR using click and tone-burst stimuli from neonates were immature and more prevalent in the latency range of ABRs than for AMLRs. The ABR-BI component was equally prominent for click and tonal stimuli. However, clicks were more effective than tone-bursts in eliciting the AMLR-BI component. McPherson, Tures, and Starr (1989) observed that the binaural interaction of AMLR was greatest at N20 in term infants.

The area under the curve (AUC) is a simple way of quantifying the maturing AMLR response and may be a more accurate index than latency and amplitude. The AUC reflects the total neural activity in the Pa waveform. Pynchon, Tucker, Ruth, Barrett, and Herr (1998) measured the AUC in five groups, namely, infants, children, preteens, teens, and adults, using ipsilateral and contralateral recordings of the AMLR at two stimulus levels (70 and 40 dB nHL) and at two stimulus rates (11.3 and 3.3 per second). They did not find a significant difference between the AUC of the AMLR waveform in subjects of different age groups.

Auditory Late Responses (ALRs)

Introduction to the Family of ALRs

More than a dozen specific components or responses can be recorded within the general latency region included within the rather vague term "auditory late responses." Over the years, a variety of terms have been coined to refer to the responses in the ALR time frame, including the N1–P2 complex. The general "late response" timeframe extends approximately from 50 ms until 1000 ms (one second) after the presentation of the stimuli. Not surprisingly, a rather vast literature consisting of thousands of papers has accumulated since the discovery of the auditory late response in 1939. The focus of the following review is the ALR waveform consisting of an N1 and P2 component elicited with simple tonal or speech stimuli. The majority of the many publications on responses within the late latency region pertain to other components or responses, ranging from variations of the N1 component (e.g., N1a, N1b, N1c), the N150, N250, Nc, Nd, N400, or positive peaks beyond the P2 component (e.g., later than 200 ms), among them the P3 and P3a waves, as well as the mismatch negativity (MMN) response. For more detailed information on these many and varied responses, the reader is referred to the textbooks of Hall (2007) and Burkard et al., (2007) and also recent review articles, such as "Speech Evoked Potentials from the Laboratory to the Clinic" (Martin, Tremblay, & Korczak, 2008).

Measurement and Analysis

A clinical protocol for recording the ALR N1 and P2 components is summarized in Table 21–4. The literature contains many variations in the protocols for ALR measurement, in part due to development of more sophisticated instrumentation and evolution of measurement strategies over the past 70 years. Although as many as 20 or even 30 electrodes are often utilized in recordings conducted in laboratory experiments, ALR measurement is feasible with as few as three electrodes. A handful of clear differences between the protocols for measurement of AMLR versus ALR are readily apparent. When recorded with the protocols summarized here, both the AMLR and the ALR are generated by the onset of stimuli (tonal or speech). Of course, analysis time is about five times longer for the ALR than the AMLR because latencies of the major ALR peaks are four or five times later than the Pb component of the AMLR. Stimulation differs considerably and in several ways for the ALR versus AMLR. Speech stimuli are now rather popular for elicitation of the ALR (e.g., Martin et al., 2008), whereas click or tone burst stimuli are commonly used to elicit the AMLR. The rate of stimuli must be relatively slow (< 1 stimulus per second) for the ALR, even when recording the response from older children and adults.

Table 21–4 Guidelines for an Auditory Late Response (ALR) Test Protocol

Parameter	***Suggestion***	***Rationale/Comment***
Stimulus Parameters		
Transducer	ER-3A	Supra-aural earphones can be used for ALR measurement. Insert earphones are more comfortable for longer AER recording sessions and they attenuate background sound.
Type	Tone-Burst	Longer duration tonal signals are preferred for ALR elicitation.
	Speech	The ALR can be effectively elicited with speech signals. Various features of speech signals, e.g., voice onset time, can be used in ALR stimulation.
Duration		
Rise / Fall	~ 10 ms	Longer signal onset times are feasible and desirable to elicit the ALR.
Plateau	~ 50 ms	Extended plateau durations are effective in eliciting the ALR.
Rate	≤ 1.1/second	A slow rate of signal presentation is essential for the ALR, due to the long refractory time of cortical neurons.
Polarity	Variable	Signal polarity is not an important parameter for ALR measurement.
Intensity	≤ 70 dB HL	Modest signal intensity levels are typical for ALR measurement.
Number	≤ 200	Signal repetitions vary depending on size of response and background noise. Averaging may require as few as 20 to 50 signals at high-intensity levels for a very quiet and normal hearing patient.
Presentation ear	Variable	Monaural or binaural signals are often used to elicit the ALR.
Masking	Variable	Masking is rarely required with insert earphones, and not needed for stimulus intensity levels of ≤ 70 dB HL.
Acquisition Parameters		
Amplification	×50, 000	Less amplification is required for larger responses such as the ALR.
Sensitivity	25 or 50 volts	Smaller sensitivity values are equivalent to higher amplification.
Analysis time	500 to 600 ms	An analysis epoch long enough to encompass the entire N1, P2, N2 sequence.
Prestimulus time	100 ms	A prestimulus time provides a stable estimate of background noise and a baseline for calculation of the amplitudes for negative and positive waveform components (N1, P2, P3).
Data points	≤ 512	
Sweeps	1,000	See comments above for signal number.
Filters		
Band-pass	0.1 to 100-Hz	The ALR consists of low frequency energy within the spectrum of the EEG.
Notch	None	Notch filtering in the region of 60 Hz should be avoided with ALR measurement because important frequencies in the response will be removed.
Electrodes		
Type	Disk or disposable	Disk electrodes applied with paste (versus gel) are useful to secure the noninverting electrodes on the scalp. Red and blue colored electrode leads for the right and left hemisphere locations, respectively, are suggested. Disposable electrodes or a multiple-electrode cap are also appropriate with ALR measurement.

continues

Table 21–4. *continued*

Parameter	Suggestion	Rationale/Comment
Electrode Sites		
	Noninverting	The Fz or Cz sites are appropriate for recording the ALR clinically. Many published studies include 20 or more electrode sites.
	Inverting	Linked earlobes are commonly used for inverting electrodes. A non-cephalic electrode site (e.g., nape of the neck) is also appropriate.
	Other	Ocular electrodes (located above and below or to the side of an eye) are required for the detection of eye blinks, and rejection of averages contaminated by eye blinks.
	Ground (Fpz)	The common (ground) electrode can be located anywhere on the body. A low forehead (Fpz) or nasion, i.e., Nz (between the eyes) location is convenient and effective.

Source: Adapted from Hall (2007).

Nonpathologic Factors

Major nonpathologic, or subject, factors influencing the ALR that must be taken into account in the analysis and interpretation of findings include:

- Age and neurologic maturation
- Attention
- Sleep
- Effects of intervention.

Given their importance in analysis of the ALR, these factors are reviewed in some detail in the following sections of the chapter. As with AMLR measurement, subject state of arousal is an important factor in ALR measurement. The strategy noted in the AMLR section (encouraging the patient to view a video or DVD during measurement) applies also when recording the ALR from young children. A typical auditory late response (ALR) waveform with the P1, N1, and P2 components evoked with a tone burst or speech signal and recorded with a single channel electrode array is depicted in Figure 21–2.

ALR in Pediatric Populations

Introduction

Morphology of the auditory late latency responses (ALRs) differs significantly for children versus adults. In addition, throughout childhood there are substantial maturational changes in ALR latency, amplitude, and morphology. The obligatory components within the ALRs, such as the P1, N1, and P2, are generated by portions of the auditory pathway beyond the medial geniculate body, more specifically the thalamocortical and corticocortical pathways, primary auditory cortex, and different association cortices (e.g., Čeponienè, Cheour, & Näätänen, 1998; Eggermont & Ponton, 2003; Näätänen & Picton, 1987; Ponton, Eggermont, Khosla, Kwong, & Don, 2002; Ponton, Eggermont, Kwong, & Don, 2000; Sharma, Dorman, & Spahr, 2002a, 2002b). Axons of the geniculocortical system, an obligatory link in the ascending auditory pathway, mature between the ages of 6 months and 5 years. These centers are important for basic central auditory processing in childhood (Illing, 2004). The fibers of the corticocortical systems which link the auditory cortex to other areas within the temporal, parietal, and prefrontal lobes may not reach maturity until the age of 12 years or more (Illing, 2004). Besides the process of maturation of the axons themselves, synaptic maturation also plays a part in the scalp recorded auditory responses from these generator sites. Hence, it is not surprising that the ALRs show significant changes with age and mature well into the teenage years. The differences between ALRs recorded at different stages of childhood and in adults are seen not simply in terms of the latency, amplitude and relative amplitude of different components, but also in terms of refractoriness and the emergence of certain components only after a certain age (e.g., Gilley, Sharma, Dorman, & Martin, 2005; Moore, 2002) and complex changes in morphology and scalp distribution (e.g., Stapells, 2002). These morphologic differences are important to know as they

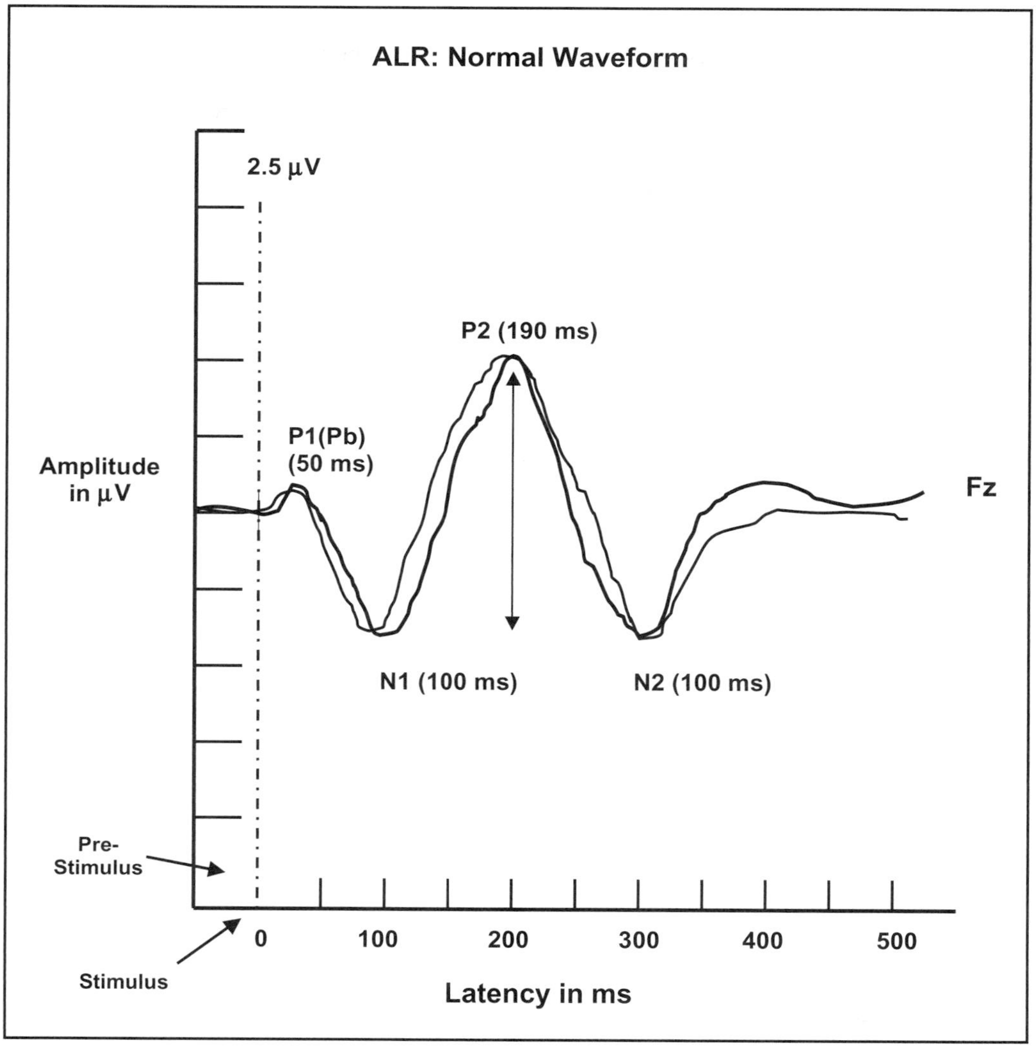

FIGURE 21–2. A typical auditory late response (ALR) waveform with the P1, N1, and P2 components evoked with a tone burst or speech signal and recorded with a single channel electrode array with the noninverting electrode located at the Fz or Cz midline location, and the inverting electrode on the nape of the neck.

govern our selection of test protocols, stimuli, acquisition parameters, and collection of normative data.

ALR in Children with Normal Hearing

The development of the obligatory subcomponents of the ALR has been studied by several researchers. The results vary across studies probably due to methodological variables known to affect the waveform, such as the type of stimuli used (tones versus syllables), number of repetitions, rate and interstimulus interval, and acquisition parameters, for example, recording electrode site (Hall, 2007). The developmental course of the P1, N1, and P2 components of the ALR can be studied with respect to their latencies, absolute and relative amplitudes and morphology. As the ALR components are obligatory, they are easy to record even in young children who are not voluntarily responding to the stimulus. Because the P1, N1, and P2 components are objective measures of cortical auditory functioning, they are valuable in the audiologic test battery. ALR components have in recent years gained importance as markers of neuromaturation (e.g., Čeponienè et al., 1998; Sharma et al., 2005b; Sharma, Kraus, McGee, & Nicol, 1997) in contrast to their historical application as objective measures of hearing threshold (Barnet & Lodge, 1967; Rapin, Reuben, & Lyttle, 1970; Taguchi, Picton, Orpin, & Goodman, 1969).

General Developmental Changes in the ALR

In general, the P1 component of the ALR de-creases in latency with increasing age. The latencies appear to decrease rapidly in the first decade of life, and then more gradually in the second decade of life (Cunningham, Nicol, Zecker & Kraus, 2000; Ponton et al., 2000; Sharma et al., 2002a; Sharma et al., 1997). The ALR in children is characterized by prominent P1 and N2 waves. In adults, however, the N1-P2 complex is prominent (Gilley et al., 2005; Hall, 2007). The P1 component first appears developmentally, followed by an almost adultlike P2 and a clear and often robust N2 by the age of 3 to 6 years (Hall, 2007). In contrast, other studies, such as Ponton et al. (2000) suggest that the P2 does not emerge before the age of 10 years.

Although the latency of all ALR components decreases, and amplitude increases, with age, the age related differences are not the same for all the waves. The P2 wave matures at a faster rate than the N1 wave. The latency of the P1 wave decreases from 96 ms at the age of 3 to 4 years to 76 ms at the age of 11 to 12 years for an inter-stimulus interval of 2000 ms (Gilley et al., 2005). Barnet, Ohlrich, Weiss, and Shanks (1975) and Ohlrich, Barnet, Weiss, and Shanks (1978) reported latency changes during the age range of 15 days to 3 years. Specifically, the latency of P2 shortens from 230 to 150 ms, N2 latency decreases from 535 to 320 ms, and P3 decreases from 785 to 635 ms. These latencies are highly prolonged compared to adult values for N1 (just under 100 ms), P2 (about 200 ms) and P3 (300 ms). Ponton et al. (2000) reported an increase in the latency of N2 with increasing age at some cephalic electrode locations. The N1/N2 amplitude ratio increases significantly with age (Čeponienè, Rinne, & Näätänen, 2002).

The ALR N1 (N100) wave is actually a wave complex (Hall, 2007). Parameters of the N1 component, including its presence, latency, and amplitude, and the presence of subcomponents or other negative waves within the same timeframe are determined by the physical properties of the stimulus and other factors such as alertness of the subject, attention and memory (Alain, Woods, & Covarrubias, 1997; Picton, Woods, Baribeau-Braun, & Healy, 1977). The negativity of the N1 wave is enhanced when a subject attends to it or listens for a specific stimulus (Hall, 2007). Most studies (e.g., Čeponienè et al., 2002; Gilley et al., 2005; Ponton et al., 2000; Sussman, Steinschneider, Gumenyuk, Grushko, & Lawson, 2008) report that the N1 is not apparent in very young children and in older children it is only observed at very slow stimulus rates. Eggermont and Ponton (2003) suggested that the emergence of the N1 component is reflective of the "maturation of the axons in layer II and upper layer III of the auditory cortex" (p. 249).

Cunningham et al. (2000) found that the N1 latency appeared adultlike by the age of 13 to 15 years with little additional age-related change. ALR N1 amplitude increased from age 5 years to well into the teenage years, and then was stable by adulthood. These researchers also found that N2 was measureable in 95% of children, 80% of young adults, and 20% of senior adults. Its latency decreased significantly between the ages of 5 and 10 years, was stable from 10 to 15 years and decreased again in young adulthood. As the amplitude and latencies of the ALR components are highly affected by state of arousal and sleep, stimuli used, stimulus and recording parameters, data across studies may vary depending on the measurement conditions prevalent in a particular study.

Developmental Changes in Scalp Distribution

According to Čeponienè et al. (2002), in adults and in children, the N1 and N2 components of the ALR are generated by anatomically distinct generators. The scalp distributions of both N1 and N2 change with maturation. In adults and older children, the neural sources of the N1 and N2 appear to be the superior aspects of the temporal lobe. The sources for N1 are posterior to the sources for N2 (Čeponienè et al., 2002). Ponton et al. (2000) measured the ALR from 30 different scalp-electrode locations in 118 subjects between the ages of 5 and 20 years of age. For analysis, the subjects were divided into groups so cross-sectional data for each year in between could be analyzed. Around the age of 10 years, the authors found sudden changes in P1, P1-N1b, and N2 peak amplitudes at the electrodes C3 and C4. No such changes were reported at the midline electrodes Cz and Fz. There were inter-hemispheric amplitude differences for the N1b peak. In all the age groups tested, except the 9-year-olds and 15-year-olds, the contralateral N1b measured at C4 was on average negative compared to the prestimulus baseline. The ipsilateral N1b amplitude did not become negative until the age of 16 years. The P2 also showed age-related difference in amplitude as a function of electrode location. Up to the age of 10 years, the P2 component was more clearly visible at electrode location Pz compared to more anterior locations such as Cz and Fz. For older children, the P2 became more prominent at anterior locations and less prominent at posterior locations. The N2 latency increased significantly as a function of age at electrodes Cz, C3, and C4, but showed no changes with age at the frontal electrode Fz. Ponton et al. (2000) speculated that the N2 might have several source components and that, "if the neural generators underlying N2 have different orientations toward the scalp, the distinct patterns of N2 maturation observed at central and frontal electrode locations may reflect the differential maturation of the generators contributing to this peak" (p. 232). These investigators also pointed out that differences in maturation observed for the components of ALR depended on recording electrode placement or the locations on the scalp. This is an important point to consider for the application of ALR in clinical populations such as children with hearing impairment, learning problems or auditory processing disorders.

Finally, Gomes et al. (2001) studied the spatiotemporal maturation of the central and lateral N1 components to tones in children ranging from 6 to 12 years of age and in adults. They found that in children, the central N1 exhibits developmental decrease in latency, but not in amplitude. The lateral N1 shows developmental changes in terms of both latency and amplitude. They postulated that probably the central component matures earlier as its generators are closer in proximity to the primary auditory areas, which mature before the association areas.

Developmental Changes in Morphology and Refractoriness.

Every neuron has a refractory period, that is, the time required for it to revert to its preconduction state. During this recovery period, the neuron's capacity to fire again is limited. The refractoriness of a neuron changes developmentally with factors such as myelination. The formation of myelin on the axon directly influences the speed of transmission (conduction velocity) of a neuron and thus can affect the ability of the neuron to conduct successive stimuli at a high rate (e.g., Sabatini & Regehr, 1999). Neural refractory periods (recovery times) for the ALR are relatively long. Hence, the interstimulus interval (ISI) rather than number of stimuli per second should be used to describe the rate factor for the ALR (Hall, 2007). Some of the early ALR studies confirmed that longer ISIs produced larger amplitudes of the N1 and P2 components, but did not have a significant effect on the latencies (e.g., Davis, Mast, Yoshie, & Zerlin, 1966; Fruhstorfer, Soveri, & Jarvilehto, 1970; Hari, Kaila, Katila, Tuomisto, & Varpula, 1982; Keidel & Spreng, 1965; Nelson & Lassman, 1968; Picton et al., 1977; Rothman, Davis, & Hay, 1970). This effect on the ALR was interpreted as a reflection of the time required by neurons to recover after being activated by a stimulus. However, refractory periods of individual neurons are significantly shorter than those for the N1 and P2 components of the ALR (Hall, 2007).

Gilley et al. (2005) studied developmental changes in refractoriness of responses within the ALR timeframe. The "cortical auditory evoked potentials" (CAEPs) for ISI conditions (offset to onset) of 2000, 1000, 560, and 360 ms were studied for 50 normal hearing children in the age range of 3 to 12 years and 10 adults ranging from 24 to 26 years of age. Results showed that for the children between the ages of 3 to 6 years, P1 dominated the cortical response with a latency of about 100 ms for all the ISI conditions. In the 7- to 8-year-olds, a "slight invagination" in the waveform began to emerge in the slowest ISI condition. This was labeled the N1. In the 11- to 12-year-olds, the N1-P2 complex was detected at all ISIs, although it was most robust in the slower ISI conditions. At the shortest ISI, the N1-P2 complex was seen only in 20% of the 3- to 4-year-olds. In the adult group, Gilley et al. (2005) found the N1-P2 complex to be the most dominant regardless of the ISI condition. The study reported by Gilley and colleagues (2005) highlighted the importance of examining the interaction between stimulation rate and age related development of the ALR. The finding that the N1 is only generated in children at ISIs of 1 second or longer has been observed in other studies as well.

According to Sussman et al. (2008), slow stimulus rates may result in better ALR amplitude, but they do not reflect the rates that occur in normal speech. Recording the ALR at higher rates may be more useful for understanding how the auditory system would cope in a realistic auditory environment. These researchers studied the effect of ISI on the elicitation of the P1–N1–P2–N2 components to stimulus onset asynchrony (SOA) of 200, 400, 600, and 800 ms (onset to onset) in children at ages 8, 9, 10, and 11 years, in adolescents at age 16 years, and in young adults at ages 22 to 40 years. Their findings showed that in their youngest age group, the P1 and N2 components were the most robust of all components irrespective of stimulus rates. N1, the dominant component in adults, emerged as a separate component only in adolescence. Although Sussman et al. (2008) described the P1–N1–P2 components as being more "adultlike" than "childlike" in the adolescent subjects, the N2 component that is typical of the child obligatory response, was still present.

Čeponienè et al. (2002) attributed this developmental change in N1 to its longer recovery cycle and its resulting overlap by the robust P1 and N2 peaks.

The authors proceeded to record the ALR at different SOAs filtering out the slow N2 activity. Despite this maneuver, the N1 was only revealed at short SOAs in the 9-year-old children that they tested but not in the 4-year-olds. The sensitivity of the N1 wave to stimulation rates is reflected by the changes in amplitude of the components that occur with changes in stimulation rate (Näätänen & Picton, 1987). Components 2 and 3 of the N1 appear to be affected by attention and orienting responses respectively. Unlike the N1, the N2 in children is largely unaffected by stimulus rate (Čeponienè et al., 1998).

Agung King et al. (2009) studied ALRs elicted by speech stimuli with different voice onset times in 10 children between the ages of 4 and 8 years. They compared their results with those obtained on previous studies with adult subjects. The authors described a "double on" pattern of the N1 response elicited by longer voice onset times in adults (from earlier literature), whereas they reported that the responses of their pediatric subjects only showed latency changes in the P1 and N2 components when stimulus voice onset times were changed. They concluded that although changes in voice onset times are reflected in the cortical responses of children in the age group of 2 to 8 years, they are represented by markers that are different from those in adults.

Anatomic and Physiologic Correlates of ALR Maturation

It would be plausible to assume that maturation of any neurologic component and the corresponding behavior should correlate with anatomic and physiologic changes that occur developmentally. Several researchers have described the neuromaturation of the auditory cortex in normal hearing children and clinical populations by means of histologic findings (e.g., Huttenlocher & Dabholkar, 1997; Kral, 2007; Moore, 2002; Moore & Guan, 2001; Moore & Linthicum, 2007; Shepherd & Hardie, 2001). Moore and Guan (2001) studied the maturation of the auditory cortex posthumously from the second trimester of gestation to young adulthood using histologic and immunohistochemic data. They found a deep-to-surface sequence of maturation of the axons of the auditory cortex (deeper layers mature first). Moore and Guan (2001) reported that, although axons are present in superficial layers of the cortex at a young age, their maturation (appearance of neurofilaments and development of a true axonal plexus) actually begins as late as age 5 years and continues as late as age 11 to 12 years. Maturation of the neurofilaments increases the conduction velocity of the axon. Moore and Guan (2001) suggest that the late onset of neurofilament maturation and myelination in the superficial layers and the continued expansion of commissural and association pathways account for the changes in auditory processing abilities with age in children.

Enhanced skills of auditory processing in degraded acoustic environments are observed in normal-hearing children beyond the age of seven years. Eggermont and Ponton (2003) point out that considering the timeline of development, it is not surprising that for children under the age of 7 years the N1 is not recordable except at very slow stimulus rates (under 1 per second). The age related alteration of the ALR and the appearance of the N1 coincide with maturation of the upper cortical layers (Moore & Linthicum, 2007). The N1 component as already mentioned matures well into adolescence and seems to be originating from the upper layer II of the cortex (Eggermont & Ponton, 2003). Synaptogenesis data reported by Huttenlocher and Dabholkar (1997) indicated that maturational differences persist for a shorter period in lower (deeper) than in upper (superficial) layers of the cortex. Also, cortical layers that receive primary afferent input (layer 4) and those that contain the neurons giving rise to the efferent pathways (layers 5 and 6) develop faster than the areas responsible for information processing (layers 2 and 3).

Eggermont and Ponton (2003) provided a detailed description of the structural, electrophysiologic, and behavioral indexes of cortical maturation. Briefly, maturation of the neuronal structure continues nearly into the early teenage years. In infants below the age of 4.5 months, only axons of layer I are mature. Neural activity at this stage is sufficient for generation of the ABR, P2, and N2. With behavioral measurement of auditory function, infants at this age are capable of responding differentially to changes in sounds. Between early infancy and 5 years of age, Eggermont and Ponton reported that the axons in layers IV, V, and VI start to mature. Electrophysiologically, this contributes to the generation of higher auditory responses such as the mismatch negativity, the T-complex, and the AMLR. Behaviorally, the auditory abilities that result from this neuronal development enable the child to develop verbal language through the auditory mode. Between the age of 5 and 12 years, layer II and III show maturation of axons with evidence of differentiation according to function. This level of neural maturation enhances the child listening performance in increasingly challenging auditory environments. Above the age of 12 years, all cortical axons reach maturity, and the rate of further change in behavioral and electrophysiologic correlates, slows down, and finally reaches a plateau.

Clinical Applications of ALR in Pediatric Populations

Introduction

There is increasing evidence that ALRs are effective noninvasive and objective tools for assessing central auditory nervous system maturation and processing (e.g., Arehole, 1995; Cunningham et al., 2000; Jerger et al., 2002; Jerger, Martin, & McColl, 2004; Ponton et al. 2000; Purdy, Kelly, & Thorne, 2001; Sharma et al., 1997, 2002a). Consequently, the ALR shows promise as a vital part of the audiologic test battery. Numerous studies have examined the differences between ALRs in normal hearing individuals and clinical populations using both life span (longitudinal) as well as cross-sectional experimental approaches. Differences are described in terms of the latencies, the presence versus absence of different components, and the relative amplitude of different components. As with other objective tests, such as the auditory brainstem response or otoacoustic emissions, their "objectivity" makes electrophysiological measures very attractive test tools for assessing in children the integrity of auditory processing in the central nervous system and, specifically for the ALR, the auditory cortex. Besides their use in diagnostic evaluation, ALRs also have been used as outcome measures of successful hearing aid fitting or cochlear implantation (e.g., Ponton, Don, Eggermont, Waring, & Masuda, 1996a; Ponton et al., 1996b; Sharma et al., 2002b; 2004, 2005a, 2005b) and auditory training in children with auditory processing disorders and learning problems (e.g., Jirsa, 1992; Warrier, Johnson, Hayes, Nicol, & Kraus, 2004).

Auditory Processing Disorders (APDs)

Introduction. According to technical reports of two American Speech-Language and Hearing Association task forces (ASHA, 1996; ASHA, 2005):

> Central auditory processing (C)AP, includes the auditory mechanisms that underlie the following abilities or skills: sound localization and lateralization; auditory discrimination; auditory pattern recognition; temporal aspects of audition, including temporal integration, temporal discrimination (e.g., temporal gap detection), temporal ordering and temporal masking; auditory performance in competing acoustic signals (including dichotic listening); and auditory performance with degraded acoustic signals. (ASHA, 1996; Bellis, 2003; Chermak & Musiek, 1997, cited by ASHA, 2005, p. 2)

According to the definition by the ASHA (2005) working group on (C)APD, "narrowly defined, (central) auditory processing refers to the perceptual processing of auditory information in the central nervous system and the neurobiologic activity that underlies that processing and gives rise to electrophysiologic auditory potentials" (p. 2). It is clear from this definition that the rationale for the use of objective measures such as the ALRs or event related potentials (ERPs) to diagnose APD is that every auditory behavior (or lack of it) should logically have a correlate in terms of presence or absence of a particular brain activity. As mentioned earlier, the obligatory components of the ALR are generated by the auditory thalamocortical and corticocortical pathways, primary auditory cortex, and different association cortices. These areas play an important role in central auditory processes. Measurement of the ALR (P1, N1, and P2 components) is recommended by these groups as part of the comprehensive test battery for diagnosing APD. This recommendation highlights the need for electrophysiologic assessment of young children for whom behavioral measures of APD may not always yield reliable or valid findings.

Correlations between auditory processing deficits and brain activity have been elegantly demonstrated through studies using topographic brain mapping. This strategy involves the measurement of cortical responses from surface electrodes on multiple scalp locations, hence enabling a study of brain regions that were active while certain tasks were being performed by the subject (Estes, Jerger, & Jacobson, 2002; Jerger et al., 2002, 2004; Jerger, Moncrieff, Greenwald, Wambacq, & Seipel, 2000). Jerger and colleagues reported their findings on a pair of fraternal twins, one of whom showed behaviors consistent with APD on the mother's as well as schoolteacher's responses on the Children's Auditory Performance Scale, or CHAPS (Smoski, Brunt, & Tannahill, 1998). The other twin was essentially normal. Both twins were evaluated with the same audiological test battery. The findings were reported in two parts (Jerger et al., 2002, 2004). The twin with symptoms of APD showed normal findings on traditional behavioral tests of APD.

In the study by Jerger et al. (2002), ERP topographies for both girls were constructed from electrophysiologic data obtained from 32 scalp locations during the performance of the tasks of visual gap detection, within-channel auditory gap detection, across channel auditory gap detection, dichotic listening for an acoustic target and dichotic listening for a phonemic target. The twins had comparable findings on the visual gap detection task, consistent with processing problems limited to the auditory system. For within-channel auditory gap detection, the nonaffected twin showed activation over both hemispheres, with more activation on the left side whereas the affected twin showed only a limited activation pattern in the temporoparietal region on the left side. For across-channel gap detection, the nonaffected twin showed activation over both hemispheres with slightly greater activation over the right hemisphere whereas the affected twin showed only a limited activation pattern in the C4 electrode (Jasper, 1958) region on the right side. For a dichotic listening task involving an acoustic target (saw tooth noise) with both right as well as left ear presentation, the nonaffected twin had an activation pattern that was asymmetric to the right of the midline (greater activity on the right side). In contrast, the pattern was attenuated and asymmetric to the left of the midline for the affected twin. For a dichotic listening task involving a phonemic target, the nonaffected twin had an activation pattern that was asymmetric to the left of the midline (greater activity on the left side). In contrast, the pattern was asymmetric to the right of the midline for the affected twin.

In other words, the results of the dichotic tasks suggested a reversal of hemispheric asymmetry and deficits in interhemispheric transfer of information via the corpus callosum. Interestingly, these researchers did not find any significant pattern of differences in the latencies of the corresponding ERPs between the twins. Hence, the brain activation patterns, rather than just latencies, brought out the differences between the twins. Jerger et al. (2002) concluded that activation patterns of ERPs for certain auditory tasks such as gap detection and dichotic listening may be especially effective in identifying auditory processing disorders.

For the second study on the same set of twins, Jerger et al. (2004) analyzed their brain maps in response to presentation of dichotic stimuli. Three of the conditions involved the processing of real words for either phonemic, semantic, or spectral targets, while one condition involved the processing of a nonword acoustic signal. The authors found marked differences in the cross-correlation functions between the twins. For the nonaffected twin, cross-correlation functions were uniformly normal across both hemispheres. For the affected twin the findings suggested "poorly correlated neural activity over the left parietal region during the three word processing conditions and over the right parietal area in the nonword acoustic condition" (p. 79). Jerger and colleagues (2004) also analyzed the results on diffusion tensor magnetic resonance imaging (DTI). The affected twin (in comparison with the nonaffected twin) showed "reduced anisotropy over the length of the midline corpus callosum and adjacent lateral structures" (p. 79) and concluded that these findings indicated "reduced myelin integrity" (p. 84). Jerger and colleagues (2004) concluded that at least some children with APD may be unable to perform adequately on tasks involving activity in both hemispheres and where the ability to perform the task is dependent on interhemispheric transfer of information through the corpus callosum.

Changes in parameters of the ALR P1, N1, and P2 waves reflect neuromaturation (e.g., Gilley, et al., 2005; Illing, 2004; Kraus & McGee, 1994; Sharma et al., 2002b). Jirsa and colleagues reported significant differences in the mean latencies of ALR N1 and P2 components, and the P3 response, in children with and without symptoms of auditory processing difficulties (Jirsa, 1992; Jirsa & Clontz, 1990). Jirsa (1992) found that the mean latencies of the components were significantly longer in children with behaviors consistent with processing problems. Jirsa and Clontz (1990) studied ALRs in children with auditory processing deficits and compared the findings with a control group of children with normal hearing, matched for age, intelligence, and gender. There was a significant latency increase for the ALR N1 and P2 waves, and the P3 response, in the group with auditory processing disorder. In addition, the interpeak latency interval for P2-P3 was significantly longer in the APD group. Among the amplitude measures, only P3 amplitude differed significantly between the groups. It is possible, then, that children with APD may be reflecting the effect of an immature auditory nervous system. Findings of abnormalities in ALR were reported even in adults with auditory problems consistent with the presence of APD (Jutras, Lagacé, Lavigne, Boissonneault, & Lavoie, 2007). In contrast, however, other studies have found no relationship between ALR P1/N1/P2 parameters and fine-grained speech sound perception (e.g., Cunningham et al., 2000).

ALR as an Index of Improvement in Central Auditory Processing. If the ALR indices of amplitude, latency, and morphology could be used to assess auditory cortical functioning and developmental plasticity, then it should follow that the ALR could be an effective tool in the objective assessment of change in cortical functioning as a result of a training program targeted at improving auditory processing at the level of the cortex. The large sample study by Warrier et al. (2004) was described in the subsection on ALRs in children with learning disabilities. These investigators documented changes in the cortical auditory evoked responses and corresponding improvements in speech perception in noise following training on the Earobics program (a commercially available software based program for auditory training in processing deficits).

Hayes, Warrier, Nicol, Zecker, and Kraus (2003) examined changes in the central auditory pathways and cognitive skills of children with learning problems (LP) as a result of training. The subject sample consisted of children between the ages of 8 and 12 years. The group of 27 children with learning problems was subdivided into two groups: one group that underwent the training program, and one that did not. In addition to the LP controls, data from seven age-matched children without learning problems were collected for comparison. Some children were on medication for ADHD (one of the control group and four in the trained LP group). The LP group that underwent training attended 35 to 40 one-hour training sessions over an 8-week period. The program consisted of the Step I and II of the Earobics computer-based program for development of auditory and pre-reading skills. The program uses interactive computer-based games to develop and improve skills such as phonological awareness and auditory language processing through interactive games, which are geared to give the child practice on skills like phoneme discrimination, auditory memory, rhyming, auditory attention, and so forth. Behavioral measures for cognitive and perceptual performance were administered. ABR was recorded with click stimuli as well as the syllable /ga/, and cortical auditory responses (the ALR) were elicited in quiet and in noise using the syllables /ga/ and /da/, respectively. Following intervention with the experimental group, all behavioral and electrophysiologic measures were repeated. On the behavioral sound blending test, the trained group showed significant improvements compared to the control group. This improvement was seen irrespective of the subject's pretraining performance on the same test. The ABR showed no changes as a result of training. However, components of the ALR showed significant improvements in association with improvement on behavioral measures.

Cunningham et al. (2001) studied the effect of "cue enhancement" on behavioral auditory performance as well as electrophysiologic measures in a sample of normal children and children with learning problems (LP). They studied the effects of enhancing specific speech cues at the syllable level in order to examine which cues resulted in better auditory perception of the stop consonants /d/ and /g/ incorporated in the syllables /ada/ and /aga/. Also studied were the corresponding differences in the auditory evoked responses (ABR, frequency following response [FFR] and ALRs). Cunningham and colleagues (2001) reported that the differences between the normal control and the LP group on ALRs were eliminated by the use of cue enhanced stimuli. This is an encouraging finding as it implies that such studies can help in designing of better therapy techniques and strategies supported by research evidence.

Language and Learning Disorders. Several studies have examined the performance of children with language and learning disabilities on difficult auditory processing tasks and corresponding auditory evoked responses (e.g., Arehole, 1995; Jerger, Martin, & Jerger, 1987; Kraus, 2001; Kraus et al., 1996; McArthur & Bishop, 2004; Moncrieff, Jerger, Wambacq, Greenwald, & Black, 2004; Warrier et al., 2004). Findings point to a possibility of altered auditory processing in at least some cases of learning disabilities (Wible, Nicol, & Kraus, 2002). Children with language-based learning problems show abnormalities in central auditory maturation (Gilley, Sharma, Dorman, & Martin, 2006). Gilley et al. (2006) studied the cortical auditory evoked potentials (ALRs) recorded from 26 children with learning problems. The authors reported that a majority of the children had abnormal responses. Gilley and colleagues (2006) identified three atypical categories of responses in children with learning problems: category 1 with delayed P1 latencies and absent N1/P2 components; category 2 with a normal P1 component but delayed N1 and P2 responses; and category 3 with overall low amplitude of all responses. A fourth subgroup had normal ALR responses. This research raises the possibility that differences in the obligatory ALRs between normal and learning-impaired children are evident only in difficult listening situations. A study by Cunningham et al. (2000) found no significant difference in the development of P1/N1 and N2 latency between normal children and children with learning problems. These authors did however note that scores on auditory processing tests correlated better with latencies of the ALR N2 component indicating the possible value of the speech-evoked N2 response in identifying auditory processing deficits.

Tonnquist-Uhlén, Borg, Persson, and Spens (1996) studied topographic maps of 20 children with learning impairment (LI) between the ages of 9 and 15 years and 20 normal age-matched children. The stimulus used was a 500-Hz tone presented with an inter-stimulus interval (ISI) of 1 second. Focusing mainly on the ALR N1 response, these researchers found that the latencies of N1 were longer in the LI group and there was no decrease in latency with increase in age. Tonnquist-Uhlén and colleagues (1996) speculated that the lack of improvement in latencies with age in the LI group might indicate the persistence of a processing disturbance, rather than just a delay in maturation. They further reported that the diagnostic sensitivity of N1 latency, amplitude, and topography in identifying LI subjects was 40% and the specificity was 90%.

Listening in noise is a difficult auditory processing task involving "auditory-figure ground" discrimination. Comparison of a given child's electrophysiologic responses to auditory stimuli in quiet versus in noise may provide a direct estimate of the effects of noise on auditory processing. Cunningham, Nicol, Zecker, Bradlow, and Kraus (2001) studied the ALRs of normal hearing children and children described as learning impaired in quiet and noise. These researchers found that the two groups had similar responses for the quiet situation, but in noise children with learning problems exhibited neurophysiologic abnormalities at both cortical and subcortical levels for auditory responses elicited by speech in noise. The authors also reported significantly lower amplitude of the ALR P1-N1 and P1'-N1' components in children with learning problems for speech in background noise. This reduction in the presence of noise was larger for the P1'-N1'. This difference between the normal and learning impaired group was eliminated when the same stimulus /da/ was presented in quiet or with cue enhancement.

Large sample studies, though difficult to design and conduct, are a good experimental approach for establishing a link among auditory evoked responses, behavioral auditory processing performance, and clinical entities involving the central nervous system. Warrier et al. (2004) conducted a relatively large sample study with children between the ages of 8 and 13 years. Eighty of the subjects had learning problems (LP) and 32 were essentially normal (NL), as determined by standard tests. Cortical auditory responses to the syllable /da/ were collected in quiet and noise conditions. The correlation of each individual subject's response in quiet versus that in noise was examined by shifting the waveforms for the latter with respect to time in order to achieve what the authors describe as a "best fit." Warrier et al. (2004) found some children in the LP group whose correlation scores fell below the lowest NL score. Based on the cross correlation of responses of the LP versus NL group, the LP group was further subdivided. The "LP-out" group consisted of those with poor correlation scores (below the mean –1SD of the NL group's correlation scores) and the remaining were grouped under "LP-in." In the quiet condition, the NL and LP groups were similar in terms of the morphology of the ALR P2-N2 complex, but in the noise condition the LP-out group had highly degraded morphology (compared to the NL and LP-in groups), particularly in the N2 region.

Warrier and colleagues (2004) postulated that the primary difference between the cortical responses of the NL and LP group was in terms of neural timing. Specifically, the difference between the groups was found for the ALR N2 component. In noise, the overall response activity in the LP group decreased to almost the same extent as the NL group, but in approximately one fourth of the LP group, the timing of the morphologic features of the waveform was altered due to noise. The latency of the N2 response in noise was earlier in the LP children. Since only a small portion (later portion) of the waveform conflicted morphologically with that obtained in a quiet condition, latency shift continued to produce a low quiet-to-noise correlation. In a second part of the experiment, some children from the LP group underwent intensive auditory training for eight weeks on the Earobics (http://www.cogcon.com) program. Importantly, the ALRs showed post-intervention improvement. The authors suggested that the LP subjects with poor quiet to noise response correlations are especially able to benefit from auditory training and reported that the LP subjects, who previously demonstrated abnormal cortical responses in noise, showed improvement to the extent that their posttraining responses fell within the normal range. This improvement was reflected in improved speech perception scores.

Brain Lesions and Injury. Auditory late responses in known cases of brain lesions are a valuable approach for exploring the generators of different wave components. However, brain pathology may be diffuse and not localized to a small region, making it very difficult to attribute the presence, absence, or abnormality of the response to deficits in a particular cortical region. As pointed out by Näätänen and Picton (1987), a lesion in one location of the brain can result in loss or change of functions of other areas of the brain. Lesions may also alter the conductivity of the brain such that the electric fields produced by an active or unaffected neural generator are distorted. The effect of brain injury on the ALRs has been studied less for children than for adults. Also, components widely studied in adults, such as the N1 component, are difficult to study in children with brain lesions because the N1 component does not mature until late childhood and is often not recorded in younger children except at very slow stimulation rates.

One of the biggest problems in studying the immediate effects of brain injury is that the patient may be sedated or even in coma at the time of the initial electrophysiologic measurement. The reduced state of arousal can seriously affect ALRs that are dependent on the state of consciousness. Young, Wang, and Connolly (2004) recommended the use of electrophysiologic techniques such as the ABR and "cognitive" event related potentials as prognostic indicators of recovery in patients who have been in coma. Liasis, Boyd, Gaxiola, and Towell (2003) recorded auditory event-related potentials (ERPs) elicited by pure tones and syllables and detected with a 51-channel electrode array concentrated over the functional hemisphere. Subjects were 17 children (mean age 14.2 years) who had undergone hemispherectomy surgical procedures for intractable seizures of which eight had congenital brain damage and seven had acquired brain damage at or after the age of 1 year. The control group consisted of 10 children with a mean age of 13.5 years. These authors reported that topography of the ALRs in the children with hemispherectomy was localized to the centrotemporal regions of the functioning hemisphere as against the midline localization observed in the normal hearing group. Regardless of the side of hemispherectomy, the clinical group showed longer latencies for cortical responses to syllables compared to tones. This finding was consistent with the pattern in the normal hearing group. Furthermore, children with a left hemispherectomy showed delayed N1 and P2 responses to syllables while those with right hemispherectomy did not. The authors suggested that the left hemisphere may be more efficient than the right hemisphere in processing tones as well as syllables. Furthermore, they surmised it may be more efficient than both hemispheres together when processing tones and syllables.

Klein et al. (1995) studied the ALR and the P3 response elicited with tones as well as consonant vowel stimuli (in an oddball paradigm) in six young adults who had verbal auditory agnosia since childhood. The ABRs and AMLRs of these subjects were normal. ALRs of the subjects with agnosia showed a delayed N1 component over the lateral temporal cortex. This was observed for both tones and speech sounds. The N1 component over the frontocentral region of the scalp was normal in latency. According to the authors, the findings indicate that processing of both speech as well as nonspeech stimuli was slower and that the abnormality is in the secondary auditory cortex.

Landau Kleffner syndrome (LKS) is a childhood-acquired epileptic aphasia. Most patients show complete recovery of epilepsy but persist in showing extinction of the ear contralateral to the affected hemisphere on dichotic tasks (Wioland, Rudolf, & Metz-Lutz, 2001). This syndrome and its associated auditory deficits have been documented in several studies (e.g. Baynes, Kegl, Brentari, Kussmaul, & Poizner, 1998; Metz-Lutz et al., 1997; Plaza, Rigoard, Chevrie Muller, Cohen, & Picard, 2001; Seri, Cerquiglini & Pisani, 1998; Wioland et al., 2001).

Wioland et al. (2001) studied the ABRs, AMLRs, and ALRs of six children who had recovered from LKS. The recordings were compared with those of five normal children of the same ages. All five children with LKS were found to have normal MLR and early potentials. However, they did find abnormalities in the long-latency potentials. The amplitude of N1c, reportedly arising from the association auditory areas, was significantly lower in amplitude in the temporal region on the side contralateral to the ear which showed extinction. On the other hand, the N1b was within normal limits in terms of both latency and amplitude. The authors concluded that since these children had been medically declared "recovered" from the epilepsy, this persistence of an abnormal pattern of extinction in brain areas previously known to have been involved in the epileptic focus, suggested that the damage to the association auditory cortex was permanent in these children. The behavioral correlate of this dysfunction is the unilateral dichotic extinction. In an earlier study, Metz-Lutz et al. (1997) had also found that dichotic deficits and unilateral extinction in individuals with LKS persist several years after recovery from the epilepsy and normalization of the EEG.

Anatomical and Physiological Changes in Auditory Deprivation. Shepherd and Hardie (2001) reviewed several studies on the effects of auditory deprivation. Studies that have looked at histological effects of hearing loss on the cochlea and nervous system largely have been animal studies. In humans, the effects of deprivation on behavioral and electrophysiologic measures have been more often studied (Eggermont, Ponton, Don, Waring, & Kwong, 1997; Kral, Hartmann, Tillein, Heid, & Klinke, 2001; Ponton et al., 1996b; Sharma et al., 2002a; Sharma, Gilley, Dorman, & Baldwin, 2007). Posthumous (postmortem) studies are more rare (Huttenlocher & Dabholkar, 1997; Moore & Guan, 2001; Moore & Linthicum, 2007) for obvious reasons. Huttenlocher and Dabholkar (1997) suggested that early synaptogenesis is intrinsically controlled and, therefore, largely independent of a child's auditory experiences. They did point out however that the formation of synapses in later life is affected by learning and memory and that onset of functions of the cerebral cortex seems to occur during the late phase of rapid synaptogenesis. Hence, cortical level auditory processing and the evoked responses that are their correlates (e.g., ALRs) should logically be dependent on auditory experience or lack of it (due to unintervened hearing impairment).

Long periods of deafness can cause structural changes in the auditory system. A review of studies on the subject by Shepherd and Hardie (2001) highlights some of these changes. Permanent sensorineural hearing loss causes "rapid and extensive loss of unmyelinated peripheral dendrites within the organ of Corti" (Terayama et al., 1997 cited by Shepherd & Hardie, 2001, p. 305). Following these changes, there is a slow degeneration of myelinated dendrites in the osseous spiral lamina and cell bodies of the Type I spiral ganglion (Shepherd & Hardie, 2001, p. 305). Auditory nerve fiber responses to brief stimuli are affected, showing loss of temporal resolution by exhibiting bursting or chopping activity and periods of inactivity in response to a train of current pulses (Shepherd & Javel, 1997, cited by Shepherd & Hardie, 2001). Furthermore, based on their review of literature, these authors reported that neurons at the level of the brainstem and, specifically, the cochlear nucleus, are not susceptible to degeneration all throughout life, in contrast to the spiral ganglion cells. With a period of stimulation before the onset of hearing loss, there is no loss of neurons in the brainstem. Cortical changes occurring as a result of deafness generally tend to affect postprocessing (secondary) auditory areas rather than the primary auditory area (Giraud, Truy, & Frackowiak, 2001).

At the level of the cortex, cross-modal remapping can occur (reorganization leading to the takeover of one sensory area by another). Remapping after visual or auditory deprivation has been extensively studied in animal models. In humans, higher order sensory areas are also capable of cross-modality remapping (e.g., Giraud et al., 2001; Kral et al., 2001). When inputs to one sensory area of the brain are lost due to deprivation, they are perhaps replaced by inputs from other sensory systems (Kral et al., 2001). Kral and colleagues (2001) also suggested that in congenital hearing loss, continued deprivation may result in the "unused or unstimulated" higher auditory areas in the cortex being taken over by other sensory systems. "Congenitally deaf patients, implanted in adulthood show deficits in temporal auditory processing such as gap detection and auditory counting abilities" (Busby et al., 1992, 1993; Busby & Clark, 1999 cited in Kral et al., 2001, p. 348). Temporal processing difficulties may cause speech processing difficulties even in individuals with normal hearing sensitivity (e.g., Tallal, 1980). Effective amplification and cochlear implantation can induce maturation of the auditory cortex, if it is done within a sensitive period (e.g., Kral et al., 2001; Ponton et al., 1996a, 1996b; Sharma et al., 2002a, 2002b, 2005a, 2005b, 2007). The ALR is the electrophysiological measure that has been maximally used in these studies to understand the effects of auditory deprivation in the auditory cortex and reorganization and plasticity of the cortex following re-introduction of sensory stimulation after a period of deprivation.

Effects of Audiologic Intervention on ALR in Children with Hearing Impairment. Sharma et al. (2002b) studied the ALRs of 22 prelingually deaf children with cochlear implants. The children who ranged in age from 1.25 to 5.65 years were divided into groups depending on the duration of stimulation with the implant. The authors found that in congenitally deaf children who underwent implantation early, the cortical responses improved in the first 6 to 8 months postimplant and reached age-appropriate latencies within 8 months. There now is general agreement that there is a sensitive period for the development of the cortex. If adequate auditory experience is provided at an early age, either through hearing aids or cochlear implants (when required), the cortex can be adequately recruited for processing.

On the other hand, late intervention may result in irreversible effects on the ALRs and their auditory behavioral correlates (Eggermont & Ponton, 2003; Ponton et al., 1996a, 1996b; Ponton, Moore, & Eggermont, 1999; Sharma et al., 2002a; Sharma Dorman, & Kral, 2005a; Sharma et al., 2007). Sharma et al. (2002a) suggested that the first 3.5 years of life are the most sensitive. During this time period the human auditory cortex is most plastic. Between the ages of 3.5 and 7 years, the degree of plasticity is variable across children. Beyond this age plasticity is greatly reduced. The age-related decrease in plasticity also holds true when the second ear is implanted late in sequential bilateral implantation (Sharma et al., 2005a). Not only does the ALR P1 not reach normal latencies, the morphology of the waveform of the later developing ALR N1-P2 component also is affected.

The same general findings were reported by Eggermont and Ponton (2003). These investigators also noted that the absence or immaturity of the ALR N1 indicates an "arrest or alteration in the maturation of the layer II axon neurofilaments" (p. 251). They further suggested that maturation of these layers coincides with improved processing of degraded and masked speech in normal children. The late-implanted children in their study reportedly had good to excellent open set word recognition in quiet, but they persisted in having difficulties in speech recognition in noise. Gordon, Tanaka, Wong, and Papsin (2008) studied the ALR using tone bursts of different frequencies, in 16 children with cochlear implants. They found differences in the morphology of their P1-N1 response compared to children with normal hearing. The positive wave dominated in all the participants of their study.

Also, in the participants who had fair speech perception skills, the N1 response, though present, did not show age-appropriate changes in amplitude with change in stimulus frequency.

Dinces, Chobot-Rhodd, and Sussman (2009) studied event-related potentials in three late-implanted children and correlated the results with findings on behavioral tasks involving auditory discrimination of frequency, intensity and duration. They found that the child who was the best user of the cochlear implant device showed better ability to discriminate these contrasts behaviorally in comparison with another child who was a poor user. Similarly, there was faster improvement in the corresponding event-related potentials of this child compared to the poor user.

We must note that the clarity and/or quality of the auditory signal, and specifically the speech signal, that a particular child receives through a cochlear implant is significantly dependent on other factors that have no connection with central auditory processing. Some of these factors include the type of cochlear implant device, the number of functioning channels, the presence of cochlear deformities, the type of processing strategy used, the programming and in general the fact that contemporary speech processing strategies are not necessarily able to provide 100% speech recognition in all including adverse listening situations, even to postlingually deafened adults who have not had long periods of auditory deprivation.

Based on findings of studies such as those mentioned already, ALRs are finding application in the testing of efficacy of hearing aid fittings. Dillon (2005) recommended that speech stimuli could be used to assess the adequacy of amplification in different frequency regions. The phonemes /m/, /g/, and /t/ were chosen for their representation of the low-, mid-, and high-frequency regions in anticipation that the ALRs elicited for these sounds would reflect the child's perception of the sounds. Agung et al. (2004) investigated the objective verification of speech perception using cortical auditory evoked responses, including the ALR. These researchers found significant differences in the ALR (P1-N1-P2) for different speech stimuli, and concluded that cortical auditory evoked responses may be used to objectively measure perception of different speech sounds. The reader is referred to a recent review by Martin et al. (2008) of the applications of speech evoked responses, including the ALR, in documenting performance with hearing aids and cochlear implants.

Attention Deficit (Hyperactivity) Disorder (ADHD). According to the Department of Health and Human Services, Center for Disease Control and Prevention, ADHD is one of the most common neurobehavioral disorders of childhood, persisting through adolescence and into adulthood. According to the American Psychiatric Association's *Diagnostic and Statistical Manual-IV, Text Revision*, 2004 (DSM-IV-TR), an estimated 3% to 7% of children suffer from ADHD. ADHD is classified into three subtypes: predominantly inattentive type, predominantly hyperactive-impulsive type and the combined type. Inattention to sensory stimuli is a hallmark of ADHD. It is generally thought that attention is the primary explanation for why an individual's auditory performance may be poorer than normal. In fact, when diagnosing (C)APD, ruling out ADHD is mandatory because both groups may present with the symptom of poor ability to attend to sound (Bellis, 2003). In ADHD, however, the inattention is generalized irrespective of the sensory modality, whereas for a child with (C)APD inattention occurs specifically for auditory tasks. Most of the research on cortical auditory evoked responses in children with ADHD has focused on event-related responses such as the P300 and the mismatch negativity (MMN) response (e.g., Brown et al., 2005; Gumenyuk et al., 2005; Jonkman, et al., 1997; Kemner et al., 2004; Oades, Dittmann-Balcar, Schepker, Eggers, & Zerbin, 1996; Winsberg, Javitt, & Shanahan/Silipo, 1997). The reason for this wide interest in event-related responses rather than the obligatory components of ALR most likely is because event-related responses such as the P300 are highly dependent on attention. Inattentiveness is a distinguishing feature of ADHD.

Oades (1998) reported that one of the striking findings in cases with ADHD was a larger ALR P2 component, but also pointed out that other previous studies actually reported a smaller P2 component that normalized after drug treatment. The discrepancy in outcomes among studies was attributed to the subgroups seen in children with ADHD, that is, children with ADHD are not a homogeneous group. Oades suggested that large P2 amplitudes were consistent with impulsivity. Hyperactivity is often treated medically. One of the drugs used in the therapy of ADHD is methylphenidate. Some researchers have measured ALRs and event-related responses before and after treatment with methylphenidate in an attempt to document objective evidence of neurophysiologic changes. Winsberg et al. (1997) investigated the P300 response and earlier occurring event related responses (potentials) in children with ADHD who had been treated with methylphenidate. These researchers did not find any changes in the ALR components, before the P3 response, as a result of the treatment. They did report an increase in the amplitude of the P3 response suggesting that methylphenidate affects attention regulation.

Brown et al. (2005) studied auditory and visual event-related responses in the predominantly inattentive subtype of ADHD. They used an intermodal oddball task in which the target was a 2000-Hz tone and the nontarget stimulus was a counterphasing checkerboard. They considered two subgroups within the "predominantly inattentive type" of ADHD based on underlying EEG activity—cortically hypoaroused and maturationally lagged (with EEGs resembling those of younger children). Their sample consisted of 27 children identified as "cortically hypoaroused," 27 identified as "maturationally lagged," and 27 age-matched controls. They reported that the task successfully differentiated the children with ADHD from the age-matched controls with the former showing smaller amplitudes for ALR N1 and P2 components and for the P3 response elicited with the auditory targets. The only difference Brown et al. (2005) found between the subtypes of ADHD was a relative increase in the left-frontal N1 amplitude in the cortically hypoaroused group. The authors concluded that in the group with maturational lag, the frontal lateralization of N1 was reduced. This supports the label for this group. The authors also observed that the cortical hypoaroused group showed abnormal lateralization of the ALR. There is very little published research on the obligatory components of the ALR in children with ADHD in comparison to the numerous papers on event-related responses elicited by auditory and visual signals. Application of the ALR as an electrophysiologic index of auditory functioning in ADHD is a topic that warrants more research.

Autism Spectrum Disorder. Autism, now more properly referred to as autism spectrum disorder, is another condition often characterized by sensory inattention despite normal peripheral hearing abilities. One of the challenges encountered in conducting behavioral audiometry in populations with autism spectrum disorders is the tendency of these individuals to ignore auditory stimuli presented to them, and to demonstrate "selective attention" to sounds that they prefer. Faced with a child showing symptoms of autism spectrum disorder, an audiologist is well advised to ask the caregivers about the type of sounds the child usually ignores or consistently attends to. Autism is currently described as a "spectrum of disorders" in which the manifested behaviors range from mild to severe. Autism spectrum disorder is also characterized by communication problems and atypical language development. Considering the type of auditory behaviors shown by these children, it would be logical to consider a neurobiological basis, and to explore this possible etiology through the measurement of electrophysiologic measures (e.g., cortical auditory evoked responses).

Bruneau, Bonnet-Brilhault, Gomot, Adrien, and Barthelemy (2003) investigated the relation between ALRs recorded at temporal sites (the N1c wave or Tb) and verbal and nonverbal abilities in children with autism spectrum disorders. Subjects were 26 mentally retarded children with autism between the ages of 4 and 8 years. The researchers elicited ALRs with tone-burst stimuli presented at slow stimulation rates (interstimulus intervals of 3 to 5 seconds), and compared the findings for the autistic group with 16 normal hearing children. ALRs recorded from both left and right temporal sites were smaller in amplitude for children with autism than for the normal subject group. Bruneau and colleagues (2003) reported a correlation between the amplitude of the right temporal N1c responses and the verbal and nonverbal communication abilities. The authors suggested that, in autism, there is an aberrant reorganization of the functions of the right and left hemispheres with activation of the right hemisphere for tasks in which the left hemisphere should be activated normally. This is especially so for tasks involving the secondary auditory areas, whose activation is reflected by the N1c and Tb wave components. One of the difficulties in such studies is the differential diagnosis of mental retardation versus autism spectrum disorders due to overlapping behavioral characteristics in both groups. Although mental retardation and autism spectrum disorders can co-exist, it is often difficult to separate the effects of both when diagnosing a child with one or the other condition.

Seri, Cerquiglini, Pisani, and Curatolo (1999) studied ALRs in 14 children with tuberous sclerosis complex (TSC), seven of whom fulfilled the DSM IV criteria for autistic disorder. TSC, also known as Bournville's disease, is typified by a classic triad of symptoms, namely, seizures, mental retardation, and adenoma sebaceum (Moe & Seay, 1993). This syndrome, which is genetically transmitted, has been documented as being associated with autism (Smalley & Henske, 2005). Children with TSC additionally show symptoms such as tumors in many body locations such as the skin, heart, brain, kidney, and retina (Smalley & Henske, 2005). Since TSC is associated with autism (in 60% of the cases as reported by Seri et al., 1999) and also with cortical and subcortical lesions of the temporal lobe, Seri and colleagues (1999) designed a study to explore the link between anatomic lesions of the TSC and functional mechanisms as exhibited by ALRs and event-related responses to auditory stimuli. All the subjects underwent high-resolution magnetic resonance imaging (MRI) and EEG. The cortical responses to different frequencies of sounds presented with different probabilities were recorded using 21 scalp electrodes. The same procedures were conducted on both groups of TSC children (the group with and without autism spectrum disorder). Results indicated that the N1 component of the ALR had a significantly prolonged latency, and lower amplitude, in all the children with autism spectrum disorder. These children, as opposed to the nonautistic children, had MRI documentation of lesions on one or both temporal lobes. The MMN had a longer latency in the autistic subgroup.

Orekhova et al. (2009) studied event-related potentials to novel temporal gaps, in 21 children with autism and 21 typically developing children. They concluded that the cortical responses of children with autism indicated impairment in the right hemisphere tasks of processing temporally novel information. They also suggested that such findings are indicative of the neurobiological basis of autism.

Echolalia is a common behavior seen in individuals with autism spectrum disorder. One of the goals in speech and language therapy is to reduce echolalia, a meaningless "echo" rather than communicative behavior. Wetherby, Koegel, and Mendel (1981) studied central auditory processing abilities through behavioral tests in six echolalic autistic individuals in the age range of 8 to 24 years. The subjects had a wide range of language abilities and different degrees of severity of echolalia. The researchers found in the subjects with echolalia, normal performance on monaural tests, but indications of central auditory dysfunction in the language dominant hemisphere on the dichotic tests (Staggered Spondaic Word Test and Competing Environmental Sound Test). Children who previously were diagnosed as autistic but no longer had echolalia yielded essentially normal findings. Considering the close link between auditory behavior and electrophysiology, it would be interesting to study topographic brain maps of cortical auditory evoked responses when subjects of any clinical group are engaged in a behavioral task (studies such as those described earlier, e.g., Estes et al., 2002; Jerger et al., 2000, 2002, 2004).

Auditory Neuropathy Spectrum Disorder. One condition documented rather recently, and gaining remarkably more attention, is "auditory neuropathy." Also referred to as "auditory dys-synchrony" (Berlin, Hood, & Rose, 2001), and more recently "auditory neuropathy spectrum disorder" (ANSD), "auditory neuropathy is a form of hearing impairment in which cochlear outer hair cell function is spared, but afferent neural transmission is disordered" (Rance, Cone-Wesson, Wunderlich, & Dowell, 2002, p. 239). Imprecise use of the term, varying sites of dysfunction among children who are labeled with auditory neuropathy, and the considerable likelihood of nonauditory neurologic disorders within this clinical entity have led to some debate and confusion regarding diagnosis and management (see Rapin & Gravel, 2003). As auditory neuropathy by strict definition is limited to dysfunction of the auditory nerve, the effects on the cortex and cortical evoked potentials are more likely due to deprivation rather than a reflection of the pathology itself. The hallmark of this condition is the absence of the ABR and presence of robust otoacoustic emissions and cochlear microphonics (e.g., Berlin et al., 2001; Hall, 2007; Hood, 1998). Individuals with auditory neuropathy form a highly heterogeneous group (Berlin et al., 2001; Hall, 2007). However, multiple studies confirm that despite an absent ABR, cortical auditory evoked potentials at conversational intensity levels are often recordable in infants, children and adults with auditory neuropathy (e.g., Cone-Wesson & Wunderlich, 2003; Michelewski, Starr, Nguyen, Kong, & Zeng, 2005; Pearce, Golding, & Dillon, 2007; Rance et al., 2002).

In order to examine whether cortical event-related responses could be recorded in children with AN and to determine the relationship between the presence of these responses and speech perception, Rance et al. (2002) conducted a study of 18 children with the diagnosis of auditory neuropathy. Children were evaluated with speech perception measures in unaided and aided conditions (PBK words), and also with cortical auditory evoked responses. Out of the 18 children, formal speech perception testing could be conducted only on 15. They found that based on their speech perception performance, the children could be classified into two categories: one which showed no open-set speech perception ability (7 out of 15), and the other (8 out of 15) in which performance levels were comparable to children with a similar degree of sensorineural hearing loss. Rance and colleagues reported that approximately 50% of the children with AN had cortical responses within normal limits with respect to latency, amplitude and morphology. They also found a direct relation between presence versus absence of the ALR and speech perception abilities. Children with poor speech perception had absent cortical auditory evoked responses while the responses of children with better speech perception abilities were normal in latency.

Rance and colleagues (2002) concluded that approximately 50% of children with auditory neuropathy benefit from amplification and show significant improvements in open-set speech perception performance. They suggested that obligatory cortical auditory evoked response test results "may offer a means of predicting perceptual skills" (p. 239) in young children diagnosed with AN, as the presence of normal cortical auditory evoked responses seemed to predict degree of benefit with amplification and achievement of some degree of open set speech recognition. On the other hand, absent cortical auditory evoked responses indicated "profound hearing disability evidenced by profound hearing loss and/or extremely poor speech perception" (p. 239).

Miscellaneous Populations. There are a handful of studies on populations such as Down syndrome (e.g., Seidl, et al., 1997) and Fragile X syndrome (Castrén, Pääkkönen, Tarkka, Ryynänen, & Partanen, 2003) that have found abnormalities in the latency and amplitude of the N1 component of the ALR. More systematic investigation of ALR in these populations is needed.

Future Directions for Clinical Research

From the foregoing review, it is apparent that these two cortical auditory evoked responses, AMLR and ALR, could play an important role in the diagnosis of central auditory dysfunction in children, and also in documenting the effectiveness of specific intervention strategies. Clearly, more research is warranted in general, and particularly in specific populations, such as children with carefully defined and diagnosed patterns of auditory processing disorders (APD). Unfortunately, to date, most of the research findings have been generated in experimental investigations with sophisticated laboratory instrumentation, rather than clinical studies with commercially available equipment available to practicing audiologists. What is needed to facilitate the transition of cortical auditory evoked response measurement from the laboratory to the clinical setting?

A handful of technologic advances and types of information would probably contribute to the inclusion of cortical auditory evoked responses into the clinical test battery, at least for selected patient populations. First, consensus is needed on accepted test protocols for the measurement of cortical auditory evoked responses. Studies reported in the literature are characterized by diverse test protocols that consist of a wide range of stimulus and acquisition parameters. There is stated disagreement among authors on basic test parameters required for measurement of cortical auditory evoked responses, such as the minimum number of electrodes required for valid detection of major components. Also, importantly, hearing scientists conducting research on cortical auditory evoked responses invariably utilize complex and expensive instrumentation that is neither user friendly nor appropriate for clinical application. It would be very helpful to incorporate techniques, protocols, stimuli, and algorithms that have worked well in the laboratory into equipment that is accessible and clinically feasible for the clinical audiologist. Clinical instrumentation, for example, must include certain new features, such as software for producing an assortment of stimuli (including speech signals) and multiple channels (e.g., 4 to 8) for the minimum number of hemisphere electrodes, and the mandatory eye blink electrode(s).

For measurement of cortical auditory evoked responses in children undergoing diagnostic assessment for APD, a major clinical application of auditory neurophysiology, protocols and algorithms are needed for measurement of the AMLR and ALR elicited with a speech-in-noise stimulus paradigm, with dichotically presented stimuli, and with stimuli with modified temporal features (e.g., a gap detection paradigm) to assess temporal auditory processing. The option for rigorous, yet user-friendly statistical analysis of ALR findings would be very helpful, and contribute importantly to the acceptance by clinical audiologists of cortical auditory evoked responses. Statistical calculation and confirmation of major response parameters (e.g., latency, amplitude, area under the curve) should be available for the traditional components of the AMLR and ALR, with the possibility of statistically assessing differences in these parameters for cortical auditory evoked responses recorded under various measurement conditions (e.g., left versus right hemispheres). And, finally, regular and confident clinical application of cortical auditory evoked responses is dependent on access to large sample and age-matched normative data collected with clinical instrumentation and various types of stimuli, and including maturational data on the AMLR and ALR from infancy to adulthood (0 to 20 years).

We confidently predict that research on clinical applications of cortical auditory evoked responses will expand considerably within the next few years, and that technologic advances in clinical instrumentation, as just outlined, will begin to catch up with the accelerating proliferation of research findings. The offspring of this marriage of laboratory and clinical technology and techniques may well be an internationally universal electrophysiologic auditory test battery that can be employed in pediatric populations with unprecedented sensitivity and specificity for the identification, diagnosis, and treatment-related documentation of cortical auditory dysfunction and auditory processing.

References

Agung King, K., Campbell, J., Sharma, A., Martin, K., Dorman, M., & Langran, J. (2008). The representation of voice onset time in the cortical auditory evoked potentials of young children. *Clinical Neurophysiology, 119*(12), 2855–2861.

Agung, K., Purdy, S., McMohan, C., Dillon, H., Katsch, R., & Newall, P. (2004). Objective verification of speech perception using cortical auditory evoked potentials. *National Acoustics Laboratories: Research and Development Annual Report 2003–2004*, pp. 15–17.

Alain, C., Woods, D. L., & Covarrubias, D. (1997). Activation of duration-sensitive auditory cortical fields in humans. *Electroencephalography and Clinical Neurophysiology, 104*(6), 531–539.

American Speech-Language and Hearing Association (ASHA). (1996). *Central auditory processing: Current status of research and implications for clinical practice* [Technical report]. Retrieved August 23, 2008, from http://www.asha.org/policy

American Speech-Language and Hearing Association (ASHA). (2005). *(Central) Auditory processing disorders* [Technical report]. Retrieved August 23, 2008, from http://www.asha.org/policy

Arehole, S. (1995). A preliminary study of the relationship between long latency response and learning disorder. *British Journal of Audiology, 29*(6), 295–298.

Arehole, S., Augustine, L. E., & Simhadri, R. (1995). Middle latency response in children with learning disabilities: Preliminary findings. *Journal of Communication Disorders, 28*(1), 21–38.

Barnet, A., & Lodge, A. (1967). Diagnosis of hearing loss in infancy by means of EEG audiometry. *Clinical Proceedings of Children's Hospital in Washington, DC, 23*, 1–18.

Barnet, A., Ohlrich, E. S. Weiss, I. P., & Shanks, B. (1975). Auditory evoked potentials during sleep in normal children from ten days to three years of age. *Electroencephalography and Clinical Neurophysiology, 39*, 29–41.

Baynes, K., Kegl, J. A., Brentari, D., Kussmaul, C., & Poizner, H. (1998). Chronic auditory agnosia following Landau-Kleffner syndrome: A 23 year outcome study. *Brain and Language, 63*(3), 381–425.

Bellis, T. J. (2003). *Assessment and management of central auditory processing disorders in the educational setting: From science to practice* (2nd ed.). Clifton Park, NY: Thomson Delmar Learning.

Berlin, C. I., Bordelon, J., St John, P., Wilensky, D., Hurley, A., Kluka, E., & Hood, L. J. (1998). Reversing click polarity may uncover auditory neuropathy in infants. *Ear and Hearing, 19*(1), 37–47.

Berlin, C. I., Hood, L., & Rose, K. (2001). On renaming auditory neuropathy as auditory dyssynchrony: Implications for a clearer understanding of the underlying mechanisms and management options. *Audiology Today, 13*, 15–17.

Brown, C. R., Clarke, A. R., Barry, R. J., McCarthy, R., Selikowitz, M., & Magee, C. (2005). Event-related potentials in attention-deficit/ hyperactivity disorder of the predominantly inattentive type: An investigation of EEG-defined subtypes. *International Journal of Psychophysiology, 58*(1), 94–107.

Bruneau, N., Bonnet-Brilhault, F., Gomot, M., Adrien, J. L., & Barthélémy, C. (2003). Cortical auditory processing and communication in children with autism: Electrophysiological/behavioral relations. *International Journal of Psychophysiology, 51*(1), 17–25.

Burkard, R. F., Don, M., & Eggermont, J. J. (2007). *Auditory evoked potentials: Basic principles and clinical applications*. Baltimore, MD: Lippincott Williams & Wilkins.

Cacace, A. T., & McFarland, D. J. (2002). Middle-latency auditory evoked potentials: Basic issues and potential applications. In J. Katz, R. F. Burkard, & L. Medwetseky (Eds.), *Handbook of clinical audiology* (5th ed., pp. 349–377). Baltimore, MD: Williams and Wilkins.

Castrén, M., Pääkkönen, A.,Tarkka, I. M., Ryynänen, M., & Partanen, J. (2003). Augmentation of auditory N1 in children with Fragile-X syndrome. *Brain Topography, 15*(3), 165–171.

Čeponienè, R., Cheour, M., & Näätänen, R. (1998). Interstimulus interval and auditory event-related potentials in children: Evidence of multiple generators. *Electroencephalography and Clinical Neurophysiology, 108*(4), 345–354.

Čeponienè, R., Rinne, T., & Näätänen, R. (2002). Maturation of cortical sound processing as indexed by event-related potentials. *Clinical Neurophysiology, 113*(6), 870–882.

Collet, L., Duclaux, R., Challamel, M. J., & Revol, M. (1988). Effect of sleep on middle latency response (MLR) in infants. *Brain and Development, 10*(3), 169–173.

Cone-Wesson, B., Kurtzberg, D., & Vaughan, H. G. Jr. (1987). Electrophysiologic assessment of auditory pathways in high risk infants. *International Journal of Pediatric Otorhinolaryngology, 14*(2–3), 203–214.

Cone-Wesson, B., Ma, E., & Fowler, C. G. (1997). Effect of stimulus level and frequency on ABR and MLR binaural interaction in human neonates. *Hearing Research, 106*(1–2), 163–178.

Cone-Wesson, B., & Wunderlich, J. (2003). Auditory evoked potentials from the cortex: Audiology applications. *Current Opinion in Otolaryngology and Head and Neck Surgery, 11*(5), 372–377.

Cottrell, G., & Gans, D. (1995). Auditory-evoked response morphology in profoundly-involved multi-handicapped children: Comparisons with normal infants and children. *International Journal of Audiology, 34*(4), 189–206.

Cunningham, J., Nicol, T., Zecker, S., Bradlow, A., & Kraus, N. (2001). Neurobiologic responses to speech in noise in children with learning problems: Deficits and strategies for improvement. *Clinical Neurophysiology, 112*(5), 758–767.

Cunningham, J., Nicol, T., Zecker, S., & Kraus, N. (2000). Speech-evoked neurophysiologic responses in children with learning problems: Development and behavioral correlates of perception. *Ear and Hearing, 21*(6), 554–568.

Davis, H. (1976). Brainstem and other response audiometry. *Annals of Otology, Rhinology and Laryngology, 85*, 3–14.

Davis, H., Mast, T., Yoshie, N., & Zerlin, S. (1966). The slow response of the human cortex to auditory stimuli: Recovery process. *Electroencephalography and Clinical Neurophysiology, 21*(2), 105–113.

Davis, P. A. (1939). Effects of acoustic stimuli on the waking human brain. *Journal of Neurophysiology, 2*, 494–499.

Diaz, F., & Zuron, M. (1995). Auditory evoked potentials in Down syndrome. *Electroencephalography and Clinical Neurophysiology, 96*(6), 526–537.

Dillon, H. (2005). So, baby, how does it sound? Cortical assessment of infants with hearing aids. *Hearing Journal, 58*(10), 10. Retrieved August 23, 2008, from http://www.audiologyonline.com/theHearingJournal/pdfs/HJ2005_10_pg10-17.pdf

Dinces, E., Chobot-Rhodd, J., & Sussman, E. (2009). Behavioral and electrophysiological measures of auditory change detection in children following late cochlear implantation: A preliminary study. *International Journal of Pediatric Otorhinolaryngology, 73*(6), 843–851.

Drake, M. E., Jr., Weate, S. J., & Newell, S. A. (1996). Auditory evoked potentials in postconcussive syndrome. *Electromyography and Clinical Neurophysiology, 36*(8), 457–462.

Eggermont, J. J., & Ponton, C. W. (2003). Auditory-evoked potential studies of cortical maturation in normal hearing and implanted children: Correlations with changes in structure and speech perception. *Acta Oto-Laryngologica, 123*(2), 249–252.

Eggermont, J. J., Ponton, C. W., Don, M., Waring, M. D., & Kwong, B. (1997) Maturational delays in cortical evoked potentials in cochlear implant users. *Acta Oto-Laryngologica, 117*(2) 161–163.

Estes, R. I., Jerger, J. & Jacobson, G. (2002). Reversal of hemispheric asymmetry on auditory tasks in children who are poor listeners. *Journal of the American Academy of Audiology, 13*(2), 59–71.

Fifer, R. C. (1985). *The MLR and SSEP in neonates.* Houston, TX: Baylor College of Medicine.

Frizzo, A. C. F., Funayama, C. A. R., Isaac, M. L., & Colafêmina, J. F. (2007). Auditory middle latency responses: A study of healthy children. *Brazilian Journal of Otorhinolaryngology, 73*(3), 398–403.

Fruhstorfer, H., Soveri, P., & Järvilehto, T. (1970). Short term habituation of the auditory evoked response in man. *Electroencephalography and Clinical Neurophysiology, 28*(2), 153–161.

Gaetz, M., & Weinberg, H. (2000). Electrophysiological indices of persistent post-concussion symptoms. *Brain Injury, 14*(9), 815–832.

Geisler, C. D., Frishkopf, L. S., & Rosenblith, W. A. (1958). Extracranial reponses to acoustic clicks in man. *Science, 128*(3333), 1210–1211.

Gilley, P. M., Sharma, A., Dorman, M., & Martin, K. (2005). Developmental changes in refractoriness of the cortical auditory evoked potential. *Clinical Neurophysiology, 116*(3), 648–657.

Gilley, P. M., Sharma, A., Dorman, M., & Martin, K. (2006). Abnormalities in central auditory maturation in children with language-based learning problems. *Clinical Neurophysiology, 117*(9), 1949–1956.

Giraud, A. L., Truy, E., & Frackowiak, R. (2001). Imaging plasticity in cochlear implant patients. *Audiology and Neuro-Otology, 6*(6), 381–393.

Goldstein, R., & Rodman, L. B. (1967). Early components of averaged evoked responses to rapidly repeated auditory stimuli. *Journal of Speech and Hearing Research, 10*(4), 697–705.

Gomes, H., Dunn, M., Ritter, W., Kurtzberg, D., Brattson, A., Kreuzer, J., & Vaughan, H. G., Jr. (2001). Spatiotemporal maturation of the central and lateral N1 components to tones. *Developmental Brain Research, 129*(2), 147–155.

Gordon, K. A., Papsin, B. C., & Harrison, R. V. (2004). Thalamocortical activity and plasticity in children using cochlear implants. *International Congress Series, 1273*, 76–79.

Gordon, K. A., Papsin, B. C., & Harrison, R. V. (2005). Effects of cochlear implant use on the electrically evoked middle latency response in children. *Hearing Research, 204*(1–2), 78–89.

Gordon, K. A., Tanaka, S., Wong, D. D. E., & Papsin, B. C. (2008). Characterizing responses from auditory cortex in young people with several years of cochlear implant experience. *Clinical Neurophysiology, 119*(10), 2347–2362.

Groenen, P., Snik, A., & van den Broek, P. (1997). Electrically evoked auditory middle latency responses versus perception abilities in cochlear implant users. *Audiology, 36*(2), 83–97.

Gumenyuk, V., Korzyukov, O., Escera, C., Hämäläinen, M., Häyrinen, T., Oksanen, H., . . . Alho, K. (2005). Electrophysiological evidence of enhanced distractibility in ADHD children. *Neuroscience Letters, 374*(3), 212–217.

Hall, J. W. III (1992). Overview of auditory evoked responses: Past, present and future. In *Handbook of auditory evoked responses* (pp. 3–40). Needham Heights, MA: Allyn and Bacon.

Hall, J. W. III. (2007). *New handbook of auditory evoked responses.* Boston, MA: Allyn and Bacon.

Hall, J. W. III, Brown, D. P., & Mackey-Hargadine, J. R. (1985). Pediatric applications of serial auditory brainstem and middle-latency evoked response recordings. *International Journal of Pediatric Otorhinolaryngology, 9*(3), 201–218.

Hall, J. W. III, Huang-fu, M., & Gennarelli, T. A. (1982). Auditory function in acute severe head injury. *Laryngoscope, 92*(8 Pt. 1), 883–890.

Hall, J. W. III, & Mueller, H. G. III. (1997). *Audiologist's desk reference. Volume I.* San Diego, CA: Singular.

Hari, R., Kaila, K., Katila, T., Tuomisto, T., & Varpula, T. (1982). Interstimulus interval dependence of the auditory vertex response and its magnetic counterpart: Implications for their neural generation. *Electroencephalography and Clinical Neurophysiology, 54*(5), 561–569.

Hayes, E. A., Warrier, C. M., Nicol, T. G., Zecker, S. G., & Kraus, N. (2003). Neural plasticity following auditory training in children with learning problems. *Clinical Neurophysiology, 114*(4), 673–684.

Huttenlocher, P. R., & Dabholkar, A. S. (1997). Regional differences in synaptogenesis in human cerebral cortex. *Journal of Comparative Neurology, 387*(2), 167–178.

Illing, R. B. (2004). Maturation and plasticity of the central auditory system. *Acta Otolaryngolgica Suppl., 552*, 6–10.

Jasper, H. (1958). The 10–20 electrode system of the International Federation. *Electroencephalography and Clinical Neurophysiology, 10*, 371–375.

Jerger. J., Martin, J., & McColl, R. (2004). Interaural cross correlation of event-related potentials and diffusion tensor imaging in the evaluation of auditory processing disorder: A case study. *Journal of the American Academy of Audiology, 15*(1), 79–87.

Jerger, J., Moncrieff, D., Greenwald, R., Wambacq, I., & Seipel, A. (2000). Effect of age on interaural asymmetry of event-related potentials in a dichotic listening task. *Journal of the American Academy of Audiology, 11*(7), 383–389.

Jerger, J., Thibodeau, L., Martin, J., Mehta, J., Tilman, G., Greenwald, R., & Overson, G. (2002). Behavioral and electrophysiologic evidence of auditory processing disorder: A twin study. *Journal of the American Academy of Audiology, 13*(8), 438–460.

Jerger, S., Martin, R. C., & Jerger, J. (1987). Specific auditory perceptual dysfunction in a learning disabled child. *Ear and Hearing, 8*(2), 78–86.

Jirsa, R. E., (1992). The clinical utility of the P3 AERP in children with auditory processing disorders. *Journal of Speech and Hearing Research, 35*(4), 903–912.

Jirsa, R. E., & Clontz, K. B. (1990). Long latency auditory event-related potentials from children with auditory processing disorders. *Ear and Hearing, 11*(3), 222–232.

Joint Committee on Infant Hearing (JCIH). (2007). Year 2007 position statement: Principles and guidelines for early hearing detection and intervention programs. *Pediatrics, 120*, 898–921.

Jonkman, L. M., Kemner, C., Verbaten, M. N., Koelega, H. S., Camfferman, G., vd Gaag, R., . . . van Engeland, H. (1997). Event-related potentials and performance of attention-deficit hyperactivity disorder: Children and normal controls in auditory and visual selective attention tasks. *Biological Psychiatry, 41*(5), 595–611.

Jutras, B., Lagacé, J., Lavigne, A., Boissonneault, A., & Lavoie, C. (2007). Auditory processing disorders, verbal disfluency and learning difficulties: A case study. *International Journal of Audiology, 46*(1), 31–38.

Keidel, W. D., & Spreng, M. (1965). Neurophysiological evidence for the Steven's power function in man. *Journal of the Acoustical Society of America, 38*, 191–195.

Kemner, C., Jonkman, L. M., Kenemans, J. L., Böcker, K. B. E., Verbaten, M. N., & van Engeland, H. (2004). Sources of auditory selective attention and the effects of methylphenidate in children with attention-deficit/hyperactivity disorder. *Biological Psychiatry, 55*(7), 776–778.

Kemner, C., Oranje, B., Verbaten, M. N., & van Engeland, H. (2002). Normal P50 gating in children with autism. *Journal of Clinical Psychiatry, 63*(3), 214–217.

Kileny, P. R., Kemink, J. L, & Miller, J. M. (1989). An intrasubject comparison of electric and acoustic middle latency responses. *American Journal of Otology, 10*(1), 23–27.

Klein, S. K., Kurtzberg, D., Brattson, A., Kreuzer, J. A., Stapells, D. R., Dunn, M. A. . . Vaughan, H. G., Jr. (1995). Electrophysiologic manifestations of impaired temporal lobe auditory processing in verbal auditory agnosia. *Brain and Language, 51*(3), 383–405.

Kral, A. (2007). Unimodal and cross-modal plasticity in the 'deaf' auditory cortex. *International Journal of Audiology, 46*(9), 479–493.

Kral, A., Hartmann, R., Tillein, J., Heid, S., & Klinke, R. (2001). Delayed maturation and sensitive periods in the auditory cortex. *Audiology and Neuro-Otology, 6*(6), 346–362.

Kraus, N. (2001). Auditory pathway encoding and neural plasticity in children with learning problems. *Audiology and Neuro-Otology, 6*(4), 221–227.

Kraus, N., Kileny, P., & McGee, T. (1994). Middle latency auditory evoked potentials. In J. Katz, W. L. Gabbay, S. Gold, L. Medwetsky, & R. A. Ruth (Eds.), *Handbook of clinical audiology* (4th ed., pp. 387–405). Baltimore, MD: Williams and Wilkins.

Kraus, N., & McGee, T. J. (1994). Mismatch negativity in the assessment of central auditory function. *American Journal of Audiology, 3*, 39–51.

Kraus, N., McGee, T. J., Carrell, T. D., Zecker, S. G., Nicol, T. G., & Koch, D. B. (1996). Auditory neurophysiologic responses and discrimination deficits in children with learning problems. *Science, 273*(5277), 971–973.

Kraus, N., McGee, T., & Comperatore, C. (1989). MLRs in children are consistently present during wakefulness, stage 1, and REM sleep. *Ear and Hearing, 10*(6), 339–345.

Kraus, N., Özdamar, O., Hier, D., & Stein, L. (1982). Auditory middle latency responses (MLRs) in patients with cortical lesions. *Electroencephalography and Clinical Neurophysiology, 54*(3), 275–287

Kraus, N., Reed, N., Smith, D. I., Stein, L., & Cartee, C. (1987). High-pass filter settings affect the detectability of MLRs in humans. *Electroencephalography and Clinical Neurophysiology, 68*(3), 234–236.

Kraus, N., Smith, D. I., Reed, N. L., Stein, L. K., & Cartee, C. (1985). Auditory middle latency responses in children: Effects of age and diagnostic category. *Electroencephalography and Clinical Neurophysiology, 62*(5), 343–351.

Lamas, F. A., López-Herce, J., Sánchez, P. L., Mencía, B. S., Borrego, D. R., & Carrillo, A. A. (2006). Middle latency auditory evoked potentials in critical care children: Preliminary study. *Annals of Pediatrics (Barc), 64*(4), 354–359. Abstract retrieved August 25, 2008, from http://www.ncbi.nlm.nih.gov/pubmed/16606573

Liasis, A., Boyd, S., Rivera-Gaxiola, M., & Towell, A. (2003). Speech and nonspeech processing in hemispherectomised children: An event-related potential study. *Cognitive Brain Research, 17*(3), 665–673.

Martin, B. A., Tremblay, K. L., & Korczak, P. (2008). Speech evoked potentials: From the laboratory to the clinic. *Ear and Hearing, 29*(3), 285–313.

Mason, S. M., & Mellor, D. H. (1984). Brain-stem, middle latency and late cortical evoked potentials in children with speech and language disorders. *Electroencephalography and Clinical Neurophysiology, 59*(4), 297–309.

McArthur, G. M., & Bishop, D. V. M. (2004). Which people with specific language impairment have auditory processing deficits? *Cognitive Neuropsychology, 21*(1), 79–94.

McGee, T., & Kraus, N. (1996). Auditory development reflected by middle latency response. *Ear and Hearing, 17*(5), 419–429.

McPherson, D. L., Tures, C., & Starr, A. (1989). Binaural interaction of the auditory brain-stem potentials and middle latency auditory evoked potentials in infants and adults. *Electroencephalography and Clinical Neurophysiology, 74*(2), 124–130.

McRandle, C. C., Smith, M. A., & Goldstein, R. (1974). Early averaged electroencephalic responses to clicks in neonates. *Annals of Otology, Rhinology and Laryngology, 83*(5), 695–702.

Mendel, M. I., Adkinson, C. D., & Harker, L. A. (1977). Middle components of the auditory evoked potentials in infants. *Annals of Otology, Rhinology and Laryngology, 86*(3 Pt.1), 293–299.

Mendelson, T., & Salamy, A. (1981). Maturation effects on the middle components of the averaged encephalic response. *Journal of Speech and Hearing Research, 24*(1), 140–144.

Metz-Lutz, M. N., Hirsch, E., Maquet, P., De Saint Martin, A., Rudolf, G., Wioland, N., & Marescau, C. (1997). Dichotic listening performances in the follow-up of Landau and Kleffner syndrome. *Child Neuropsychology, 3*(1), 47–60.

Michalewski, H. J., Starr, A., Nguyen, T. T., Kong, Y. Y., & Zeng, F. G. (2005). Auditory temporal processes in normal-hearing individuals and patients with auditory neuropathy. *Clinical Neurophysiology, 116*(3), 669–680.

Miliciç, D, Alçada, M. N., Pais, C. L., Vecerina-Voliç, S., Jurkoviç, J., & Pais, C. M. (1998). A study of auditory afferent organization in children with dyslalia. *International Journal of Pediatric Otorhinolaryngology, 46*(1–2), 43–56.

Moe, P. G., & Seay, A. R. (1993). Neurologic and muscular disorders. In W. E. Hathaway, W. W. Hay, J. R. Groothuis, & J. W. Paisley (Eds.), *Current pediatric diagnosis and treatment* (pp. 674–747). East Norwalk, CT: Appleton and Lange.

Moncrieff, D., Jerger, J., Wambacq, I., Greenwald, R., & Black, J. (2004). ERP evidence of a dichotic left-ear deficit in some dyslexic children. *Journal of the American Academy of Audiology, 15*(7), 518–534.

Moore, J. K. (2002). Maturation of human auditory cortex: Implications for speech perception. *Annals of Otology, Rhinology and Laryngology Suppl. 189*, 7–10.

Moore, J. K., & Guan, Y. L. (2001). Cytoarchitectural and axonal maturation in human auditory cortex. *Journal of the Association for Research in Otolaryngology, 2*(4), 297–311.

Moore, J. K., & Linthicum, F. H., Jr. (2007). The human auditory system: A timeline of development. *International Journal of Audiology, 46*(9), 460–478.

Musiek, F. E, Geurkink, N. A., Weider, D. J., & Donnelly, K. (1984). Past, present, and future applications of the auditory middle latency response. *Laryngoscope, 94*(12 Pt. 1), 1545–1553.

Näätänen, R., & Picton, T. (1987). The N1 wave of the human electric and magnetic response to sound: A review and an analysis of the component structure. *Psychophysiology, 24*(4), 375–425.

Naveen, K. V., Srinivas, R., Nirmala, K. S., Nagarathna, R., Nagendra, H. R., & Telles, S. (1998). Differences between congenitally blind and normally sighted subjects in the P1 component of middle latency auditory evoked potentials. *Perceptual and Motor Skills*, 86 (3 Pt. 2), 1192–1194.

Nelson, D. A., & Lassman, F. M. (1968). Effects of intersignal interval on the human auditory evoked response. *Journal of the Acoustical Society of America, 44*(6), 1529–1532.

Oades, R. D. (1998). Frontal, temporal and lateralized brain function in children with attention-deficit hyperactivity disorder: A psychophysiological and neuropsychological viewpoint on development. *Behavioural Brain Research, 94*(1), 83–95.

Oades, R. D., Dittman-Balcar, A., Schepker, R., Eggers, C, & Zerbin, D. (1996). Auditory event-related potentials (ERPs) and mismatch negativity (MMN) in healthy children and those with attention-deficit or tourette/tic symptoms. *Biological Psychology, 43*(2), 163–185.

Ohlrich, E. S., Barnet, A. B., Weiss, I. P., & Shanks, B. L. (1978). Auditory evoked potential development in early childhood: A longitudinal study. *Electroencephalography and Clinical Neurophysiology, 44*(4), 411–423.

Okitsu, T. (1984). Middle components of the auditory evoked response in young children. *Scandinavian Audiology, 13*(2), 83–86.

Orekhova, E. V., Stroganova, T. A., Prokofiev, A. O., Nygren, G., Gillberg, C., & Elam, M. (2009). The right hemisphere fails to respond to temporal novelty in autism: Evidence from an ERP study. *Clinical Neurophysiology, 120*(3), 520–529.

Pasman, J. W., Rotteveel, J. J., de Graaf, R., Maassen, B., & Notermans, S. L. (1991). Detectability of auditory evoked response components in preterm infants. *Early Human Development, 26*(2), 129–141.

Pearce, W., Golding, M., & Dillon, H. (2007). Cortical auditory evoked potentials in the assessment of auditory neuropathy: Two case studies. *Journal of the American Academy of Audiology, 18*(5), 380–390.

Picton, T. W., Hillyard, S. A., Krausz, H. I., & Galambos, I. (1974). Human auditory evoked potentials. I. Evaluation of components. *Electroencephalography and Clinical Neurophysiology, 36*(2), 179–190.

Picton, T. W., Woods, D. L., Baribeau-Braun, J., & Healy, T. M. G. (1977). Evoked potential audiometry. *Journal of Otolaryngology, 6*, 90–119.

Plaza, M., Rigoard, M. T., Chevrie-Muller, C., Cohen, H., & Picard, A. (2001). Short-term memory impairment and unilateral dichotic listening extinction in a child with Landau-Kleffner syndrome: Auditory or phonological disorder? *Brain and Cognition, 46*(1–2), 235–240.

Poblano, A., Muñoz-Hernández, S. E., Arias-Aranda, I., Castro Cue-De Carpizo, L., Montes de Oca-Fernández, E., & de la Vega-De Teyssier, G. (1991). Brain-stem auditory evoked potentials and median latency in children with Down syndrome. *Boletín médico del Hospital Infantil de México*, 48(11), 793–799. Retrieved August 25, 2008 from http://www.ncbi.nlm.nih.gov/pubmed/1837461

Ponton, C. W., Don, M., Eggermont, J. J., Waring, M. D., Kwong, B., & Masuda, A. (1996b). Auditory system plasticity in children after long periods of complete deafness. *NeuroReport, 8*(1), 61–65.

Ponton, C. W., Don, M., Eggermont, J. J., Waring, M. D., & Masuda, A. (1996a). Maturation of human cortical auditory function: Differences between normal-hearing children and children with cochlear implants. *Ear and Hearing, 17*(5), 430–437.

Ponton, C. W., Eggermont, J. J., Khosla, D., Kwong, B., & Don, M. (2002). Maturation of human central auditory system activity: Separating auditory evoked potentials by dipole source modeling. *Clinical Neurophysiology, 113*(3), 407–420.

Ponton, C. W., Eggermont, J. J., Kwong, B., & Don, M. (2000). Maturation of human central auditory system activity: Evidence from multi-channel evoked potentials. *Clinical Neurophysiology, 111*(2), 220–236.

Ponton, C. W., Moore, J. K., & Eggermont, J. J. (1999). Prolonged deafness limits auditory system developmental plasticity: Evidence from an evoked potentials study in children with cochlear implants. *Scandinavian Audiology Suppl., 51*, 13–22.

Prosser, S., & Arslan, E. (1985). Does general anaesthesia affect the child's auditory middle latency response (MLR)? *Scandinavian Audiology, 14*(2), 105–107.

Purdy, S. C., Kelly, A. S., & Davies, M. G. (2002). Auditory brainstem response, middle latency response, and late cortical evoked potentials in children with learning disabilities. *Journal of the American Academy of Audiology, 13*(7), 367–382.

Purdy, S. C., Kelly, A. S., & Thorne, P. R. (2001). Auditory Evoked potentials as measures of plasticity in humans. *Audiology and Neuro-Otology, 6*(4), 211–215.

Pynchon, K. A., Tucker, D. A., Ruth, R. A., Barrett, K. A., & Herr, D. G. (1998). Area- under-the-curve measure of the auditory middle latency response (AMLR) from birth to early adulthood. *American Journal of Audiology, 7*(2), 45–49.

Rance, G., Cone-Wesson, B., Wunderlich, J., & Dowell, R. (2002). Speech perception and cortical event-related potentials in children with auditory neuropathy. *Ear and Hearing, 23*(3), 239–253.

Rapin, I., & Gravel, J. (2003). "Auditory neuropathy": Physiologic and pathologic evidence calls for more diagnostic specificity. *International Journal of Pediatric Otorhinolaryngology, 67*(7), 707–728.

Rapin, I., Ruben, R. J., & Lyttle, M. (1970). Diagnosis of hearing loss in infants using auditory evoked responses. *Laryngoscope, 80*(5), 712–722.

Rodríguez Holguín, S., Corral, M., & Cadaveira, F. (2001). Middle-latency auditory evoked potentials in children at high risk for alcoholism. *Clinical Neurophysiology, 31*(1), 40–47.

Rogers, S. H., Edwards, D. A., Henderson-Smart, D. J., & Pettigrew, A. G. (1989). Middle latency auditory evoked responses in normal term infants: A longitudinal study. *Neuropediatrics, 20*(2), 59–63.

Rothman, H. H., Davis, H., & Hay, I. S. (1970). Slow evoked cortical potentials and temporal features of stimulation. *Electroencephalography and Clinical Neurophysiology, 29*(3), 225–232.

Rotteveel, J. J., Colon, E. J., de Graaf, R., Notermans, S. L., Stoelinga, G. B., & Visco, Y. M. (1986). The central auditory conduction at term date and three months after birth. III. Middle latency responses (MLRs). *Scandinavian Audiology, 15*(2), 75–84.

Rotteveel, J. J., Stegeman, D. F., de Graaf, R., Colon, E. J., & Visco, Y. M. (1987). The maturation of the central auditory conduction in preterm infants until three months post term. III. The middle latency auditory evoked response (MLR). *Hearing Research, 27*(3), 245–256.

Sabatini, B. L., & Regehr, W. G. (1999). Timing of synaptic transmission. *Annual Review of Physiology, 61*, 521–542.

Schochat, E., & Musiek, F. E. (2006). Maturation of outcomes of behavioral and electrophysiologic tests of central auditory function. *Journal of Communication Disorders, 39*(1), 78–92.

Seidl, R., Hauser, E., Bernert, G., Marx, M., Freilinger, M., & Lubec, G. (1997). Auditory evoked potentials in young patients with Down syndrome. Event-related potentials (P3) and histaminergic system. *Cognitive Brain Research, 5*(4), 301–309.

Seri, S., Cerquiglini, A., & Pisani, F. (1998). Spike induced interference in auditory sensory processing in Landau-Kleffner syndrome. *Electroencephalography and Clinical Neurophysiology/Evoked Potentials Section, 108*(5), 506–510.

Seri, S., Cerquiglini, A., Pisani, F., & Curatolo, P. (1999). Autism in tuberous sclerosis: Evoked potential evidence for a deficit in auditory sensory processing. *Clinical Neurophysiology, 110*(10), 1825–1830.

Sharma, A., Dorman, M. F., & Kral, A. (2005a). The influence of a sensitive period on central auditory development in children with unilateral and bilateral cochlear implants. *Hearing Research, 203*(1–2), 134–143.

Sharma, A., Dorman, M. F., & Spahr, A. J. (2002a). A sensitive period for the development of the central auditory system in children with cochlear implants: Implications for age of implantation. *Ear and Hearing, 23*(6), 532–539.

Sharma, A., Dorman, M. F., & Spahr, A. J. (2002b). Rapid development of cortical auditory evoked potentials after early cochlear implantation. *NeuroReport, 13*(10), 1365–1368.

Sharma, A., Gilley, P. M., Dorman, M. F., & Baldwin, R. (2007). Deprivation-induced cortical reorganization in children with cochlear implants. *International Journal of Audiology, 46*(9), 494–499.

Sharma, A., Kraus, N., McGee, T. J., & Nicol, T. G. (1997). Developmental changes in P1 and N1 central auditory responses elicited by consonant-vowel syllables. *Electroencephalography and Clinical Neurophysiology, 104*(6), 540–545.

Sharma, A., Martin, K., Roland, P., Bauer, P., Sweeney, M. H., Gilley, P., & Dorman, M. (2005b). P1 latency as a biomarker for central auditory development in children with hearing impairment. *Journal of the American Academy of Audiology, 16*(8), 564–573.

Sharma, A., Tobey, E., Dorman, M., Bharadwaj, S., Martin, K., Gilley, P., & Kunkel, F. (2004). Central auditory maturation and babbling development in infants with cochlear implants. *Archives of Otolaryngology-Head and Neck Surgery, 130*(5), 511–516.

Shepherd, R. K., & Hardie, N. A. (2001). Deafness-induced changes in the auditory pathway: Implications for cochlear implants. *Audiology and Neuro-Otology, 6*(6), 305–318.

Smalley, S. L., & Henske, E. P. (2005). In M. L. Bauman & Kemper, T. L. (Eds.), *The neurobiology of autism* (2nd ed., pp. 265–275). Baltimore, MD: John Hopkins University Press.

Smoski, W., Brunt, M., & Tannahill, C. (1998). *C.H.A.P.S. Children's Auditory Performance Scale instruction manual.* Tampa, FL: Educational Audiology Association.

Stapells, D. R. (2002). Cortical event-related potentials to auditory stimuli. In J. Katz, R. F. Burkard, & L. Medwetsky (Eds.), *Handbook of clinical audiology* (5th ed., pp. 378–406). Baltimore, MD: Lippincott Williams & Wilkins.

Sussman, E., Steinschneider, M., Gumenyuk, V., Grushko, J., & Lawson, K. (2008). The maturation of human evoked brain potentials to sounds presented at different stimulation rates. *Hearing Research, 236*(1–2), 61–79.

Taguchi, K., Picton, T. W., Orpin, J. A., & Goodman, W. S. (1969). Evoked response audiometry in newborn infants. *Acta Otolaryngologica Suppl., 252,* 5–17.

Tallal, P. (1980). Auditory temporal perception, phonics and reading disabilities in children. *Brain and Language, 9*(2), 182–198.

Tonnquist-Uhlén, I., Borg, E., Persson, H. E., & Spens, K. E. (1996). Topography of auditory evoked cortical potentials in children with severe language impairment: The N1 component. *Electroencephalography and Clinical Neurophysiology, 100*(3), 250–260.

Tucker, D. A., & Ruth, R. A. (1996). Effects of age, signal level, and signal rate on the auditory middle latency response. *Journal of American Academy of Audiology, 7*(2), 83–91.

Vandana, & Tandon, O. P. (2006). Auditory evoked potential responses in chronic malnourished children. *Indian Journal of Physiology and Pharmacology, 50*(1), 48–52.

Warrier, C. M., Johnson, K. L., Hayes, E. A., Nicol, T. G., & Kraus, N. (2004). Learning impaired children exhibit timing deficits and training-related improvements in auditory cortical responses to speech in noise. *Experimental Brain Research, 157*(4), 431–441.

Wetherby, A. M., Koegel, R. L., & Mendel, M. (1981). Central auditory nervous system dysfunction in echolalic autistic individuals. *Journal of Speech and Hearing Research, 24*(3), 420–429.

Wible, B., Nicol, T., & Kraus, N. (2002). Abnormal neural encoding of repeated speech stimuli in noise in children with learning problems. *Clinical Neurophysiology, 113*(4), 485–494.

Winsberg, B. G., Javitt, D. C., & Shanahan/Silipo, G. (1997). Electrophysiological indices of information processing in methylphenidate responders. *Biological Psychiatry, 42*(6), 434–445.

Wioland, N., Rudolf, G., & Metz-Lutz, M. N. (2001). Electrophysiological evidence of persisting unilateral auditory cortex dysfunction in the late outcome of Landau and Kleffner syndrome. *Clinical Neurophysiology, 112*(2), 319–323.

Wolf, K. E., & Goldstein, R. (1978). Middle component averaged electroencephalic responses to tonal stimuli from normal neonates. *Archives of Otolaryngology, 104*(9) 508–513.

Wolf, K. E., & Goldstein, R. (1980). Middle component AERs from neonates to low-level tonal stimuli. *Journal of Speech and Hearing Research, 23*(1), 185–201.

Young, G. B., Wang, J. T., & Connolly, J. F. (2004). Prognostic determination in anoxic-ischemic and traumatic encephalopathies. *Journal of Clinical Neurophysiology, 21*(5), 379–390.

22

Behavioral Audiometry With Infants

Judith E. Widen

Introduction

The first section of this chapter describes the development of behavioral audiometric assessment procedures for infants and toddlers, including some of the data that support our current practices. With the advent of universal hearing screening and the subsequent increase in the number of infants seen for audiologic assessment, the need for accurate and efficient behavioral assessment methods is greater than ever. In the later sections, we refer back to this as we describe the details of current practices of behavioral audiometry with infants.

History of Behavioral Assessment of Infants

Fifty or sixty years ago, before we had auditory brainstem response (ABR), otoacoustic emissions (OAE) and immittance measures, audiologists had to rely on their observations of an infant's behavioral responses to sound to estimate the audiogram. If changes such as a startle, arousal from sleep, grimaces, changes in sucking, eye widening, or localization toward the sound source were time-locked with presentation of a sound stimulus, the observer assumed the change was a response to sound. Noting that behavioral responses varied depending on stimulus type (speech, noise, and tones), stimulus level, and the infant's age, Downs (1967) tabulated these observations into the Auditory Behavior Index. The index showed the typical soundfield minimum response levels (MRL) for normal hearing children from birth to 24 months of age, indicating that the levels required for a minimum response were higher for younger than older infants, and that the minimum response level for pure tones was higher than noise, which was still higher than speech. The index was subsequently published in five editions of *Hearing in Children* (Northern & Downs, 1974, 1978, 1984, 1991, 2002). Cartoon drawings that summarized the findings also were included in that venerable text. Both the index and the cartoon drawings found their way into audiology test rooms around the country and were used as guides for comparing an infant's behavior being tested with that of normal-hearing infants.

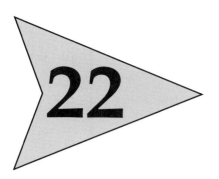

This observational procedure was called behavioral observation audiometry (BOA). Efforts were made by researchers to quantify responses from normal hearing infants as a guide for comparing abnormal responses to sound. Investigators such as Thompson and Thompson (1972), Eisenberg (1976), and Muir, Abraham, Forbes, and Harris (1979) described the range of behaviors to a variety of stimuli at varying loudness levels associated with auditory development within the first months and years of life. The results confirmed the observations of Downs (1967) that the MRLs of normal-hearing and typically developing infants vary as a function of age, stimulus type, and stimulus level. Studies by Thompson and Weber (1974) showed the intersubject variability was great with the BOA procedure. In addition, evidence that infants habituate quickly to test stimuli resulted in considerable intrasubject variability as well. Another problem with BOA was that of examiner bias. Knowledge of the stimulus level or knowledge of previous test results sometimes resulted in under- or overestimating the degree of hearing loss (Gans & Flexer, 1982; Ling, Ling, & Doehring, 1970; Weber, 1969).

For the reasons stated above, BOA has serious limitations as an audiometric method. The most frequency-specific signals, those used for audiometry, especially at low stimulus levels near threshold, are the least likely to result in responses from infants. With normal-hearing infants showing such a wide range of responsiveness, the usefulness of BOA in detecting mild and moderate degrees of hearing loss was limited. Largely for this reason, Jerger and Hayes (1976) introduced the pediatric cross-check principle in which an electrophysiologic measure such as immittance audiometry or ABR is employed to verify behavioral results. The auditory behavior index has its place, not as an index of sensitivity but rather as an index of responsivity. It has been misused and misinterpreted for audiometry.

Operant Conditioning Audiometry

Suzuki and Ogiba (1961) are credited with the first published description of an operant conditioning procedure for audiometry. They called the procedure conditioned orientation reflex (COR). As the name implies, the infant was required to orient to the sound source, which was one of two speakers at each corner of the test room. Correct orientation was rewarded by the lighting of a doll on top of the speaker. Later in Sweden, Liden and Kankkunen (1969) reported another conditioning procedure that did not require localization but rewarded changes in behavior that occurred when a test signal was presented. They called their procedure visual reinforcement audiometry (VRA).

Aspects of each of these procedures were used in subsequent studies at the University of Washington that systematically investigated the use of operant conditioning for audiometry with infants and toddlers. A systematic series of studies on operant conditioning audiometry began that documented its usefulness and laid the foundation for the procedures we use today. Thompson and Thompson (1972) documented the tenets of the auditory behavior index, showing that speech elicited responses at lower levels than noise, which in turn elicited responses at lower levels than tones. They also showed that older children responded at lower levels than did younger children. Next, the study by Thompson and Weber (1974) confirmed the wide inter- and intrasubject variability of BOA. Moore, Thompson, and Thompson (1975) then investigated the strength of different types of reinforcers and found that a lighted, animated toy kept infants on task for nearly 30 stimulus trials. Further study showed that this type of reinforcer was effective for infants as young as 5 months of age (Moore, Wilson, & Thompson, 1977). Encouraged by these findings, investigators proceeded to show that infant thresholds to a complex noise stimulus approximated those of adults tested under the same conditions and, more importantly that infants were no more variable than adults in their responses (Wilson, Moore, & Thompson, 1976). Likewise, using audiometric stimuli (pure tones of 500, 2000, and 4000 Hz), infant responses were found to approximate adults tested using the same paradigm (10 dB step size, reinforcement provided as feedback). Then came the comparison of soundfield thresholds for infants and adults versus earphone thresholds for infants and adults (Wilson & Moore, 1978). It was concluded that VRA yielded results that were remarkably similar to adults (Wilson & Thompson, 1984). The sequence of the studies described here are included as classic articles in the Behavioral Methodology section of Bess and Gravel's *Foundations of Pediatric Audiology* (2006).

Numerous other studies followed but perhaps the most important in terms of general applicability to pediatric audiology was the study by Thompson and Folsom (1985), which documented that once a child is under stimulus control, VRA threshold is not influenced by stimulus type; that is, broadband noise, narrowband noise, and pure tones were equally effective in eliciting responses from infants. Details of conditioning and response strength were addressed by Thompson and Folsom (1984) and Primus and Thompson (1985).

Other studies focused on the use of VRA for infants with or at-risk for developmental delay. Initial studies indicated that a developmental age of 10 months might be necessary for successful VRA with infants with Down syndrome (Greenberg, Wilson, Moore, & Thompson, 1978; Thompson, Wilson, & Moore, 1979), but scrutiny of the data suggest that only a few infants under 10 months were included in the study sample. Later studies of graduates of neonatal intensive care units (NICU), many of whom were at risk for developmental delay, indicated that when age was corrected for prematurity, most could be tested successfully with VRA at 6 to 8 months corrected age (Moore, Thompson, & Folsom, 1992; Widen, 1990). Overall, these studies documented that developmental age is the primary determinant of a child's ability to do VRA. Of course, there is a range of abilities. Thus, in hopes of getting a successful test on the first return visit, two later large-scale multicenter studies using VRA to validate newborn test results aimed to provide the VRA follow-up testing once the infants reached a corrected age of 8 months (Widen et al., 2000, 2005).

Besides the studies conducted at University of Washington, numerous others have documented that VRA is a valid measure of hearing sensitivity in infants. In 1988, Olsho, Koch, Carter, Halpin, and Spetner summarized several existing studies and added data from their own subset of infants to show that infant thresholds generally fall within 10 dB of adult thresholds obtained with comparable methods. A particularly valuable study is one by Talbott (1987) that retrospectively reviewed the records of children with hearing loss seen within her private audiology practice. She compared the audiograms obtained with VRA to the children's later audiograms obtained using play audiometry and found that VRA thresholds were highly consistent with later play audiograms and that there were no statistically significant differences between the thresholds found with the two approaches. From these studies it was apparent that even slight deviations from normal could be detected when using operant audiometry. Later studies compared tone burst ABR with pure-tone VRA thresholds showing good correspondence between the two measures (Stapells, Gravel, & Martin, 1995).

Visual Reinforcement Audiometry in Clinical Practice

The purpose of behavioral audiometry in infants is the same as it is in adults: to describe the hearing status of each ear according to type, degree, and configuration. Hearing testing of infants is really no different than testing adults. Instead of verbal instructions, infants are shown what is expected of them through a process of operant conditioning. As with adults, the primary test stimuli are pure tones presented through earphones and a bone oscillator. A speech detection threshold is obtained to confirm the accuracy of the pure-tone thresholds. Instead of a hand raise or a button push, the expected response is a head turn. Feedback about correct responses is provided by a visual reward that also acts to reinforce continued responding.

The Instructions: Operant Conditioning

Operant conditioning is a process in which the frequency of occurrence of a particular behavior is modified by the consequences of that behavior (Widen, 1990). In VRA, the frequency of the head-turn responses is increased because the behavior of head-turning results in a pleasurable visual event. VRA employs an operant paradigm in which the auditory test signal serves as a discriminative stimulus that cues the infant that a response (head turn) will produce reinforcement or a desirable event (in this case, the lighting and activation of the toy). Figure 22–1 depicts the basic tenets of operant conditioning as applied to infant audiometry.

Conditioning refers to the process of training or shaping the desired behavior. This is usually accomplished by pairing the reinforcer with a signal that is presumed to be audible to the infant. Because localization toward sounds, particularly novel ones, is a natural response for most infants, conditioning often occurs rapidly and may not require the simultaneous pairing of discriminative and reinforcing stimuli. When the

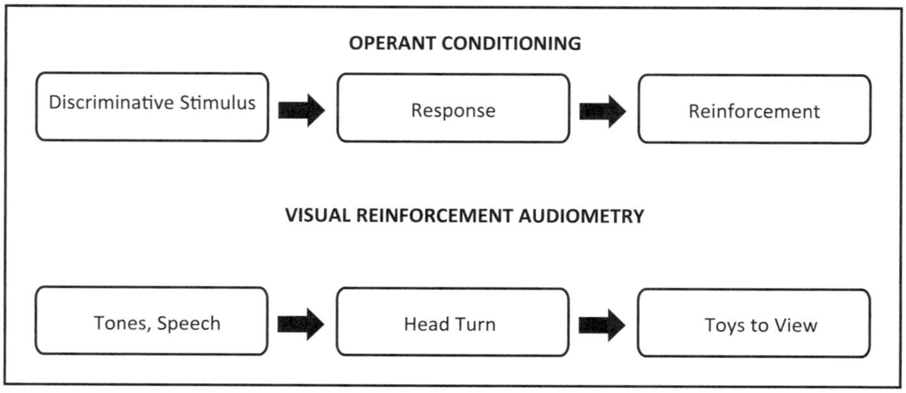

FIGURE 22–1. The basic tenets of operant conditioning as related to VRA.

infant turns consistently (usually twice consecutively) to the test signal before the presentation of reinforcement, it is assumed that the auditory signal is acting as the discriminative stimulus cuing the infant of the availability of reinforcement. It is imperative that the stimulus used during initial "instructions" is audible, or at least *perceptible* to the infant. If severe hearing loss is suspected then a vibrotactile stimulus, such as a low-frequency bone-conducted stimulus, should be used for the pairing.

Stimulus control refers to the strength of the discriminative stimulus in producing the desired response. Stimulus control is compromised when a test signal that previously resulted in the head turn no longer results in the response or when the head turn occurs when the signal is not present. Stimulus control can be assessed by using probe and control trials.

Probe trials are suprathreshold stimulus presentations presented at a level at which the infant has previously responded. They are used to demonstrate understanding of the task before descending in level to determine threshold and throughout the test to determine if the infant is still "on task."

Control trials are observation intervals in which the examiner judges whether a head turn occurs in the absence of sound stimulation. The primary purpose for control trials is to determine if the responses (head turns) being judged are truly responses to the test stimuli and not just random head turns. If the child turns as often during control trials as during stimulus trials, then the test is not valid.

Test Stimuli

There are two considerations for selecting test stimuli. First, what type of stimulus is best for conditioning? And, once conditioning is established, what type of stimulus should be used for threshold testing?

For conditioning, many clinicians use complex signals such as speech or noise, since they are the more "alerting" according to the auditory behavior index. In one of our multisite studies, the protocol allowed the audiologists to choose the stimulus they preferred for conditioning (Widen et al., 2005). Of the seven sites, five chose to begin with pure tones, two with speech. When the results were analyzed at the end of the study, it appeared that the type of stimulus used for conditioning had little to do with ultimate success in completing VRA.

Theoretically, the stimuli used for infant testing can be the same pure tones that are used for adults. Thompson and Folsom (1985) demonstrated that once infants are under stimulus control, they will continue to respond (and work for the reward of seeing the reinforcer) despite the stimulus bandwidth. However, most audiologists choose to add a little interest to the conventional pure-tone stimuli, by pulsing or warbling them. This practice is probably a holdover from the days of reliance on the auditory behavior index or just good intuition that "complex" signals are more alerting. Some audiologists prefer to use the narrow bands of noise designated for masking as test stimuli. This should be done with caution, as their wider bandwidth might stimulate adjacent frequency regions of better hearing if not filtered appropriately, and thus result in erroneous thresholds.

Just as in pure-tone audiometry with adults (ANSI, 2004; Carhart & Jerger, 1959), a short signal duration (one to two seconds) is important for infants as well. Students and audiologists who are not experienced testers of infants, tend to extend the duration of signals to infants. Just like adults, some infants will respond to the onset of the test signal while others respond to the offset. If the signal is not discontinued, the infant will keep waiting. Or, more likely given typical infant curiosity, an infant who has to wait too long will turn toward the reinforcer even when the test signal was not heard.

With respect to the sequence of tones, just as in adult audiometry (ANSI, 2004; ASHA, 2005) the sequence will depend on the referral question and the case history. If a normal result is expected, we usually start at 2000 Hz (perhaps the most important frequency for the understanding of spoken English, as well as a frequency that is easy to detect in a background of infant wiggling noise). On the other hand, if previous information suggests a probable high frequency hearing loss, then the test sequence should begin in the lower frequencies where normal hearing is expected. Once stimulus control is assured, then the pertinent high frequencies can be tested. An excellent discussion of clinical VRA protocols is provided in Gravel and Hood (1999).

Speech is used as a test stimulus for infants as well as adults and for the same reason: to confirm the accuracy of the pure-tone thresholds. Speech should NOT be used as the primary stimulus to estimate amount of hearing loss. We continue to be amazed at the number of audiograms we see from audiologists in nonpediatric settings who report that a child's hearing is "within the normal range" based on a speech awareness threshold alone! On the other hand, because of its inherent interest to many infants, speech may be a good stimulus for initial conditioning and probe trials, as described above.

Tranducers

The transducers used for infant audiometry are the same type as those used with adults. Earphones are needed if the goal is to obtain information about each ear. Unfortunately, many audiologists, especially in the past, settle for sound-field stimulus presentation, assuming that infants will object to wearing earphones. This is such a common assumption that we often hear audiologists from nonpediatric settings interchange the terms "VRA" and "sound-field" when referring to infant thresholds. However, "VRA" refers to the procedure used to obtain thresholds and "sound-field" refers to the transducer used to present the signal. Insert earphones that have come into routine use are of great benefit to infant testing because they are lightweight and relatively unobtrusive. I fondly remember the remark of my mentor, Wes Wilson, who when asked, "How do you get infants to wear earphones?" would reply, "I'm bigger than they are."

Nonetheless, the same questions we posed under Test Stimuli above are also pertinent here. Should conditioning begin in the soundfield or with earphones? Many clinicians opt for sound-field conditioning for a couple of reasons. First, if the infant ultimately objects to earphones, then at least the audiologist has gained some information, although about the better ear. Second, intuitively, the natural headturn toward a sound source seems more robust in a localization condition than in a lateralization one. Widen et al. (2005) in their multisite study found that beginning in the soundfield or with earphones did not make a difference in a clinic site's ultimate success in obtaining pure-tone earphone data for the group of infants in this clinical study.

Successful ear-specific testing of infants is well documented. In fact, the early study by Liden and Kankkunen (1969) reported ear-specific thresholds for infants, obtained not by using earphones but by occluding one ear and presenting the test signals in the sound field (occluding one ear of an infant should not be any less objectionable than wearing an earphone!). Many research studies that use operant head-turn procedures for studying various aspects of infant auditory behavior (beyond sensitivity) have used earphones (cf. Nozza & Wilson, 1984). Clinical reports of VRA testing with earphones include those of Talbott (1987), Gravel and Traquina (1992) and Day, Bamford, Parry, Shepherd, and Quigley (2000). The multisite studies of Widen et al. (2000, 2005) documented the successful use of insert phones with several thousand infants. With the advent of universal newborn hearing screening and subsequent increase in the numbers of infants on the audiology caseload, clinicians sometimes use the child's custom earmold for threshold assessment, especially during hearing aid fitting procedures (Gravel, 1994).

There are some questions posed by clinical audiologists about the use of earphones with infants. Does the smaller ear canal size significantly change the sound pressure level in the infant ear canal? Do we need to make corrections for age? Is the variation in SPL greater than that found in the differing size canals of adults? Is the variation greater than that provided by test-retest reliability for the standard step size? What about the other standard transducer, the bone conduction oscillator? Chapter 25 provides a thorough discussion of the impact of small ear canals on sound pressure level measured at the eardrum.

Response

For VRA, the expected response is a head turn, something that infants do naturally and a movement that is clear and can be easily observed by examiners. With many research protocols, the judgments of two examiners are required for reinforcement of the head-turn response. Intra and interjudge agreement is reported as over 96% for each (Moore et al., 1975, 1977; Wilson et al., 1976).

The ease with which a head turn can be judged will be influenced by the placement of the reinforcers relative to the child. Placement of the reinforcers at a 90-degree angle to the child's midline should require a headturn that is easy to observe. When speakers are mounted in the corners of test booths (at 45-degree angles) the reinforcer is often placed on top of the speakers. This placement can create at least a couple of problems. A robust head turn is not required for children to see the reinforcer making the audiologist's determination of a response more difficult. Second, given that speakers are typically mounted at ear level for the child, the reinforcer can be quite high relative to the infant's line of vision.

Pediatric audiologists do not all agree on whether reinforcement should be provided in just one location or two (on each side of the child). VRA does not require localization as Suzuki and Ogiba's (1961) COR procedure did. It makes sense that VRA does not require the infant to correctly locate the sound source. The task is one of detection of the test signal. Adults are not asked to detect the signal AND indicate where it is heard. In fact, at low signal levels localization is not particularly good, even with normal hearing listeners. For those with hearing impairment, localization skills are typically poorer than those with normal hearing (Gatehouse & Cox, 1972). This has been demonstrated in infants as well in studies of localization with simulated unilateral hearing loss (Auslander, Lewis, Schulte, & Stelmachowicz, 1991).

A study by Primus (1992b) provides convincing evidence that although VRA is not dependent on localization, inaccurate localization cues can reduce VRA performance significantly. He showed that infants can perform VRA with reinforcement on just one side or both sides, but in terms of conditioning success and time required, there may be clinical advantages of placing toys on each side so that reinforcement is adjacent to the sound source. In a master's thesis at the University of Kansas, Moran (1995) investigated the role of lateralization in VRA under earphones. She too found that infants could do the VRA task in either condition, with reinforcement on one side or on each side of stimulation, and that it was not unusual for an infant to turn to the side that was stimulated even when there was no reinforcer on that side. The studies of Primus and Moran are convincing that it is preferable to have reinforcement available to each side, so that correct responses can be rewarded no matter which way the infant turns.

Threshold Procedure

Before discussing the procedure for determining threshold in infants, we need to address some terminology. In audiometry, the term "threshold" refers to the level at which the listener detects the test stimulus 50% of the time. Because it is assumed that infants do not respond to signals at their detection threshold, the term "minimum response level" (MRL) may be more appropriate. We agree that for unconditioned responses, MRL is the appropriate term. Also, when threshold is not sought, but responses are detected at a specified stopping level within a normal range, then MRL is also an appropriate term. Nonetheless, the term, "VRA threshold" is a good one to define the 50% response level when VRA is employed.

The standard threshold procedure for audiometry in adults (ANSI, 2004; ASHA, 2005) is based on the modified Hughson-Westlake procedure described by Carhart and Jerger in 1959 and employs a familiarization period at suprathreshold levels, followed by signals presented at descending levels of 10 dB until there is no response, then ascending in 5 dB steps. Some studies and some clinicians use this same procedure for infants. Others have used a 10 dB step-size (down 20, up 10) largely to save time and avoid multiple test sessions. Of course, when step size is increased, test-retest reliability also increases. Simulation studies by Eilers, Miskiel, Ozdamar, Urbano, and Widen (1991a), Eilers, Widen, Urbano, Hudson, and Gonzales (1991b), and Tharpe and Ashmead (1993) may be reviewed to see how factors such as starting level and step size may influence the ultimate estimation of threshold.

As explained in the previous section on Test Stimuli, the test order of frequencies should be determined by the referral question and case history. The suggested order of 1000, 2000, 4000 Hz, then 500 and 250 Hz with adults assumes that the entire sequence will be completed. However with infants, this assumption cannot be made as they might not cooperate for the full sequence. Therefore, one must decide which frequencies are most important to assess on a case-by-case basis.

Just as with adults, it is important with infants to avoid a regular pattern of stimulus presentation that can lull them into a similar pattern of response. The insertion of probe and control trials has been used in VRA to assure the validity of infant's responses. One element of a reliable test is a high percentage of correct control trials. Experience and simulation studies suggest that if correct control trials fall below 70%, the accuracy of the test may be affected by more than the measurement step size (i.e., the VRA "threshold" you obtain may be 10 dB better than "true threshold"). Some false positives are allowed, just as they are in standard audiometry so long as the testing pattern is modified so the examiner is comfortable judging the response accurately. It is not true, however, that 100% correct control trials necessarily indicate a valid test, since the child who never responds to stimulus trials would not respond to control trials either.

Control trials are particularly critical in the shortest of test sessions, when the child is trained rapidly to the task and responds repeatedly at the lowest levels of stimulation. In these instances, the number of reinforced stimulus trials will be high compared to the total number of stimulus trials, and it is particularly important that the percentage of correct control trials is also high. When a child turns during a control trial, the examiner at the audiometer should insert an additional control trial to ensure response accuracy. In longer test sessions, when the child does not respond at the 20 dB HL and VRA "threshold" is determined, the lack of responses at lower levels serves as a type of control as well.

Test Environment

The standard sound-treated test environment works for VRA as long as it is large enough to seat two adults and an infant. One adult serves as in-room examiner and one adult (usually the parent) serves as infant holder. Typically, the infant is held in the parent's lap or if the infant is seated in a high chair, the parent is seated nearby.

Reinforcement

Three-dimensional toys that can be lighted and animated typically are housed in smoked plexiglass boxes. Some pediatric clinics are equipped with several toys that can be presented randomly to help maintain the infant's interest and attention in either a stacked grouping (Gravel, 1989; Gravel, Seewald, & Buerkli-Halevy, 1997) or on each side of the infant. Most reinforcement equipment provides for lighting and animation separately. Recently some clinics have installed monitors that can be activated for short glimpses of cartoons or pictures from a DVD. These animated images have been found to be either equally effective or superior to conventional animated toy reinforcers (Lowery, von Hapsburg, Plyler & Johnstone, 2009; Schmida, Peterson, & Tharpe, 2003). As discussed in the section on transducers, the location of the reinforcement, whatever it is, should be at the child's eye level and 90 degrees to the side of the child.

Number of Examiners

Traditionally, VRA employs two examiners: one at the audiometer to control the test stimuli and reinforcement, the other in the test room with child and parent. The role of the in-room examiner is important in achieving a valid and reliable audiogram (Figure 22–2). It takes skill and practice to keep the child in what we assume is a listening posture, so that the child wants to see the reinforcer toy more than anything else while still allowing the attention to be drawn away so that a head turn can be easily judged. The examiner and the examiner's actions must not be more interesting than the reinforcer toys. The examiner should refrain from talking or smiling at the infant, except to provide praise for correct responses. A secondary role of the in-room examiner is to maintain a quiet environment and rapport with the parent, as well as to be available for quick insertion (and possibly reinsertion) of earphones. The in-room examiner's role is deemed so important that several investigators have refined procedures and equipment so that one examiner can do it all: control the stimuli and reinforcement while located within the exam room with the child and parent (Gravel et al., 1997; Widen, 1990, 1993). Another alternative includes the use of a centering toy. Some clinicians report good success training the parent to perform the in-room examiner duties, especially when the child is seated in a high chair where they can see the parent (Madell, 2008).

Practical Considerations

Although similarities between testing infants and adults have been noted, clearly there are differences as well. The primary difference is time. Verbal explanation of the purpose of procedures and the expected time they will take is usually enough to keep adults attentive and cooperative. Not so with infants. The infant decides how long testing will last. Thus, when testing infants we strive to save time. We want to select an efficient protocol, one that minimizes the number of required responses from the infant. As stated earlier, a larger step size can be employed with VRA as compared to that used with traditional pure-tone audiometry. Furthermore, it is less likely or necessary to seek thresholds below a "normal" level (i.e., 15 or 20 dB HL).

There are ways to delay habituation. If the examination is scheduled for the infants' "best time" (after a nap, for example), they are likely to cooperate longer than if they are tired or hungry. Many clinicians begin the presentation of reinforcement by simply lighting the toys, adding animation as the test session progresses. The use of many different distracting toys seems to contribute to longer test sessions, as does the provision of a variety of visual reinforcements. Other possibilities for extending test time have been reported: intermittent reinforcement, duration of intermittent reinforcement, varying test frequency, or changing ears (Culpepper & Thompson, 1994; Primus, 1987, 1992a; Thompson, Thompson, & McCall, 1992). Some of these studies are ones that have focused on the best way to test 2-year-olds who are notorious for their short attention spans, their fast-changing preferences and their love of the word, "No!"

Reasonable Expectations of VRA

In the past two decades, two multicenter research studies have been conducted in which VRA was used to validate hearing status of infants who had been

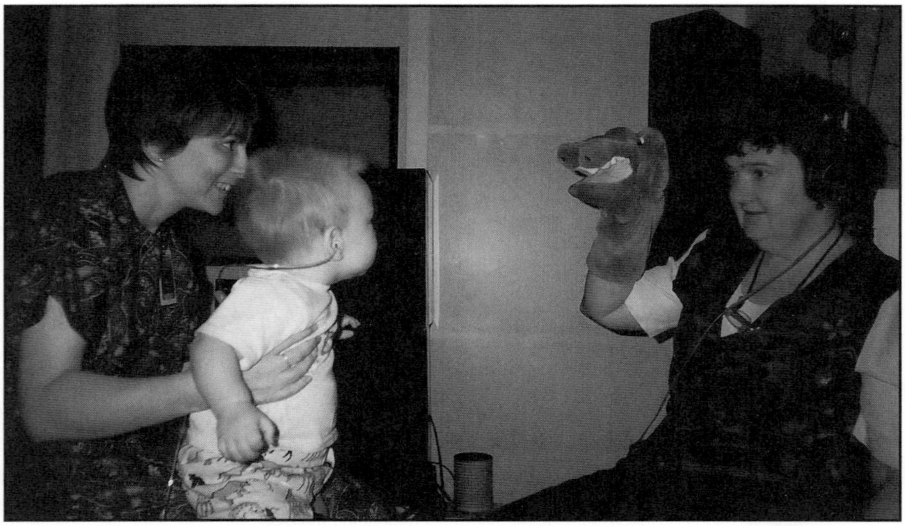

A

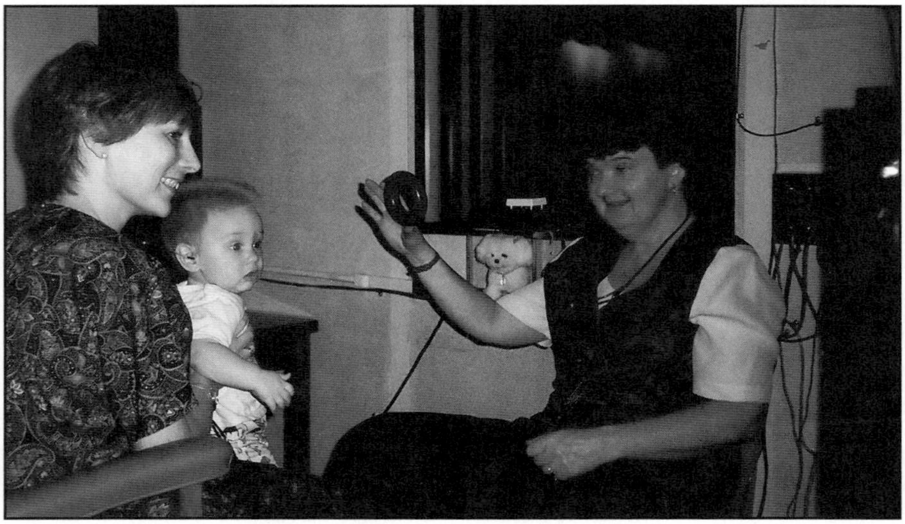

B

FIGURE 22–2. A. The in-room examiner plays an important role in VRA. As shown in this photo, the child is interested in the examiner's distraction toy. **B.** The child turns readily to see the reinforcer with each stimulus presentation, demonstrating stimulus control and the positive nature of the reinforcement.

tested as newborns using ABR and/or OAEs (Johnson et al., 2005a, 2005b; Norton et al., 2000). VRA protocols were developed to ensure that infants were tested in a comparable manner across sites. Both studies have been published in a series of articles, each with a detailed description of the protocol and the results of VRA testing on large groups of infants (Widen et al., 2000, 2005). The data from the studies cited and described in this chapter were the foundation for the protocols used in the multicenter studies. These studies provided an opportunity to not only implement the protocols, but also to study their performance. Some of the interesting things that were learned are shared below.

In the National Institute on Deafness and Other Communication Disorders (NIDCD) Multicenter Consortium on Identification of Neonatal Hearing Impairment (Norton et al., 2000), VRA was attempted on 3134 infants (mean corrected age of 10 months, SD 2.5). Ninety-six percent of the infants could be conditioned for VRA and provided at least one threshold; whereas 92% completed a test (three pure-tone frequencies and a speech detection threshold for each ear). Fifty-six percent of the infants were tested in one test session, 30% within two tests sessions, and 14% required three sessions. The primary reason for repeat visits, accounting for 44%, was habituation prior to completion of the protocol (VRA thresholds for 4 test signals for each ear). Additional reasons for repeat visits were failure to condition (32%), fussiness (30%), and poor test reliability (19%). Twenty-nine percent had abnormal tympanograms and elevated VRA thresholds and had to return for repeat testing when the ears were free of fluid. Only 7% of infants were recalled for repeat testing because they refused to wear earphones.

The average length of a test session was 15 minutes. The standard deviation of 10 minutes indicated that some sessions were terminated quickly (often because conditioning was unsuccessful) and others extended beyond half an hour. The average number of reinforced stimulus trials was 45, suggesting that there was plenty of opportunity to bracket threshold for a number of test signals. On average, only two to three stimulus trials were required prior to beginning the threshold search, and often the "instructions" (conditioning) had to be repeated during the test session (often when the test for the second ear was begun).

Another interesting finding was the difference between the time it took to test infants with hearing loss compared to infants with normal hearing. Related to this was an indication that examiners tended to lack confidence in the results that indicated hearing loss. In the second multisite study by Johnson et al. (2005a, 2005b), it was found that examiners had greater confidence in the results with 20 dB MRLs than with higher MRLs (Widen et al., 2005).

Clinicians might argue that research protocols do not always translate to useful clinical tools. However, we argue that the participants in these studies *were* actual patients. Most of the infants were at higher risk for hearing loss than the general population. In best clinical practice these infants should be monitored for possible changes in hearing status in the period between newborn screening and beginning school age.

Variations of Operant Conditioning Audiometry

Beyond Pure-Tone Authority

Obtaining the pure-tone audiogram is just the beginning in adult audiometry. Speech or word recognition testing is a regular part of the basic audiologic test battery for adults and older children. Such testing supplements the pure tone audiometry for medical diagnosis and plays an even more important role in the treatment of the communication problems resulting from hearing loss. Likewise, measures of speech perception in infants and young children can be equally useful. Most speech tests rely on knowledge of language; however, the ability to discriminate one speech sound from another does not require knowledge of language, but simply the ability to tell the difference. Discrimination tasks have been used in studies of infant speech perception for years, but only minimally for clinical work. Modifications of the head turn technique have been used to determine speech discrimination abilities in infants, and are referred to as visually reinforced infant speech discrimination (VRISD; Eilers, Wilson, & Moore, 1977; Gravel, 1989; Nozza, 1987b; Nozza, Rossman, Bond, & Miller, 1990). The concept is receiving more attention from researchers and clinicians now because of the increase in the number of children with hearing loss identified in infancy and the interest in determining their speech perception skills.

Beyond Infancy

As infants approach 2 years of age, the test procedure of choice is less clear-cut and in large part depends on a child's overall developmental level, attention and motivation for certain tasks. Many toddlers are ready for more active involvement in the test procedure than what VRA affords. They may be taught to push a button in response to a sound, which in turn activates reinforcement toys or a video display. This technique is sometimes referred to as visually reinforced operant conditioning audiometry (VROCA) to distinguish it from VRA, in which the conditioned head turn is assumed to be the response. The reward also may be changed to a more tangible one, such as food (cereal, raisins, etc.) or tokens that can be exchanged for prizes. In this case, the term tangible reinforced operant conditioning audiometry (TROCA) is used. These techniques tend to be available in clinics that specialize in testing children and are especially useful for years 2 to 3 (Thompson, Thompson, & Vethivelu, 1989).

Later, play audiometry (often called "conditioned" play audiometry) becomes the standard. For this procedure, the response and the reward are combined. That is, it is really no different from standard raise-your-hand procedures except that the response is a motor act with toys, putting a peg in a pegboard, or a block in a bucket, for example. The toy or game can be changed repeatedly to accommodate attention span and keep the child on task. The motor task can be almost anything that is easy and fun (i.e., reinforcing) for the child to do and also easy for the examiner to judge. Chapter 23 in this text covers behavioral audiometry in children.

Behavioral Assessment When Operant Conditioning Audiometry Does Not Work

Despite its success with most typically developing infants, there are limitations to VRA and its alternative operant conditioning techniques. There are several reasons why an infant might not condition. Besides the most common one (disposition, i.e., not being in the mood), infants might be too young, developmentally delayed, or physically incapable of providing a head-turn response or seeing the visual reinforcers, or the reinforcement could simply not be reinforcing to some infants. So what can we do if our attempts to condition are not successful?

Many audiologists have abandoned the use of BOA in any formal sense and the pediatric assessment guidelines from one of our national organizations has recommended against its use for determining hearing thresholds (ASHA, 2004; Diefendorf & Gravel, 1996). BOA can be appropriately used to observe auditory behavior especially when used in conjunction with electrophysiologic measures.

An alternative option to BOA is the use of functional scales, which can be completed by parents, early interventionists (speech-language pathologists, teachers of the deaf, early childhood specialists), and/or audiologists. Tools such as the Developmental Index of Audition and Listening (DIAL) or the Infant-Toddler Meaningful Auditory Integration Scale (IT-MAIS) can be used to quantify behavioral observations and determine if infant behavior is consistent with the electrophysiologic test results (Robbins, Svirsky, Osberger, & Pisoni, 1998; Zimmerman-Phillips, Osberger, & Robbins, 1997). The Auditory Behavior Index can serve as a guide for functional use of hearing by providing information about a child's listening and speaking behaviors in outside settings.

Conclusion

Recalling the advice of Jerger and Hayes (1976) that the results on one test measure should be cross-checked with another, comprehensive audiologic assessment of infants and toddlers should include physiologic measures of auditory function as well as behavioral assessment of hearing. The ASHA Guidelines for Audiological Assessment of Infants and Children Birth to 5 Years of Age (2004) recommend that for infants from birth to 6 months, the primary measures will be physiologic ones (auditory evoked potentials, otoacoustic emissions, immittance measures) supplemented by behavioral observations by parents and professionals of the infants' behavioral responses to sound. For the developmental ages 6 months to 2 years, VRA is the primary method to assess hearing sensitivity, supplemented by tympanometry and acoustic reflexes, evoked otoacoustic emissions, and ABR (when necessary). Beside these guidelines of ASHA, details of the behavioral assessment in procedures described in this chapter can be found in protocols from the province of Ontario, Canada (2008), the American Academy of Audiology (2000), and the Joint Committee on Infant Hearing (2007).

References

American Academy of Audiology (AAA). (2000). *Clinical practice algorithms and statements*. Retrieved January 28, 2010, from http://www.audiology.org/resources/documentlibrary/Pages/PediatricDiagnostics.aspx

American National Standards Institute (ANSI). (2004). *Method for manual pure-tone threshold audiometry*. ANSI S3.21-2004. New York, NY: Author.

American Speech-Language-Hearing Association (ASHA). (2004). *Guidelines for the audiologic assessment of children from birth to 5 years of age*. Retrieved January 28, 2010, from http://www.asha.org/docs/html/GL2004-00002.html

American Speech-Language-Hearing Association. (2005). *Guidelines for manual pure-tone audiometry*. Retrieved January 28, 2010, from http://www.asha.org/docs/html/GL2005-00014.html

Auslander, M. C., Lewis, D. E., Schulte, L., & Stelmachowicz, P. G. (1991). Localization ability in infants with simulated unilateral hearing loss. *Ear and Hearing, 12*, 371–376.

Bess, F. H., & Gravel, J. S. (Eds). (2006). *Foundations of pediatric audiology.* San Diego, CA: Plural.

Carhart, R., & Jerger, J. (1959). Preferred method for clinical determination of pure-tone thresholds. *Journal of Speech and Hearing Disorders, 24,* 330–345.

Culpepper, B., & Thompson, G. (1994). Effects of reinforcer duration on the response behavior of preterm 2-year-old in visual reinforcement audiometry. *Ear and Hearing, 15,* 161–167.

Day, J., Bamford, J., Parry, G., Shepherd, M., & Quigley, A. (2000). Evidence on the efficacy of insert earphone and sound field VRA with young infants. *British Journal of Audiology, 34,* 329–334.

Diefendorf, A. O., & Gravel, J. S. (1996). Behavioral observation and visual reinforcement audiometry. In S. E. Gerber (Ed.), *The handbook of pediatric audiology* (pp. 55–83). Washington, DC: Gallaudet Press.

Downs, M. P. (1967). Testing hearing in infancy and early childhood. In F. McConnell & P. H. Ward (Eds.), *Deafness in childhood.* Nashville, TN: Vanderbilt University Press.

Eilers, R. E., Miskiel, E., Ozdamar, O., Urbano, R., & Widen, J. E. (1991a). Optimization of automated hearing test algorithms: Simulations using an infant response model. *Ear and Hearing, 12,* 191–198.

Eilers, R. E., Widen, J. E., Urbano, R., Hudson, T., & Gonzales, L. (1991b). Optimization of automated hearing test algorithms: A comparison of data from simulations and young children. *Ear and Hearing, 12,* 199–204.

Eilers, R. E., Wilson, W. R., & Moore, J. M. (1977). Developmental changes in speech discrimination in infants. *Journal of Speech and Hearing Research, 20,* 766–780.

Eisenberg, R. B. (1976). *Auditory competence in early life—The roots of communicative behavior.* Baltimore, MD: University Park Press.

Gans, D., & Flexer, C. (1982). Observer bias in the hearing testing of profoundly involved multiply handicapped children. *Ear and Hearing, 3,* 309–313.

Gatehouse, R. W., & Cox, W. (1972). Localization of sound by completely monaural deaf subjects. *Journal of Auditory Research, 12,* 179–183.

Gravel, J. S. (1989). Behavioral assessment of auditory function. *Seminars in Hearing, 10,* 216–228.

Gravel, J. S. (1994). Auditory assessment of infants. *Seminars in Hearing, 15,* 100–113.

Gravel, J. S., & Hood L. J. (1999). Pediatric audiologic assessment. In F. E. Musiek & W. R. Rintleman (Eds.), *Contemporary perspectives in hearing assessment* (pp. 305–316). Boston, MA: Allyn & Bacon.

Gravel, J. S., Seewald, R. C., & Buerkli-Halevy, O. (1997). Pediatric hearing assessment. *Phonak Focus. "Sound beginnings"* Videotape series. Stäfa, Switzerland: Phonak AG.

Gravel, J. S., & Traquina, D. N. (1992). Experience with the audiologic assessment of infants and toddlers. *International Journal of Pediatric Otorhinolaryngology, 23,* 59–71.

Gravel, J. S., & Wallace, I. F. (2000). Effects of otitis media with effusion on hearing in the first 3 years of life. *Journal of Speech and Hearing Research, 43,* 651–644.

Greenberg, D. B., Wilson, W. R., Moore, J. M., & Thompson, G. (1978). Visual reinforcement audiometry (VRA) with young Down syndrome children. *Journal of Speech and Hearing Disorders, 4,* 448–458.

Jerger, J. F., & Hayes, D. (1976). The cross-check principle in pediatric audiology. *Archives of Otolaryngology, 102,* 614–620.

Johnson, J. L., White, K. R., Widen, J. E., Gravel, J. S., James-Trychel, M., Kennalley, T., . . . Holstrum, J. (2005a). A multicenter evaluation of how many infants with permanent hearing loss pass a two-stage OAE/A-ABR newborn hearing screening protocol. *Pediatrics, 116,* 663–672.

Johnson, J. L., White, K. R., Widen, J. E., Gravel, J. S., Vohr, B. R., James, M., . . . Meyer, S. (2005b). A multisite study to examine the efficacy of the otoacoustic emission/automated auditory brainstem response newborn hearing screening protocol: Introduction and overview of the study. *American Journal of Audiology, 14,* S178–S185.

Joint Committee on Infant Hearing (JCIH). (2007). Year 2007 Position Statement: Principles and guidelines for early hearing detection and intervention programs. *Pediatrics, 120,* 898–921.

Liden, G., & Kankkunen, A. (1969). Visual reinforcement audiometry. *Acta Oto-Laryngologica, 67,* 281–292.

Ling, D. A., Ling, A. H., & Doehring, D. G. (1970). Stimulus response and observer variables in the auditory screening of newborn infants. *Journal of Speech and Hearing Research, 13,* 9–18.

Lowery, K. J., von Hapsburg, D., Plyler, E. L., & Johnstone, P. (2009). A comparison of video versus conventional visual reinforcement in 7- to 16-month-old infants. *Journal of Speech and Hearing Research, 52,* 723–731.

Madell, J. R. (2008). Using behavioral observation audiometry to evaluate hearing in infants from birth to 6 months. In J. R. Madell & C. Flexer (Eds), *Pediatric audiology: Diagnosis, technology, and management* (pp. 54–64). New York, NY: Thieme.

Moore, J. M., Thompson, G., & Folsom, R. C. (1992). Auditory responsiveness of premature infants utilizing visual reinforcement audiometry (VRA). *Ear and Hearing, 13,* 187–194.

Moore, J. M., Thompson, G., & Thompson, M. (1975). Auditory localization of infants as a function of reinforcement conditions. *Journal of Speech and Hearing Disorders, 40,* 29–34.

Moore, J. M, Wilson, W. R., & Thompson, G. (1977). Visual reinforcement of head-turn responses in infants under 12 months of age. *Journal of Speech and Hearing Disorders, 42,* 328–334.

Moran, M. (1995). *The role of lateralization in visual reinforcement audiometry.* Unpublished masters thesis. University of Kansas.

Muir, D., Abraham, W., Forbes, B., & Harris, L. (1979). The ontogenesis of an auditory localization response from birth to four months of age. *Canadian Journal of Psychology, 33,* 320–333.

Northern, J. L., & Downs, M. P. (1974, 1978, 1984, 1991). *Hearing in children* (1st, 2nd, 3rd, 4th eds.). Baltimore, MD: Williams & Wilkins.

Northern, J. L., & Downs, M. P. (2002). *Hearing in children* (5th ed.) Philadelphia, PA: Lippincott Williams & Wilkins.

Norton, S., Gorga, M., Widen, J., Folsom, R., Sininger, Y., Cone-Wesson, B., . . . Fletcher, K. (2000). Identification of neonatal hearing impairment: Evaluation of transient evoked otoacoustic emission, distortion product otoacoustic emission, and auditory brain stem response test performance. *Ear and Hearing, 21*, 508–528.

Nozza, R. J. (1987a). The binaural masking level difference in infants and adults: Developmental change in binaural hearing. *Infant Behavior and Development, 10*, 105–110.

Nozza, R. J. (1987b). Infant speech-sound discrimination testing: Effects of stimulus intensity and procedural model on measures of performance. *Journal of Acoustical Society of America, 81*, 1928–1939.

Nozza, R. J., Rossman, R. N., Bond, L. C., & Miller, S. L. (1990). Infant speech sound discrimination in noise. *Journal of Acoustical Society of America, 87*, 339–350.

Nozza, R. J., Wagner, E. F., Crandell, M. A. (1988). Binaural release from masking for a speech sound in infants, preschoolers and young children. *Journal of Speech and Hearing Research, 31*, 212–218.

Nozza, R. J., & Wilson, W. R. (1984). Masked and unmasked pure-tone thresholds of infants and adults: Development of auditory frequency selectivity and sensitivity. *Journal of Speech and Hearing Research, 27*, 613–622.

Olsho, L. W., Koch, E. G., Carter, E. A., Halpin, C. F., & Spetner, N. B. (1988). Pure-tone sensitivity of human infants. *Journal of Acoustical Society of America, 84*, 1316–1324.

Ontario Infant Assessment Program. (2008). *Audiologic assessment protocol.* Version 3.1. Retrieved January 28, 2010, from http://www.mountsinai.on.ca/care/infant-hearing-program/ihp

Primus, M. A. (1987). Response and reinforcement in operant audiometry. *Journal of Speech and Hearing Disorders, 52*, 294–299.

Primus, M. A. (1992a). Operant response in infants as a function of time interval following signal onset. *Journal of Speech and Hearing Research, 35*, 1422–1425.

Primus, M. A. (1992b). The role of localization in visual reinforcement audiometry. *Journal of Speech and Hearing Research, 35*, 1137–1141.

Primus, M. A., & Thompson, G. (1985). Response strength of young children in operant audiometry. *Journal of Speech and Hearing Research, 28*, 539–547.

Robbins, A. M., Svirsky, M., Osberger, M. J., & Pisoni, D. B. (1998). Beyond the audiogram: The role of functional assessments. In F. H. Bess (Ed.), *Children with hearing impairment: Contemporary trends* (pp. 105–116). Nashville, TN: Vanderbilt Bill Wilkerson Press.

Schmida, M. J., Peterson, H. J., & Tharpe, A. M. (2003). Visual reinforcement audiometry using digital video disc and conventional reinforcers. *American Journal of Audiology, 12*, 35–40.

Stapells, D. R., Gravel, J. S., & Martin, B. A. (1995). Thresholds for auditory brain stem responses to tones in notched noise from infants and young children with normal hearing or sensorineural hearing loss. *Ear and Hearing, 16*, 361–371.

Suzuki, T., & Ogiba, Y. (1961). Conditioned orientation reflex audiometry. *Archives of Otolaryngology, 74*, 192–198.

Talbott, C. B. (1987). A longitudinal study comparing responses of hearing-impaired infants to pure tones using visual reinforcement and play audiometry. *Ear and Hearing, 8*, 175–179.

Tharpe, A. M., & Ashmead, D. H. (1993). Computer simulation technique for assessing pediatric test protocols. *Journal of the American Academy of Audiology, 4*, 80–90.

Thompson, G., & Folsom, R. C. (1984). A comparison of two conditioning procedures in the use of visual reinforcement audiometry (VRA). *Journal of Speech and Hearing Disorders, 49*, 241–245.

Thompson, G., & Folsom, R. C. (1985). Reinforced and non-reinforced head-turn responses of infants as a function of stimulus bandwidth. *Ear and Hearing, 6*, 125–129.

Thompson, G., Thompson, M., & McCall, A. (1992). Strategies for increasing response behavior of one-and two-year-old children during visual reinforcement audiometry (VRA). *Ear and Hearing, 13*, 236–240.

Thompson, G., & Weber, B. (1974). Responses of infants and young children to behavior observation audiometry (BOA). *Journal of Speech and Hearing Disorders, 39*, 140–147.

Thompson, G., Wilson, W. R., & Moore, J. M. (1979). Application of visual reinforcement audiometry (VRA) to low-functioning children. *Journal of Speech and Hearing Disorders, 44*, 80–90.

Thompson, M., & Thompson, G. (1972). Response of infants and young children as a function of auditory stimuli and test methods. *Journal of Speech and Hearing Research, 15*, 699–707.

Thompson, M., Thompson, G., & Vethivelu, S. (1989). A comparison of audiometric test methods for 2-year-old children. *Journal of Speech and Hearing Research, 54*, 174–179.

Vander Werff, K. R., Prieve, B. A., & Georgantas, L. M. (2009). Infant air and bone conduction tone burst auditory brain stem responses for classification of hearing loss and the relationship to behavioral thresholds. *Ear and Hearing, 30*, 350–368.

Weber, B. A. (1969). Validation of observer judgments in behavioral observation audiometry. *Journal of Speech and Hearing Disorders, 34*, 350–355.

Widen, J. E. (1990). Behavioral screening of high-risk infants using visual reinforcement audiometry. *Seminars in Hearing, 11*, 342–356.

Widen, J. E. (1993). Adding objectivity to infant behavioral audiometry. *Ear and Hearing, 14*, 49–57.

Widen, J. E., Folsom, R. C., Cone-Wesson, B., Carty, L., Dunnell, J. J., Koebsell, K., . . . Norton, S. J. (2000). Identification of neonatal hearing impairment: Hearing status at 8–12 months corrected age using a visual reinforcement audiometry protocol. *Ear and Hearing, 21*, 471–487.

Widen, J. E., Johnson, J. L., White, K. R., Gravel, J. S., Vohr, B., James, M., . . .Meyer, S. (2005). A multisite study to examine the efficacy of the otoacoustic emission/automated auditory brainstem response newborn hearing screening protocol: Results of visual reinforcement audiometry. *American Journal of Audiology, 14*(2), S200–S216.

Wilson, W. R. (1978). Behavioral assessment of auditory function in infants. In F. D. Minifie & L. L. Lloyd (Eds.), *Communicative and cognitive abilities—Early behavioral asssessment* (pp. 37–59). Baltimore, MD: University Park Press.

Wilson, W. R., Lee, K., Owen, G., & Moore, J. M. (1976). *Instrumentation for operant infant auditory assessment*. Seattle, WA: Child Development and Mental Retardation Center.

Wilson, W. R., & Moore, J. M. (1978). *Pure-tone earphone thresholds of infants utilizing visual reinforcement audiometry (VRA)*. Paper presented at ASHA Convention, San Francisco, CA.

Wilson, W. R., Moore, J. M., & Thompson, G. (1976). *Sound-field auditory thresholds of infants utilizing visual reinforcement audiometry (VRA)*. Paper presented at ASHA Convention, Houston, TX.

Wilson, W. R., & Thompson, G. (1984). Behavioral audiometry. In J. Jerger (Ed.), *Pediatric audiology* (pp. 1–44). San Diego, CA: College-Hill Press.

Zimmerman-Phillips, S., Osberger, M. J., & Robbins, A. H. (1997). *Infant-Toddler: Meaningful Auditory Integration Scale (IT-MAIS)*. Indianapolis, Indiana University School of Medicine, Dept. of Otolaryngology-Head and Neck Surgery.

23

Behavioral Audiometry With Children

Allan O. Diefendorf

> *Experience gained in the field of audiology for children during its rapid development in the past few decades has made it clearly evident that auditory disorders in children require more differential diagnosis than was formerly considered necessary, and that the earlier this diagnosis is established the better. The pedagogic program that should be planned for the development of speech and put into effect from the first most formative years demands the detailed charting of the auditory range made possible by modern pure tone audiometry.*
>
> Bengt Barr, 1955, p. 5

Introduction

The importance of assessing hearing in children was recognized in 1928 when Alexander William Gordon (A.W.G.) Ewing advocated, "that the hearing of all children suspected of aphasia should be tested" (Ewing, 1930, p. 12). A.W.G. Ewing further recommended that reliable methods of testing young children's response to sound are needed in the diagnosis of congenital aphasia and of other forms of defects that call for speech therapy (Ewing, 1930). This emphasis on threshold audiometry challenged clinicians to pursue the goal of developing valid and reliable techniques with young children. As such, the application of classical conditioning and instrumental conditioning facilitated the development of pediatric audiology as a subspecialty of audiology. Conditioned techniques would be pursued over the next 30 years with both "objective" (psychogalvanic skin response [PSR] audiometry) and "subjective" (play audiometry) techniques evolving as approaches to hearing assessment in children.

Although other "objective" approaches (auditory evoked potentials, acoustic reflexes, evoked otoacoustic emissions) to hearing assessment have supplanted GSR audiometry, play audiometry and conventional audiometry with children have been (Barr, 1955; Dix & Hallpike, 1947; I. Ewing, 1943; Ewing & Ewing, 1944; O'Neill, Oyer, & Hillis, 1961; Shimizu & Nakamura, 1957; Statten & Wishart, 1956), and continue to be (Diefendorf, 2009), the most utilized behavioral techniques in audiology to monitor and verify the audiologic record of children's threshold responses to auditory stimuli.

This chapter aims to detail the application and outcomes of behavioral audiometry with children. To achieve this outcome, this chapter addresses those issues that directly influence operant behavior (i.e., instrumental [operant] conditioning and reinforcement) and those that exert a secondary influence on behavioral audiologic outcomes (e.g., acoustic and other environmental factors, procedural adaptations, and resourcefulness of audiologists).

Respondent Behavior

Behavior elicited by a stimulus is considered *respondent* behavior. Respondent behavior can be achieved through *classical* (or Pavlovian) *conditioning*, or through *instrumental* (or operant) *conditioning*.

Classical Conditioning

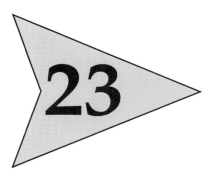

In the classical model, the response is *elicited* by the conditioned stimulus. The most familiar example of this paradigm is Pavlov's experiments in the 1880s in which he conditioned a dog to salivate at the sound of a bell. The bell initially is considered a neutral stimulus (NS), while food is considered the unconditioned stimulus (UCS). It is possible to transfer the power of an unconditioned stimulus to a neutral stimulus to elicit a conditioned response (salivation). That is, by pairing the sound of a bell with the presentation of food, Pavlov, after several trials, conditioned the dog to salivate in response to the bell. In classical conditioning, the neutral stimulus becomes the conditioned stimulus (NS→CS), and the unconditioned response becomes the conditioned response (UCR→CR). The power of the conditioned stimulus (the bell) to continue to elicit a conditioned response (salivation) diminishes over time through repeated trials unless the conditioned stimulus is restrengthened by occasional re-pairing with the unconditioned stimulus (food).

The application of the classical conditioning paradigm to the measurement of hearing in young children was achieved through the GSR technique (Bordley, Hardy, & Richter, 1948). In an attempt to measure hearing in young children, an auditory stimulus (neutral stimulus) and electric shock (unconditioned stimulus) are paired while measuring the amplitude and/or frequency of change in skin resistance (unconditioned response). In the initial trials of this procedure, the auditory stimulus is neutral and will not, of itself, elicit a response. However, after repeated trials, the response-eliciting power of the unconditioned stimulus (the electric shock) will be transferred to the neutral stimulus (the auditory stimulus). At this point, the neutral stimulus becomes the conditioned stimulus (NS→CS) and the resulting response (changes in skin resistance) becomes a conditioned response (UCR→CR). The GSR was used in the early evolution of pediatric audiology as an alternative to play audiometry for measuring hearing in children (Barr, 1955; O'Neill et al., 1961; Statten & Wishart, 1956). However, the GSR was phased out of use when it was clearly demonstrated that the audiometric results and outcomes with children were less accurate, more time consuming, and traumatic when compared to the use of instrumental (operant) conditioning techniques.

Instrumental (Operant) Conditioning

Operant behavior is frequently spoken of as willful or purposeful behavior. In the instrumental model, a behavioral response elicited by a stimulus is *controlled* by the consequences of the behavior. Skinner (1953) stated, "the term 'operant' emphasizes the fact that the behavior *operates* upon the environment to generate consequences" (p. 65).

It is convenient to approach the behavioral assessment of hearing in young children through an operant conditioning paradigm, specifically, through use of an operant discrimination procedure. In the operant conditioning paradigm, an auditory stimulus is introduced as a contingency to indicate the time interval during which an appropriate response will have a consequence. Thus, the auditory stimulus serves as a discriminative stimulus. In this paradigm, a response is defined as a single example of the appropriate behavior; an *operant* is defined as a range of responses that are controlled by their consequences. The consequence is an appropriately selected and appropriately applied reinforcement (Figure 23–1).

When a behavior generates a reinforcing consequence, there is an increased probability that similar behavior will reoccur. Operant behavior is increased or decreased in frequency by the changes it brings about in an organism's environment. The events in an environment may be classified as positive reinforcers, negative reinforcers, and neutral events. Neutral events have little or no specific effect on behavior. Depending on the application of negative or positive reinforcement, the response probability effect can be either increased or decreased (Table 23–1). In behavioral audiometry with children, behavioral responses (operants) are strengthened by positive reinforcement. This approach recognizes a view of young children as active receptors of auditory stimuli who, when given the opportunity, will interact with their auditory environment to control subsequent consequences.

Behavioral Audiometric Measurements

Behavioral audiometric measurements include those which require volitional responses on the part of the listener (responder). The traditional response in standard pure tone audiometry with children involves the raising of a finger or hand, or pressing a button. Furthermore, the instructions are usually presented orally. When the listener cannot understand verbal (oral) instructions, some modification in the form of demonstration or conditioning is employed. The former is commonly referred to as conventional pure tone audiometry. The latter modification employs some form of "play" activity (pegs in a board, stacking blocks, placing blocks in a can) in establishing the conditioned

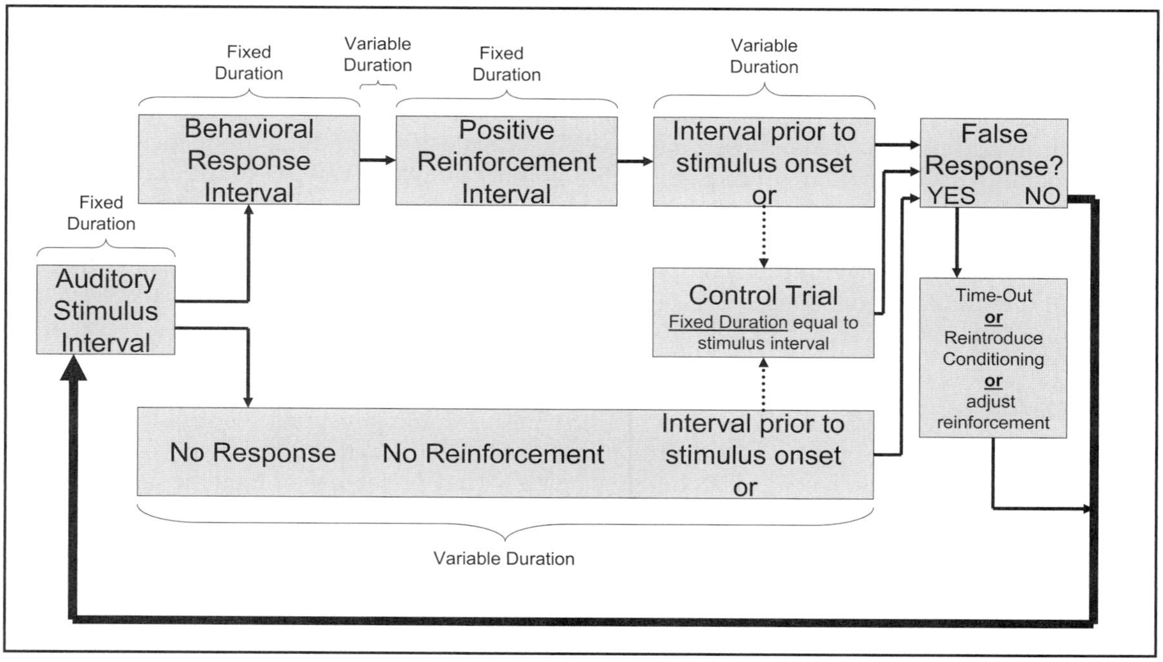

FIGURE 23–1. Required intervals in an operant discrimination procedure.

Table 23–1. Influence of Reinforcement on Operant Behavior

	Present	***Remove***
Positive Reinforcement	(Reinforcement) (Increases) Response Probability	(Punishment) (Decreases) Response Probability
Negative Reinforcement	(Punishment) (Decreases) Response Probability	(Reinforcement) (Increases) Response Probability

response. In the literature, this procedure is referred to as play audiometry.

Conventional and play audiometry are accomplished through the operant discrimination procedure. In the operant discrimination paradigm, the auditory stimulus is introduced as a contingency to indicate the time interval during which an appropriate response (finger or hand raising; a play activity) will have a consequence, that is, reinforcement. Operant behavior is strengthened by the application of positive reinforcement. Thus, it is possible to increase the rate of response when a positive reinforcer is identified and presented. As audible signals of the type used in assessing auditory function (pure tones) are known to have little reinforcing value in children, it is best to use a test procedure in which the signal and reinforcer are separate and the signal serves only to cue the youngster that a correct response will result in reinforcement.

Stages in Operant Conditioning

Multiple stages make up the process of an operant discrimination procedure. It is important to note from Figure 23–1 that in addition to the identified components of the operant discrimination procedure, each component (interval) is defined by a temporal duration. Thus, examiners who employ the operant discrimination paradigm must be familiar with each component of the process, the examiner's role in each component and the recommended time duration for each interval.

Auditory Stimulus

Reliable audiometric data depends on the degree to which the stimulus being used to test a child's hearing can be specified and controlled. Although familiar sounds such as speech or noise-band stimuli that are filtered may attract the attention of a child more so than pure tones, a pure tone is more easily specified in terms of its frequency and intensity calibration. The American National Standards Institute (ANSI) provides the explicit standards (ANSI, S3.6-2004) for the calibration of pure-tone stimuli.

Narrow bands of noise and filtered speech have been advocated as substitutes for pure tones in threshold assessment for difficult-to-test children and pediatric patients. However, if the child has a remnant of better hearing sensitivity, as is often seen in the lower test frequencies, there is a significant concern of underestimating the degree of hearing loss with broadband stimuli (Matkin, 1977a).

Studies by Stephens and Rintelmann (1978) have demonstrated some of the limitations associated with narrow bands as test stimuli. Their results indicated that, for individuals with sloping sensory-neural hearing losses, narrowband noise thresholds tended to underestimate the degree of high-frequency hearing loss by more than 20 dB as a result of side-band effects. Stephens and Rintelmann concluded that listeners with sloping audiometric contours probably were responding to energy adjacent to the test stimulus. That is, the individual's response was based on a perception of energy in the noise band that coincided with a frequency region where hearing was more sensitive than it was in the range presumed to be under test. The disparity between narrow band noise and pure-tone stimuli increased with the steepness of the slope. Similar differences did not exist between pure-tone and warble-tone stimuli. Orchik and Mosher (1975) stated that this disparity was dependent on the width of the narrow band and the rejection rate of the filter; the wider the noise band the more hearing was underestimated.

Additional and similar concerns have been expressed about speech-band stimuli. Surr, Seidman, Schwartz, and Mueller (1982) demonstrated that speech-band thresholds substantially underestimated the degree of hearing loss in the high frequencies for individuals with sloping audiometric configurations.

There are two alternatives to stimulus presentation methods: single-tone presentation (continuous mode) and pulsed-tone presentations (pulsed mode). Although little research data are available on differences in response behavior from children between these two modes, close observation on the part of the audiologist may facilitate which mode is most effective in maintaining stimulus-response control with children.

Some children can be categorized as "off responders." They prefer to wait until the stimulus has stopped prior to completing the task. For these children, utilizing a continuous tone can often assist them in feeling more confident in responding because there is a definite "off" to the signal.

The major consideration for controlling the stimulus, regardless of mode, is the duration of the stimulus itself. The stimulus should be activated for at least two seconds and should remain on for no more than four seconds. Thompson, Thompson, and Vethivelu (1989) have demonstrated the effectiveness of a two-second duration signal with young children engaged in play audiometry. In either presentation mode, latency factors help to validate a response; if the response occurs too early or too late it is unacceptable.

In the operant discrimination paradigm, the auditory stimulus serves as a contingency to indicate that an appropriate response will have a consequence. That is, in operant conditioning theory the discriminative stimulus (auditory signal) serves only to cue the availability of reinforcement. Thus, it follows that the nature of the auditory stimulus should have no effect on response behavior. In the operant discrimination paradigm, the reinforcement of appropriate behavior is the key to maintaining response behavior. When reinforcement is appropriately selected for the child under study, the discriminative stimulus (the pure tone) is only serving to cue the child that a conditioned response will result in reinforcement. Therefore, in conventional and play audiometry techniques with children, a pure tone stimulus, presented in either continuous or pulsed mode for a minimum of two seconds and a maximum of four seconds, is considered the optimal discriminative stimulus.

Behavioral Response

Selecting an appropriate response for children is critical to the success of conventional and play audiometry. A selected behavior must be clearly defined as the behavioral response and the criteria limits of that behavior must be established. The response definition must explicitly differentiate the behavior from other random behavior. Additionally, the motor response must easily facilitate the procedure of operant conditioning and responding. If the physical demands are too great, the task will distract the child from maintaining a listening posture. If the task is too simple, the child will have less motivation to participate and will tire of the task.

In conventional audiometry the response may be selected from finger-raising, to hand-raising, to button-pushing depending on the comfort level and physical capabilities of the child to easily comply with the selected response behavior. In play audiometry, the response may be selected from toys geared to different developmental ages: plain blocks for building a tower to a more simplified placing (throwing) of blocks into a bucket. Graduated ring towers have been utilized in play audiometry, as well as peg boards with colored pegs. Putting together simple puzzles also may be selected as a response, as long as the number of puzzle pieces does not compromise the latency of response behavior.

Usually, a single task requiring a motor behavior to complete the response is sufficient to complete the acquisition of an audiogram. However, audiologists must be ready to switch to another play activity at the first sign of boredom. The learning of play-conditioning techniques starts at 2 years of age. Hodgson (1985) observed however, "for successful play audiometry with a 2-year-old, an exceptional child (and audiologist) is required." Northern and Downs (2002) commented, "one should not be deceived by the bright, talkative 2-year-old who appears certain to be able to learn the procedure" (p. 183). That is, great care needs to be taken when differentiating "skill at completing the motor response" from "developmentally appropriate behavior and consistency within the operant conditioning paradigm."

In conventional and play audiometry, a response is defined as performance of the desired motor behavior within three seconds after stimulus onset of the auditory signal, and no later than 4 seconds after stimulus onset. The rigorous definition of response latency (3- to 4- seconds after stimulus onset) is to minimize false response behavior accepted as true response behavior. By comparing the response behavior during the stimulus interval with response behavior during a control trial (see Figure 23–1), audiologists engage in a systematic protocol of comparing response behavior between the two intervals, leading to a quantification of false response behavior.

Reinforcement

Careful examination of Table 23–1 is important in understanding the concepts of reinforcement and punishment. Response probability can be increased by either a positive reinforcement (presenting a desired consequence when the required response is completed) or negative reinforcement (removing an undesired consequence when the required response is completed). Additionally, response probability can be decreased by either of two punishment procedures: presenting an undesired consequence for completion of a required response; or removing a desired consequence for completion of a required response. It is important to understand the distinction between presenting and removing consequenting stimuli on response behavior/probability.

Decreasing unwanted behavior by removing the opportunity for receiving a desired stimulus is called *time-out*. Time-out is an effective punishment procedure for decreasing response probability. For example, if an unwanted behavior (false responding) from a child results in a delay (time-out) in the opportunity to receive positive reinforcement, the child will decrease the frequency of the unwanted behavior.

Because of a long-standing commitment to human/patient rights and to protecting patients through informed decision-making, positive reinforcement procedures are preferred to increase response behavior, and the removal of a desired consequence (time out) is the preferred punishment to decrease unwanted behaviors. In conventional and play audiometry procedures both positive reinforcement and time-out (punishment) are employed to shape and control response behavior (see Figure 23–1).

Many different types of reinforcement have been used with children during play audiometry. Dix and Hallpike (1947) introduced the "peep show" procedure where pictures were illuminated following a correct button-press response. Statten and Wishart (1956) adapted the peep-show idea of showing pictures by constructing a "movie screen" within an attractively colored doll's house. Rather than using single pictures, they used a color movie projector to show familiar animals and scenes from a farm. For young children who were frightened by the activity of a movie, Statten and Wishart also used a slide projector to show colored still pictures. Shimizu and Nakamura (1957) also adapted their picture reinforcement from the peep-show idea. Their concern about the peep-show was that children must look at a picture in a box through a peephole; under Shimizu and Nakamura's technique, "no such complicated equipment is necessary and the children can enjoy the lantern slides in an easy and free posture"

(p. 395). Miller (1963) also used slides as positive reinforcement. However, Miller recommended slide sets that tell a story as opposed to unrelated pictures. The Pediacoumeter is similar in principle to the peep-show. The basic difference is that instead of being rewarded for response to sound by a peep-show, the child may see any one of seven jack-in-the-box figures emerge from the testing apparatus (Guilford & Haug, 1952).

A common form of positive reinforcement used for young children is verbal praise ("that's good"; "good listening") and/or social reinforcement (pat-on-the-back; a smile and nod of the head; applause). Verbal praise and social reinforcement must be delivered naturally and meaningfully so that the child under test embraces this "consequenting event" as positive reinforcement. If not viewed as positive reinforcement, the child eventually will become disinterested in the response behavior. In addition to verbal praise and social reinforcement, other forms of reinforcement have been suggested with children. Tokens that can be traded for small toys or stickers at the end of the test session, unsweetened cereal, or a changing computer display screen, all have been used successfully with play audiometry.

Importantly, play audiometry is not difficult to implement, but its successful application demands certain personal characteristics in the examiner. Examiners must be interested in children, comfortable with their actions and behavior, and able to relate to them well when delivering verbal praise and/or social reinforcement.

Reinforcement Schedules

In general, a 100% reinforcement schedule (reinforcement for every correct response) results in more rapid conditioning, yet more rapid habituation. Conversely, an intermittent reinforcement schedule produces slower conditioning but also a slower rate of habituation. Consequently, most clinicians recommend a protocol that begins with a 100% reinforcement schedule and then gradually shifts to an intermittent reinforcement schedule.

Intermittent reinforcement may be a fixed-ratio schedule, in which the child is required to complete a predetermined number of behavioral responses to receive reinforcement. Or reinforcement may be delivered on a variable-ratio schedule, in which the child receives reinforcement for a continuously varying number of responses. Certainly, the child's developmental level, motivation, enthusiasm, boredom, indifference, and shyness must be considered in presenting an appropriate schedule of reinforcement.

Reinforcement should be withheld when clinicians are uncertain about reinforcing delayed or ambiguous behavioral responses. The risk of reinforcing a false response is that it may lead to confusion for a child under stimulus control. Failure to reinforce a correct response, however, does not degrade performance. In this situation, withholding reinforcement is viewed as intermittent reinforcement, which will not interfere with subsequent behavioral responses.

Interval Between Response and Reinforcement

Reinforcement is time-related. That is, reinforcement should be presented immediately upon completion of the desired behavioral response. Delays in reinforcement may suggest to the child that more than a single response is necessary to receive reinforcement. In turn, this behavior will increase false responding if the child receives reinforcement after an additional response has been initiated.

Conditioning Operant Behavior

In the event a child cannot understand verbal (oral) instructions, some modification generally in the form of demonstration or conditioning is required. That is, children must be taught to perform the motor task (e.g., building a block tower; placing colored rings on a spindle; putting pegs in a pegboard) that represents the defined response behavior. Conditioning then, refers to the process of training or shaping the response behavior.

The audiologist is responsible for getting the child into a proper ready state (listening while holding a ring or peg next to the ear) and for teaching the child to respond (placing the ring on spindle or putting the peg in the board) at the onset of the auditory stimulus. Response shaping is critical to the success of the operant procedure. Moreover, this phase of testing is completely under the examiner's control. Thus, the examiner must be skilled in interacting with children, and response training, delivering positive reinforcement, and familiar with the process of response acquisition.

Phase One of behavioral audiometry with children is the conditioning process which consists of auditory stimulus → behavioral response → presenting reinforcement. This description is accurate, but it minimizes the actual complexity of the process. In the operant paradigm, the auditory stimulus is introduced as a contingency to indicate the boundaries of the interval during which the response will result in reinforcement. The stimulus must be selected based on the acoustic characteristics for which the audiologist desires to obtain relevant audiometric information. Additionally, the stimulus must comply with an established signal duration, and meet the necessary calibration standards regardless of the signal transducer used. Individual circumstances in hearing assessment may dictate the use of various starting intensities. Typically, the most efficient test is one that uses a low starting level (e.g., 30-40 dB HL).

The behavioral response requires the examiner to teach and engage the child to perform a motor task in response to the auditory signal. The examiner may use both verbal instruction ("put it on" or "drop the block") and physical assistance (taking the child's hand and helping the child perform the desired motor task) to guide the child. The response must be deliberate, consistent with the child's motor skill, and time efficient. A response is defined as performance of the desired motor behavior within three to four seconds after the onset of the auditory stimulus. Immediately following the required response, positive reinforcement is presented to strengthen subsequent responses. Once again, the duration of reinforcement should be short, but effective.

A brief interval (see Figure 23–1) prior to a subsequent stimulus is essential to ready the child for the next trial. During this period, it is necessary for the child to sit quietly, listen carefully, and be prepared to respond quickly.

Following several training (conditioning) trials, probe trials are used to determine if conditioning has been established. It is generally accepted that if the child responds appropriately during probe trials (e.g., two times out of three stimulus presentations), conditioning criteria have been met. If a child fails to meet the conditioning criteria, additional conditioning trials are employed until the conditioning criterion is met. It is recommended that when additional conditioning trials are required to teach the response, the stimulus intensity is raised to ensure that the child hears the stimulus. Failure to condition rapidly should alert the examiner to a potential calibration or auditory problem or other important factors (physical, cognitive, social) that may affect the child's behavior. After repeated unsuccessful attempts to condition a child to what is considered an age-appropriate behavioral technique (conventional or play audiometry), it may be necessary and prudent to drop back to a more developmentally appropriate behavioral technique (e.g., visual reinforcement audiometry).

Children who meet the conditioning criterion move to Phase Two of the operant procedure, which is threshold exploration. Depending on response outcome during the test phase, signal intensity is either attenuated after every "yes" response or increased after every "no" response. An adaptive threshold search is initiated until a stopping criterion is met. For example, stimulus intensity is attenuated in 10 dB steps until the child makes the first "no" response to a signal trial. A "no" response is followed by an increase in signal (5 dB). A correct response is followed by a decrease in signal level. After a specific number of reversals, the threshold search has ended for that particular stimulus.

Interval Prior to Stimulus Onset

If a false response occurs during this interval, it may be necessary to implement time-out, reintroduce conditioning (depending on which phase of the operant procedure the examiner is engaged in), or adjust reinforcement. Responses during this interval (the nonauditory stimulus interval) should be consequated by time out (punishment by delaying opportunity for next auditory signal). This strategy provides differential consequation of the two intervals: auditory stimulus interval and nonauditory stimulus (interval prior to stimulus onset) interval. When it is demonstrated that the desired response occurs during the presentation of the auditory stimulus and does not occur at other times, the child is considered to be under "stimulus control." At this time in the operant procedure, two levels of control actually have been demonstrated. The level of reinforcement control has been demonstrated (the response is under control of the reinforcer and an effective reinforcer has been established) and the level of stimulus control has been demonstrated (the stimulus controls discriminative responding).

Control Trials

The "interval prior to stimulus onset" is almost always longer in duration than the "auditory stimulus interval." Thus, a direct comparison between responses observed during these two periods is unequated. Therefore, false positive responses must be monitored by control trials when assessing children's hearing. Both signal trials (signal presented) and control trials (no signal presented) occur during threshold estimation. Either trial initiates an observation interval of approximately four seconds during which behavioral responses are judged. If the required behavioral response occurs during, or just after a signal trial it is considered a correct detection, and reinforcement is presented. A behavioral response occurring during a control trial, however, is considered a false positive response. Control trials are interspersed within the operant discrimination procedure to examine systematically the child's false-alarm rate. That is, the presence or absence of false-positive responses during control trials allows the audiologist to calculate the percentage of false-positive responses. The assumption is that children will produce a comparable number of incorrect behavioral responses during both signal and control trials. Therefore, it is possible to estimate chance responding (false responses during signal trials) during stimulus trials by monitoring false response rate during control trials.

The purpose of the control trial is to assess the reliability of responses during behavioral audiometry. Test results on any child who reaches an unacceptable false response rate (greater than 25 to 30% is suggested) should be excluded or interpreted with caution. If the criterion for false response behavior is exceeded during conventional or play audiometry, audiologists should focus on four factors to rectify clinical outcomes: (1) reconditioning the desired behavioral response; (2) changing the desired behavioral response; (3) reconsidering the positive reinforcement utilized to maintain response behavior; and (4) increasing the duration of time-out as a form of punishment.

Behavioral Audiologic Outcomes

Barr (1955) and Thompson and Weber (1974) tested children between the ages of 2 and 6 years and 2 and 5 years, respectively by play audiometry and found that the percentage of success was directly related to age. When data between the two studies are compared based on similarities in subject demographics, conditioning procedures, and subject exclusion criteria, the outcomes are remarkably similar. In both studies, children age 3 years and older were successfully tested by play audiometry greater than 95% of the time. Thompson and Weber reported successful tests on 2½ to 3-year-olds 90% of the time, whereas Barr reported success 61% of the time. For the 2- to 2½-year-olds Thompson and Weber reported success 70% of the time, whereas Barr reported success 20% of the time. Differences between the two studies at the two age levels may be attributed to differences between the two studies relative to stimuli used, earphone (Barr) versus sound field testing (Thompson and Weber), and the use of one examiner (Barr) versus the use of two examiners (Thompson and Weber) during conditioning and threshold measurements. Both studies support the use of play audiometry with children at developmental ages of 3 years, and carefully selected children beginning at age 2 years. When 2-year-olds are proficient with play audiometry, they are more likely to provide more responses before habituation than they would if tested by visual reinforcement audiometry (Thompson, et al., 1989). However, visual reinforcement audiometry (VRA) has a greater likelihood of success as a test procedure in the sense that almost all typically developing 2-year-olds are certain to comply and learn the VRA procedure.

Eagles and Wishik (1961) demonstrated that in a sample public school system population conventional pure tone audiometry was successful down to at least 3 years of age. The total study sample consisted of 3,882 children ranging in age from 3 to 17 years. The significant points from this study included: (1) hearing sensitivity from 0 dB to 10 dB (corrected to current American National Standards Institute [ANSI], 2004, standards) for the frequencies 250 Hz through 8000 Hz, for the ages of children represented in the study; and (2) the auditory sensitivity in children below 6 years of age and as young as 2½ to 3 years of age is not different from older, school-age children.

Experience with play audiometry indicates that reliable responses can be obtained when auditory stimulus → response control has been established and response criterion is maintained. Results from a clinical study (Diefendorf, 1981) of 40 preschool children, aged 30 to 48 months, revealed thresholds at an audiometric level of 10 dB HL or better. These findings were in close agreement with other 4-year-old children (Gerwin & Glorig, 1974).

Additional Factors to Consider in Audiologic Assessment

Acoustic and Other Environmental Factors

Audiometric testing as part of an audiologic assessment must be done in a room free of high levels of ambient noise or intermittent noises (cafeteria noise, noise from a hallway, telephone, pagers). Importantly, the environment in which the test is to be carried out must be evaluated. ANSI S3.1-1999 (ANSI, 1999) provides criteria for permissible ambient noise during audiometric testing. ANSI S3.1-1999 provides acceptable ambient noise values for threshold estimation at 0 dB HL, for one- and third-octave bandwidths, for use with supra-aural and insert earphones, and for sound field and bone conduction testing.

In addition to controlling the acoustic aspects, the test environment also should be free of distracting visual stimulation. Young children easily can be distracted by items such as pictures on the walls, games stored in the test area, and equipment stored in the room. Test rooms free of distraction help children focus on the conditioning task and subsequent response behavior.

Prior to selecting the behavioral response activity and shaping stimulus-response behavior, it can be extremely helpful to position the child, if physically appropriate, in a student desk. The structure of the student desk assists the child in focusing on the task. If the child is enrolled in a school-based program, the desk may be a familiar reminder to pay attention and listen.

Procedural Adaptations

For some children, a period of pre-play may be advisable to help comfort the child within a new environment, put the child at ease with unfamiliar faces, and to see to which toys the child may be naturally drawn. Once a toy is identified, it becomes the selected motor response for use in play audiometry.

Initial training can often be most easily accomplished with the audiologist seated directly beside the child. Importantly, the audiologist must be in close proximity to the child and maintain direct eye contact. Occasionally, instructions and/or demonstrations may be facilitated by the mother, a sibling, or familiar caregiver. Use of pantomime, demonstration, and exaggerated gestures enhance teaching a child the desired task.

For some children, having the parent play an active role in the play audiometry task is often very helpful in encouraging the child's behavior. The parent may need to play the game to encourage the child's participation and to model the correct response. Occasionally, some children prefer to use their parent's hand to play the game. Additionally, the parent may need to alternate taking turns with the child until the child is more comfortable in the test situation.

When two audiologists are used during testing (one with the child, one operating the equipment from the control room), the audiologist with the child must be able to hear all stimuli presented either by wearing an auxiliary intercom earphone or by wearing the bone oscillator with simultaneous presentation to the child (earphone) and audiologist (bone oscillator). In two-person play audiometry, precise timing of the stimulus presentation and resultant response is essential. Presenting reinforcement for correct responses is facilitated when the audiologist in the exam room is aware of signal trials versus control trials.

Resourcefulness of the Audiologist

Play audiometry can be readily accomplished with only one examiner. The audiologist can position the child in a desk or chair next to the audiometer. All monitors and talkback microphones are turned off. The audiologist then manages the stimulus presentation, response and social reinforcement independently and with total control. Having the child and the audiologist in the same room gives the audiologist an even better sense of when the child is truly in a listening posture, the time intervals for the stimulus presentation, the intensity level of the stimulus presentation, whether or not the response is reliable and consistent, and which responses should receive reinforcement.

Some children can certainly be categorized as "false responders." When confronted with false responders, the audiologist may place an open hand just in front of, or resting against the child's hand holding the response peg or block. The child then has to go around or through the audiologist's hand to complete the task once the sound is heard. This gentle visual and tactile reminder to wait is often sufficient to dramatically decrease a child's tendency to offer false positive responses.

Another difficulty encountered using play audiometry is the "reluctant responder." These children frequently wait until they are visually prompted to complete the task despite numerous training trials and reinforcement. In this event, the audiologist may want to identify if there is a definite facial response or reaction when the tone is presented. Some children look up at the audiologist for approval every time the tone is presented. The audiologist can then assist the child in completing the play task and watch for the child's reaction to the next stimulus.

For the child who is reluctant to respond, sometimes changing the game to something slightly more fun will be beneficial. If manual dexterity would suggest that placing a block in a large bucket might be the play activity of choice, then the play activity can be made more fun by moving the bucket away slightly and having the child "shoot a basket."

Speech Perception

Since the range of sounds important for functional hearing is represented by words, phrases, and sentences, tests utilizing speech stimuli are desirable for the evaluation of all children suspected of, and diagnosed with hearing loss. Determination can be made of the extent to which hearing loss affects the ability to perceive, recognize, and discriminate speech stimuli. Such information is useful both in the diagnosis of the type and degree of hearing loss, and in the approach to assessing the development of auditory skills and subsequent functional listening behavior.

Audiologists concerned with assessing speech perception skills in children must consider several variables, both internal and external. Internal or subject factors include the child's developmental age, vocabulary, language competency, and cognitive abilities. External factors include the designation of an appropriate response task, the effective utilization of reinforcement, and controlling the memory load inherent in the task that can influence test performance.

Efforts to develop materials for testing speech perception in children date back to the late 1940s. Haskins (1949) developed *phonetically balanced* (PB) word lists based on the receptive vocabulary skills of children in kindergarten (PB-K). As such, clinicians must exercise caution in administering the PB-K words to children under the age of 6 years (Matkin, 1977b) because of limitations in word vocabulary. Clearly, test items must be in the vocabularies of the children tested. If not, the PB-K scores may be depressed reflecting vocabulary deficits, language deficits, or both, as well as deficits in speech perception. Sanderson-Leepa and Rintelmann (1976) indicated that normal-hearing preschoolers at 3½ years of age yielded scores substantially lower on the PB-K words than did older children. Therefore, it is recommended that audiologists exercise caution in administering the PB-K test unless there is good assurance that the receptive vocabulary age of the child under test approaches at least that of a kindergarten-age child.

Verbal responses, as required by PB-K word presentation, may be limited not only by vocabulary deficits, but also by articulation deficits or lack of motivation. Yet, written responses on measures of speech perception are essentially out of the question for most young children. To bypass these problems and still test speech perception skills in children, picture discrimination tests may be used.

Ross and Lerman (1970) developed the Word Intelligibility by Picture Identification (WIPI) test which takes into consideration children who have restricted receptive vocabulary and cannot read. The WIPI test includes picture plates with six illustrations per plate. Four of the illustrations have words that rhyme, and the other two illustrations are presented as distractors to decrease the probability of a correct guess. The use of pictures rather than printed words adapts the test to those who cannot read.

Sanderson-Leepa and Rintelmann (1976) demonstrated that normal-hearing children at 3½ years of age manifest a significant number of errors on the WIPI test due to words not being in their recognition vocabulary. Thus, the use of WIPI materials is appropriate for those children with receptive vocabulary ages of 4 years and greater. Moreover, Ross and Lerman concluded that the WIPI test is suitable for children with moderate hearing losses from ages 5 or 6 years and for children with severe hearing losses from ages 7 or 8 years.

Hodgson (1973) investigated the relationship between the WIPI words used as an open-set and as a closed-set test for normal-hearing children. Open-set tests are those in which the subject theoretically has an unlimited number of response possibilities. Upon hearing the test item, no response alternatives are given and, therefore, the listener is free to make any response. Closed-set tests restrict the subject to one of a fixed number of possible responses (e.g., as in a multiple-choice test).

In the open-set version, children repeated the WIPI words. The closed-set version required the usual picture identification response task. Children also repeated the words of a PB-K list administered in the conventional open-set fashion. Although there was no reported difference between the intelligibility of the WIPI and PB-K words presented in the open-set format, use of the WIPI as a closed-set test improved the intelligibility scores by about 10%. Because the number of potential responses is limited, closed-set tests are easier and yield higher scores than open-set test procedures. Therefore, it is recommended that the audiologic record include intelligibility scores, the specific test materials used, and whether the test was presented in an open-set or closed-set format.

The Northwestern University Children's Perception of Speech (NU-CHIPS) test by Elliott and Katz (1980) was developed as a speech perception test appropriate for younger children, and as a test designed to utilize a closed-set, picture-pointing response. The test items are representative of the most frequently occurring phonemes of English, with the exception of initial /r/. Additionally, test materials are limited to monosyllabic words that are documented to be in the recognition vocabulary of children with normal hearing as young as 3 years of age.

Children with hearing loss and a receptive language of at least 2.6 years demonstrate familiarity with the words and pictures of NU-CHIPS. Children with language skills better than the target group for which NU-CHIPS was developed achieve higher scores on NU-CHIPS than on the WIPI test (Elliott & Katz, 1980). These findings are expected on the basis of the somewhat more difficult vocabulary on the WIPI test.

The development of the Pediatric Speech Intelligibility (PSI) monosyllabic word test by Jerger, Lewis, Hawkins, and Jerger (1980) was undertaken to create an instrument for use with children as young as 3 years of age. Initially, 30 monosyllabic words were chosen to represent an array of English phonemes in the initial and final positions. The responses to the 30 words by children sampled (normal hearing children ranging in ages from 3 to 7 years) did not differ as a function of chronologic age, vocabulary skill, or receptive language ability. However, for 20 words, a correct response was observed in more than 95% of the children. Thus, only those 20 words were selected for the PSI monosyllabic word test. The words are depicted on four response plates (five pictures per plate) in a closed-set format, and the child uses a picture-pointing response.

Finitzo-Hieber, Gerling, Matkin, and Cherow-Skalka (1980), investigated the use of familiar environmental sounds as an alternative to speech stimuli for assessing auditory perception skills in children with very limited verbal abilities who are not capable of discriminating verbal stimuli. A measure of sound effects recognition is a unique approach to using environmental sounds to measure auditory recognition and perception.

The Sound Effects Recognition Test (SERT) incorporates a closed-set format with a picture-pointing response. The SERT is composed of three equivalent sets, each containing 10 familiar environmental sounds (i.e., 30 different sounds, most of which are broadband in spectral content). The authors reported that by age 3 years, a child should be able to identify an average of 25 to 30 environmental test sounds. By the age of 5 years, a mean score of 29 of the 30 test sounds should be obtained.

The test contains four pictures on each of 10 response plates. Three of the pictures are foils, with one target item per page. The forms are equivalent in terms of item difficulty for children between the ages of 3 and 6½ years. The SERT may be too easy for a large number of children with hearing losses who have measurable speech recognition. However, the SERT should be considered when other tests using verbal materials are inappropriate.

Conventional yet dated measures of word recognition in children provide descriptive information about word recognition performance, but yield limited information about the nature of underlying perceptual mechanisms contributing to word recognition. As traditional measures have considered receptive vocabulary and word similarity, a more systematic approach to speech perception may be achieved by identifying targets with similar acoustic-phonetic patterns, and selecting targets that occur with different word frequency.

Lexical characteristics, such as word frequency (i.e., the frequency of occurrence of words in the language) and lexical similarity (i.e., the number of phonetically similar items), have been shown to affect the accuracy of spoken word recognition in listeners with normal hearing. A measure of lexical similarity is the number of phonetically similar words or "lexical neighbors" that differ by one phoneme from the target word (Greenberg & Jenkins, 1964; Landauer & Streeter, 1973). For example, the following words are all lexical neighbors of the target word *cat*: bat, cap, cut, and scat. Words that occur frequently and have few lexical neighbors are considered "easy" words and are identified with greater accuracy than words that occur less frequently and have many lexical neighbors (i.e., "hard" words; Cluff & Luce, 1990; Elliot, Clifton, & Servi, 1983; Luce, Pisoni, & Goldinger, 1990).

The Lexical Neighborhood Test (LNT) and the Multisyllabic Lexical Neighborhood Test (MLNT) were developed by Kirk, Pisoni, and Osberger (1995) to assess word recognition and lexical discrimination in children with hearing loss. A primary goal in the development of the LNT and MLNT was to select words that were likely to be within the vocabulary of children with profound hearing losses. An initial pool of potential words was identified that are produced by children between the ages of 3 and 5 years of age with normal hearing. From the database, "easy" and "hard" word lists were developed for both the LNT and MLNT based on word occurrence and lexical density.

The LNT contains two lists of "easy" and two lists of "hard" monosyllabic words, while the MLNT contains one "easy" list and one "hard" list of two-to three-syllable words. The tests use an open-set response format, and are scored as the percentage of words and phonemes correctly identified as a function of lexical difficulty.

Kirk et al. (1995) assessed a group of pediatric cochlear implant users on the LNT and MLNT and compared their performance with individual scores from the PB-K word test. Results for both the LNT and MLNT demonstrated that word recognition was significantly better on the "easy" lists than on the "hard" lists, indicating that pediatric cochlear implant users are sensitive to acoustic-phonetic similarities among words. Moreover, these data suggest these children with cochlear implant organize words into similarity neighborhoods in long-term memory, consistent with children who have normal hearing. Additionally, word recognition was significantly higher on the lexically controlled lists than on the PB-K. Only 30% of the words on the PB-K are contained within the original database of words used for constructing the LNT and MLNT word lists. A reasonable explanation of these findings may be that restrictions imposed by creating phonetically balanced word lists such as the PB-K word lists result in the selection of test items that are unfamiliar to children with hearing loss.

Conclusion

The importance of assessing hearing in young children has been recognized for over 80 years. Adherence to two principles has been consistent during that period: balancing physiologic and behavioral approaches to hearing assessment results in the most optimal audiologic outcomes; and utilizing age-appropriate (based on developmental age) test techniques with children fosters efficiency and accuracy in audiologic measurement.

Consistent with these two principles is the recognition that behavioral test outcomes provide the audiologist with data that reflect what children are actually "hearing." Therefore, the validity and reliability of behavioral test findings is of utmost importance. When principles of operant conditioning are maximized and when the operant discrimination protocol is applied to "hearing" assessment, audiometric data meet the high expectation of our patients, our health care colleagues, and our profession. Moreover, when operant principles are followed, the objectivity of our audiologic outcomes is quantified to the same level of "objective" precision achieved with our battery of physiologic measures.

References

American National Standards Institute. (1999). *Maximum permissible ambient noise for audiometric test rooms. ANSI S3.1-1999*. New York, NY: Author.

American National Standards Institute (ANSI). (2004). *About ANSI overview*. Available at: http://ansi.org/about.ansi/overview.aspx?menuid=1.

Barr, B. (1955). Pure tone audiometry for preschool children. *Acta Oto-Laryngologica Suppl., 121*, 5.

Bordley, J. E., Hardy, W. G., & Richter, C. P. (1948). Audiometry with use of galvanic skin-resistance response; Preliminary report. *Bulletin of Johns Hopkins Hospital, 82*, 569.

Cluff, M. S., & Luce, P. A. (1990). Similarity neighborhoods of spoken two-syllable words: Retroactive effects on multiple activation. *Journal of Experimental Psychology: Human Perception and Performance, 16*, 551–563.

Diefendorf, A. O. (1981). *The effect of a pre-play period on play audiometry*. Paper presented at the annual convention of the Tennessee Speech-Language-Hearing Association, April. Memphis, TN.

Diefendorf, A. O. (2009). Assessment of hearing loss in children. In J. Katz, L. Medwetsky, R. Burkard, & L. Hood (Eds.), *Handbook of clinical audiology* (6th ed., pp. 545–562). Baltimore, MD: Lippincott Williams & Wilkins.

Dix, M. R., & Hallpike, C. S. (1947). The Peep Show: A new technique for pure-tone audiometry in young children. *British Medical Journal, 2*, 719–723.

Eagles, E. L., & Wishik, S. M. (1961). A study of hearing in children. *Transactions of the American Academy of Ophthalmology and Otology, 65*, 261–282.

Elliot, L. L., Clifton, L. B., & Servi, D. G. (1983). Word frequency effects for a closed-set word identification task. *Audiology, 22*, 229–240.

Elliott, L. L., & Katz, D. (1980). *Development of a new children's test of speech discrimination* [Technical manual]. St. Louis, MO: Auditec.

Ewing, A. W. G. (1930). *Aphasia in children*. Oxford, UK: Oxford Medical.

Ewing, I. R. (1943). Deafness in infancy and early childhood. *Journal of Laryngology and Otology, 58*, 137–142.

Ewing, I. R., & Ewing, A. W. G. (1944). The ascertainment of deafness in infancy and early childhood. *Journal of Laryngology and Otology, 59*, 309–333.

Finitzo-Hieber, T., Gerling, I. J., Matkin, N. D., & Cherow-Skalka, E. (1980). A sound effects recognition test for the pediatric audiological evaluation. *Ear and Hearing, 1*(5), 271–276.

Gerwin, K. S., & Glorig, A. (Eds.). (1974). *Detection of hearing loss and ear disease in children*. Springfield, IL: Charles C. Thomas.

Greenberg, J. H., & Jenkins, J. J. (1964). Studies in the psychological correlates of the sound system of American English. *Word, 20*, 157–177.

Guilford, R., & Haug, O. (1952). Diagnsosis of deafness in the very young child. *American Medical Association Archives of Otolaryngology, 55*, 101–106.

Haskins, H. (1949). *A phonetically balanced test of speech discrimination for children*. Master's thesis, Northwestern University, Evanston, Illinois.

Hodgson, W. R. (1973). *A comparison of WIPI and PB-K discrimination test scores*. Paper presented at the ASHA Convention, Detroit, MI.

Hodgson, W. R. (1985). Testing infants and young children. In J. Katz (Ed.), *Handbook of clinical audiology* (3rd ed., pp. 642–663). Baltimore, MD: Williams and Wilkins.

Jerger, S., Lewis, S., Hawkins, J., & Jerger, J. (1980). Pediatric speech intelligibility test 1: Generation of test materials. *International Otorhinolaryngology, 2*, 217–230.

Kirk, K. I., Pisoni, D. B., & Osberger, M. J. (1995). Lexical effects on spoken word recognition by pediatric cochlear implant users. *Ear and Hearing, 16*, 470–481.

Landauer, T. K., & Streeter, L. A. (1973). Structural differences between common and rare words: Failure of equivalence assumptions for theories of word recognition. *Journal of Verbal Learning and Verbal Behavior, 12*, 119–131.

Luce, P. A., Pisoni, D. B., & Goldinger, S. D. (1990). Similarity neighborhoods of spoken words. In G. M. Altman (Ed.), *Cognitive models of speech processing: Psycholinguistic and computational perspectives*. Cambridge, MA: MIT Press.

Matkin, N. D. (1977a). Assessment of hearing sensitivity during the preschool years. In F. Bess (Ed.), *Childhood deafness: Causation, assessment and management* (pp. 127–134). New York, NY: Grune & Stratton.

Matkin, N. D. (1977b). Hearing aids for children. In W. Hodgson & P. Skinner (Eds.), *Hearing aid assessment and use in audiologic habilitation* (pp. 145–149). Baltimore, MD: Williams & Wilkins.

Miller, A. L. (1963). The use of slide projectors in pure tone audiometric testing. *Journal of Speech and Hearing Disorders, 28*, 94–96.

Northern, J. L., & Downs, M. P. (2002). *Hearing in children* (5th ed). Baltimore, MD: Lippincott Williams & Wilkins.

O'Neill, J., Oyer, H. J., & Hillis, J. W. (1961). Audiometric procedures used with children. *Journal of Speech and Hearing Disorders, 26*, 61–66.

Orchik, D. J., & Mosher, N. L. (1975). Narrow-band noise audiometry: Effects of filter slope. *Journal of the American Auditory Society, 1*, 50–53.

Ross, M., & Lerman, J. (1970). Picture identification test for hearing-impaired children. *Journal of Speech and Hearing Research, 13*, 44–53.

Sanderson-Leepa, M. E., & Rintelmann, W. F. (1976). Articulation function and test-retest performance of normal-learning children on three speech discrimination tests: WIPI, PBK50, and NU auditory test no. 6. *Journal of Speech and Hearing Disorders, 41*, 503–519.

Shimizu, H., & Nakamura, F. (1957). Pure-tone audiometry in children: Lantern-Slides Test. *Annals of Otology, Rhinology, and Laryngology, 66*, 392–398.

Skinner, B. B. (1953). *Science and human behavior*. New York, NY: Macmillan.

Statten, P., & Wishart, D. E. S. (1956). Pure-tone audiometry in young children: Psychogalvanic-skin resistance and peep-show. *Annals of Otology, Rhinology, and Laryngology, 65*, 511–534.

Stephens, M. M., & Rintelmann, W. F. (1978). The influence of audiometric configuration on pure-tones, warbled-tone and narrow-band noise thresholds of adults with sensorineural hearing losses. *Journal of the American Auditory Society, 3*, 221–226.

Surr, R. K., Seidman, J. H., Schwartz, D. M., & Mueller, H. G. (1982). Effects of audiometric configurations on speech-band thresholds in sensorineural hearing loss subjects. *Ear and Hearing, 3*(5), 246–250.

Thompson, G., & Weber, B. A. (1974). Responses of infants and young children to behavioral observation audiometry (BOA). *Journal of Speech and Hearing Disorders, 39*, 140–147.

Thompson, M. D., Thompson, G., & Vethivelu, S. (1989). A comparison of audiometric test thresholds for 2-year-old children. *Journal of Speech and Hearing Disorders, 54*, 174–179.

24

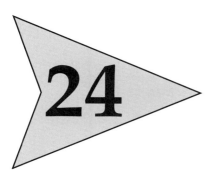

Putting It All Together: Assessment Protocols

Diane L. Sabo and Patti F. Martin

Introduction

Since the pioneering days of audiologist Marion Downs, audiology has benefited from advances in technology and the endeavors of other disciplines. Current initiatives in systems of care, health care policy, medical home, newborn screening, evidence-based practice and family-driven outcomes have enhanced both the "art" and the "science" of pediatric audiology.

A new paradigm in pediatric audiology has been suggested that conceptualizes diagnostic and management outcomes across three broad categories, including: (a) systems, (b) clinical, and (c) experiential considerations (Nicholson & Martin, 2009). As an example, within early hearing detection and intervention (EHDI) programs, a systems conceptualization focuses on the structure and organization of EHDI and highlights how the processes are operationalized. Clinical considerations form the "science" of service delivery, including evidence-based practices, protocol development and test selection, as well as individual professional competencies. Experiential aspects of the EHDI process include considerations such as cultural sensitivity, environment of care, and family-centered practices. Pediatric audiologists need to recognize the impact of these relational components, or potentially miss opportunities for improving outcomes and ensuring continuity of care and patient/family satisfaction. Positive outcomes result from understanding the multifaceted aspects of service delivery in pediatric audiology, as well as understanding the necessity of multidisciplinary care when hearing loss is identified in childhood. This chapter provides a comprehensive overview of pediatric audiology clinical assessment and management in the context of a systems approach that embraces culturally sensitive and family-centered care.

Systems Overview

Looking back 20 years the typical scenario for a family with a child with hearing loss would culminate with a diagnosis between the ages of 18 and 36 months. Parents would report an ever growing concern: "Robbie does not speak as well as the other children at his birthday party"; "I am frustrated that Lily doesn't pay attention when she is playing in the park and I call her"; "Dale isn't learning to talk as fast as his sister Jamie did, but our pediatrician said it's because he's a boy." Parents who expressed alarm when their children were very young often encountered an uphill battle to convince health care providers about the validity of their concerns and access appropriate services in a timely manner.

Fortunately, newborn hearing screening has changed this scenario, allowing families to be the beneficiaries of the implementation of EHDI systems of care. Beyond newborn hearing screening, EHDI encompasses diagnostic audiology, early intervention, family support, medical home, legislation, data management, program evaluation, and ongoing childhood screening (National Center for Hearing Assessment & Management [NCHAM], 2009). Benefits of this systems approach include: an increased public awareness of hearing and hearing loss; improved likelihood of parental follow-through; recognition by primary care physicians of the need to manage the referral process and respond to parental concerns; decreased age of identification; and awareness of options for families and development of family support networks. By design, EHDI systems should provide entry into a seamless system of care for children who are deaf/hard of hearing and their families, as well as lay a foundation for parental/self-efficacy, empowerment, and advocacy.

Furthermore, with the implementation of newborn hearing screening as a standard of care, the Centers for Disease Control (CDC) in the United States (U.S.) has established a timeline for determination of hearing sensitivity and implementation of intervention services. This time line is often referred to as the 1-3-6 plan: screening by 1 month of age, diagnosis by 3 months of age and initiation of intervention by 6 months of age, and it provides a benchmark for those working with this young population (CDC, 2009). As more audiologists develop the skills necessary to evaluate this population, the potential for a 1-2-3 plan is feasible, including diagnosis by 2 months of age and implementation of habilitation by 3 months of age.

> ***Parent Reaction to Newborn Hearing Screening Results***
>
> When we were on our way out of the hospital, after my husband had the car pulled around and I was on my way out the door, they said that our baby didn't pass her hearing exam and that I needed to take her to a specialist to make sure her hearing was fine. They said that since she was a C-section baby, she probably had fluid in her ear and that caused her to fail. When I got home with my baby, I thought "Surely she can hear, because she would be in her bassinet crying and I would walk up the stairs and into her room and I'd say, 'Mommy is here,' and before she could see me, she would start to quiet." I didn't realize at the time that she only felt the vibrations of my feet on the floor, and that's how she knew I was coming. She had us fooled for a good long while.
>
> —Parent

> ***Parent Advice***
>
> One of the most important things to remember is that time is so valuable. You don't have any time to waste. When they diagnose your child, you need to hit the ground running.
>
> —Parent

Clinical Considerations in Assessment

For pediatric assessment, the cross-check principle, originally developed by Jerger and Hayes (1976), serves to guide our test selection and interpretation. Use of the cross-check principle helps to minimize mistakes in diagnosis and develop an audiometric profile that best represents the child's auditory abilities. This principle relies on a combination of behavioral and physiologic tests to provide a comprehensive picture of hearing sensitivity and auditory status. Behavioral tests, although usually considered more subjective because of their reliance on patient participation, are combined with the results of objective physiologic tests that do not require active participation by the child or infant. At very young ages, or in the case of significant developmental delay, electrophysiologic test findings (e.g., auditory brainstem response [ABR]) often prevail in the initial decision making about the management of the child who is deaf or hard of hearing. As the child develops and can participate in behavioral testing, the behavioral findings serve to validate the electrophysiological findings, as well as document sequential development of auditory skills. For older children with developmental skills adequate for behavioral testing, audiologic findings with or without ABR are used to determine management of the hearing loss.

The pediatric audiologic evaluation, in comparison to the adult evaluation where hearing loss can be defined in one clinic visit, often requires repeated visits scheduled in close proximity before the exact configuration, degree, and sometimes nature of the hearing loss is defined. The audiologic assessment of children in general, but in particular for the very young infant with a hearing loss, is a time-intensive and ongoing process. Although a comprehensive audiometric profile is always the goal and is necessary before the hearing aid fitting process can be completed, reliable threshold estimates of sensitivity at critical frequencies can be used to initiate the amplification and habilitation process. Refinements and adjustments of the hearing aid fitting occur as more and more precise information is obtained. Delays in habilitation are not acceptable even when only partial audiologic information is available, and valuable time should not be wasted waiting for complete audiometric profiles. Diagnostic and habilitative management is an ongoing process with a young child who is deaf or hard of hearing and must be conveyed to parents in a manner that promotes their understanding and enlists their co-operation. For diagnostic testing, parents can be taught to understand what is involved and the number of sessions that it might take to obtain sufficient information. In addition, parents need to be informed from the start that the components necessary for optimal intervention in young children will entail a process of refinement, enhancement, and confirmation throughout early childhood.

What follows are brief descriptions of the behavioral and electrophysiologic tests that are appropriate for the young pediatric patient. The detail of these test methods can be found in the other chapters of this book. The intent of this chapter is to present the tests as they collectively contribute to the profile of a child's hearing. Using evidence-based protocols should be the basis of all audiologic evaluations. When working with children, adjustments during the test session are often necessary, and the adage "monitor and adjust" should be taken to heart. Most protocol modifications are driven by problems with maintaining the optimal condition needed to achieve the desired test results. Protocol modification is aimed at adjusting to the changing situation often encountered with children. For example, natural sleep for an ABR evaluation in infants may not last, an infant's reaction to sedation may not be as expected, or infant state during behavioral testing may not be maintained. Anticipating these possibilities ensures that the integrity of the evaluation session is not compromised and that adequate information can be obtained. One must be cognizant though of the impact that altering protocols has on test findings. The decision to modify a protocol requires quick thinking and is usually honed through experience and with a good understanding of the science behind the test methods.

Audiologic Assessment of Young Children

Typically, the selection of an appropriate assessment protocol is linked to a child's developmental age. Therefore, infants under 6 months developmental age need physiologic testing as the primary means of estimating threshold, due to their limited ability to participate in behavioral testing for threshold purposes. Although 6 months is the average developmental age when reliable behavioral test results can be obtained, physiologic testing is often also completed on children older than this to provide confirmation of hearing loss, to determine type of hearing loss, or to avoid repeated behavioral test sessions (Joint Committee Infant Hearing [JCIH], 2007).

Physiologic Measures

The physiological assessment of hearing for infants or young children can include either ABR, auditory steady state response (ASSR), or both. Currently, there is a paucity of literature on ASSR relative to the wealth of information on ABR, and ASSR has limited widespread use at this time. That being said, ASSR is being used in clinics, but often to supplement information obtained from tone-burst ABR.

Although the use of ABR and ASSR to estimate the audiogram has some limitations, the benefits far outweigh the limitations. The goal of ABR and ASSR with children is to determine ear- and frequency-specific information at 500, 1000, 2000, and 4000 Hz in

> ***Parent Reactions to Audiologic Evaluation***
>
> I remember looking at my sweet baby girl who looked so tiny on a big hospital bed with all those wires. I am a professional person who is comfortable with technology so I stared at the monitor with all these squiggles moving around on the screen trying to figure out what they meant and wondering what that had to do with how our baby could hear. Was she "doing good" on the test? Was it bad or good that it was taking so long?
>
> —Parent
>
> We live almost three hours away from the audiology center. My instructions were to keep Ben awake on the drive down so he would sleep through the test. Have you ever tried to drive to an unfamiliar place, miles away, with a 2-month-old in the back seat who is used to nursing on demand?
>
> —Parent
>
> The minute we walked through the front entrance with Grace Ann, it was apparent that we were in a place that knew about babies and families! Even though we had been to two other places about her hearing since she was born, and even though we were scared and nervous, my mom and I both felt like we had found the place that was going to help us get Grace Ann figured out. It was a huge relief.
>
> —Parent

order to responsibly fit amplification. Therefore, a prioritization of the sequence of the frequencies used during testing is necessary to proceed with amplification. Prioritization improves the efficiency of the testing situation, which is needed while testing infants in natural sleep or under sedation. The knowledge and skills required to obtain these responses quickly cannot be stressed enough to ensure a full understanding of the nature and extent of the hearing loss.

The optimal time to conduct an ABR or ASSR on a child is during sleep. Unfortunately, children will not sleep on demand and therefore, sedation will need to be considered. In a hospital setting, policy and procedure manuals might already delineate the sedation protocol, or consultation with an anesthesiologist can assist with proper protocol development. In a nonmedical setting, the recommended guidelines established by the American Academy of Pediatrics (2002, 2006) should be followed.

Factors such as the child's disposition, other health conditions, chronologic versus adjusted age, family travel time, wait time for appointment, and other practicalities all influence the need for sedation. However, patient safety takes priority over these practicalities. Protocols for sedation should be clearly stated with allowance for exceptions and mitigating circumstances evaluated on a case-by-case basis. For example, an infant with a 27-week gestation who is now 6 months chronologically should be considered to have a corrected age of 3 months and should not need to have sedation. On the other hand, for a 4-month-old infant who has waited two months for an evaluation and lives three hours away, arranging for sedation can help to minimize the number of visits that may be needed, as well as maximize the quantity and quality of the information obtained in one session. Having flexibility in meeting the family's and child's needs provides quality care, as well as sets the stage for a partnering relationship that can be beneficial for years to come.

Audiologists working with young children must bear in mind that auditory evoked potentials and behavioral tests provide information on different aspects of a child's auditory function and are used to complement, not substitute for, each other. That is, the ABR or ASSR cannot independently provide sufficient information essential for adequate decision-making about management of hearing loss (ASHA, 2004; Turner, 2003). Therefore, in keeping with the crosscheck principle, the evaluation also needs to include a thorough case history, acoustic immittance measures, and otoacoustic emissions measurements. At the end of this comprehensive diagnostic evaluation, information on the nature and extent of hearing loss will be used to determine habilitative and counseling needs, as well as additional referrals.

Otoacoustic emissions (OAEs) are sensitive to hearing loss and can be absent with as little as a 20 to 30 dB HL hearing loss. The absence of OAEs must be viewed within the context of the status of the middle ear as both the stimulus and the response pass through the middle ear. That is, the absence of an OAE is diagnostically significant for sensorineural hearing loss only when middle ear function is relatively normal. The presence of an OAE can rule out a conductive component as a mitigating issue. Therefore, acoustic immittance measures, using the appropriate probe tone, need to round out the battery of tests used to obtain an accurate picture of a young child's hearing abilities.

Ongoing monitoring for changes in middle ear status during early childhood is needed because of the high incidence of otitis media in young children. Even transient conductive hearing loss secondary to effusion impacts auditory access available to a child, and this is

Parent Reaction to Diagnosis

The lyrics to one of my favorite songs are, "Life is a roller coaster." I remember when our daughter was diagnosed at about 2 months old, but we didn't have her hearing aids yet. I didn't know if she was hearing me or not. And I remember thinking, "If she can't hear what I'm saying, then maybe she can feel it." So, I would lay her on her side with her ear up against my chest, so she could feel my heartbeat and my throat moving when I was singing or talking and I thought, "Okay, maybe she can get some of what I'm saying." For me, as a parent, that was a low point, because I didn't really understand much about hearing loss.

—Parent

Parent Response to Follow-Up

I just didn't understand why they kept repeating the same ol' test every time we went in. Obviously, Mikah was not going to pass it. Why didn't they do something different rather than keep having us come back time after time? In hindsight, it makes me mad that we lost a little bit of time there.

—Parent

particularly detrimental for children who are focused on communication development through auditory access.

Although acoustic immittance and otoacoustic emissions testing provides data necessary for completion of a child's hearing profile, it might not be necessary to obtain the results of those tests prior to obtaining evoked potentials or behavioral evaluation. Furthermore, the findings of one test do not always preclude conducting other tests in the battery. For example, a tympanogram that demonstrates reduced middle ear mobility should not prevent conducting the ABR. Delaying the ABR might not be necessary because abnormal middle ear function does not always predict the presence of conductive hearing loss, and bone-conduction ABR can determine the nature of the hearing loss. Likewise, the presence of an otoacoustic emission cannot ensure normal hearing across the frequency range (see Chapters 18 through 21 for detailed information about physiologic assessments in young children).

Case 1

Brandi was referred for an audiologic evaluation as follow-up to her newborn hearing screen that she did not pass. Brandi was seen at 7 weeks of age and her mother was instructed to keep her awake and wait to feed her until time for the ABR, which was being conducted during natural sleep. As with most babies, Brandi fell asleep in her car seat on the way to the hospital but did arrive quite hungry. After registering and filling out forms, Brandi and her mother were seated in a rocker/recliner where Brandi's mother proceeded to feed her while the audiologist prepared Brandi's skin for electrode placement. Four sites were cleaned, enabling two channel recording (Note that electrode placement is a practical consideration for bone-conduction testing. Electrodes cannot be placed on the mastoid when bone-conduction testing is being done because of the small mastoid area in children and the electromagnetic interference that can occur when the electrode is close to the bone vibrator. Moving the electrode off the mastoid to the earlobe or in front of the tragus in very young infants is necessary. Use of insert earphones permits placement of the bone vibrator and masking earphone on a small child's head, among other advantages).

After about 40 minutes, Brandi fell asleep in her mother's arms but could not be moved as she awakened each time her mother tried to put her into a crib. Therefore, testing was initiated with the mother holding her daughter. An insert earphone was inserted in only one ear as her other ear was against her mother. The testing was started with a 2000 Hz stimulus at 40 dB nHL, and no response was obtained. Intensity was increased to 70 dB and what was thought to be a response was obtained (replicated × 1). In order to verify the presence of a response at 70 dB nHL, the intensity was increased to 80 dB nHL, and two well-formed responses that were replicable were obtained. Two responses at 60 dB nHL yielded no response. The stimulus was then changed to a 500-Hz tone burst and testing was initiated at 80 dB nHL. A questionable (low amplitude) response was obtained at this level so the intensity was increased to 90 dB nHL where a clearer response was obtained. The stimulus was then dropped to 70 dB, where no response was observed. All response levels were replicated. Testing proceeded to 4000 Hz (responses at 90 dB nHL) and 1000 Hz (responses at 75 dB nHL) on the same side. Brandi awoke from her nap while attempting to reposition her for testing of the other ear. After attempting to have Brandi fall back to sleep without success, the ABR session was ended. Distortion product otoacoustic emissions (DPOAEs) from 1500 to 8000 Hz were obtained and showed no difference between the noise floor, which was low, and the emission amplitude, consistent with absent emissions for both ears. Tympanometry using a 1000-Hz probe tone was conducted and produced well-formed peaked tympanograms in both ears and absent 1000 Hz ipsilateral acoustic reflexes. Brandi's mother was given the test findings to date, showing a severe hearing loss of about 65 to 95 dB in at least the ear that was tested. Brandi's mother, while distressed with the news, scheduled a follow-up test for the following week, this time for a morning appointment as this was when Brandi takes her longer nap. Brandi's mother was encouraged to make an appointment with a pediatric otolaryngologist for a medical evaluation of the hearing loss and medical clearance to wear hearing aids.

Lessons learned: inform parents prior to the test session what is going to happen on the day of the appointment, and schedule appointments at times that coincide with the child's schedule.

The following week, Brandi, her mother, father, and grandmother (who was visiting from out of town) all came to the appointment. As Brandi's mother was aware of what was going to happen and the consequence of having her daughter awaken, she kept Brandi alert on the way to the hospital. The results for the second ear showed worse levels than for the ear previously tested (90 dB or greater) and no response to bone conduction click stimuli. Because hearing levels were a bit worse in the second ear tested, a quick check of the first ear was conducted to ensure that hearing was stable. Bone conduction testing using a click stimulus showed no response and tympanometric finding showed normal findings for a 1000-Hz probe tone. After completion of the audiologic assessment, the audiologist proceeded to explain the results of Brandi's evaluation. The details of the hearing loss were not even described before Brandi's grandmother expressed doubt, as no other family members have had hearing loss, and Brandi's dad wanted to know what could be done to correct the hearing loss. Brandi's mother just sat quietly, holding Brandi with tears in her eyes. The audiologist provided them with written materials to take home, explained the audiogram by plotting Brandi's hearing thresholds, told the family to return for earmold impressions, and instructed them to see their doctor for a hearing aid clearance before returning for the next appointment. The family's emotions ranged from shock to grief to denial, but were never acknowledged or addressed by the audiologist. Rather than follow the family's lead, the audiologist opted to pursue her preset agenda.

Lessons learned: These differing emotions are not uncommon as each family and each family member will bring their own thoughts, feelings, and reactions to the clinic. If the same "script" was used with each family, the individual family member's needs and the family unit's needs would not be addressed, ultimately impacting long-term outcomes for both the child and family.

Behavioral Assessment

Although behavioral observation audiometry (BOA) is not an acceptable approach for estimating hearing sensitivity in infants, observing an infant's behavioral responses to sound can provide useful information for audiologists. Early behavioral responses likely will not match the physiologic response levels, although they can provide baseline information on the child's listening skills and provide teaching opportunities. These teaching opportunities are for both the parent and clinician. The audiologist can help with the parents' understanding of how their child responds to sound, as well as to teach parents how to expand the child's listening range. For audiologists, it allows them to estimate where the child is in their hierarchy of developing listening skills. Learning to recognize auditory behaviors in young children provides the baseline from which auditory skill development can be monitored once amplification has been introduced. However, and importantly, BOA results should be interpreted cautiously with an understanding that the presence of unconditioned responses to auditory stimuli cannot be used to estimate hearing levels or predict speech and language development.

For children between about 6 and 24 months developmental age, the preferred behavioral test technique is visual reinforcement audiometry (VRA). Prior to the availability of insert earphones, VRA was often of limited use in the sound field, as it did not allow for determining hearing levels for each ear. That is, a child's ability to localize or not localize to a sound source when testing in the sound field cannot be used to predict hearing for each ear, as numerous variables affect localization ability. Use of earphones is the only way to determine ear-specific information, and today, best practice is to use insert earphones for VRA.

Because not all children will complete testing for both ears at all frequencies in one visit, the order of stimuli presentation should be prioritized to provide information about the degree and configuration of the hearing loss. This will maximize the quantity of information obtained during the test. Alternating between the presentation of a high- and low-frequency stimulus will yield an audiogram that provides some, if not all, information necessary to predict the contour of the audiogram and the impact on the audibility of speech, should the child stop responding before all of the frequencies have been tested. In the case of a severe-to-profound hearing loss, if there is a lack of responsiveness at higher frequencies, this should trigger the clinician to move quickly to a stimulus at 500 Hz or below to determine if there is residual hearing in the lower frequencies. In addition, when conditioning to tonal stimuli cannot be achieved, the use of a bone vibrator with a low frequency stimulus at high intensity levels should be attempted. If a child can be conditioned to the task with this technique, it validates the presence of a significant hearing loss. If the child cannot be conditioned with this technique, the implication is that the task is not appropriate for assessing hearing for that child.

Behavioral audiologic testing of the young child yields reliable results when proper procedures are followed during the test session (e.g., adequate conditioning, effective reinforcers, and booth arrangement). If the child is able to be conditioned, the child's maturational or developmental level does not influence the threshold level and thresholds obtained using VRA do not differ substantially from adults (Nozza, 1995; Olsho, Koch, Carter, Halpin, & Carter, 1987). That is, a decrease in threshold level is not observed with an increase in age, as long as conditioning is achieved (Wilson & Moore, 1978). Unlike unconditioned behavioral responses, VRA not only allows for assessment of threshold, but also provides information on the integrity of the auditory pathway and the child's ability to detect or discriminate auditory stimuli. Chapter 22 provides more detail about the VRA procedure.

For children between about 2 and 5 years developmental age, one can use conditioned play procedures for assessing hearing. These behavioral tests typically are accompanied by other physiologic measures such as OAEs and immittance testing. However, ABR or ASSR are not typically used with children in this age range unless one is attempting to determine etiology of hearing loss (e.g., auditory neuropathy) or behavioral testing is considered unreliable. Chapter 23 provides a thorough review of play audiometric techniques.

Experimental Components in Management

The identification of hearing loss in infants and young children is often the least challenging aspect of service delivery. The true challenges usually lie in the ongoing management and habilitation following confirmation of the hearing loss and addressing the concomitant impact on the family.

Historically, audiologists have been most comfortable in the role of diagnostician. With childhood hearing loss being identified at younger ages than ever before, audiologists who choose to work with children are required to rethink their roles and expand beyond that of only diagnostician. That is, they must broaden their repertoire of skills to meet the ongoing management and habilitative needs of children and their families. The pediatric audiologist's role is multifaceted (e.g., see ASHA document "Roles, Knowledge and Skills: Audiologists Providing Clinical Service to Infants and Young Children Birth to 5 Years of Age," 2006) and includes not only a focus on the hearing loss of the identified child, but on the impact and implications for the entire family.

Patient and family encounters form the crux of the relationship between the audiologist and families. Meeting the needs of families when they are perhaps at

Parent Reactions to Hearing Aids

I was so proud of our big girl the first time we went in the sound room. I could tell she was "listening" to the sounds, and even though I couldn't tell how loud they had to be for her to respond, I could tell she knew what she was supposed to do. It was an important milestone for us, and I put it in her baby book, just like the first time she rolled over and when she cut her first tooth.

—Parent

My dad was having a hard time believing that his first grandson needed to wear hearing aids. He had a complete turnaround after he went to an appointment with me and got to sit in the booth and watch Jarod respond—it was like he finally got it. It was such a load off my mind because it was one of those times in my adult life when I really needed my dad to be there for me, and inviting him to the audiology appointment did the trick. Now he is the proudest grandpa and has even learned how to use the Internet so he can help me figure everything out.

—Parent

Parent Realization

When they finally diagnosed her with a moderate to severe hearing loss, I was devastated. I watched my child whom I thought was so perfect playing on the floor, realizing for the first time that she wasn't hearing anything that was going on in the room.

—Parent

their most vulnerable remains an often elusive, occasionally daunting and ultimately rewarding challenge, even in the hands of the most seasoned audiologist. Management of hearing loss in children might be easier if it could be broken down into discreet steps beginning with counseling, moving onto the fitting of amplification, and finally referring for early intervention. In this simplified scenario, the audiologist would complete the tests, counsel the family on the "verdict" of the tests, assign a follow-up appointment and make the required referral to the state early intervention program. Although these steps are important, the overlap and interrelationship of each component cannot be discounted. To do so fails to recognize the role of management as a multifaceted, evolving process. In addition, discrete steps discount the ever-changing needs of families. In a more experiential-focused scenario, following confirmation of hearing loss, the primary responsibility of the audiologist becomes assisting the family in understanding the diagnosis and in the garnering and investigation of resources—physical, emotional and family-specific—in order to promote sound decision-making (Table 24–1).

The audiologist plays a large role in the management process and needs to understand the complexity of the family and their emotions and impressions. Families arrive for an initial audiology encounter, regardless of the age of the child, with a range of emotions that can include anxiety, fear, nonchalance, hope, and anger. In the waiting room of a busy pediatric practice, it would not be unusual to find parents of newborn twins stressed about arriving on time because even routines getting out of the house with one baby, much less two, are not yet well established. Another parent might have searched to find convenient parking, and then struggled to unlatch the infant from the car seat and transfer the baby into the stroller. An additional parent might have grabbed the hand of a sibling, thrown a purse or backpack and bulging baby bag over the shoulder, and then balanced the infant carrier with the other hand before ever getting to the front door. Emotionally, families of infants might be very apprehensive, as they have had little time to observe their child and form a solid opinion one way or the other as to whether they think their child can hear, or conversely, they might appear unconcerned or indif-

Table 24–1. Suggestions for Clinical Practice That Should Be Implemented as Quickly as Possible

1. There should be good and detailed information for parents, written in an easily accessible form.
2. Services should be well coordinated with clear procedures for exchange of information between different aspects of the services.
3. Parents should be treated as equal partners in the management of their child with hearing impairment.
4. It is important to involve the wider family (e.g., grandparents) in the audiologic management decisions.
5. Identification of children with permanent bilateral hearing impairment should be early and followed by fast and thorough audiologic assessment with the minimum of delays.
6. Hearing aid fitting should take place without delay and should be appropriate and guided by a prescription procedure.
7. Services should adopt appropriate service targets and should audit their performance against these targets on a regular basis.
8. Families of children with hearing impairments with complex needs require audiologic assessment that is sensitive to the implications of these complex needs.
9. Parents of children with hearing impairments should be involved in service planning and policy discussions.

From: Bamford, J., Davis, A., Hind, S., McCracken, W., and Reeve, K. (2000). Evidence on very early service delivery: What parents want and don't always get. In R. Seewald (Ed.), *A sound foundation through early amplification: Proceedings of an international conference* (p. 156). Stäfa, Switzerland: Phonak AG. Reprinted with permission.

ferent because a solid night of sleep has eluded them for many weeks.

The families' perceptions are formed from the moment a family enters the office or clinic—does the space look welcoming to children and families? Does the front desk staff convey competence and warmth? Are there helpful books and materials displayed? Is the check-in and registration process prompt? Are delays explained to the family? These and other external factor can influence not only a parent's initial impressions, but also the parent's confidence in the professionalism and competency of the audiologist. The initial introduction when the family first meets the audiologist lays the groundwork for building a trusting relationship that will be the cornerstone for effective counseling and collaboration. While it may not be possible or appropriate to bring the child's grandmother, the best friend, the favorite aunt, and the neighbor who drove the family to the appointment into the test area, attempting to include them in the process by acknowledging each of them and establishing their relationship to the child is a first step in establishing rapport with the family.

Even the most seasoned audiologist could feel less than confident when looking into the eyes of anxious family members when the time to convey the results of an evaluation session is at hand. Research shows that audiologists find themselves ill-prepared to deliver life-changing and generally unwelcomed news, although relatively recent changes in graduate education may help remedy this situation (English, Mendel, Rojeski, & Hornak, 1999; Martin, Barr, & Berstein, 1992; McCarthy, Culpepper, & Lucks, 1986). Informing a family that their child has a hearing loss is a serious undertaking and is more than information delivery. Rather, it places the audiologist in the position to offer a family the unique balance of facts and results with empathy and compassion.

Two aspects of counseling parents of children with newly diagnosed hearing loss include providing information as well as support, with the challenge of individualizing the right balance for each family. Although sharing information the family needs in order to understand the diagnosis is often of primary importance from the audiologist's point of view, this might not be what the family needs (e.g., see Harrison & Roush, 2001). The audiologist needs to acknowledge and respond to the complex array of emotions that the diagnosis may evoke. Parental reactions are not predictable, nor tied to the degree of hearing loss—parents of children who have milder degrees of hearing loss experience the same spectrum of emotions as parents of children with hearing in the severe-to-profound range (see Chapters 38 and 39 in this volume) (Table 24–2).

Families of infants who have had difficulties during the pre- or perinatal period or have other congenital conditions may be prepared emotionally to receive an unwelcome diagnosis or, conversely, the "latest" diagnosis of hearing loss may be the "straw that breaks the camel's back." Furthermore, as more than 90% of children who are deaf or hard of hearing are born to parents with typical hearing, most parents of young infants have not even considered the possibility that

Management Decisions

We had to travel to several different places in the United States to learn about different opinions—we were very confused as to what to do.

—Parent

The advice that I would give to new parents is to be strong advocates for your children. Never allow anybody to pigeonhole them. Each child is an individual child with his or her own gifts, and no one should ever, ever stereotype or put any roadblocks in his or her path because of a hearing loss.

—Parent

Another mom told me that the most important teacher for the child early on is the parent. So the parents need to educate themselves, and then they can educate their child. That was great advice and it's made all the difference for us with Haley.

—Parent

He's not even 1 now and so he is under one state program, but when he turns 3 he is no longer under the health co-op program, and they'll send him to something like a pre-school . . . I think . . . that's what I'm trying to still figure out myself. I'm not sure why it is so complicated for parents.

—Parent

I told my friends at church that we want the same thing for Dominic that they want for their children. We want him to be independent and do everything, to socialize, to be able to fit in and to always feel like he belongs.

—Parent

Table 24–2. Comparison of Priorities for Parents of Children With Mild-To-Moderate Hearing Loss, Parents of Children With Severe-To-Profound Hearing Loss, and Audiologists

Mild-to-Moderate	*Severe-to-Profound*	*Pediatric Audiologists*
Causes of hearing loss	Causes of hearing loss	Emotional aspects
Understand audiogram	Emotional aspects	Causes of hearing loss
Understand ear & hearing	Learn to listen and speak	Understand audiogram
Realistic timelines for learning to listen and speak	Understand ear and hearing	Understand ear and hearing
Emotional aspects		

Note: Data from Harrison, M., & Roush, J. (2001). Information for families with young deaf and hard of hearing children: Reports from parents and pediatric audiologists. In R. Seewald & J. Gravel (Eds.), *A sound foundation through early amplification 2001—Proceedings of the second international conference* (pp. 233–249). Stäfa, Switzerland: Phonak AG.

Case 2

Jackson, now 4 months of age, was referred by another audiologic facility after several rescreens were done and he continued to show no OAEs. The first rescreen (1 month of age) showed abnormal tympanometric findings, as well as absent emissions, and the primary care physician/practioner (PCP) treated him for middle ear effusion. The second rescreen (3 months) continued to show absent emissions but normal tympanometric findings (Note that the time delay occurred because of the lag time in appointments, as well as the treating of the middle ear condition. JCIH [2007] recommends that a diagnostic evaluation occur after the second failed screen).

The ABR showed bilateral mild sloping to moderate SNHL. DPOAEs showed no response, and tympanometric findings showed normal acoustic reflexes present at 500 Hz. The family expressed disbelief as Jackson seemed to react to most sounds around the home.

Much of the counseling session was used to help the family understand hearing loss and to simulate their child's hearing loss so that they could understand that their child does hear, but is not hearing all sounds normally. Jackson's family was instructed to see a pediatric otolaryngologist to obtain medical clearance to wear hearing aids, as well as to investigate the etiology of the hearing loss. Jackson was fitted with hearing aids from the state loaner hearing aid bank while the parents investigated financial options and procured payment of the hearing aids. Continued surveillance of the hearing loss occurred with behavioral testing every 3 to 4 months at the time of the making of new earmolds.

Lesson learned: In the United States, some states have hearing aid loaner banks, and some states offer different types of financial assistance for the purchase of hearing aids. Knowing how (even having necessary forms available) to obtain proper help can expedite the process of getting services for families.

their child's hearing status would be in question. Regardless, parents continue to report that they digest very little of what is said after hearing the words that their child has a hearing loss. They also report remembering how they felt about the person who delivered the news to them: "Our audiologist had taken the electrode wires off my baby and put her in my arms before she told me the news. I just remember being so glad that I could just hold her tight"; "She seemed very business-like, as if this was just another part of her day and something that was 'old hat' for her to do"; "The best thing our audiologist did was reassure me that I didn't have to 'get it' all today—and offer me some tissues!" Even parents of older children experience a grab bag of emotions—they may feel guilty, or alternately relief that their suspicions are confirmed, and a sense of helplessness or sadness over challenges in the future. Families value being told that having different emotions is not only "okay" but expected. Allowing families to talk about their thoughts or feelings, if they are comfortable doing so, is not as easy as it sounds for some audiologists. There can be silence from the parents, and silence can be hard to interpret. There can be anger, some of which can be directed toward the audiologist. There can be tears, and audiologists can devalue the emotions of the parent by offering well-meaning remarks, such as, "Everything will be OK" or "In this day and age, wearing a hearing aid is just like wearing a cell phone device!" Regardless of the truth that might be in these statements, parents need to feel comfortable showing and sharing their emotions, and audiologists need to feel comfortable allowing and acknowledging parental reactions. Allowing families to determine the direction of the conversation may be viewed by some audiologists as getting in the way of all the "important" information that needs to be shared, but following the lead of the parent increases understanding and acceptance, as well as builds partnerships and trust.

Because limited processing of information might occur on the day of the diagnosis, prioritizing and individualizing the informational needs for families helps bridge the gap from informational counseling to family support. Families do not need to understand everything explained to them on the day of diagnosis. A well-meaning audiologist might explain how we hear, how we plot hearing, how we measure hearing, funding sources, educational options, communications options, educational laws, how to navigate a different system, and so forth, when most parents retain very little of this type of information initially.

It is helpful to families to acknowledge that there will be many opportunities to share information about these topics through multiple mediums. Perhaps the main points parents might need to understand on the day of diagnosis includes what the child is able to hear or not hear when up close (e.g., held in their arms) or farther away (e.g., sitting on the floor or in the infant carrier), as well as whether or not the loss is permanent. Placing the diagnosis in functional terms can be helpful—"That means that Kayla can hear your voice when you talk to her if she is in your arms or on your lap, but may not recognize what she hears as speech if she is more than a few feet away from you"; "Even though Aaron has a very significant hearing loss, it is important that you continue to talk, talk, talk to him because he is able to pick up the tone, rhythm, and inflection of your voice, and that is so important for all babies"; "Because Deonte has better hearing in the left ear, try to position him in such a way that his 'good' ear is towards whoever is talking as much as possible." Understanding of the function of their child's hearing is important because initially parents might hear the term 'hearing loss' and assume 'deafness.' They do not have the knowledge yet to understand categorization of the hearing loss by degree, and practical examples can facilitate this process.

Working with infants and young children takes time. Karzon and Cho Lieu (2006) report that the average amount of time needed for a diagnostic evaluation, including adequate time for discussion with families, is approximately two hours. In addition to not bombarding them with information, it is important to make families feel comfortable and understand that they are the only priority for the moment.

After a diagnosis of hearing loss is made, the true work for the family and the audiologist begins. Although the steps involved in reaching a diagnosis may have been a major undertaking, this quickly takes a back seat to moving forward and preparing for the potential implications of the diagnosis on the family and the child's life. In the authors' experience, families want to know "what comes next?" and what they should "do" between the day of diagnosis and the next appointment. Recognizing and validating the tasks of the parent might include: discussing how to share the news with other family members and friends; considering broadly what outcomes they want for the infant; making contact with parent support networks; and/or investigating funding/insurance options for technology needs. Although audiologists often appropriately convey a sense of urgency for completing paper work for funding applications, investigating intervention options and other agencies or making prompt decisions on communication modalities, a word of caution is offered. Perhaps the greatest gift audiologists can give is reassurance to families that the most important job they have is to love and nurture their baby, focusing on the infant or toddler as a child first, who is not defined by tracings on a computer screen or Xs and Os on a chart.

The diagnosis of a permanent childhood hearing loss should trigger a series of specific steps. Audiologists should be familiar with legislation and mandates related to the identification of a hearing loss in a child. They should also understand the mechanics of notifying the state newborn hearing screening program, as well as the child's physician or primary care provider of the test results. Many primary care physicians will have had limited or no experience with a child who is deaf or hard of hearing, and making extra efforts to not only convey results, but also provide guidance and/or education on the implications should not be missed. Furthermore, in the United States, most states require referral to the appropriate early intervention agency within 48 hours of diagnosis, and informing families that they will be contacted within the next few weeks helps to avoid confusion. Additionally, considering what other referrals should be made may vary, but likely will include evaluations by a pediatric otolaryngologist, a geneticist, a speech-language pathologist, a pediatric ophthalmologist, or other professionals who can offer additional insights about the child and the hearing loss.

Information and support counseling cannot be conducted separately but are intertwined as the needs of the family can shift from session to session and over time. Believing and reinforcing the concept that parents and family members know the child best is not only a sign of respect, but is the initial step in helping families acquire self-advocacy and self-efficacy. Letting parents know that they are viewed as the "expert" for their child and that the audiologist wants to listen to their observations of and experiences with their child sends a powerful message and places them on equal footing with the "professionals." It may be helpful to provide a journal for them to keep notes about their observations of their child, as well as jot down questions and concerns to be covered at the next visit.

The reward for the hard work of the pediatric audiologist is in seeing the successful transition of the child to adolescence and adulthood and seeing a family who has helped to optimize their child's potential. It started with early identification of hearing loss from screening and continued through the accurate diagnosis of the hearing loss, the accuracy in fitting the hearing aid and good monitoring. But it was the ongoing support and effective counseling that set the stage for the family to be empowered and advocate for their child. Remembering the critical role that the pediatric audiologist plays in the family's journey with their child who has a hearing loss will keep us mindful of the knowledge, skills and expertise needed to be a pediatric audiologist. Although there are protocols and guidelines to help with diagnosis and management of hearing loss in children, just as in life, there is no recipe to follow that is foolproof. Having a solid foundation in the methodology and keeping in mind the child's needs coupled with a family-centered approach will help achieve success.

Case 3

Nevaeh was referred for an audiologic evaluation by her pediatrician at 18 months of age because she was not using any single words consistently. Nevaeh's mother was concerned but also felt that Nevaeh's older sibling was just talking for her. Nevaeh was seated in a high chair with her mother to the side and back of her, while an assistant with various distraction toys sat to the other side of her. Insert earphones were successfully inserted but even with the mother and the assistant helping, the insert earphones were pulled out numerous times with increasing agitation by Nevaeh with each reinsertion. Since reliable conditioning was not achieved with the insert earphones, sound field testing was attempted. Responses to speech stimuli were obtained at 25 dB. Some inconsistent responses to warbled pure tones and narrow bands of noise were observed, but Nevaeh's state was less than optimal for testing, even when she was taken out of the highchair and placed on her mother's lap. Testing in the booth was discontinued, and otoacoustic emission testing was attempted. Again, Nevaeh was agitated and successfully pulled out the probe and eventually testing was discontinued even though numerous distracters (bubbles, mirrors, video, and toys) were used to try to obtain a good state for testing. Tympanometry was successfully completed but acoustic reflexes could not be monitored due to too much movement.

Nevaeh was rescheduled for another day at the same time, as her mother said this was her best time of day. Over the next three months, numerous other attempts were made to obtain an audiogram by behavioral means with a mixture of results that ultimately did not any show consistency from session to session.

Lesson learned: Repeated testing that does not expand the audiometric profile or continues to yield inconsistencies is unacceptable because it may result in delay of diagnosis. Develop a strategy for return visits that includes a change in protocols, use of sedation, use of additional examiners, or referral to a regional center.

References

American Academy of Pediatrics. (2002). Committee on Drugs. Guidelines for monitoring and management of pediatric patients during and after sedation for diagnostic and therapeutic procedures: Addendum. *Pediatrics, 110*, 836–838.

American Academy of Pediatrics. (2006). American Academy of Pediatric Dentistry, Charles J. Coté, Stephen Wilson, the Working Group on Sedation for Diagnostic and Therapeutic Procedures: An Update. (2006). Guidelines for monitoring and management of pediatric patients during and after sedation. *Pediatrics, 118*, 2587–2602.

American Speech-Language-Hearing Association. (2004). *Guidelines for the audiologic assessment of children from birth to 5 years of age.* Retrieved Sept. 22, 2009, from http://www.asha.org/docs/html/GL2004-00002.html

American Speech-Language-Hearing Association (2006). *Roles, knowledge, and skills: Audiologists providing clinical services to infants and young children birth to 5 years of age.* Retrieved Sept. 22, 2009, from http://www.asha.org/docs/html/KS2006-00259.html

Bamford, J., Davis, A., Hind, S., McCracken, W., & Reeve, K. (2000). Evidence on very early service delivery: What parents want and don't always get. In R. Seewald (Ed.), *A sound foundation through early amplification: Proceedings of an international conference* (pp. 151–158). Stäfa, Switzerland: Phonak AG.

Centers for Disease Control and Prevention (CDC). (2009). *National EHDI goals.* Retrieved September 22, 2009, from www.cdc.gov/NCBDDD/EHDI/nationalgoals.htm

Coats, A., & Martin, J. (1977). Human auditory nerve action potentials and brainstem evoked responses: Effects of audiogram shape and lesion location. *Archives of Otolaryngology, 103*, 605–622.

English, K., Mendel, L. L., Rojeski, T., & Hornak, J. (1999) Counseling in audiology, or learning to listen: Pre- and post-measures from an audiology counseling course. *American Journal of Audiology, 8*(1), 34–39.

Harrison, M., & Roush, J. (2001). Information for families with young deaf and hard of hearing children: Reports from parents and pediatric audiologists. In R. Seewald & J. Gravel (Eds.), *A sound foundation through early amplification 2001—Proceedings of the second international conference* (pp. 233–249). Stäfa, Switzerland: Phonak AG.

Jerger, J., & Hayes, D. (1976). The cross-check principle in pediatric audiometry. *Archives of Otolaryngology, 102*, 614–620.

Joint Committee on Infant Hearing (JCIH). (2007). Year 2007 position statement: Principles and guidelines for early hearing detection and intervention programs. *Pediatrics, 120*, 898–921.

Karzon, R., & Cho Lieu, J. (2006). Initial audiologic assessment of infants referred from well baby, special care, and neonatal intensive care unit nurseries. *American Journal of Audiology, 15*, 14–24.

Martin, F. N., Barr, M. M., & Bernstein, M. (1992). Professional attitudes regarding counseling of hearing-impaired adults. *American Journal of Otology, 13*, 279–287.

McCarthy, P., Culpepper, B., & Lucks, L. (1986). Variability in counseling experiences and training among ESB-accredited programs. *ASHA, 28*, 49–52.

National Center for Hearing Assessment & Management (NCHAM). (2009). *National resource center for the implementation and improvement of comprehensive and effective early hearing detection and intervention (EHDI) systems.* Retrieved Sept 22, 2009, from: http://www.infanthearing.org

Nicholson, N., & Martin, P. (2009). *Diagnostic and management outcomes: A new paradigm in pediatric audiology.* Presentation at Neurotology Conference, University of Arkansas for Medical Sciences, Little Rock, AR.

Nozza, R. (1995). Estimating the contribution of nonsensory factors to infant-adult differences in behavioral thresholds. *Hearing Research, 91*, 72–78.

Olsho, L., Koch, E., Carter, E., Halpin, C., & Carter, E. (1987). An observer based psychoacoustic procedure for use with young infants. *Developmental Psychology, 23*, 627–641.

Turner, R. (2003). Double checking the cross-check principle. *American Journal of Audiology, 15*, 269–277.

Wilson, W., & Moore, J. (1978). *Pure-tone earphone thresholds of infants utilizing visual reinforcement audiometry (VRA).* Paper presented at the American Speech and Hearing Association Convention, San Francisco, CA.

VI

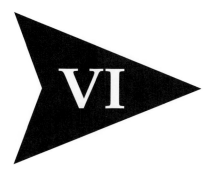

Hearing Technologies

25

Current Approaches to the Fitting of Amplification to Infants and Young Children

Marlene Bagatto and Susan Scollie

Introduction

Many infants and children who have hearing loss use hearing aids to hear spoken language, and this is often their primary mode of communication. Early hearing detection and intervention programs allow us to assist families with hearing aid fitting even during infancy. In this chapter, we will present current theories and practices that link hearing assessment to hearing aid fitting, with the goal of providing beneficial hearing aids to children of all ages.

Infants and young children bring unique qualities to hearing aid fitting, in at least three important ways. First, children who are born with hearing loss, or develop it early in life, have different listening needs from adults. In the context of universal hearing screening, a child's first hearing aid fittings may occur while in the process of learning speech and language during a critical period for the development of these skills (i.e., birth to 2 years of age). We therefore focus on providing full access to sound to support speech and language learning. Second, the ear canals of small children differ, acoustically, from those of the average adult and change as the child grows. We therefore focus on strategies to measure ear canal acoustics because they impact the level of sound delivered to the ear canal by the hearing aid. Finally, an infant or young child is dependent upon a parent or other caregiver for their hearing aid use, monitoring, and maintenance. We therefore focus on child-friendly, family-friendly, evidence-based techniques for pediatric hearing aid fitting, so that the caregiver's efforts to mediate hearing aid use are supported by a beneficial and comfortable fitting.

This chapter is organized into sections that follow *the first three* of the five sequential stages that clinical audiologists follow when providing hearing aids to infants and children. The fourth and fifth sequential stages are covered in subsequent chapters of this volume. These sections follow the framework originally suggested by the Pediatric Working Group (PWG) in 1996:

1. The *assessment* provides information about the degree and configuration of the hearing loss in each ear from which candidacy for amplification is determined.
2. During *selection*, numerical values for the electroacoustic performance of the hearing aids are calculated, and the physical attributes of the hearing aid (size, shape, coupling to the ear) are chosen. A particular make and model of device (and typically, a custom earmold) is specified that meets both the electroacoustic and physical requirements.
3. *Verification* of the hearing aids is conducted to ensure that the desired electroacoustic performance is achieved.
4. In the *information and instruction* stage, hearing aid orientation is provided and hearing aid use is monitored.
5. *Outcome evaluation* occurs in the final stage where the child's aided auditory performance is assessed and compared with habilitative goals.

Each stage of this process provides feedback to previous and subsequent stages. This allows clinicians to continuously monitor the patient in a systematic way (Figure 25–1).

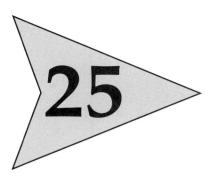

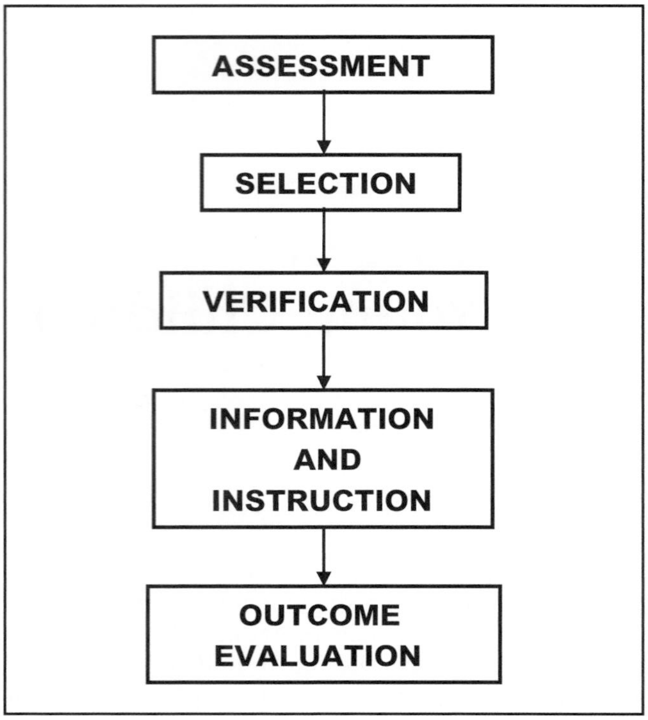

FIGURE 25–1. The five sequential stages involved in providing hearing aids to infants and children with hearing loss as suggested by the Pediatric Working Group (1996).

Assessment

Before we can determine whether a child is a candidate for hearing aids, we need a clear description of the child's hearing status in each ear. Therefore, audiological assessment precedes determination of hearing aid candidacy for patients of all ages. At the assessment stage, two variables affect directly the hearing aid prescription: (1) hearing thresholds and (2) ear canal acoustics. In the following sections, we review current knowledge of assessment considerations for infants or children who are possible hearing aid candidates. We also provide clinical strategies for ensuring that complete and valid assessment data are available for accurate pediatric hearing aid fittings.

Hearing Assessment in Infants and Young Children

A description of the degree, configuration and type of hearing loss for each ear is necessary prior to proceeding with hearing aid fitting in young patients (American Speech Language Hearing Association [ASHA], 2004; Joint Committee on Infant Hearing [JCIH], 2007; Pediatric Working Group [PWG], 1996). Proceeding with amplification before these factors are known can result in improper assessment of candidacy and/or improper hearing aid recommendations, such as hearing aid provision rather than medical referral for medically treatable conductive hearing loss, or binaural amplification for monaural hearing loss (Gravel, 2002). Complete audiometric assessment is therefore an essential first step, including estimation of thresholds with air- and bone-conducted stimuli for *at least* two frequencies per ear, along with case history, otoscopic examination, immittance measures and diagnostic otoacoustic emissions. When a clear audiologic picture is available, hearing aid candidacy evaluation and hearing aid prescription can begin. We refer the reader to Chapters 18 through 24 of this text for detailed information on hearing assessment in infants and children.

Clinical Application: Using Electrophysiologic Threshold Estimates for Hearing Aid Fitting in Early Infancy

In order to facilitate early assessment and intervention, electrophysiologic estimates of hearing sensitivity may be used as part of a complete audiologic test battery. These tests may come from the auditory brainstem response (ABR) or the auditory steady state response (ASSR) in combination with ABR (see Chapter 20). Either approach can support the provision of hearing aids in early infancy.

The ABR may be measured for brief yet frequency-specific stimuli, allowing the results from frequency-specific ABR (FS-ABR) to be used as the basis for infant hearing aid fitting. Threshold estimates from FS-ABR have been shown to be highly correlated with behavioral thresholds, both for infants with normal hearing and with hearing loss (Gorga, Kaminski, Beauchaine, & Bergman, 1993; Stapells, 2000a; Stapells, Gravel, & Martin, 1995). However, FS-ABR threshold estimates overestimate the behavioral audiogram by five to 30 dB across frequencies, depending upon the patient's age and the calibration and stimulus parameters used. Some FS-ABR and ASSR procedures include this factor in their calibration (Gorga et al., 1993; Stapells, Herdman, Small, Dimitrijevic, & Hatton, 2005). Other FS-ABR procedures require correction of this overestimation prior to hearing aid prescription or fitting (Bagatto et al., 2005; Stapells, 2000b). As FS-ABR threshold estimates (nHL) are typically *higher* than behavioral thresholds (HL), the correction is *subtracted* from the nHL value

dB nHL – correction = dB eHL

FIGURE 25–2. A frequency-specific correction is subtracted from the threshold estimation, in dB nHL, obtained from the ABR system. The result is a dB eHL value that better predicts a behavioral threshold and denotes that the ABR (nHL) value has been corrected.

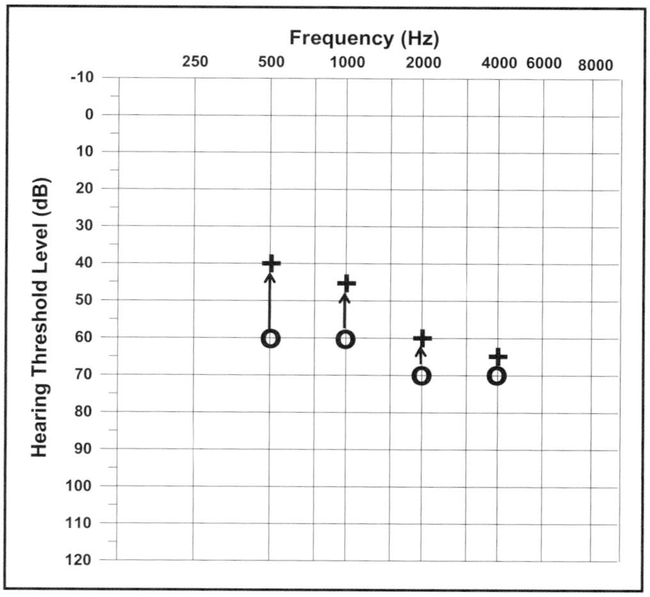

FIGURE 25–3. Correcting ABR threshold estimations in nHL to an estimated behavioral threshold in eHL. The circles (o) represent the nHL values obtained from the ABR system. The plus signs (+) represent the corrected ABR values that are now referenced in eHL.

to estimate behavioral thresholds (eHL; Figure 25–2). This correction process is important for hearing aid prescription, because the prescribed targets will be too high (i.e., require too much gain in the hearing aid) if the corrections are inadvertently omitted. This could occur, for example, if one clinician conducts the FS-ABR evaluation and another prescribes the hearing aid, yet neither corrects the FS-ABR results to eHL. We recommend that correction protocols be in place to ensure that corrections are applied once, *and only once*. Otherwise, substantial over- or underamplification may occur.

The correction values are frequency-specific and are generally larger in the low frequencies than in the high frequencies (Stapells, 2000a; Stapells et al., 1995; Bagatto et al., 2005). Clinics that follow Stapells' calibration and stimulus parameters (see http://www.audiospeech.ubc.ca/haplab) may use the following correction values: 20 dB at 500 Hz, 15 dB at 1000 Hz, 10 dB at 2000 Hz, and 5 dB at 4000 Hz. Figure 25–3 shows an example of applying these corrections to the results of an FS-ABR assessment. This FS-ABR correction approach is incorporated within the Desired Sensation Level (DSL®) Method for hearing aid prescription and fitting (Bagatto et al., 2005; Scollie et al., 2005).

Clinical Application: Obtaining Ear-Specific Thresholds in Behavioral Audiometry

In hearing assessments of infants and children, we place a high priority on obtaining ear-specific thresholds. For example, if using visual reinforcement audiometry (VRA) or conditioned play audiometry (CPA), we can obtain ear-specific thresholds under headphones or insert earphones. Insert earphones typically are preferred for their lighter weight and improved attenuation of sound from the room and between ears (ASHA, 2004). Some clinicians report difficulty in having young children accept insert earphones during hearing assessment, or that the insert earphones fall out of child's ears during the VRA procedures. Erber (1973) suggested that a child's own button receiver earmold could be used during audiometry, within procedures for obtaining in situ estimates of thresholds in real-ear sound pressure level (SPL). Today, we maintain this general philosophy, by coupling the child's behind-the-ear (BTE) earmold to insert earphones during VRA, CPA, or standard audiometry (Moodie & Moodie, 2004). In our experience, this unusual but helpful step permits better acceptance and retention of the insert earphones (Bagatto & Moodie, 2007). This approach may facilitate early assessment and intervention, by supporting the measurement of ear-specific behavioral thresholds earlier and more consistently. A few clinical tips can help when using this strategy. First, clipping the insert earphones to the back of the child's shirt can help to keep the tubing and transducers out of view and reach. Second, if the BTE earhook has stretched the earmold tubing, the insert earphone may not couple well to the earmold. In these cases, a small amount of thin tubing from a standard insert earphone foam tip may be temporarily attached to the insert earphone, permitting a tight seal to the earmold. An example of this strategy is shown in Figure 25–4. Third, the use of a custom earmold is not the standard coupling type for insert earphone calibration. Therefore, the use of individualized HL to SPL transforms (discussed below) is

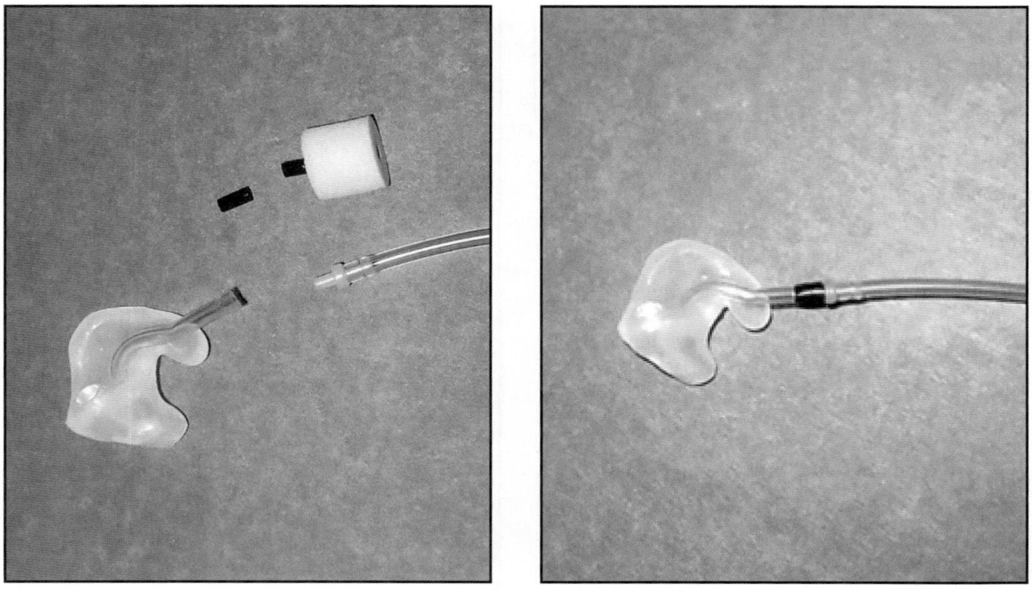

A B

FIGURE 25–4. A technique for securely connecting an insert earphone to an earmold. **A.** A small portion is cut from the tubing of an insert earphone foam tip. **B.** The tubing is connected to the tip of the insert earphone and then inserted into the earmold tubing.

of interest, to convert the resulting thresholds to either real-ear SPL or equivalent adult HL. Both scales have earmold acoustics removed in their calculations, allowing accurate comparisons to normative data over time.

Individual Ear Canal Acoustics

Accounting for the individual child's ear canal acoustics is the next step in improving the accuracy of pediatric hearing aid fitting. This affects both the assessment results and the hearing aid prescription and fitting. Individual ear canal acoustics vary by as much as 36 dB SPL, even in adults (Valente, Potts, Valente, Vass, & Goebel, 1994). Studies with children have shown a similarly large range of individual variability within and across age groups (Bagatto, Scollie, Seewald, Moodie, & Hoover, 2002; Feigin, Kopun, Stelmachowicz, & Gorga, 1989; Lewis & Stelmachowicz, 1993). To summarize, individual children of the same age vary substantially in their individual ear canal acoustics. Also, a given child's ear canal acoustics will change significantly over time as the ears grow and develop (Kruger, 1987). In general, smaller ear canal volumes are associated with larger resonant peaks in the ear canal's response, and these peaks may occur at higher frequencies. Larger ear canal resonances associated with smaller volumes have been demonstrated in the literature for both infants and children, with values generally maturing when the pinna reaches adult size, at around age 5 or 6 years. The next section defines three clinical measurements of external ear canal acoustics, and review their normative properties in the pediatric population.

Clinical Measurements of External Ear Canal Acoustics

Three clinical measurements of external ear canal acoustics are available to capture the effects of individual ear canal acoustics in audiometry and/or hearing aid fitting. These are the real-ear unaided gain (REUG), the real-ear-to-coupler difference (RECD), and the real-ear-to-dial difference (REDD; ANSI S3.46, 2007; Mueller, 2001). The REUG is a derived measurement of the acoustic response of the *unoccluded ear canal,* with a characteristic 17 dB resonant peak that occurs just below 3000 Hz in the average adult (Shaw & Vaillancourt, 1985). Individual REUGs vary considerably from one another, particularly when the ear canal volume is small or the middle ear system is either stiff or flaccid. REUGs from young infants tend to peak at a higher frequency (up to 6000 Hz) and reach adult values by two years of age (Kruger, 1987); see Figure 25–5A.

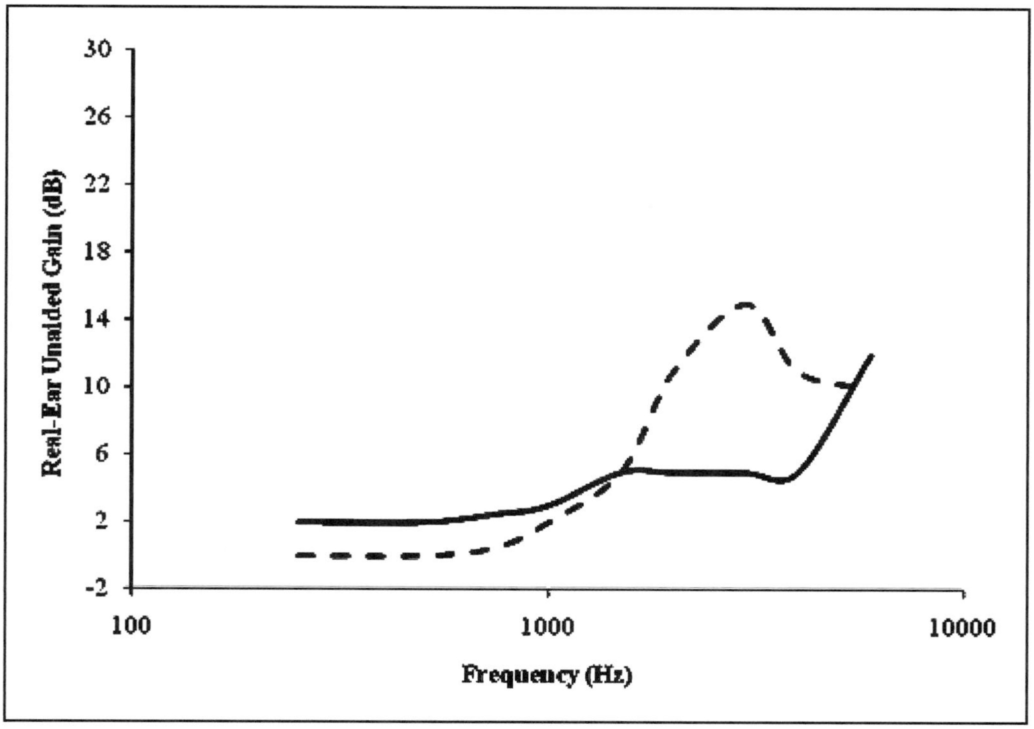

A

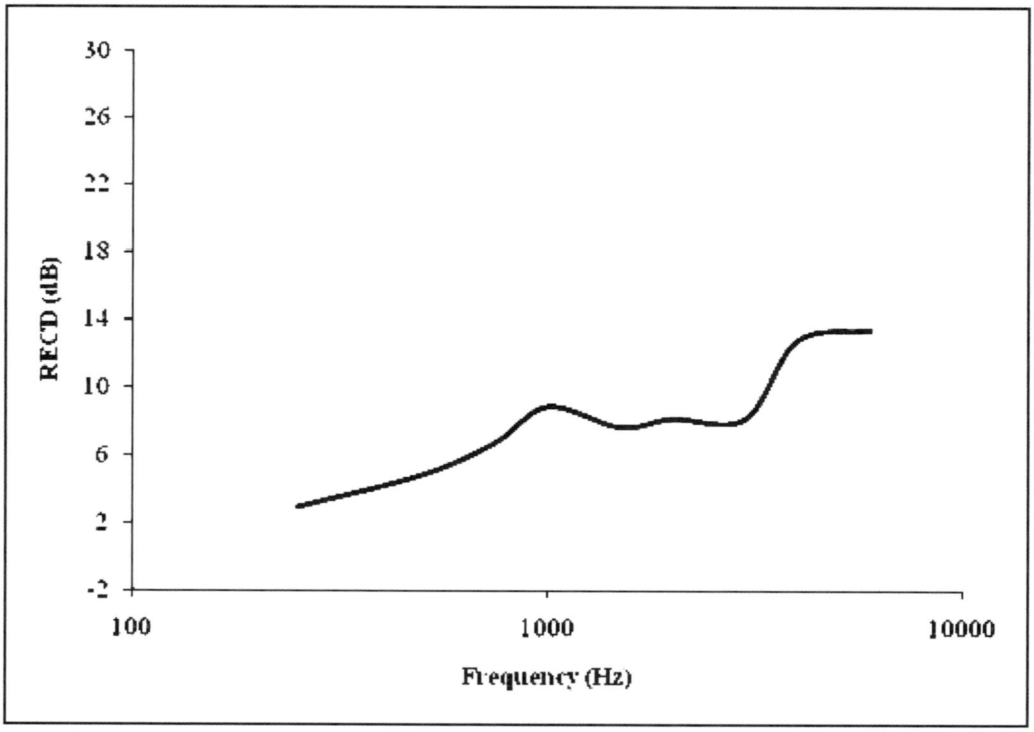

B

FIGURES 25–5. Examples of real-ear measurements. **A.** Real-ear unaided gain (REUG) across frequency for an infant (*solid line*) and an adult (*dashed line*). **B.** Real-ear-to-coupler difference (RECD) for an infant across frequency.

Finally, the REUG varies with signal azimuth: the average adult REUG peaks at a higher frequency when the source signal is to the side rather than to the front of the listener. In fact, this important variation provides one of the primary cues for localization of sound.

The RECD and REDD are measures of the acoustic response of the *occluded ear canal*. The RECD is measured with an insert earphone transducer, coupled either to a standard audiometric eartip or to the hearing aid wearer's earmold, and is referenced to the 2-cc coupler. The RECD is the *difference* between the real-ear SPL of a signal from the insert earphone transducer and the SPL of the same signal measured in a 2-cc coupler, across frequency. Typically, RECD values are positive and increase with increasing frequency (Figure 25–5B). Early investigations of age-related differences in the RECD demonstrated that pediatric RECDs were significantly higher than average adult RECDs, likely due to the smaller volume of the child's ear canal (Feigin et al., 1989). Test-retest reliability of the RECD is good, ranging from 0-2 dB in adults (Munro & Davis, 2003; Sinclair et al., 1996) to 1 to 4 dB in infants and children (Sinclair et al., 1996; Tharpe, Sladen, Huta, & Rothpletz, 2001).

In theory, the REDD could be measured as a comparison of the ear canal levels to those in a 6-cc coupler, rather than a 2-cc coupler. If this measurement was clinically feasible, it could serve a function as an audiometric transform for use with TDH headphones (discussed in detail in the next section). However, clinics do not typically have a 6-cc coupler. Therefore, the REDD was developed as an alternative measure of individual ear canal acoustics as they occur under TDH headphones. The REDD is the difference between the real-ear SPL produced by the audiometer and TDH phones and the dial level that produced it.

A key component of real-ear measurements is proper placement of the probe tube microphone in the child's ear canal. The goal is to place the probe tube far enough in the ear canal to represent the high frequencies accurately while avoiding standing waves. Placing the probe tube to within 5 mm of the eardrum is the typical clinical guideline (Dirks & Kincaid, 1987; Moodie, Seewald, & Sinclair, 1994). Although there are several methods for ensuring placement of the probe tube to the appropriate depth in the ear canal, a constant insertion depth strategy has been shown to be less time consuming and avoids contact with the tympanic membrane (Tharpe et al., 2001), which is preferred when working with the pediatric population. When measuring the RECD, different techniques can be used for young infants versus older infants and children.

For young infants, align the probe tube along the bottom of the earmold so the medial end of the tube extends 3 mm beyond the sound bore, and mark the tube on the portion of the earmold corresponding to the intertragal notch (Figure 25–6A). With young infants, it is often helpful to couple the probe tube to the foam eartip or earmold with plastic wrap or soft surgical tape (Figure 25–6B). This technique is helpful in coordinating insertion and ensuring a constant length of the probe tube remains at the tip edge, especially for active toddlers and very young infants with small ear canals (Bagatto, Seewald, Scollie, & Tharpe, 2006). The combined earmold/probe tube assembly is then inserted into the ear for the real-ear portion of the RECD measurement. Prior to the measurement, otoscopy is necessary to ensure that the ear canal is clear of debris. During the measurement, visual distraction of the infant (if awake) is often helpful.

For older infants and young children, the earmold can also be used as a guide. Align the probe tube along the bottom of the earmold so the medial end of the tube extends 5 mm beyond the sound bore and mark the tube on the portion corresponding to the intertragal notch (see Figure 25–6A). General insertion depth guidelines are 20 to 25 mm for children, with the mark meeting the intertragal notch (Moodie et al., 1994). The child's earmold is lubricated and inserted into the ear, taking care not to move the probe tube, and the real-ear portion of the RECD is measured. During probe insertion and measurement, the child is allowed to watch in a mirror or play with an engaging toy (Figure 25–6C).

Effects of the External Ear on Audiometry

The section above defined the REUG, RECD, and REDD as three different measures of individual ear canal resonance. All of these transforms vary across individuals, and some vary with development due to ear growth. This development has an impact on audiometry. Specifically, if the patient's hearing thresholds are stable, the real-ear SPL at threshold will remain the same across subsequent hearing tests. However, as the external ear grows, the HL required to generate a given real-ear SPL level will increase. Therefore, it is important to consider the impact of changing ear canal acoustics when comparing hearing assessment results at different ages for the same child. This issue occurs whether the assessment results were obtained using electrophysiologic or behavioral techniques. Two methods exist for addressing this issue: (1) conversion of audiometric data from HL to real-ear SPL; and (2) conversion of audiometric data from observed HL to equivalent adult HL.

Regardless of which method is used, understanding the corrections requires a review of how audiometric calibration relates to the HL values obtained during audiometry. Audiometric calibration sets the levels

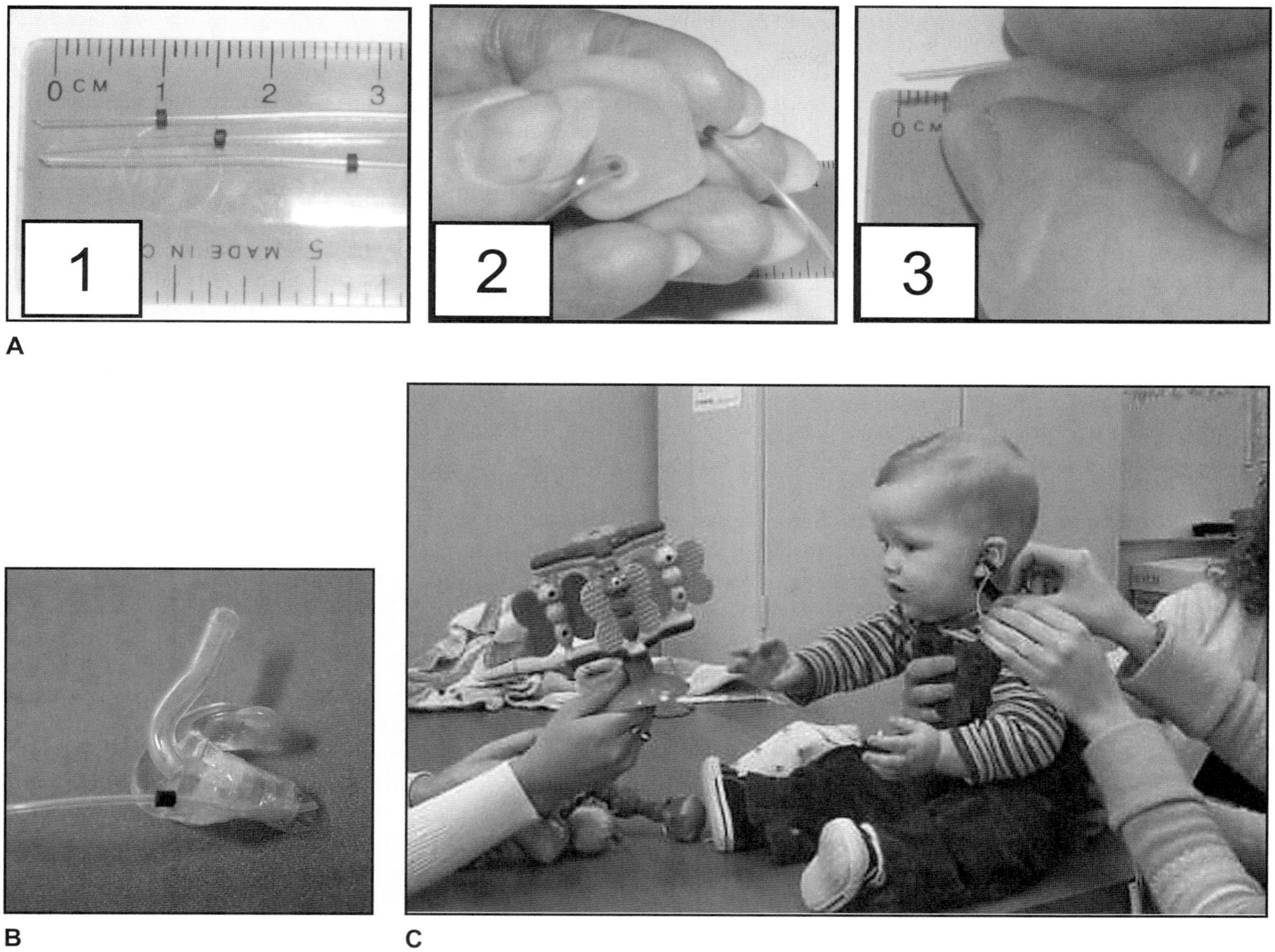

FIGURE 25–6. Customized probe tube insertion depth. **A.** (1) A constant insertion depth can be marked by using a ruler and following suggested insertion depth guidelines. (2) Or, lay the probe tube microphone along the bottom of the earmold. (3) Ensure the end of the tube extends a few millimeters beyond the sound bore and mark the tube at the point corresponding to the intertragal notch. **B.** Attach the probe tube to the earmold with plastic wrap (*shown here*) or soft surgical tape for simultaneous insertion during RECD measures. **C.** Keep the child engaged during probe tube insertion.

from each audiometric transducer so that a level of 0 dB HL approximates the normal threshold of hearing. These levels are the reference equivalent threshold sound pressure levels (RETSPLs) specified for each audiometric transducer (ANSI S3.6, 2004). The RETSPL values are defined by studies of the average normal hearing *adult* population, and are often defined in a fixed test location (i.e., 6-cc coupler for TDH phones, 2-cc coupler for insert earphones and sound field for loudspeakers). Therefore, for any value of HL we can compute precisely the 6-cc, 2-cc, or sound field SPL, but we cannot know the exact real-ear SPL unless further measures are made.

When a calibrated transducer is placed onto a human ear during audiometry, sound is delivered in different ways depending on the style of transducer. For instance, testing using sound field loudspeakers leaves the ear unoccluded whereas assessment using insert earphones occludes the ear. The resulting SPL at the eardrum will differ according to the specific combination of the transducer and the individual's external ear. Theoretically, a direct measure of the real-ear SPL during audiometry would be the preferred option to account for these factors (Gagné, Seewald, Zelisko, & Hudson, 1991; Hawkins, 1987; Keissling, 1987, 1993). However, ambient and/or probe tube microphone noise floor, which can be higher than normal or near-normal threshold levels, and probe tube retention during audiometric assessment makes this technique impractical. A more clinically feasible approach is to *predict* these values using an HL-to-SPL transform.

Clinical Application: HL-to-SPL Transforms

Since each audiometric transducer is calibrated differently, and uses a different set of RETSPL values, there is a different HL-to-SPL transform for each transducer. When insert earphones are used, the transform equals the 2-cc RECD plus the 2-cc RETSPLs for insert earphones (see Table 25–1 for case example calculations). When TDH headphones are used, the transform equals the 6-cc RECD plus the 6-cc RETSPL for TDH headphones. This is equivalent to the REDD. When loudspeakers are used, the transform equals the azimuth-dependent REUG plus the azimuth-dependent RETSPL for sound field. In summary, each HL-to-SPL transform has a real-ear component and a calibration component. These are summed together with the audiogram to calculate the child's thresholds in predicted real-ear SPL. This HL-to-SPL approach is incorporated within the DSL Method for hearing aid prescription and fitting (Bagatto et al., 2005; Scollie et al., 2005). Several studies have found the HL-to-SPL transform approach, as implemented for insert earphones, to be valid for clinical use (Bentler & Pavlovic, 1989; Munro & Davis, 2003; Revit, 1997; Scollie, Seewald, Cornelisse, & Jenstad, 1998).

An alternative to the HL-to-SPL approach is the *equivalent adult HL* approach (Ching & Dillon, 2003; Marcoux & Hansen, 2003; Seewald, Ramji, Sinclair, Moodie, & Jamieson, 1993; Seewald et al., 1997). This approach corrects the audiogram for the difference between the child's ear canal and that of an average adult. It provides the HL audiogram that would have been measured on the ear of the average adult, assuming the same hearing sensitivity. The measured ear canal properties required for this correction are identical to the insert earphone, TDH, and sound field requirements described for HL-to-SPL transforms. The main difference is that the equivalent adult HL approach does not convert the audiogram to real-ear SPL, and therefore does not make use of the calibration values, or RETSPLs. The equivalent adult HL approach is incorporated within the NAL-NL1 prescriptive software (Ching & Dillon, 2003), and the DSL Method (Scollie et al., 2005).

Regardless of the signal transducer used during audiometry, individual measurement of the real-ear component (e.g., RECD, REUG) is recommended to accurately define hearing thresholds for hearing aid fitting (Bagatto et al., 2002; Bentler, 1989). Sometimes, we cannot measure the real-ear component, such as when the child is too active or ear canal conditions prevent probe tube insertion (i.e., cerumen requiring management, discharge, objects requiring removal). In these cases, age-related normative values are available for both insert earphone and soundfield transforms (Bagatto et al., 2002, 2005; Kruger, 1987). Detailed information on normative data for the RECD is presented below. Transforms for TDH headphones exist on average, but evidence for age-related normative values do not exist (Lewis & Stelmachowicz, 1993).

Insert earphones are the only transducer that is calibrated in the 2-cc coupler. This allows a single real-

Table 25–1. HL-to-SPL Calculations for a 4-Month-Old Infant

	500 Hz	1000 Hz	2000 Hz	4000 Hz
dB eHL Threshold	40	45	60	65
+	+	+	+	+
Insert Earphone RETSPL	6	1	6	2
+	+	+	+	+
Measured RECD	8	13	15	23
=	=	=	=	=
dB SPL Threshold	54	59	81	90

ear measurement, the RECD, to be used for the HL-to-SPL transform and also for hearing aid transforms (discussed separately below). This, combined with improved interaural attenuation, lightweight and ear-specificity, makes insert earphones the preferred and recommended transducer type for use in assessments of children with hearing loss (ASHA, 2004). Therefore, the measurement of the RECD is more clinically relevant, in most cases, than measurement of the other real-ear transforms described above.

Clinical Application: Comparing Different Audiometric Test Sessions

The sections above have described two approaches that account for the effects of individual ear canal acoustics during audiometry. In pediatric audiology, it is common, and important, to see children for repeated assessments over time, and to compare results over time in order to evaluate stability of hearing thresholds. Sometimes, these results are compared across multiple assessment techniques and time points. For example, an infant whose hearing was assessed using FS-ABR techniques at the age of 4 months may have thresholds of 40, 45, 60, and 65 dB eHL at 500, 1000, 2000, and 4000 Hz, respectively. A behavioral hearing test session five months later, when the infant is 9 months of age, may show thresholds of 45, 55, 70, and 80 dB HL at the same frequencies in the right ear (Figure 25–7A). A common misconception may be that the child's hearing loss has progressed. However, it is important to consider the change in ear canal acoustics from 4 to 9 months of age. This can be accomplished by measuring or predicting (using age-appropriate norms, as discussed in the following section) the RECD at the different audiometric test sessions. The thresholds from each session can be converted to real-ear SPL (or equivalent adult HL) for a more accurate comparison. This will account for the ear canal growth that occurred in the five months between test sessions (Figure 25–7B).

The example shown in Figure 25–7 reveals that a higher level of SPL was required to elicit a response in HL at age 9 months, compared to the assessment of eHL at 4 months of age. The likely cause of this change was ear canal growth, which was likely substantial between these two ages. Both sets of audiometric data were measured using insert earphones, so the relevant measure of ear canal acoustics for both is the RECD. By measuring or predicting the infant's RECDs at both points in time and applying them to each set of thresholds or threshold estimates, a more accurate comparison is available for interpretation. In this example, the

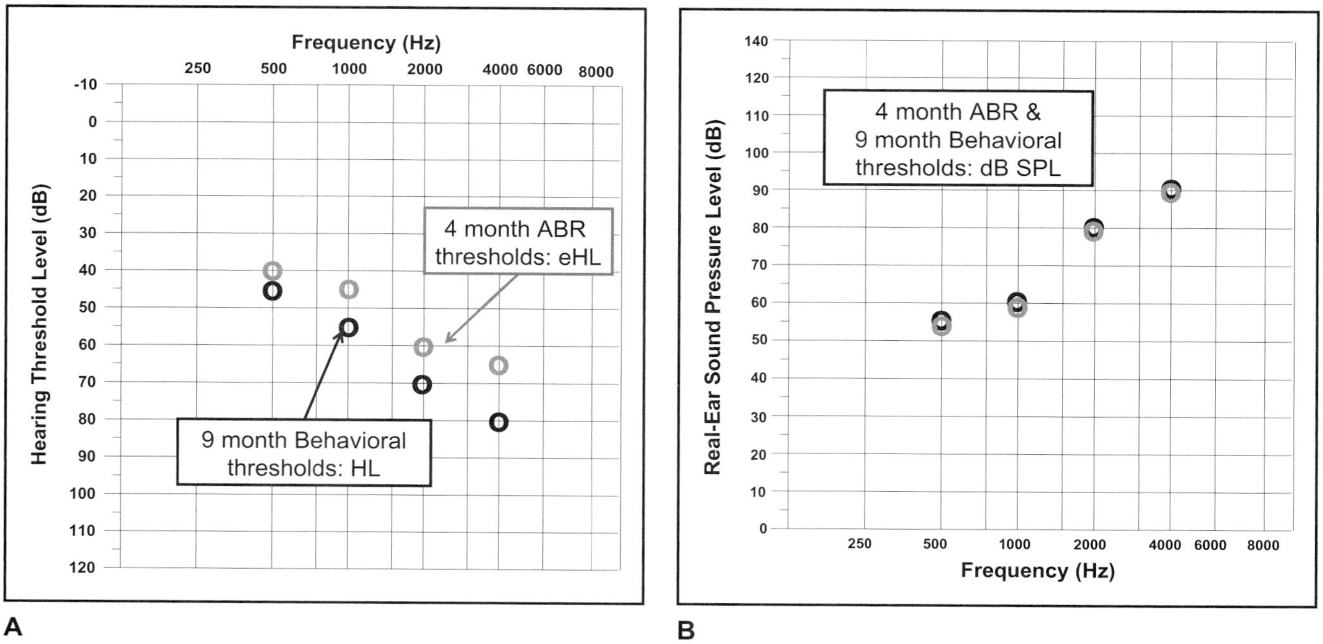

FIGURE 25–7. When comparing HL thresholds for the two test sessions, an elevation in hearing levels from the ABR to behavioral assessments is noted **(A)**. When the RECD is measured and used to convert the HL thresholds to real-ear SPL, thresholds are more similar because ear canal growth has been accounted for in the comparison **(B)**.

real-ear SPL thresholds were 54, 59, 81, and 90 dB SPL at the test frequencies for the ABR assessment and 56, 62, 82, and 92 dB SPL for the behavioral assessment at the same frequencies. Therefore, the increase in HL level was not due to a progression in hearing but a change in individual ear canal acoustics over time. The absence of progression, in this case, is clarified by accounting directly for the acoustic effects of ear canal growth via the RECD.

For some clinicians, it may be preferable to account for ear canal acoustics in the dB HL scale when comparing audiometric test sessions in young children over time. This allows plotting of the test results over time on a standard audiogram, and is easily accomplished by converting the infant's thresholds to equivalent adult HL. We have shown the required calculations for use with insert earphones in Table 25–2 for this case example. This calculation is implemented in some real-ear measurement systems by changing the scale from SPL to HL. This procedure may be helpful, in some cases, to account for the child's growing ear when comparing audiograms at different stages of the child's development to avoid inaccurate conclusions about the child's hearing sensitivity.

For these reasons, repeated measurements of a child's external ear canal acoustics over time are an important component of providing ongoing accurate care. In most cases, we can accomplish this by re-measuring the RECD using the child's own earmold, every time the earmold is re-made. This earmold RECD can be used as an HL-to-SPL transform as well as a 2cc-to-real-ear transform (discussed further below), maximizing the customization of the prescription and fitting.

Normative RECD Values

There are times when individual measurement of the RECD is not possible on a young patient during a particular clinical appointment. An active toddler may not sit still for probe tube placement or debris in the ear canal may prevent appropriate probe tube insertion. In these circumstances, age-appropriate normative values for the RECD are a reasonable alternative to individualized measures.

One current set of RECD normative data are available for infants through adulthood, and are implemented in the DSL Method, version 5.0 (Bagatto et al., 2002, 2005). These norms were derived from RECDs collected in the clinical environment, from infants and children of varying ages and are provided for both foam eartip and earmold coupling types. However, these values were derived from infants and children with normal middle ear status. Therefore, the predicted values may not reflect any acoustic changes that a fluid filled middle ear or perforated eardrum will display, in the individual ear. For infants and children with normal ear status, tested with eartips, one can expect RECD prediction errors to fall within a range of ± 5.6 dB (at 500 Hz) at best and ± 10.9 dB (at 6000 Hz)

Table 25–2. Equivalent Adult HL Audiogram Calculations for the Same Infant at 4 and 9 Months of Age

	500 Hz		*1000 Hz*		*2000 Hz*		*4000 Hz*	
	4 mos	*9 mos*	*4 mos*	*9 mos*	*4 mos*	*9 mos*	*4 mos*	*9 mos*
Measured RECD	8	5	13	7	15	9	23	12
–	–		–		–		–	
Average Adult RECD	4		5		5		13	
+	+		+		+		+	
dB (e)HL Threshold	40	45	45	55	60	70	65	80
=	=		=		=		=	
Equivalent Adult HL Threshold	44	46	53	57	70	74	75	79

at worst for children 24 months of age and younger. Predictions of earmold RECDs can span a range of accuracy from ± 6.7 dB (at 2000 Hz) to ± 12.4 dB (at 6000 Hz) for children 36 months of age and younger. Therefore, it is important to attempt an RECD measurement on an infant or child whenever possible.

Summary: Importance of Accurate Assessment Information

To this point, our chapter has described key factors to consider in the assessment stage of the hearing aid fitting process to infants and young children. The pediatric population differs from the adult population in several ways, and these differences warrant careful consideration. First, the hearing of infants is often assessed using electrophysiological techniques (i.e., ABR), which provides an estimate of behavioral thresholds if the appropriate correction is applied prior to the calculation of the hearing aid prescription. In addition, the ear canal acoustics of infants and young children are substantially different from the average adult and therefore will have an impact on the interpretation of HL thresholds if not accounted for. Finally, the acoustic characteristics of infant ear canals can be measured and applied regularly in the early stages of the hearing aid fitting process. Such dynamic and unique features are part of what make fitting hearing aids to infants and young children a challenge. Individualizing the fitting for each child supports successful intervention with amplification. If key steps in the process are eliminated, error may be introduced into the fitting. Table 25–3 summarizes the procedures required for the assessment stage of the hearing aid fitting process, and the potential error introduced if each is eliminated.

Selecting Hearing Aids

Following the identification of a permanent hearing loss in an infant or child, hearing aids are a common device choice among families as part of a larger intervention program. The goal of amplification is to improve functional auditory capacity and participation in hearing- and communication-specific situations. Several published reports indicate that early improvement in hearing can facilitate the development of sensory and perceptual skills, receptive and expressive language, speech production and literacy, academic performance, and social-emotional growth (e.g., Carney & Moeller, 1998; Ching, Dillon, Day, & Crowe, 2007; Moeller, 2000; Vohr et al., 2008).

The specific objectives of early amplification are to: (1) provide an amplified speech signal that is consistently audible across varying input levels; (2) avoid distortion of varying inputs at prescribed settings; (3) ensure amplification of sounds in as broad a frequency range as possible; and (4) include sufficient electroacoustic flexibility to allow for changes in the required frequency/output characteristics related to ear growth or changes in the auditory characteristics of the infant (JCIH, 2007; PWG, 1996). Calculation of prescriptive targets based on accurate, ear-specific assessment information and the selection of the physical and electroacoustic elements of hearing aids are key aspects of the fitting process.

The prescription includes a specification of the type of hearing aid and earmold to be fitted, and appropriate settings and applications that will result in an amplification system that addresses the evolving needs of the individual infant and family. Prescription is followed by verification to ensure that the prescribed listening levels

Table 25–3. Procedures Used for the Assessment Stage of the Hearing Aid Fitting Process and the Potential Error Introduced if Eliminated

Clinical Procedure	*Potential Error If Not Applied*
Audiometry with insert earphones	TDH uses 6-cc coupler for calibration; probe microphone systems do not allow for 6-cc coupler measures. Sound field not ear specific.
nHL to eHL correction	Threshold estimates will be 5 to 20 dB higher, depending on frequency.
Measure the RECD	Up to 20 dB if average adult values are assumed.
Predict RECD using age-appropriate values	± 15 dB

are produced by the hearing aids. This important step confirms that the real-ear performance of the selected hearing aid(s) provides output levels that are comfortable, safe, and without feedback. A scientifically based, generic fitting algorithm that takes into consideration the unique characteristics of infants and young children with hearing loss will provide fitting targets that, when matched appropriately, aim to meet these goals.

Prescriptive Algorithms

Prescriptive algorithms provide the foundation on which the hearing aid performance characteristics are selected for the infant to be fitted. Infants will wear their hearing aids at settings determined by their clinician for several months or years before being able to reliably express their preferences about the fitting (Scollie, 2004). It therefore is important to use a valid approach to selecting the hearing aid settings in order to facilitate speech and language development and maintain consistent treatment across children, clinicians, and clinics. The use of a systematic, objective prescriptive strategy has been recommended by several consensus statements (American Academy of Audiology [AAA], 2003; JCIH, 2007; PWG, 1996). Prescriptive algorithms provide objective and consistently derived targets for electroacoustic hearing aid performance that are acceptable and provide consistent benefit across patients. They are typically based on the hearing levels of the wearer to prescribe specific amplification characteristics. The resulting targets provide electroacoustic settings for the hearing aids that should result in appropriate detection, loudness, and intelligibility of amplified speech.

Generic Versus Proprietary Prescriptive Algorithms

Currently available prescriptive algorithms can be divided into two classifications: generic and proprietary. *Generic* prescriptive algorithms are based on published scientific evidence and are intended for use with any hearing aid. *Proprietary* prescriptive algorithms incorporate calculations developed by hearing aid manufacturers and are used with their specific brand of hearing aids. The lack of published information regarding the development of proprietary algorithms makes it difficult for clinicians to make an informed decision about which procedure will be best for their young patient.

Several investigators have compared different proprietary prescriptive algorithms to generic algorithms within manufacturer software. Differences in the amount of gain prescribed for adults were as much as 10 dB (Keidser, Brew, & Peck, 2003) and prescribed output ranged from 90 to 109 dB SPL (re: 2-cc coupler) for the same audiogram (Mueller, Bentler, & Wu, 2008). A study with pediatric algorithms from five different hearing aid manufacturers revealed differences of as much as 20 dB in the simulated real-ear aided response and 30 dB for the simulated real-ear saturation response (Seewald, Mills, Bagatto, Scollie, & Moodie, 2008). These large differences in prescriptions point to the importance of using an evidence-based prescriptive algorithm so that consistent amplification characteristics are applied across patients, regardless of the hearing aid being prescribed.

Current pediatric amplification guidelines recommend the use of a generic prescriptive algorithm that contains appropriate elements for use with infants and children (AAA, 2003; JCIH, 2007). Two prescriptive approaches have been suggested for use in deriving targets for pediatric hearing aid fittings: the DSL Method and the National Acoustics Laboratories' (NAL) prescription. Both formulae contain specific characteristics that are important for application with the pediatric population.

Characteristics of a Pediatric Prescriptive Method

There are several psychoacoustic and electroacoustic variables that impact the outcome of a hearing aid fitting for an infant or child with hearing loss. Relevant variables that should be included in a pediatric prescriptive algorithm include: (1) implementation of auditory thresholds estimated from electrophysiological tests of hearing; (2) accounting for external ear canal acoustics in assessment data; (3) access to age-specific normative data for predicting ear canal acoustics; and (4) the methods to conduct coupler-assisted verification. Key functions of a prescriptive formula for pediatrics ensure that these variables are handled appropriately and are discussed in the following sections.

The prescriptive method should be able to compute targets based only on thresholds, and to handle partial audiometric data. Hearing thresholds, in dB HL, are the primary source used for computing gain and output targets. Although there can be large between-subject variability, loudness discomfort levels (LDLs) can be predicted from auditory thresholds (Bentler & Cooley, 2001; Dillon & Storey, 1998; Seewald, 1991) and used to define the auditory area for the listener. Predictions of LDL are computed conservatively when used with the pediatric population (Seewald, 1991) and typically are the only option when fitting hearing aids to an infant who cannot perform suprathreshold assessments. Therefore, a pediatric prescriptive formula should provide a prediction of the LDL for use in the common case that the LDL cannot be measured.

Hearing aid fitting should proceed based on electrophysiologic tests of hearing and not be postponed to obtain behavioral thresholds. For some electrophysiologic procedures, corrections are applied to facilitate an accurate estimation of behavioral thresholds (see Assessment section of this chapter). A prescriptive algorithm intended to be used with infants should have the capability to handle electrophysiologic assessment data appropriately and provide appropriate corrections, if necessary, prior to calculating targets.

The targets should account for the external ear canal acoustics. This is required in the assessment data, using HL-to-SPL transforms prior to calculating the prescription or by using the RECD to correct the assessment data to equivalent adult HL (see Assessment section). Additionally, the smaller size of the infant ear canal means that less coupler gain is required from the hearing aids, but also that the gain requirements must be revised as the ear grows. Therefore, target calculations should account for the child's RECD. Some clinical situations will prevent measurement of the RECD on a young patient, in which case the prescriptive formula should provide age-appropriate external ear normative data (Bagatto et al., 2002, 2005). Both the DSL and NAL prescriptive approaches integrate the child's RECD into target calculations, thereby updating the prescription as the child grows. Both accurately incorporate ear canal acoustics within prescription calculations, and make the prescribed targets available in 2-cc coupler format. This supports measurement and adjustment of the hearing aid response on the 2-cc coupler (see Verification section, below). Overall, these pediatric-friendly approaches to prescription ensure accuracy and consistency in the fitting for infants and young children.

Listening Needs of Infants and Children with Hearing Loss

In addition to accounting for the variables mentioned above, a pediatric prescriptive approach should take into consideration the specific listening needs of the population. Since children acquire hearing loss either before or during a period of speech and language learning, they must learn these skills through aided hearing rather than from prior experience with the language. This is different from adults who acquire hearing loss after many years of experience with language. Many investigators have demonstrated that children with hearing loss require more speech audibility than adults or children with normal hearing in order to perceive all speech sounds (Elliott, 1979; Elliott et al., 1979; Gravel, Fausel, Liskow, & Chobot, 1999; Hnath-Chisholm, Laipply, & Boothroyd, 1998; Kortekaas & Stelmachowicz, 2000; Nábûlek & Robinson, 1982; Neuman & Hochberg, 1982). Age-related interactions with level, bandwidth, and sensation level in the perception of fricatives or the use of context for word recognition have been shown between children with normal and impaired hearing (Pittman, 2008; Pittman & Stelmachowicz, 2000; Pittman, Stelmachowicz, Lewis, & Hoover, 2003; Stelmachowicz, Hoover, Lewis, Kortekaas, & Pittman, 2000; Stelmachowicz, Pittman, Hoover, & Lewis, 2001, 2002). Therefore, children with hearing loss require more gain, a higher signal-to-noise ratio and a broader audible bandwidth of speech in order to have a better chance at acquiring speech and language. Currently there are two prescriptive procedures that are actively recommended for use in pediatric fitting because they take into account these variables: the Desired Sensation Level Multistage Input/Output Method (DSL *m*[i/o]) v5.0a and the National Acoustics Laboratories Nonlinear Algorithm (NAL-NL1). The characteristics of each are described in the following sections.

The Desired Sensation Level Multistage Input/Output Algorithm (DSL m[i/o]) v5.0a

Dr. Richard Seewald and his colleagues developed the original DSL Method in 1985. Their review of research with adults and children with hearing loss indicated that speech must be amplified to a certain sensation level (SL) to maximize comfort and intelligibility (Erber & Witt, 1977; Kamm, Dirks, & Mickey, 1977; Macrae, 1986; Pascoe, 1978, 1988). The findings from these studies were used to define target SLs for amplified speech for children with hearing loss (Seewald, Ross, & Spiro, 1985) for various hearing levels. A longstanding goal of this prescriptive method is to amplify speech to these "desired sensation levels" across as broad a frequency range as possible to support auditory learning via audibility of speech cues. This has been described as an habilitative audibility approach (Scollie, 2004). Another goal of the DSL Method has been to provide targets that limit the maximum output, while still providing appropriate headroom and comfort for loud sounds. During this era, hearing aids with linear circuitry were available; therefore, the resulting DSL version 3.0 targets were developed for this type of processing.

With the advent of wide dynamic range compression (WDRC) circuitry in hearing aids, an updated version of the DSL Method was developed. In 1995, Leonard Cornelisse and his colleagues designed the "input/output formula" (DSL [i/o]) by using Steven's Power Law to map a wide range of input levels to target hearing aid output levels across various frequencies. The DSL [i/o] Method Version 4.1 prescribed targets for gain, output limiting and compression ratios for use with both linear and WDRC hearing aids. The average speech SLs were equivalent to those recommended by earlier versions of the DSL Method (Cornelisse, Seewald, & Jamieson, 1995). A key feature of the DSL Method has been to display the characteristics of the hearing aid output together with the child's auditory characteristics in an "SPLogram" format. The SPLogram uses a real-ear SPL reference scale across frequencies to permit direct comparison of the performance of the hearing aid with the listener's thresholds and LDLs.

Several validation studies of the DSL [i/o] v4.1 algorithm were conducted in the late 1990s. The work showed that the preferred listening levels (PLLs) of children were 2 dB higher than the listening levels recommended by DSL, with about 70% of the PLLs falling within 5 dB of the DSL target (Scollie, Seewald, Moodie, & Dekok, 2000). In addition, WDRC hearing aids fitted to DSL [i/o] targets achieved comfort, intelligibility and the perception of normal loudness of speech across a range of speech input levels (Jenstad, Pumford, Seewald, & Cornelisse, 2000; Jenstad, Seewald, Cornelisse, & Shantz, 1999). These studies indicate that the DSL algorithm: (1) improves speech recognition scores in children over unaided performance; (2) improves low-level speech recognition and normalize loudness when paired with WDRC; and (3) more closely approximates children's PLLs.

In 2005, we released the DSL Multistage Input/Output (DSL *m*[i/o]) v5.0a. Although the habilitative audibility goals are the same as previous versions of the DSL Method, DSL *m*[i/o] v5.0a provides compatibility with ABR data, updated RECD normative data for infants and children, infant-friendly RECD measurement techniques, targets for quiet and noisy environments, adjustments for conductive losses and binaural fittings and accounts for multichannel compression characteristics of modern hearing aids. Detailed descriptions of these modifications and additions can be found in Scollie et al. (2005) and Bagatto et al. (2005). This version of DSL is widely implemented in hearing aid fitting and verification systems.

The National Acoustics Laboratories Nonlinear Algorithm (NAL-NL1)

The National Acoustics Laboratories (NAL) originally developed a prescriptive formula for fitting hearing aids to adults by amplifying all bands of speech to the most comfortable level. Following a series of studies, it was noted that the NAL prescription did not achieve this goal and the algorithm was revised (Byrne, 1986a, 1986b). The revised formula, NAL-R, was evaluated and found to be superior to the original formula for measures of speech recognition and preference. However, the authors noted that the gain and frequency response may not be suitable for listeners with severe-to-profound hearing loss (Byrne & Dillon, 1986; Byrne & Murray, 1986). The PLLs of adults with severe-to-profound hearing loss wearing linear BTE hearing aids led to the release of NAL-RP (Byrne, Parkinson, & Newall, 1990). This formula was recommended for use with adult listeners wearing linear hearing aids whose thresholds exceed 95 dB HL at 2000 Hz.

More recent versions of the NAL formula advocate an effective audibility approach which attempts to limit the loudness of the fitting while optimizing speech recognition (Ching, Dillon, & Byrne, 1998). This approach assumes that additional high-frequency gain may not further improve word recognition performance in adults; therefore, provision of audibility across the full frequency range is not always a goal for this algorithm (Ching, Dillon, Katsch, & Byrne, 2001). In 2001, Drs. Byrne, Ching, Dillon, and colleagues released the NAL-NL1 prescriptive approach for fitting nonlinear amplification. This version prescribes targets for nonlinear hearing aids using an effective audibility approach. Current versions use appropriate corrections for the acoustic properties of children's ear canals, including measured RECDs and age-appropriate averages. The limits to prescribed bandwidth derived from effective audibility predictions are applied for both adults and children, on the assumption that the limits of effectiveness in the adult population also apply to infants and children (Ching et al., 2001).

Comparisons of NAL-NL1 and DSL Prescriptive Formulae

Because both NAL and DSL currently offer similar ranges of software support for pediatric hearing aid fitting, the clinician might debate over the choice between the two. In general, the choice of prescription for children might be informed by evidence, and by consideration of the theoretical principles of each prescription. The evidence for prescriptive difference may evolve as new information accrues. At the time of this writing, several sources of evidence exist. Older studies have compared children's listening preferences to prescribed listening response shapes and/or listening levels, but consistent findings have not been measured (Ching, Hill, Birtles, & Beacham, 1999; Ching, Newall,

& Wigney, 1997; Ching et al., 2001; Scollie et al., 2000). In general, studies of children who were DSL users were more likely to prefer DSL, and studies of NAL users were more likely to prefer NAL, leading the authors to speculate that acclimatization may play a role in preferences. Older studies also compared the actual hearing aid frequency responses of successful pediatric hearing aid users to various targets. In general, these studies found that used gain was within ± 5 dB of both the NAL and DSL prescriptions for speech-level inputs, and for the DSL targets for output limiting (Snik & Stollman, 1995; Snik, van den Borne, Brokx, & Hoekstra, 1995).

More recently, a collaborative study between the authors of the NAL and DSL prescriptions compared the performance of DSL[i/o] v4.1 and NAL-NL1 for a group of 48 school-aged children with up to moderately-severe hearing losses. These children participated in a double-blind crossover study that evaluated both laboratory and real-world outcomes (Ching, Scollie, Dillon, & Seewald, 2010a). The fittings in this study employed coupler-based verification and individualized measurement of RECDs, achieving a 7 dB difference in gain, overall, between the two prescriptions at an input level of 70 dB SPL (Ching, Scollie, Dillon, Seewald, Britton, & Steinberg, 2010b). With these fittings, children carried out an eight-week trial with one prescription, then again with the other, and then completed another eight-week trial in which they wore both and compared the two. Loudness ratings for the two fittings changed significantly after the single-prescription trials, showing acclimatization-related changes that removed most of the baseline differences in loudness between prescriptions (Scollie et al., 2010a). Speech recognition measures in quiet indicated a high level of performance (average scores greater than 85% correct for nonsense syllables) across sites and prescriptions (Scollie, et al., 2010a). Performance on this task varied with test level for the NAL prescription but not the DSL prescription. Real world ratings from the single-prescription trials found that children have significantly more listening difficulty in noisy environments (Ching et al., 2010c). These same performance ratings in noise were higher for the NAL fitting than for the DSL fitting. Australian children were more likely to prefer the NAL fitting overall in these trials. In the real-world trials comparing the two prescriptions, children at both sites rated the DSL fitting as preferable for speech in quiet and/or from behind (Scollie et al., 2010b). Children's preferences fell into two factors: quiet or low level situations versus noisy and/or reverberant situations. Canadian children were more likely to prefer DSL overall in these trials. Many children expressed a preference for using both programs in a multimemory fitting, and described their strategic use of two memories in ways that were appropriate to each listening environment. The use of less gain to control excessive loudness and/or noisiness, and the use of more gain to enhance clarity of speech and perceived closeness of the talker were both important in many environments. Overall, of the objective and subjective measures in this study, individual children varied in whether they would perform best with or prefer the DSL or NAL prescription. Even when no difference existed on average, individual children demonstrated significant individual performance or preference advantages with one of the fittings.

Overall, this collaborative study provides strong evidence that hearing aid benefit is high when a systematic hearing aid prescription and fitting method is used with school-aged children. It also provides some insight into: (a) the relative performance of DSL and NAL in different real world environments; (b) children's ability to use a multimemory strategy reliably and rationally; (c) the importance of evaluating outcome at the individual level; and (d) the importance of allowing a period of acclimatization prior to evaluation of outcome.

With some exceptions, the studies above have primarily evaluated children with up to moderately-severe hearing losses: less information is available about children with severe to profound hearing losses. The studies mentioned above may also have been constrained, to some degree, by hearing aid flexibility in meeting precisely the prescriptive targets (Ching et al., 2010b). Clinicians practicing hearing aid fitting today may frequently treat infants with severe to profound hearing loss, using instruments that are now capable of a more faithful representation of the prescriptions, and perhaps employing revised versions of these prescriptions. Therefore, current practice should consider the evidence for prescription choice, in addition to theoretical factors. First, if fitting an infant, is the prescription designed to compute targets based on electrophysiologic estimates of threshold? Second, if the fitting is steeply sloping and/or severe to profound, does the clinician wish to take a habilitative audibility approach or an effective audibility approach in fitting? Third, once fitted, does the infant or child's behavior indicate an experience of sound awareness, comfortable loudness, and clear reception of speech cues? Although answers to this final question may take some time to obtain, we end this section by stressing the needs of the individual over the initial prescription. Fitting to a well-calculated target is an excellent beginning, but all prescriptive targets are best used within a larger program of care in which the child's responses and development are carefully considered.

Clinical Application: Deriving Prescriptive Targets

Prescriptive algorithms are available in real-ear measurement systems and hearing aid manufacturer's software so that clinicians can have easy access to the target calculations. This allows the clinician to determine the gain and output characteristics of the hearing aid based on the child's auditory thresholds and ear canal acoustics. Information to be entered into the applications typically consists of: (1) hearing thresholds at each frequency for each ear, with an indication of the format (nHL, eHL, HL); (2) age of the child to be fitted; (3) type of transducer used during the assessment; (4) measured or predicted RECD values; and (5) style of the hearing aid to be fitted. Each piece of data is used in the calculation of targets for the individual.

Figure 25–8 shows the SPLogram for the case example shown in Figure 25–7. This includes targets for average conversational speech (large +) and maximum power output (small +) that were generated based on the hearing thresholds (o) and measured RECD from the child in this example. The graph also shows the patient's audiometric thresholds plotted against unaided average conversational speech (shaded region), all of which are referenced to real-ear SPL. In this case, when hearing aids are provided and adjusted to match the suggested targets, the child will have clear and safe access to speech at various levels. This explanation, in combination with the SPLogram display, becomes a useful counseling tool for parents to help them understand the goals of the hearing aid fitting.

Electroacoustic Characteristics

When choosing hearing aids for a young patient, consideration should be given to select devices that: (1) avoid distortion; (2) allow frequency/output shaping and flexibility to provide audibility and prevent

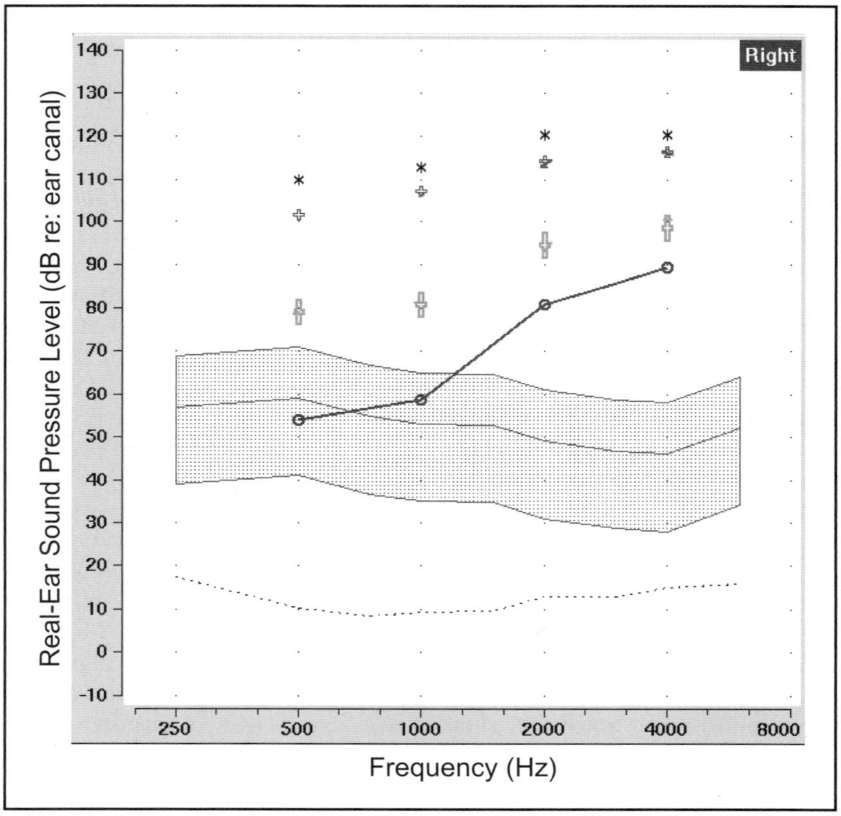

FIGURE 25–8. An SPLogram displaying the recommended targets for average speech (large +) and maximum power output (small +) for the infant in this case example. The circles (o) represent the child's hearing thresholds in real-ear SPL and the shaded region represents unaided average conversational speech.

loudness discomfort; (3) apply wide dynamic range compression for most hearing losses (Jenstad et al., 1999, 2000); and (4) apply compression output limiting. Advanced signal processing schemes (e.g., expansion, multiple channels, frequency lowering, feedback cancellation/management, noise reduction, directional microphones and frequency lowering) are considered for each infant and child on an individual basis. For example, some feedback cancellation/management systems work effectively to control feedback without reducing high frequency output. This may be a better option for controlling feedback while ensuring access to sound, compared to alternatives that reduce high-frequency output.

Audibility of high-frequency sounds may be limited by the bandwidth of conventional hearing aids, possibly impacting high-frequency speech sound recognition and production (see review in Stelmachowicz, Pittman, Hoover, Lewis, & Moeller, 2004). Possible solutions include the fitting of hearing aids with extended high-frequency bandwidths, or the use of frequency lowering signal processing either via frequency transposition or frequency compression. Recent studies of both forms of frequency lowering suggest that this technology can amplify high-frequency sounds (e.g., /s/, /ʃ/) for listeners who would otherwise have difficulty accessing such sounds (Auriemmo et al., 2009; Glista et al., 2009; Kuk, Keenan, Korhonen, & Lau, 2009; Miller-Hansen, Nelson, Widen, & Simon, 2003; Wolfe, Caraway, John, Schafer, & Nyffeler, 2009). Frequency transposition and frequency compression provide different degrees and forms of frequency lowering. However, the specific audiometric range for frequency lowering, and for choosing among frequency lowering strategies is not yet entirely clear. Our knowledge in this area is rapidly evolving as new research emerges. Advantages of frequency lowering include improved detection and/or recognition of high frequency speech sounds, and, in some cases, improved speech production. Some early evidence indicates that children and adults may respond differently to this type of signal processing, with children having stronger candidacy, at least for nonlinear frequency compression (Glista et al., 2009).

Noise reduction algorithms have not been extensively evaluated in the pediatric population. Adult focused literature suggests that noise reduction algorithms may help to provide comfort and/or acceptance for listening in noisy environments (e.g., restaurant, vehicle) if the technology is activated and deactivated appropriately (see Bentler, 2005; Bentler, Yu-Hsiang, Kettel, & Hurtig, 2008; Mueller & Ricketts, 2005; and Palmer, 2006 for informative data and reviews). However, we should also consider the potential effects on a child's awareness of nonspeech sounds in the environment. The selection of a digital noise reduction (DNR) scheme that preserves audibility of speech and environmental sounds while reducing noisiness and/or loudness may help to provide comfort for children in a wider range of situations.

Directional microphones have been shown to provide benefit to older children and adults in noisy listening situations (Gravel et al., 1999; Ricketts & Tharpe, 2004). However, directional benefit is typically associated with communication situations in which the talker of interest is located in front of the listener. Infants and children do not always communicate in this situation, and may choose to manipulate their orientation to the talker or multiple talkers within a given situation. Some studies indicate that children can and do orient their heads at least some of the time to a talker of interest (Ching et al., 2009; Ricketts & Galster, 2008). Maintaining correct orientation in a classroom context may be challenging, particularly when taking notes while a teacher is speaking (Ricketts & Galster, 2008). Current research suggests that directional microphones provide a deficit for signals arising from the side or behind the child (Ching et al., 2009). This can cause a directional deficit in the frequent case where a child has not oriented toward the signal of interest (Ching et al., 2009). Importantly for the school environment, directional microphones provide less benefit than an FM system in simulated classroom environments (Ricketts, Galster, & Tharpe, 2007). Therefore, use of a directional microphone does not replace the FM system for management of room acoustics and/or classroom noise effects.

For infants or very young children, auditory access to the target talker and the potential contribution of overhearing on an infant's speech and language development should be considered along with the need for noise management. For many children, the most appropriate processing strategy may vary with the listening environment, just as it does for adults. An issue of controversy is how best to access this listening program, in order to avoid an inappropriate choice that could prevent the child from being aware of signals in the environment. Children who are about age 7 years and older may be able to take responsibility for the use of multiple hearing aid memories. In one study, children used two memories reliably and appropriately, indicating that children who can monitor their own listening performance can and do make technology choices that will benefit them in terms of communication performance (Scollie et al., 2010b). For younger children, a proxy strategy is required if noise management is to be utilized. Can we consider signal processing schemes that automatically enable directionality and/or noise reduction, and do they function appropriately? Can caregivers take responsibility for program manipulation?

Strong evidence for either of these strategies is currently unavailable for the infant/toddler population. Clinicians are therefore advised to consider each child and each technology individually on respective needs and merits, applying solutions with caution, monitoring, and verifying of their effects electroacoustically. Empirical data regarding their effectiveness in the infant population are rare, and likely will continue to be rare, due to the challenges of evaluating such technologies in infants. Clinicians may choose to infer the possible needs, benefits, and limitations associated with these technologies from studies conducted on children in the absence of research on infants. In practice, consultation with the caregivers prior to introducing these technologies to the infant is critical to ensure accurate use and informed reporting of outcomes associated with the technology's use.

Physical Characteristics

The style of the hearing aid(s), monaural versus binaural fitting, deactivation of unnecessary signal processing, FM system compatibility, locking mechanism for the volume control, and tamper-resistant battery doors are important considerations when providing hearing aids to infants and young children (Table 25–4).

Behind-the-ear (BTE) hearing aids are the recommended style for infants and children for several reasons. Acoustic feedback is less of an issue and greater electroacoustic flexibility is offered with this style of hearing aid. In addition, BTEs have direct audio input capabilities that are more compatible with the pediatric population. Finally, should the BTE aid require repairs from the manufacturer, a similar device from the loaner hearing aid stock can be coupled to the personal earmold so the infant is not without amplification while the device is being repaired.

A pediatric earhook is recommended to support secure retention on the ear. Unfiltered earhooks will add resonant peaks to the output response of the hearing aid, possibly causing feedback and making adjustment to maximum power output (MPO) targets difficult. A filtered earhook will smooth the response and allow for a better match to targets with less chance of feedback (Scollie & Seewald, 2002). Tamper resistant battery doors should also be included on hearing aids for infants and children and a deactivation or locking system for the volume control and other automatic features should be available.

Direct audio input (DAI) should be included on the selected devices. This will enable coupling of assistive technology, such as FM systems, to the hearing aids. FM system use will enhance the benefits of hear-

Table 25-4. Physical Characteristics of Hearing Aids Provided to Infants and Children

Characteristic	***Benefit***
Behind-the-ear (BTE) style	Reduces acoustic feedback Provides greater electroacoustic flexibility Provides direct audio input capabilities Allows loaner device to be easily used if needed Durable
Pediatric-sized filtered earhook	Supports secure retention on ear Reduces resonant peaks Allows for better match to targets
Tamper-resistant battery door	Prevents accidental ingestion of batteries
Deactivation or locking system for volume control	Prevents inadvertent increases or decreases to hearing aid output
Deactivation of advanced features	Allows for flexibility in the application of advanced technologies
Direct audio input (DAI)	Enables coupling of FM system
Choice of bright colors	For enjoyment

ing aids in infants and children and can be provided as an option to families for consideration. Other types of personal amplification such as implantable devices are considered on an individual basis. Further discussion regarding the use of other hearing technologies in the pediatric population can be found in Chapters 26 through 29 of this text.

Summary: Selecting Hearing Aids

Deriving electroacoustic targets and selecting the physical characteristics of hearing aid(s) is the second step in the hearing aid fitting process, following the collection of assessment information. When the hearing aid(s) have been received, confirmation that they are performing close to the prescriptive targets is the next essential step. The following sections describe the verification stage of the hearing aid fitting process for infants and children.

Verification of Electroacoustic Performance

Once we have defined the auditory thresholds, the acoustic characteristics of the ear canal, and the electroacoustic and nonelectroacoustic specifications of the hearing aid, we can proceed to verification of electroacoustic performance. In the verification stage, we adjust the hearing aids to match a set of targets for electroacoustic performance. This process provides a fitting that is expected to be comfortable, safe, and wearable without feedback. The following sections describe options and clinical procedures for the verification of hearing aids for infants and young children.

Real-Ear Measurements

Hearing aids can be measured in the context of the child's auditory area in order to evaluate the hearing aid fitting for audibility and comfort. This type of evaluation uses the SPLogram, on which we plot the thresholds and predicted LDLs, prescribed targets, and measured hearing aid responses in real-ear SPL as a function of frequency on the same graph (Figure 25–9). The advantage of using an SPLogram display for verification is that it allows electroacoustic evaluation of the hearing aid to serve as a proxy for the child's feedback regarding audibility and comfort of amplified sounds. This supports the fittings of hearing aids that provide a broad audible band of speech, yet avoids loudness discomfort. The primary verification format for an SPLogram is therefore the real-ear aided response (REAR). The REAR format is chosen over other real-ear measurement formats such as real-ear insertion gain (REIG). Most REIG insertion gain calculations assume average adult real-ear unaided responses (REUR), whereas measured insertion gain is calculated using the patient's measured REUR. Infants and young children are not likely to have average adult REURs, therefore significant error is likely to be introduced into the hearing aid fitting if the insertion gain approach to verification is used. Even when these errors are removed by computing the REIG target using a child's own REUG, the measurement is made without any perceptual context: the REIG measurement cannot be directly compared to the patient's auditory thresholds or loudness discomfort levels.

There are two options for obtaining REAR measures using real-ear measurement equipment. One is to directly measure the output of the hearing aid while it is on the patient's ear. *Real-ear verification* protocols involve placement of a probe tube microphone in the ear canal prior to placing the hearing aid on the ear. While the patient faces a loudspeaker, stimuli of various input levels are delivered, and the output is measured directly in the ear canal. The hearing aid is adjusted using hearing aid fitting software in order to better approximate the prescriptive targets. Although this approach offers the advantage of directly measuring the output of the hearing aid in the ear canal and displays it within the context of the patient's auditory characteristics, there are some limitations of this approach for use with infants and children. First, care must be taken when selecting the levels of the test signals. Verification of the MPO of the hearing aid requires the use of a high intensity (90-100 dB SPL) narrowband signal in order to saturate the hearing aid. This test level may be startling to the child and, depending on how the hearing aid was set prior to running the signal, may be uncomfortable for the listener. Second, passive cooperation is required during real-ear verification. The patient is required to sit still and quiet during the several minutes required to adequately adjust the hearing aid to meet targets. This typically is a challenge for children who are vocal and active. Young infants who do not have the head and neck control to face the loudspeaker without the assistance of a parent or caregiver will provide additional challenges for this approach. Their random head movements will introduce variability into the measurement.

For these reasons, an alternative strategy for measuring the real-ear performance of the hearing aid has been developed. This alternative approach requires

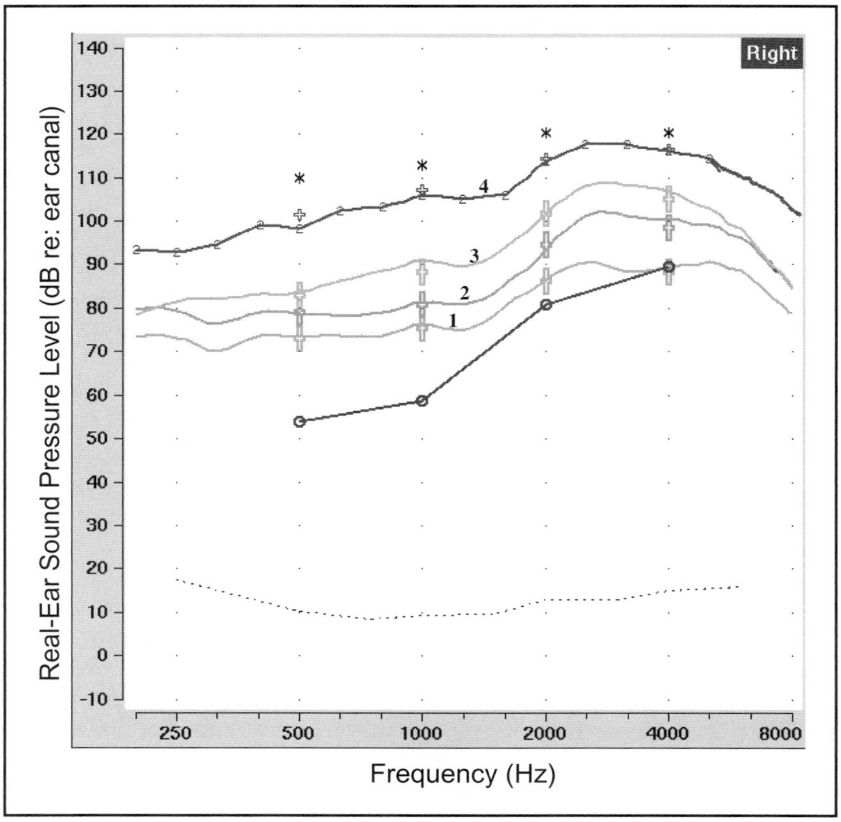

A

FIGURE 25–9. Verification of hearing aid performance displayed on an SPLogram. The solid lines represent the output of the hearing aid at soft (1), average (2), and loud (3) speech input levels as well as the MPO (4). These are compared to the targets represented by the plus (+) signs or asterisks (*) **(A)**. *continues*

measurements of coupler output, rather than the REAR. Then, the RECD is used, together with predictions of the acoustic effects of the hearing aid microphone's location (behind the ear or at various locations in the ear), to predict the REAR based on the coupler measures. This may be done using a measured or predicted age-appropriate set of RECD values. This *simulated or coupler* approach to real-ear verification generally is more compatible with the pediatric population, the details of which are described below.

Simulated Real-Ear Measurements

In the assessment stage, the RECD is used to convert HL thresholds to SPL. The same RECD values are used to convert real-ear gain and output requirements to 2-cc coupler targets for the purposes of selection. The third use of the RECD is to convert 2-cc coupler measurements of hearing aid output to predicted real-ear measurements. Simulated or coupler-based verification has the primary advantage of allowing clinicians to perform all electroacoustic response shaping of the hearing aid using an SPLogram format within the highly controlled acoustic conditions of a test box.

Simulating the REAR involves two main components: RECD values and coupler measures of hearing aid output. The RECD captures the child's individual ear canal acoustics across frequency and is applied to the coupler measures to *predict* the REAR, rather than measure it directly (Moodie et al., 1994; Seewald, 1991). Measuring the RECD takes little time and is unaffected by head movement, making it more accurate and reliable for the pediatric population than measuring the

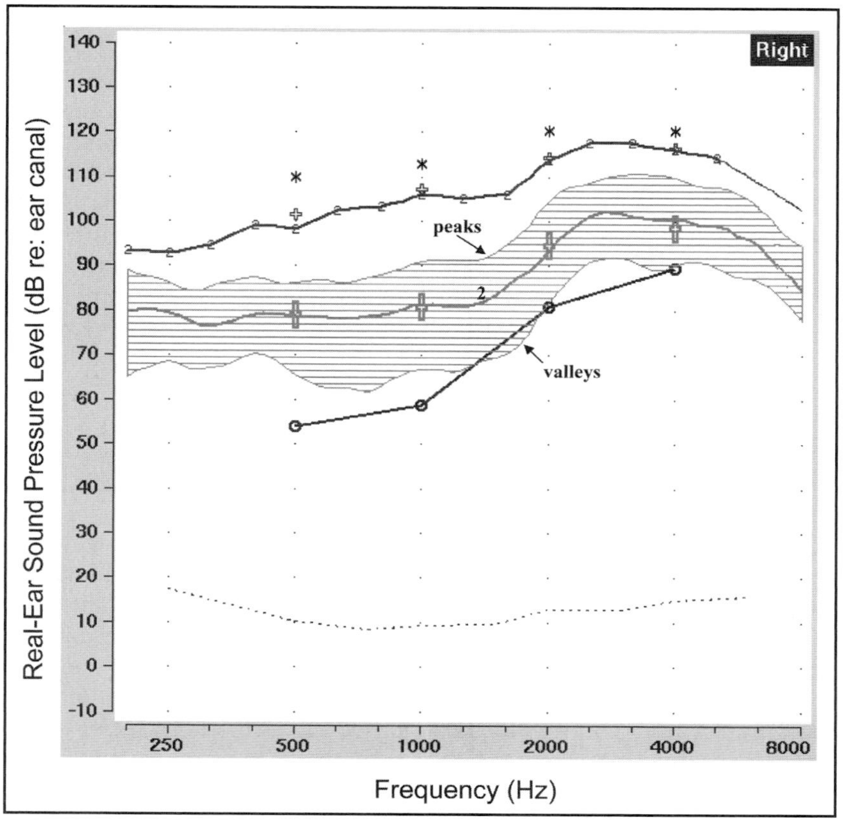

B

FIGURE 25–9. *continued* Alternatively, the peaks and valleys of the output of average conversational speech can be viewed in this format **(B)**.

REAR (Seewald, Moodie, Sinclair, & Scollie, 1999; Sinclair et al., 1996).

In the coupler approach to real-ear verification, targets are generated for the 2-cc coupler. The hearing aid is attached to the 2-cc coupler and placed in a test box, and verification of hearing aid performance is conducted at various input levels representing soft, average, and loud speech (i.e., 55 to 70 dB SPL) in order to evaluate fit to targets and determine audibility of speech. The hearing aid's MPO is verified using high-level narrowband stimuli. In addition, a loud speech stimulus (75–80 dB SPL) may be measured to ensure that the peaks of speech fall at or below the upper limits of comfort (Scollie & Seewald, 2002). Figure 25–9A displays one example of this procedure. The solid lines represent the output of the hearing aid at various input levels. These are compared to the targets represented by the plus (+) signs or asterisks (*). Approximation of the output of the hearing aid to the calculated targets is important to ensure that speech is audible and loud sounds are not uncomfortable, across a broad frequency range. Figure 25–9B displays the same hearing aid fitting with the peaks and valleys for average conversational speech displayed.

The predicted REAR and RESR are plotted on an SPLogram so that performance of the hearing aid can be directly compared to thresholds, upper limits of comfort, and prescriptive targets. Using this display, the clinician can evaluate audibility, appropriate output limiting levels and acoustic headroom across frequencies.

Following simulated real-ear verification, the hearing aids are placed on the infant or child and the fit is checked for physical comfort and to ensure that they can be worn at the recommended settings without feedback. This is an essential step with coupler-based verification because the real-ear fit and the acoustic seal of the hearing aids are not assessed during coupler measures. It also does not assess any earmold venting that may be present in the fitting.

With these limitations in mind, simulated real-ear measurements are still the approach of choice when verifying hearing aids for infants and young children. Seewald and his colleagues (1999) examined the predictive validity of using the RECD to predict the REAG and real-ear saturation response (RESR) of hearing aids. They measured and predicted the REAG for 14 participants and results indicated that, on average, the REAG values were predicted using RECD values to within ± 2.3 dB across frequency for 95% of cases. In addition, the average error for the predictions of the RESR was 4.4 dB. Similar findings were also noted in a study by Munro and Hatton (2000).

However, more recent studies have reported errors associated with this procedure due to impedance differences between hearing aids and some transducers used to measure the RECD (Munro & Salisbury, 2002; Munro & Toal, 2005). Resulting errors are exacerbated when the tubing in the custom earmold is longer, as it would be for adult earmolds, and/or when the earhook is unfiltered (Bagatto et al., 2005; Munro & Toal, 2005). In general, earmold tubing lengths typical of infants and young children, coupled with the use of filtered earhooks, result in accuracy of the RECD-based coupler verification procedure to within a clinically acceptable range (Bagatto et al., 2005).

Other Approaches to Verification

Behavioral evaluation (i.e., aided audiogram, functional gain measures) and insertion gain measures may be viewed as alternatives to the real-ear verification procedures for infants and young children discussed in the previous sections. With advances in hearing aid technology, real-ear measurement systems, and pediatric-friendly hearing aid fitting protocols, several limitations to these alternative approaches to verification have been noted.

Behavioral verification of the electroacoustic performance of the hearing aid is not compatible with young infants identified through early hearing and communication development (EHCD) programs. The first fitting of the hearing aid(s) is targeted to occur by 6 months of age, at which age many infants cannot perform conditioned tasks for behavioral tests of hearing. Therefore, relying on behavioral thresholds for hearing aid fitting is likely to delay the first fitting, thereby delaying intervention. In addition, aided soundfield measures require prolonged cooperation from the infant, provide information at only a few frequencies, and have poor test-retest reliability (Stuart, Durieux-Smith, & Stenstrom, 1990). Additionally, the narrowband stimuli used for aided soundfield measures are not representative of speech nor do they provide an estimate of the MPO of the hearing aid. Finally, the validity of aided soundfield thresholds is poor, especially with severe to profound hearing losses, or when nonlinear signal processing is used (Humes & Kirn, 1990; Macrae & Frazier, 1980; Seewald, Moodie, Sinclair, & Cornelisse, 1996; Stelmachowicz & Lewis, 1988). Aided soundfield threshold testing can be useful as an outcome measure and for counseling and educational purposes, but is not the recommended procedure for use when verifying and fine tuning hearing aids for infants and children.

Summary

This chapter has described key considerations in the assessment, selection, and verification stages of providing hearing aids to infants and young children with hearing loss. Details regarding the use of ABR threshold estimates for hearing aid fitting, the importance of accounting for ear canal acoustics, the use of evidence-based generic prescriptive formulas and pediatric-friendly electroacoustic verification procedures are just a few of the topics discussed. A systematic approach to the provision of amplification provides a framework with which clinicians can continuously monitor their young patients. This is especially important given the unique qualities that infants and young children bring to the hearing aid prescription process. The information and instruction, and outcome evaluation stages are important aspects of the hearing aid fitting process and are addressed in subsequent chapters of this volume.

References

American Academy of Audiology. (2003). *Pediatric amplification guidelines.* http://www.audiology.org/resources/documentlibrary/Documents/pedamp.pdf

American National Standards Institute. (1996). *Specification for audiometers.* ANSI S3.6–1996 (R 2004). New York, NY: Acoustical Society of America.

American National Standards Institute. (1997). *Methods of measurement of real-ear performance characteristics of hearing aids.* ANSI S3.46-1997 (R 2007). New York, NY: Acoustical Society of America.

American Speech-Language-Hearing Association. (2004). *Guidelines for the audiologic assessment of children from birth to 5 years of age.* Retrieved July 2, 2010, from http://www.asha.org/docs/html/GL2004-00002.html

Auriemmo, J., Kuk, F., Lau, C., Marshall, S., Thiele, N., Pikora, M., ... Stenger, P. (2009). Effect of linear frequency transposition on speech recognition and production of school-age children. *Journal of the American Academy of Audiology, 20*(5), 289–305.

Bagatto, M. P., & Moodie, S. T. (2007). Learning the art to apply the science: Common questions related to pediatric hearing instrument fitting. *Audiology Online.* Retrieved July 2, 2010, from http://www.audiologyonline.com/articles/article_detail. asp?article_id=1886

Bagatto, M. P., Moodie, S. T., Scollie, S., Seewald, R. C., Moodie, S., Pumford, J., & Liu, K. P. R. (2005). Clinical protocols for hearing instrument fitting in the Desired Sensation Level Method. *Trends in Amplification, 9*(4), 199–226.

Bagatto, M. P., Scollie, S. D., Seewald, R. C., Moodie, K. S., & Hoover, B. M. (2002). Real-ear-to-coupler difference predictions as a function of age for two coupling procedures. *Journal of the American Academy of Audiology, 13*(8), 407–415.

Bagatto, M. P., Seewald, R. C., Scollie, S. D., & Tharpe, A. M. (2006). Evaluation of a probe-tube insertion technique for measuring the real-ear-to-coupler difference (RECD) in young infants. *Journal of the American Academy of Audiology, 17*, 573–581.

Bentler, R. A. (1989). External ear resonance characteristics in children. *Journal of Speech and Hearing Research, 54*(2), 265–268.

Bentler, R. A. (2005). Effectiveness of directional microphones and noise reduction schemes in hearing aids: A systematic review of the evidence. *Journal of the American Academy of Audiology, 16*, 473–484.

Bentler, R. A., & Cooley, L. J. (2001). An examination of several characteristics that affect the prediction of OSPL90 in hearing aids. *Ear and Hearing, 22*(1), 58–64.

Bentler, R. A., & Pavlovic, C. V. (1989). Transfer functions and correction factors used in hearing aid evaluation and research. *Ear and Hearing, 10*, 58–63.

Bentler, R., Yu-Hsiang, W., Kettel, J., & Hurtig, R. (2008). Digital noise reduction: Outcomes from laboratory and field studies. *International Journal of Audiology, 47*(8), 447–460.

Byrne, D. (1986a). Effects of bandwidth and stimulus type on most comfortable loudness levels of hearing-impaired listeners. *Journal of the Acoustical Society of America, 80*(2), 484–493.

Byrne, D. (1986b). Effects of frequency response characteristics on speech discrimination and perceived intelligibility and pleasantness of speech for hearing-impaired listeners. *Journal of the Acoustical Society of America, 80*(2), 494–504.

Byrne, D., & Dillon, H. (1986). The National Acoustic Laboratories' (NAL) new procedure for selecting the gain and frequency response of a hearing aid. *Ear and Hearing, 7*(4), 257–265.

Byrne, D., & Murray, N. (1986). Predictability of the required frequency response characteristic of a hearing aid from the pure-tone audiogram. *Ear and Hearing, 7*(2), 63–70.

Byrne, D., Parkinson, A., & Newall, P. (1990). Hearing aid gain and frequency response requirements for the severely/profoundly hearing impaired. *Ear and Hearing, 11*(1), 40–49.

Carney, A. E., & Moeller, M. P. (1998). Treatment efficacy hearing loss in children. *Journal of Speech, Language and Hearing Research, 41*, S61–S84.

Ching, T. C., & Dillon, H. (2003). Prescribing amplification for children: Adult-equivalent hearing loss, real-ear aided gain, and NAL-NL1. *Trends in Amplification, 7*(1), 1–9.

Ching, T. Y., Dillon, H., & Byrne, D. (1998). Speech recognition of hearing-impaired listeners: Predictions from audibility and the limited role of high-frequency amplification. *Journal of the Acoustical Society of America, 103*(2), 1128–1140.

Ching, T., Dillon, H., Day, J., & Crowe, K. (2007). The NAL longitudinal study on outcomes of hearing-impaired children: Interim findings on language of early and later-identified children at six months after hearing aid fitting. In R. C. Seewald, & J. M. Bamford (Eds.), *A sound foundation through early amplification: Proceedings of an international conference* (pp. 185–199). Stäfa, Switzerland: Phonak AG.

Ching, T. Y., Dillon, H., Katsch, R., & Byrne, D. (2001). Maximizing effective audibility in hearing aid fitting. *Ear and Hearing, 22*, 212–224.

Ching, T. Y. C., Hill, M. Birtles, G., & Beacham, L. (1999). Clinical use of paired comparisons to evaluate hearing aid fitting of severely/profoundly hearing impaired children. *Australian and New Zealand Journal of Audiology, 21*(2), 51–63.

Ching, T. Y. C., Newall, P., & Wigney, D. (1997). Comparison of severely and profoundly hearing-impaired children's amplification preferences with the NAL-RP and the DSL 3.0 prescriptions. *International Journal of Audiology, 26*(4), 219–222.

Ching, T. Y. C., O'Brien, A., Dillon, H., Chalupper, J., Hartley, L., Hartley, D., Raicevich, G., & Hain, J. (2009). Directional effects on infants and young children in real life: Implications for amplification. *Journal of Speech, Language, and Hearing Research, 52*(5), 1241–1254.

Ching, T. Y. C., Scollie, S. D., Dillon, H., & Seewald, R. C. (2010a). A cross-over, double-blind comparison of the NAL-NL1 and the DSL v4. 1 prescriptions for children with mild to moderately severe hearing loss. *International Journal of Audiology, 49*(Suppl. 1), S4–S15.

Ching, T. Y. C., Scollie, S. D., Dillon, H., Seewald, R. C., Britton, L., & Steinberg, J. (2010b). Prescribed real-ear and achieved real-life differences in children's hearing aids adjusted according to the NAL-NL1 and the DSL v. 4. 1 prescriptions. *International Journal of Audiology, 49*(Suppl. 1), S16–S25.

Ching, T. Y. C., Scollie, S. D., Dillon, H., Seewald, R. C., Britton, L., Steinberg, J., . . . & King, K. (2010c). Evaluation of the NAL-NL1 and the DSL v. 4.1 prescriptions for children: Paired-comparison judgments and functional performance ratings. *International Journal of Audiology, 49*(Suppl. 1), S35–S48.

Cornelisse, L. E., Seewald, R. C., & Jamieson, D. G. (1995). The input/output formula: A theoretical approach to the fitting of personal amplification devices. *Journal of the Acoustical Society of America, 97*(3), 1854–1864.

Dillon, H., & Storey, L. (1998). The National Acoustic Laboratories' procedure for selecting the saturation sound pressure level of hearing aids: Theoretical derivation. *Ear and Hearing, 19*(4), 255–266.

Dirks, D., & Kincaid, G. (1987). Basic acoustic considerations of ear canal probe measurements. *Ear and Hearing, 8*(5), 60S–67S.

Elliott, L. L. (1979). Performance of children aged 9 to 17 years on a test of speech intelligibility in noise using sentence material with controlled word predictability. *Journal of the Acoustical Society of America, 66*(3), 651–653.

Elliott, L. L., Connors, S., Kille, E., Levin, S., Ball, K., & Katz, D. (1979). Children's understanding of monosyllabic nouns in quiet and in noise. *Journal of the Acoustical Society of America, 66*(1), 12–21.

Erber, N. P. (1973). Body-baffle and real-ear effects in the selection of hearing aids for deaf children. *Journal of Speech and Hearing Disorders, 38*, 224–231.

Erber, N. P., & Witt, L. H. (1977). Effects of stimulus intensity on speech perception by deaf children. *Journal of Speech and Hearing Disorders, 42*, 271–278.

Feigin, J. A., Kopun, J. G., Stelmachowicz, P. G., & Gorga, M. P. (1989). Probe-tube microphone measures of ear canal sound pressure levels in infants and children. *Ear and Hearing, 10*(4), 254–258.

Gagne, J. P., Seewald, R. C., Zelisko, D. L., & Hudson, S. P. (1991). Procedure for defining the auditory area of hearing-impaired adolescents with a severe/profound hearing loss. II: Loudness discomfort levels. *Journal of Speech-Language Pathology, 12*, 27–32.

Glista, D., Scollie, S., Bagatto, M., Seewald, R., Parsa, V., & Johnson, A. (2009). Evaluation of nonlinear frequency compression: Clinical outcomes. *International Journal of Audiology, 48*(9), 632–644.

Gorga, M. P., Kaminski, J. R., Beauchaine, K., L., & Bergman, B. M. (1993). A comparison of auditory brain stem response thresholds and latencies elicited by air- and bone-conducted stimuli. *Ear and Hearing, 14*, 85–94.

Gravel, J. (2002). Potential pitfalls in the audiological assessment of infants and young children. In R. C. Seewald, & J. S. Gravel (Eds.), *A sound foundation through early amplification 2001: Proceedings of the second international conference* (pp. 85–101). Stäfa, Switzerland: Phonak AG.

Gravel, J. S., Fausel, N., Liskow, C., & Chobot, J. (1999). Children's speech recognition in noise using omni-directional and dual-microphone hearing aid technology. *Ear and Hearing, 20*, 1–11.

Hawkins, D. B. (1987). Clinical ear canal probe tube measurements. *Journal of Speech and Hearing Research, 8*(Suppl), 74–81.

Hnath-Chisolm, T. E., Laipply, E., & Boothroyd, A. (1998). Age-related changes on a children's test of sensory-level speech perception capacity. *Journal of Speech Language and Hearing Research, 41*, 94–106.

Humes, L. E., & Kirn, E. U. (1990). The reliability of functional gain. *Journal of Speech and Hearing Disorders, 55*, 193–197.

Jenstad, L. M., Pumford, J., Seewald, R. C., & Cornelisse, L. E. (2000). Comparison of linear gain and wide-dynamic-range compression (WDRC) hearing aid circuits II: Aided loudness measures. *Ear and Hearing, 21*(2), 32–44.

Jenstad, L. M., Seewald, R. C., Cornelisse, L. E., & Shantz, J. (1999). Comparison of linear gain and wide-dynamic-range compression hearing aid circuits: Aided speech perception measures. *Ear and Hearing, 20*(2), 117–126.

Joint Committee on Infant Hearing (JCIH). (2007). Year 2007 Position Statement: Principles and guidelines for early hearing detection and intervention programs. *Pediatrics, 120*(4), 898–921.

Kamm, C., Dirks, D., & Mickey, M. R. (1977). Effect of sensorineural hearing loss on loudness discomfort level and most comfortable loudness judgements. *Journal of Speech and Hearing Research, 21*, 668–681.

Keisder, G., Brew, C., & Peck, A. (2003). How proprietary fitting algorithms compare to each other and to some generic algorithms. *Hearing Journal, 56*(3), 28–38.

Kiessling, J. (1987). In situ audiometry (ISA): A new frontier in hearing aid selection. *Hearing Instruments, 38*, 28–29.

Kiessling, J. (1993). Current approaches to hearing aid evaluation. *Journal of Speech-Language Pathology, 16*(Suppl.), 39–49.

Kortekaas, R. W. L., & Stelmachowicz, P. G. (2000). Bandwidth effects on children's perception of the inflectional morpheme /s/. *Journal of Speech, Language and Hearing Research, 43*, 645–660.

Kruger, B. (1987). An update on the external ear resonance in infants and young children. *Ear and Hearing, 8*(6), 333–336.

Kuk, F., Keenan, D., Korhonen, P., & Lau, C. (2009). Efficacy of linear frequency transposition on consonant identification in quiet and in noise. *Journal of the American Academy of Audiology, 20*(8), 465–479.

Lewis, D. E., & Stelmachowicz, P. G. (1993). Real-ear to 6-cm^3 coupler differences in young children. *Journal of Speech and Hearing Research, 36*(1), 204–209.

Macrae, J. (1986). *Relationships between the hearing threshold levels an aided speech discrimination of severely and profoundly deaf children*. NAL Report No. 107. Canberra: Australian Government Publishing Service.

Macrae, J., & Frazier, G. (1980). An investigation of variables affecting aided thresholds. *Australian Journal of Audiology, 2*, 56–62.

Marcoux, A., & Hansen, M. (2003). Ensuring accuracy of the pediatric hearing aid fitting. *Trends in Amplification, 7*(1), 11–27.

Miller-Hansen, D. R., Nelson, P. G., Widen, J. E., & Simon, S. D. (2003). Evaluating the benefit of speech recoding hearing aids in children. *American Journal of Audiology, 12*, 106–113.

Moeller, M. P. (2000). Early intervention and language development in children who are deaf and hard of hearing. *Pediatrics, 106*, e43.

Moodie, S., & Moodie, S. (2004). An approach to defining the fitting range of hearing instruments children with severe-to-profound hearing loss. In R. C. Seewald, & J. M. Bamford (Eds.), *A sound foundation through early amplification: Proceedings of the third international conference* (p. 247–254). Stäfa, Switzerland: Phonak AG.

Moodie, K. S., Seewald, R. C., & Sinclair, S. T. (1994). Procedure for predicting real-ear hearing aid performance in young children. *American Journal of Audiology, 3*, 23–31.

Mueller, H. G. (2001). Probe microphone measurements: 20 years of progress. *Trends in Amplification, 5*, 35–68.

Mueller, H. G., Bentler, R., & Wu, Y. (2008). Prescribing maximum hearing aid output: Differences among manufacturers found. *Hearing Journal, 61*(3), 30, 32, 34, 36.

Mueller, H. G., & Ricketts, T. A. (2005). Digital noise reduction: Much ado about something? *Hearing Journal, 58*(1), 10–18.

Munro, K. J., & Davis, J. (2003). Deriving the real-ear SPL of audiometric data using the "coupler to dial difference" and the "real ear to coupler difference." *Ear and Hearing, 24*, 100–110.

Munro, K. L., & Hatton, N. (2000). Customized acoustic transform functions and their accuracy at predicting real-ear hearing aid performance. *Ear and Hearing, 21*(1), 59–69.

Munro, K. J., & Salisbury, V. A. (2002). Is the real-ear-to-coupler difference independent of the measurement earphone? *International Journal of Audiology, 41*, 408–413.

Munro, K. J., & Toal, S. (2005). Measuring the RECD transfer function with an insert earphone and a hearing instrument: Are they the same? *Ear and Hearing, 26*, 27–34.

Nábělek, A. K., & Robinson, P. K. (1982). Monaural and binaural speech perception in reverberation for listeners of various ages. *Journal of the Acoustical Society of America, 71*(5), 1242–1248.

Neuman, A. C., & Hochberg, I. (1982). *The effect of reverberation on the phoneme discrimination of children.* Paper presented at the 1982 American Speech and Hearing Association convention, Toronto, ON.

Pascoe, D. P. (1978). An approach to hearing aid selection. *Hearing Instruments, 29*, 12–16.

Pascoe, D. P. (1988). Clinical measurements of the auditory dynamic range and their relation to formulas for hearing aid gain. In J. H. Jensen (Ed.), *Hearing aid fitting: Theoretical and practical views* (pp. 129–151). Copenhagen, Amsterdam: Stougaard/Jensen.

Palmer, C. V. (2006). Amplification with digital noise reduction and the perception of annoying and aversive sounds. *Trends in Amplification, 10*(2), 95–104.

Pediatric Working Group. (1996). Conference on Amplification for Children with Auditory Deficits. Amplification for infants and children with hearing loss. *American Journal of Audiology, 5*(1), 53–68.

Pittman, A. L. (2008). Short-term word-learning rate in children with normal hearing and children with hearing loss in limited and extended high-frequency bandwidths. *Journal of Speech, Language and Hearing Research, 51*, 785–797.

Pittman, A. L., & Stelmachowicz, P. G. (2000). Perception of voiceless fricatives by normal-hearing and hearing-impaired children and adults. *Journal of Speech, Language and Hearing Research, 43*, 1389–1401.

Pittman, A. L., Stelmachowicz, P. G., Lewis, D. E. & Hoover, B. M. (2003). Spectral characteristics of speech at the ear: Implications for amplification in children. *Journal of Speech, Language and Hearing Research, 46*, 649–657.

Revit, L. J. (1997). The circle of decibels: Relating the hearing test, to the hearing instrument, to the real-ear response. *Hearing Review, 4*, 35–38.

Ricketts, T. A., & Galster, J. (2008). Head angle and elevation in classroom environments: Implications for amplification. *Journal of Speech, Language and Hearing Research, 51*(2), 516–525.

Ricketts, T., Galster, J., & Tharpe, A. M. (2007). Directional benefit in simulated classroom environments. *American Journal of Audiology, 16*(2), 130–144.

Ricketts, T., & Tharpe, A. M. (2004). Potential for directivity-based benefit in actual classroom environments. In R. C. Seewald & J. M. Bamford (Eds.), *A sound foundation through early amplification: Proceedings of the third international conference* (pp. 143–153). Stäfa, Switzerland: Phonak AG.

Scollie, S. D. (2004). Prescriptive procedures for infants and children. In R. C. Seewald, & J. M. Bamford (Eds.), *A sound foundation through early amplification: Proceedings of the third international conference* (pp. 91–104). Stäfa, Switzerland: Phonak AG.

Scollie, S. D., Ching, T. Y. C., Seewald, R. C., Dillon, H., Britton, L., Steinberg, J., & King, K. (2010a). Children's speech perception and loudness ratings of children when fitted with hearing aids using the DSL v. 4.1 and the NAL-NL1 prescriptions. *International Journal of Audiology, 49*(Suppl. 1), S26–S34.

Scollie, S. D., Ching, T. Y. C., Seewald, R. C., Dillon, H., Britton, L., Steinberg, J., & Corcoran, J. (2010b). Evaluation of the NAL-NL1 and DSL v4. 1 prescriptions for children: Preference in real world use. *International Journal of Audiology, 49*(Suppl. 1), S49–S63.

Scollie, S. D., & Seewald, R. C. (2002). Evaluation of electroacoustic test signals I: Comparison with amplified speech. *Ear and Hearing, 23*(5), 477–487.

Scollie, S. D., Seewald, R. C., Cornelisse, L. C., & Jenstad, L. M. (1998). Validity and repeatability of level-dependent HL to SPL transforms. *Ear and Hearing, 19*(5), 407–413.

Scollie, S. D., Seewald, R. C., Cornelisse, L. C., Moodie, S. T., Bagatto, M. P., Laurnagaray, D., . . . Pumford, J. M. (2005). The Desired Sensation Level Multistage Input/Output Algorithm. *Trends in Amplification, 9*(4), 159–197.

Scollie, S. D., Seewald, R. C., Moodie, K. S., & Dekok, K. (2000). Preferred listening levels of children who use hearing aids: Comparison to prescriptive targets. *Journal of the American Academy of Audiology, 11*(4), 230–238.

Seewald, R. C. (1991). Hearing aid output limiting considerations for children. In J. Feigin & P. Stelmachowicz (Eds.), *Pediatric amplification: Proceedings of the 1991 national conference* (pp. 19–35). Omaha, NE: Boys Town National Research Hospital Press.

Seewald, R. C., Cornelisse, L. E., Ramji, K. V., Sinclair, S. T., Moodie, K. S., & Jamieson, D. G. (1997). *A software implementation of the Desired Sensation Level (DSL[i/o]) Method for fitting linear gain and wide-dynamic-range compression hearing instruments, Version 4.1.* Hearing Health Care Research Unit, University of Western Ontario, London, ON.

Seewald, R., Mills, J., Bagatto, M., Scollie, S., & Moodie, S. (2008). A comparison of manufacturer-specific prescriptive procedures for infants. *Hearing Journal, 61*(11), 26–34.

Seewald, R. C., Moodie, K. S., Sinclair, S. T., & Cornelisse, L. E. (1996). Traditional and theoretical approaches to selecting amplification for infants and young children. In F. H. Bess, J. S. Gravel J. S., & A. M. Tharpe, (Eds.), *Amplification for children with auditory deficits* (pp. 161–191). Nashville, TN: Bill Wilkerson Center Press.

Seewald, R. C., Moodie, K. S., Sinclair, S. T., & Scollie, S. D. (1999). Predictive validity of a procedure for pediatric hearing instrument fitting. *American Journal of Audiology, 8*(2), 143–152.

Seewald, R. C., Ramji, K. V., Sinclair, S. T., Moodie, K. S., & Jamieson, D. G. (1993). *A computer-assisted implementation of the Desired Sensation Level Method for electroacoustic selection and fitting in children: Version 3.1*. Hearing Health Care Research Unit Technical Report #02. London, ON: University of Western Ontario.

Seewald, R. C., Ross, M., & Spiro, M. K. (1985). Selecting amplification characteristics for young hearing-impaired children. *Ear and Hearing, 6*(1), 48–53.

Shaw, E. A. G., & Vaillancourt, M. M. (1985). Transformation of sound pressure level from the free field to the eardrum presented in numerical form. *Journal of the Acoustical Society of America, 78*(3), 1120–1123.

Sinclair, S. T., Beauchaine, K. L., Moodie, K. S., Feigin, J. A., Seewald, R. C., & Stelmachowicz, P. G. (1996). Repeatability of a real-ear-to-coupler-difference measurement as a function of age. *American Journal of Audiology, 5*, 52–56.

Snik, A. F., van den Borne, S., Brokx, J. P., & Hoekstra, C. (1995). Hearing-aid fitting in profoundly hearing impaired children. *Scandinavian Audiology, 24*, 225–230.

Snik, A. F. M. & Stollman, M. H. P. (1995). Measured and calculated insertion gains in young children. *British Journal of Audiology, 29*, 7–11.

Stapells, D. R. (2000a). Threshold estimation by the tone-evoked auditory brainstem response: A literature meta-analysis. *Journal of Speech-Language Pathology and Audiology, 24*, 74–83.

Stapells, D. R. (2000b). Frequency-specific evoked potential audiometry in infants. In: R. C. Seewald (Ed.), *A sound foundation through early amplification: Proceedings of an international conference* (pp. 13–32). Stäfa, Switzerland: Phonak AG.

Stapells, D. R., Gravel, J. S., & Martin, B. E. (1995). Thresholds for auditory brainstem responses to tones in notched noise from infants and young children with normal hearing or sensorineural hearing loss. *Ear and Hearing, 16*, 361–371.

Stapells, D. R., Herdman, A., Small, S. A., Dimitrijevic, A. & Hatton, J. (2005). Current status of the auditory steady-state responses for estimating an infant's audiogram. In R. C. Seewald, & J. M. Bamford (Eds.), *A sound foundation through early amplification: Proceedings of the third international conference* (pp. 43–59). Stäfa, Switzerland: Phonak AG.

Stelmachowicz, P. G., Hoover, B. M., Lewis, D. E., Kortekaas, R. W. L., & Pittman, A. L. (2000). The relation between stimulus context, speech audibility, and perception for normal-hearing and hearing-impaired children. *Journal of Speech, Language and Hearing Research, 43*, 902–914.

Stelmachowicz, P. G., & Lewis, D. E. (1988). Some theoretical considerations concerning the relation between functional gain and insertion gain. *Journal of Speech and Hearing Research, 31*, 491–496.

Stelmachowicz, P. G., Pittman, A. L., Hoover, B. M., & Lewis, D. E. L. (2001). Effects of stimulus bandwidth on the perception of /s/ in normal- and hearing-impaired children and adults. *Journal of the Acoustical Society of America, 110*(4), 2183–2190.

Stelmachowicz, P. G., Pittman, A. L., Hoover, B. M., & Lewis, D. E. L. (2002). Aided perception of /s/ and /z/ by hearing-impaired children. *Ear and Hearing, 23*(4), 316–324.

Stelmachowicz, P. G., Pittman, A. L., Hoover, B. M., Lewis, D. E., & Moeller, M. P. (2004). The importance of high-frequency audibility in the speech and language development of children with hearing loss. *Archives of Otolarygology–Head and Neck Surgery, 130*, 556–562.

Stuart, A., Durieux-Smith, A., & Stenstrom, R. (1990). Critical differences in aided sound field thresholds in children. *Journal of Speech and Hearing Research, 33*(9), 612–615.

Tharpe, A. M., Sladen, D., Huta, H. M., & Rothpletz, A. M. (2001). Practical considerations of real-ear-to-coupler difference measures in infants. *American Journal of Audiology, 10*, 41–49.

Valente, M., Potts, L. G., Valente, M., Vass, W., & Goebel, J. (1994). Intersubject variability of real-ear sound pressure level: conventional and insert earphones. *Journal of the American Academy of Audiology, 5*, 390–398.

Vohr, B., Jodoin-Krauzyk, J., Tucker, R., Johnson, M. J., Topol, D., & Ahlgren, M. (2008). Early language outcomes of early-identified infants with permanent hearing loss at 12 to 16 months of age. *Pediatrics, 122*(3), 535–544.

Wolfe, J., Caraway, T., John, A., Schafer, E. C. & Nyffeler, M. (2009). Study suggests that non-linear frequency compression helps children with moderate loss. *Hearing Journal, 62*, 32–37.

26

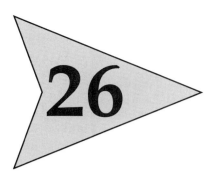

FM Systems and Communication Access for Children

Dawna Lewis and Leisha Eiten

Introduction

With the expansion of newborn hearing screening programs, infants with hearing loss are being identified at very early ages. Once hearing loss has been identified, an essential goal for pediatric audiologists is to provide children with communication access across a wide variety of listening environments. Although there are many factors that may impact communication access, audibility of the signal of interest is of primary importance. In addition to degree and configuration of hearing loss and amplification issues, audibility will be affected by distance between the sound source and listener, background noise, and reverberation.

Communication Access

As the distance between listeners and talkers varies throughout the day, the audibility of speech also will vary. This affects both the level of the primary signal reaching the listener's ears and the level of that signal relative to background noise. For example, the overall level of a classroom teacher's voice one meter from the listener is approximately 71 dB SPL and at four meters is approximately 61 dB SPL (Pearsons, Bennett, & Fidell, 1977). The level of average conversational speech at one meter is approximately 60 dB SPL (Cox & Moore, 1988). Instances of "conversational speech at one meter" may not be as common for children as for adults. Any parent of a young child will be quick to report that the distance between a talker and a young listener can vary considerably in a very short period of time. In addition, there will be many times when the talker and listener will not be face-to-face. For infants and young children, there will be times when the level of speech reaching their ears will be higher than that of speech at one meter. The level of speech at the near ear of an infant held in the cradle position is approximately 68 dB SPL and at the near ear of a young child held on the hip is approximately 76 dB SPL (Stelmachowicz, Mace, Kopun, & Carney, 1993). At other times the level of speech reaching an infant or young child's ears may be lower, such as when the talker is farther away or the orientation of talkers is not face-to-face. For example, in the United States infants up to 20 pounds or one year of age are placed in rear-facing infant seats in the back seat of cars. Even when they move to front-facing car seats, it is recommended that they remain in the back seat until they are 12 years of age (American Red Cross, 2007). In this environment, the combined effects of distance, orientation, and car noise may significantly impact the audibility of speech.

For school-age children, the ability to hear and understand verbal information is critical to learning in the classroom. However, in many schools poor classroom acoustics may impact this ability. Background noise can be defined as unwanted sounds that interfere with the primary signal. Noise can come from sources outside the school building (e.g., traffic, playground noise), inside the building but outside the classroom (e.g., sounds from the hallway, a nearby music class), or in the classroom (e.g., heating and air conditioning systems, the students themselves). Reverberation is the repeated reflection of sound and typically is reported in terms of the time it takes for a sound to decrease 60 dB from its original intensity once the sound stops (reverberation time). Long reverberation times may negatively impact perception of the primary speech signal.

In 2002, the American National Standards Institute (ANSI) published guidelines for classroom acoustics. These guidelines recommended maximum background noise levels of 35 dB(A) and maximum reverberations times of 0.6 to 0.7 seconds (ANSI, 2002) for typical classrooms. However, many classrooms fail to meet these criteria (Crandell, 1991; Crandell & Smaldino, 1994; Finitzo-Heiber, 1981). For example, Knecht, Nelson, Whitelaw, and Feth (2002) evaluated background noise levels and reverberation times in 32 elementary classrooms in three different school districts. Noise levels ranged from 34 to 66 dB(A), with only four classrooms having noise levels below the ANSI recommended levels. Reverberation times ranged from 0.2 to 1.27 seconds, with 13 classrooms exceeding the ANSI recommendations.

The deleterious effects of noise, distance and reverberation on the speech perception of listeners with hearing loss are well known (e.g., Johnson, Stein, Broadway, & Markwalter, 1997; Ross & Giolas, 1971). Finitzo-Heiber and Tillman (1978) examined word recognition for 12 children with hearing loss and 12 children with normal hearing under various conditions of noise and reverberation. In all conditions, children with hearing loss performed more poorly than their peers with normal hearing. In adverse listening conditions, children with minimal hearing loss perform more poorly than their peers with normal hearing on tasks of speech perception in noise, especially when speech is directed to the poor ear and noise to the good ear for those with unilateral hearing loss (Bess, Klee, & Culbertson, 1986; Crandell, 1993; Kenworthy, Klee, & Tharpe, 1990; Ruscetta, Arjmand, & Pratt, 2005).

The effects of distance, noise, and reverberation also may negatively impact some groups of children with normal hearing (e.g., Bradley & Sato, 2004; Crandell & Smaldino, 1996; Jamieson, Kranjc, Yu, & Hodgetts, 2004; Nelson, Kohnert, Sabur, & Shaw, 2005). Over 25 years ago, Zentall and Shaw (1980) compared the performance of children who had been identified as hyperactive with children who were not hyperactive on classroom tasks in the presence of background noise with a high linguistic content. When the task was familiar, the hyperactive children performed more poorly in high noise levels than the other children. When the task was unfamiliar, both groups performed poorly in high noise levels. More recently, Bradlow, Kraus, and Hayes (2003) showed that children with normal hearing who have learning disabilities (LD) also may experience difficulties understanding speech in adverse environments. They compared sentence perception in noise (–4 and –8 dB signal-to-noise ratio) for children with and without LD. Children with LD performed more poorly than their peers and were more adversely affected by decreasing signal-to-noise ratio. Children with normal hearing sensitivity who may be negatively impacted in adverse listening environments include young children and children who are English language learners, as well as those with the following:

- Attention deficit disorders,
- Auditory processing disorders,
- Developmental delays,
- Dyslexia,
- Recurrent middle-ear dysfunction,
- Speech and language disorders,
- History of conductive hearing loss,
- Hyperactivity.

Challenges experienced by children with hearing loss in adverse listening environments may negatively impact development/performance in a number of areas. For example, difficulties perceiving speech in noise may impede a listener's ability to follow conversations with multiple talkers. In addition, because most communication takes place in environments where noise is present, children with hearing loss may experience difficulties following conversations from a distance or acquiring information via overhearing. These difficulties may, in turn, affect speech and language development as well as social-emotional functioning. Subtle difficulties in language abilities might be expected to have an impact on advanced language skills, such as social reasoning (e.g., emotion understanding, theory of mind), discourse participation, complex narratives (justifying opinion, explanations), complex syntax (cohesive ties, complementation), and complex vocabulary. Difficulties in advanced language skills may, in turn, negatively affect psychosocial development. Numerous studies have suggested that children with hearing loss experience difficulties in areas such as self-esteem, stress, energy, peer relations, and social confidence (e.g., Bess, Dodd-Murphy, & Parker, 1998; Cappelli, Daniels, Durieux-Smith, McGrath, & Neuss, 1995; Loeb & Sarigiani, 1986; Oyler, Oyler, & Matkin, 1988).

Educational performance also may be affected since the acoustic conditions in typical classroom environments are less than ideal (Blair, Peterson, & Viehweg, 1985; Brookhouser, Worthington, & Kelly, 1991; Culbertson & Gilbert, 1986; English & Church; 1999). Oyler et al. (1988) reported results of teacher questionnaires completed for children with unilateral hearing loss in a large school district. Twenty-four percent of these students had repeated at least one grade (compared to a district average of 2%) and 41% were receiving special services (compared to a district average of 8.6%).

Listeners with hearing loss also may need to exert more effort than their peers with normal hearing in the same listening environment (Bess et al., 1998). Hicks and Tharpe (2002) found that children (5–11 yrs.) with mild-to-moderate or high-frequency hearing loss expended more listening effort than children with normal hearing in both easy and difficult classroom listening situations.

In 2006, the National Institute on Deafness and Other Communication Disorders at the National Institutes of Health sponsored a workshop on outcomes in research in children with mild-severe hearing loss. Among the outcomes from that workshop was a series of papers on the current state of knowledge regarding this population of children. Topics included psychosocial development (Moeller, 2007), language and literacy (Moeller, Tomblin, Yoshinaga-Itano, Connor, & Jerger, 2007), perceptual processing (Jerger, 2007), speech recognition and production (Eisenberg, 2007), as well as research considerations (Tomblin & Hebbeler, 2007) and implications for future research (Eisenberg et al., 2007). These papers provide an overview of many of the challenges experienced by children with hearing loss as well as directions for future research.

Communication Solutions

When hearing loss is first identified, hearing instruments typically are the most common technology option for achieving auditory access. Cochlear implants also are an option available for children with severe to profound hearing loss. Although these devices provide communication access in many situations, access will continue to be negatively impacted by noise, distance and reverberation (Anderson & Goldstein, 2004; Anderson, Goldstein, Colodzin, & Iglehart, 2005; Schafer & Thibodeau, 2006). Leavitt and Flexer (1991) used the Rapid Speech Transmission Index (RASTI) to examine the integrity of a speechlike signal at multiple seating positions in a classroom in relationship to a sound source at the front of the room. Perfect reproduction of the signal was only obtained 6 inches from the sound source. The integrity of the signal reaching typical seating positions in the classroom was far from ideal. Although direct correlations between RASTI scores and speech perception were not examined, these results reveal that the signal reaching a hearing instrument or cochlear implant microphone will be significantly degraded at all but the closest listening distances. One way to ensure a high quality speech input to the hearing instrument or cochlear implant is to maintain a close distance between the talker and listener; a solution that is neither practical nor desirable. A more feasible solution is to place a microphone on the talker, transmitting the signal directly to a receiver worn by the listener.

Remote microphone technologies can provide reproduction of close, un-degraded input signals with no reverberation effects and reduced impact of noise. A variety of remote-microphone hearing assistance technology (HAT) choices are available for classroom and home use. Large area systems are often used for educational and public venue applications. They may utilize induction loops/mats, sound-field FM (frequency modulation) or IR (infrared) transmission. Personal systems can be adapted to both in-school and out-of-school use. Personal remote-microphone systems include portable desktop FM or IR systems and individual FM systems.

Expansion of the use of wireless connections has resulted in many questions about the use of Bluetooth technology as a remote-microphone HAT. Wikipedia defines Bluetooth as:

> A wireless protocol utilizing short-range communications technology facilitating data transmission over short distances from fixed and/or mobile devices, creating wireless personal area networks. The intent behind the development of Bluetooth was the creation of a single digital wireless protocol, capable of connecting multiple devices and overcoming problems arising from synchronization of these devices. (Wikipedia, 2008)

A number of factors impact the application of Bluetooth technology as a remote microphone HAT option (Fabry, 2008). These include:

- High power consumption,
- Limited transmission range,
- Latency (delay) in signal transmission.

Although not a direct remote-microphone HAT, Bluetooth technology is being used as a means of connecting the listener to other electronic accessories such as cell phones, MP3 players, and computers.

FM Solutions to Enhance Communication Access

Frequency-modulated (FM) systems are an effective solution to the problems of noise, distance, and reverberation because they use a microphone near a talker's mouth to maintain a close listening distance between the talker and the listener. FM systems use a low-power radio transmitter to send FM radio signals from this remote microphone to a miniature receiver worn by the listener. The FM transmitter/microphone is worn by the primary talker who is often a parent or teacher. The use of a remote microphone provides an advantage because the transmitted signal preserves a consistent input level even if the distance between the talker and the listener changes. Because the speech signal is picked up inches from the talker's mouth, the transmitted signal maintains a positive signal-to-noise ratio advantage above the level of background noise without reverberation effects.

FM Developments

The changes in FM technology in the last 20 years have been significant. Prior to the mid 1990s most FM systems transmitted in the 72- to 76-mHz frequency range. Transmission in this range was prone to interference and required strong antennae. Many FM systems used one dedicated transmission channel that could not be changed. FM receivers were body-worn units that originally required the hearing instruments to be removed entirely, and later could be connected to a child's personal hearing instrument(s) via direct audio input cords. Environmental (local) microphones on these body-worn receivers used linear amplification circuits with limited frequency-response adjustability. Prior to 1982, the local microphone was always on the body-worn receiver, which resulted in its placement at chest level (P. Henry, personal communication, May 30, 2008).

One of the most significant changes in wireless technology has been the introduction of smaller and more flexible FM receiver options (Figure 26–1).

Unlike the previous body-worn FM systems that had fixed receiver channels, today's FM receivers have a large number of channels that can be easily changed or synchronized with different transmitters. Federal Communications Commission approval of additional FM channels in the 216- to 217-mHz bands (Federal Communications Commission, 1996) reduced the need for large antennae on the receiver. This, along with increased miniaturization of integrated circuitry, has allowed smaller FM receivers to be built. FM receivers are now designed to be ear-level devices that can be worn with a child's personal hearing instruments or cochlear implants. Because of the change to ear-level FM receivers, the hearing instrument or cochlear implant microphone acts as the local microphone for the system. One advantage of ear-level FM systems is that the advanced circuitry and signal processing of digital hearing instruments or cochlear implants can be available to the child at the same time as the benefits of a remote (FM) microphone system. With the availability of ear-level receivers, the FM system has moved away from serving only as a classroom "auditory trainer" and now is utilized as hearing assistance technology (HAT) in many areas of the child's home and family life. In any listening situation where background noise and reverberation or distance from the

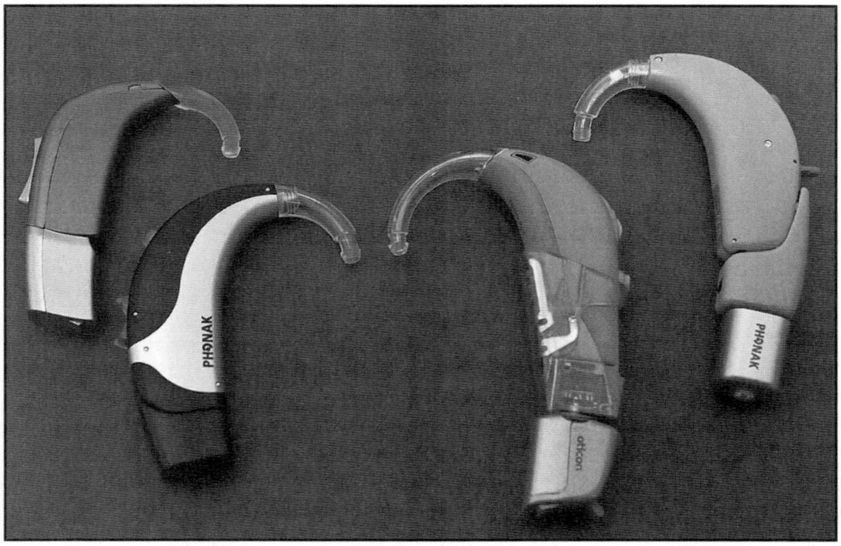

FIGURE 26–1. Examples of ear-level FM receivers coupled to behind-the-ear hearing instruments.

talker makes understanding difficult, an FM system can be used. Conversations in the car, family trips to the zoo and recreational activities can all be enhanced.

Current state-of-the-art FM receivers allow the audiologist to adjust or program the output level of the FM signal in relation to the local microphone signal to accommodate an individual child's needs. In addition, a teacher or parent can quickly change or synchronize FM receiver channels as the child moves from classroom to classroom or from classroom to home. A range of integration options are available, including FM receivers fully integrated into the hearing instrument, modular or dedicated receivers for specific hearing instruments or cochlear implant models, and universal receivers that can be switched between hearing instrument and cochlear implant models and manufacturers. Ear-level FM-only devices also are now available for children with normal hearing who have special listening needs and may benefit from an improved signal-to-noise ratio, such as those populations previously listed in this chapter.

Changes in FM transmitters also have improved their flexibility. Current FM transmitters incorporate features such as directional microphones, cheek or boom microphone placement options, digital noise reduction circuitry and Bluetooth wireless compatibility for integration with cell phones, computers, and MP3 (e.g., iPod™) players. The choice of directional microphone settings allows flexibility in using the FM system in a variety of settings outside traditional classrooms. Some examples include using the transmitter as a conference microphone to hear a number of talkers in a group activity, or choosing a narrow directional setting to use the transmitter as a hand-held "pointer" microphone in a family gathering or party setting, where the main talker frequently changes. Recent advances in FM system technology include transmitters that incorporate adaptive FM levels to maintain ideal signal-to-noise ratios, as well as technology to adjust for varying voice levels and microphone placements. Talker networks can be activated to improve team-teaching with multiple FM transmitters active in a classroom. More functions are becoming available to assist teachers and families with troubleshooting and daily monitoring of FM system use. Audiologists who evaluate FM systems should be knowledgeable about current transmitter features and how those features impact daily use.

Developmental Aspects of FM System Use

Although FM systems have been utilized outside the classroom for a number of years (Benoit, 1989; Madell, 1992; Moeller, Donaghy, Beauchaine, Lewis, & Stelmachowicz, 1996), body-worn FM systems were considered bulky and cumbersome, limiting their use beyond classroom environments. The introduction of the first integrated FM/hearing instrument combination in 1992 (Sonovation, 2008) and, more significantly, the miniaturization of FM receivers coupled directly to hearing instruments (Phonak, 2008) had a tremendous impact on the extension of FM system use beyond classroom environments and on their use with infants and young children.

With the miniaturization of FM receivers, it has become more common for audiologists to recommend FM systems for infants and young children with hearing loss. Gabbard (2005) reported preliminary findings from a loaner FM project in the state of Colorado. Parents of nine children between the ages of 15 and 30 months completed a questionnaire designed to provide information regarding use and benefit from hearing instruments and FM systems. On average, hearing instruments were used 10 hours per day and FM systems were used four hours per day. Both were rated as easy to operate and comfortable for the children. Comments from parents suggested that the FM system benefits were seen in the expected areas of distance and noise and that they helped the children attend to speech in those environments.

As stated earlier in this chapter, while very young infants spend much of their time in close proximity to talkers, there will be many situations where noise, distance, and reverberation become factors in their ability to hear and understand speech. Once the child is mobile, these situations become even more common. Also, unlike adults, children (especially young children) are in the process of learning speech and language. As such, they require good audibility to develop adequate speech and language skills. Thus, a primary reason for using FM systems with infants and young children is to provide them with a consistently audible signal during this crucial period of speech and language development.

Anecdotally, concerns occasionally are expressed regarding a possible negative impact of FM system use on the development of localization abilities in infants and young children as well as on their ability to learn to understand speech in noise. Currently, no research exists to support either of these concerns. There also are practical reasons to question such concerns. It is important to remember that FM systems typically are not worn 100% of the time. There will be many situations in which infants and young children will be using only their hearing instruments. During those times, they will be receiving inputs from many directions, providing information about the location of the sound source. In addition, the signal of interest will arrive at the ears embedded within any background noises within the environment. Even when the infant uses the FM system, it is most common that both the FM system and hearing instrument microphones are active simultaneously. Thus, the only input signal that would not be providing information about sound-source location would be that of the person wearing the FM microphone. Although the signal from the FM microphone will be received at a better SNR than it would through the hearing instruments alone, background noise is not eliminated completely. It also is important to remember that there are many adverse listening environments where practice will not be able to improve speech understanding for an individual with hearing loss. Recall the Leavitt and Flexer (1991) data presented previously in this chapter. If the signal reaching the ear has been severely degraded by noise, distance, and reverberation, even a hearing instrument that perfectly reproduces the signal will be presenting that severely degraded signal to the listener.

As children grow, and before they reach school age, the potential benefit of FM system use enlarges as their listening experiences expand. Adverse listening environments where FM systems may improve audibility include car trips, family outings and group activities (e.g., dance lessons, children's sports teams). As parents of children seen in our clinics have reported, the FM system increases the language learning opportunities the child experiences in daily life.

When children reach school age, listening environments continue to expand. Although the ability to hear and understand verbal information is critical to learning in most classrooms, acoustics may impede audibility for many children with hearing loss and some groups of children with normal hearing. FM systems can improve audibility of the teacher's voice, the voices of other students if they use the FM microphone, and audibility of the audio signal from televisions, videos, and computers. FM systems also may be used in extracurricular activities such as sports, dance, or drama. As they reach adolescence, students may be involved in after-school jobs or in volunteer organizations where utilizing FM systems can improve communication access in a variety of adverse listening environments. Especially in adolescence, the ability to couple a small FM receiver to a personal hearing instrument or to have the FM receiver incorporated into a BTE hearing instrument case makes utilization in a variety of listening environments much more feasible and attractive to users.

As high school students transition to college or full-time employment, FM systems can continue to play a role in communication access. Those individuals who have benefited from FM system use for many years may be more likely to continue using the devices into adulthood, viewing them as an integral part of their hearing assistance technology. Audiologists can remain a vital resource in helping to examine technology options and funding sources for changing needs.

FM System Verification

The development of ear-level FM receivers has meant that the hearing instrument microphone acts as the local microphone of the FM system. This allows the FM system user to hear other talkers and sounds in the environment and monitor one's own voice, while still receiving a consistent input from the main talker using the FM microphone/transmitter. With most current hearing instrument circuits incorporating some type of nonlinear compression processing, verification of FM systems has been significantly impacted. Any verification of the function of the FM system is dependent on accurate evaluation of the hearing instrument processing. Hearing instrument processing options may include multiple channels, frequency compression/transposition and active noise-reduction. Previous FM system verification guidelines (ASHA, 1994, 2002) assumed local microphones functioned with single-channel linear circuitry. It has become clear in recent years that the rapid advances in hearing instrument and FM technology require a re-examination of FM system fitting and verification procedures.

Another technological advance that has impacted FM system verification is the availability of hearing instrument test systems that offer speech-mapping using real speech inputs, rather than broadband noise or pure-tone inputs. As an input signal, real speech allows more accurate evaluation of how hearing instruments and FM systems respond to typical inputs. Speech is one of the primary signals that both FM systems and hearing instruments are designed to transmit and amplify. Advanced compression and noise reduction processing react differently to rapidly changing speech than they do to constant-level signals. Current guidelines recommend the use of calibrated real-speech inputs for the evaluation of hearing instrument and FM microphone responses.

Electroacoustic FM System Verification

There are three assumptions that guide current verification processes and assist in prioritizing testing (American Academy of Audiology [AAA], 2008a, 2008b).

1. Ear-level FM systems use the microphone of the hearing instrument as the local microphone, and the input from the FM microphone is processed by the hearing instrument circuitry. All verification measures of the relationship between the FM and hearing instrument microphones are based on the assumption that the hearing instrument processing has been adjusted to provide appropriate audibility and output for the individual user (AAA, 2004). Before verifying FM system performance, the audiologist must first verify that the hearing instrument is set appropriately and is meeting chosen prescriptive targets for a variety of speech input levels. True estimates of maximum output are obtained from input to the hearing instrument microphone, not the FM microphone. High compression ratios in the FM microphone/transmitter likely will prevent the hearing instrument from reaching its maximum output in response to FM input. The audiologist must also confirm that the hearing instrument is able to accept an FM input.

2. Most FM systems are worn with both the FM microphone and hearing instrument microphone(s) active at the same time. Therefore, all verification should be completed with the FM system and hearing instrument microphones active simultaneously. The FM system output level can then be adjusted in relationship to the hearing instrument response so as to preserve as much of a speech-to-noise benefit as possible. Traditionally, it has been recommended that the signal from the FM system maintain a 10 dB advantage over other signals coming to the local microphone.

3. Because of the nonlinear characteristics of current hearing instrument and FM system circuitry, different input levels to the two microphones will result in changing compression and gain results. This will create problems during electroacoustic verification measures as testing *only* can be completed sequentially, meaning that the hearing instrument microphone response is evaluated, followed by the FM microphone response. Current test systems do not allow for simultaneous inputs to both the hearing instrument and FM system microphones with separate outputs for the two inputs. Therefore, *if* the FM microphone response is evaluated using input levels that are typical for close microphone placements (80–95 dB SPL) and the hearing instrument microphone response is evaluated separately for conversational input levels (60–65 dB SPL), the compression parameters in response to these input signals will be significantly different than they will be when those signals reach both microphones simultaneously. Consequently, no valid comparisons could then be made between the FM system and hearing instrument responses if different input levels were tested sequentially. A thorough discussion of the impact of nonlinear compression characteristics and the use of sequential versus simultaneous measurements can be found in Platz (2004, 2006).

Because current test systems do not allow simultaneous measures of hearing instrument and FM system microphones, electroacoustic verification protocols require that input levels to the FM microphone be less than actual use inputs. This is required to ensure that the hearing instrument response to an FM system input has the same compression characteristics as its response to input from the hearing instrument microphone. Verification of the relationship between FM system and hearing instrument responses can be completed with equal inputs to the FM system and hearing instrument microphones. The input level to both systems must be sufficiently low so that input compression in the FM transmitter is not activated, and compression in the hearing instrument will act equally on both the FM and hearing instrument test signals. The goal is to achieve equal outputs for equal inputs to the two microphones. This new approach to FM system verification is defined as transparency.

With the FM receiver set at its default FM system gain position of +10 dB, the AAA Guidelines (AAA, 2008b) recommend a 65 dB SPL input to the hearing instrument microphone and a 65 dB SPL input to the FM microphone (in the HA+FM position) to evaluate for transparency (Figure 26–2).

If the FM system output at this +10 dB setting is more than ±2 dB different from the hearing instrument output, adjustments (offsets) are made to the FM system level to achieve equal outputs, or transparency. When verified in this manner, the FM system has been shown to maintain a 10 dB signal-to-noise advantage in relationship to the hearing instrument when typical use inputs are presented simultaneously to both microphones (Platz, 2006). This 10 dB recommendation is offered as a general starting point for selecting the FM system level. It is based on the relationship between typical use inputs to the FM and hearing instrument microphones and the kneepoint for compression in the FM microphone/transmitter. For step-by-step verification procedures, see AAA (2008b).

Because of the nonlinear nature of current hearing instrument and FM system technology, functional gain or amplified sound field threshold (ASFT) testing should never be used to verify FM system function. With the changing compression characteristics of both FM and hearing instrument microphones, no predictable relationship exists between amplified threshold information and FM system performance at typical use input levels.

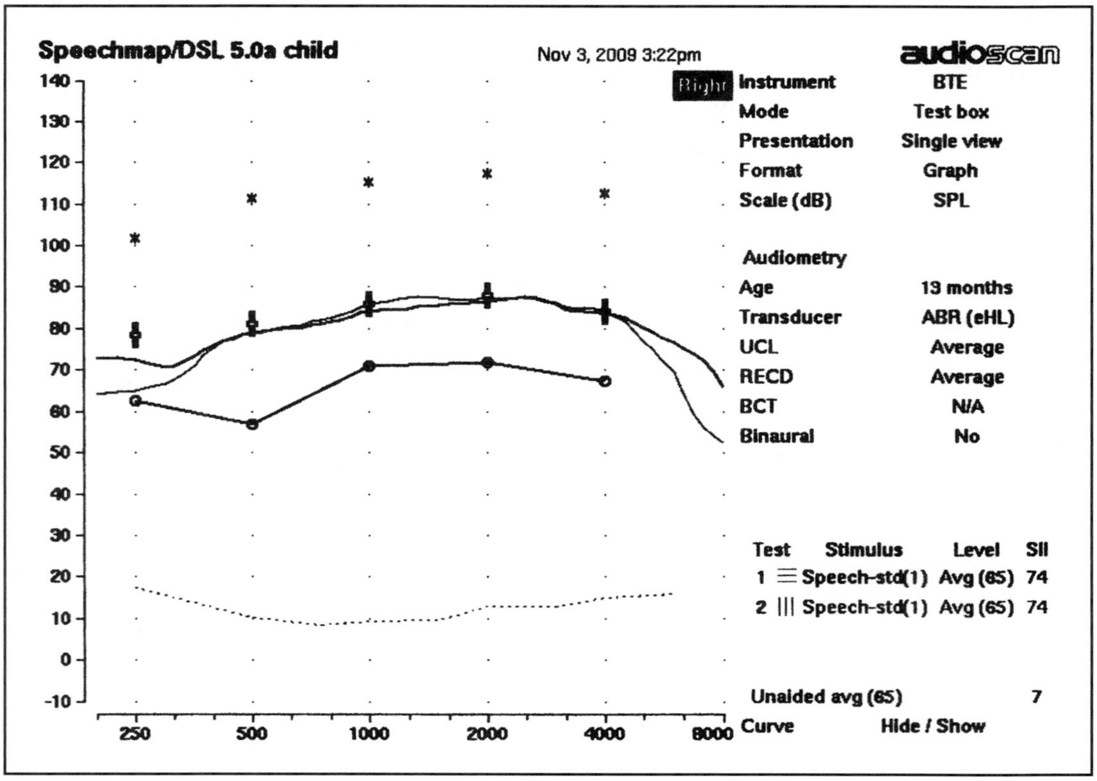

FIGURE 26–2. SPLogram graph illustrating transparency measures with 65 dB SPL input to the hearing instrument (test 1) and 65 dB SPL input to the FM microphone (test 2). Circles are hearing thresholds, crosses are long-term average speech spectrum targets, and asterisks are maximum output targets.

Real-Ear FM System Verification

Real-ear verification of FM systems can be completed for any hearing instrument + FM or FM-only combination. Due to the number of measures and possible adjustments needed when verifying FM receivers coupled to hearing instruments, electroacoustic verification in a test box is typically the more efficient approach. However, verification of ear-level FM-only systems requires special considerations. Ear-level FM-only fittings are primarily used with children/students who have normal or near-normal hearing. The child's ability to hear oneself and others needs to be preserved; therefore, ear-level FM-only fittings are designed to be nonoccluding. Electroacoustic verification in a test box with the FM receiver coupled to a 2 cc coupler does not provide accurate information about how the system functions on the child's ear when open-ear acoustics are preserved. In addition to open-ear acoustic considerations, the FM-only receiver is not coupled to personal hearing instruments and has no local microphone that amplifies other talkers. Using the same transparency approach previously described for FM receivers coupled to hearing instruments is not appropriate when verifying ear-level FM-only receivers.

When verifying any nonoccluding fitting, two sound pathways must be considered (Figure 26–3): (1) the amplified sound pathway, which is the transmitted signal from the FM system. This is the primary signal of interest for verification; and (2) the direct or unamplified sound pathway, which includes unamplified portions of the main talker's voice, other talkers, the FM user's own voice and background noise. In a nonoccluding fitting, unamplified signals can move freely into and out of the ear canal. At the same time, much of the low-frequency regions of the amplified input signal leak out of the open ear canal (Hoover, Stelmachowicz, & Lewis, 2000). This will affect the expectations and targets for the FM system response in the child's nonoccluded ear (Figure 26–4).

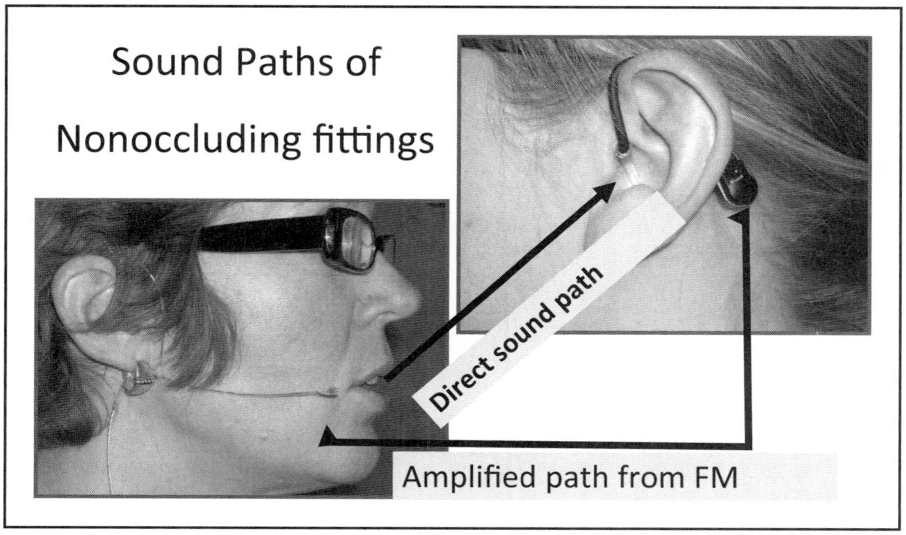

FIGURE 26–3. Two sound paths into the ear when wearing a nonoccluding FM system.

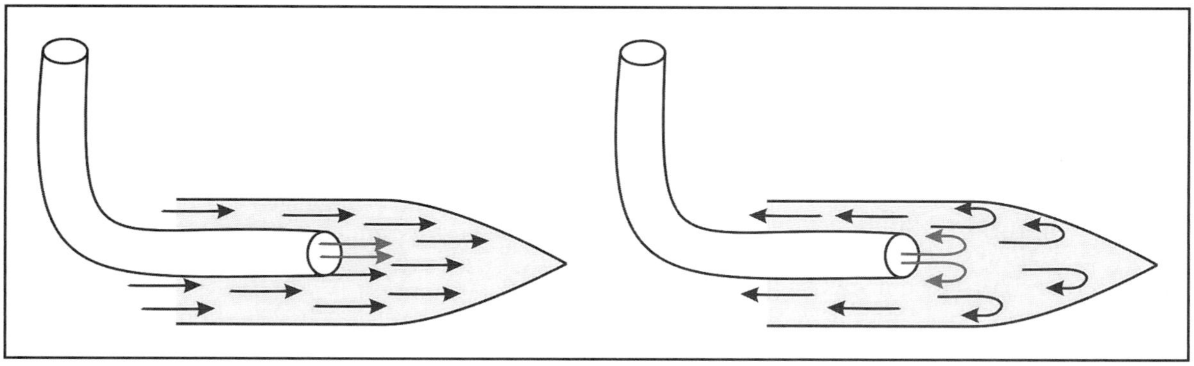

FIGURE 26–4. Graphic representation of amplified (*gray arrows*) and direct (*black arrows*) sound as it enters (*left*) and leaves (*right*) the nonoccluded ear canal.

Verification priorities for ear-level FM-only fittings are two-fold. First, maximum output should be confirmed in the child's ear. Because most FM-only devices are fitted on normal-hearing ears, it is critical to verify the maximum output of the system using a high-level pure-tone input. Output or volume control adjustments may be needed to prevent exposure to excessive sound pressure levels. Second, the FM system should maintain consistent audibility and comfort for the main talker's voice. Recommended use settings are determined based on the response of the FM-only system to close speech inputs (1-6″ from talker's mouth).

Specific procedures for real-ear verification of FM-only receivers will vary depending on the real-ear test system that is utilized. These procedures will be influenced by how the real-ear reference microphone is used during testing and whether FM specific inputs and targets are available in the test system (AAA, 2008b; Eiten, 2008; Eiten & Lewis, 2008). For step-by-step real-ear verification procedures, see AAA (2008b).

Behavioral FM System Verification

Behavioral verification of FM systems using speech perception measures is a recommended option when an appropriate sound-field test environment is available (AAA, 2008b). Although behavioral verification is not a substitute for electroacoustic verification for HA+FM and FM-only systems, it remains the primary method of verification for FM systems coupled to cochlear implants. When using speech perception tasks to verify FM system performance, testing should be completed under listening conditions that are representative of the child's typical listening environments. Priority is given to testing in noise. The child's performance when the FM microphone is not active (unaided, hearing instrument only, cochlear implant only) is compared to performance with the FM microphone active under the same noise conditions. The vocabulary and language level of the child must be considered when choosing this verification option.

Testing with adaptive or variable noise and/or speech levels is not recommended as part of the behavioral verification of FM systems. When testing is conducted with varying speech levels and a fixed noise level, the input to the FM microphone will most likely be significantly lower than that found in normal use (Boothroyd & Iglehart, 1998). Similarly, when testing is conducted with varying noise levels and a fixed speech level at the FM microphone, the resulting noise levels may exceed typical classroom noise levels. For these reasons, the use of such testing to determine a threshold signal-to-noise ratio is not recommended for behavioral FM system verification. These types of procedures *are* appropriate when evaluating performance with personal hearing instruments or cochlear implants alone for determining HAT candidacy. Some currently available speech-in-noise tests that use adaptive or variable speech and/or noise levels include the BKB-SIN (Bamford-Kowal-Bench Speech-In-Noise test; Etymotic Research, 2005) and HINT-C (Hearing-In-Noise Test-Child; Nilsson, Soli, & Gelnett, 1996).

Conclusions

Research continues to support the need for hearing assistance technology in poor acoustic environments for children with hearing loss and for children with normal hearing who have special listening needs. Developments in FM system technology have expanded their use and now provide audiologists with many options for addressing communication access needs. Miniature, ear-level FM receivers are appropriate for children of all ages both in and out of school. Fitting and verification techniques have evolved to keep pace with technological developments in both hearing instruments and FM systems. It is important for audiologists who work with children to understand current methods for selecting and fitting FM systems in order to address the specific communication needs of each child. Audiologists must also incorporate appropriate verification guidelines into their clinical practice and be aware of future advances as they become available.

References

American Academy of Audiology. (2004). Pediatric amplification guideline. *Audiology Today*, *16*(2), 46–53.

American Academy of Audiology. (2008a). *AAA Clinical Practice Guidelines: Remote microphone hearing assistance technologies for children and youth birth–21 years.* Retrieved July 1, 2008, from http://www.audiology.org/NR/rdonlyres/3C5FE1CC-3536-45B3-A4DF-9EB835A6BB07/0/HATGuideline042208.pdf

American Academy of Audiology. (2008b). *Supplement A. Fitting and verification procedures for ear-level FM.* Retrieved July 1, 2008, from http://www.audiology.org/NR/rdonlyres/E4BD5693-68BB-4866-B24D-4A14C39A1935/0/HATSup042208.pdf

American National Standards Institute. (2002). *Acoustical performance criteria, design requirements, and guidelines for schools* [ANSI s12.60-2002]. New York, NY: Acoustical Society of America.

American Speech-Language-Hearing Association. (1994). Guidelines for fitting and monitoring FM systems. *ASHA*, *36*(Suppl.), 1–9.

American Speech-Language-Hearing Association. (2002). Guidelines for fitting and monitoring FM systems. *ASHA Desk Reference*.

American Red Cross. (2007). *Health and safety tips: Car safety.* Retrieved December 21, 2007, from http://www.redcross.org/services/hss/tips/carsafety.html.

Anderson, K., & Goldstein, G. (2004). Speech perception benefits of FM and infrared devices to children with hearing aids in a typical classroom. *Language, Speech, and Hearing Services in Schools, 35,* 169–184.

Anderson, K., Goldstein, H., Colodzin, L., & Iglehart, F. (2005). Benefit of S/N enhancing devices to speech perception of children listening in a typical classroom with hearing aids or a cochlear implant. *Journal of Educational Audiology, 12,* 14–28.

Benoit, R. (1989). Home use of FM amplification systems during the early childhood years. *Hearing Instruments, 40,* 8–12.

Bess, F., Dodd-Murphy, J., & Parker, R. (1998). Children with minimal sensorineural hearing loss: Prevalence, educational performance, and functional status. *Ear and Hearing, 19*(5), 339–354.

Bess, F., Klee, T., & Culbertson, J. (1986). Identification, assessment, and management of children with unilateral sensorineural hearing loss. *Ear and Hearing, 7*(1), 43–51.

Blair, J., Peterson, M., & Viehweg, S. (1985). The effects of mild sensorineural hearing loss on academic performance of young school-age children. *Volta Review, 87,* 87–93.

Boothroyd, A., & Iglehart, F. (1998). Experiments with classroom FM amplification. *Ear and Hearing, 19*(3), 202–217.

Bradley, J., & Sato, H. (2004). *Speech recognition by grades 1, 3 and 6 children in classrooms.* Institute for Research in Construction. Retrieved July 1, 2008, from http://irc.nrc-cnrc.gc.ca/pubs/fulltext/nrcc46871/nrcc46871.pdf

Bradlow, A., Kraus, N., & Hayes, E. (2003). Speaking clearly for children with learning disabilities. Sentence perception in noise. *Journal of Speech Language Hearing Research, 46*, 80–97.

Brookhouser, P., Worthington, D., & Kelly, W. (1991). Unilateral hearing loss in children. *Laryngoscope, 101*(12 Pt. 1), 1264–1272.

Cappelli, M., Daniels, T., Durieux-Smith, A., McGrath, P., & Neuss, D. (1995). Social development of children with hearing impairments who are integrated into general education classrooms. *Volta Review, 97*, 197–208.

Cox, R., & Moore, J. (1988). Composite speech spectrum for hearing aid gain prescriptions. *Journal of Speech and Hearing Research, 31*, 102–107.

Crandell, C. (1991). Classroom acoustics for normal-hearing children: Implications for rehabilitation. *Educational Audiology Monograph, 2*(1), 18–38.

Crandell, C. (1993). Speech recognition in noise by children with minimal degrees of sensorineural hearing loss. *Ear and Hearing, 14*(3), 210–216.

Crandell, C., & Smaldino, J. (1994). An update of classroom acoustics for children with hearing impairment. *Volta Review, Fall*, 291–306.

Crandell, C., & Smaldino, J. (1996). Speech perception in noise by children for whom English is a second language. *American Journal of Audiology, 5*, 47–51.

Culbertson, J., & Gilbert, L. (1986). Children with unilateral sensoirneural hearing loss: Cognitive, academic, and social development. *Ear and Hearing, 7*(1), 38–42.

Eisenberg, L. (2007). Current state of knowledge: Speech recognition and production in children with hearing impairment. *Ear and Hearing, 28*(6), 766–772.

Eisenberg, L., Widen, J., Yoshinaga-Itano, C., Norton, S., Thal, D., Niparko, J., & Vohr, B. (2007). Current state of knowledge: Implications for developmental research—key issues. *Ear and Hearing, 28*(6), 773–777.

Eiten, L. (2008). *Assessing open-ear Edulink fittings.* Online presentation, First Phonak Virtual FM Conference: ACCESS 2, February, 2008.

Eiten, L., & Lewis, D. (2008). FM verification for the 21st century. *Perspectives on Hearing and Hearing Disorders in Childhood, 18*(1), 4–9.

English, K., & Church, G. (1999). Unilateral hearing loss in children: An update for the 1990's. *Language, Speech and Hearing Services in Schools, 30*, 26–31.

Etymotic Research. (2005). *BKB-SIN Test, Version 1.03* (Compact disk). 61 Martin Lane, Elk Grove Village, IL 60007.

Fabry, D. (2008). *Something old, something new, something borrowed, something blue: The marriage of FM technology with consumer electronics.* Online presentation, First Phonak Virtual FM Conference: ACCESS 2, February, 2008.

Federal Communications Commission. (1996). *Amendment of the commission's rules concerning low power radio and automated maritime telecommunications system operations in the 216–217 MHz Band* (FCC 96-315, ET Docket NO. 95-96), July 25.

Finitzo-Hieber T. (1981). Classroom acoustics. In R. Roeser & M. Downs (Eds.), *Auditory disorders in school children: The law, identification, remediation* (pp. 250–262). New York, NY: Thieme-Stratton.

Finitzo-Hieber, T., & Tillman, T. (1978). Room acoustics effects on monosyllabic word discrimination ability for normal and hearing impaired children. *Journal of Speech and Hearing Research, 21*, 440–458.

Gabbard, S. (2005). The use of FM technology for infants and young children. In R. C. Seewald & J. M. Bamford (Eds.), *A sound foundation through early amplification* (pp. 155–162). Stäfa, Switzerland: Phonak AG.

Hicks, C., & Tharpe, A. (2002). Listening effort and fatigue in school-age children with and without hearing loss. *Journal of Speech Language Hearing Research, 45*(3), 573–584.

Hoover, B., Stelmachowicz, P., & Lewis, D. (2000). Effect of earmold fit on predicted real ear SPL using a real ear to coupler difference procedure. *Ear and Hearing, 21*(4), 310–317.

Jamieson, D., Kranjc, G., Yu, K., & Hodgetts, W. (2004). Speech intelligibility of young school-aged children in the presence of real-life classroom noise. *Journal of the American Academy of Audiology, 15*, 508–517.

Jerger, S. (2007). Current state of knowledge: Perceptual processing by children with hearing impairment. *Ear and Hearing, 28*(6), 754–765.

Johnson, C., Stein, R., Broadway, A., & Markwalter, T. (1997). "Minimal" high-frequency hearing loss and school-age children: Speech recognition in a classroom. *Language, Speech, and Hearing Services in Schools, 28*, 77–85.

Kenworthy, O., Klee, T., & Tharpe, A. (1990). Speech recognition ability of children with unilateral sensorineural hearing loss as a function of amplification, speech stimuli, and listening condition. *Ear and Hearing, 11*(4), 264–270.

Knecht, H., Nelson, P., Whitelaw, G., & Feth, L. (2002). Background noise levels and reverberation times in unoccupied classrooms: Predictions and measurements. *American Journal of Audiology, 11*, 65–71.

Leavitt, R., & Flexer, C. (1991). Speech degradation as measured by the Rapid Speech Transmission Index (RASTI). *Ear and Hearing, 12*, 115–118.

Loeb, R., & Sarigiani, P. (1986). The impact of hearing impairment on self-perceptions of children. *Volta Review*, Feb/Mar, 89–100.

Madell J. (1992). FM systems for children birth to age five. In M. Ross (Ed.), *FM auditory training systems: Characteristics, selection and use* (pp. 157–174). Timonium, MD: York Press.

Moeller, M. (2007). Current state of knowledge: Psychosocial development in children with hearing impairment. *Ear and Hearing, 28*(6), 729–739.

Moeller, M., Donaghy, K., Beauchaine, K., Lewis, D., & Stelmachowicz, P. (1996). Longitudinal study of FM system use in nonacademic settings: Effects on language development. *Ear and Hearing, 17*(1), 28–41.

Moeller, M., Tomblin, J. B., Yoshinaga-Itano, C., Connor, C. M., & Jerger, S. (2007). Current state of knowledge:

Language and literacy of children with hearing impairment. *Ear and Hearing, 28*(6), 740–754.
Nelson, P., Kohnert, K., Sabur, S., & Shaw, D. (2005). Classroom noise and children learning through a second language: Double jeopardy? *Language, Speech, and Hearing Services in Schools, 36*, 219–229.
Nilsson, M., Soli, S., & Gelnett, D. (1996). *Development and norming of a hearing in noise test for children.* House Ear Institute Internal Report.
Oyler, R., Oyler, A., & Matkin, N. (1988). Unilateral hearing loss: Demographics and educational impact. *Language, Speech, and Hearing Services in Schools, 19*, 191–210.
Pearsons, K., Bennett, R., & Fidell, S. (1977). *Speech levels in various noise environments* (Report No. EPA-600/1-77-025). Washington, DC.
Phonak. (2008). *Inspiro guide for parents and teachers.* Stäfa, Switzerland: Author.
Platz, R. (2004). SNR advantage, FM advantage and FM fitting. In D. Fabry & C. DeConde Johnson (Eds.), *ACCESS: Achieving Clear Communication Employing Sound Solutions, 2003.* Proceedings of the First International FM Conference. (pp. 147–154). Stäfa, Switzerland: Phonak AG.
Platz, R. (2006). *New insights and developments in verification of FM systems*. Paper presented at the American Academy of Audiology Convention, Minneapolis, MN. Available from http://www.phonak.com/com_professionals_eschool desk_aaa_rainerplatz_handout.pdf
Ross, M., & Giolas, T. (1971). Effects of three classroom listening conditions on speech intelligibility. *American Annals of the Deaf, 116*, 580–584.
Ruscetta, M., Arjmand, E., & Pratt, R., Sr. (2005). Speech recognition abilities in noise for children with severe-to-profound unilateral hearing impairment. *International Journal of Pediatric Otorhinolaryngology, 69*(6), 771–779.
Schafer, E. C., & Thibodeau, L. M. (2006). Speech recognition in noise in children with cochlear implants while listening in bilateral, bimodal, and FM system arrangements. *American Journal of Audiology, 15*, 114–126.
Sonovation. (2008). *Logicom FM products*. Retrieved July 1, 2008, from http://www.avrsono.com/
Stelmachowicz, P., Mace, A., Kopun, J., & Carney, E. (1993). Long-term and short-term characteristics of speech: Implications for hearing aid selection for young children. *Journal of Speech and Hearing Research, 36*, 609–620.
Tomblin, B., & Hebbeler, K. (2007). Current state of knowledge: Outcomes research in children with mild to severe hearing impairment—approaches and methodological considerations. *Ear and Hearing, 28*, 715–728.
Wikipedia. (2008). *Bluetooth*. Retrieved September 8, 2008, from http://en.wikipedia.org/wiki/Bluetooth .
Zentall, S., & Shaw, J. (1980). Effects of classroom noise on performance and activity of second grade hyperactive and control children. *Journal of Educational Psychology, 8*, 830–840.

27

Cochlear Implants for Children: Promoting Auditory Development With Electrical Pulses

Karen A. Gordon

Introduction to Cochlear Implants

Cochlear implants allow individuals with severe to profound hearing loss to hear because they bypass any dysfunction in the inner ear (cochlea) and directly stimulate the auditory nerve with electrical pulses. Electrical stimulation of the auditory nerve was first attempted in an adult patient in the 1950s by surgeons Djourno and Eyries (1957; Djourno, Eyries, & Vallancien, 1957a, 1957b). Their work sparked scientific and clinical endeavors culminating in the development of commercial cochlear implants. The early recipients were almost entirely adults who had lost their hearing, and cochlear implants were first approved for adults in the United States in 1985.

Once the adult cochlear implant recipients began to show hearing benefits, children with acquired or even congenital deafness were considered for implantation. One hesitation in implanting children was the question of whether the completely abnormal auditory input from a cochlear implant would promote auditory development. Indeed, there were some who felt that cochlear implants could never represent speech sounds clearly enough to allow children to develop oral speech and language. In 1990, cochlear implants were approved for children in the United States. Now, almost two decades later, it is clear that children with early onset deafness can learn to hear and understand speech with their cochlear implants and many have developed age appropriate speech and language skills (e.g., Geers, 2006; Uziel et al., 2007). Not all children achieve the same outcomes of cochlear implantation, however, and most require considerable therapy and effort to learn to hear and speak. These facts support the continuing efforts of current research, which seek to better understand both the effects of the many types of deafness that can occur in childhood and how we might best promote development of the auditory system in children with hearing loss. This chapter briefly summarizes what is known presently.

Basics of Cochlear Implant Structure and Function

Cochlear implants are designed to stimulate activity in the auditory nerve. This is done using electrical pulses delivered by electrodes that are typically placed in the cochlea as close to the auditory neurons as possible. Stimulation of the auditory nerve is normally accomplished by cochlear hair cells that send signals to auditory neurons regarding the frequency (pitch) and the intensity (loudness) of the incoming acoustic sound over time. Deafness is most commonly the result of dysfunction of the hair cells or the hair cell-neuron synapse and, consequently, the auditory nerve receives little or no information regarding the sounds passing through the ear. Current research has been focused on which types of dysfunction occur in the hair cells and hair cell-neuron synapses and why these abnormalities occur.

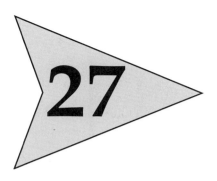

As discussed in Chapter 2, sound causes displacement of the tympanic membrane and middle ear ossicles. The last bone of the ossicular chain, the stapes, presses upon the round window causing fluid displacement in the cochlear, which, in turn, results in movement of the basilar membrane. The stiffness gradient of the basilar membrane sets up an organized arrangement of frequencies; high frequencies cause displacement at the base of the cochlea with progressively lower frequencies displacing the basilar membrane at more apical cochlear locations. The arrangement of frequencies by "place" provides an important basis for hearing pitch differences. Cochlear implants attempt to mimic this organization by sending electrical pulses from electrodes located in basal areas of the cochlea to represent high frequencies and from more apical electrodes for lower frequency sounds. In a normal auditory system, the displacement of the basilar membrane activates a signaling pathway between hair cells and auditory neurons in the area of displacement. This signaling can occur in phase with the frequency of the incoming acoustic sound (when < 4 kHz), allowing auditory neurons to fire at the same rate. The ability to hear frequency (pitch) changes are based on these "phase" cues in addition to the "place" cues. Cochlear implants are limited in their ability to provide phase cues because they deliver electrical pulses at one fixed and limited rate. Thus, cochlear implant users rely primarily on place cues to hear pitch differences. Acoustic amplitude cues, normally coded by the amplitude of basilar membrane movement, are converted to a range of current levels which represent very soft to loud sounds.

A typical cochlear implant, both internal and external components, is shown in Figure 27–1. In brief, the external components pick up and analyze acoustic sound and send this information to the internal components. Instructions are sent to an array of electrodes that are implanted in the scala tympani and these electrodes deliver pulses of electricity. At present, the internal component has no power source and cannot work without the external equipment.

A more detailed schematic of how cochlear implants function is shown in Figure 27–2. Sounds are picked up by the microphone and sent to the speech processor, as depicted in Figure 27–2A. At any one time, speech sounds are made up of a number of frequencies (pitches), each with its own intensity (amplitude). As shown in Figure 27–2B, the cochlear implant processor divides the sound into specific bands of frequencies and then analyzes the intensity within each band. Although Figure 27–2 shows four bands and four electrodes, the number of bands and electrodes varies across different cochlear implant devices. Each frequency band typically is assigned to one implanted electrode. The intensity information for each frequency band is sent through FM wave transmission to the internal receiver-stimulator, which provides instructions to the cochlear implant electrodes (depicted in Figure 27–2A). Each electrode is programmed to deliver pulses with a dynamic range of current intensity spanning from threshold of audibility to a percept of comfortably loud. The cochlear implant analyzes the quick changes in frequency and amplitude of running speech in real time. The plot in Figure 27–2C shows an example of how speech is converted into electrical pulses by the cochlear implant. Most implant users can track the rhythmic changes in amplitude of the incoming sound and learn to discriminate between different sound frequencies. With these cues, they can learn to understand speech sounds. For children, this means that the cochlear implant provides access to sounds that they could not have received through conventional hearing aids and enables oral speech and language development.

Awakening the Deprived Auditory System

Electrical stimulation of the auditory nerve initiates a relay of activity along auditory pathways, that might not have been active for a long period of time or that might never have been stimulated before. Cochlear implant stimulation therefore provides a unique opportunity to study the functional consequences of deafness in both humans and in animal models. The responses obtained in a naïve auditory system (one that has not been active before) are very important because they: (a) confirm that neural pathways are present, can be stimulated electrically and are organized in an expected way; (b) provide a measure of the effects of deafness; and (c) are a baseline for any changes realized with ongoing cochlear implant use.

Electrophysiologic Responses Evoked by Initial Cochlear Implant Stimulation in Children

Even on the first day of cochlear implant activation in a child born with profound bilateral sensorineural hearing

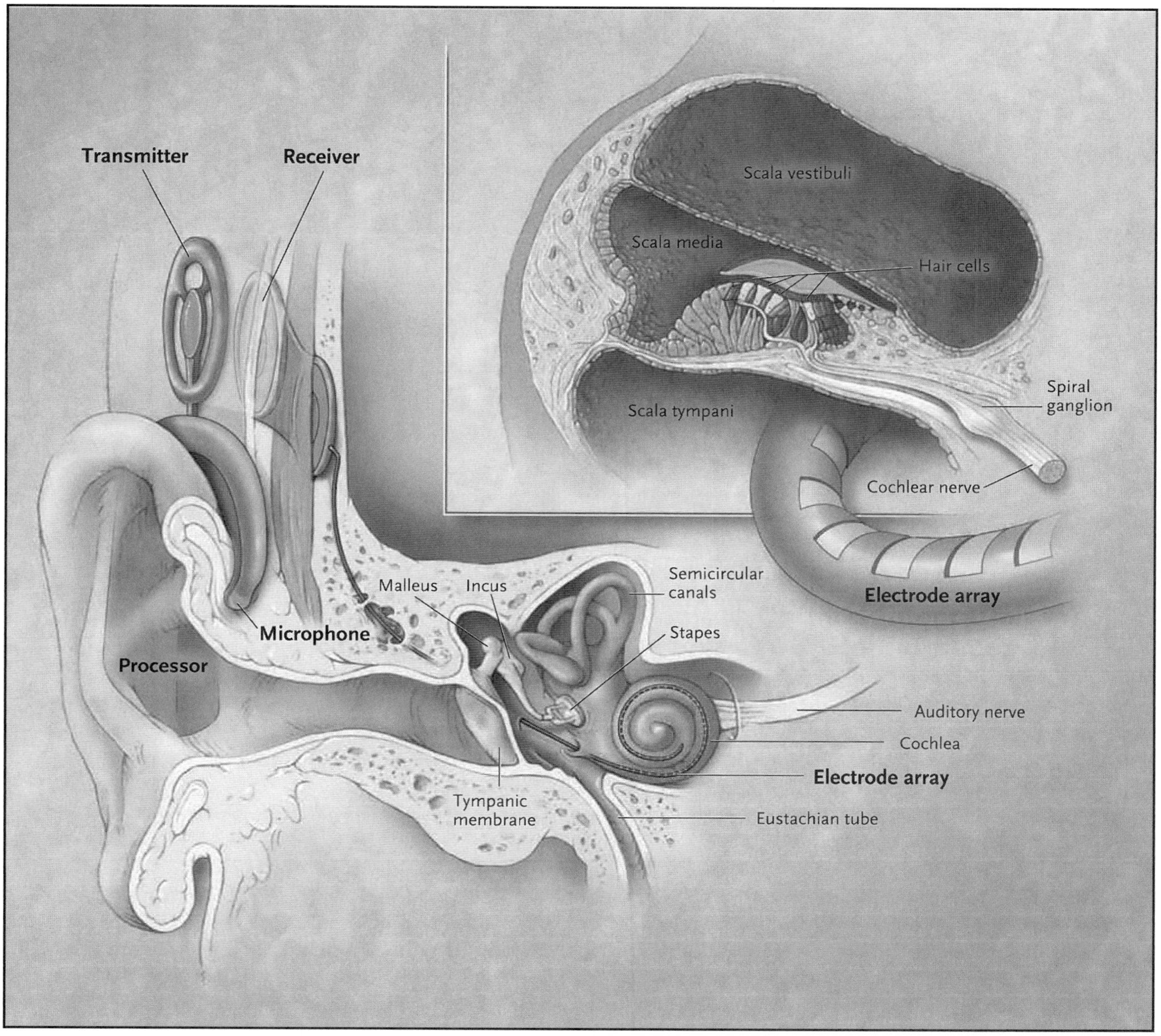

FIGURE 27–1. The cross-section of the cochlea shows the electrode array surgically placed in the scala tympani. The implant converts acoustic sound to electrical pulses that stimulate the auditory nerve. Acoustic input enters the microphone, which is worn on the ear, and is sent to the speech processor for analysis of intensity in a number of set frequency bands. The resulting information is sent from the externally worn transmitting coil to the subcutaneous receiver-stimulator through FM waves. These components are held together by a pair of magnets so that they are separated only by the thickness of the skin flap. Each frequency band is assigned to a particular electrode along the implanted array (mimicking the normal basal-to-apical organization of high to low frequencies in the cochlea). If instructed, this array will provide a biphasic electrical pulse to stimulate the auditory nerve. The current level for the pulse provided by any one electrode will depend on the intensity of the frequency band and the dynamic range of the current level (minimum to maximum) programmed for that electrode. Reprinted with permission from Papsin, B. C., and Gordon, K. A. (2007). Cochlear implants for children with severe-to-profound hearing loss. *New England Journal of Medicine, 357*(23), 2380–2387. Copyright 2007 Massachusetts Medical Society.

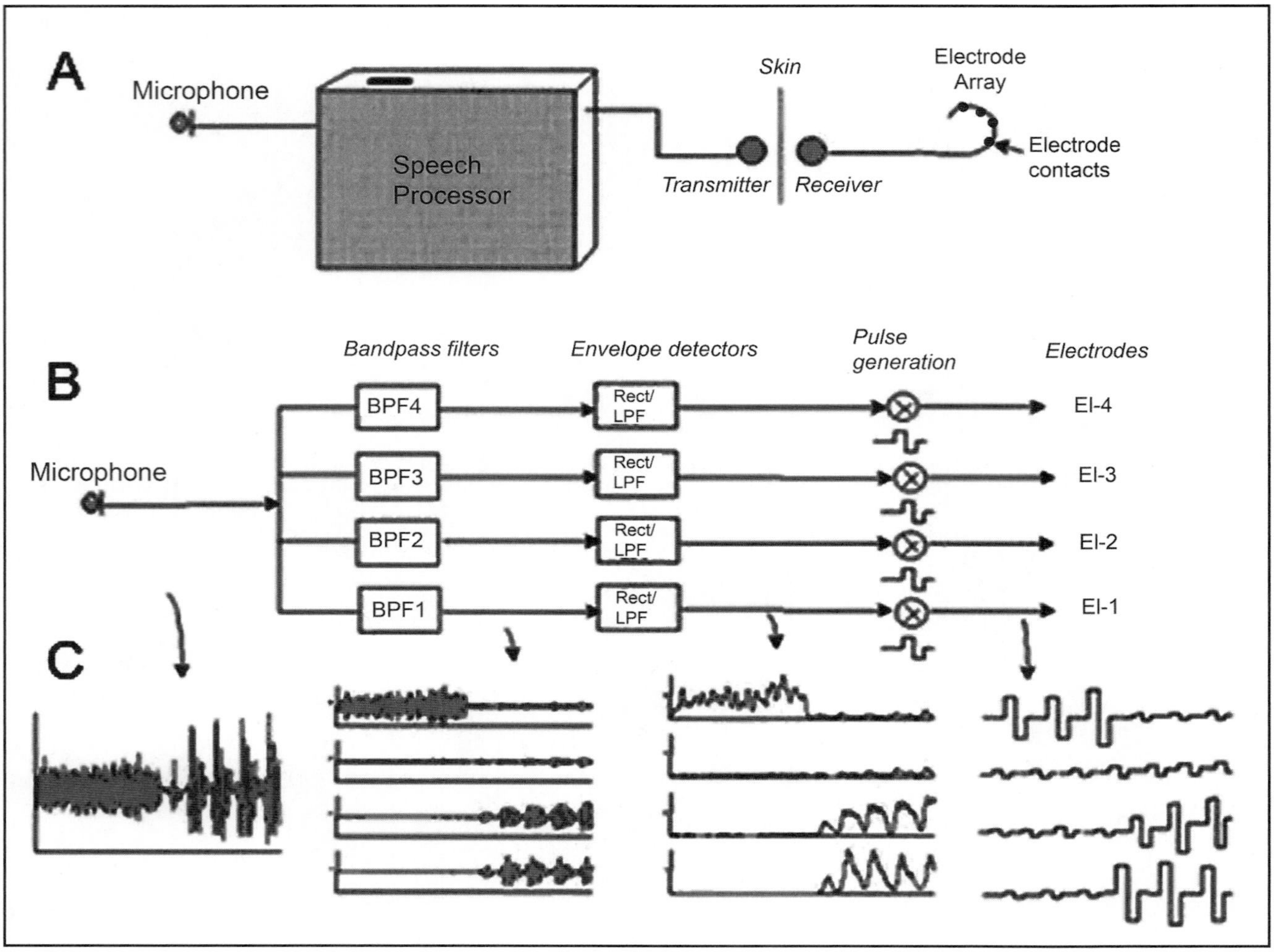

FIGURE 27–2. A. Sound is picked up by the microphone and sent to the speech processor for analysis. The transmitting coil (worn externally) sends this information to the receiver-stimulator (implanted under the skin) and provides instructions to the electrodes implanted in the cochlea. **B.** Further details of the speech processor analyses are shown. The frequency components of the sound are divided into a number of frequency ranges (bandwidths) using bandpass filters (BPFs). The intensity of each bandwidth over time (the envelope) is extracted by rectifying (Rect) and low pass filtering (LPF) the signal. This information is then converted into electrical pulses delivered by one implant electrode (El). High frequency bandwidths are assigned to electrodes at the basal end of the array and lower frequencies to more apical electrodes. The current level is customized for each implant user from very soft to comfortably loud. **C.** The process is shown for a particular sound. In this example, sound is divided into four bandwidths (BPFI, BPFZ, BPF3, BPF4) and four electrodes (E-1, E-2, E-3, E-4) are available. There is little intensity in one of the four bandwidths and thus the electrode assigned to this frequency range remains inactive while the others deliver biphasic electrical pulses. In current cochlear implants, electrical pulses are delivered by up to 22 electrodes. Reprinted with permission from Loizou, P. (1998). Mimicking the human ear. *IEEE Signal Processing Magazine, 15*(5), Figure 4. Copyright 1998 NANOBIO.

loss, we can record electrophysiologic responses from discrete areas of the auditory system. The cochlear implant is used to stimulate the auditory pathways; examples of responses are shown in Figure 27–3, with a rough approximation of where along the auditory pathways each is generated. The amplitude peaks of the

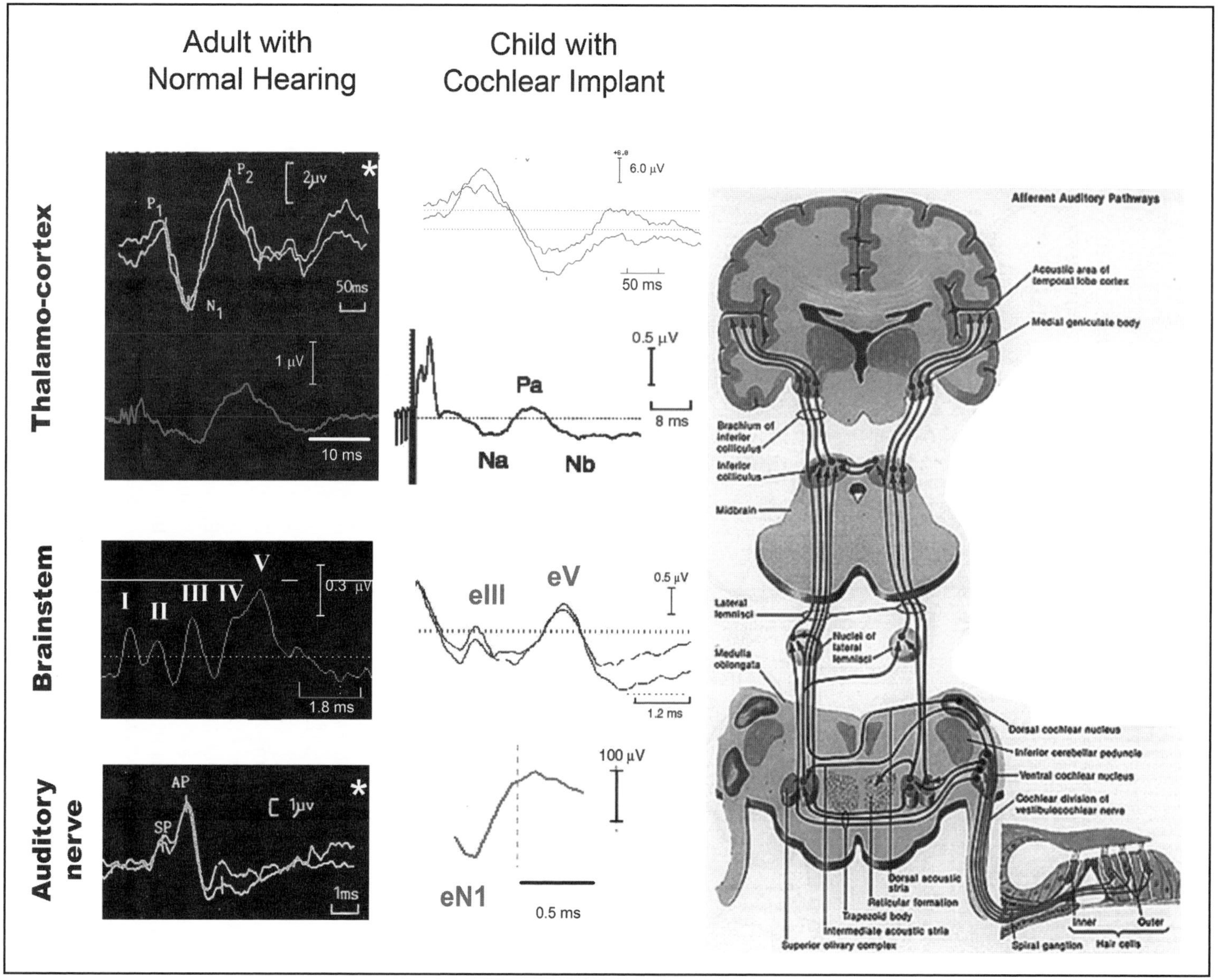

FIGURE 27–3. Electrophysiologic responses evoked by acoustic stimuli in a normal hearing adult and evoked by electrical pulses in a child using a cochlear implant. The responses are shown alongside the approximate areas at which they are generated in the central auditory system (as illustrated by Netter). The cortical response and auditory nerve response from the normal hearing adult (*) are from Hall (1992). *Handbook of auditory evoked responses* (p. 4). Copyright 1992 Reprinted with permission by Pearson Education, Inc.

responses evoked in children using cochlear implants are somewhat different than those recorded from individuals with normal hearing. These differences can be explained to some extent by the direct stimulation of the auditory pathways with an electrical pulse. Direct stimulation results in shorter latencies of response peaks that are most evident in the early latency responses. Also, the rapid onset of the electrical pulse may result in an increase in the numbers of neurons that respond at the same time (neural synchrony) (van den Honert & Stypulkowski, 1984) and measured as larger and sharper response peaks than those generated by acoustic pulses. The effects of deafness might also play a role in some of the differences between the cochlear implant and normal hearing responses.

Responses From the Auditory Nerve and Brainstem

The electrically evoked compound action potential (ECAP) of the auditory nerve can be recorded via the telemetry system of the cochlear implant, using a subtraction method to minimize stimulus artifact (Abbas et al., 1999). Electrodes along the cochlear implant array act to both stimulate and record, whereas responses occurring at longer latencies (as shown in Figure 27–3) are measured by recording electrodes placed on the head. The ECAP typically has a negative peak (eN1) at a very short latency (~0.30 ms) reflecting the direct stimulation of the auditory nerve. In a normal hearing individual, the auditory nerve is stimulated at ~1.5 ms, and the response can be recorded along with cochlear responses (see Figure 27–3) or as waves I and II of the normal auditory brainstem response (ABR; Moller & Jannetta, 1982; Moller, Jannetta, Bennett, & Moller, 1981). As shown in Figure 27–3, the ABR is characterized by five to six positive amplitude peaks (I, II, III, IV, V, VI). The electrically evoked brainstem response (EABR) typically occurs at latencies < 5 ms and has three to four characteristic peaks (eII, eIII, eIV, eV) following the initial stimulus artifact. EABRs in our laboratory are often evoked using current levels at the upper part of the dynamic range in children. Waves eIII and eV are most commonly observed, and wave eIV is rarely found. Comparisons between the ABR and EABR wave latencies and interwave latencies suggest that wave eII comes from the auditory nerve (Gordon et al., 2006). The EABR has shorter interwave latencies compared to the ABR. In particular, eII-eIII and eIII-eV are shorter than the ABR II-III and III-V, respectively. These measures indicate that neural activity is relayed more quickly through the electrically stimulated than the acoustically stimulated auditory brainstem. This may be due to the high degree of neural synchrony evoked by the electrical pulse and/or that the EABR is generated by different populations of brainstem neurons than the ABR (Gordon et al., 2006).

Responses from Auditory Thalamus and Cortex

The electrically evoked middle latency response (EMLR) ranges in latency from ~15 to 60 ms and is generated by thalamocortical pathways. The most commonly found peaks are eNa, ePa, and eNb. As shown in Figure 27–3, this response is very similar to the middle latency response (MLR) recorded in a normally hearing adult. At this level of the auditory system, differences in peak latencies are no longer clear. The MLR in children below approximately 9 years of age is known to be obscured when the child is asleep (McGee & Kraus, 1996; McGee, Kraus, Killion, Rosenberg, & King, 1993), but is typically present when the child is awake or in REM sleep (Rotteveel, Stegeman, de Graaf, Colon, & Visco, 1987). In contrast, we have found that detection of the EMLR at cochlear implant activation in children is variable even though all children were awake at the time of testing (Gordon, Tanaka, & Papsin, 2005). These differences suggest an immaturity of the thalamocortical pathways in children who are deaf. A normal late latency response is shown in the upper left of Figure 27–3 and reflects cortical activity. This response typically is characterized by three peaks (P1, N1, and P2) in normally hearing teenagers and adults, as well as in adults who received a cochlear implant after postlingual onset of deafness (Ponton & Eggermont, 2001). A typical cortical response in a child with early onset deafness is dominated by a large positive peak of variable latency (100–300 ms) (Gordon et al., 2005). Henkin et al., 2004; Ponton, 2006; Sharma, Dorman, & Kral, 2005). A similar response is found in children younger than about 9 years of age (Pang & Taylor, 2000; Ponton, Eggermont, Khosla, Kwong, & Don, 2002; Sharma, Kraus, McGee, & Nicol, 1997). We have shown that the late latency response in children using cochlear implants can deviate substantially from the more typical waveform shown in Figure 27–3 (Gordon, Tanaka, Wong, & Papsin, 2008) and that this deviation might be particularly true at device activation. We are currently investigating the atypical peaks recorded in children using cochlear implants with an aim to better understand where they are generated in the cortex and how they differ from normal responses of the auditory cortex.

Bilateral Deafness in Childhood Changes the Auditory System Over Time

Electrophysiological measures recorded at initial cochlear implant activation provide a rare glimpse into the deaf auditory system and can be used to ask questions about the effects of deafness in childhood. We and several other investigators have shown that responses from the auditory nerve, brainstem, and cortex can be evoked in most children receiving cochlear implants at the first cochlear implant stimulation. This is true even for children who had severe to profound hearing loss from infancy or birth, which suggests that the central auditory pathways form depite the absence of normal auditory experience. These findings are consistent with recordings of electrically evoked auditory activity in the auditory nerve (Miller, Abbas, & Robinson, 1993; van den Honert & Stypulkowski, 1984), brainstem (Moore, Vollmer, Leake, Snyder, & Rebscher, 2002; Snyder, Rebscher, Leake, Kelly, & Cao, 1991; van den Honert & Stypulkowski, 1986; Vollmer et al., 1999), thalamus, and cortex (Hartmann, Shepherd, Heid, & Klinke, 1997; Klinke, Kral, Heid, Tillein, & Hartmann, 1999; Kral, Hartmann, Tillein, Heid, & Klinke, 2000) in deaf animals. The auditory nerve and brainstem respond in a very regular and predictable way, as shown by clear recording of ECAPs and EABRS at cochlear implant activation in most children who receive cochlear implants (Gordon, Papsin, & Harrison, 2004a, 2000b). Even children who have been bilaterally deaf from birth and implanted as teenagers can show clear ECAPs and EABRs at cochlear implant activation (Gordon et al., 2003, 2007). Remarkably, ECAP and EABR amplitude and latency measures do not appear to be affected by the period of auditory deprivation (Gordon et al., 2006, 2007). At the same time, the auditory nerve and brainstem pathways do not mature during the period of deafness and remain at the same developmental stage in both older and younger children.

In contrast, thalamocortical responses are affected by an extended period of deafness in childhood. Although EMLRs were detected in the majority of older children with longer periods of early onset bilateral deafness, they were poorly detected in younger children (Gordon et al., 2005). Work by Sharma and colleagues has shown some interesting parallels in late latency responses. "Late implanted" children showed earlier latency cortical responses than "early implanted" children (Sharma et al., 2005). Shortened response latencies typically reflect a more mature system because latencies decrease as developing pathways become myelinated and as neural connections (synapses) become more efficient. Thus, both the EMLR and late latency responses suggest that the auditory thalamus and cortex undergo change during the period of bilateral deafness. It is possible that these changes are due to competitive influences from nonauditory systems. Lee and colleagues have shown that the auditory cortex in children who are deaf is abnormally quiet but that it becomes more active as the period of deafness increases (Lee et al., 2001, 2007). The authors suggest that the changes are driven by nonauditory activity in a process referred to as crossmodal plasticity. In support, cortical responses after long-term bilateral or unilateral deafness have been shown to be generated in nonauditory areas of the brain such as the parietal cortex (Gilley, Sharma, & Dorman, 2008; Gordon, Wong, & Papsin, 2010). The visual system plays a role in reorganization of the deaf auditory cortex as evidenced by abnormally high activity in the auditory cortex when visual signals are shown to individuals who were deaf from an early age (Finney, Clementz, Hickok, & Dobkins, 2003; Finney, Fine, & Dobkins, 2001).

Do Different Types of Childhood Deafness Affect the Auditory Pathways?

Responses from initial implant stimulation can be useful for studying effects of different types of deafness in children. The discoveries of multiple genetic mutations associated with hearing loss (see the Hereditary Hearing Loss Homepage at http://webh01.ua.ac.be/hhh/) have provided a major advance in our understanding of why some children are born without hearing. Each of these genetic changes might cause unique effects on the central auditory system. We have been interested in effects of homozygous *GJB-2* gene mutations that lead to the disruption of the connexin 26 protein in the cochlea. The ECAP response recorded at initial device activation, as shown in Figure 27–4, indicates that response amplitudes evoked at the apical and basal ends of the array are more similar to one another in children with homozygous *GJB-2* mutations than in children with no such mutations (Propst, 2006). We suggest that the disruption to cochlear gap junctions by a loss of connexin 26 is likely to occur randomly along the length of the basilar membrane. Any changes to the spiral ganglia as a result of connexin 26 depletion should then also be independent of cochlear location. In contrast, primary nerve responses in children without *GJB-2* mutations show more variable effects of deafness by place of electrical stimulation. Specifically, basal electrodes evoked lower amplitude

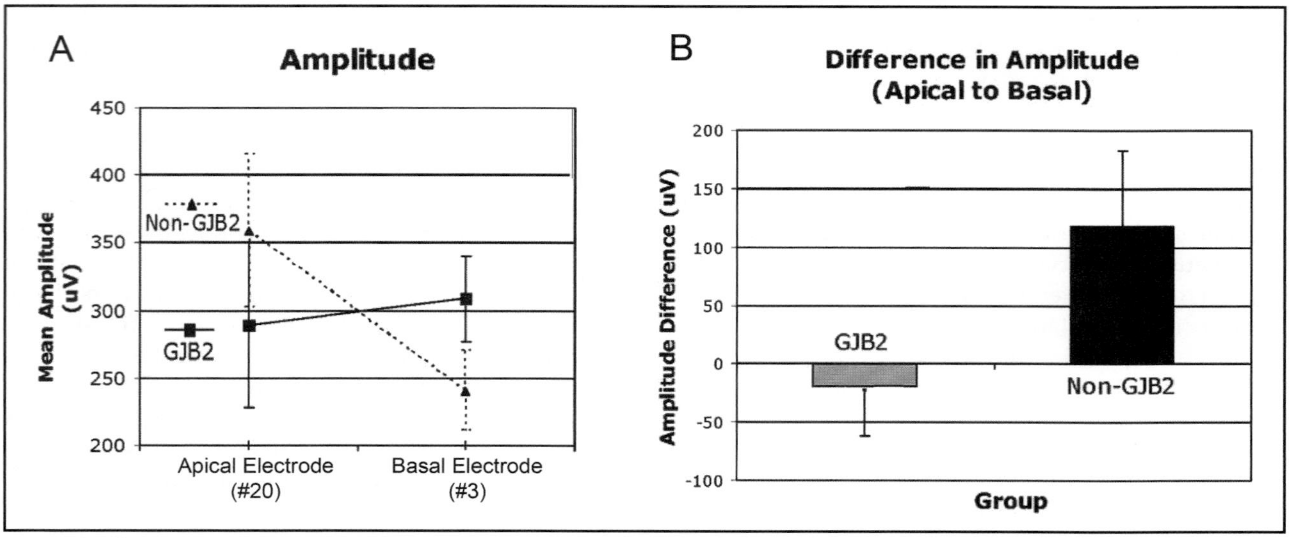

FIGURE 27–4. A. Estimated marginal mean amplitudes across electrodes for *GJB2* groups. **B.** The difference in amplitude from apical to basal electrodes tended to be smaller in the *GJB2* group as compared with the non-*GJB2* group. Reprinted with permission from Propst, E. J., Papsin, B. C., Stockley, T. L., Harrison, R. V., and Gordon, K. A. (2006). Auditory responses in cochlear implant users with and without GJB2 deafness. *Laryngoscope*, 116(2), p. 323. Copyright 2006 John Wiley & Sons.

responses with shallower amplitude growth than those evoked byapical electrodes. We have also found this pattern of response in the auditory brainstem. As shown in Figure 27–5, a large group of children with early onset deafness of primarily unknown etiology had reduced amplitudes and shallower amplitude growth of EABRs when evoked by a basal implant electrode compared to responses evoked by an apical electrode (Gordon et al, 2007). These findings suggest that, when the etiology of deafness is largely unknown, neural integrity is poorer in the basal than apical ends of the implanted array. This is consistent with evidence from temporal bone analyses that show lower spiral ganglion counts in the basal versus apical ends of the cochlea (Nadol, 1997) and perhaps with the tendency for poorer residual hearing in the high versus low frequencies. Understanding subtle changes between different etiologies of childhood deafness is important as we strive to best promote auditory development in all children with hearing loss.

Clinical Use of Initial Electrophysiologic Responses

The responses shown in Figure 27–3 can be used both to evaluate the auditory system and to determine the current levels required to stimulate these pathways. Because no behavioral responses are required to record the responses, they might help to determine appropriate cochlear implant stimulation levels in children who provide limited or no reliable behavioral reactions to cochlear implant stimulation. Each child must be tested because the levels of current required for one implant user to hear can be quite different from another. In order to provide a dynamic range of intensities (loudness), current from the implant should range from the minimum level required to hear a very soft sound (threshold) to a maximum level that must be loud but comfortable for the user. Behavioral measures of thresholds remain the gold standard to determine these levels, but electrophysiologic measures could help to predict these values (Kileny, 1991; Shallop, 1993). ECAP and EABR thresholds do show significant correlations with behavioral measures of threshold, but these relationships are not exact (Gordon et al., 2004a, 2004b; Hughes, Brown, Abbas, Wolaver, & Gervais, 2000) and thus cannot be used to accurately predict optimal stimulus levels in all children (Brown, 2003). We have pointed out that maximum current levels are difficult to determine using behavioral responses in children with limited hearing prior to cochlear implantation (Gordon et al., 2004a, 2004b). The stapedius reflex provides a helpful alternative given that it is known to be elicited at loud levels in normal hearing individuals; that it can be evoked by electrical pulses in cochlear implant

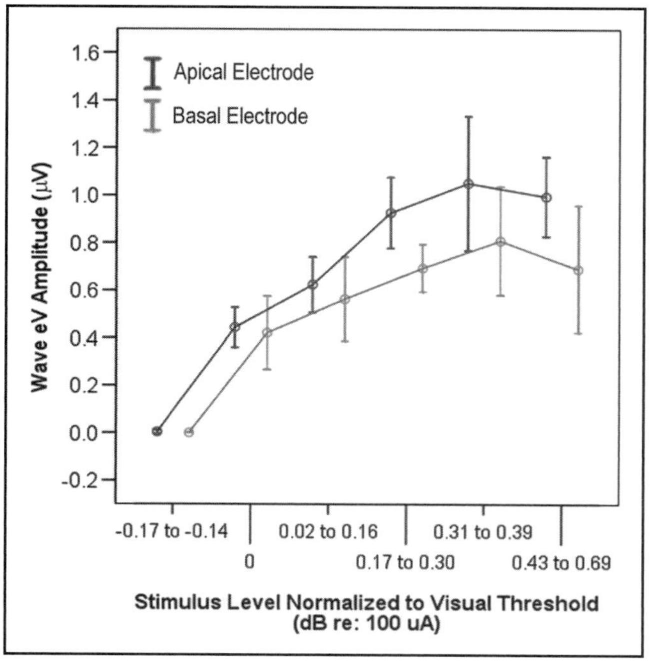

FIGURE 27–5. Mean (1SE) wave eV amplitude obtained at initial stimulation in 50 children is plotted with respect to intensity (dB re:100 uV). Intensity is normalized to visual response thresholds; negative intensities are below visual threshold, 0 dB is equal to visual threshold and positive values are suprathreshold measures. Amplitude growth appears slightly steeper when evoked by the apical versus basal electrode. Reprinted with permission from Gordon, K. A., Papsin, B. C., and Harrison, R. V. (2007). Auditory brainstem activity and development evoked by apical versus basal cochlear implant electrode stimulation in children. *Clinical Neurophysiology, 118*(8), p. 1676. Copyright 2007 Elsevier.

users (Almqvist, Harris, & Shallop, 2000; Shallop, 1993; Stephan, Welzl-Muller, & Stiglbrunner, 1990; van den Borne, Snik, Mens, Brokx, & van den Broek, 1996); and that the threshold of the reflex correlates with perceived loudness in adult cochlear implant users who acquired deafness after having normal hearing (Polak, Hodges, & Balkany, 2005; Shallop & Ash, 1995). In our clinic we typically do not provide stimulation levels that exceed the stapedius reflex threshold so that the children do not experience these reflexes as part of their daily listening.

We have found that ECAP and/or EABR measures taken at the time of implantation in the operating room are very helpful for initial device activation. When clear responses have been recorded, we can be confident that the device is working and that the auditory system will respond. The stapedius reflex thresholds, measured by watching the stapedius muscle contract to electrical stimulation in the operating room, can be used to define the upper limits of this stimulation. Often children will only tolerate a limited dynamic range at initial stages of device use. As they become accustomed to the sound, however, we aim to increase the range of current intensities based on both objective and behavioral responses.

Objective measures might also be used to track changes in speech perception abilities over time. Cortical responses have been identified as the most likely candidates for this, and there has been some interest in measuring whether the auditory cortex can discriminate between two auditory inputs. Both the mismatched negativity response (MMN; Groenen, Snik, & van den Broek, 1996; Kelly, Purdy, & Thorne, 2005; Kraus et al., 1993; Ponton & Don, 1995; Ponton et al., 2000; Roman, Canevet, Marquis, Triglia, & Liegeois-Chauvel, 2005) and the cortical "change" response (Brown et al., 2008; Friesen & Tremblay, 2006; Martin, 2007) have been recorded in individuals who use cochlear implants. These measures might thus help to monitor how the auditory cortex deals with changes in electrical input and to track improvements in hearing abilities (Cone-Wesson & Wunderlich, 2003; Singh, Liasis, Rajput, & Luxon, 2006; Wable, van den Abbeele, Gallego, & Frachet, 2000). Again, this is important for children who are not able to give reliable behavioral reactions to stimulation from their cochlear implant.

Summary of Findings at Initial Cochlear Implant Activation in Children

In general, the cochlear implant is very effective in stimulating the auditory nerve even immediately following implant surgery, although the responses might vary subtly with different types of deafness. The activity evoked by cochlear implant stimulation in the primary auditory nerve is relayed through pathways that form in the absence of significant auditory experience but remain immature without auditory experience. Responses in children using implants can occur at shorter latencies than responses evoked by acoustic stimuli in normal hearing children and can have different amplitude peaks. These differences reflect the unique effects of electrical versus acoustical stimulation of the auditory pathways and also effects of deafness in the central auditory system. As the period of bilateral deafness lengthens, the thalamocortical areas of the pathways are vulnerable to competitive influences from nonauditory areas including the visual system. Responses from discrete areas of the auditory pathways, regardless of how they might differ from normal, indicate that the auditory system is responding to electrical pulses from the cochlear implant. They thus are useful for approximating the current levels required for an individual child to hear. When behavioral responses are not available this information is particularly valuable.

Stimulating Auditory Development With a Cochlear Implant

The value of electrophysiologic responses in children extends beyond the initial stimulation. As the child continues to wear and use the cochlear implant, responses can be monitored for change. The normal auditory system changes and develops throughout childhood (for review see Moore & Linthicum, 2007). Myelin forms around neural projections (axons) and some of the connections (synapses) between neurons are strengthened (Ponton, Moore, & Eggermont, 1996) and others are pruned away (Huttenlocher & Dabholkar, 1997). The auditory nerve and brainstem are normally mature by 1 to 2 years of life whereas the thalamocortical pathways take longer to develop. In the auditory cortex, axonal density increases over many years. As shown in Figure 27–6 from Moore and Guan (2001), deep cortical layers show maturity by ~6 years of age while superficial layers gain axons for another ~6 years. Children using cochlear implants allow us to explore whether this development requires activity or experience. The changes in auditory responses in children using cochlear implants reflect not only the ability of the auditory system to change in response to new input (auditory plasticity), but also the importance of activity in development. As discussed in the previous section, the auditory brainstem is formed, but does not mature in children who are deaf. Moreover, cortical responses provide evidence of immaturity and even abnormal cortical organization after a period of bilateral deafness. This implies that auditory development does require stimulation, but a number of questions arise: (1) Can auditory development be promoted with cochlear implant stimulation? (2) Can the effects of deafness be overcome by cochlear implant use? and (3) Is electrically evoked auditory development different from normal?

Children using cochlear implants do learn to perceive speech with their cochlear implants over time (i.e., Geers, Brenner, & Davidson, 2003; Nikolopoulos, Archbold, & O'Donoghue, 1999; Papsin, Gysin, Picton, Nedzelski, & Harrison, 2000; Pulsifer, Salorio, & Niparko, 2003; Zeitler et al., 2008), although some children learn to hear better and more quickly than others (i.e., Connor, Craig, Raudenbush, Heavner, & Zwolan, 2006; Geers, 2006; Harrison, Gordon, & Mount, 2005; Papsin, 2005). There may be many factors that affect how one child uses a cochlear implant compared with another, but the basis for any improvements in hearing are developmental changes that are promoted by the cochlear implant along the auditory pathways. We have used electrophysiologic responses to detect small changes occurring at discrete areas of the auditory system in children using cochlear implants. These measures are also useful because they can be obtained in children of any age and done repeatedly without the use of sedation.

Figure 27–7 shows a typical example of ECAP and EABR recordings measured in one child over the first year of cochlear implant use. Responses are evoked by stimulation from an apical and a basal cochlear implant electrode. The auditory brainstem shows clear decreases in wave latencies over the first year of cochlear implant use. In a group of children, these changes are statistically significant and are not affected by the duration of bilateral deafness (Gordon et al., 2003, 2006, 2007). This has been confirmed by Thai-Van and colleagues (2007) who also showed that a period of normal hearing before the onset of deafness results in shorter EABR wave eV latency. Decreasing EABR wave and interwave latencies reflect increasingly rapid neural conduction through the auditory brainstem with ongoing cochlear implant use. The ABR undergoes similar latency decreases over the first year of life in normal hearing infants (Beiser, Himelfarb, Gold, & Shanon, 1985; Jiang, 1995; Ponton, Moore, & Eggermont, 1996; Ponton, Eggermont, Coupland, & Winkelaar, 1992). These changes have been explained by increased myelination and improved synaptic efficiency (Eggermont, 1985, 1988). The EABR changes suggest that, once the auditory brainstem receives stimulation, similar processes can occur in children using cochlear implants. The developmental time course for decreasing EABR eIII-eV interwave latency in children with early onset deafness spans over the first year of implant use (Gordon et al., 2006). This means that the unilaterally electrically stimulated auditory brainstem should be approaching maturation at the first anniversary of implant activation.

Thalamocortical responses in children also show change with ongoing cochlear implant use, however, these changes were not consistent for all children (unlike the EABR latency decreases); (Gordon et al., 2005). Children implanted at older ages, who also had longer periods of bilateral deafness, showed slower and more subtle changes in both EMLRs (Gordon et al,

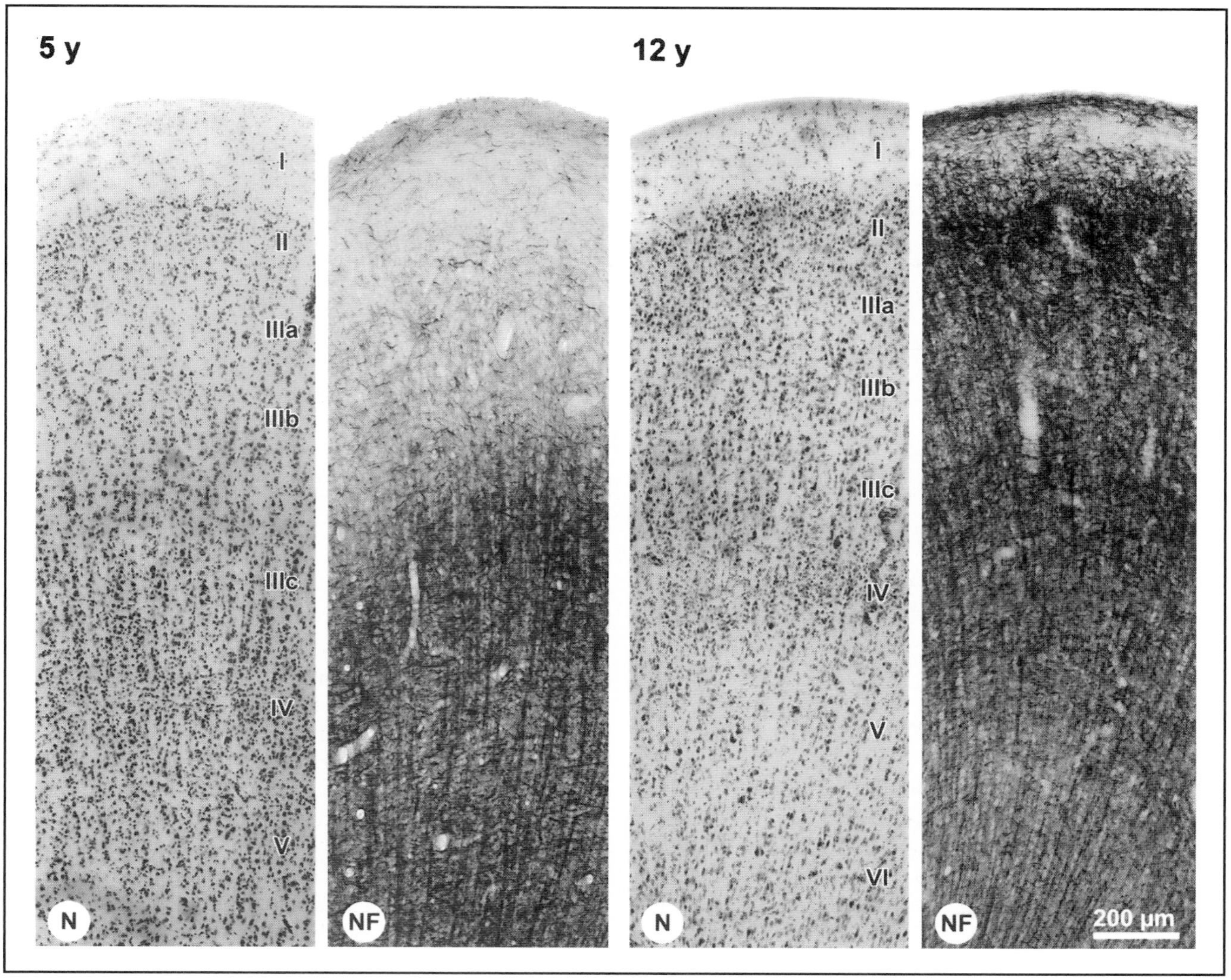

FIGURE 27–6. Cytoarchitecture and axonal maturation in later childhood: Roman numerals indicate cortical layers I-VI. At ages 3 and 12 years (3 y, 12 y), the Nissle material (N) indicates that cortical depth and cytoarchitecture are similar to that seen at ages 1 to 3 years. NF immunostaining at 5 years (5 y, NF) showed that axonal density in layers VI-IIIc is greater than at ages 1 to 3 years. By 12 years of age, layers IIIb, IIIa, and II have become filled with a grid of horizontal and vertical immunostained axons (12 y, NF). At both 5 and 12 years, a limited number of NF-positive axons are present near the surface of the marginal layer. Reproduced with permission from Moore, J. K., and Guan, Y. L. (2001). Cytoarchitectural and axonal maturation in human auditory cortex. *Journal of the Association for Research in Otolaryngology, 2*(4), p. 306. Copyright 2001 Association for Research in Otolaryngology.

2005) and late latency responses (Sharma et al., 2005) than their younger peers who demonstrated rapid changes in both responses during the first 6 months of implant use. Any limitations to change (or plasticity) of auditory responses in such children could be related to the changes found at initial stimulation. As discussed above, the EMLR was found to be better detected in late than early implanted children (Gordon et al., 2005), late latency peaks were observed at shorter latencies (Sharma et al., 2005), and the auditory cortex was more active in children with longer periods of deafness likely due to crossmodal reorganization (Lee et al., 2001; Lee et al., 2007). It is possible that changes in thalamocortical areas of the auditory pathways, occurring during

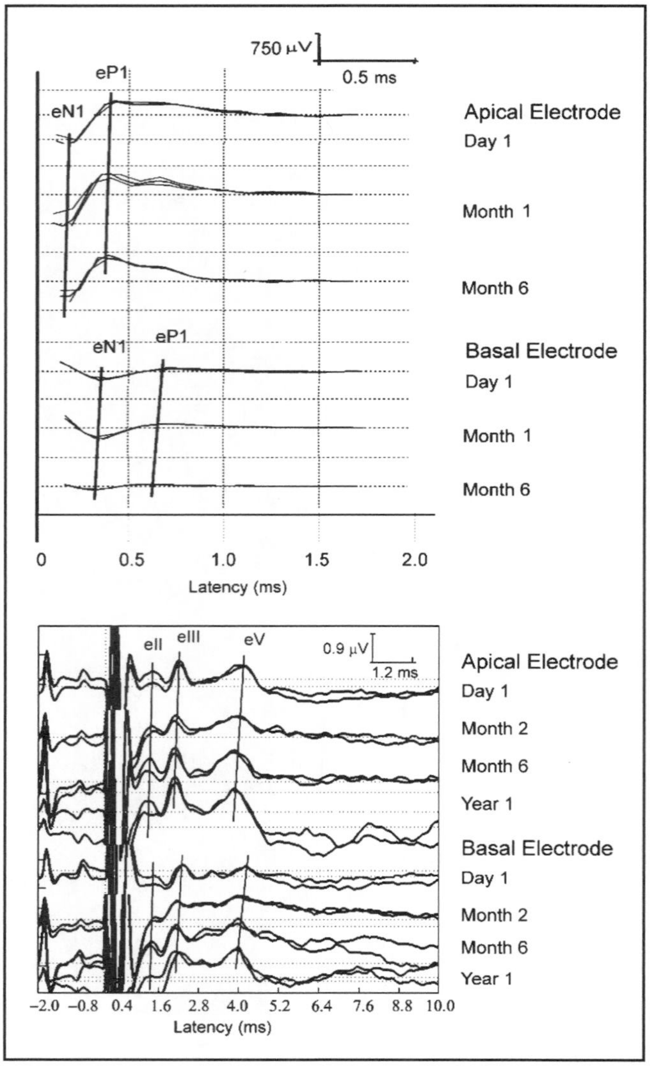

FIGURE 27–7. Measures completed over the first year of implant use in a child with prelingual deafness implanted at 3 years of age. The electrically evoked compound action potential is shown in the top panel and the electrically evoked auditory brainstem response in the panel below. Responses evoked by apical electrodes have noticeably shorter latencies than those evoked by basal electrodes. Decreasing latencies with implant use can also be seen. Reprinted with permission from Gordon, K. A., Papsin, B. C., and Harrison, R. V. (2007). Auditory brainstem activity and development evoked by apical versus basal cochlear implant electrode stimulation in children. *Clinical Neurophysiology, 118*(8), p. 1679. Copyright 2007 Elsevier.

the period of deafness, are not reversible or cannot be revised in a way that is meaningful for development of hearing. It has been suggested that this permanent effect of deafness is most likely to occur in children implanted after aged 7 years and least likely to occur in children implanted before 3.5 years of age (Sharma, 2007; Sharma, Dorman, & Spahr, 2002). Based on these findings, the period of 0 to 3.5 years of age has been proposed to be a sensitive period in auditory development. What is not clear, however, is whether this age cutoff is related to the duration of bilateral deafness or the age of the child or both. Children born with bilateral deafness age at the same rate as their duration of deafness lengthens, which makes it difficult to separate these issues. The answer to this is yet unknown but it will be important to fully understand the effects of increasing age and longer periods of deafness as we explore the optimal timing of bilateral cochlear implantation. We must also ask whether children who are implanted at young ages will experience normal auditory development. Given the long-term development of the normal auditory cortex (at least 12 years) and the heterogeneity of childhood deafness, we will need to follow children implanted at young ages over long periods of implant use in order to fully answer this question.

In sum, developmental change can be promoted with cochlear implant stimulation. Clear changes occur after very short periods of cochlear implant use (≤ 12 months) in the auditory nerve, brainstem, and thalamocortical pathways as measured by electrophysiological responses. Thalamocortical responses showed more restricted degrees of change in children with early onset deafness and implanted at ages older than 7 years. This could be related to an inability to reverse the changes experienced by these areas of the pathway during the period of deafness. How this development compares to normal development of the auditory system remains a subject of ongoing research.

Limitations to Auditory Development in Children Using Cochlear Implants

There are a number of reasons why children using cochlear implants might develop different listening skills than their hearing peers:

1. Current cochlear implants do not replace normal hearing and cannot perfectly code acoustic sounds;
2. Effects of deafness in the auditory system may not be reversible;
3. One cochlear implant provides unilateral stimulation only;

These issues are familiar to clinicians involved in cochlear implantation. In our program, parents and children receive counseling prior to implantation to expect that listening will be challenging, and all children implanted in our program are required to enroll in auditory training therapy.

Limitations of Cochlear Implant Devices

Electrical pulses from a cochlear implant are highly effective in providing auditory percepts, but they cannot perfectly represent or code acoustic sound. For children, this means that, although they are using the best signal currently available, they will not be able to hear as well as their normal hearing peers. Because electrical pulses from a cochlear implant are presented at a fixed rate, the implant user has no access to the fine timing cues in speech. Efforts to increase the fine timing cues available have included the delivery of electrical pulses at rates of 4,000 pulses or greater. Unfortunately, higher rates of electrical stimulation do not appear to benefit speech perception (Verschuur, 2005) and cause degraded perception of auditory cues (Galvin & Fu, 2005; Pfingst, Xu, & Thompson, 2007). This might be related to neural adaptation that occurs in the auditory brainstem in response to high electrical pulse rates (Davids, Valero, Papsin, Harrison, & Gordon, 2008). In an attempt to mimic normal cochleotopic organization of place cues, cochlear implants assign low frequencies to apical electrodes and higher frequencies to progressively more basal electrodes. However, even the place cues are degraded relative to the normal cochlea because: (1) there are a limited number of electrodes on each array; (2) most electrodes are located in the first basal turn of the cochlea; and (3) electrical current from one electrode can overlap with current from a neighboring electrode limiting the independence of each electrode (Cohen, Richardson, Saunders, & Cowan, 2003; Hughes & Abbas, 2006).

Limitations Related to Deafness

As discussed above, the type and duration of deafness in childhood might promote changes in the auditory system that cannot be reversed by cochlear implant stimulation. Although the genetic origins of hearing loss in children are becoming clearer, there is still much to be learned about the mechanisms and effects of these abnormal changes. A better understanding of the effects of different types of deafness might help to improve the interface between the implant and the primary auditory nerve. One such effort, studied in animal models, has been to release growth factors from the cochlear implant to induce peripheral processes of auditory neurons to grow toward the implanted electrode array (Pettingill, Richardson, Wise, O'Leary, & Shepherd, 2007). The growth factors show some promise, however, neural growth may be too random at this stage to provide the place cues that implant users rely on to hear pitch changes.

Limitations Related to Unilateral Stimulation

Hearing with a cochlear implant is further compromised by the lack of binaural cues available when only one cochlear implant is provided. With only unilateral auditory input available, even through a normally hearing ear, auditory processing is limited, resulting in poorer than normal speech and language development and impaired educational outcomes (Bess, Tharpe, & Gibler, 1986; Klee & Davis-Dansky, 1986; Lieu, 2004). Problems may stem from the inability to localize sound and detect speech in noisy environments. Binaural integration, beginning at the level of the brainstem, mediates these functions by assessing interaural intensity cues (in the lateral superior olive) and interaural timing cues (in the medial superior olive). Children with bilateral severe to profound deafness can achieve very good speech and language perception in quiet situations using unilateral cochlear implants; however, they have difficulties hearing in noise (Battmer, Reid, & Lenarz, 1997; Luntz, Shpak, & Weiss, 2005), localizing sound (Ching et al., 2005; Figueiredo, Abel, & Papsin, 2001), and understanding emotion in speech (Hopyan-Misakyan, Gordon, Dennis, & Papsin, 2009).

Auditory Development in a Growing Child

Recently there have been efforts to understand outcomes of cochlear implantation in context with the overall development of the child as a member of a family and society (Eisenberg et al., 2006; Fink et al., 2007). The picture in Figure 27–8 is drawn by a child using bilateral cochlear implants who, when asked to draw a picture of himself, includes the color of his hair, the color of his eyes, his cochlear implants (also the correct color!), and other members of his family. He has also drawn his brother's bilateral cochlear implants. It is important to remember that, although the primary goal of cochlear implantation in children is to promote auditory development so that speech and language skills can develop, these changes will happen in a

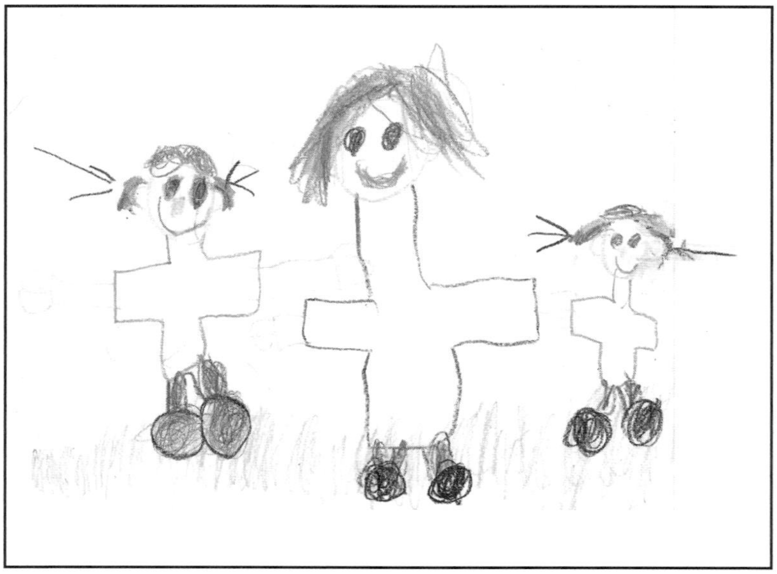

FIGURE 27–8. A portrait by a seven-year-old boy of himself, his mother, and his brother. All the main character traits are shown including the boys' bilateral cochlear implants (*arrows*).

growing and changing child. The child's educational, emotional, and social development must press on with or without auditory input. Language development is closely intertwined in all of these areas and thus the child could suffer delays in many areas if language is not attained.

Summary of Limitations to Auditory Plasticity in Children Using Implants

There are a number of factors that set up potential challenges to auditory development in children using unilateral cochlear implants. These include: (1) limitations of the cochlear implant and of electrical stimulation; (2) effects of deafness in the auditory system; and (3) a lack of binaural cues. Children using cochlear implants are thus forced to expend greater than normal effort and attention to hear and understand speech in everyday listening environments including school. These issues are important to keep in mind when assessing cochlear implant candidacy and counseling children and families regarding cochlear implant outcomes. Moreover, this means that the role of therapy, which emphasizes listening and speech-language skills and the use of supportive devices and personnel in school, continue to be vital for children using cochlear implants.

Bilateral Cochlear Implants

Of the issues raised in the previous section, one has a potentially viable solution in the short term. We may be able to provide binaural cues and stimulate bilateral auditory development by implanting both ears. Bilateral cochlear implantation is becoming more common in both adults and children. Data from adults who had normal bilateral hearing prior to becoming deaf and who received bilateral cochlear implants indicate that the use of the second device provides increased loudness of auditory input due to the summation of input between the ears (Litovsky, Parkinson, Arcaroli, & Sammeth, 2006). They also experience normal-like processing of level differences between the ears (Grantham, Ashmead, Ricketts, Haynes, & Labadie, 2008), which enables some improvements in sound localization (Litovsky et al., 2004) and speech perception in noise (Tyler, Dunn, Witt, & Noble, 2007). Unfortunately, these adults are not able to use interaural timing cues as effectively as normal-hearing adults (Grantham, Ashmead, Ricketts, Haynes, & Labadie, 2008; van Hoesel, 2007).

Bilateral cochlear implantation in children presents unique difficulties (Papsin & Gordon, 2008) because: (a) processing of bilateral input may be complicated by the immaturity of the deprived central auditory system; (b) young children with limited auditory experience often cannot describe what they hear through the implant/s (Gordon, et al., 2004a, 2004b); and (c) the two cochlear implants must be individually programmed and customized for each child, but as yet there are no methods to "balance" or "calibrate" level, timing, and pitch information provided by the two devices. Nonetheless, bilateral cochlear implantation is rapidly becoming the desired standard of care for bilateral deafness in both adults and children as indicated in position statements from American (Balkany et al., 2008), British (http://www.bcig.org.uk/downloads/pdfs/BCIG%20position%20statement%20-%20Bilateral%20Cochlear%20Implantation%20May%2007.pdf), and Canadian (in preparation) groups. One of the strongest arguments for bilateral implantation in children is that there may be a sensitive period for bilateral auditory brainstem development that could be missed if bilateral implants are not available for children with deafness in both ears (Gordon, Valero, van Hoesel, & Papsin, 2008). Cortical responses also suggest that older children with long periods of unilateral implant use prior to bilateral implantation may experience activation of nonauditory areas of the brain and limited auditory plasticity (Bauer, Sharma, Martin, & Dorman, 2006; Gordon et al., 2010; Wong, Papsin, & Gordon, 2010). Behavioral data indicate that children using two cochlear implants are better able to understand speech in quiet and in particular noise conditions (Galvin, Mok, & Dowell, 2007; Gordon & Papsin, 2009) and to discriminate between sound locations (Litovsky et al., 2006) than when using only one implant. Early data from children receiving bilateral implants simultaneously suggest that they are developing skills more like normal-hearing children (Beijen, Snik, & Mylanus, 2007; Gordon & Papsin, 2009) than children who had a long period of unilateral implant use prior to bilateral implantation (Mok, Galvin, Dowell, & McKay, 2007). Children with bilateral implants perceive interimplant level cues better than interimplant timing cues (Salloum, Valero, Papsin, van Hoesel, & Gordon, 2010) and thus likely use amplitude cues between the implants to achieve functional benefits. Long-term outcomes of bilateral cochlear implantation in children still need to be collected.

Conclusions

Cochlear implants allow children who otherwise would be almost completely isolated from sound to hear. Remarkably, cochlear implants have enabled such children to achieve excellent speech perception skills and to develop oral speech and language. We must realize, however, that these outcomes are variable and come with considerable effort on the part of child and family through therapy and educational support. There are multiple factors that contribute to successful cochlear implant use in children. Some issues relate specifically to the input provided by the implant and the auditory system as reviewed in this chapter. Some important factors related to the former set of issues have been addressed in this chapter.

The basic aim of cochlear implants is to effectively stimulate the auditory nerve. However, electrical hearing through a cochlear implant cannot be equated to normal hearing because the implants bypass normal processing by the external and middle ears and the cochlea; use fixed rate electrical pulses from limited cochlear locations; stimulate auditory systems that may have been affected by deafness; and are often provided unilaterally. Bilateral cochlear implantation aims to provide easier hearing for children and adults by addressing the latter point and making binaural cues available. The extent to which binaural processing can be provided by two independent devices may relate to a number of issues, including effects of bilateral deafness, effects of unilateral stimulation, and the age of the child. Moreover, we do not yet know how best to program the two devices to allow children to have access to binaural cues.

The effects of deafness in childhood and developmental plasticity of the auditory system are important factors to understand in order to achieve successful cochlear implant use in children. Interestingly, much of what we know about these issues has been afforded through electrical stimulation and cochlear implantation itself. Through both animal and human studies, we have learned that rudimentary auditory pathways develop independent of input but need stimulation to mature. Neural development or survival might depend on the etiology of deafness. When the pathways are deprived of stimulation, development in the auditory brainstem is virtually arrested, whereas crossmodal changes are allowed to occur in the auditory cortex. Sensitive periods in auditory development reflect the time point at which these changes are limited or irreversible. We suggest that a period of unilateral stimulation will cause reorganization through the auditory pathways including the brainstem that could compromise development of contralateral pathways after bilateral implantation. Thus, there may be at least two sensitive periods in auditory development.

Going forward, cochlear implant research strives to provide the most effective input at optimal periods in order to promote auditory development which follows a normal auditory trajectory. Clearly, this is the first step for children who need this access to sound to acquire oral speech and language skills that they can use to pursue any educational, vocational, or other avenues of their choosing.

References

Abbas, P. J., Brown, C. J., Shallop, J. K., Firszt, J. B., Hughes, M. L., Hong, S. H., & Staller, S. J. (1999). Summary of results using the nucleus CI24M implant to record the electrically evoked compound action potential. *Ear and Hearing, 20*(1), 45–59.

Almqvist, B., Harris, S., & Shallop, J. K. (2000). Objective intraoperative method to record averaged electromyographic stapedius muscle reflexes in cochlear implant patients. *Audiology, 39*(3), 146–152.

Balkany, T., Hodges, A., Telischi, F., Hoffman, R., Madell, J., Parisier, S., . . . Litovsky, R. (2008). William House Cochlear Implant Study Group: Position statement on bilateral cochlear implantation. *Otology and Neurotology, 29*, 107–108.

Battmer, R. D., Reid, J. M., & Lenarz, T. (1997). Performance in quiet and in noise with the Nucleus Spectra 22 and the Clarion CIS/CA cochlear implant devices. *Scandinavian Audiology, 26*(4), 240–246.

Bauer, P. W., Sharma, A., Martin, K., & Dorman, M. (2006). Central auditory development in children with bilateral cochlear implants. *Archives of Otolaryngology-Head and Neck Surgery, 132*(10), 1133–1136.

Beijen, J. W., Snik, A. F., & Mylanus, E. A. (2007). Sound localization ability of young children with bilateral cochlear implants. *Otology and Neurotology, 28*(4), 479–485.

Beiser, M., Himelfarb, M. Z., Gold, S., & Shanon, E. (1985). Maturation of auditory brainstem potentials in neonates and infants. *International Journal of Pediatric Otorhinolaryngology, 9*(1), 69–76.

Bess, F. H., Tharpe, A. M., & Gibler, A. M. (1986). Auditory performance of children with unilateral sensorineural hearing loss. *Ear and Hearing, 7*(1), 20–26.

Brown, C. J. (2003). Clinical uses of electrically evoked auditory nerve and brainstem responses. *Current Opinions in Otolaryngology, Head and Neck Surgery, 11*(5), 383–387.

Brown, C. J., Etler, C., He, S., O'Brien, S., Erenberg, S., Kim, J. R., . . . Abbas, P. J. (2008). The electrically evoked auditory change complex: Preliminary results from nucleus cochlear implant users. *Ear and Hearing,* 29, 704–717.

Ching, T. Y., Hill, M., Brew, J., Incerti, P., Priolo, S., Rushbrook, E., & Forsythe, L. (2005). The effect of auditory experience on speech perception, localization, and functional performance of children who use a cochlear implant and a hearing aid in opposite ears. *International Journal of Audiology, 44*(12), 677–690.

Cohen, L. T., Richardson, L. M., Saunders, E., & Cowan, R. S. (2003). Spatial spread of neural excitation in cochlear implant recipients: Comparison of improved ECAP method and psychophysical forward masking. *Hearing Research, 179*(1–2), 72–87.

Cone-Wesson, B., & Wunderlich, J. (2003). Auditory evoked potentials from the cortex: Audiology applications. *Current Opinions in Otolaryngology, Head and Neck Surgery, 11*(5), 372–377.

Connor, C. M., Craig, H. K., Raudenbush, S. W., Heavner, K., & Zwolan, T. A. (2006). The age at which young deaf children receive cochlear implants and their vocabulary and speech-production growth: Is there an added value for early implantation? *Ear and Hearing, 27*(6), 628–644.

Davids, T., Valero, J., Papsin, B. C., Harrison, R. V., & Gordon, K. A. (2008). Effects of stimulus manipulation on electrophysiological responses of pediatric cochlear implant users. Part II: Rate effects. *Hearing Research, 244*, 15–24.

Djourno, A., & Eyries, C. (1957). Auditory prosthesis by means of a distant electrical stimulation of the sensory nerve with the use of an indwelt coiling. *La Presse Médicale, 65*(63), 1417.

Djourno, A., Eyries, C., & Vallancien, B. (1957a). Electric excitation of the cochlear nerve in man by induction at a distance with the aid of micro-coil included in the fixture [in French]. *Comptes Rendus des Seances de la Societe de Biologie et de Ses Filiales, 151*(3), 423–425.

Djourno, A., Eyries, C., & Vallancien, P. (1957b). Preliminary attempts of electrical excitation of the auditory nerve in man, by permanently inserted micro-apparatus [in French]. *Bulletin de Academie Nationale de Medecine, 141*(21–23), 481–483.

Eggermont, J. J. (1985). Evoked potentials as indicators of auditory maturation. *Acta Otolaryngologica Suppl (Stockh), 421*, 41–47.

Eggermont, J. J. (1988). On the rate of maturation of sensory evoked potentials. *Electroencephalography and Clinical Neurophysiology, 70*(4), 293–305.

Eisenberg, L. S., Johnson, K. C., Martinez, A. S., Cokely, C. G., Tobey, E. A., Quittner, A. L., . . . Niparko, J. K.; CDaCI Investgative Team. (2006). Speech recognition at 1-year follow-up in the childhood development after cochlear implantation study: Methods and preliminary findings. *Audiology and Neuro-Otology, 11*(4), 259–268.

Figueiredo, J. C., Abel, S. M., & Papsin, B. C. (2001). The effect of the audallion BEAMformer noise reduction preprocessor on sound localization for cochlear implant users. *Ear and Hearing, 22*(6), 539–547.

Fink, N. E., Wang, N. Y., Visaya, J., Niparko, J. K., Quittner, A., Eisenberg, L. S., . . . Tobey, E. A.; CDaCI Investigative Team. (2007). Childhood development after cochlear implantation (CDaCI) study: Design and baseline characteristics. *Cochlear Implants International, 8*(2), 92–116.

Finney, E. M., Clementz, B. A., Hickok, G., & Dobkins, K. R. (2003). Visual stimuli activate auditory cortex in deaf subjects: Evidence from MEG. *NeuroReport, 14*(11), 1425–1427.

Finney, E. M., Fine, I., & Dobkins, K. R. (2001). Visual stimuli activate auditory cortex in the deaf. *Natural Neuroscience, 4*(12), 1171–1173.

Friesen, L. M., & Tremblay, K. L. (2006). Acoustic change complexes recorded in adult cochlear implant listeners. *Ear and Hearing, 27*(6), 678–685.

Galvin, J. J., 3rd, & Fu, Q. J. (2005). Effects of stimulation rate, mode and level on modulation detection by cochlear implant users. *Journal of the Association for Research in Otolaryngology, 6*(3), 269–279.

Galvin, K. L., Mok, M., & Dowell, R. C. (2007). Perceptual benefit and functional outcomes for children using sequential bilateral cochlear implants. *Ear and Hearing, 28*(4), 470–482.

Geers, A. E. (2006). Factors influencing spoken language outcomes in children following early cochlear implantation. *Advances in Oto-Rhino-Laryngology, 64*, 50–65.

Geers, A., Brenner, C., & Davidson, L. (2003). Factors associated with development of speech perception skills in children implanted by age five. *Ear and Hearing, 24*(1 Suppl), 24S–35S.

Gilley, P. M., Sharma, A., & Dorman, M. F. (2008) Cortical reorganization in children who are deaf. *Brain Research, 1239*, 56–65.

Gordon, K. A., & Papsin, B. C. (2009), Benefits of short interimplant delays in children receiving bilateral cochlear implants. *Otology and Neurotology, 30*(3), 319–331.

Gordon, K. A., Papsin, B. C., & Harrison, R. V. (2003). Activity-dependent developmental plasticity of the auditory brainstem in children who use cochlear implants. *Ear and Hearing, 24*(6), 485–500.

Gordon, K. A., Papsin, B. C., & Harrison, R. V. (2004a). Programming cochlear implant stimulation levels in infants and children with a combination of objective measures. *International Journal of Audiology, 43*(Suppl 1), S28–S32.

Gordon, K. A., Papsin, B. C., & Harrison, R. V. (2004b). Toward a battery of behavioral and objective measures to achieve optimal cochlear implant stimulation levels in children. *Ear and Hearing, 25*, 447–463.

Gordon, K. A., Papsin, B. C., & Harrison, R. V. (2005). Effects of cochlear implant use on the electrically evoked middle latency response in children. *Hearing Research, 204*(1–2), 78–89.

Gordon, K. A., Papsin, B. C., & Harrison, R. V. (2006). An evoked potential study of the developmental time course of the auditory nerve and brainstem in children using cochlear implants. *Audiology and Neuro-Otology, 11*(1), 7–23.

Gordon, K. A., Papsin, B. C., & Harrison, R. V. (2007). Auditory brainstem activity and development evoked by apical versus basal cochlear implant electrode stimulation in children. *Clinical Neurophysiology, 118*(8), 1671–1684.

Gordon, K. A., Tanaka, S., & Papsin, B. C. (2005). Atypical cortical responses underlie poor speech perception in children using cochlear implants. *NeuroReport, 16*(18), 2041–2045.

Gordon, K. A., Tanaka, S., Wong, D. D. E., & Papsin, B. C. (2008). Characterizing responses from auditory cortex in young people with several years of cochlear implant experience. *Clinical Neurophysiology, 119*, 2347–2362.

Gordon, K. A., Valero, J., van Hoesel, R., & Papsin, B. C. (2008). Abnormal timing delays in auditory brainstem responses evoked by bilateral cochlear implant use in children. *Otology and Neurotology, 29*(2), 193–198.

Gordon, K. A., Wong, D. D. E., & Papsin, B. C. (2010) Cortical function in children receiving bilateral cochlear implants simultaneously or after a period of inter-implant delay. *Otology and Neurotology*, Epub July 15.

Grantham, D. W., Ashmead, D. H., Ricketts, T. A., Haynes, D. S., & Labadie, R. F. (2008). Interaural time and level difference thresholds for acoustically presented signals in postlingually deafened adults fitted with bilateral cochlear implants using CIS+ processing. *Ear and Hearing, 29*(1), 33–44.

Groenen, P., Snik, A., & van den Broek, P. (1996). On the clinical relevance of mismatch negativity: Results from subjects with normal hearing and cochlear implant users. *Audiology and Neurotology, 1*(2), 112–124.

Hall, J. W. (1992). *Handbook of auditory evoked responses*. Needham Heights, MA: Allyn and Bacon.

Harrison, R. V., Gordon, K. A., & Mount, R. J. (2005). Is there a critical period for cochlear implantation in congenitally deaf children? Analyses of hearing and speech perception performance after implantation. *Developmental Psychobiology, 46*(3), 252–261.

Hartmann, R., Shepherd, R. K., Heid, S., & Klinke, R. (1997). Response of the primary auditory cortex to electrical stimulation of the auditory nerve in the congenitally deaf white cat. *Hearing Research, 112*(1–2), 115–133.

Henkin, Y., Kishon-Rabin, L., Tatin-Schneider, S., Urbach, D., Hildesheimer, M., & Kileny, P. R. (2004). Low-resolution electromagnetic tomography (LORETA) in children with cochlear implants: A preliminary report. *International Journal of Audiology, 43*(Suppl. 1), S48–S51.

Hopyan-Misakyan, T. M., Gordon, K. A., Dennis, M., & Papsin, B. C. (2009). Recognition of affective speech prosody and facial affect in deaf children with unilateral right cochlear implants. *Child Neuropsychology, 15*, 136–146.

Hughes, M. L., & Abbas, P. J. (2006). The relation between electrophysiologic channel interaction and electrode pitch ranking in cochlear implant recipients. *Journal of the Acoustical Society of America, 119*(3), 1527–1537.

Hughes, M. L., Brown, C. J., Abbas, P. J., Wolaver, A. A., & Gervais, J. P. (2000). Comparison of EAP thresholds with MAP levels in the nucleus 24 cochlear implant: Data from children. *Ear and Hearing, 21*(2), 164–174.

Huttenlocher, P. R., & Dabholkar, A. S. (1997). Regional differences in synaptogenesis in human cerebral cortex. *Journal of Comprehensive Neurology, 387*(2), 167–178.

Jiang, Z. D. (1995). Maturation of the auditory brainstem in low risk-preterm infants: A comparison with age-matched full term infants up to 6 years. *Early Human Development, 42*(1), 49–65.

Kelly, A. S., Purdy, S. C., & Thorne, P. R. (2005). Electrophysiological and speech perception measures of auditory processing in experienced adult cochlear implant users. *Clinical Neurophysiology, 116*(6), 1235–1246.

Kileny, P. R. (1991). Use of electrophysiologic measures in the management of children with cochlear implants: Brainstem, middle latency, and cognitive (P300) responses. *American Journal of Otology, 12*(Suppl.), 37–42; discussion, 43–37.

Klee, T. M., & Davis-Dansky, E. (1986). A comparison of unilaterally hearing-impaired children and normal-hearing children on a battery of standardized language tests. *Ear and Hearing, 7*(1), 27–37.

Klinke, R., Kral, A., Heid, S., Tillein, J., & Hartmann, R. (1999). Recruitment of the auditory cortex in congenitally deaf cats by long-term cochlear electrostimulation. *Science, 285*(5434), 1729–1733.

Kral, A., Hartmann, R., Tillein, J., Heid, S., & Klinke, R. (2000). Congenital auditory deprivation reduces synaptic activity within the auditory cortex in a layer-specific manner. *Cerebral Cortex, 10*(7), 714–726.

Kraus, N., Micco, A. G., Koch, D. B., McGee, T., Carrell, T., Sharma, A., . . . Weingarten, C. Z. (1993). The mismatch negativity cortical evoked potential elicited by speech in cochlear-implant users. *Hearing Research, 65*(1–2), 118–124.

Lee, D. S., Lee, J. S., Oh, S. H., Kim, S.-K., Kim, J.-W., Chung, J.-K., . . . Kim, C. S. (2001). Deafness: Cross-modal plasticity and cochlear implants. *Nature, 409*(6817), 149–150.

Lee, H. J., Giraud, A. L., Kang, E., Oh, S. H., Kang, H., Kim, C. S., & Lee, D. S. (2007). Cortical activity at rest predicts cochlear implantation outcome. *Cerebral Cortex, 17*(4), 909–917.

Lieu, J. E. (2004). Speech-language and educational consequences of unilateral hearing loss in children. *Archives of Otolaryngology-Head and Neck Surgery, 130*(5), 524–530.

Litovsky, R., Parkinson, A., Arcaroli, J., & Sammeth, C. (2006). Simultaneous bilateral cochlear implantation in adults: A multicenter clinical study. *Ear and Hearing, 27*(6), 714–731.

Litovsky, R. Y., Johnstone, P. M., Godar, S., Agrawal, S., Parkinson, A., Peters, R., & Lake, J. (2006). Bilateral cochlear implants in children: Localization acuity measured with minimum audible angle. *Ear and Hearing, 27*(1), 43–59.

Litovsky, R. Y., Parkinson, A., Arcaroli, J., Peters, R., Lake, J., Johnstone, P., & Yu, G. (2004). Bilateral cochlear implants in adults and children. *Archives of Otolaryngology-Head and Neck Surgery, 130*(5), 648–655.

Loizou, P. (1998). Mimicking the human ear. *IEEE Signal Processing Magazine, 15*(5), 101–130.

Luntz, M., Shpak, T., & Weiss, H. (2005). Binaural-bimodal hearing: Concomitant use of a unilateral cochlear implant and a contralateral hearing aid. *Acta Otolaryngologica, 125*(8), 863–869.

Martin, B. A. (2007). Can the acoustic change complex be recorded in an individual with a cochlear implant? Separating neural responses from cochlear implant artifact. *Journal of the American Academy of Audiology, 18*(2), 126–140.

McGee, T., & Kraus, N. (1996). Auditory development reflected by middle latency response. *Ear and Hearing, 17*(5), 419–429.

McGee, T., Kraus, N., Killion, M., Rosenberg, R., & King, C. (1993). Improving the reliability of the auditory middle latency response by monitoring EEG delta activity. *Ear and Hearing, 14*(2), 76–84.

Miller, C. A., Abbas, P. J., & Robinson, B. K. (1993). Characterization of wave I of the electrically evoked auditory brainstem response in the guinea pig. *Hearing Research, 69*(1–2), 35–44.

Mok, M., Galvin, K. L., Dowell, R. C., & McKay, C. M. (2007). Spatial unmasking and binaural advantage for children with normal hearing, a cochlear implant and a hearing aid, and bilateral implants. *Audiology and Neuro-Otology, 12*(5), 295–306.

Moller, A. R., & Jannetta, P. J. (1982). Auditory evoked potentials recorded intracranially from the brain stem in man. *Experimental Neurology, 78*(1), 144–157.

Moller, A. R., Jannetta, P., Bennett, M., & Moller, M. B. (1981). Intracranially recorded responses from the human auditory nerve: New insights into the origin of brain stem evoked potentials (BSEPs). *Electroencephalography and Clinical Neurophysiology, 52*(1), 18–27.

Moore, J. K., & Guan, Y. L. (2001). Cytoarchitectural and axonal maturation in human auditory cortex. *Journal of the Association for Research in Otolaryngology, 2*(4), 297–311.

Moore, J. K., & Linthicum, F. H., Jr. (2007). The human auditory system: A timeline of development. *International Journal of Audiology, 46*(9), 460–478.

Moore, C. M., Vollmer, M., Leake, P. A., Snyder, R. L., & Rebscher, S. J. (2002). The effects of chronic intracochlear electrical stimulation on inferior colliculus spatial representation in adult deafened cats. *Hearing Research, 164*(1–2), 82–96.

Nadol, J. B., Jr. (1997). Patterns of neural degeneration in the human cochlea and auditory nerve: Implications for cochlear implantation. *Otolaryngology-Head and Neck Surgery, 117*(3 Pt. 1), 220–228.

Nikolopoulos, T. P., Archbold, S. M., & O'Donoghue, G. M. (1999). The development of auditory perception in children following cochlear implantation. *International Journal of Pediatric Otorhinolaryngology, 49*(Suppl. 1), S189–S191.

Pang, E. W., & Taylor, M. J. (2000). Tracking the development of the N1 from age 3 to adulthood: An examination of speech and non-speech stimuli. *Clinical Neurophysiology, 111*(3), 388–397.

Papsin, B. C. (2005). Cochlear implantation in children with anomalous cochleovestibular anatomy. *Laryngoscope, 115*(1 Pt. 2 Suppl. 106), 1–26.

Papsin, B. C., & Gordon, K. A. (2007). Cochlear implants for children with severe-to-profound hearing loss. *New England Journal of Medicine, 357*(23), 2380–2387.

Papsin, B. C., & Gordon, K. A. (2008). Bilateral cochlear implants should be the standard for children with bilateral sensorineural deafness. *Current Opinions in Otolaryngology-Head and Neck Surgery, 16*(1), 69–74.

Papsin, B. C., Gysin, C., Picton, N., Nedzelski, J., & Harrison, R. V. (2000). Speech perception outcome measures in prelingually deaf children up to four years after cochlear implantation. *Annals of Otology, Rhinology and Laryngology Suppl., 185*, 38–42.

Pettingill, L. N., Richardson, R. T., Wise, A. K., O'Leary, S. J., & Shepherd, R. K. (2007). Neurotrophic factors and neural prostheses: Potential clinical applications based upon findings in the auditory system. *IEEE Trans Biomed Eng, 54*(6 Pt. 1), 1138–1148.

Pfingst, B. E., Xu, L., & Thompson, C. S. (2007). Effects of carrier pulse rate and stimulation site on modulation detection by subjects with cochlear implants. *Journal of the Acoustical Society of America 121*(4), 2236–2246.

Polak, M., Hodges, A., & Balkany, T. (2005). ECAP, ESR and subjective levels for two different nucleus 24 electrode arrays. *Otology and Neurotology, 26*(4), 639–645.

Ponton, C. W. (2006). Critical periods for human cortical development: An ERP study in children with cochlear implant. In S. G. Lomber & J. J. Eggermont (Eds.), *Reprogramming the cerebral cortex: Plasticity following central and peripheral lesions* (pp. 213–228). Oxford, UK: Oxford University Press.

Ponton, C. W., & Don, M. (1995). The mismatch negativity in cochlear implant users. *Ear and Hearing, 16*(1), 131–146.

Ponton, C. W., & Eggermont, J. J. (2001). Of kittens and kids: Altered cortical maturation following profound deafness and cochlear implant use. *Audiology and Neuro-Otology, 6*(6), 363–380.

Ponton, C. W., Eggermont, J. J., Coupland, S. G., & Winkelaar, R. (1992). Frequency-specific maturation of the eighth nerve and brain-stem auditory pathway: Evidence from derived auditory brain-stem responses (ABRs). *Journal of the Acoustical Society of America, 91*(3), 1576–1586.

Ponton, C. W., Eggermont, J. J., Don, M., Waring, M. D., Kwong, B., Cunningham, J., & Trautwein, P. (2000). Maturation of the mismatch negativity: Effects of profound deafness and cochlear implant use. *Audiology and Neurootology, 5*(3–4), 167–185.

Ponton, C., Eggermont, J. J., Khosla, D., Kwong, B., & Don, M. (2002). Maturation of human central auditory system activity: Separating auditory evoked potentials by dipole source modeling. *Clinical Neurophysiology, 113*(3), 407–420.

Ponton, C., Moore, J. K., & Eggermont, J. J. (1996). Auditory brain stem response generation by parallel pathways: Differential maturation of axonal conduction time and synaptic transmission. *Ear and Hearing, 17*(5), 402–410.

Propst, E. J., Papsin, B. C., Stockley, T. L., Harrison, R. V., & Gordon, K. A. (2006) Auditory responses in cochlear implant users with and without GJB2 deafness. *Laryngoscope, 116*(2), 317–327.

Pulsifer, M. B., Salorio, C. F., & Niparko, J. K. (2003). Developmental, audiological, and speech perception functioning in children after cochlear implant surgery. *Archives of Pediatric and Adolescent Medicine, 157*(6), 552–558.

Roman, S., Canevet, G., Marquis, P., Triglia, J. M., & Liegeois-Chauvel, C. (2005). Relationship between auditory perception skills and mismatch negativity recorded in free field in cochlear-implant users. *Hearing Research, 201*(1–2), 10–20.

Rotteveel, J. J., Stegeman, D. F., de Graaf, R., Colon, E. J., & Visco, Y. M. (1987). The maturation of the central auditory conduction in preterm infants until three months post term. III. The middle latency auditory evoked response (MLR). *Hearing Research, 27*(3), 245–256.

Salloum, C., Valero, J., Papsin, B. C., van Hoesel, R., & Gordon, K. A. (2010) Lateralization of inter-implant timing and level differences in children who use bilateral cochlear implants. *Ear and Hearing, 31*(4), 441–456.

Shallop, J. K. (1993). Objective electrophysiological measures from cochlear implant patients. *Ear and Hearing, 14*(1), 58–63.

Shallop, J. K., & Ash, K. R. (1995). Relationships among comfort levels determined by cochlear implant patient's self-programming, audiologist's programming, and electrical stapedius reflex thresholds. *Annals of Otology, Rhinology and Laryngology Suppl., 166*, 175–176.

Sharma, A. (2007). Special issue on central auditory system development and plasticity. *International Journal of Audiology, 46*(9), 459.

Sharma, A., Dorman, M. F., & Kral, A. (2005). The influence of a sensitive period on central auditory development in children with unilateral and bilateral cochlear implants. *Hearing Research, 203*(1–2), 134–143.

Sharma, A., Dorman, M. F., & Spahr, A. J. (2002). A sensitive period for the development of the central auditory system in children with cochlear implants: Implications for age of implantation. *Ear and Hearing, 23*(6), 532–539.

Sharma, A., Kraus, N., McGee, T. J., & Nicol, T. G. (1997). Developmental changes in P1 and N1 central auditory responses elicited by consonant-vowel syllables. *Electroencephalography and Clinical Neurophysiology, 104*(6), 540–545.

Singh, S., Liasis, A., Rajput, K., & Luxon, L. (2006). Event related potentials—are they useful in pediatric cochlear implant patients? *Clinical Otolaryngology, 31*(3), 248–249.

Snyder, R. L., Rebscher, S. J., Leake, P. A., Kelly, K., & Cao, K. (1991). Chronic intracochlear electrical stimulation in the neonatally deafened cat. II. Temporal properties of neurons in the inferior colliculus. *Hearing Research, 56*(1–2), 246–264.

Stephan, K., Welzl-Muller, K., & Stiglbrunner, H. (1990). Stapedius reflex growth function in cochlear implant patients. *Audiology, 29*(1), 46–54.

Thai-Van, H., Cozma, S., Boutitie, F., Disant, F., Truy, E., & Collet, L. (2007). The pattern of auditory brainstem response wave V maturation in cochlear-implanted children. *Clinical Neurophysiology, 118*(3), 676–689.

Tyler, R. S., Dunn, C. C., Witt, S. A., & Noble, W. G. (2007). Speech perception and localization with adults with bilateral sequential cochlear implants. *Ear and Hearing, 28*(2 Suppl.), 86S–90S.

Uziel, A. S., Sillon, M., Vieu, A., Artieres, F., Piron, J. P., Daures, J. P., & Mondain, M. (2007). Ten-year follow-up of a consecutive series of children with multichannel cochlear implants. *Otology and Neurotology, 28*(5), 615–628.

van den Borne, B., Snik, A. F., Mens, L. H., Brokx, J. P., & van den Broek, P. (1996). Stapedius reflex measurements during surgery for cochlear implantation in children. *American Journal of Otology, 17*(4), 554–558.

van den Honert, C., & Stypulkowski, P. H. (1984). Physiological properties of the electrically stimulated auditory nerve. II. Single fiber recordings. *Hearing Research, 14*(3), 225–243.

van den Honert, C., & Stypulkowski, P. H. (1986). Characterization of the electrically evoked auditory brainstem response (ABR) in cats and humans. *Hearing Research, 21*(2), 109–126.

van Hoesel, R. J. (2007). Sensitivity to binaural timing in bilateral cochlear implant users. *Journal of the Acoustical Society of America, 121*(4), 2192–2206.

Verschuur, C. A. (2005). Effect of stimulation rate on speech perception in adult users of the Med-El CIS speech processing strategy. *International Journal of Audiology, 44*(1), 58–63.

Vollmer, M., Snyder, R. L., Leake, P. A., Beitel, R. E., Moore, C. M., & Rebscher, S. J. (1999). Temporal properties of chronic cochlear electrical stimulation determine temporal resolution of neurons in cat inferior colliculus. *Journal of Neurophysiology, 82*(6), 2883–2902.

Wable, J., van den Abbeele, T., Gallego, S., & Frachet, B. (2000). Mismatch negativity: A tool for the assessment of stimuli discrimination in cochlear implant subjects. *Clinical Neurophysiology, 111*(4), 743–751.

Wong, D. D. E., Papsin, B. D., & Gordon, K. A. (2010) *Hemispheric lateralization of cortical responses in children using bilateral cochlear implants*. Poster presentation at the Association for Research in Otolaryngology, Anaheim, CA, February 5–10.

Zeitler, D. M., Kessler, M. A., Terushkin, V., Roland, T. J., Jr., Svirsky, M. A., Lalwani, A. K., et al. (2008). Speech perception benefits of sequential bilateral cochlear implantation in children and adults: A retrospective analysis. *Otology and Neurotology, 29*(3), 314–325.

28

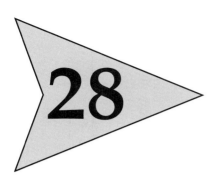

Other Implantable Devices: Bone-Anchored Hearing Aids

Bill Hodgetts

Overview

In the hearing sciences, two types of hearing are often described: air conduction (AC) and bone conduction (BC). Air conduction hearing involves the entire auditory system. Tiny acoustic vibrations in the air molecules are funneled down the ear canal where they induce vibrations on the tympanic membrane. The tympanic membrane then vibrates the ossicular chain, which results in a traveling wave of fluid displacement in the cochlea. Sufficient displacement of the basilar membrane begins the electrochemical cascade from the inner hair cells through the auditory nerve, brainstem, and eventually the cortex where the sound is interpreted. Bone conduction hearing largely bypasses the external and middle ear, delivering the mechanical vibrations directly to the cochlea. To hear by bone conduction, no matter how complex the actual physiology, vibrations from some location on the skull need to be sufficiently intense to generate a traveling wave in the cochlea. If that traveling wave is of sufficient magnitude, the cochlea-to-cortex pathway will be stimulated and the perception of sound will occur. When we speak, we are actually hearing a blend of air conducted and bone conducted sounds. Some of our perception will come from the acoustic vibration of air molecules from our mouths that travel around our heads to the ear canals (air conduction). However, a portion of our speech will generate a mechanical vibration of the skull bones of sufficient magnitude to also contribute to our perception of our own voice (Reinfeldt, 2009). This phenomenon is why we seldom recognize (and often dislike) our own voices on a recording such as voicemail, where only the air conducted sound is available.

In recent years, increasing attention has been given to how we hear by bone conduction. Figure 28–1 shows the numbers of publications on the bone-anchored hearing aid (Baha®) from 1980 to 2009. Over this period much has been learned about the value of this treatment approach for individuals who are not able to wear regular air conduction hearing aids. The aim of this chapter is to share what is known about the candidacy criteria and the audiologic and surgical considerations of the present Baha system. Additionally, attention will be given to the entire Baha fitting process including assessment, selection/prescription, verification, and validation (Seewald, Moodie, Sinclair, & Cornelisse, 1996).

Indications for Bone Conduction Amplification

The Baha was originally indicated only for individuals with bilateral conductive hearing loss. The Baha was developed as a replacement for traditional bone conduction devices that were held in place by a steel tension headband or by the arms of eyeglasses. These traditional bone conduction technologies had three major limitations: (1) the tension from the headband or the arms of the eyeglasses was very uncomfortable and would often result in pressure sores and depressions in the skull bone; (2) there was a less predictable

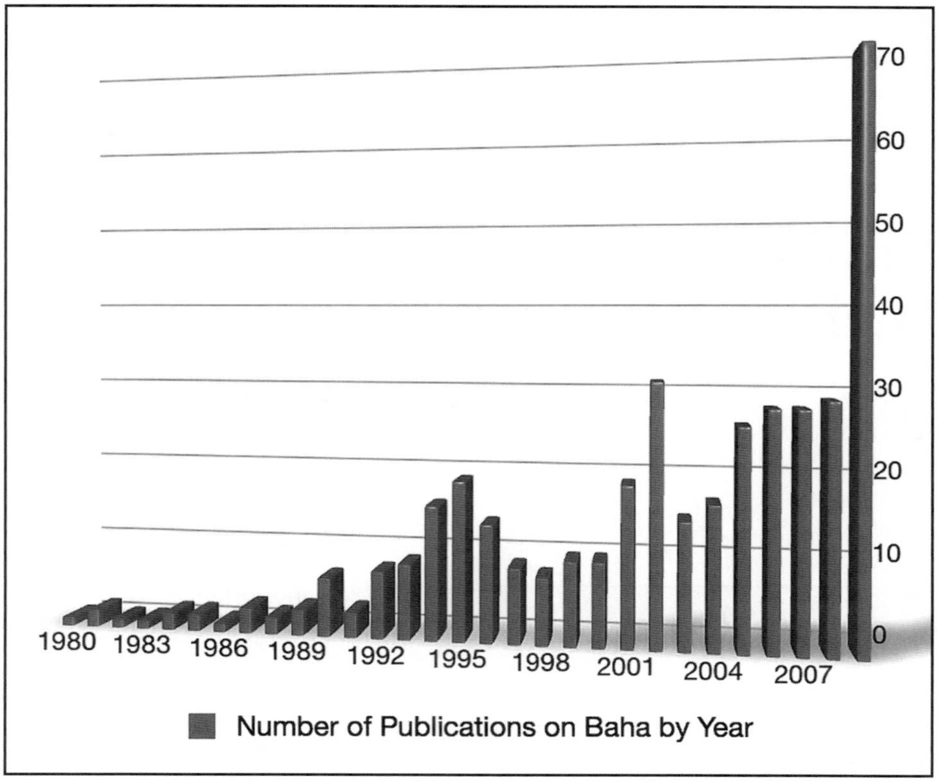

FIGURE 28–1. Number of peer-reviewed publications on the Baha by year.

and less efficient connection between the bone vibrator and the skull due to the presence of the skin and subcutaneous tissue in the vibrations pathway (more on this below); and (3) the esthetics of the device were poor. In recent years, indications for Baha candidacy have expanded to include individuals with unilateral conductive, mixed and sensorineural hearing loss. Baha candidates can be broadly grouped into three categories:

1. those with conductive or mixed hearing loss who cannot wear an air conduction hearing aid;
2. those with conductive or mixed hearing loss for whom surgery has been unsuccessful and/or future surgery is contraindicated; and
3. those with unilateral conductive, mixed or sensorineural hearing loss.

A summary of candidacy criteria and indications for Baha use related to these groups of patients is presented in Table 28–1.

Given the variety of etiologies and the associated difficulties with hearing in the unaided condition, not all Baha candidates can be expected to receive the same amount of benefit from the Baha (Dumper, Hodgetts, Liu, & Brandner, 2009). However, the Baha is now a viable option for many individuals who would have otherwise gone untreated in the past.

Implantable Bone Conduction Hearing Devices (Baha)

In the 1960s, Professor Per-Ingvar Brånemark discovered that living bone would connect to titanium through a process he coined "osseointegration" (Albrektsson & Wennerberg, 2005). Osseointegration was first applied to the field of dentistry. Titanium screws were implanted into the mouths of patients, and, after a period of healing, teeth could be connected to the implants. Researchers soon speculated that these same implants could possibly be used outside of the mouth to anchor facial prosthetics and Bahas.

Broadly speaking, Baha processors are very similar to air conduction hearing aids. They contain a microphone, battery, and internal digital signal processing (DSP) chips. The main difference between air conduction hearing aids and all bone conduction hearing aids

Table 28–1. Otologic and Audiologic Conditions That May Have Indications for Baha Use Divided Into Categories for Baha Candidacy

1. Air-Conduction Hearing Aid Contraindicated	*2. Canal or Middle Ear Surgery Contraindicated*	*3. Unilateral Hearing Loss*
Congenital bilateral atresia	Repeated surgery fails to close air-bone gap; Baha reliably closes air-bone gap	Congenital unilateral atresia
Chronic draining ears that are unresponsive to treatment	Conductive or mixed hearing loss in only hearing ear. Risk of damaging only remaining ear; Baha is a safe alternative	Acquired unilateral conductive or mixed hearing loss
External ear canal irritation	Total absence of ossicular chain and/or insufficient tissue to reconstruct ossicular chair	Congenital unilateral profound unilateral sensorineural hearing loss (often called single sided deafness in the Baha literature)
Large mastoid cavity resulting from mastoidectomy		Single-sided deafness resulting from VIIIth nerve tumor or tumor resection
Postoperative ear defects (absence of pinna, closure of ear canal) resulting from temporal bone resection		Sudden unilateral sensorineural hearing loss
Excessive occlusion effect		

(including the Baha) is the type of output delivered from each device. Air conduction hearing aids deliver acoustic vibrations while bone conduction devices deliver mechanical vibrations. The main difference between the Baha and other traditional bone conduction devices is the method by which the processor is connected to the patient. There are three main components to the Baha system: The bone-anchored implant (usually a 4-mm titanium screw), the bone conduction processor and the skin-penetrating abutment (the interface between the implant and the processor). These components can be seen in Figure 28–2.

Today, very few manufacturers offer traditional bone conduction hearing devices on a headband. This can be attributed to two factors: (1) the practical limitations of the headband mentioned above and (2) the superior benefit derived from the direct connection of the Baha to the skull bone.

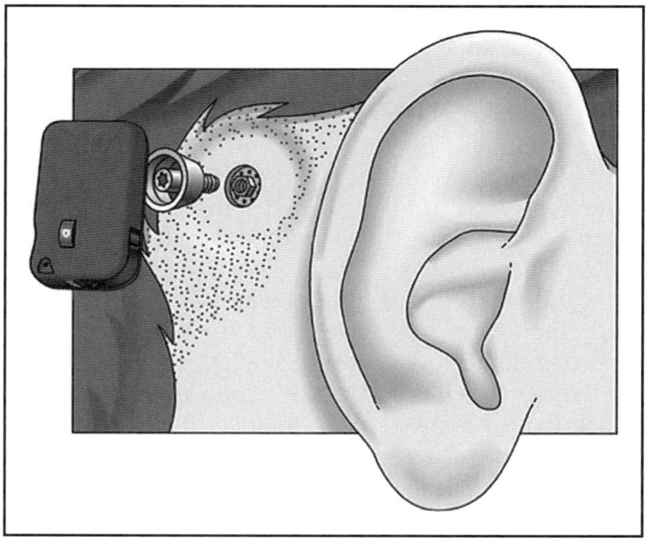

FIGURE 28–2. Exploding diagram showing all three components of the Baha system: implant, skin-penetrating abutment, and processor. Reprinted with permission © Cochlear Bone-Anchored Solutions 2009. All rights reserved.

Comparisons of Baha and Traditional Bone Conduction Devices

In the early stages of development, the majority of comparison studies were between traditional bone conduction hearing aids and the Baha. The Baha has better high frequency output capabilities and lower distortion compared to traditional bone conduction hearing aids (Cremers, Snik, & Beyon, 1992). Significant improvements on sound field-aided warble tone threshold tests, speech in quiet, and speech-in-noise tests have all been found with the Baha system. These findings apply to both adults and children (Powell, Burrell, Cooper, & Proops, 1996; Tietze & Papsin, 2001; Tjellström & Håkansson, 1995). Long-term studies have also concluded that the majority of Baha users were still using their Baha system daily and were quite satisfied with the device even five to 10 years after the Baha fitting (Håkansson et al., 1990; van der Pouw, Snik, & Cremers, 1999). From an outcomes perspective, the Baha represents a superior audiologic option compared to traditional bone conduction hearing aids (Snik et al., 2005).

Comparisons of Baha and Traditional Air Conduction Hearing Devices

Bone conduction hearing aids are often prescribed for individuals suffering from chronic otitis media. With chronic otitis media, air conduction hearing aids may: (1) prevent adequate aeration of the ear canal, (2) result in feedback or insufficient gain due to the large air vents, and (3) continue or exacerbate the infection/inflammation. Chronic otitis media may lead to additional sensorineural hearing loss if the infection invades the cochlea (Papp, Rezes, Jokay, & Sziklai, 2003). In spite of these drawbacks, many individuals still choose to use air conduction hearing aids instead of bone conduction hearing aids. Several studies have assessed the outcomes for individuals who have switched from an air conduction hearing aid to a Baha. In audiologic terms, the majority of these studies are equivocal. Some patients perform better with the Baha, whereas others perform better with their air conduction hearing aid (Snik, Bosman, Mylanus, & Cremers, 2004). Questionnaire data reveal similar subjective preference between the two technologies (McDermott, Dutt, Reid, & Proops, 2002). Mylanus, van der Pouw, Snik, and Cremers (1998) reported an interesting relationship that emerged from their data. They concluded that if the air-bone gap exceeded 30 dB, better results could be expected with the Baha than with the air conduction hearing aid. The wider the air-bone gap, the higher the gain requirement in order for the air conduction hearing aid to "push through" the conductive component of the hearing loss. Consequently, air conduction hearing aid users will experience greater feedback problems and reduced sound quality as the high frequencies begin to roll off with the widening air-bone gap. Furthermore, several studies have shown that despite the ambiguous audiological results, the vast majority of Baha users with chronic otitis media have safe, dry ears once the air conduction hearing aids are removed from their ear canals (Macnamara, Phillips, & Proops, 1996; McDermott et al., 2002; Mylanus et al., 1998).

Bilateral Baha

In the past, bilateral Baha was debated because it was assumed that the interaural attenuation by bone conduction was roughly 0 dB. There were legitimate concerns about "cross hearing." However, a number of studies have shown that the bilateral Baha can lead to improved sound localization, improved diotic summation and improved speech recognition in noise (Bosman, Snik, van der Pouw, Mylanus, & Cremers, 2001; Dutt et al., 2002; Priwin, Stenfelt, Granstrom, Tjellstrom, & Håkansson, 2004). Most studies have used individuals with symmetrical cochlear function. The literature has not fully addressed how much asymmetry can be tolerated before bilateral benefits disappear.

Baha Surgical Procedures

Adults and Children

The surgical procedures for Baha have been described in detail by Tjellstrom, Håkansson, and Granstrom (2001) and have not changed dramatically from this publication. A thin flap of skin is lifted and then a significant portion of subcutaneous tissue is removed so that the skin flap will ultimately rest flush to the skull. The titanium screw is carefully inserted into the skull and an abutment is attached to the screw. Finally, a hole is punched through the skin flap so that the Baha can be connected to the abutment. In adult patients, implant survival is achieved in 90 to 98% of cases and approximately 90% of implant sites remain free of serious skin reactions (Granstrom, Bergstrom, Odersjo, & Tjellstrom, 2001; Tjellstrom et al., 2001; van der Pouw, Mylanus, & Cremers, 1999). The majority of adult Baha surgeries take place under local anesthesia in a one-stage operation. Patients are advised to wait anywhere between 6 weeks to 3 months before the processor is connected to allow sufficient time for osseointegration.

Children are more complicated than adults with respect to the Baha surgery. The skull is often very thin until children are at least 3 to 4 years old (Granstrom et al., 2001; Snik, Leijendeckers, Hol, Mylanus, & Cremers, 2008). Additionally, the skull bone of infants and young children is softer and less suitable for osseointegration (Tjellstrom et al., 2001). Although the age of implantation for children in many countries is entirely at the discretion of the Baha surgical team, in the United States, the Food and Drug Administration requires that children reach the age of 5 years before they are allowed to proceed with Baha surgery. The majority of surgeries for children occur over two-stages under general anesthesia. In the first stage of surgery, the Baha implant is installed. The second stage of surgery, when the Baha abutment is installed and punched through the skin, does not usually occur until at least

3 months after the first implant (Snik et al., 2005). Consensus statements indicate that most surgeons recommend a two stage Baha procedure for children until they are 10 years old (Snik et al., 2005). Typically, the processor can be connected to the child two weeks after the second surgery, once enough time has passed for the soft tissues around the abutment to heal. Children are much more susceptible to trauma than adults. A recent evaluation in a cohort of children in Nijmegen, the Netherlands, indicated that as many as 16.3% of children either lost their implant or had it removed (deWolf, Hol, Huygen, Mylanus, & Cremers, 2008). Some have recommended placing a second implant (sleeper implant), in the same region as the first surgery in children in case the primary implant does not integrate well or is lost to trauma (Snik et al., 2005).

Alternative to Surgery in Young Children: The Baha Softband

For children too young or medically fragile (e.g., compromised airway) to undergo implant surgery, the Baha can be attached to a small plastic disk held in place by an elastic headband known as the Baha Softband (Figure 28–3). As the Baha, connected in this way, still delivers the vibrations through the skin and subcutaneous tissue, there will be a loss of output, especially in the high frequencies. In terms of aided sound field thresholds and language development, researchers have found that results with the Baha Softband are comparable to the results obtained with traditional bone conduction hearing aids connected to a steel tension headband (Hol, Cremers, Coppen-Schellekens, & Snik, 2005). The Baha Softband is easier to wear and more comfortable than traditional bone conduction hearing aids. Additionally, as long as at least 2 to 3 newtons of pressure (approximately 200 to 300 grams of pressure) is applied, the tension of the Baha Softband is not a critical factor in the vibrations received by the child (Hodgetts, Scollie, & Swain, 2006). Verhagen, Hol, Coppens-Schellekens, Snik, and Cremers (2008) reported that aided sound field thresholds with the Baha Softband are typically in the range of 25 to 30 dB HL. It is broadly accepted that any hearing loss in excess of 15 dB HL constitutes a handicap for children (Northern & Downs, 1991). Aided sound field thresholds improve with direct bone conduction offered by the Baha implant. Therefore, while the Baha serves an important function in providing some early amplification for children, parents should be advised to consider the Baha surgery as soon as the child is old enough or medically ready for the implant.

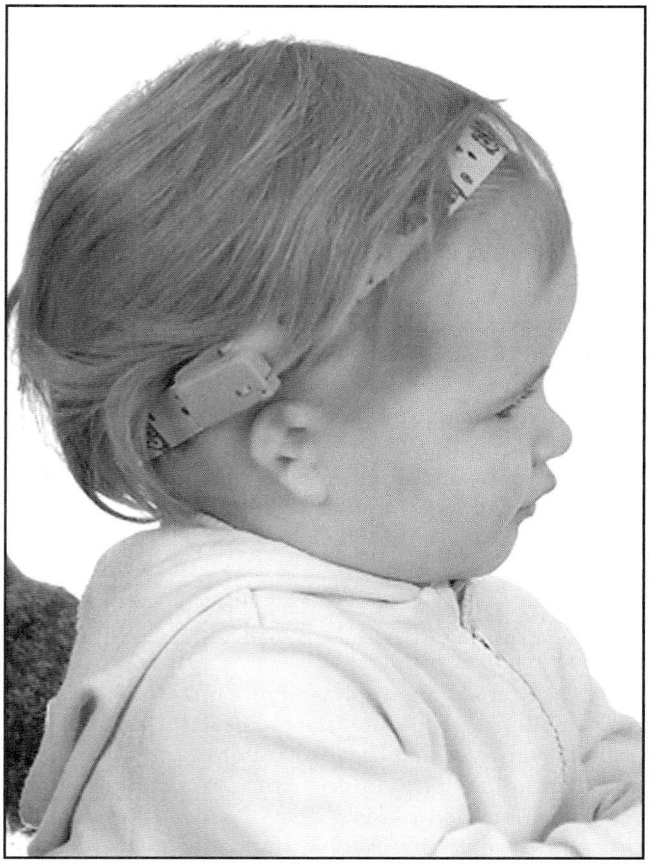

FIGURE 28–3. Baha Softband connected to a young child.

Hearing Aid Fitting Considerations for Baha

The goal for selecting and fitting amplification should be to match, as closely as possible, the amplification characteristics of a hearing aid(s) to the unique auditory characteristics of the person with the hearing loss so that person can use his or her residual hearing to its maximum potential (Cornelisse, Seewald, & Jamieson, 1995). This goal should not change depending on what type of hearing aid is being fitted (air conduction versus bone conduction). How one arrives at meeting the goal, however, does vary slightly.

Consensus documents have recommended that hearing aid fitting be done in a systematic way (AAA, 2003; ASHA, 1998; Pediatric Working Group, 1996). The recommended approach typically follows a series of stages from assessment to validation. Accurate information obtained during the assessment phase is used to guide the selection or prescription of appropriate output characteristics for a given individual with a given device. Next, the hearing aid output is determined to verify the appropriateness of the aided output to the electroacoustic parameters determined in the selection phase. Finally, if the hearing aid output has been verified to be acceptable, the individual's performance with the device is validated through outcome measurement (Seewald et al., 1996).

The same rules for validating a hearing aid fitting (e.g., aided speech recognition in noise, subjective benefit, satisfaction) are applicable to both air conduction hearing aids and Bahas. Validation results from these types of studies have been reported above. However, assessment procedures, selection or prescriptive methods and verification approaches differ slightly for the Baha compared to air conduction hearing aids. These will be considered below.

Assessment Considerations

During the assessment phase, information is gathered to define the type and degree of hearing loss as well as patient perceived handicap. The thresholds of hearing and thresholds of discomfort are two critical measures typically obtained (ASHA, 1998). Current assessment procedures for Baha involve threshold testing with a standard audiometric bone oscillator. Unfortunately, this coupling method is inherently unsatisfactory. The Baha functions by direct bone conduction. The processor is rigidly anchored to the skull (percutaneous connection), and there is no loss of energy through the skin and subcutaneous tissues (transcutaneous connection). The section below outlines why transcutaneous thresholds offer limited information as a baseline for aided Baha output. The thresholds of interest for Baha users should be those obtained directly through the Baha abutment.

Transcutaneous Versus Percutaneous Hearing Thresholds

One of the most common questions asked by patients when being assessed for Baha candidacy is "how much better will I hear with this implant compared to my previous bone conduction aid or to the trial device I used on a headband?" A number of researchers have attempted to answer this question (Håkansson, Tjellstrom, & Rosenhall, 1984, 1985; Mylanus, Snik, & Cremers, 1994; Stenfelt & Håkansson, 1999). There are three methods that have been used to estimate the differences between transcutaneous and percutaneous bone conduction. If a given subject's hearing thresholds are used, one can determine the difference (in dB) at threshold between: (1) the electrical voltage or current delivered to the bone conduction transducer, (2) the acceleration off of the skull, and (3) the force required to vibrate the skull. For example, Håkansson et al. (1984) used Békèsy audiometry to investigate the difference in voltage (dB) required to stimulate bone conduction thresholds with a conventional bone conduction transducer pressed against the skin or rigidly connected to a Baha abutment. On the 10 subjects tested, they found almost no difference in transcutaneous versus percutaneous bone conduction thresholds in the low frequencies. However, they discovered a mean threshold improvement with the direct bone conduction of between 10 and 20 dB in the mid to high frequencies. Håkansson et al. (1985) found an even more dramatic improvement in thresholds by direct bone conduction when measuring the acceleration level at threshold. This time the differences were large at all frequencies especially at 1000, 1500, and 2000 Hz, where the threshold improvements on the seven subjects averaged 27, 25.5, and 27.5 dB, respectively. Stenfelt and Håkansson (1999) measured the voltage to the transducer for trans- and percutaneous thresholds and then converted these voltages to force as a reference quantity on 9 subjects. They found that, at 250, 500, and 1500 Hz, the force level required to generate a threshold was actually lower through the skin than when measured directly through the abutment (likely due to a skin resonance). At all other frequencies the direct bone conduction thresholds required a lower force level. However, this time the average differences were only 7 dB or less. The threshold level shifts (±1 SD) for these three studies are graphed in Figure 28–4. Two things should be fairly obvious to the reader: (1) there are considerable differences in thresholds shifts depending on the study and the method used to measure the threshold differences, and (2) the variability in responses at a given frequency appears to be fairly large. In fact, Håkansson et al. (1985) noted that, "The shapes and the absolute values of each threshold curve are highly individual and do not give any universally valid information" (p. 245).

In spite of this conclusion more than 20 years ago, it is often noted in journal articles, at conferences and symposia, in company literature and most likely in the Baha candidacy clinics, that a given user can expect an improvement of somewhere between 10 and 20 dB with the Baha compared to traditional bone conduction through the skin and subcutaneous tissue. It is not that this is necessarily an incorrect statement; however, given the differences between studies and the

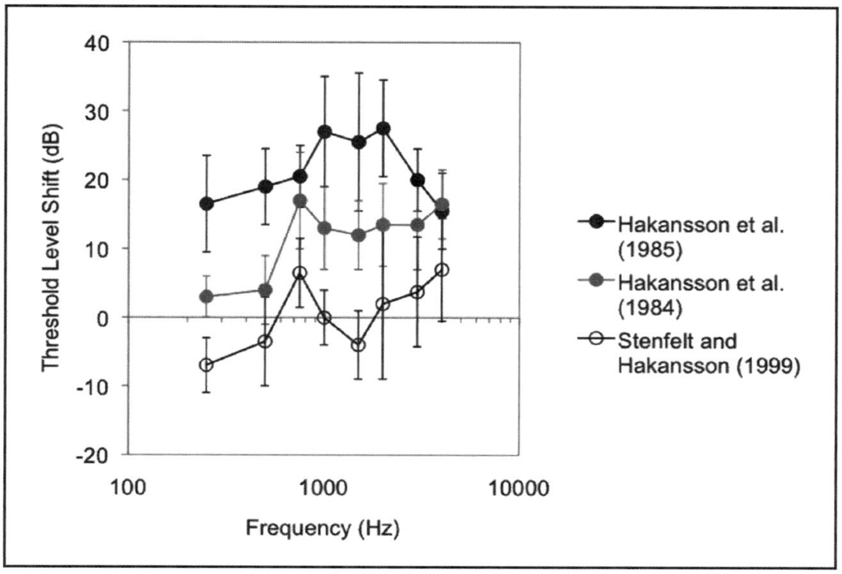

FIGURE 28–4. Difference in threshold level shifts measured three ways in three different studies (error bars = ±1 SD).

variability in subject responses, this conclusion may be somewhat misleading for a given individual.

To make matters worse, the differences in transcutaneous and percutaneous thresholds from subject to subject appear to be unrelated to what would seem to be an obvious variable. Mylanus et al. (1994) found no correlation between the thickness of the skin and subcutaneous tissue and the pure tone average (PTA) threshold shift. An individual was just as likely to display a threshold shift of 10 dB with only 2 mm of skin and tissue as was an individual with 9 mm of skin and tissue. Conversely, they found an individual with only 2 mm of thickness had a PTA threshold shift of 16 dB, whereas someone else had 13 mm of thickness but a PTA threshold shift of only 3 dB (Figure 28–5).

What do these results mean to the Baha clinician? The reality is, from an assessment perspective, Baha clinicians are always dealing with a degree of uncertainty with respect to how a patient will ultimately hear by direct bone conduction compared to their transcutaneous hearing. Until the patient has a Baha abutment, the clinician will not know how much better their patient is able to hear by direct bone conduction. It is often wise to recommend a trial with a Baha on a headband to any individual who may be a borderline candidate based on their transcutaneous bone conduction thresholds (see discussion below). I also recommend that, after surgery, the subject should be tested again through the Baha abutment to determine their actual thresholds of importance for the Baha fitting.

Selection/Prescriptive Considerations

Output Targets for Aided Speech

The goal of the selection or prescription stage of the fitting process is to generate output targets of a desired hearing aid for a particular individual. A component of the selection/prescription phase for Baha will always involve choosing an appropriate device (discussed below). However, underpinning that choice are two fundamental considerations: (1) what is that individual's dynamic range of hearing in direct mechanical quantities (such as force level or acceleration level) through the Baha abutment? and (2) what targets will ensure that the majority of important aided speech information will be available to that Baha user's residual auditory area. This is an important point. No matter how complex the actual physiology of bone conduction and no matter how complicated the perception of sound by bone and air conduction may be, defining the individual's dynamic range of hearing by bone conduction in direct mechanical quantities facilitates prescription by producing a residual area into which aided speech can be mapped. In our lab we have used a modified version of the Desired Sensation Level (DSL[i/o]) prescriptive algorithm (Cornelisse et al., 1995; Scollie et al., 2005) to "map" targets for amplified

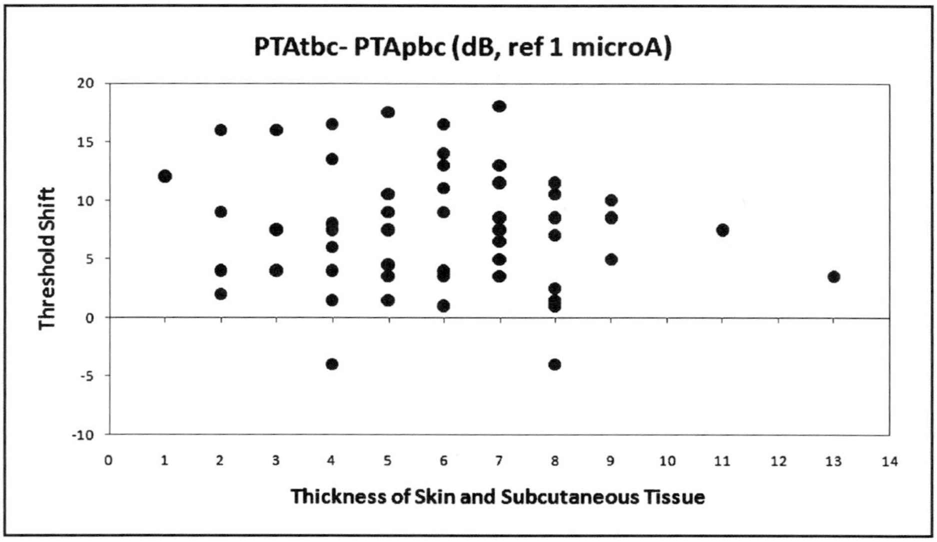

FIGURE 28–5. Pure tone average threshold shift between trans- and percutaneous thresholds as a function of skin thickness in mm.

speech within the dynamic range of a given user (Hodgetts, Hagler, Håkansson, & Soli, in press). We have used both force level targets and acceleration level targets Figure 28–6 shows sample targets for a hypothetical individual using acceleration as the direct mechanical quantity. These targets serve as a guide for subsequent verification of hearing aid output on an individual basis.

Although most clinics do not yet have the facilities or capacity to accomplish this type of advanced selection and prescription, there are signs that this type of approach will be available in the not too distant future. The new Baha BP-100 has the capacity to measure force level thresholds in situ through the Baha abutment. Once the force level thresholds are known, it will be critical to select a Baha that has the capacity to generate sufficient force levels to ensure audibility of speech for each user.

Current Baha Devices

At the time of writing, there are two manufacturers of Baha devices: Cochlear Corporation and Oticon Medical. Cochlear manufacturers 4 models of Baha: The BP-100, Divino, Intenso, and Cordelle II. Oticon Medical has released the Ponto that can be configured to be a more basic device or a more advanced device depending on the chosen configuration. All devices contain DSP chips with the exception of the Cordelle II. The BP-100, Ponto and Divino all have directional microphones. The Intenso and Cordelle have only omnidirectional microphones. The Intenso and Divino are linear devices with output compression. The BP-100, Ponto and Cordelle II can all be set to linear or wide dynamic range compression (WDRC); Cordelle II has a K-amp inside). The BP-100 and Ponto have advanced multichannel compression, multiple program options and are software programmable. The Intenso, Divino, and Cordelle II are all controlled with potentiometers (Figure 28–7).

Fitting Ranges of Baha Devices

Manufacturer recommendations for the BP-100, Divino and Ponto are displayed in Figure 28–8. Individuals with dB HL bone conduction thresholds up to approximately 35 dB HL are good candidates for any of these three Bahas. Between 35 and 45 dB HL the patient may still do well with one of these three devices. However, given the inherent variability in patients mentioned above, those with thresholds in the 35 to 45 dB HL range may be better suited to the Intenso. The Intenso has a fitting range up to 45 dB HL (and possibly as high as 55 dB HL). The Cordelle II is better suited for individuals with bone conduction thresholds between 50 and 65 dB HL.

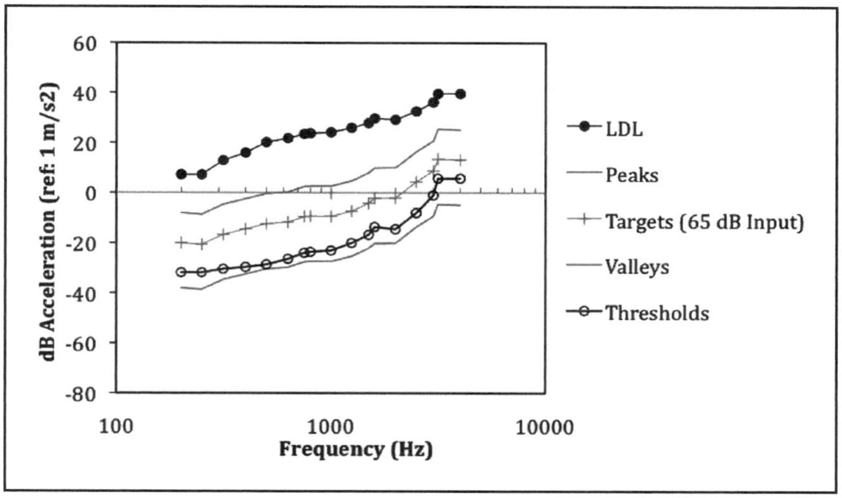

FIGURE 28–6. Residual auditory area measured in direct mechanical quantities through the Baha abutment. The plus signs indicate prescriptive targets for aided speech with a Baha.

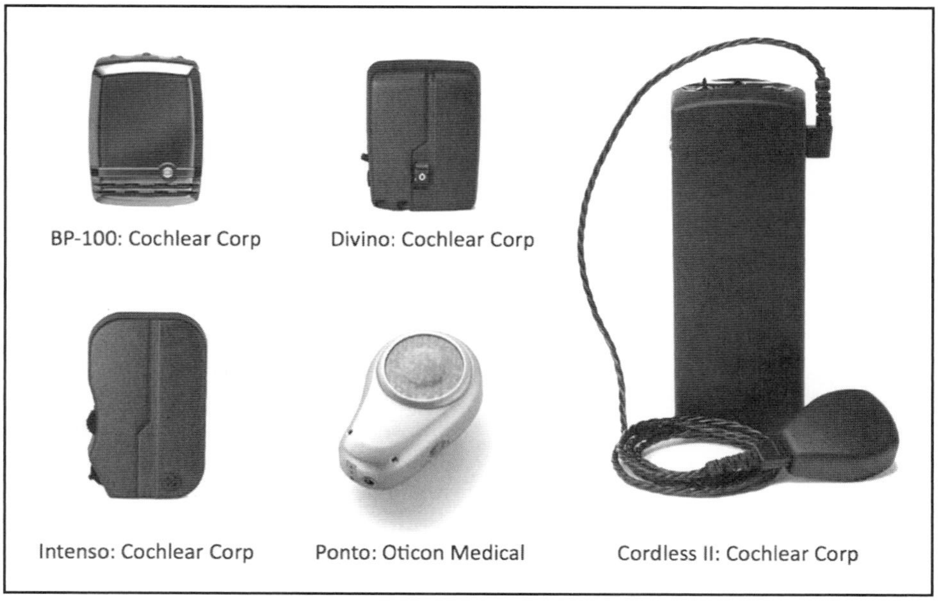

FIGURE 28–7. Baha processors available at the time of writing. Reprinted with permission © Cochlear Bone-Anchored Solutions 2009. All rights reserved.

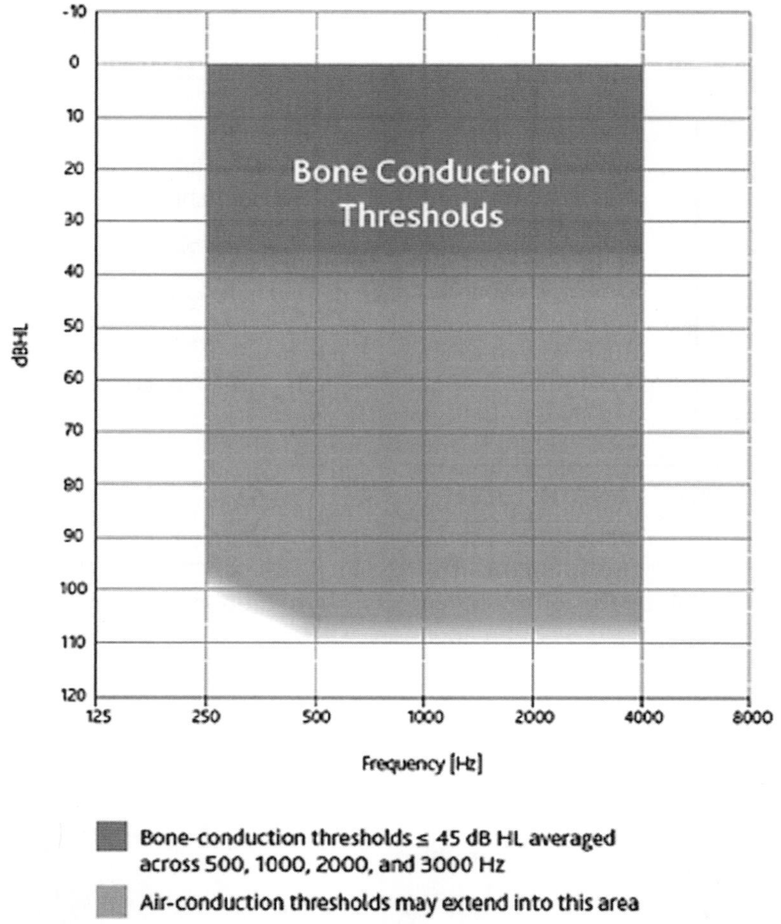

FIGURE 28–8. Fitting range of Baha Divino, BP-100, and Ponto. Reprinted with permission © Cochlear Bone-Anchored Solutions 2009. All rights reserved.

Verification Considerations

Limitations of Current Baha Verification Approaches

During the verification stage, the actual hearing aid output characteristics are compared to the prescribed characteristics determined during the selection or prescription stage. For the verification of Baha, traditional approaches have used functional gain via aided sound field threshold measures to verify the in situ performance of the device. Functional gain is defined as the difference in dB between unaided thresholds obtained in the sound field (dB HL) and aided thresholds obtained in the sound field with the Baha connected (dB HL). The rationale for calculating functional gain reflects the idea that, so long as the Baha is functioning within the linear range, the gain estimate achieved at threshold will reflect the gain of the device for higher level inputs (e.g., conversational speech). This is not necessarily a valid assumption. First, the functional gain will always overestimate the gain by the size of the air-bone gap (difference between air conduction and bone conduction thresholds). Second, gain estimated from threshold calculations will be incorrect because of nonlinearity often associated with higher-level inputs. The limited maximum power output (MPO) of some current Bahas results in output compression even in response to conversational level inputs of 65 to 70 dB SPL.

Aided sound field thresholds have other significant limitations as a verification tool. For example, there are noise floor effects (mostly due to microphone noise), test-retest reliability issues and confusion about the definition of the speech spectrum in dB HL. Also, they only inform the clinician about the hearing aid response to low level inputs (a challenge for WDRC aids) and provide no information regarding the MPO of the device (see Seewald et al., 1996 and Hawkins, 2004 for excellent reviews of these issues). Real-ear measures have supplanted the aided sound field threshold approach for verifying the majority of air conduction hearing aid fittings. Similar approaches for verifying Baha are beginning to emerge.

Alternative Baha Verification Approaches

One such in situ approach proposed by Hodgetts, Håkansson, Hagler, and Soli (2010) used accelerometers placed on the backside of a special transducer known as the Balanced Electromagnetic Separation Transducer (BEST; Håkansson, 2003). The BEST transducer is rigid through its entire vibrating core. So vibrations delivered to the patients are reflected in the acceleration response on the transducer. Instead of ear canal SPL measured by a probe microphone (as in the case of air conduction hearing aids), acceleration (in dB) was used as a reference for direct bone conduction dynamic range of hearing and aided Baha responses. Figure 28–9 shows the average acceleration responses (Accelogram) for the 23 Baha subjects used in this study. This approach facilitates a direct comparison of all measures in the same units at a common reference point.

The audibility of aided speech using this approach was compared to the audibility of aided speech using the aided sound field approach (Hodgetts et al., 2010; Figure 28–10). At all frequencies, the aided sound field approach overestimated the audibility of aided speech in comparison to the in situ accelerometer approach. As both approaches were supposed to estimate the same thing, and the same hearing aid was used on the same patient, equivalent results would have indicated that no one approach is necessarily better than the next. However, significant differences were found between approaches, illustrating how different procedures can provide different answers to the same clinical question (Seewald, Hudson, Gagné, & Zelisko, 1992).

Although acceleration is the most direct method of measuring the vibratory response on a given patient, there are limitations for this approach in terms of clinical uptake. As the current models of Baha do not use the BEST transducer, it is not possible at this time to use this approach with patients. We currently are validating

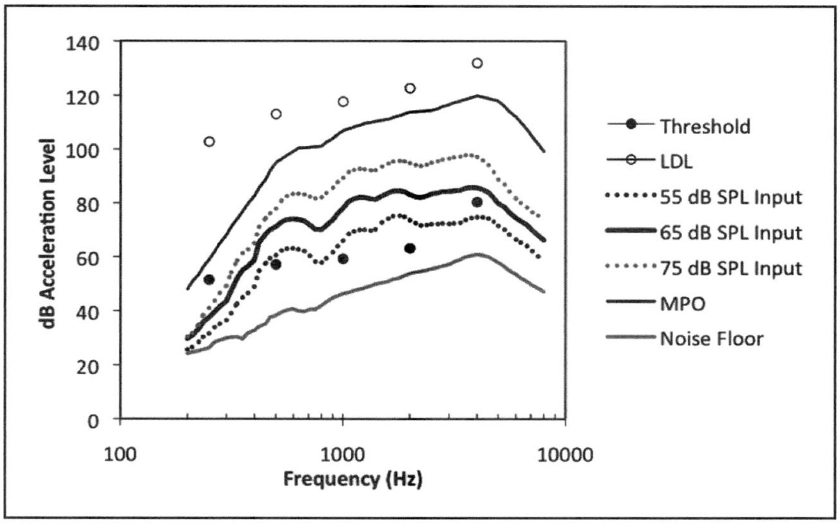

FIGURE 28–9. In situ acceleration responses (Accelogram) showing all hearing information and aided Baha output in acceleration level at the Baha abutment.

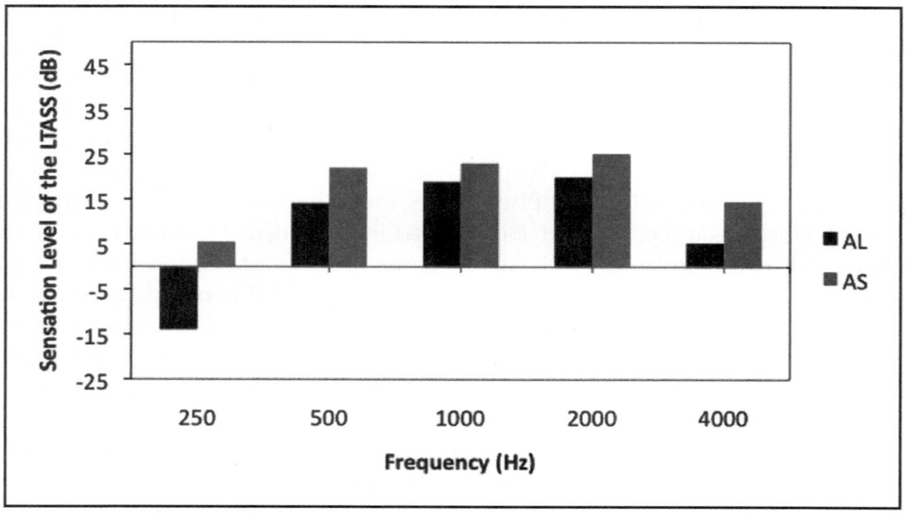

FIGURE 28–10. Sensation level estimates derived using two different verification approaches for Baha in response to 65 dB SPL speech input. With the exception of 250 Hz, the Aided Soundfield (AS) approach routinely overestimated the sensation level of speech compared to the accelerometer approach (AL).

an alternative approach that uses "Force" (in dB) referenced to a skull simulator (Håkansson & Carlsson, 1989) that could be used with current real ear systems to measure Baha. If this approach proves valid (and early indications are promising), then it may be as easy for clinicians to measure Baha as it is for them to measure air conduction hearing aids in a 2-cc coupler.

Final Thoughts on Baha Fitting Procedures

Thresholds from a standard bone conduction oscillator are not an ideal reference for the direct bone conduction hearing used with the Baha system, and aided sound field thresholds do little to inform the clinician about the appropriateness of the fitting. All assessment information should be obtained in direct mechanical quantities (force or acceleration level) through the Baha abutment. For the prescription of aided output, a necessary starting point would be to prescribe targets that ensure that the majority of aided speech falls within the individual's residual auditory area. All Bahas should be verified using some sort of in situ approach (either accelerometers or skull simulator) to ensure that aided speech is at least audible (if not meeting some sort of prescriptive target). Although some of the work summarized in the previous sections may not quite be ready for direct clinical uptake, audiologists seeking alternatives to the current Baha fitting and verification approaches should be optimistic that researchers (and the manufacturers of Baha) are not far from making clinically deliverable alternatives a reality.

Conclusions

The Baha has become the standard of care for individuals with sufficient residual cochlear function, but who cannot wear air conduction hearing aids. Outcomes are better with the Baha compared to traditional bone conduction amplification and comparable outcomes are obtained in comparison to air conduction hearing aids. However, in cases of chronic otitis media, the Baha keeps the ear canal open and allows for a safer, drier ear. Bilateral Baha offers bilateral hearing to individuals with symmetric cochlear loss.

In spite of the large number of promising outcome studies that show the effectiveness of the Baha, it is this author's opinion that even greater outcomes are possible with more careful attention paid to the entire fitting process including assessment, prescription, and verification of Baha. These additional measures may still be in the formative stages and may seem complicated for what is often a simple device. However, the field of Baha is entering a phase comparable to the gradual uptake of probe microphone measures in the 1990s that has led to better fittings for air conduction hearing aids. If a better outcome is available to Baha patients by applying more accurate and reliable fitting approaches, we owe it to them to provide it.

References

Albrektsson, T., & Wennerberg, A. (2005). The impact of oral implants—Past and future, 1966–2042. *Journal of the Canadian Dental Association, 71*(5), 327.

American Academy of Audiology (AAA). (2003). *Pediatric amplification protocol, draft.* Reston, VA: Author. Retrieved August 2009, from http://www.audiology.org

American Speech and Hearing Association. (ASHA). (1998). Guidelines for hearing aid fitting for adults: ASHA ad hoc committee on hearing aid selection and fitting. *American Journal of Audiology, 7*(1), 5–13.

Bosman, A. J., Snik, A. F. M. van der Pouw, C. T. M., Mylanus, E. A. M., & Cremers, C. W. R. J. (2001). Audiometric evaluation of bilaterally-fitted bone anchored hearing aids. *Audiology, 40*, 158–167.

Cornelisse, L. E., Seewald, R. C., & Jamieson, D. G. (1995). The input/output formula: A theoretical approach to the fitting of personal amplification devices. *Journal of the Acoustical Society of America, 97*(3), 1854–1864.

Cremers, C. W. R. J., Snik, A. F. M., & Beyon, A. J. (1992). Hearing with the bone-anchored hearing aid compared to a conventional bone conduction hearing aid. *Clinical Otolaryngology, 17*, 275–279.

deWolf, M. J. F., Hol, M. K. S., Huygen, P. L. M., Mylanus, E. A. M., & Cremers, C. W. R. J. (2008). Clinical outcome of the simplified surgical technique for Baha implantation. *Otology and Neurotology, 29*(8), 1100–1108.

Dumper, J. D., Hodgetts, W. E., Liu, R., & Brandner, N. (2009). Indications for BAHA®: A functional outcomes study. *Journal of Otolaryngology-Head and Neck Surgery, 38*(1), 96–105.

Dutt, S. N., McDermott, A. L. Burrell, S. P. Cooper, H. R., Reid, A. P., & Proops, D. W. (2002). Speech intelligibility with bilateral bone anchored hearing aids. *Journal of Laryngology and Otology Suppl., 28*, 47–51.

Granstrom, G., Bergstrom, K., Odersjo, M., & Tjellstrom, A. (2001). Osseointegrated implants in children: Experience from our first 100 patients. *Otolaryngology-Head and Neck Surgery, 125*, 85–92.

Håkansson, B., & Carlsson, P. (1989). Skull simulator for direct bone conduction hearing devices. *Scandinavian Audiology, 18*(2), 91–98.

Håkansson, B., Liden, G., Tjellstrom, A., Ringdahl, A., Jacobsson, M., Carlsson, P., & Erlandson, B. E. (1990). Ten years of experience with the Swedish bone-anchored hearing system. *Annals of Otology, Rhinology, and Laryngology Suppl., 151*, 1–16.

Håkansson, B., Tjellstrom, A., & Rosenhall, U. (1984). Hearing thresholds with direct bone conduction versus conventional bone conduction. *Scandinavian Audiology, 13*(1), 3–13.

Håkansson, B., Tjellstrom, A., & Rosenhall, U. (1985). Acceleration levels at hearing threshold with direct bone conduction versus conventional bone conduction. *Acta Oto-Laryngologica, 100*(3–4), 240–252.

Håkansson, B. E. V. (2003). The balanced electromagnetic separation transducer a new bone conduction transducer. *Journal of the Acoustical Society of America, 113*(2), 818–825.

Hawkins, D. B. (2004). Limitations and uses of the aided audiogram. *Seminars in Hearing, 25*(1), 51–62.

Hodgetts, W. E., Hagler, P., Håkansson, B. E. V., & Soli, S. (In press). Technology-limited and patient-derived versus audibility-derived fittings in Baha users: An efficacy study. *Ear and Hearing*.

Hodgetts, W. E., Håkansson, B. E. V., Hagler, P., & Soli, S. (2010). A comparison of three approaches to verifying aided Baha output. *International Journal of Audiology, 49*(4), 286–295.

Hodgetts, W. E., Scollie, S. D., & Swain, R. (2006). The BAHA® Softband: Effects of the applied contact force and volume control setting on output force level. *International Journal of Audiology, 45*, 301–308.

Hol, M. K. S., Cremers, C. W. R. J., Coppen-Schellekens, W., & Snik, A. F. M., (2005). The BAHA Softband: A new treatment for young children with bilateral congenital aural atrisia. *International Journal of Pediatric Otolaryngology, 69*, 973–980.

Macnamara, M., Phillips, D., & Proops, D. W. (1996). The bone-anchored hearing aid (BAHA) in chronic suppurative otitis media (CSOM). *Journal of Laryngology and Otology Suppl., 21*, 38–40.

McDermott, A. L., Dutt, S. N., Reid, A. P., & Proops, D. W. (2002). An intra-individual comparison of the previous conventional hearing aid with the bone anchored hearing aid: The Nijmegen Group questionnaire. *Journal of Laryngology and Otolaryngology, Suppl., 28*, 15–19.

Mylanus, E. A., Snik, A. F., & Cremers, C. W. (1994). Influence of the thickness of the skin and subcutaneous tissue covering the mastoid on bone-conduction thresholds obtained transcutaneously versus percutaneously. *Scandinavian Audiology, 23*(3), 201–203.

Mylanus, E. A., van der Pouw, K. C., Snik, A. F., & Cremers, C. W. (1998). Intraindividual comparison of the bone-anchored hearing aid and air-conduction hearing aids. *Archives of Otolaryngology-Head and Neck Surgery, 124*(3), 271.

Northern, J. L., & Downs, M. P. (1991). *Hearing in children*. Baltimore, MD: William and Wilkins.

Papp, Z., Rezes, S. Jokay, I., & Sziklai, I. (2003) Sensorineural hearing loss in chronic otitis media. *Otology and Neurotology, 24*, 141–144.

Pediatric Working Group. (1996). Amplification for infants and children with hearing loss. *American Journal of Audiology, 5*(1), 53–68.

Powell, R. H., Burrell, S. P., Cooper, H. R., & Proops, D. W. (1996). The Birmingham bone anchored hearing program:

Pediatric experience and results. *Journal of Laryngology and Otology Suppl.*, *21*, 21–29.

Priwin, C., Stenfelt, S., Granstrom, G., Tjellstrom, A., & Håkansson, B. (2004). Bilateral bone anchored hearing aids: An audiometric evaluation. *Laryngoscope*, *114*, 77–84.

Reinfeldt, S. (2009). *Bone conduction hearing in human communication: Sensitivity, transmission and application*. Doctoral dissertation, Chalmers University of Technology at Goteborg, Sweden.

Scollie, S. D., Seewald, R. C., Conelisse, L., Moodie, S., Bagatto, M, Laurnagaray, D. & Pumford, J. (2005). The desired sensation level multistage input/output algorithm. *Trends in Amplification*, *9*(4), 159–197.

Seewald, R. C., Hudson, S. P., Gagné, J. P., & Zelisko, D. L. (1992). Comparison of two methods for estimating the sensation level of amplified speech. *Ear and Hearing*, *13*(3), 142.

Seewald, R. C., Moodie, K. S., Sinclair, S. T., & Cornelisse, L. E. (1996). Traditional and theoretical approaches to selecting amplification for infants and young children. In F. H. Bess, J. S. Gravel, & A. M. Tharpe (Eds.), *Amplification for children with auditory deficits* (pp. 161–191). Nashville, TN: Bill Wilkerson Press.

Snik, A. F. M., Bosman, A. J., Mylanus, E. A. M., & Cremers, C. W. R. J. (2004). Candidacy for the bone anchored hearing aid. *Audiology and Neurotology*, *9*, 190–196.

Snik, A. F. M., Leijendeckers, J., Hol, M., Mylanus, E. A. M., & Cremers, C. W. R. J. (2008). The bone-anchored hearing aid for children: Recent developments. *International Journal of Audiology*, *47*, 554–559.

Snik, A. F. M., Mylanus, E. A. M., Proops, D. W., Wolfaardt, J. F., Hodgetts, W. E., Somers, T., . . . Tjellstrom, A. (2005). Consensus statements on the BAHA system: Where do we stand at present? *Annals of Otology, Rhinology and Laryngology, Suppl.*, *195*, 1–12.

Stenfelt, S. P., & Håkansson, B. E. (1999). Sensitivity to bone-conducted sound: Excitation of the mastoid vs the teeth. *Scandinavian Audiology*, *28*(3), 190–198.

Tietze, L., & Papsin, B. (2001). Utilization of bone anchored hearing aids in children. *International Journal of Pediatric Otolaryngology*, *58*, 75–80.

Tjellström, A., & Håkansson, B. (1995). The bone-anchored hearing aid: Design principles, indications, and long-term clinical results. *Otolaryngologic Clinics of North America*, *28*(1), 53–72.

Tjellstrom, A., Håkansson, B., & Granstrom, G. (2001). Bone-anchored hearing aids: Current status in adults and children. *Otolaryngologic Clinics of North America*, *34*, 337–364.

van der Pouw, C. T. M., Mylanus, E. A. M., & Cremers, C. W. R. J. (1999). Percutaneous implants in the temporal bone for securing a bone conductor: Surgical methods and results. *Annals of Otology, Rhinology and Laryngology*, *108*, 532–536.

van der Pouw C. T. M., Snik, A. F. M., & Cremers, C. W. R. J. (1999). The BAHA HC200/300 in comparison with conventional bone conduction hearing aids. *Clinical Otolaryngology in the Allied Sciences*, *24*, 171–176.

Verhagen, C. V. M., Hol, M. K. S., Coppens-Schellekens, W., Snik, A. F. M., & Cremers, C. W. R. J. (2008). The Baha Softband. A new treatment for young children with bilateral congenital aural atresia. *International Journal of Pediatric Otorhinolaryngology*, *72*(10), 1455–1459.

29

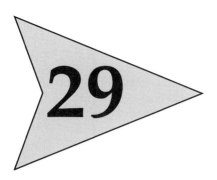

Hearing Instrument Orientation for Children and Their Families

Anne Marie Tharpe and Hollea M. Ryan

Introduction

As established in previous chapters, the purpose of early identification of hearing loss in infants and children is the implementation of early intervention. And, the foundation of early intervention for children with hearing loss is the accurate and timely fitting of amplification. However, the fitting of amplification is only the first step. If families do not understand the importance of hearing aids or are not confident placing the devices on their children, our best efforts will be thwarted. Only when families are comfortable with and understand the importance of hearing aids will they be carefully cared for and worn consistently. Therefore, effective hearing aid orientation is fundamental to the long-term goals of consistent hearing aid use and care, and the development of auditory and speech-language skills. This chapter describes the family support and education needed from audiologists throughout the hearing aid orientation process. Hearing aid orientation is referred to as a process because it does not occur only at the time when the child is first fitted with hearing aids. Rather, audiologists continue to educate families and children about hearing technology after the first fitting as technology options change and as the child's hearing needs change over time. This education extends to the child's other caregivers via interactions with daycare workers, educational audiologists, teachers, and other qualified interventionists. Furthermore, although in many instances adults are the intended targets of the orientation information, as a child gets older and is able to participate in the care of and decisions about hearing technology, children also become direct recipients of this information.

Family Counseling and Education

A number of variables contribute to a family's ability to cope with the challenges of raising a child who has hearing loss. One of these variables is the level of support and education provided to the family by their audiologist throughout the various stages of intervention and management. The hearing aid orientation provides an opportunity for families to gain knowledge and thus, confidence about the technology that can contribute to significant changes in their child's life. In other words, this knowledge can reinforce a family's confidence that they are making effective contributions toward their child's success.

Family Education

Following initial diagnosis of hearing loss in children, it is typical for there to be a two- to three-week delay in the fitting of hearing aids after earmold impressions are made. This period of time can be an anxious one for families who want to start helping their newly diagnosed child. During this time parents can either begin to grow in the knowledge that they are competent parents for their child with hearing loss or can begin to doubt themselves and their ability to parent their child effectively. This can be a key time for audiologists to contribute to parental confidence-building. In 2002, Robbins published a list of things that parents can do in the weeks and months following the diagnosis of hearing loss in their child; things that are likely to build confidence in parents by keeping them actively involved in their child's development. This information can be shared with parents at the time earmold impressions are made. Specifically, Robbins divided the time period after diagnosis into three phases with recommendations of actions parents can take in each phase. These phases and recommendations are outlined in Table 29–1.

Active participation in such activities prevents parents from spending time waiting for "professionals" to tell them what to do. Parents can proceed with the act of parenting, thus gaining confidence in their own abilities and reducing family stress.

It is also during these early stages of hearing aid fitting that it is important to explain to family members how influential their attitudes are to their child's ultimate acceptance of hearing aids. If parents are obviously stressed during the process of making earmold impressions or during the hearing aid fitting, their child might interpret those signs as a reflection of their parents' attitudes about the hearing aids themselves. Recall that young children with hearing loss are likely to have language delays at the time of the hearing aid fitting and will be interpreting facial expressions as one way of communicating with their parents. Therefore, one responsibility of audiologists during this time is to maintain a calm, pleasant attitude and atmosphere: inform families beforehand that most children are reluctant to readily embrace wearing hearing aids for the first time, but assure them that they will be instructed on how to maximize their child's acceptance and hearing aid wearing time. Audiologists can remind parents to maintain pleasant facial expressions and demeanor while attempting to insert their child's earmolds and position the hearing aids.

Households today can be quite diverse with some consisting of a single parent and child, and others having multiple generations living under one roof. Audiologists can increase the likelihood that the information relayed during hearing aid orientation is heard and understood by inviting all of those directly involved in a child's care to participate—what one family member does not hear or remember, another might. The information conveyed can also be reinforced by the provision of written materials, including manufacturer's user guides. However, one must consider the clarity, complexity, organization, appearance, and cultural appropriateness of educational materials provided to families. Using tools such as the Flesch Reading Ease Formula (FRE), one can ensure that educational materials are

TABLE 29–1. Recommendations for Family Involvement Immediately Following Diagnosis

Phase I—From time of diagnosis to hearing aid fitting
∞ Continue to talk to your child—Play gesture games, sing songs, be animated
∞ Begin a journal of your experiences
∞ Contact the John Tracy Clinic—they provide correspondence courses for families in more than 20 languages
Phase II—Early weeks just following the hearing aid fitting
∞ Keep a weekly hearing aid calendar
∞ Refer to your child by name—always have a purpose for calling your child
∞ Use a hand-to-ear response when a sound is heard
∞ Tell your interventionists of changes in vocalizations as well as auditory responses
Phase III—After the initial adjustment to hearing aids until formal intervention
∞ Imitate your child's vocalizations, using intonation, patterns and sound
∞ Encourage an anticipatory response to sound—make clear to your child that you expect a response and wait for that response
∞ Select three common sounds in your home for your child to learn

Reprinted from Robbins, A. M. (2002). Empowering parents to help their newly diagnosed child gain communication skills. *Hearing Journal*, *55*(11), 55–59, with permission of *The Hearing Journal* and Lippincott Williams & Wilkins.

written at a reading level appropriate for that of the average adult in the United States (eighth grade level).

One of the first skills that parents must learn is the insertion and removal of the earmold and hearing aid from their child's ear. Parents should practice while with the audiologist and should demonstrate the ability to insert/remove the hearing aid and earmold for each ear before leaving the clinic with the hearing aids for the first time. Helpful insertion tips, such as using a thin layer of water-based lubricant on the canal portion of the earmold, can be useful for parents. Parents, and children if they are old enough, should be discouraged from removing the earmold by the tubing. Overtime, this practice can result in the tubing being pulled loose from the mold or in tears in the tubing. Either of these problems can result in feedback. Furthermore, if the earmold is not placed correctly, irritation and sores could develop in the child's ear. If possible, provide the parents with a photo, perhaps with the parent's camera phone, of how the earmold should look when properly inserted.

In addition to the expected benefits to a child upon receiving hearing aids, limitations of hearing aid use must be explained to families. Such discussions assist in setting appropriate and reasonable expectations, thus, reducing disappointment in families. Potential limitations, even temporary, that might warrant discussion include:

- Background noise—although current hearing aids have circuits, microphones and other features that can reduce the impact of background noise, it cannot be totally eliminated. The amount of difficulty one has listening in the presence of background noise is dependent on many factors including the degree and configuration of the loss, specific hearing aid features, and child-specific features such as age and language ability.
- Acoustic feedback—there are numerous reasons for feedback from hearing aids, especially in infants and young children whose pinnae and external auditory canals continue to grow until approximately 9 years of age. This problem can be addressed by feedback reduction technology, changes in hearing aid settings, new earmolds, or behavioral changes initiated by parents and children. However, parents can expect to experience the irritation of acoustic feedback on at least a temporary or occasional basis.
- Alternative strategies—despite the significant benefits that hearing aids can provide, additional strategies will likely be needed. These include: (1) facing the child when speaking so facial expressions and gestures can be seen for speech reading purposes; (2) whenever possible, finding a quiet place to communicate away from background noise like televisions, and high-traffic areas in restaurants; (3) when background noise is problematic, considering alternative technologies like FM systems for use in classrooms or for recreational activities; and (4) depending on the degree of hearing loss, considering assistive devices such as amplified or lighted alerting devices (e.g., door bells, fire alarms, and alarm clocks). See Chapter 26 for additional information about FM technologies.

Child Education

As children get older, it becomes necessary and appropriate to include them in the hearing aid orientation process. This might start with something as simple as letting them select the color of their earmolds or hearing aids. Later, as they become more dependable, they can be taught care tasks such as removing and inserting their own earmolds/hearing aids, changing hearing aid batteries, cleaning earmolds, and putting their hearing aids in drying kits.

A curriculum aimed at empowering school-age children by learning more about their hearing loss and hearing technology is the Knowledge is Power Curriculum (KIP; Mississippi Bend Area Educational Agency). KIP focuses on moving children along a continuum of knowledge from understanding the basics of anatomy and physiology of the ear to self-reliance and personal responsibility. Specifically, the following areas are reviewed in the KIP curriculum:

- Anatomy and physiology of the ear
- Causes of hearing loss
- Hearing measurement
- Hearing technology
- Coping with hearing loss
- Rational emotive education
- Stories
- Legislation
- Transition
- Resources

KIP can be used with any school-age student with hearing loss if content and presentation adjustments are made to match the student's ability and language development. Worksheets and other handouts can be used to carry over information to parents and other family members.

The Physical Fit

Earmolds

As with adults, the earmold serves as a means to direct sound emitting from a behind-the-ear (BTE) or body-worn hearing aid down the ear canal towards the tympanic membrane. Well-selected and well-fitted earmolds also accomplish several other important objectives. First, a good earmold minimizes feedback by providing an acoustic seal. This seal primarily occurs at the first bend of the ear canal necessitating an earmold impression that extends beyond that point. Second, a good earmold helps to retain the hearing aid behind the ear. Third, a well-fitted earmold should be comfortably worn by the child for the duration of the day. Finally, earmold filters can be used to alter the acoustics of the amplified signal. Procedures that can be applied to account for the effects of earmold features on the acoustics of the amplified signal are discussed in detail in Chapter 25.

Earmold Material

Many considerations should be taken into account when selecting an earmold for infants or children. One of the first considerations is proper material for the earmold. Traditionally, a soft material is selected, both for a comfortable fit as well as for safety concerns. Soft materials, such as a polyvinyl or silicone, typically provide a comfortable fit and a strong acoustic seal, are often hypoallergenic (if not colored), and are useful when fitting high-powered hearing aids, as the material can help minimize feedback. For infants, a hypoallergenic material should be selected to minimize the risks of an allergic reaction, typically seen as redness in the concha and/or ear canal. Despite these positive reasons for using a soft material, there are some negative considerations including:

- Difficulty modifying—It can be difficult to buff down and smooth off areas of a soft earmold that are creating pressure points or a poor fit, thus, requiring the entire earmold to be remade.
- Difficulty getting glue to adhere—Cement used for adhering the tubing is traditionally not effective on soft material, resulting in the tubing being easily disconnected from the earmold. Retention rings, or tube locks, on the tubing can be used and help secure the tubing into the earmold. However, brass retention rings can reduce the high frequency signals being emitted by the hearing aid (Ingrao, 1999). A compromise might be achieved by consulting the earmold laboratory and finding a balance between softness and ability to secure the tubing.
- Earmold color—Often, the type of material used will dictate what color options are available. Many parents initially select flesh-colored or clear earmolds to minimize the appearance of the molds. Children should be given the opportunity to select earmold colors once they are capable of making that decision. Allowing the child to select from colored, multicolored, swirled, or even glittered earmold options provides the child with ownership of the fitting process.

Earmold Tubing

The length of the tubing is also important during the fitting of the hearing aid. In addition to acoustic effects, the length of tubing affects the placement of the hearing aids behind the ears. Proper placement ensures that the microphones are in the desired planes. In addition, the proper length of the tubing is essential to prevent sores or blisters resulting from too tight a fit of the hearing aid. Conversely, tubing cut too long will result in a loose fit and the hearing aid could end up dangling to the side of the ear rather than fitting snugly and comfortably behind the ear.

Earmold Venting

A final consideration during the selection of the earmold is venting. Venting is provided to patients for pressure equalization between the ear canal and the environment and as a means of affecting low frequency response. For infants, or children with very small ear canals, it might be impossible for any size vent to be added. When possible without introducing feedback, a small pressure vent can be appropriate even for severe losses. For those with milder losses, a medium or small vent can be appropriate.

Care and Maintenance

Care and maintenance of the hearing aid and earmold should be reviewed with parents at the time of dispensing, and as often as needed thereafter. As the child matures and is capable of keeping the hearing aid and earmold clean, the responsibility should be moved from the parent to the child, with parental supervision as needed. The primary components of the hearing aid should be noted and a demonstration provided on how to clean and protect those features. Caution should be advised when cleaning near the microphone and the receiver. A daily "wipe down" with a soft lint-free cloth is recommended with periodic detailed cleaning as necessary. The difference between the vent and the sound bore of the earmold should be clearly defined. On a regular basis, the earmold should be cleaned in warm soap and water, never alcohol as it can dry out some materials. Parents must be reminded that the earmold should be removed from the hearing aid prior to cleaning with water and allowed to dry thoroughly (usually overnight) prior to being reattached to the hearing aid.

Often, when hearing aids are ordered for a child, a care kit is also provided by the manufacturer. Typically, this kit includes a listening stethoscope, battery tester, blower, a cleaning tool, and some form of desiccant container. If a kit does not come from the hearing aid manufacturer, the dispensing audiologist should encourage the purchase of these items by the parent. Effective use of each item in the kit should be reviewed with the parents and with the child when appropriate. When possible, an extra care kit should be provided to a school-age child's classroom teacher. Parents should review with the teacher key signs that the hearing aid might not be working properly (e.g., child's attention has noticeably changed; child does not respond to name; child asks for things to be repeated; or child pulls at ear or takes hearing aid off).

A listening check via a stethoscope should also be demonstrated at the initial orientation. Parents should be encouraged to listen to all programs (if applicable), and shown how to verify the t-coil function and any assistive listening devices. Parents also should be instructed on how and why to conduct the Ling-Six-Sound Test (Ling 1976, 1989). The Ling-Six-Sound Test is a behavioral listening check to determine the functionality of amplification. The sounds /ah/, /ee/, /oo/, /sh/, /s/, and /m/ are presented and the child indicates the ability to detect them. Obviously, this listening task cannot be completed with infants or very young children.

Hearing aids should be kept in their case or in a drying kit overnight with battery doors left at least partially open. Even if the hearing aids are removed temporarily, they should be kept in either a soft or hard case and out of a small child's, or pet's, reach. To prolong the life of the hearing aid, the use of a storage case is recommended when the device is not worn. The hearing aids should not be kept loose in the bottom of a parent's purse, backpack, diaper bag, or pocket. A brief hearing aid orientation checklist is included in Appendix 29–A.

The importance of routine troubleshooting became apparent during the 1970s when several investigators examined the functionality of hearing aids in schools. Based on visual inspections and listening checks, a 20 to 60% range of inadequate hearing aid function was documented (Bess, 1997; Riedner, 1978; Ross, 1977; Zink, 1972). As a result of these studies, hearing aid monitoring programs in schools were implemented to address these problems. The documented number of hearing aids with problems in classroom settings appeared to decrease (Kemker, McConnell, Logan, & Green, 1979). A more recent study showed that 17% of hearing aids (all behind-the-ear models) in a large metropolitan school system with a stringent monitoring program were defective, affecting roughly 27% of the hearing aid users. Improper earmold tubing (i.e., loose or torn tubing) and dead batteries accounted for the majority of the problems (Smitherman, 2005).

Another topic to review with parents during the initial fitting is extended hearing aid warranties. For the pediatric population, the chances are high that a hearing aid will be damaged or lost at some point. It is not unusual for children's hearing aids to be thrown out car windows, flushed down toilets, dropped into cereal bowls, eaten by family pets, stepped on, and so on. Thus, the family might find it beneficial to purchase a warranty that covers both loss and damage.

Safety Features and Issues

Overamplification

Overamplification has been a long-standing concern among audiologists who work with young children (Berry, 1939; Humes & Bess, 1981; Jerger & Lewis, 1975; Kinney, 1961; Rintelman & Bess, 1988). Although the primary responsibility for avoiding overamplification will occur during the verification stage (see Chapter 25), there is an additional safety feature that can be implemented during hearing aid orientation. A volume control cover is a thin piece of plastic that fits over the volume control wheel. While in place, such a cover keeps the volume control wheel from being accidentally adjusted or moved by a small child playing with the wheel. The cover can be removed for volume adjustment as needed. With current technology, hearing aids can be ordered without a volume control wheel. In some cases, one might want to order a remote control (available with certain brands) allowing for volume changes when desired but with a reduced risk for accidental changes in volume level.

Battery Ingestion

In addition to overamplification, audiologists should demonstrate an appropriate level of concern about battery ingestion. Battery ingestion occurs at an estimated rate of 2,000 to 3,000 per year in the United States (National Capital Poison Center [NCPC], 2006; Martin, 2009). Children under the age of 5 years, and particularly those between one and two years, are particularly prone to swallowing batteries, contributing to 62% of the reported battery ingestion cases per year in the United States (NCPC, 2006). Although "button batteries" are found in many items, such as toys and watches, 49% of ingested batteries are hearing aid batteries and of those swallowed by children, 33% come from their own hearing aids (Dire, 2009; NCPC, 2006).

At one time, hearing aid batteries were made out of mercury. Although most hearing aid batteries are currently made of alkaline, a potentially less hazardous material, it is still important to avoid battery ingestion. Batteries can be dangerous even without leaking chemicals into the human system. Even more alarming is the fact that at least one infant death as a result of battery ingestion has been documented (Bronstein et al., 2007). Thus, for young children, it is important to consider ordering a locking mechanism on the battery door to reduce the likelihood of accidental battery ingestion. Different methods for locking the battery door are offered by different hearing aid manufacturers. It is important for audiologists to review with parents how to lock and unlock the tamper-proof battery door. The National Capital Poison Center within the United States or one's local poison control center should be contacted immediately if one suspects that a child has swallowed a battery.

Proper Placement

Additional consideration needs to be given to ensure that each hearing aid is worn on the intended ear. Although many children diagnosed with bilateral hearing loss will have symmetric loss, this is not always the case. The first time a child is fitted with a hearing aid, it is useful for the parents to have the right and left hearing aids differentiated, usually with stickers or tabs that are affixed to the hearing aids. Traditionally, a blue sticker is placed on the left hearing aid and a red on the right hearing aid. If a sticker or tab is not provided with the hearing aid from the manufacturer, a simple solution is to place a small red dot of fingernail polish, for the right hearing aid, on the side positioned against the head or on the bottom of the battery door. Likewise, it is important to remind parents that if they remove the earmold from the hearing aid for any reason, to do so one at a time until they are able to differentiate the left and right earmolds. This helps to ensure that the correct earmold is connected to its hearing aid.

Retention

Behavioral Retention

One of the most common exclamations by parents on the day that their child first receives a hearing aid is, "How in the world am I going to keep that in?!" This is when audiologists explain to parents that children are taught to wear hearing aids in much the same way as they learn to wear their shoes and their clothes. No new techniques are needed. Families have their own philosophies about following rules and their own forms of discipline. They already should have the skills and instincts to gain compliance from their children. If not, a discussion about behavioral modification techniques or even a referral to parenting classes might be appropriate. In any case, parents will need some assistance on determining wearing schedules.

When a child first receives a hearing aid, it is helpful if it is taken home on a day and at a time when the family can provide close supervision. In other words, one would not want to dispense a hearing aid to a child in the morning only to have the child dropped off at daycare for the rest of the day with those who have not been instructed in the care and retention of the device. The following guidelines might be useful to a family receiving the child's first hearing aid:

- Insert and remove the hearing aid while the child is on a soft surface like a bed or carpeting. If the hearing aid should drop, it is not likely to be damaged.
- For infants and young children, adult caregivers should be the only ones who insert or remove the hearing aid. If the child purposefully or accidentally removes the hearing aid, the caregiver should immediately re-insert it, even if it is about time to remove the aid anyway. Like all other routines in a child's life, if an exception is made, the child is likely to remember it and might be encouraged to "challenge" the routine of caregiver control. This re-insertion is likely to be required over and over again for the first few days after the initial fitting. However, with caregiver patience and consistency, most children will stop removing the hearing aid after two to three days.
- It generally is a good idea to insert the new hearing aids at a time when a child can be distracted and not as likely to investigate the aids. For example, a

parent might insert the hearing aids right before sitting down to a meal, reading a book, or playing a game with the child.

- Unlike getting accustomed to wearing contact lenses, hearing aids do not require a graduated wearing time period. That is, if a child is willing to wear the hearing aids all day right after they are received, that is fine. However, more important than the length of time that the child initially wears the aids is learning to wear the hearing aids without trying to take them off. To accomplish that, for example, parents might determine that their child is willing to wear the aids for about an hour before getting fussy or restless. In that case, the parents might remove the hearing aids after an hour and then re-insert them after a short period of time, extending that time period throughout the course of the first several days after receiving the aids. It should not be necessary to have a child adjust to wearing one hearing aid and then introduce the second hearing aid at a later time. We do not have children wear one shoe for a while and then introduce a second shoe. By the end of one to two weeks, a child should be wearing the hearing aids during all waking hours removing them only rarely, if at all.

Physical Retention and Protection

Even when all behavioral techniques for retention have been implemented, sometimes the physical fit of the hearing aid is difficult to maintain, especially if the child is young and resistant to the aids or if the child is involved in activities that require considerable physical movement (e.g., sports activities). Devices have been created that help secure hearing aids under these conditions. For the smallest patients, sometimes the pinnae are not sturdy enough to support hearing aids. A pediatric-sized earhook will help maintain the hearing aid behind the ear. Additionally, double-sided tape, such as wig or toupee tape, can be used to adhere the hearing aid to the head so that it will not fall off from behind the ear and dangle from the earmold.

Even if a hearing aid stays in place during most typical child activities, at some point parents might face a time when their child is purposely pulling the hearing aids out of their ears. To help prevent the loss of hearing aids, the use of a clip and cord (Figure 29–1A) will help. Essentially, the clip has a small plastic ring that slides onto the hearing aid. This ring is attached to a cord that is connected to a clip and is fastened to the upper back or shoulder area of the child's shirt, out of reach of the child. Thus, if the hearing aids fall or are pulled out, they are still attached to the child. A single clip can be used to secure one hearing aid whereas a "Y" clip will secure two hearing aids.

When children are older, it might become necessary to secure the hearing aid(s) when participating in some sort of physical activity. Specifically, children participating in sports like gymnastics need to have a means of keeping the hearing aid(s) from falling off from behind the ear. A recently introduced retention tool has a plastic seat in which a hearing aid is snapped. Connected to the bottom of this seat is a flexible wire that can be bent around the bottom of the ear (Figure 29–1B) to secure the hearing aid(s) behind the ear. This also is an effective way to minimize movement of the hearing aid(s) during sporting events.

Another security device is a retention ring (Figure 29–1C). The retention ring consists of two small plastic rings that slide around the hearing aid. These thick, small rings are attached to a thinner, larger ring that is wrapped around the ear. The sizes of retention rings vary, accommodating infants to adults.

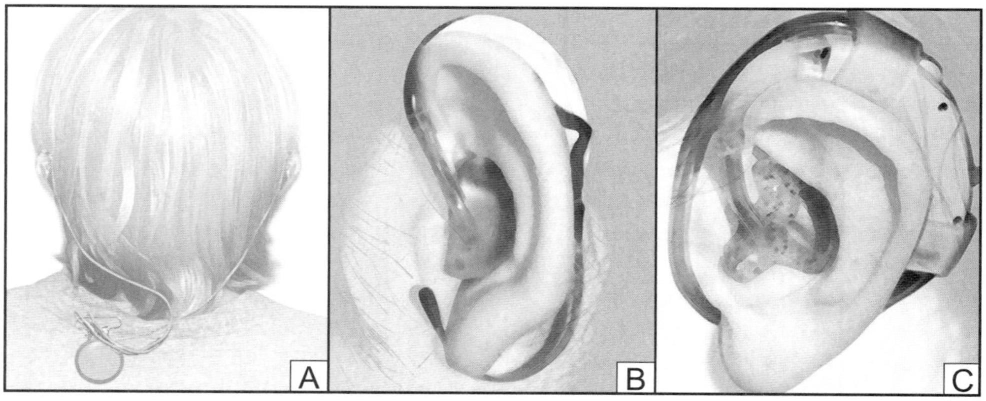

FIGURE 29–1. Hearing aid retention devices including a clip with Y-cord, **(A)**, a wrap-around wire **(B)**, and a retention ring **(C)**.

An additional method to help reduce the likelihood of hearing aids being removed from the ear is to include a helix lock on the earmold. Although the addition of the helix lock makes the earmold slightly more difficult to properly insert, this modification provides a tighter, more secure fit that can make it just slightly more difficult for the infant or toddler to remove.

Finally, for children who need to protect their hearing aids from excessive moisture, such as perspiration generated during sports activities, there are options that completely cover the hearing aid, thus, preventing or minimizing the amount of moisture that can penetrate the hearing aid. These items, which function much like a slip cover for a hearing aid, are typically made of spandex or latex to reflect moisture or acoustically-transparent fabric to absorb or repel moisture from the hearing aid (Figure 29–2 presents illustrative examples of such devices).

Validation

Validation of hearing aid performance involves a demonstration of the benefits and limitations of aided hearing abilities and can begin during orientation. As part of the follow up and monitoring of hearing technologies, audiologists obtain measures of aided performance in clinical settings and functional auditory assessments in real world environments. Functional assessment tools are typically questionnaires designed for administration to parents and other caregivers, such as teachers. The goal of functional assessments is to tell us not only *what* a child hears but, more importantly, how the child *uses* what is heard in everyday situations. In addition, information can be obtained about how listening behavior might change in different settings, under different conditions, or with different speakers. This information can then be used to guide our management plans for infants and children with hearing loss.

Insofar as families are the primary observers of behavior of their infants and young children, part of the orientation process should include teaching families how to observe their child's speech/language and auditory behavior with and without amplification. Such instruction should include warnings about potential visual cues that might be perceived by children that can result in a misinterpretation of what a child can actually hear. Functional assessments, many of which rely on these observations, are available for infants and children of all ages and with all degrees of hearing loss. Appendix 29–B lists commonly used functional assessment tools for children with varying degrees of hearing loss.

Follow-Up and Monitoring

It is reasonable to expect that families will not remember all of the information provided to them on the day that hearing aids are dispensed. Furthermore, it is likely, and desirable, that an audiologist will not explain everything that families ultimately need to know about hearing aids at the first visit. Audiologists will provide the type and amount of information needed based on their interactions with the parents at the time. Therefore, it is important to review information already provided and add new information as needed on subsequent follow-up visits with families. As recommended by the American Academy of Audiology (2003), follow-up visits should occur quarterly (i.e., every three months) for the first 2 years of life. After 2 years of age, appoint-

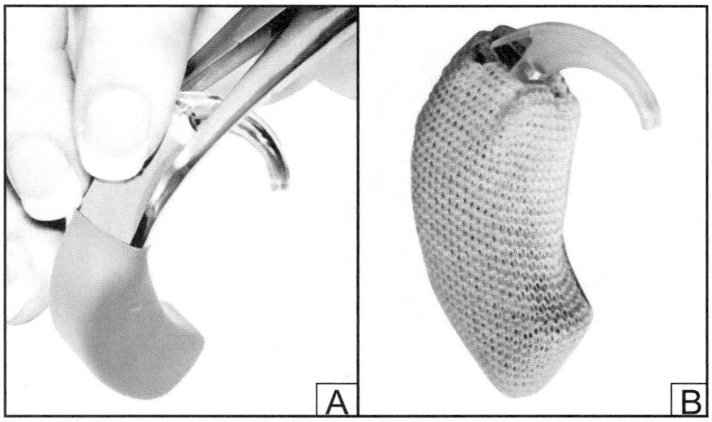

FIGURE 29–2. Protective covers for hearing aids that are designed to reflect moisture **(A)** or wick moisture **(B)**.

ments should be scheduled every 4 to 6 months. Naturally, this schedule of appointments assumes that the parents, teachers, and/or child have not noticed a change in hearing ability, which would necessitate an immediate visit to the audiologist.

The allotted appointment times should allow for the following activities to be completed:

- Re-evaluation of hearing function—This is especially important for infants and young children who are unable to report changes in their hearing.
- Re-making of earmolds—Especially for infants and young children, growth of the ear might necessitate new earmolds as often every other month, but typically about every four to six months for children under the age of 5 years.
- Visual inspection of the ear—The audiologist should ensure at every follow-up visit that there are no sore spots in the child's concha, helix area, or ear canal resulting from the earmold or hearing aid. In addition, it is important to remember that properly cut tubing might become too short if the child experiences a growth spurt. Therefore, it is important to visually inspect the fit of the earmold and the hearing aid to ensure the best fit for the child.
- Electroacoustic analysis of the hearing aid(s)—Only through electroacoustic analysis can we verify appropriate hearing aid function. Electroacoustic analysis should be completed before the hearing aid is dispensed to ensure that it meets the specifications and desired settings. Electroacoustic analysis should also be completed at follow-up visits to verify hearing aid function and to confirm listening checks.
- Listening check of hearing aid(s)—Although audiologists will be conducting electroacoustic analyses of hearing aids, listening checks can reveal the presence of poor sound quality that might not be otherwise detected.
- Acquisition of real-ear-to-coupler differences (RECD)—Whenever a new earmold is received, it is necessary to remeasure the child's RECD. If a change is noted from the previous measurement, adjustments to hearing aid settings will need to be made.

During these follow-up visits, the audiologist will also focus on ensuring that parents or caregivers have the necessary information and skills to care for the child's hearing needs. Table 29–2 provides information that should be shared with families about troubleshooting hearing aids when problems arise.

Table 29–2. Troubleshooting Common Hearing Aid Issues

Complaint	***What to Do***
"I don't hear any sound"	∞ Ensure device is turned on ∞ Ensure that the battery door is closed ∞ Ensure volume control wheel is set to desired level ∞ Check battery function via battery tester ∞ Check that battery contacts are clean ∞ Check that earmold bore is free of debris
"Hearing aid has feedback"	∞ Ensure volume control wheel is set to desired level ∞ Check that earmold bore is free of debris ∞ Determine if earmold and/or tubing has a tear and needs to be replaced ∞ Verify that hearing aid casing does not have any damage ∞ Make sure microphone and receiver are free of debris
"HA is weak or intermittent"	∞ Check battery function via battery tester ∞ Verify that HA casing doesn't have any damage ∞ Check that earmold and tubing are free of moisture ∞ Re-check function of hearing aid after overnight use with desiccant container ∞ Check that earmold bore is free of debris ∞ Check that microphone and receiver are free of debris

Conclusion

The day a child receives a first hearing aid can be one of the most memorable times in a family's experience. They come to this appointment with a myriad of emotions: anxiety, uncertainty, and, in all likelihood, great hope and expectation. Audiologists can execute their finest work in this moment, families can find their greatest ally, and a new relationship can flourish.

Acknowledgment. The authors appreciate the graphic services of the Vanderbilt Kennedy Center for Research on Human Development, supported in part by NICHD Grant P30 HD15052.

References

American Academy of Audiology (AAA). (2003). *Pediatric amplification protocol*. Washington, DC: Author.

Anderson, K. L. (1989). *Screening Instrument for Targeting Educational Risk (SIFTER)*. http://www.hear2learn.com

Anderson, K. L., & Matkin, N. (1996). *Screening Instrument for Targeting Educational Risk in Preschool Children (Age 3–Kindergarten) (Preschool SIFTER)*. http://www.hear2learn.com

Anderson, K. L, & Smaldino, J. J. (2000). *Children's Home Inventory for Listening Difficulties (CHILD)*. http://www.hear2learn.com

Berry, G. (1939). The use and effectiveness of hearing aids. *Journal of Laryngology, 49*, 912–921.

Bess, F. H. (1997). *Condition of hearing aids worn by children in a public school setting*. (Publication No. OE 77-05002); Washington, DC: DHEW.

Bronstein, A. C., Spyker, D. A., Cantilena, L. R., Green, J., Rumack, B. H., & Heard, S. E. (2007). 2006 Annual report of the American Association of Poison Control Centers' national poison data system. *Clinical Toxicology, 45*, 815–917.

Ching, T. C., Hill, M., & Psarros, C. (2000). *Strategies for evaluation of hearing aid fitting for children*. Paper presented at the International Hearing Aid Research Conference, August 23, Lake Tahoe, CA. http://www.nal.gov.au

Dire, D. J. (2009). *Disk battery ingestion: Treatment and medication*. Retrieved from http://members.medscape.com/article/774838-treatment

Grimshaw, S. (1996). *The extraction of listening situations which are relevant to young children, and the perception of normal-hearing subjects of the degree of difficulty experienced by the hearing impaired in different types of listening situations*. Nottingham, UK: MRC Institute of Hearing Research.

Humes, L., & Bess, H. (1981). Tutorial on the potential deterioration in hearing due to hearing aid usage. *Journal of Speech and Hearing Science, 46*, 3–15.

Ingrao, B. (2005, Nov. 8). Stick it in your ear: A systematic approach to earmold selection. *Asha Leader, 30–31*, 6–7.

Jerger, J. F., & Lewis, N. (1975). Binaural hearing aids: Are they dangerous for children? *Archives of Otolaryngology, 101*, 480–483.

Kemker, F. J., McConnell, F., Logan, S. A., & Green, B. W. (1979). A field study of children's hearing aids in a school environment. *Language, Speech and Hearing Services in Schools, 10*, 47–53.

Kinney, C. E. (1961). Further destruction of partially deafened children's hearing by use of powerful hearing aids. *Annals of Otology, Rhinology and Laryngology, 70*, 828–835.

Kopun, J., & Stelmachowicz, P. G. (1998). Perceived communication difficulties of children with hearing loss. *American Journal of Audiology, 7*, 30–38.

Küehn-Inacker, H., Weichbold, V., Tsiakpini, L. Coninx, S., & D'Haese, P. (2003). *LittlEARS Auditory questionnaire: Parents questionnaire to assess auditory behavior*. Retrieved February 8, 2010, from http://www.medel.com/english/img/PDF/reha/MKT1070E_r20.pdf

Ling, D. (1976). *Speech and the hearing-impaired child: Theory and practice*. Washington, DC: Alexander Graham Bell Association for the Deaf.

Ling, D. (1989). *Foundations of spoken language for the hearing-impaired child*. Washington, DC: Alexander Graham Bell Association for the Deaf.

Martin, R. L. (2009). In case of battery ingestion, act fast! *Hearing Journal, 62*(3), 64.

Mississippi Bend Area Educational Agency, Special Education Division. (n.d.). *Knowledge is power*. Retrieved December 8, 2009, from http//:www.edaud.org/storelistitem.cfm?itemnumber=18

National Capital Poison Center (NCPC). (2006). *Swallowed a battery button? Battery button in the nose or ear?* Retrieved December 8, 2009, from http://www.hearingoffice.com/download/Swallowed_a_Button_Battery_Battery.pdf

Purdy, S., Farrington, D. R., Moran, C. A., Chard, L. L., & Hodgson, S-A. (2002). ABEL: Auditory behavior in everyday life. *American Journal of Audiology, 11*, 72–82.

Riedner, E. D. (1978). Monitoring of hearing aids and earmolds in an educational setting. *Journal of the American Auditory Society, 4*(1), 39–43.

Rintelman, W., & Bess, F. (1988). High level amplification and potential hearing loss in children. In F. Bess (Ed.), *Hearing impairment in children* (pp. 278–309). Timonium, MD: York Press.

Robbins, A. M. (2002, November). Empowering parents to help their newly diagnosed child gain communication skills. *Hearing Journal, 55*(11), 55–59.

Robbins, A. M., Renshaw, J. J., & Berry, S. W. (1991). Evaluating meaningful integration in profoundly hearing impaired children. *American Journal of Otolaryngology, 12*(Suppl), 144–150.

Robbins, A. M. Renshaw, J. J., & Berry, S. W. (1998). Meaningful auditory integration scale. In W. Estabrooks (Ed.), *Cochlear implants for kids* (pp. 373–386). Washington, DC: A.G. Bell Association for the Deaf, Inc.

Ross, M. (1977). *A review of studies on the incidence of hearing aid malfunctions*. Publication No. OE 77-05002); Washington, DC: DHEW.

Smitherman, S. (2005). *Evaluating amplification used by public school children: Hearing aids, fm systems, and cochlear implants.* Unpublished Au.D. capstone project. Vanderbilt University, Nashville, Tennessee.

Tharpe, A. M., & Flynn, T. S. (2005). *Incorporating functional auditory measures into pediatric practice: An introductory guide for pediatric hearing professionals*. Copenhagen, Denmark: Oticon A/S.

Williams, C. (2003) The Children's Outcome Worksheets—An outcome measure focusing on children's needs (ages 4–12). *News from Oticon*, January 2005. http://www.oticon.com

Zimmerman-Phillips, S., Osberger, M. F., & Robbins, A. M: (1997). *Infant-toddler: Meaningful auditory integration scale (IT-MAIS)*. Sylmar, CA: Advanced Bionics Corp. www.agbell.org8

Zink, G. D. (1972). Hearing aids children wear: A longitudinal study of performance. *Volta Review, 74*(1), 41–51.

APPENDIX 29–A

Hearing Aid Orientation Checklist

1. Components of the hearing aid and earmold
   - ☐ Microphone, receiver, program switch, on/off control, volume control, battery door, earhook, tubing, sound bore, and venting

2. How to operate a hearing aid
   - ☐ Turn on/off, switch between programs, operate battery door, especially if tamper proof, and how to connect/disconnect earmold tubing from earhook
   - ☐ Insertion and removal of hearing aid and earmold

3. Retention of hearing aids
   - ☐ use of retention devices
   - ☐ behavioral retention strategies

4. How to differentiate the left from the right
   - ☐ use of a sticker on one or both hearing aids
   - ☐ use of red paint or permanent marker on only the right hearing aid
   - ☐ orientation of earmold

5. Appropriate hearing aid settings
   - ☐ Volume control wheel setting
   - ☐ How to switch between programs and how to confirm those settings
   - ☐ How to connect to assistive listening devices, when appropriate

6. How to care for hearing aid and earmold
   - ☐ Daily activities, including wiping hearing aids and earmolds off with soft cloth, opening battery door overnight, how to store hearing aids and earmolds especially overnight, use of desiccant container
   - ☐ Weekly cleaning of earmolds in soapy water

7. Troubleshooting guidelines
   - ☐ Troubleshooting kit for parents, and if possible, one for school use (by either teacher or child)
   - ☐ Demonstrate procedure, including how to do Ling-Six-Sound Test, to parents

8. Battery information
   - ☐ Battery size
   - ☐ How and how often to replace
   - ☐ How to check battery function with and without a battery tester
   - ☐ Storage of batteries
   - ☐ Dangers of battery ingestion
   - ☐ Safe disposal of batteries

9. Warranty info
   - ☐ Regarding earmolds
   - ☐ Regarding hearing aids
     - i. Manufacturer
     - ii. Extended warranty purchases

10. Clinical procedure for addressing hearing aid issues
    - ☐ Walk-in clinic schedule
    - ☐ Options offered by clinic if hearing aids need to be sent in for repair (e.g., loaner bank, etc.)

11. Additional information
    - ☐ Issuance of brochures from hearing aid and earmold manufacturer on care, maintenance, etc.
    - ☐ Troubleshooting tips for parents
    - ☐ Local, regional, and national organization and support group information
    - ☐ Web sites pertaining to troubleshooting, pediatric hearing loss, etc.
    - ☐ Use and coupling of assistive listening devices

APPENDIX 29–B

Functional Auditory Assessment Tools

Test Name:	ABEL: Auditory Behavior in Everyday Life
Age Range:	2–12 years
Purpose:	Twenty-four item questionnaire with three subscales (Aural-Oral, Auditory Awareness, Social/Conversational skills) which evaluates auditory behavior in everyday life.
Reference:	Purdy, S. et al. 2002. ABEL: Auditory Behaviour in Everyday Life. *American Journal of Audiology, 11*, 72–82.

Test Name:	CHILD: Children's Home Inventory for Listening Difficulties
Age Range:	3–12 years
Purpose:	Questionnaire for the child and for the parent with 15 situations which rate how well the child understood speech.
Reference:	Anderson K. L., & Smaldino, J .J. (2000). *Children's Home Inventory for Listening Difficulties (CHILD)*. http://www.hear2learn.com

Test Name:	COW: Children's Outcome Worksheets
Age Range:	4–12 years
Purpose:	Three worksheets (child, parent, and teacher) are requested to specify 5 situations where improved hearing is desired.
Reference:	Williams, C. (2003). *The Children's Outcome Worksheets—An outcome measure focusing on children's needs (Ages 4–12)*. News from Oticon, January 2005. http://www.oticon.com

Test Name:	ELF: Early Listening Function
Age Range:	5 months–3 years
Purpose:	Twelve listening situations in which the parent and audiologist observe the child and record the distance the child responds to the auditory stimuli.
Reference:	Anderson, K. L. (2000). *Early Listening Function (ELF)*. http://www.hear2learn.com

Test Name:	IT-MAIS: Infant Toddler Meaningful Auditory Integration Scale
Age Range:	Birth to 3 years
Purpose:	Parental interview with ten questions that evaluates the meaningful use of sound in everyday situations (vocal behavior, attachment with hearing instrument, ability to alert to sound, ability to attach meaning to sound).
Reference:	Zimmerman-Phillips, S., Osberger, M. F., & Robbins, A. M. (1997). *Infant-Toddler: Meaningful Auditory Integration Scale (IT-MAIS)*. Sylmar, CA: Advanced Bionics Corp. http://www.agbell.org8

Test Name:	LIFE: Listening Inventory for Education
Age Range:	6 years and up.
Purpose:	Questionnaire that identifies classroom situations that are challenging for the child. There are two formats of the questionnaire: a teacher questionnaire with 16 items and a child questionnaire with 15 items.
Reference:	Anderson K. L., & Smaldino, J. J. (1996). *Listening Inventory for Education; An efficacy tool (LIFE).* http://www.hear2learn.com

Test Name:	Little Ears
Age Range:	0 years and up
Purpose:	Questionnaire for the parent with 35 age-dependent questions that assesses auditory development.
Reference:	Küehn-Inacker, H., Weichbold, V., Tsiakpini, L. Coninx, S., & D'Haese, P. (2003). *Questionnaire for the parent with 35 age-dependent questions that assesses auditory development.* Little Ears: Auditory Questionnaire. Innsbruck, MED-EL.

Test Name:	Little Ears: Auditory Questionnaire. Innsbruck, MED-EL LSQ: Listening Situations Questionnaire
Age Range:	7 years and up
Purpose:	Questionnaire for the parent and child with eight situations. Responses focus on help of amplification, difficulty of understanding, and satisfaction of amplification.
Reference:	Grimshaw, S. (1996). *The extraction of listening situations which are relevant to young children, and the perception of normal-hearing subjects of the degree of difficulty experienced by the hearing-impaired in different types of listening situations.* Nottingham: MRC Institute of Hearing Research.

Test Name:	MAIS: Meaningful Auditory Integration Scale
Age Range:	3 to 4 years and up.
Purpose:	Parental interview with ten questions that evaluates meaningful use of sound in everyday situations (attachment with hearing instrument, ability to alert to sound, ability to attach meaning to sound).
Reference:	Robbins, A. M. Renshaw, J. J., & Berry, S. W. (1991). Evaluating meaningful integration in profoundly hearing-impaired children. *American Journal of Otolaryngology, 12*(Suppl.), 144–150. Robbins, A. M., Renshaw, J. J., & Berry, S. W. (1998). Meaningful auditory integration scale. In W. Estabrooks (Ed.), *Cochlear implants for kids* (pp. 373–386) Washington DC, A. G. Bell Assoc. for the Deaf, Inc.

Test Name:	PEACH: Parents' Evaluation of Aural/oral performance of Children
Age Range:	Preschool to 7 years
Purpose:	Interview with parent with 15 questions targeting the child's everyday environment. Includes scoring for 5 subscales (Use, Quiet, Noise, Telephone, Environment)
Reference:	Ching, T. C., Hill, M., & Psarros, C. (2000). *Strategies for evaluation of hearing aid fitting for children.* Paper presented at the International Hearing Aid Research Conference, August 23, Lake Tahoe, USA. http://www.nal.gov.au
Test Name:	P-APHAB: Pediatric Abbreviated Profile of Hearing Aid Benefit
Age Range:	10 to 15 years
Purpose:	Questionnaire with 24 situations completed by the child in regard to use of a hearing aid and no use of a hearing aid. It includes scoring for four subscales (ease of communication, background noise, reverberation and aversion)
Reference:	Kopun, J., & Stelmachowicz, P. G. (1998). Perceived communication difficulties of children with hearing loss. *American Journal of Audiology, 7,* 30–38.
Test Name:	Preschool SIFTER: Preschool Screening Instrument For Targeting Educational Risk
Age Range:	3 to 6 years
Purpose:	Questionnaire with 15 items completed by the teacher that identifies children at risk for educational failure with five subscales (academics, attention, communication, participation, behavior).
Reference:	Anderson, K. L., & Matkin, N. (1996). *Screening Instrument for Targeting Educational Risk in Preschool Children (Age 3–Kindergarten) (Preschool SIFTER).* http://www.hear2learn.com
Test Name:	SIFTER: Screening Instrument For Targeting Educational Risk
Age Range:	6 years and above.
Purpose:	Questionnaire with 15 items completed by the teacher that identifies children at risk for educational failure with five subscales (academics, attention, communication, participation, behavior).
Reference:	Anderson, K. L. (1989). *Screening Instrument for Targeting Educational Risk (SIFTER).* http://www.hear2learn.com
Test Name:	TEACH: Teachers' Evaluation of Aural/oral performance of Children
Age Range:	preschool to 7 years
Purpose:	Interview with teacher with 13 questions targeting the child's everyday environment. Includes scoring for five subscales (Use, Quiet, Noise, Telephone, Environment)
Reference:	Ching, T. C., Hill, M., & Psarros, C. (2000). *Strategies for evaluation of hearing aid fitting for children.* Paper presented at the International Hearing Aid Research Conference, August 23, Lake Tahoe, California. http://www.nal.gov.au

VII

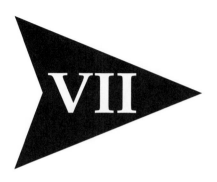

Management Considerations

30

History of the Management of Hearing Loss in Children

Andrée Durieux-Smith and Elizabeth Fitzpatrick

Deaf Children: Historical Perspective

Permanent bilateral hearing loss, if undetected, can lead to significant delays in the development of speech, language and literacy, which in turn can limit educational and occupational options. The consequences of hearing loss have been known for centuries although not clearly understood. Misconceptions abounded particularly in relation to individuals with severe to profound hearing loss. One such misconception concerning "the deaf" was that these individuals could not speak because they had no vocal folds (Davis & Silverman, 1970). This inaccurate information led to the unfortunate term of "deaf mute" suggesting that deafness and muteness depended on some common organic abnormality. In addition, it was acknowledged even at that time that speech was the vehicle to transmit thought and was essential for education. The term "deaf and dumb" reflected the belief that the deaf could not be educated because they could not hear or speak. This implied that the deaf had limited mental capacity that in turn influenced their legal and civil status. Roman law (Silverman, 1970) classified individuals who were deaf with those who were considered mentally incompetent.

Deafness was clearly seen as an educational barrier since hearing was the normal channel through which speech is perceived and was considered essential for learning. Although information on the education of the deaf is relatively sparse prior to the 15th century, it is clear that during this period, some thought was given to providing the deaf with other means so that they could express their thoughts. Agricola wrote a book that was not published until the 16th century in which he proposed that the deaf could express themselves by putting their thoughts down in writing (Silverman, 1970). Little information is available on the method that was used to achieve this goal. In the 16th century as well, Cardano, an Italian physician and father of a deaf child became interested in Agricola's work and promoted the notion that the deaf could be taught to comprehend written symbols by using pictures (Silverman, 1970). At this time, the belief that the deaf could learn to express themselves using words or gestures was introduced. This was a turning point as it was realized that deafness was a barrier to communication and not an intellectual deficit. The key therefore was to find ways to help the deaf communicate and learn.

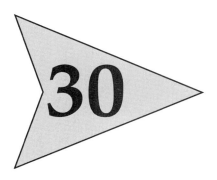

In 1555, the first school for the deaf was established in Spain by Pedro Ponce de Leon, a Catholic monk. The goal of this school was to teach "deaf mutes" to speak. The first book exclusively on the deaf was produced by Juan Pablo Bonet in 1620 (Silverman, 1970) and promoted the teaching of language and articulation supplemented by sign language and a manual alphabet. Several other books followed and it is clear that, in this period, there was recognition that the deaf could be educated and that they were equal to normal hearing individuals. In the latter part of the 17th century, two individuals in particular developed different methods to educate deaf children and both made significant contributions to this field. In France, the Abbe de l'Epee founded the first public school for the deaf in Paris, and students were educated using sign language. In Germany, Heinicke founded a public school for the deaf and advocated for the use of speech and speech reading. De l'Epee and Heinicke disagreed about the merits of sign language and oralism as methods of instruction, a controversy that was repeated in many countries and still persists today. Regardless of the methods used, by the end of the 17th century, it was clear that the deaf were capable of instruction and it was also recognized that this was a legal and moral obligation. In the United States, the first permanent school for the deaf was founded in 1817 in Hartford Connecticut, by Thomas Hopkins Gallaudet who had travelled to France and learned the methods of de l'Epee. The school at Hartford was known as the American Asylum for the Education and Instruction of the Deaf and Dumb, which later became the American School for the Deaf. In 1872, a Canadian educator of the deaf and inventor, Alexander Graham Bell opened a training school for teachers of the deaf in Boston. Bell was a strong believer of lipreading and speech in the education of deaf children.

Technologic developments were taking place at this time that eventually had a great impact on the management of hearing loss in children. This was also the era of the advent of electricity and Bell started experimenting with ways to make speech visible and audible to the deaf. This led to the invention of the telephone that laid the firm foundation for the electrical transmission of sound. The development of devices that had the potential to increase the audibility of sound for the deaf was a critical milestone in the management of deaf children. Bell founded the Volta Bureau in 1887 to disseminate information about deafness. In 1897, Max Goldstein, an otologist who was also a strong advocate for the importance of residual hearing founded the St. Joseph's School for the Deaf in St. Louis Missouri. Instruction included a series of exercises to give children practice with sound stimulation. In 1924, Goldstein established the Central Institute for the Deaf in St. Louis. In the late 19th century and at the beginning of the 20th century, deafness was viewed as a problem that belonged to the field of education. Many schools for the deaf developed programs predominantly for school age children. Over the years, with the advent of electricity and the development of technology, a better understanding of deafness took place.

Technologic Developments That Have Influenced the Management of Hearing Loss in Children

The Profession of Audiology

Prior to the advent of electricity and the development of the audiometer, it was very difficult to obtain precise information on the degree, configuration, and nature of hearing loss. The importance of obtaining information about a child's hearing loss was recognized and methods using various environmental sounds and speech were used. Itard in the 19th century (Silverman & Lane, 1970) developed a classification based on children's responses to bells, drums, and flutes. Urbantschitsch (Silverman & Lane, 1970) used a harmonica with specific frequency ranges and known intensities for the same purpose. These efforts led to classifications of types of hearing loss based on children's responses that were not unlike those used a half century later.

In 1929, the National Research Council in the United States sponsored a conference to address the problems of the deaf and hard of hearing (Hirsh, 1952). The need to accurately measure the degree and type of hearing loss was identified as an important priority together with the standardization of methods.

During World War II, audiology became the recognized profession with expertise in the science of hearing. Audiology was best defined by its multidisciplinary origins as it included knowledge from physics, psychology, education, and otolaryngology. This new specialty was created because of the numerous war casualties who suffered from hearing loss and deafness. Audiology provided a much needed professional service that had not been available. Since the work of Hirsh (1952), considerable information has been collected about sound and hearing measurement. The developments of the electric audiometer and audiometric standards have made it possible to measure auditory thresholds at frequencies important for speech perception. In addition, the medical field of otology contributed to the identification of the site of lesion and to the medical management of hearing loss in children. Hearing aids were developed and could provide some deaf children with access to sound. In these early days of technologic developments, the professions of audiology, otology, and education worked together to develop the most appropriate rehabilitation and educational programs for children with hearing loss.

The ability to measure hearing led to some interesting classifications of hearing loss in children. The terms deaf and hard-of-hearing were based predominantly on the degree of hearing loss and age of onset, and were used to guide the educational process and also, indirectly, to set expectations. It also was recognized that some children who had developed speech and language prior to the onset of severe to profound deafness had very different needs and therefore fell into the hard-of-hearing category. The deaf child was defined as one who did not have sufficient residual hearing to enable him or her to understand and develop speech even with a hearing aid, without special instruction. The sense of hearing for the deaf child was thought to be nonfunctional for everyday functioning. Systematic and laborious procedures were necessary in order for the deaf child to learn to communicate (Silverman & Lane, 1970). As in North America, a similar trend took place in England under the School Health Regulations, whereby children were described as deaf and partially deaf (Ewing & Ewing, 1954). The deaf had no "naturally" acquired speech when they were admitted to school, whereas the hard-of-hearing had begun to talk naturally although with some imperfections. The hard-of-hearing child was thought to have a sense of hearing which, although defective, was also functional with or without a hearing aid. Deaf children were described as having pure-tone average hearing losses of 91 dB or greater, and as not being able to rely on the auditory channel as a primary avenue of communication. It was believed that hearing losses of such severity could not be overcome. Although the terms "deaf" and "hard of hearing" were used extensively at that time, the need to define children with hearing loss in terms of their educational and psychological potential was also identified. In fact, it came to be recognized that some "totally deaf" individuals could benefit from the use of appropriate amplification (Silverman & Lane, 1970).

Early Identification

Although the technologic developments of the 1940s to the 1960s clearly contributed to enhancing the management of children with hearing loss, many challenges still needed to be addressed. One such challenge was the late identification of hearing loss in children. The importance of early education of children with hearing loss had been identified and it was recognized that infants needed to be exposed to sound. The period from birth to the age of 5 years was identified as being particularly critical to learning. At the same time, however, it was acknowledged that it was difficult to evaluate a young child's hearing reliably and there was a lack of awareness by physicians of hearing loss in children. The average age of identification for hearing impairment in children was reported as 3 to 4 years (Bess, 2000; Wong & Shah, 1979) and there were significant delays between identification of hearing loss and hearing aid fitting. In addition, there was a difference of opinion on when a child was ready to wear a hearing aid and whether hearing aids could damage hearing.

Several individuals and events influenced the developments of early identification initiatives. In the United Kingdom, the Ewings (Ewing, 1957), who stressed the importance of early identification, parental involvement, and early amplification had an enormous impact on the management of hearing loss in children. In 1964, an international conference, "The Deaf Child" took place in Toronto, Canada, bringing together more than 30 experts from North America, Great Britain, Scandinavia and the Netherlands (Davis, 1965). Participants at this workshop were already sensitized to the importance of the early identification and early management of hearing loss in children. The purpose of the meeting was to find ways to alleviate the handicap to auditory communication imposed by early hearing loss. Considerable discussion took place on definitive tests of hearing for the very young, which were not available at that time. Systematic reviews of available tests were presented at the meeting and these included new electrical techniques that detected cortical evoked responses to sound in young children. This was seen as a breakthrough that might make it possible to eventually identify hearing loss in newborns and infants. Neonatal tests of hearing and the age at which reliable, reasonably valid, and definite tests of hearing could be performed were seen as crucial but the technology was not yet available. For this reason, the screening of high-risk groups of infants was recommended although the concept of universal neonatal screening in fact, was also discussed. Participants felt that it was too early to form an opinion about auditory evoked cortical responses as a test, and some were sceptical that an inexpensive, uncomplicated instrument could be developed to satisfy the requirements for clinical applications. All felt that more research was needed to determine the validity and reliability of tests to identify hearing loss early. Interestingly, at this conference, consensus was not reached on the age at which the use of amplified sound should be initiated and opinions ranged from two weeks to two months. The majority agreed, however, that two years was the maximum acceptable delay. Generally, participants felt that it would be ideal if hearing impairment were detected and confirmed by six months of age.

In 1969, in the United States, the Joint Committee on Infant Hearing (JCIH) was established and included representatives from audiology, otolaryngology, pediatrics, and nursing. The committee was mandated to make recommendations with regard to early identification of hearing loss. Over the years, several statements were issued by the Joint Committee on newborn screening (JCNS, 1970) and the JCIH (1982, 1990, 1994, 2000, 2007) and addressed the populations to be screened and the methods to be used for screening. In the first statement (JCNS, 1970), after reviewing the data from a small number of controlled studies on the screening of infants for hearing loss, the committee did not recommend the routine screening of newborns because of a lack of accurate screening methods. At that time, screening methods were limited to behavioral responses to the presentation of relatively loud broadband stimuli (Mencher, 1976). This kind of testing had evolved from the behavioral responses obtained to auditory stimuli by Ewing and Ewing (1944) and Wedenberg (1956) to name a few. At the same time, and similar to the recommendations made by the 1964 Conference on the Deaf Child, the JCIH started to identify certain children who were at significant risk of developing hearing loss. This gave rise to the use of the high risk register, which was introduced as a supplement to the 1970 JCNS statement (Joint Committee on Infant Screening, 1976). Between 1982 and 1994, the high risk register was further refined to include additional factors (JCIH, 1982, 1990, 1994). The approach was therefore to screen children who fell on the high risk register since it was felt this would lead to the identification of the majority of children with a permanent hearing loss. At the same time, it became more and more evident that behavioral screening, even in its most sophisticated and automated form such as the Crib-O-Gram (Simmons & Russ, 1974), was not reliable nor valid (Durieux-Smith, Picton, MacMurray, & Goodman, 1987; Wright & Rybak, 1983).

In the last 30 years, considerable technologic developments have taken place, making it possible to accurately identify abnormal auditory function in newborns and infants. Two physiological measures, the auditory brainstem response (ABR) and otoacoustic emissions (OAEs) have clearly revolutionized early hearing detection and have led to the early identification and intervention of children with permanent hearing loss. In the late 1970s, Schulman-Galambos and Galambos (1979) recommended the ABR for newborn hearing assessment. Subsequently, several studies continued to investigate the usefulness of the ABR, particularly with high risk infants (Durieux-Smith, Picton, Edwards, Goodman, & MacMurray, 1985; Galambos, Hicks, & Wilson, 1982, 1984; Hyde, Riko, & Malizia, 1990; Kileny, 1987). Follow up studies of infants screened by this technique also showed good validity (Durieux-Smith et al., 1987; Hyde et al., 1990). The 1982 Position Statement of the JCIH recommended that the initial screening include the observation of behavioral or electrophysiological responses to sound, although the committee did not recommend any specific testing method. In the 1990 Position Statement, the JCIH recommended the use of ABR using clicks as the screening method for high-risk neonates. One of the problems at the time was that the equipment used to assess the ABR was costly, required considerable expertise to operate, and was not readily portable and therefore not really appropriate for screening. In the late 1980s and early 1990s, another technique, OAEs, was introduced as a promising method to assess cochlear function in newborns and infants. In 1978, Kemp in England was the first to show that OAEs could be detected in the human external ear in response to stimulation with clicks. The recording of these OAEs was viewed as evidence of normal cochlear function and more specifically of outer hair cell integrity (Kemp, 1980). Kemp's discovery and the development of equipment to record OAEs gave rise to an entire new approach to newborn and infant screening (Bonfils, Uziel, & Pujol, 1988; Kennedy et al., 1991; Stevens et al., 1989, 1990; White & Behrens, 1993). Studies that followed infants screened with this technique reported that OAEs could identify infants with hearing loss of approximately 30 dB HL and greater (Kennedy et al., 1991).

In 1993, the National Institute of Deafness and other Communication Disorders (one of the National Institutes of Health [NIH]) held a consensus development conference, "Early Identification of Hearing Impairment in Infants and Young Children," in the United States (NIH, 1993). The objective of this conference was to develop an improved approach to identifying hearing loss in infants. The 1993 Consensus Statement recommended that all infants be screened for hearing loss by 3 months of age. This recommendation was made after reviewing compelling evidence that clearly demonstrated that screening infants on a high risk register missed 50% of children who had a permanent hearing loss (Jacobson & Jacobson, 1990; Mauk, White, Mortensen, & Behrens, 1991; Watkin, Baldwin, & McEnery, 1991); this was subsequently confirmed by other studies (Durieux-Smith & Whittingham, 2000; Korres et al., 2005; Uus & Bamford, 2006). This was the first recommendation for universal newborn hearing screening. In addition, a screening protocol was proposed that included a two-stage screening process, namely, OAEs followed by ABRs for children who were referred by the OAE screen. In 1994, the JCIH gave careful consideration to the recommendations of the NIH conference and endorsed universal hearing screening while recommending additional research on the evaluation of the electrophysiological techniques that were now established to assess auditory function in newborns and infants. Since 1994, several investigators (Finitzo, Albright, & O'Neal, 1998; Mason & Hermann, 1998; Prieve & Stevens, 2000; Vohr, Carty, Moore, & Letourneau, 1998) have documented the validity, reliability and effectiveness of both electrophysiological measures for universal newborn hearing screening. In 2000, the JCIH issued a new position statement describing the principles underlying effective Early

Hearing Detection and Intervention (EHDI) programs and providing guidelines for their successful implementation. In 2007, the JCIH reiterated its support for universal hearing screening, recommending that all infants be screened by one month of age, have a complete audiological evaluation by 3 months of age and receive appropriate intervention no later than six months of age. The definition of the target disorder was refined together with protocols for screening, diagnostic audiologic evaluation and medical evaluation.

In addition to technologic advances in screening for auditory function in newborns and infants, considerable progress has also taken place in methods for audiologic diagnosis (Ackley & Decker, 2006). Tone pip ABRs have supplemented click ABR and can now yield clinically acceptable estimates of pure tone thresholds by air conduction (Stapells, 2000). Bone conduction (BC) frequency-specific ABR threshold estimates can be obtained although the dynamic range of BC stimulation is limited and the possibility of error still exists (Campbell, Harris, Hendricks, & Sirimanna, 2004; Stapells & Oates, 1997). An assessment of infant middle ear systems using high frequency probe tones also can contribute to differential diagnosis (Alaerts, Lutz, & Woulters, 2007; Meyer, Jardine, & Deverson, 1997). Technologic developments in the last 30 to 40 years now make it possible to accurately identify hearing loss in infants and proceed with management for those with a permanent hearing loss.

Amplification

One of the preoccupations in the management of permanent hearing loss in children has been to expose the deaf child to sound stimulation through the use of amplification. Before the advent of electricity, mechanical hearing devices were developed. The ear trumpet dating from the seventeenth century was initially used by sailors to communicate with each other over long distances. Only in the 19th century did this device become an option for the deaf together with smaller versions known as cornets and auricles (Niemoller, Silverman, & Davis, 1970). The first electric hearing aid was designed in the late 1800s and it is thought that this invention was related to Alexander Graham Bell's work on the development of the telephone. This first prototype amplified sounds by mechanically funnelling sound to the ear by electronic magnification. The first amplification device contained a battery operated carbon transmitter and earphones, and subsequently a carbon transmitter model hearing aid became commercially available. In the 1920s, the carbon transmitter was replaced by the vacuum tube. The device now consisted of a microphone, an ear receiver, amplifier, and two batteries. Batteries only lasted for one day. One of the main challenges of the early hearing aids was to deliver sufficient energy. Over the next several decades, improvements were made with batteries becoming smaller, and in 1947 a major breakthrough came with the development of the transistor (Northern & Downs, 1991). Silicon transistors allowed hearing aids to shrink in size so that they could become "body aids." Even with these developments, early hearing aids were still very large, unattractive, provided limited bandwidth, and produced high levels of harmonic distortion (Killion, 1997). During that time, hearing aids primarily were designed for adults and not children. Binaural fittings were impossible with these cumbersome instruments and monaural fittings became an established practice. Because hearing aids were so large, a single Y-cord was often used to provide "binaural" amplification.

The main difficulty with these early electrical instruments continued to be the high power requirements and the size. Nevertheless, these early electronic aids revolutionized opportunities for deaf children as they provided sound stimulation. Due to their large size, the earliest electric models were not portable and were used exclusively in classrooms. The portable or desk type hearing aid was used as it had more power and provided a better quality signal (Niemoller et al., 1970). The teacher spoke into a free-standing microphone and the hearing-impaired listener received the amplified sound through headphones. This type of system required that the child remain in one place. The microphone and headphones were connected to an amplifier by means of cables and the child's movements were restricted by the radius of the cord connecting the amplifier and the headphones. This system was used for individual speech training. Systems were capable of reproducing a wider range of frequencies than individual hearing aids, few of which could provide significant amplification beyond 3500 Hz (Ling & Ling, 1978). For some children, hard wire systems helped to provide acoustic cues not available through personal hearing aids.

Another type of system was the group hearing aid with one or more microphones, an amplifier and as many as 10 pairs of over-the-ear or insert receivers. The use of electromagnetic transmission eliminated the need for connecting wires from amplifier to the listeners. Because the speaker wore the microphone, a better signal to noise ratio (S/N) was achieved. Another method used an induction loop around the classroom that received electric energy from the amplifier of the group hearing aid. The magnetic field created by the loop current was sensed by a telephone pick up. This allowed the child to receive speech at the same level anywhere within the loop. In addition, the movements of the child were not restricted and loops could be used in settings outside of the classroom such as the child's home. One of the disadvantages was that loops could not be used in adjacent classrooms because of overspill whereby the electromagnetic field would extend outside the loop area. Group hearing aids were used in schools for the deaf and the technology at that time required that the management of children with permanent hearing loss take place predominantly in an educational setting. Today, special amplification systems such as radio frequency modulated systems (FM) make it possible for children to wear their personal hearing aids with an FM system. This ensures teacher/child mobility, and consistent favorable signal levels and has facilitated the inclusion of children with a permanent hearing loss in the regular school system (Sanders, 1993). Furthermore, the use of such systems is not restricted to the classroom setting.

With the advent of transistor circuitry and resulting miniaturization of hearing aids, it became recognized that the greatest advantage of personal hearing aids was that the child could have access to amplification at all times. It was acknowledged that the management of hearing loss should not only take place in the classroom setting but that children should benefit from auditory experience in everyday life. In the early 1950s, it became possible to wear two body aids and by 1955 hearing aids were worn in a harness around the body worn over clothing. The superiority of true binaural fittings was recognized as providing an increased directional sense and better perception of speech in noise (Carhart, 1958; Harris, 1965; Jordan, Greisen, & Bentzen, 1967; Ross, 1969). Furthermore, it became recognized that in most instances binaural hearing aids should be the standard treatment in every case of bilateral hearing loss. It also was acknowledged that it was more natural to receive sound at ear level and since the early 1960s ear level hearing aids have become more widely used (Northern & Downs, 1974). Because behind-the-ear aids were not as powerful as body hearing aids, it was recommended that behind–the-ear aids be fitted on all hearing losses less than below 80 dB HL and that two body aids be used for children with hearing losses greater than 80 dB HL (Jordan et al., 1967). The other advantage of body hearing aids was the separation of microphone and receiver that diminished the probability of acoustic feedback.

Tremendous technologic advances have been made with regard to hearing aids in the past four decades. Digital technology developments have led to signal processing that allows the provision of a uniform and high quality signal, but is beyond the scope of this chapter to review all of these in detail. Furthermore, there have been advances in hearing aid selection and verification methods. Much research and discussion have taken place addressing the appropriate selection of frequency responses, gain and output characteristics of hearing aids for children (Stelmachowicz, 2005). In the 1970s and early 1980s, systematic hearing aid fitting algorithms began to emerge although these were based solely on average adult data. One major development has been the use of clinical probe-microphone systems in the 1980s which facilitated the fitting of hearing aids to children. Through the use of these systems, Seewald and colleagues (Moodie, Seewald, & Sinclair, 1994) developed the innovative real ear to coupler difference (RECD) procedure that facilitates real-ear measures in infants as young as a few weeks of age (see Chapter 25 of this volume).

Despite these developments with hearing aids, there remained a population of profoundly deaf children who received very limited auditory information with conventional amplification. Cochlear implants were developed on the premise that in sensorineural deafness although hair cells are damaged or depleted, some cochlear neurons could be stimulated directly by the application of an externally produced electric current. Cochlear implants were developed from a single channel analog device in the 1960s and in the 1980s, multichannel implants were introduced (Owens & Kessler, 1989). Initially, the use of cochlear implants was restricted to adults who were postlingually deafened. In 1990, cochlear implants were approved by the Federal Drug and Administration (FDA) for use with children. The signal analog channel cochlear implant such as the 3M/House single channel implant provided little more than sound awareness, prosody or rhythm of speech. Improvements also were observed in speech recognition as determined on closed-set auditory only tests. Multichannel cochlear implants, with each channel uniquely programmable, provide sufficient frequency discrimination capability to facilitate speech perception and understanding (Thoutenhoofd et al., 2005). Language and literacy improvements in children with cochlear implants have been reported as being comparable to the results obtained with children who use hearing aids and who have less severe hearing loss (Moog & Geers, 2003). In fact, language scores of some children with implants have been documented as being within the range of children with normal hearing (Geers, Nicholas, & Sedley, 2003). Consequently, cochlear implants have become the standard of care for children with bilateral severe to profound hearing loss (Berg, Ip, Hurst, & Herb, 2007).

Recent advances in technology have fundamentally altered the way we think of the development of communication skills in deaf children. The early, appropriate fitting of hearing aids was probably the single most important tool in the management of the child with permanent hearing loss (Ross, 1977). Technologies for early identification and audiologic diagnosis of permanent hearing loss have made it possible to fit amplification to babies. Technologies for digital and programmable hearing aids and cochlear implants have made it possible for children with profound hearing losses to have access to sound and to spoken language. These advances have significantly altered our expectations of spoken language development for deaf children. These technologies have had a major impact on the development of different types of intervention. On their own, however, they are of little use if not followed by intervention programs.

Intervention for Children With Hearing Loss

Educational Options

Historically, there has been considerable difference of opinion about the most effective methods for developing communication. However, there is a consensus that the overall goal of (re)habilitative and educational management for children with hearing loss is to overcome or minimize the barriers to communication imposed by hearing loss in order to enable learning and participation in society. The extent to which permanent hearing loss affects typical spoken communication development and the need for specialized management will depend on characteristics of the hearing loss, such as time of onset and severity as well as characteristics specific to the child, family, and learning environment. These factors undoubtedly influence decisions related to language learning and educational approaches for facilitating communication development. However, it is clear that over the years management approaches have also been extensively influenced by technologic limitations, practitioners' experiences and philosophical views of what constitutes appropriate communication for a child with hearing loss (Beattie, 2006; Marschark & Spencer, 2006). It is perhaps these views, more than empirical data, that have contributed to the rich history of the (re)habilitation and education of children with hearing loss, one characterized by a mosaic of intervention methods.

As outlined in the previous sections of this chapter, prior to the advent of modern day hearing aids and particularly cochlear implant technology, children with hearing loss fell essentially into two broad categories based on hearing potential; those who had considerable access to acoustic speech signals and those who had limited or no access to speech despite the best available hearing technology. Two parallel (re)habilitation and educational management philosophies evolved, both with a focus on equipping the child with communication skills. One philosophy described as a manual approach supported the development of communication through a visual-based sign language system as the natural language of individuals who were deaf. In contrast, the oral philosophy adopted spoken communication and participation in the hearing community as a primary goal of intervention. Numerous variants of these two primary philosophies were developed throughout the world. A detailed review of the many approaches are beyond the scope of this chapter but a brief description of some of the most common intervention methods that fall under the manual and oral philosophies will be described briefly in the following sections. The interested reader is referred to more comprehensive historical perspectives and critical reviews in such writings as Spencer and Marschark (2006), Schick, Marschark, and Spencer (2005), and Lynas, Huntington, and Tucker (1989).

Although hearing loss begins as a health issue, the management of children with hearing loss has its roots in education and historically, service provision was viewed as the "field of education of the hearing-impaired" with teachers of the deaf responsible for educating children (Clark, 1997). This was likely due to the fact that most children were not identified with hearing loss until late and there were no or limited intervention programs in the preschool years. As audiologic services and better technology became available, earlier identification and early intervention services provided the foundations for changes in practice. Accordingly, responsibilities for the management of children expanded to include not only educators but also speech-language pathologists, audiologists, and other specialists in the management of children with hearing loss.

Traditionally, the educational system for children with hearing loss consisted primarily of special schools for the deaf that provided services in either sign language or oral communication methods. Two important notions underlie the support for manual communication. One fundamental concept is that sign language systems such as American Sign Language (ASL) or its international counterparts constitute the natural language of individuals who are deaf. Accordingly, ASL is viewed as a visual language comprised of signs with its own grammatical structure that is distinctly different from that of spoken English grammar. Visual-manual systems such as ASL are consistent with a cultural view of deafness in which the Deaf individual is viewed as belonging to a linguistic minority with a distinct language and culture (Lynas, 2005). Essentially, ASL and other manual languages are structured for visual rather than auditory learning. The second important concept that led to support for sign language, particularly for children with profound deafness (prior to cochlear implantation), is that strong visual input is a requirement to overcome the barriers to communication imposed by reduced access to the acoustic patterns of speech.

More recently, programs referred to as bilingual-bicultural or sign-bilingualism (Lynas, 2005) have also emerged. The premise of these educational methods is that from the time of diagnosis of hearing loss, children should be exposed to a language such as ASL as their first language in an educational model that meets not only their linguistic but also their cultural needs as a participant in the Deaf community. Subsequently, written English is taught as a second language. These programs may also teach spoken English as a second language to enable the child to participate in everyday situations as a bilingual child (Lynas, 2005).

In contrast to visual-based approaches, the oral communication philosophy has been supported on the basis that more than 90% (Marschark, Lang, & Albertini, 2002) of children with permanent hearing loss have normal hearing parents who participate in a hearing society where spoken communication is central to the child's development, education, and employment opportunities. Central to this philosophy is the notion that despite reduced auditory access to the natural acquisition of spoken language, children can learn verbal communication through systematic teaching methods.

As noted previously, prior to the widespread availability of hearing instruments, access to hearing through vacuum tube hearing aids and group amplification systems was necessarily limited to classroom settings. Oral educational options therefore consisted primarily of special schools with special classroom programs for children with hearing loss. Unquestionably, a major breakthrough occurred with the availability of small transistorized hearing aids in the 1950s to 1960s. Wearable hearing instruments dramatically affected the variety of educational environments that became available for children with hearing loss (Clark, 1997), ranging from special schools to special classrooms in schools for normal-hearing children and eventually to integration into typical classrooms with normal hearing peers (Clark, 1997; Northcott, 1990).

The limited and part-time access to the sounds of spoken communication dictated the methods that evolved for teaching children spoken communication. Until the 1960s, oral communication methods consisted primarily of oral-visual methods with a strong focus on speech-reading and a related spoken language curriculum that concentrated on didactic methods of teaching through the teaching of words and sentence patterns (Clark, 1997). Speech skill teaching developed as a separate activity aimed at improving the quality of the child's articulation. Certain practitioners also believed that the written text was an effective method for teaching children spoken language, thus structured writing approaches as a visual means to teaching spoken communication supplemented traditional oral methods to provide the learner with increased access to communication (Clark, 1997; Marschark & Spencer, 2006).

As hearing technology and early identification services progressed and as new knowledge was acquired about speech and language development, traditional oral communication methods were modified. Several variants of the oral communication philosophy were developed to capitalize on these new opportunities. Overall, the ultimate goal of oral education of children with hearing loss remained the development of speech and language as similar to hearing models as possible. The oral approaches are based on the premise that despite reduced input, the overwhelming majority of children have residual hearing and essentially acquire language along the same developmental trajectory as children with normal hearing, although they may reach milestones at a slower pace. Improved access to hearing led to the development of models of rehabilitation that differed in their focus on audition, and natural language acquisition, inclusion with hearing peers, and parental involvement. Known under terms such as auditory-oral or aural-oral and auditory-verbal therapy, the defining difference between these variants of the oral philosophy to rehabilitation appears to relate primarily to the emphasis on the use of residual hearing.

As noted above, traditional oral methods involved significant emphasis on speech-reading. At the other end of the spectrum, lies auditory-verbal therapy, an approach that gained momentum in the 1980s and continued to grow as hearing technologies improved. The approach, which is fundamentally based on the premise that even small amounts of hearing can be tuned to acquire spoken language, has grown in popularity with the increased access to hearing provided by cochlear implants for children with severe to profound hearing loss. The approach relies heavily on language learning through the development of residual hearing. Characteristics of auditory-verbal practice include individual teaching of language via a primary caregiver and the early inclusion of children with hearing loss with their normal hearing peers. However, until the advent of cochlear implants, a significant proportion of children with profound hearing loss who required specialized care had minimal access to acoustic speech signals (Boothroyd, 2008). Therefore, support continued for auditory-oral methods that also use speech-reading in teaching spoken language. The primary differences between auditory-verbal and other oral-based approaches are related to the emphasis placed on audition as the primary learning channel for speech reception and on the view that optimal development of communication and social functioning requires that children with hearing loss interact in group learning situations with children with normal hearing.

The assumption of all these oral language approaches is that exposure of the child to visual-based systems will delay or prevent the acquisition of spoken communication skills. In addition to the auditory-based learning methods, other teaching approaches have evolved that can be viewed as aligned with manual or oral communication methods depending on the ultimate communication development goals of the rehabilitation program. Cued speech is one method that is consistent with the oral philosophy but involves the addition of a systematic system of hand signals or cues to facilitate speech-reading and therefore speech reception. Cued speech involves the use of hand cues to code the phonemes of speech (Cornett, 1967).

Total communication is another teaching method that gained widespread recognition, particularly in the United States in the 1970s and 1980s. The method promotes the use of all input modalities including audition, speech-reading, and signs in order to enhance comprehension of speech. The approach essentially involves manually coded speech with visual symbols intended to compensate for reduced access to speech sounds through hearing. Other terms such as simultaneous communication and the combined approach have been used to describe manually coded speech systems. These multimodal communication approaches were promoted by some experts as a response to improve the low language and academic outcomes documented for children with hearing loss educated through oral communication approaches (Babbidge, 1965; Geers & Moog, 1989; Schildroth & Karchmer, 1986).

New Influences on (Re)Habilitation

As described above, developments in newborn hearing screening, hearing aid, and cochlear implant technology have had a significant impact on current thinking and management approaches. Cochlear implantation has had a significant impact on the quantity and quality of auditory information available to children with profound hearing loss and represents the single most important development in auditory (re)habilitation for these children in recent years. Early and appropriate hearing aid fitting or cochlear implants coupled with early identification of hearing loss resulting from universal newborn hearing screening initiatives have created a dramatic shift in the approaches and expectations for all children with hearing loss. Early identification through newborn hearing screening combined with advanced hearing technology has shifted rehabilitation from a remedial to a developmental model whether the choice of rehabilitation is sign language or oral language. Early access to spoken language patterns has created opportunities for children to acquire language in more naturalistic contexts and to participate in the educational system with hearing peers. Previous rehabilitation models such as auditory-verbal therapy emphasized spoken language acquisition following typical language developmental models, and efforts were made to develop spoken language in natural home and learning environments (Simser, 1993). However, due to late identification and limited access to auditory information, particularly for children with severe to profound hearing loss, many approaches included structured speech and language teaching that included remedial components particularly as children grew older (Ling, 2002).

The possibilities afforded by early identification, management through hearing technology and the developmental model are aligned with a model of family-centred care. The notion of family-centered care has dominated the management of children with hearing loss for many years, but is now growing due to the need to manage hearing loss in infancy and the new opportunities for enhancing language development in more natural and everyday contexts (Tattersall & Young, 2006; Young & Tattersall, 2007). Studies indicate that families want to be involved as partners in the process of language development and to make informed choices (Fitzpatrick, Angus, Durieux-Smith, Graham, & Coyle, 2008; Robinshaw & Evans, 2003).

There is a body of research documenting that children with various degrees of hearing loss who receive early intervention have the potential to develop spoken communication (Fitzpatrick, Durieux-Smith, Eriks-Brophy, Olds, & Gaines, 2007; Kennedy et al., 2006; Yoshinaga-Itano, Sedley, Coulter, & Mehl, 1998). In particular, a large body of research in cochlear implantation has documented positive outcomes in children with severe to profound hearing loss (Thoutenhoofd et al., 2005). Nevertheless, despite the many technologic advances and improvement in communication outcomes, studies continue to show that children with hearing loss, as a group, have spoken language abilities significantly below their hearing peers (Kennedy et al., 2006; Wake, Poulakis, Hughes, Carey-Sargeant, & Rickards, 2005). These findings suggest that management through hearing technology alone is insufficient to attain age-appropriate skills. Accordingly, children with hearing loss continue to require professional management in developing communication and parents are required to make decisions about which intervention approach is best suited to their needs and desired outcomes.

In summary, there is a wide range of management approaches for children with hearing loss. Many of these constitute different routes to a common objective, that of developing competent spoken communication. Other approaches focus on the development of a strong communication system through sign language, which is viewed by supporters as the natural language of children who are deaf. The intervention approach and type of amplification selected depend partly on the severity of the hearing impairment and on the characteristics of the child and family but also largely on the families' choice of communication mode for the child. Advances in hearing technology and newborn hearing screening, combined with research documenting the benefits of these interventions, have increased the demand for spoken communication approaches for children with hearing loss. However, there is an understanding that families should have the right to make a fully informed decision based on the best available evidence and their long-term objectives and values for their child and family (Jerger, Roeser, & Tobey, 2001; Joint Committee on Infant Hearing, 2007).

References

Ackley, R. S., & Decker, N. T. (2006). Audiological management and the acquisition of spoken language in deaf children. In P. E. Spencer & M. Marschark (Eds.), *Advances in the spoken language development of deaf and hard of hearing children* (pp. 64–84). New York, NY: Oxford University Press.

Alaerts, J., Lutz, H., & Woulters, J., (2007). Evaluation of middle ear function in young children: Clinical guidelines for the use of 226- and 1000-Hz tympanometry. *Otology & Neurotology, 28*(6), 727–732.

Babbidge, H. (1965). *Education of the deaf. A report to the Secretary of Health, Education, and Welfare by his Advisory Committee on the Education of the Deaf.* Ref. No. 0-765-119. Washington, DC: Government Printing Office.

Bamford, J., Uus, K., & Davis, A. (2005). Screening for hearing loss in childhood: Issues, evidence and current approaches in the UK. *Journal of Medical Screening, 12,* 119–124.

Beattie, R. G. (2006). The oral methods and spoken language acquisition. In P. E. Spencer & M. Marschark (Eds.), *Advances in the spoken language development of deaf and hard-of-hearing children* (pp. 103–135). New York, NY: Oxford University Press.

Berg, A. L., Ip, S. C., Hurst, M., & Herb, A. (2007). Cochlear implants in young children: Informed consent as a process and current practices. *American Journal of Audiology, 16,* 13–28.

Bess, F. (2000). Endnote address, Early amplification for children: Implementing change. In R. C. Seewald (Ed.), *A sound foundation through early amplification: Proceedings of an international conference* (pp. 247–251). Stäfa, Switzerland: Phonak AG.

Bonfils, P., Uziel, A., & Pujol, R. (1988). Screening for auditory dysfunction in infants by evoked otoacoustic emissions. In K. Gerkin & A. Amochaev (Eds.), Hearing in infants: Proceedings of the national symposium. *Seminars in Hearing, 8,* 165–168.

Boothroyd, A. (2008). The acoustic speech signal. In J. R. Madell & C. Flexer (Eds.), *Pediatric audiology: Diagnosis, technology, and management* (pp. 159–167). New York, NY: Thieme Medical.

Campbell P. E., Harris C. M., Hendricks S., & Sirimanna T. (2004). Bone conduction auditory brainstem responses in infants. *Journal of Laryngology & Otology, 118*(2), 117–122.

Carhart, R. (1958). The usefulness of the binaural hearing aid. *Journal of Speech and Hearing Disorders, 23,* 41–51.

Clark, M. (1997). An overview of educational provision for hearing-impaired children from 1950 to present day. *Seminars in Hearing, 18*(3), 229–239.

Cornett, R. O. (1967). Cued speech. *American Annals of the Deaf, 112,* 3–13.

Davis, H. (Ed.). (1965). The young deaf child: Identification and management. *Acta Oto-Laryngologica Suppl., 206*(5), 1–258.

Davis, H., & Silverman, S. R. (1970). Forward to the first edition (1947). In H. Davis & S. R. Silverman (Eds.), *Hearing and deafness* (3rd ed., pp. XV–XV1). New York, NY: Holt, Rinehart and Winston.

Durieux-Smith, A., Picton, T. W., Edwards, C. G., Goodman, J. T., & MacMurray, B. (1985). Brainstem electric-response audiometry in infants of neonatal intensive care unit. *International Journal of Audiology, 26,* 284–297.

Durieux-Smith, A., Picton, T., MacMurray, B., & Goodman, J. (1987). The Crib-o-gram in the NICU and evaluation based on brainstem electric response audiometry. *Ear and Hearing, 6,* 20–24.

Durieux-Smith, A., & Whittingham, J. (2000). The rationale for neonatal hearing screening. *Journal of Speech-Language Pathology and Audiology, 24,* 59–67.

Eriks-Brophy, A. (2004). Outcomes of auditory-verbal therapy: A review of the evidence and a call for action. *Volta Review, 104*(1), 21–35.

Ewing, A. W. G. (Ed.). (1957). *Educational guidance and the deaf child*. Washington, DC: The Volta Bureau.

Ewing, J. R., & Ewing, A. W. G. (1944). The ascertainment of deafness in infancy and early childhood. *Journal of Laryngology and Otology, 59*, 309–333.

Ewing, J. R., & Ewing, A. W. G. (1954). *Speech and the deaf child*. Washington, DC: The Volta Bureau.

Finitzo, T., Albright, K., & O'Neal, J. (1998). The newborn with hearing loss: Detection in the nursery. *Pediatrics, 102*(6), 1452–1460.

Fitzpatrick, E., Angus, D., Durieux-Smith, A., Graham, I., & Coyle, D. (2008). Parents needs following identification of childhood hearing loss. *American Journal of Audiology, 17*, 1–12.

Fitzpatrick, E., Durieux-Smith, A., Eriks-Brophy, A., Olds, J., & Gaines, R. (2007). The impact of newborn hearing screening on communication development. *Journal of Medical Screening, 14*, 123–131.

Galambos, R., Hicks, G. E., & Wilson, M. J. (1982). Hearing loss in graduates of a tertiary intensive care nursery. *Ear and Hearing, 3*, 87–90.

Galambos, R., Hicks, G. E., & Wilson, M. J. (1984). The auditory brain stem response reliably predicts hearing loss in graduates of a tertiary intensive care nursery. *Ear and Hearing, 5*, 254–260.

Geers, A. E., & Moog, J. (1989). Factors predicting the development of literacy in profoundly hearing-impaired adolescents. *Volta Review, 91*(2), 69–86.

Geers, A. E., Nicholas, J. G., & Sedley, A. L. (2003). Language skills of children with early cochlear implantation. *Ear and Hearing, 24*, 46S–58S.

Harris, J. D. (1965). Monaural and binaural speech intelligibility and the stereophonic effect based on temporal cues. *Laryngoscope, 75*, 428–446.

Hirsh, I. J. (1952). *The measurement of hearing*. New York, NY: McGraw-Hill.

Hyde, M. L. (2005). Newborn hearing screening programs: Overview. *Journal of Otolaryngology, 34*, S70–S78.

Hyde, M. L., Riko, K., & Malizia, K. (1990). Audiometric accuracy of the click ABR in infants at risk for hearing loss. *Journal of the American Academy of Audiology, 1*, 59-66.

Jacobson, C. A., & Jacobson, J. T. (1990). Follow-up services in newborn hearing screening programs. *Journal of the American Academy of Audiology, 4*, 181–186.

Jerger, S., Roeser, R. J., & Tobey, E. A. (2001). Management of hearing loss in infants: The UTD/Callier Center position statement. *Journal of the American Academy of Audiology, 12*, 329–336.

Joint Committee on Infant Hearing JCIH. (1982). Position statement 1982. *Pediatrics, 70*(3), 496–497.

Joint Committee on Infant Hearing JCIH. (1990). 1990 Position statements. *ASHA, 33*(Suppl. 5), 3–6.

Joint Committee on Infant Hearing JCIH. (1994). 1994 Position statement. *Pediatrics, 95*(1), 152–156.

Joint Committee on Infant Hearing JCIH. (2000). Year 2000 Position statement: Principles and guidelines for early hearing and intervention programs. *Pediatrics, 106*(4), 798–817.

Joint Committee on Infant Hearing JCIH. (2007). Year 2007 Position statement: Principles and guidelines for early hearing detection and intervention programs. *Pediatrics, 120*(4), 898– 921.

Joint Committee on Infant Screening JCIS. (1976). The supplementary statement of the Joint Committee on Infant Screening. In S. E. Gerber & G. T. Mencher (Eds.), *Early diagnosis of hearing loss* (Appendix 1, pp. 12–13). New York, NY: Grune and Stratton.

Joint Committee on Newborn Screening JCNS. (1970). Statement on neonatal screening for hearing impairment. In J. Northern, & M. P. Downs (Eds.), *Hearing in children* (1974, pp. 108–109). Baltimore, MD: Williams and Wilkins.

Jordan, O., Griesen, O., & Bentzen, O. (1967). Treatment with binaural hearing aids. *Archives of Otolaryngology, 85*, 319–326.

Kemp, D. T. (1980). Toward a model for the origin of cochlear echos. *Hearing Research, 2*, 533–548.

Kennedy, C. R., Kimm, L., Dees, D. C., Evans, P. I., Hunter, M., Lenton, S., & Thorton, R. D. (1991). Otoacoustic emissions and auditory brainstem responses in the newborn. *Archives of Diseases in Childhood, 66*, 1124–1129.

Kennedy, C. R., McCann, D. C., Campbell, M. J., Law, C. M., Mullee, M., Petrou, S., . . . Stevenson, J. (2006). Language ability after early detection of permanent childhood hearing impairment. *New England Journal of Medicine, 354*, 2131–2141.

Kileny, P. R. (1987). ALGO-1 automated infant hearing screener: Preliminary results. In K. P. Gerkin & A. Amochaev (Eds.), Hearing in infants: Proceedings from the National Symposium. *Seminars in Hearing, 8*, 125–131.

Killion, M. C. (1997). Hearing aids: Past, present and future: Moving toward normal conversations in noise. *British Journal of Audiology, 31*, 141–148.

Korres, S., Nikolopoulos, T. P., Komkotou, V., Balatsouras, D., Kandiloros, D., Constantinou, D., & Ferekidis, E. (2005). Newborn hearing screening: effectiveness, importance of high-risk factors, and characteristics of infants in the neonatal intensive care unit and well-baby nursery. *Otology & Neurotology, 26*(6), 1186–1190.

Ling, D. (2002). *Speech and the hearing-impaired child: Theory and practice* (2nd ed.). Washington, DC: Alexander Graham Bell Association for the Deaf.

Ling, D., & Ling, A. H. (1978). *Aural habilitation: The verbal foundations of learning in hearing-impaired children*. Washington, DC: A. G. Bell.

Lynas, W. (2005). Controversies in the education of deaf children. *Current Paediatrics, 15*, 200–206.

Lynas, W., Huntington, A., & Tucker, B. (1989). *A critical examination of different approaches to communication in the education of deaf children*. Manchester, UK: Department of Audiology, University of Manchester.

Marschark, M., Lang, H. G., & Albertini, J. A. (2002). *Educating deaf students: From research to practice*. New York, NY: Oxford University Press.

Marschark, M., & Spencer, P. E. (2006). Spoken language development of deaf and hard-of-hearing children: Historical and theoretical perspectives. In P. E. Spencer & M.

Marschark (Eds.), *Advances in the spoken language development of deaf and hard-of–hearing children* (pp. 3–21). New York, NY: Oxford University Press.

Mason, J. A., & Herrmann, K. R. (1998). Universal infant hearing screening by automated auditory brainstem response measurement. *Pediatrics, 103*(3), 670–672.

Mauk, G. W., White, K. R., Mortensen, L. B., & Behrens, T. R. (1991). The effectiveness of screening programs based on high-risk characteristics in early identification of hearing impairment. *Ear and Hearing, 2*, 312–319.

Mencher, G. (Ed.). (1976). *Early identification of hearing loss*. New York, NY: Basel, Karger.

Meyer, S. E., Jardine, C. A., & Deverson, W. (1997). Developmental changes in tympanometry: A case study. *British Journal of Audiology, 31*, 189–195.

Moodie, S., Seewald, R. C., & Sinclair, S. T. (1994). Procedure for predicting real-ear hearing aid performance in young children. *American Journal of Audiology, 3*, 23–31.

Moog, J. S., & Geers, A. E. (2003). Epilogue: Major findings, conclusions and implications for deaf education. *Ear and Hearing, 24*, 1215–1255.

National Institutes of Health (NIH). (1993). Early identification of hearing impairment in infants and young children. *NIH Consensus Statement, 11*, 1–24.

Niemoeller, A. F., Silverman, S. R., & Davis, H. (1970). Hearing aids. In H. S. Davis (Ed.), *Hearing and deafness* (3rd ed., pp. 280–317). New York, NY: Holt, Rinehart and Winston.

Northcott, W. H. (1990). Mainstreaming: Roots and wings. In M. Ross (Ed.), *Hearing-impaired children in the mainstream* (pp. 1–25). Parkton, MD: York Press.

Northern, J. L., & Downs, M. P. (1974). *Hearing in children*. Baltimore, MD: Williams and Wilkins.

Owens, E., & Kessler, D. K. (Eds.). (1989). *Cochlear implants in young deaf children*. Boston, MA: College-Hill Press.

Prieve, B., & Stevens, F. (2000). The New York State universal newborn hearing screening demonstration project: Introduction and overview. *Ear and Hearing, 21*, 85–91.

Robinshaw, H., & Evans, R. (2003). Service provision for preschool children who are deaf: Parents' perspectives. *Journal of Social Work in Disability and Rehabilitation, 2*, 3–39.

Ross, M. (1969). Changing concepts in hearing aid candidacy. *Eye, Ear, Nose and Throat Monographs, 48*, 27–34.

Ross, M. (1977). Hearing aids. In B. Jaffe (Ed.), *Hearing loss in children—a comprehensive text*. Baltimore, MD: University Park Press.

Sanders, D. A. (1993). *Management of hearing handicaps* (3rd ed.). Englewood Cliffs, NJ: Prentice-Hall.

Schick, B., Marschark, M., & Spencer, P. E. (Eds.). (2005). *Advances in the sign language development of deaf children*. New York, NY: Oxford University Press.

Schildroth, A. N., & Karchmer, M. A. (Eds.). (1986). *Deaf children in America*. San Diego, CA: College-Hill Press.

Schulman-Galambos, C., & Galambos, R. (1979). Brain stem evoked response audiometry in newborn hearing screening. *Archives of Otolaryngology, Head and Neck Surgery, 105*, 86–90.

Silverman, S. R. (1970). From Aristotle to Bell. In H. Davis & S. R. Silverman (Eds.), *Hearing and deafness* (3rd ed., pp. 375–383). New York, NY: Holt, Rinehart and Winston.

Silverman, S. R. & Lane, H. S. (1970). Deaf children. In H. Davis & S. R. Silverman (Eds.), *Hearing and deafness* (3rd ed., pp. 384–425). New York, NY: Holt, Rinehart and Winston.

Simmons, B., & Russ, F. N. (1974). Automated newborn hearing screening, the Crib-o-gram. *Archives of Otolaryngology, 100*, 1–7.

Simser, J. (1993). Auditory-verbal intervention: Infants and toddlers. *Volta Review, 95*(3), 217–229.

Spencer, P. E., & Marschark, M. (Eds.). (2006). *Advances in spoken language development of deaf and hard-of-hearing children*. New York, NY: Oxford University Press.

Stapells, D. R. (2000). Threshold estimation by tone-evoked auditory brainstem response; A literature meta-analyses. *Journal of Speech Language Pathology and Audiology, 24*, 74–83.

Stapells, D. R., & Oates, P. (1997). Estimation of the pure tone audiogram by the auditory brainstem response: A review. *Audiology & Neuro-Otology, 2*, 257–280.

Stelmachowicz, P. G. (2005). Pediatric amplification: Past, present, and future. In R. C. Seewald & J. M. Bamford (Eds.), *A sound foundation through early amplification: Proceedings of the third international conference* (pp. 27–40). Stäfa, Switzerland: Phonak AG.

Stevens, J. C., Webb, H. D., Hutchinson, J., Connell, J., Smith, M. F., & Buffin, J. T. (1989). Click evoked otoacoustic emissions compared with brain stem electric response. *Archives of Diseases in Childhood, 64*(8), 1105–1111.

Stevens, J., Webb, H., Hutchinson, J., Connell, J., Smith, M., & Buffin, J. (1990). Click evoked otoacoustic emissions in neonatal screening. *Ear and Hearing, 11*, 128–133.

Tattersall, H., & Young, A. (2006). Deaf children identified through newborn hearing: Parents' experiences of the diagnostic process. *Child: Care Health and Development, 32*, 33–45.

Thoutenhoofd, E., Arhbold, A., Gregory, S., Lutman, M., Nikilopoulos, T., & Sach, T. (2005). *Pediatrics cochlear implantation: Evaluating outcomes*. London, UK: Whurr.

Uus, K., & Bamford, J. (2006). Effectiveness of population-based newborn hearing screening in England: Ages of interventions and profile of cases. *Pediatrics, 117*(5), e887–e893.

Wake, M., Poulakis, Z., Hughes, E. K., Carey-Sargeant, C., & Rickards, F. W. (2005). Hearing impairment: A population study of age at diagnosis, severity, and language outcomes at 7–8 years. *Archives of Disease in Childhood, 90*, 238–244.

Watkin, P. M., Baldwin, M., & McEnery, G. (1991). Neonatal at risk screenings and the identification of deafness. *Archives of Disease in Childhood, 66*(10 Spec. No.), 1130–1135.

Wedenburg, E. (1956). Auditory tests on newborn infants. *Acta Otolaryngologica, 45*, 446–461.

White, K. R., & Behrens, T. R. (Eds). (1993). The Rhode Island Hearing Assessment Project: Implications for universal newborns hearing screening. *Seminars in Hearing, 14*, 1–119.

Wong, D., & Shah, C. D. (1979). Identification of impaired hearing in early childhood. *Canadian Medical Association Journal, 121*(5), 529–546.

Wright, L. B., & Rybak, L. P. (1983). Crib-o-gram (COG) and ABR effect of variables on test results. *Journal of the Acoustical Society of America, 74*, 540–544.

Vohr, B. R., Carty, L. M., Moore, P. E., & Letourneau, K. (1998). The Rhode Island Hearing Assessment Program: experience with statewide hearing screening (1993–1996). *Journal of Pediatrics, 133*(3), 353–357.

Yoshinaga-Itano, C., Sedley, A. L., Coulter, D. K., & Mehl, A. L. (1998). Language of early- and later-identified children with hearing loss. *Pediatrics, 102*, 1161–1171.

Young, A., & Tattersall, H. (2007). Universal newborn hearing screening and early identification of deafness: Parents' responses to knowing early and their expectations of child communication development. *Journal of Deaf Studies and Deaf Education, 12*, 209–220.

31

Facilitating Communication in Infants and Toddlers With Hearing Loss

Melody Harrison

Introduction

In the first decade of the 21st century, several factors have combined to dramatically alter the potential for children with hearing loss, even those with significant hearing loss, to develop spoken language. These factors include, of course, the implementation of newborn hearing screening and the development of increasingly sophisticated hearing aids and cochlear implants. The success of these innovations in early detection and management of hearing loss can be compromised or even negated, however, unless careful attention is given to development of auditory learning and subsequent language development.

Following a diagnosis of hearing loss, some families will be fortunate enough to have access to speech-language pathologists, early service providers, or teachers with excellent training in the development of audition and spoken language. Unfortunately for many families and their children, there are substantial barriers to accessing optimal services. As efforts to identify hearing loss in infants have become more and more successful and technologic innovations have occurred, stresses on early intervention programs in the United States have both increased and changed. Services for infants are being requested in rapidly increasing numbers. In some states the number of children with hearing loss enrolled in early intervention has tripled in the last few years (White, 2006). Clearly, the early age at which identification now occurs has altered the skills required of service providers who must now be knowledgeable about multiple aspects of development from the earliest months of infancy to adolescence or later. Additionally, they must have skills in working collaboratively with parents as a team. In a child's earliest years, parents play the primary role in developing their child's auditory and language abilities, thus the professionals who provide services to very young children and their families must assume the roles of coach and mentor in guiding families to acquire skills they never expected or wanted to have.

Perhaps more dramatically, the nature of services requested has altered. Given that almost 95% of children with hearing loss are born to hearing parents (Mitchell & Karchmer, 2004); identification of hearing loss is occurring by 6 months of age and earlier (Harrison, Roush, & Wallace, 2003); and amplification or implantation technology can provide audition across an increasing range of the speech spectrum (Glista et al., 2009), parents are choosing auditory/oral communication in rapidly increasing numbers. In a 10-year period the percent of parents selecting auditory/oral programs for their children in North Carolina, more than doubled from 40% in 1995 to 85% in 2005 (Brown, 2006). Unfortunately, the demand for professionals with skills in developing spoken language does not correspond with the focus within personnel preparation programs.

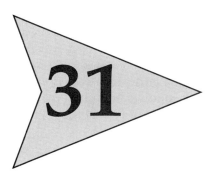

White (2006) reported that only 8% of graduates of deaf/hard of hearing teacher education programs were from programs with an emphasis on spoken language development. Speech-language pathologists in the United States are required to take only one audiology course, usually as undergraduates, but are no longer required to take even an introductory aural habilitation/rehabilitation course to qualify for ASHA certification. Few early childhood or early special education programs offer any coursework or experiences related to childhood hearing loss. The result is that in many cases, professionals providing early services have little or no education regarding the effects of hearing loss on the development of spoken language, or the knowledge and skills to develop communication based on the child's auditory abilities. In contrast, research suggests that services designed specifically for children with hearing loss result in better outcomes than general special education (Nittrouer & Burton, 2002).

When access to professionals prepared to guide families in developing spoken language is unavailable, the audiologist is likely to be the individual to whom the family, as well as other professionals, turns as the expert regarding all things related to hearing loss, including oral language development. This chapter has been designed primarily as a resource for those audiologists who find themselves in such a role. It is not a step-by-step guide to auditory, language, and speech development, but rather provides a framework the practicing audiologist can use to support others in the child's sphere, especially family members, to create an accessible and responsive communication environment that can maximize the hearing technology that has been fitted.

Working with parents to help them learn about their child's developing auditory skills provides numerous opportunities for an audiologist to develop a collaborative relationship with the family. In addition, as parents learn about their child's hearing loss they gain not only knowledge, but also acquire a sense of mastery over a body of information that initially seems alien and overwhelming. Most parents want to be actively involved in providing solutions to the challenges and limitations created by their child's hearing loss. Engaging the family in the process of habilitation, including consistent device use and maintenance, control of the child's listening environment and promotion of early communication and auditory development provides excellent opportunities for parents to understand the hearing loss and to accept and even promote device use. As clinical experience has demonstrated and research has supported, those children with the best language outcomes by school age are those whose parents have invested time and attention in early intervention and hearing loss management from the beginning (Moeller, 2000). Calderon and her colleagues have reported that early parental involvement has resulted in improved reading skills (Calderon & Naidu, 2000) and better communication between parent and child (Calderon, Bargones, & Sidmans, 1998). As the Chinese proverb states, "One parent is more valuable than a thousand schoolmasters."

This chapter is divided into two primary sections. The first covers topics related to management of the child's listening environments, which is essential to listening and spoken language development. The second is devoted to the fundamentals of how to facilitate early communication development for a child who has hearing loss.

Managing the Listening Environment

Developing Mastery of Hearing Aid Maintenance

The most important event in the development of a child's auditory and communication development is an accurate prescriptive hearing aid fitting. Even prescriptively fitted aids however, are of little benefit if they are not well maintained, or if they are not worn for most of the child's waking hours. The two most fundamental tasks in developing auditory skills and language are: (1) teaching parents to perform a daily listening check of their child's equipment, and (2) helping them understand the importance of device use. Although these tasks may seem to be too obvious to address, they are the foundation of communication development. Yet, they often receive only cursory attention when hearing aids are initially fitted and even less thereafter. Elfenbein (1994) reported that although parents were aware of the need to check their preschoolers hearing aids, they lacked the necessary equipment and skills to accomplish the task. Even when they did check the hearing aids they frequently missed cues that the device was not functioning properly. In response to questions regarding their child's hearing aid fitting, parents reported their greatest concern was the care and maintenance of the hearing aids and feeling overwhelmed by the technology provided for their child (Sjoblad, Harrison, Roush, & McWilliam, 2004). Moeller, Hoover, Peterson, and Stelmachowicz (2009) queried parents of young children regarding their early experiences with hearings aids. One of the findings was that many parents need ongoing support in the management of their child's hearing technology throughout early childhood. Most manufacturers of hearing aids and cochlear implants provide information about care and maintenance of the device at the time of purchase as well as on their Web sites. However, the old adage regarding learning a clinical skill, "Watch One, Do One, Teach One," is useful in helping a parent master a comprehensive listening and maintenance check. As described in Chapter 29 on hearing aid orientation, before sending the family home with new hearing instruments, it is important to demonstrate a maintenance and listening check. However, as important as this initial demonstration is in developing a parent's sense of comfort and competence with these instruments, it is only the first of many steps in establishing consistent use of optimally functioning devices.

After a comprehensive listening and hearing aid check has been demonstrated, ask the parent to practice it with you. It almost certainly will be necessary to provide cues the first time through. Coaching the family through a maintenance check as they begin to master the task, in addition to demonstrating it provides a multidimensional learning experience. Written instructions, preferably illustrated, will support them as they conduct the check at home. On the family's first return visit, reinforce the importance of conducting this daily task by asking them to run through the hearing aid check to confirm that they are comfortable with the process. Although this may require more time than the audiologist would like to devote to the task, the time spent assuring that parents are comfortable assessing devices function is well worth the investment. Once it is clear that one family member is knowledgable about and confident in the ability to complete a routine check, that individual should be asked to teach one other person in the household how to conduct a check. Not only is teaching a skill the final step in mastery, it ensures that more than one person in the family can complete the task.

In the future, the family will need to learn how to conduct a maintenance and listening check on each device and each combination of devices their child uses. For example, if more than one program/memory is available or an FM system is used, they must listen to each of these to check there is a clear and undistorted signal. If an FM system is used at home, instruct the family how to set the FM microphone/transmitter close to radio or television and listen to the signal as they move to different areas of the house to check for interference. As the child becomes older and begins to use the telephone, that signal will need to be tested as well. By this point, the child is old enough to become involved in monitoring their own equipment. Each time a new program or device is added to the child's array, remind the family to include it in the daily listening check.

Daily Maintenance Routine

Although a daily maintenance check may initially require more time as families are learning to master the task, they should be encouraged to anticipate that once they are familiar with it, the maintenance check typically will take less than 5 minutes a day. The daily maintenance check is most likely to become part of the family's routine if it is completed at the same time every day. For some families this may be after the child goes to sleep in the evening, for other it may be first thing in the morning or at nap time. When a family has difficulty incorporating the daily maintenance check into their routine, a demonstration of the importance of a well functioning instrument might be motivating. Some audiologists and speech pathologists have used poorly functioning hearing aids to demonstrate the differences in the signal produced by a well-maintained instrument versus one that has not been to illustrate the importance of this activity.

Daily Listening Check and Hearing Aid Use

In addition to the hearing aid maintenance check, the family should also learn how to conduct a quick listening check using the Ling-6-Sound Test (Ling, 1989). The sounds included in the Ling-6-Sound Test are /ah/, /ee/, /oo/, /s/, /sh/, and /m/. These were selected because they cover the range of speech sounds we hear and say, from the lowest frequencies in /m/ around 500 Hz, to the highest in /s/ which contains frequencies as high as 8400 Hz, depending on the vowel context and the gender of the speaker (Boothroyd & Medwetsky, 1992). Each sound should be presented at a normal conversational level. Using a stetheset, parents or other caregivers should listen for clarity with no distortion or unwanted noise in the signal as each of the sounds is presented. The Ling-6-Sound Test can be used by anyone, audiologists, speech language pathologists, teachers, and parents to conduct a listening check. It can also be used for a variety of purposes ranging from simple detection of the presence of sound, to discrimination and identification.

Initially, a parent will use a stetheset to do a daily listening check as they say each of the six sounds; however, as soon as the child is old enough to respond reliably, and this will depend on the interplay of cognitive ability, chronologic age, and to some degree personality, the child should become the listener. At approximately 18 months of age a child can begin to produce a reliable response to sounds they detect. Their response can be any of a wide variety of actions including clapping or some other physical activity such as tossing a toy in a box. Then as soon as they are able, the child should be encouraged to imitate the sounds as they are presented. Children who were prescriptively fitted with hearing aids soon after birth and are able to hear sounds across the speech spectrum are likely to begin to imitate some of the sounds by 18 months of age.

Parents should be reminded that this is an auditory-only task. The child should not be able to see their parent's mouth; however, placing a hand or an object too close to the mouth can distort the signal and so modeling the technique is helpful. Demonstrating how to conduct a daily listening check should require less than a minute, and the long-term payoff can be considerable. Whether the child is fitted with hearing aids or has cochlear implant(s), use of the Ling 6-Sound Test is an excellent way to monitor device function. Appendixes 31–A and 31–B provide additional details regarding the maintenance of hearing aids and cochlear implants, respectively.

Remind parents to: (1) practice presenting all the sounds at *relatively* equal degrees of intensity (given the frequency range the word relatively is stressed), (2) vary the order of presentation of the sounds so that the child doesn't learn a specific presentation pattern, and (3) present all sounds at the same distance from the child. When parents begin to explore the range of their child's listening abilities, sounds will be presented at varying distances; however, for the purpose of checking the working condition of the equipment, distance should be constant. Presentation of the sounds, one at a time and waiting for the child to imitate provides a check of the overall integrity of the system.

When parents are able to identify positive changes in their child's auditory behavior they may be more likely to persevere in device use (Harrison, 2000). Sharing a brief instrument such as the Infant-Toddler Meaningful Auditory Integration Scale (IT-MAIS; Zimmerman-Philips, Osberger, & Robbins, 1997) with parents may be useful in assisting them to observe and record changes in their child's auditory behaviors with hearing aid use. The questions are straightforward with a simple response format and the directions are clearly written. Although it was developed for children with cochlear implants, the IT-MAIS can be used with children who have lesser degrees of hearing loss, although it is not likely to be sensitive enough to demonstrate change among children with mild-moderate hearing loss.

Hearing aid or cochlear implant use is the foundation of successful spoken language development and creating a shared understanding of the importance of device use and a team approach (a team that will eventually include the child) to hearing device management is a cornerstone to successful device use.

The Roles of Distance and Noise in Facilitating Communication Development

Understanding how distance and noise affect audibility is a key element in developing listening and language skills in a child with hearing loss. The role of distance in relation to audibility may be one of the least abstract and therefore most easily understood by parents and the professionals who work with the child's family. The inverse square rule, known to all audiologists, states that the sound pressure of a spherical wave-front radiating from a point source decreases by 50% as the distance is doubled. Measured in dB, it decreases by 6.02 dB as the distance is doubled. The behavior actually is not inverse-square, but is inverse-proportional. Simply translated, however, it means that as a sound source moves away from the child, the more difficult it will be for the child to hear and understand the sound. As basic as this concept might seem, it is not immediately evident to most individuals. Many parents and even some professionals do not understand the importance of distance. A simple demonstration using a nonsense word and having the adult begin at a distance of 12 to 15 feet away from the sound source may assist in explaining the important role distance plays. One of the strategies employed in auditory-verbal therapy when the child fails to respond to the auditory signal is reducing the distance between the sound source and child. Reducing distance is an easy, low-tech strategy adults interacting with the child should know about and use. The pediatric audiologist may be the only person in the child's sphere who is aware of this information.

Young children typically live in very noisy environments, and listening for language can be a challenging task even for those with normal hearing. Homes are often filled with the sounds of other children, the television, radio, or video games. In child care centers and preschools the sounds and noise of childhood activities and mishaps reverberate. Providing children who have hearing loss with as many opportunities as possible to listen in situations in which the auditory signal is accessible is absolutely necessary for successful language development. Recent research at the University of Washington reported that television exposure of young children between 2 and 48 months of age was associated with significantly reduced child vocalizations. In addition, the number of words uttered to them by adults with television on was reduced. Every additional hour of television exposure resulted in further reduction in both child and adult scores. Not only does television increase noise in the environment, Christakis et al. (2009) demonstrated that when television was on, significantly less language was directed to the child by adults in the home. Thirty percent of households in the United States report that the television is on all of the time. Young children who are at risk for developing auditory-based language are even more vulnerable to the negative effects of television than children with hearing in the normal range.

Encourage families to be aware of the noise level in the child's environments, and whenever possible turn off the television and reduce extraneous noise

A useful tool to share with parents and early service providers who are less familiar with the influence noise and distance have on listening is the test of Early Listening Function (ELF), developed by Anderson (2002). The ELF was designed to obtain an estimate of a child's functional use of hearing as it relates to distance and noise. The concept that is presented and reinforced in the ELF is that of the child's "Listening Bubble." The "Listening Bubble" represents the variable area surrounding a child within which sounds with differing degrees of loudness can be heard. The "bubble" is wider for louder sounds and more restricted for those that are quieter. The ELF describes 12 specific, contrived listening activities that can easily be performed at home. Parents are asked to determine if their child exhibits a behavioral response at specified distances, in quiet and "typically noisy" conditions. As they perform the various tasks described in the ELF, parents gain knowledge about how far away their child can hear a variety of sounds under several different conditions. The activities can be conducted over a period of days or even weeks. In fact, one strategy that has been successful is to break the ELF into smaller subsets of activities. When the family completes the activities and returns for their next appointment, their observations are shared and discussed with the pediatric audiologist. The next set is then sent home. Engaging the professionals who are providing early services in administration of the ELF creates a valuable learning opportunity for those who are unfamiliar with the challenges created by hearing loss and can assist in opening communication between the audiologist and the early service providers. The results of the activities provide parents with a clear understanding of exactly how far away from a sound their child can be and what the listening conditions must be for the child to be able to hear.

Results from the ELF guide parents in discovering the role distance and noise play in their child's specific listening ability. One family may learn that although a sound is audible in quiet conditions at a distance of 9 feet, in noisy conditions the same sound is inaudible at 6 feet. Another may learn that their child's listening bubble is less than 6 feet for a sound in quiet and in noise they are unable to hear the sound at all. As parents gain expertise in estimating the size of their child's listening bubble, they begin to become knowledgeable about the conditions that must be present in the child's auditory environment for listening and language learning to occur.

Parents who have been sufficiently supported in learning about their child's listening environment and understand the importance of device use have accomplished two very important tasks. First, they have learned to provide the conditions necessary for auditory learning. Perhaps even more importantly, in the process they have acquired knowledge and learned new skills that increase their self confidence regarding management of their child's hearing loss. The role of early interventionists in "help-giving" practices is to provide opportunities for families to learn strategies and techniques for working with their young children so that they develop confidence in their own competence. DesJardin (2006) points out that the key elements of "self-efficacy," or belief in our ability to accomplish a goal, are knowledge and confidence. Whether the professional is an early services specialist, an early childhood special educator, a speech-language pathologist, or an audiologist, the essential components to developing parental self efficacy are: (1) to provide parents with knowledge, and then (2) to support them in persisting in mastering a goal until they are successful. The importance of both of these elements of self-efficacy as it relates to parent-child relationships was demonstrated by Conrad, Goss, Fogg, and Ruchala (1992) who reported that when mothers saw themselves as being less competent, an increase in knowledge alone failed to change the quality of mother-child interactions. In contrast, increased knowledge positively changed the interactions of those mothers who had perceived themselves to be more competent. Simply providing parents with information is not always sufficient. Mastery of a goal is essential to achieving self-efficacy and those parents who do not think of themselves as able to be successful need support to incrementally achieve the goals that will foster their child's development. Partnerships among audiologists, speech pathologists, early intervention specialists, and families are often necessary to accomplish mastery.

The Building Blocks of Language Learning

Linking early speech perception to later language development can be helpful in explaining the need for early and consistent device use to parents. Indirect evidence of the role speech perception plays in language and reading development can be found in studies of children with normal hearing. Much of this work comes from the area of reading and learning disabilities and is drawn from studies of children who have normal peripheral hearing but appear to be unable to use auditory information in an effective manner. Reed (1989) demonstrated that children with reading disabilities were much poorer at discriminating consonants compared to children the same age with no reading challenges. Links between deficits in speech perception abilities and reduced language skills have been strongly established in children with specific language impairment (Leonard, McGregor, & Allen, 1992). These studies are representative of a large body of work supporting the idea that a child's ability to accurately extract information from an auditory signal is directly related to later language and reading development. Hearing loss obviously creates a barrier to the acquisition of information from an auditory signal. Hearing aids and cochlear implants can, when fitted and used optimally, provide the only means to access the information essential to development of speech and language.

Recently, a relationship between babies' ability to discriminate between vowels at 6 months of age and their later vocabulary, as measured by the number of words produced, was described by Kuhl and her colleagues (Kuhl, Conboy, Padden, Nelson, & Pruitt, 2005). Six-month-old babies who were able to discriminate between two simple vowels /i/ (tea) and /u/ (two), had larger vocabularies when they were 18 and 24 months old as measured by the MacArthur Communicative Development Inventory (Fenson et al., 1993) than babies who could not. Furthermore, babies with the highest level of vowel discrimination had the largest vocabularies. Early vocabulary development is vitally important because it remains one of the strongest predictors of overall language ability at school-age. Language ability in turn, is a strong predictor of academic achievement. These findings, in conjunction with a number of supporting studies, led Kuhl and her colleagues to propose a theory of native language neural commitment (NLNC).

Simply stated, NLNC posits that language acquisition depends upon early phonetic learning in a baby's native language. Babies who are most able to capture phonemic contrasts such as those in the words "tea" and "two" are creating neural connections essential for native language development. When infants are born and for several months afterward, their phonetic discrimination is universal. That is, they are responsive to phonemes in their own language as well as to those of other, very different, languages. By the time they are a year old, however, their ability to discriminate nonnative phonemes has declined significantly. NLNC proposes that early phonetic learning alters perception, as illustrated by our rapidly changing ability to discriminate phonemic differences and thus, changes future phoneme and language learning ability. Native language neural commitment drives language learning early in a baby's life by committing neurons to phonemic discrimination tasks. This theory hypothesizes that the trajectory of language learning between 7 and 30 months of age is highly dependent on an infant's level of sophistication in learning native language phonemic structure well before the age of 12 months. In fact, in a study of 6-month-old infants Kuhl and her colleagues demonstrated that exposure to a specific language in the first half-year of life altered the infants' phonetic perception (Kuhl, Williams, Lacerda, Stevens, & Lindbolm, 1991). For professionals who work with families choosing an oral/auditory approach, this work offers support and motivation for promoting consistent use of amplification that can provide access to audition across the entire speech range. When audibility of speech cannot be achieved with hearing aid fitting, advocacy for cochlear implantation as early as feasible should occur.

Even when hearing loss is identified at birth and hearing aids are optimally fitted, children with profound hearing loss are not likely to have access to audition to the degree that they make the phonemic discriminations described above. Recent studies conducted by Stelmachowicz and her colleagues (Stelmachowicz, Pittman, Hoover, & Lewis, 2001; Stelmachowicz, Pittman, Hoover, Lewis, & Moeller, 2004; Stelmachowicz et al., 2008) have suggested that reduced audibility in the high frequencies (because of the bandwidth of hearing instruments) restricts access to important phonemes in English and thus plays a role in the delays in phonological development often exhibited by children with hearing impairment. McGowen and colleagues (2008) found that even when profoundly deaf infants were identified at birth and consistently used amplification, at the age of 12 months they had fewer multisyllabic utterances with consonants; produced fewer fricatives (/f/, /s/, and /sh/) and fewer stops with alveolar-velar stop place (/t/, /d/); and more restricted front-back tongue position for vowels. This was attributed to restricted output of hearing aids. As seen in Figure 31–1, discrimination of all of the elements of speech requires audition across a wide range of frequencies.

Most hearing aids are capable of providing audibility only to approximately 3000 Hz. However, according to Boothroyd and Medwetsky (1992) some of the phonemes that carry important information in English require audition in frequencies up to 8300 Hz, depending on age and gender of the speaker and the vowel context. It is reasonable to assume that babies are unlikely to produce phonemic content to which they have never had access. Recent advances in hearing aid technology, specifically frequency compression

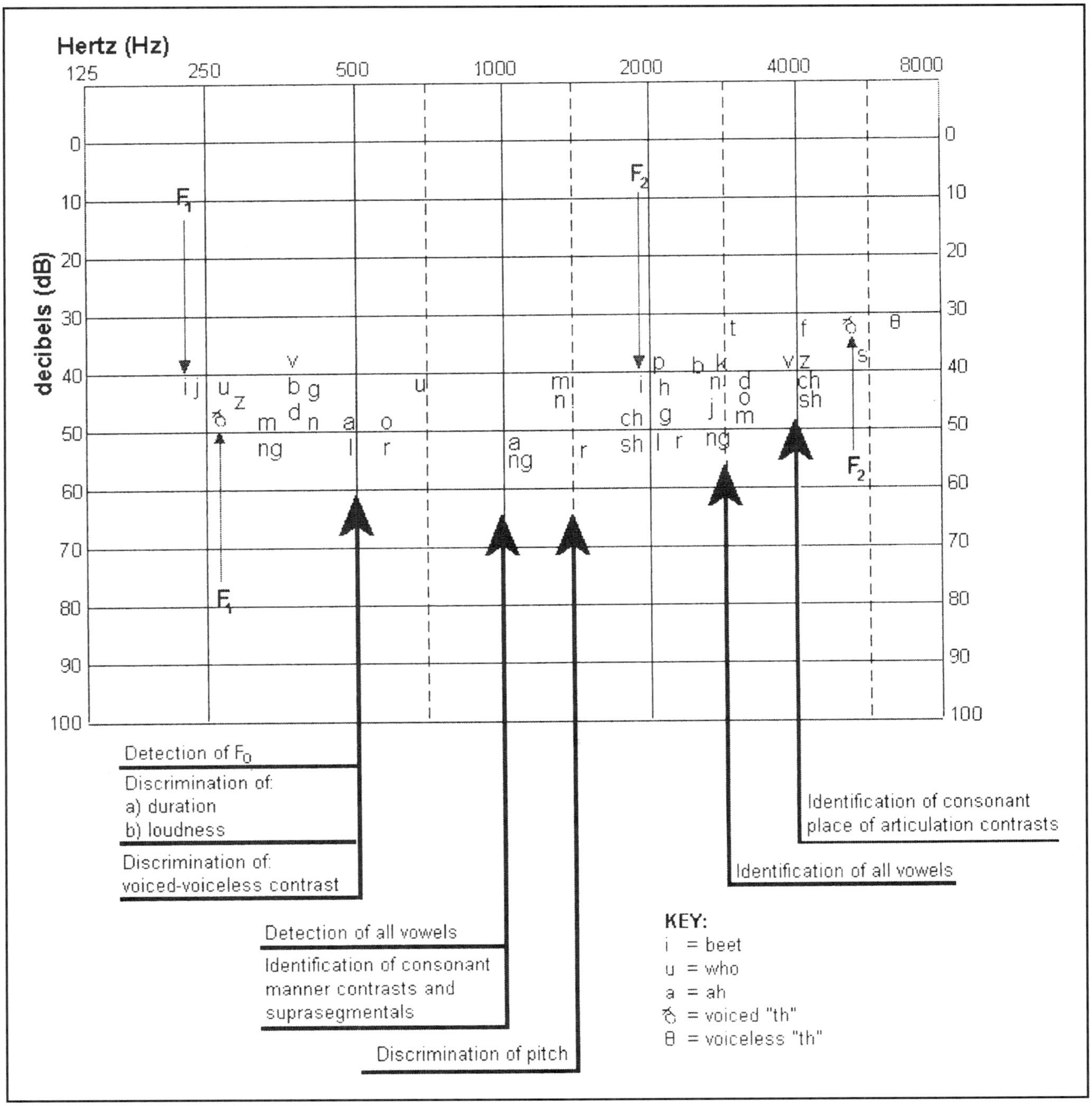

FIGURE 31–1. An audiometric representation of the suprasegmental aspects and relative intensity of the primary components of spoken English. Reprinted with permission from Edwards, C. (1988). *Seminar in educational audiology.* Auditory Management Services, Toronto, Canada.

strategies, which provide audibility of important high-frequency phonemes, may provide infants with more of the information they need to hear the high-frequency phonemes necessary for vocabulary and language acquisition (Glista et al., 2009). Later language development appears to heavily depend on acquisition of the phonemic elements of a language prior to twelve months of age. This requires exposure to language for most of a child's waking hours from birth. The consequences of failing to establish a pattern of consistent hearing aid use as early as possible in a child's life can very negatively affect later language outcomes. These effects can be seen as early as 2 years of age.

Language Facilitation Strategies

The First Few Months

Beginning in the first few days of an infant's life, parents and babies engage in mutual, reciprocal gazing. Babies only a few weeks old will attempt, often quite successfully, to imitate facial expressions. A bit later they begin to vocalize in response to an adult's simple vocal model. This interaction, although quite endearing, is also an important communication benchmark indicating the establishment of "conversational" turn-taking and the earliest steps in developing joint attention and gestural communication. At this early point, a communicative relationship has begun to develop between a parent and child. A positive communicative strategy that parents can begin to use with very young babies is *waiting*. Encourage parents to model a face or a sound for their baby and then wait . . . and wait a while longer, to allow the baby time to organize a response. The strategy of waiting is one that will be useful across the child's language acquisition years and it is never too early for adults, parents, and professionals, to learn to use it. Most adults enjoy this type of interaction with babies but few are aware of the developmental importance of the activity. Knowledge that establishing mutual gazing and attempts at imitation of facial expressions are early forms of communication and an early developmental step may promote increased interaction between parents and their infant.

Very young infants can easily be positioned so that they are supported and close enough to clearly see the parents or caregivers face. An ideal situation is to have the adult sit on the floor with their back against a wall or sturdy furniture with their legs together and knees bent so that they form an inverted "V." Place the baby so that the back rests against the parent's thighs and the feet are on the parent's chest. In this position the baby has a clear view of the adult's face, is secure and comfortable, and the adult is an ideal visual and auditory distance from the child. In addition, both of their hands are free. As the baby grows, an infant seat can be used while maintaining a similar distance, at least initially, for interactions. In the beginning, encourage parents to interact with their babies in the simplest ways. Look at them and smile, tell them they are adorable. If the baby's eyes open widely, encourage the parents to imitate. Have them smile, or open their mouths and then wait for the baby to imitate them. At this stage, the goal is to develop mutual gazing, reciprocity, and early turn-taking; thus, it is essential that the baby be able to clearly see the adult's face. Later, when the focus shifts to auditory development it may be more appropriate for the adult to position themselves beside the child some of the time.

The Value of Routines

The earliest communication between adults and babies is based on an adult successfully reading the baby's cues and then responding appropriately to those cues. If a baby is fussy, and has not been fed for several hours, the mother may interpret the behavior as hunger and feed her. The mother's behavior is a signal to the baby, who may quiet down for a few moments when she sees preparations for a feeding underway. The baby has successfully communicated a need and in turn, the parent has successfully communicated that the need has been understood. The easier a baby's cues are to read, the more successful the parents will feel in responding; and the more predictable the parent's response, the more competent the baby can become in signaling their needs or states to the parents. Successful parent-infant communication, which in the earliest weeks is similar regardless of hearing status, contributes to parents' sense of self efficacy. The fundamental aspect of this earliest communication is reciprocity. The adult reads the baby's cues and then responds with cues or behaviors that the baby can easily understand. These successful interactions provide a perfect platform for early language learning. Every daily activity, whether it is feeding, bathing, burping, or dressing, can become a routine, something that is done in about the same way, with a similar outcome and at roughly the same time every day. Routines promote predictability through repetition, which is important to language learning for all children. Listening and language development depend on providing an environment that provides a wealth of opportunities to interact with competent language users (i.e., parents, siblings, and other caregivers). Predictability, consistency, and repetition are particularly important when barriers or challenges such as hearing loss are present. The earlier a child learns that sound is meaningful and can be predictive, (the sounds of food preparation mean eating and feeling satisfied) the more likely they are to integrate a wide range of sounds, including those of their native language, into their auditory awareness.

Routines provide an ideal context for the words, phrases and sentences and other communicative acts the baby is exposed to every day, day after day in a predictable manner. Coaching parents to: (1) identify their own routines, (2) recognize the language that can be incorporated into those routines, and (3) understand the importance of repetition in the routines, allows them to incorporate language learning activities without increasing either stress or time to their day. In fact, being knowledgable about strategies that support their child's language learning will likely reduce stress. Understanding how to use everyday routines also reinforces the idea that communication goes on throughout the entire day and is not a special event during a specified period of time that has to be set aside to "work with" the child.

Early Strategies: Birth to Three Months

From birth until the baby is about 3 to 4 months of age, encourage parents to talk about the child's immediate realm of experience; what they are *feeling* or *experiencing* at that moment. "You are so tired and sleepy. It's time to go to bed." or "Oooooh, you're all clean, let's get you nice and dry." If there are any concerns about the parents' understanding of baby talk or "motherese" demonstrate speaking in a sing-song manner typical of the speech that experienced parents use. Many but certainly not all parents seem to understand that such a manner of speaking is more engaging to babies. Motherese typically has a slightly higher pitch with clearly spoken words. It is slower with longer pauses between words and phrases and vowels are slightly enlongated. The vowel stretching that is found in motherese ("Ooooooh, you're aaall cleeeean!"), is an example of acoustic highlighting, a technique for focusing the child's attention on a specific piece of auditory information. The acoustic stretching of phonetically relevant information in infant directed speech focuses the child's attention on acoustic cues and appears to play an important role in speech discrimination. Tsao, Liu, and Kuhl (2004) used vowel stretching, typical in motherese and a recognized measure of speech intelligibility, as a measure of speech clarity. They found that the degree to which mothers engaged in vowel stretching was strongly related to infant speech perception skill at six months of age. When they measured the language ability of those babies at 13, 16, and 24 months there were significant correlations between individual infant's speech perception skills and their later language abilities including word understanding, word production, and phrase understanding as measured by the MacAuthur-Bates Development Communicative Inventory years (Fenson et al., 1993). It also is the case that adults using motherese tend to repeat their utterances. Again, repetition is an important element of early language learning and for children whose access to spoken language is degraded by hearing loss, repetition should be greatly increased. When children are developing typically, motherese begins to disappear by the time the child is about 2 years of age. However, clearly articulated speech, with some acoustic highlighting, is a technique used for children with hearing loss throughout childhood and beyond. It is one of the important early strategies for developing listening and language abilities.

Three to Six Months

As babies develop, their head and neck control matures permitting them to look from left to right as well as up and down. In addition, their visual field becomes wider and deeper providing expanded visual access to their environments. As a baby's world expands, so will the objects and experiences to which they are exposed. Around the time the baby is about three months of age, parents should begin to include vocabulary and language related to events or objects the surrounding child. People or objects that reappear frequently, such as the names of siblings or other family members, pets, toys or events that occur as part of daily routines, are typical examples. Linking words to objects, people, or activities assists the baby in attaching meaning to words and phrases. Guide parents to tune into what the baby appears to be interested in and comment or describe where they are visually focused. If something interesting is occurring and the baby is unaware of it, hold or turn them so they can see, draw their attention and then comment, "There's a bird." or "Look, Mommy's home!" Family routines remain a foundation for language acquisition. If for example, weekday mornings include taking an older sibling to the school bus stop, with the family dog in tow, vocabulary and language might focus on the sibling's name, the dog's name, school bus, stroller, or articles of clothing needed to stay warm. Phrases such as, "time for the bus" or "let's go" and "bye-bye" also can be part of the language routine. Critical elements in facilitating early language learning are: (1) talk about what is in the baby's immediate experience; and (2) the language should name or describe someone or something in which they are *interested*, and (3) ideally there should be opportunities to talk about the person, object, or event repeatedly.

Six to Twelve Months

Although people and objects in the child's environments remain the primary topics of conversation for many more months, in the second half of the child's first year language topics expand to keep pace with the baby's cognitive, social, and motor development.

For example, if a fire truck roars past with sirens blazing, a parent might say, "That was a loud fire truck." Likewise, when an older brother gets on the school bus and rides away, he can no longer be seen. He is not immediately present. However, it is entirely reasonable to talk about him and say, "Bye-bye, Nick, see you later." The objects and events are no longer in the baby's immediate environment; however, because of their saliency, one because it was big, red, and noisy, the other because he is such an important person in the baby's life, they can be referenced and their existence beyond the present moment has begun to be established.

At around this time, parents' vocabulary typically begins to expand to include descriptors of people and objects. Words such as happy, soft, clean, and dirty begin to appear more frequently. Other children are described as big girl or cute baby. The more opportunities a child has to interact with adults who are able to establish responsive, mutual communication focusing on the child's feelings, experiences, and environment in a predictable manner, the more likely they are to acquire new sounds and words. Even as topics, vocabulary, and language expand it continues to be important to pay attention to how far away from a sound source the child is and the level of noise in the environment. These factors should always be considered unless an FM system is being used. Use of clear speech with characteristics of motherese and waiting for a response should be characteristic of the adults' style of interaction by this time.

Book Sharing

Picture books for babies offer an excellent resource for facilitating vocabulary and language learning. At around 6 or 7 months of age, when the baby is old enough to have developed good head control and sit up with only slight props, parents can begin to use sturdy picture books with bright, interesting pages as a platform for language learning.

The baby should be positioned so that they can easily see both the book and the parent's face. Some parents seem intuitively to understand how to share books with infants, while others require guidance. If a relationship with a speech-language pathologist or other early service provider has been established, working with them to develop book-sharing skills with the parents can provide reinforcement for what will hopefully become an enjoyable activity for both the parent and the child. With both the baby and the adult in a comfortable position, have the adult point to a picture, or if the child is already attending to the book, point to their focus of attention, and then comment about the object. "It's a cute puppy." Next, the adult should look at the baby and once eye-contact has occurred, return their gaze to the picture, point to the same object and comment on the picture again. The act of directing the child's attention through the use of eye gaze and/or pointing is strategic in developing "joint attention." Joint attention is the process by which one individual alerts another to a person, object, or event through nonverbal means, such as gazing or pointing. Joint attention occurs when two partners share attention to the same subject. Learning to engage in joint attention is critical for a child's language, cognitive and social development. Book sharing not only creates opportunities for linguistic interaction, it is an activity that perfectly supports development of joint attention (Figure 31–2).

Some adults believe they need to read all the text in a book in much the same manner an adult might read to a linguistically competent 4-year-old. Babies, particularly those with hearing loss, are unable to manage this level of interaction and will respond negatively. Parents who have employed this approach to book sharing often report that their child does not like to read books. Pointing at, describing, and commenting to the child about the pictures constitutes how book sharing is ideally conducted at this age. Adults may also incorporate gestures such as pretending to sniff the picture of a flower, or scratching behind the ear of a picture of a puppy and then actually scratching behind the baby's ear to maintain their attention. Language and vocabulary should be descriptive and responsive to the baby's focus of attention, using an engaging voice with characteristics of motherese in a relatively quiet environment. As the baby's vocabulary and language understanding expand, the complexity of the pictures in books and the language used in book sharing should always match or be slightly beyond that of the child's.

Prelinguistic Communication: The Foundation of Language

Understandably, parents of a child with a hearing loss can become so focused on speech and oral language that they are unaware of the importance of nonverbal prelinguistic foundations of communication upon which later oral language is constructed. Coaching parents to be aware of and responsive to those early communication acts is extremely important in building language competency. Two of the basic prelinguistic constructs are *intent* and *gesture*, which are intricately linked. Behavior that clearly seeks to engage an adult's attention or

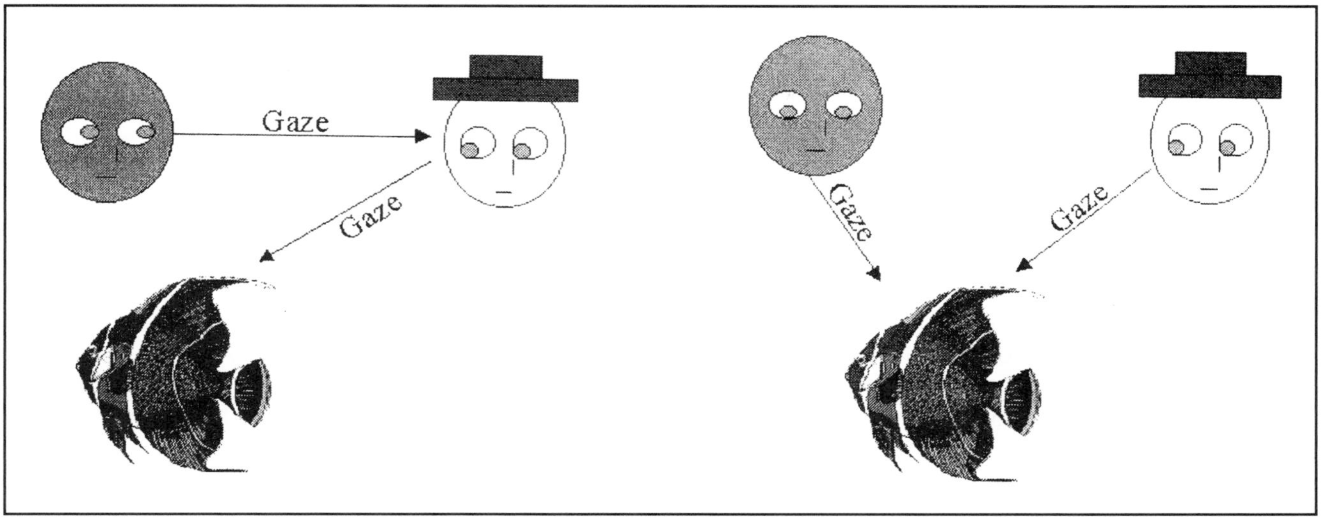

FIGURE 31–2. Joint attention: Using eye contact or gesture to show or direct the attention of another person. Reprinted with permission from http://eigsti.psy.uconn.edu/jt_attn.html by Inge-Marie Eigsti.

assistance can be called "intentional communication" and does not appear until the child understands that behavior can have an effect on the world (an adult). Learning cause and effect depends upon the cognitive and biological development of the child, as well as the types of experiences the child has had with adults. Iverson and Thal (1998) describe gestures as actions produced with the intent to communicate, typically with fingers, hands, and arms but sometimes including other parts of the body or lips. Gestures can be interpreted only in context and can involve a variety of objects and events.

More than 30 years ago, Elizabeth Bates demonstrated that infant gesture and nonverbal communicative functions or intentions provide a foundation for later verbal overlay. Prelinguistic communication is the only means of signaling early intentionality that typically developing children, regardless of their hearing status, begin to develop early in the first year of life. Not only is a child's level of prelinguistic communication an indicator of their current linguistic and cognitive development, it can serve as a predictor of later language competence (Crais, Douglass, & Campbell 2004; Mundy et al., 2007; Stoel-Gammon, 1999). Thus, being aware of and appropriately responding to prelinguistic communication reinforces the child's earliest attempts at communicating. For many years, the production of gestures by children with hearing loss was strongly discouraged as being a precursor of sign-language. Some programs went so far as to discourage toddlers from waving "bye-bye"; however, more recently the foundational role of gesture in the emergence of language has resulted in a different perspective regarding this fundamental communicative function.

The earliest gestures emerge between 7 and 9 months of age (Carpenter, Mastergeorge, & Coggins, 1983) and are referred to as "deitic gestures." Deitic gestures, which account for about 88% of the gesture repertoire in infants and toddlers, are divided into two categories, "contact" and "distal" gesture (Thal & Tobias, 1992). Contact gestures generally require physical contact between the child and an object or caregiver. Examples of deictic gestures with an object might be pushing an offered bottle away as if to say, "I don't want that." These often first appear as an open-handed gesture indicating that an object is desired or rejected. Another example of a deitic gesture is turning the head away from an object as an indication of refusal. Distal deictic gestures require no direct contact and typically involve pointing or reaching. One of the most universally recognized is a baby reaching with both arms up, indicating a desire to be picked up. Understanding the communicative value of a deitic gesture provides parents with opportunities to respond to the baby's communicative act and to provide appropriate linguistic input. For example, if a baby turns his head away from a spoonful of food it may be because he has had enough, or it might be that he does not care for strained peas. The parent's response depends on the knowledge of the context. If the baby has been eating spoonful after spoonful of peas and then turns his head, a logical interpretation of the gesture would be that he is full and the appropriate adult language something such as, "All done," "No more," or "You're full!" If the baby turns his head at the first spoonful, another interpretation is more probable.

The second major type of gesture, "representational gesture," appears near the end of the first year, around 12 months of age (Bates, Benigni, Bretherton, Camaioni, & Volterra, 1979) and typically occurs after deictic gestures emerge and are established. Representational gestures establish a reference and also indicate particular semantic or meaningful content. These gestures are used primarily to add information to a communicative exchange or to maintain the "listener's" attention. They can be "conventional" gestures that are used socially, such as blowing a kiss or waving goodbye, or they can be "object related" gestures that signify some feature of the referent, for example, pretending to give a baby doll a bottle or sniffing a flower.

Representational gestures often emerge within familiar routines and games such as peek-a-boo that parents and other caregivers use to engage children (Accredolo & Goodwyn, 1988). Representational gestures tend to require the parent's modeling of the gesture, and so, are dependent on parent practices, the amount of parental input, and the family routines. All of these are influenced by culture, beliefs, and tradition. One family may indicate "hungry" by rubbing their tummy, while another might do so by putting their fingers to the mouth. The importance of representational gestures as they relate to facilitating language development among children with hearing loss is that higher levels of gestural production have been associated with higher levels of comprehension among typically developing hearing children (Bates, Bretherton, & Snyder, 1988) and that the use of gesture is communicatively functional. Clearly, in order for gestures to provide a framework for later language learning to occur, language must be present in conjunction with gesture. Parents who react to their child's gestures with an action plus appropriate vocabulary and language are providing a rich linguistic environment that will promote language learning in a manner that responding without language cannot. Being aware of the role gesture plays in the development of communication and the opportunities gesture provides for adults to engage in meaningful, responsive, and reciprocal language can be pivotal in developing parent-child linguistic interaction in the early months of life.

Gesture Function

Understanding the function of a gesture is critical to determining an accurate response and the language to use. The function of children's prelinguistic communicative acts was first described by Bruner (1981) who identified three functional categories of prelinguistic communication including: behavior regulation, social interaction, and joint attention. Behavior regulation functions overlap both deitic and representational gestures. Behavior regulation and social interaction emerge prior to joint attention; however, they emerge in an overlapping rather than sequential manner. Crais and her colleagues (2004) and Carpenter et al. (1983) have begun to describe the emergence of gestural communicative functions.

Behavior regulation is a term used to describe a baby's attempts to manage adult behavior. Behavior regulation includes both *protesting* and *requesting* gestures and their age of emergence is the most predictable of all gestures. Protesting is commonly the first to appear at approximately 6 months of age and can be expressed by pushing an object away or turning the head, for example, deitic gestures which were discussed earlier. Requesting gestures begin at roughly the same time or shortly thereafter. These gestures include the request of either objects or actions. Object requests, which generally are observed first, typically involve the child's arm outstretched in the direction of an object, such a toy or a person, and *may* be accompanied by vocalization. "Oh, you want the red truck" might be the parent's response. Requesting an action, such as playing peek-a-boo, is more sophisticated communication and commonly emerges several months later at 8 to 9 months of age.

Social interaction gestures, Bruner's second functional category, emerge shortly after birth and develop complexity throughout infancy (Bruner, 1981). First, there is an initial period, early in life when the infant attends to social partners. This is seen first as mutual gazing and then may involve other parts of the body. Gestural greetings can be seen in 3-month-olds who smile and coo in response to an attentive adult. A bit later a social interaction gesture might take the form of a body movement, such as a 6-month-old repeatedly kicking her legs to gain attention.

The next period of development in social interaction is marked by the infant's efforts and growing ability to maintain a shared attentional focus to objects and events with social partners, often involving social games and object sharing. A 10-month-old might pull a blanket on her head as a social gesture to initiate a game of peek-a-boo. A few months later the toddler might blow a kiss or wave bye-bye and may produce a verbal approximation of "bye-bye." These conventional gestures typically promote a reciprocal gesture or utterance from the person to whom they were directed. Thus conversational turn-taking advances to the next level.

In the last 3 months of the first year of life, a prelinguistic milestone occurs when babies begin to intentionally communicate their interests and needs to others. Joint attention, initiated by the *child*, is the final prelinguistic communication function to emerge. It does so in stages, beginning as early as 9 months of age when the baby shows or gives objects directly to an adult. Within the next few months the baby will simply point to a person, object, or event often while vocalizing, in order to draw the adult's attention to the object of interest. Around 15 to 18 months of age toddlers will point in response to an adult's language prompting, "Where's the kitty?" or request information from the adult by pointing at something and then looking at the adult for comment of explanation. Finally, as oral language emerges, the toddler will use gesture to clarify a word approximation when it is not understood. For example, in an attempt to request juice the toddler might repeat "ooz," point to the refrigerator and then look back at the adult to ascertain that the adult is attending and understands the request.

Transition from Prelingusitic to Linguistic Communication

As children move from the nonverbal prelinguistic stage to the early stages of verbal language, parent strategies for supporting language acquisition must also evolve. The *Division of Early Childhood (DEC) Recommended Practices in Early Intervention* (Sandall, McLean, & Smith, 2000) notes the importance of appropriate parent responsiveness to best support language development in young children. When parents are able to fine tune their responses to their child's utterance, language development appears to occur at an optimal rate. Not surprisingly, parent response to a child's utterance should be governed by the complexity of the utterance. When children are at the one-word level, the types of parent responses recommended by the *DEC Recommended Practices* include both *imitation* and *expansion*. Imitation is simply responding to a child's utterance with the word the child has said, albeit in the adult rather than child form. If the child holds out stuffed bunny and says, "Bebe," the adult imitation should be "Bunny" or "It's Bunny," unless of course the bunny's name is Bebe. Expansion involves the simple addition of elements to the child's utterance to produce a slightly more complex model. For example, in response to "gawgee," the adult model might be, "Brown doggie" or "Yes, that's a brown doggie." or "It's a big doggie!" The adult has expanded the child's one word utterance to a two-word utterance or a simple sentence with one adjective, modeling the next level of complexity for them.

When the two- to three-word level is attained, adult responses evolve in complexity to include strategies such as *parallel talk, recasting*, and *asking open-ended questions*. Parallel talk occurs most frequently as an adult plays along with a young child in a form of parallel play during which the child and adult play with similar toys but do not engage in coordinated, cooperative play. Children from the age of 2 to 3 years are typically at the two- to three-word level and engage in parallel play with other children as well as adults. Parallel talk is related to the activities around which play is centered. It might involve description of the toys or actions of the toys. It could be suppositional, "I think my baby is hungry. I'm going to feed her." The adult does not necessarily expect the child to respond but is simply modeling appropriate linguistic content for the situation in which they are engaged. Recasting is a more complex language facilitating technique that is contingent upon the child's utterance. In recasting, the child's language is restated or "recast" in a changed sentence structure that still maintains and refers to the central meaning of the child's production. For example, if the child observes someone fall from a bike and says, "fall down" the adult recast might be, "He was going too fast. That's why he fell down."

Open-ended questions promote the most complex response the child is capable of making and is appropriate for children who are firmly into the two-word utterance stage. Asking a how, what, or why question avoids a simple yes or no response. Thus, asking, "What's Daddy doing?" supports the more elaborate and developmentally appropriate response, "Daddy singing." than if the child had simply been asked, "Is Daddy singing?"

Although the strategies and language adults use to promote the child's language development evolve continually from early infancy through toddlerhood and into early childhood, it continues to be the case that all young children learn language within the context of their daily routines and through daily interactions with their parents. Although the services of a professional with specialization in providing speech and language service to infants and toddlers with hearing loss should be available to every family, the reality is quite different. However, whether or not services with an expert are available, there is a need for proactive management with the involvement of family members and those who provide services to them. Family involvement is the key to child success in all areas of development. The information presented in this chapter should be sufficient to create a solid foundation for a child's communication development in the earliest years of life if parents are supported by a pediatric audiologist who is both knowledgeable and understanding.

References

Acredolo, L., & Goodwyn, S. (1988). Symbolic gesturing in normal infants. *Child Development, 59*, 450–466.

Anderson, K. (2002). Early Listening Function (ELF). Parent involvement: The magic ingredient in successful child outcomes: Improving parent participation using the ELF and the CHILD. *Hearing Review, 9*(11), 24–26.

Bates, E., Benigni, L., Bretherton, I., Camaioni, L., & Volterra, V. (1979). *The emergence of symbols: Cognition and communication in infancy.* New York, NY: Academic Press.

Bates, E., Bremerton, I., & Snyder, L. (1988*). From first words to grammar: Individual differences and dissociable mechanisms.* New York, NY: Cambridge University Press.

Boothroyd, A., & Medwetsky, L. (1992). Spectral distribution of /s/ and the frequency response of hearing aids. *Ear and Hearing, 13,* 150–157.

Brown, C. J. (2006). *Early intervention: Strategies for public and private sector collaboration.* Paper presented at the 2006 Convention of the Alexander Graham Bell Association for the Deaf and Hard of Hearing. Pittsburgh, PA.

Bruner, J. (1981). The social context of language acquisition. *Language and Communication, 1,* 155–178.

Calderon, R., Bargones, J., & Sidman, S. (1998). Characteristics of hearing families and their young deaf and hard-of-hearing children: Early intervention follow-up. *American Annals of the Deaf, 143,* 347–362.

Calderon, R., & Naidu, S. (2000). Further support for the benefits of early intervention for children with hearing loss. *Volta Review, 100*(5 Monograph), 53–84.

Carpenter, M., Mastergeorge, A. M., & Coggins, T. (1983). The acquisition of communicative intentions in infants eight to fifteen months of age. *Language and Speech, 26,* 101–116.

Christakis, D., Gilkerson, J., Richards, J., Zimmerman, F., Garrison, M., Xu, D., . . . Yapanel, U. (2009). Audible television and decreased adult words, infant vocalizations, and conversational turns: A population based study. *Archives of Pediatric and Adolescent Medicine, 163*(6), 554–558.

Conrad, B., Goss, D., Fogg, L., & Ruchala, P. (1992). Maternal confidence, knowledge, and quality of mother-child interactions: A preliminary study. *Infant Mental Health Journal, 13,* 353–362.

Crais, E., Douglass, D., & Campbell C. (2004). The intersection of the development of gestures and intentionality. *Journal of Speech, Language and Hearing Research, 47,* 678–694.

DesJardin, J. (2006). Family empowerment: Supporting language development in young children who are deaf or hard of hearing. *Volta Review, 106*(3 Monograph), 275–298.

Elfenbein, J. (1994). Monitoring preschooler's hearing aids: Issues in program design and implementation. *American Journal of Audiology, 3*(2), 65–70.

Fenson, L., Dale, P., Resnick, S., Thal, D., Bates, E., Hartung, J., Pethick, S., & Reilly, J. (1993). *MacArthur Communicative Development Inventories: User's guide and technical manual.* San Diego, CA: Singular.

Glista, D., Scollie, S., Bagatto, M., Seewald, R., Parsa, V., & Johnson, A. (2009). Evaluation of nonlinear frequency compression: Clinical outcomes. *International Journal of Audiology, 48*(9), 632–644.

Harrison, M. (2000). How do we know we've got it right? Observing performance with amplification. In R. Seewald (Ed.), *A sound foundation through early amplification: Proceedings of an international conference* (pp. 119–140). Chicago, IL: Phonak.

Harrison, M., Roush, J., & Wallace, J., (2003) Trends in age of identification and intervention in infants with hearing loss. *Ear and Hearing, 24,* 89–95.

Iverson, J., & Thal, D. (1998). Communication transitions: There's more to the hand than meets the eye. In A. Wetherby, S. Warren, & J. Reichle (Eds.), *Transitions in prelinguistic communication* (pp. 59–86). Baltimore, MD: Brookes.

Kuhl, P., Conboy, B., Padden, C., Nelson, T., & Pruitt, J. (2005). Early speech perception and later language development: Implications for the critical period. *Language Learning and Development, 1*(3–4), 237–264.

Kuhl, P., Williams, K., Lacerda, F., Stevens, K., & Lindbolm, B. (1991). Linguistic experience alters phonetic perception by 6 months of age. *Science, 255,* 606–608.

Leonard, L., McGregor, K., & Allen, G. (1992).Grammatical morphology and speech perception in children with specific language impairment. *Journal of Speech and Hearing Research, 35,* 1076–1085.

Ling, D. (1989). *Foundations of spoken language for the hearing-impaired child.* Washington, DC: Alexander Graham Bell Association for the Deaf.

McGowen, R., Nittrouer, S., Chenausky, K., (2008) Speech production in 12 month old children with and without hearing loss. *Journal of Speech Language and Hearing Research, 51,* 879–888.

Mitchell, R., & Karchmer, M. (2004). Chasing the mythical ten percent: Parental hearing status of deaf and hard of hearing students in the United States. *Sign Language Studies, 4*(2), 138–163.

Moeller, M. P. (2000). Early Intervention and language development in children who are deaf or hard of hearing. *Pediatrics, 106*(3), 43–50.

Moeller, M. P., Hoover, B., Peterson, B., & Stelmachowicz, P. (2009). Consistency of hearing aid use with early identified infants. *American Journal of Audiology, 18,* 14–23.

Mundy, P., Block, J., Delgado, C., Pomaes, Y., Van Hecke, A., & Parlade, M. (2007). Individual differences and the development of joint attention in infancy. *Child Development, 78,* 938–954.

Nittrouer, S., & Burton, L. (2002). The role of early language experience in the development of speech perception and language processing abilities in children with hearing loss. *Volta Review, 103*, 5–37.

Reed, M. (1989). Speech perception and the discrimination of brief auditory cues in dyslexic children. *Journal of Experimental Child Psychology, 48,* 270–292.

Sandall, S., McLean, M. E., & Smith, B. J. (2000). *DEC recommended practices: Early intervention/early childhood special education*. Denver, CO: Division for Early Childhood of the Council for Exceptional Children.

Schery, T., & Zika, G. (2003). *Supporting children with cochlear implants in educational settings*. Paper presented at the Council for Exceptional Children, Division for Communication Disabilities and Deafness. Seattle, WA.

Sjoblad, S., Harrison, M., Roush, J., & McWilliam, R. (2001). Parents' reactions and recommendations after diagnosis and hearing aid fitting. *American Journal of Audiology, 10,* 24–31.

Stelmachowicz, P., Nishi, K., Sangsook, C., Lewis, D., Hoover, B., Dierking, D., & Lotto, A. (2008). Effects of stimulus bandwidth on the imitation of english fricatives by normal-hearing children. *Journal of Speech, Language and Hearing Research, 51*(5), 1369–1380.

Stelmachowicz, P., Pittman, A., Hoover, B., & Lewis, D. (2001). Effect of stimulus bandwidth on the perception of /s/ in normal and hearing impaired children and adults. *Journal of the Acoustical Society of America, 110*(4), 2183–2190.

Stelmachowicz, P. G., Pittman, A. L., Hoover, B. M., Lewis, D. L., & Moeller, M. P. (2004). The importance of high-frequency audibility in the speech and language development of children with hearing loss. *Archives of Otolarynogology, 130*, 556–562.

Stoel-Gammon, C. (1999). Role of babbling and phonology in early linguistic development. In A. Wetherby, S. Warren, & J. Reichle, (Eds.), *Transitions in paralinguistic communication* (pp. 87–111). Baltimore, MD: Brookes.

Thal, D., & Tobias, S. (1992). Relationships between language and gesture in normally developing and late-talking toddlers. *Journal of Speech, Language, and Hearing Research, 337,* 147–170.

Tsao, F., Liu, H., & Kuhl, P. (2004).Speech perception in infancy predicts language development in the second year of life: A longitudinal study. *Child Development, 75*(4), 1067–1084.

White, K. (2006). Early intervention for children with permanent hearing loss: Finishing the EDHI revolution. *Volta Review, 106*(3 Monograph), 237–258.

Zimmerman-Philips, S., Osberger, M. J., & Robbins, A. M. (1997). *Infant-toddler: Meaningful Auditory Integration Scale (IT-MAIS)*. Sylmar, CA: Advanced Bionics Corporation.

APPENDIX 31–A

Elements of Comprehensive Hearing Aid Maintenance

If the child has severe or profound hearing loss, be sure to lower the volume setting prior to the listening check.

- First, use a battery tester to see that the battery is fully charged. Encourage parents always to replace low batteries.
- With the earmold connected to the hearing instrument, use a listening stethoscope attached to the hearing aid to listen.
- Check to see that the earmold and tubing do not have any cracks or tears that could cause feedback (whistling or squealing). Let parents know that when feedback occurs, tubing always should be checked and that if it is cracked it can easily and inexpensively be replaced.
- Check to see that the tubing has not become brittle or hard. This could reduce the diameter of the tubing and modify the signal.
- If the earmolds are dirty, wipe them with a damp cloth. Be sure not to get the hearing instruments wet.
- Check that the earmold tubing is free of moisture, as a drop of water blocking the tube can prevent sound getting to the ear. If you see moisture, detach the earmold from the hearing instrument and use an earmold blower to dry it. If the earmold has a vent, blow the air through that opening as well.
- Check to be sure the opening to the ear canal portion of the earmold is free of wax. Should you find wax there, simply wipe it with a damp cloth or use a wax loop or brush to remove it.
- Turn hearing aid on and off. Adjust the volume controls (if activated) and change between programs. There should be smooth transitions among the programs while performing these tasks.
- Gently press on the casing of the hearing aid while listening. The sound should not cut in and out.

APPENDIX 31–B

Elements of Comprehensive Cochlear Implant Maintenance

- **Batteries:** Check the batteries to determine if they are fully charged, properly inserted, or have corrosion on the contacts. Many processors have indicator lights or a display to show the charge status of the battery. Some processors are equipped with an audible alarm to indicate when the battery is running low.
- **Microphone:** Use listening earphones provided by the implant manufacturer to test the microphone. Some processors are equipped with visual displays which indicate the microphone is detecting sounds. If the microphone is suspected to be faulty, test the device with another microphone to determine whether or not the problem is located in the microphone.
- **Processor:** Check to determine that the processor has turned on, the correct program is selected, and the volume and sensitivity setting are correct. The visual display on the processor may indicate if there is a problem with the processor electronics or if a program location has been corrupted by static electricity.
- **Cables:** Particular weak points are at the ends of the cable where it attaches to the processor and the transmitting coil. Determine if the cables are twisted, frayed, or broken.
- **Transmitting coil:** In some devices, processor display lights and audible alarms indicate that the coil is not correctly transmitting information to the internal device. A signal check accessory is provided by some manufacturers.

(Adapted from Schery & Zika, 2003)

Further information regarding troubleshooting guides can be found at the following Web sites:

Advanced Bionics devices
http://www.advancedbionics.com/Products/Product_User_Guides_and_Troubleshooting/index.cfm?langid=1

Cochlear Americas devices
http://products.cochlearamericas.com/support/cochlear-implant/ci-troubleshooting

Med El devices
http://www.medel.com/int/show3/index/id/54/title/PRODUCTS?

The Illinois School for the Deaf
http://www.morgan.k12.il.us/isd/outreach_services_CISupport.html

University of Texas-Dallas
http://www.utdallas.edu/calliercenter/clinic/cochlear/faq.php

32

Toddlers and Preschool-Aged Children

Kathryn L. Beauchaine, Darcia M. Dierking, and Jack E. Kile

Introduction

During the toddler and preschool years, between infancy and kindergarten, children make gains in their development and become progressively more independent. The toddler, 12 to 36 months of age, and the preschooler, 36 to 60 months of age, typically become mobile and spend more time at greater distances from their parent or caregiver. The stage is set for academic achievement as cognitive, social, motor, language, and speech skills blossom. Adequate hearing is necessary to optimize spoken communication-skill development. The audiologist plays a key role in assessing and monitoring hearing status and hearing-instrument use. Working with this population is both challenging and rewarding.

Each aspect of development in the early childhood years affects audiologic assessment and management. With that in mind, it is important to acknowledge that approximately 20 to 40% of children who have hearing loss also have other developmental concerns (Dalzell et al., 2000). Thus, many children who have hearing loss present with exceptions to typical developmental milestones. This, in turn, modifies the audiologic approach. The purpose of this chapter is to further familiarize the reader with audiologic assessment and management issues specific to this age group, with an emphasis on protocols and guidelines, and their implementation.

Audiologic Assessment Guidelines

The *Guidelines for the Audiologic Assessment of Children from Birth to 5 Years of Age* (American Speech and Hearing Association [ASHA], 2004) detail clinical indicators, assessment objectives, procedures, and follow-up appropriate for this age group. There is overlap in test procedures for infants and *young* toddlers, those between 12 and 24 months of age. For purposes of this discussion, the procedures recommended for 25 to 60 months of age include:

- Case History
- Otoscopy
- Behavioral Assessment, which may include visual reinforcement audiometry (VRA) or conditioned play audiometry (CPA)
- Speech Perception Skills, which may include detection, discrimination, and comprehension
- Physiologic Assessment, which may include tympanometry, acoustic reflex thresholds, otoacoustic emissions (OAE), and auditory brainstem response (ABR)
- Developmental Screening and Functional Auditory Assessment

The ASHA document *Roles, Knowledge, and Skills: Audiologists Providing Clinical Services to Infants and Young Children Birth to 5 Years of Age* (ASHA, 2006) details the special knowledge base and skill set required of the audiologist to implement the guidelines. The audiologist is viewed as a diagnostician, counselor, and audiologic care coordinator. The Joint Committee on Infant Hearing (JCIH, 2007) also emphasizes the importance of audiologists' skills and knowledge as they relate to this young group of patients.

Each of the procedures is examined below, with an emphasis on the clinical implementation of each component. The reader is referred to other pertinent chapters for in-depth discussions of specific audiologic procedures.

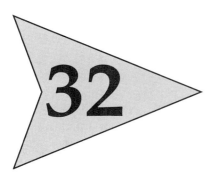

Case History

An astute clinician begins the assessment in the waiting room, or on first meeting the family. Much can be gleaned about family dynamics during those first minutes. Is the child calmly playing near the parents, crying in a stroller, or running seemingly unattended in the waiting area? Observe the child's ease when you approach the family. Does the child's development seem age appropriate? Is the 18-month-old walking? Is the child responding to sounds? Is he socially appropriate? Are vocalizations present and consistent with age expectations? What is the style of the parent-child interaction? Think about how you will use this information in your audiologic assessment, as well as during counseling. Keep in mind that this first meeting with the family sets the stage for the audiologic appointment and potentially for many follow-up appointments. At this same time, the family and child are forming opinions of the clinician.

At the beginning of the case history, determine the reason for the referral. Ask the parents what their concerns are. Developmental milestones, with a focus on communication-skill development, are important to note as part of the case history. The child already may be in an early intervention program for reasons other than hearing or communication. The child may have vision impairment or other health issues that will drive the test session and your approach to the remainder of the case history. If the child is not talking when expected and has previously passed hearing screenings, obtain a copy of those test results for review, if possible. There may be risk factors for late-onset or progressive hearing loss (JCIH, 2007). An abbreviated case history form, which includes the risk factors for permanent congenital, delayed-onset, and progressive hearing loss in childhood (JCIH, 2007) is found in Table 32–1.

Otoscopy

Prior to placing an insert earphone, tympanometry probe, OAE probe or probe-microphone tube into the child's ear, it is critical to ensure that the ear canal is free of drainage or any debris that would affect test results. During otoscopy, the audiologist is looking for the presence of ear pits or tags, and pinna or ear canal anomalies. Some young children are accustomed to otoscopy; however, it can be helpful to ask the parent how the child typically reacts to this procedure. For children who have tactile defensiveness or are extremely wary or shy, it is reasonable to defer otoscopy until later in the appointment as they may not tolerate earphones until they are more at ease. For children with a high level of wariness, behavioral testing likely will begin in the sound field. Of course, each child is unique and audiologists should adapt their interaction style to accommodate the child and family.

Behavioral Assessment

Parents usually are astute observers of their child's auditory behavior and can be helpful in the audiologic assessment process. Parental concern for hearing loss is considered a risk factor for hearing impairment (JCIH, 2007). Parent questionnaires can be helpful in assessing auditory behavior and in corroborating audiologic test results. One such questionnaire is found in Kile, Schaffmeyer, and Kuba (1994). The questionnaire, completed before the audiologic evaluation, elicits parental responses to a number of auditory behaviors observed in their child. These behaviors include: auditory alertness, response consistency, response latencies, responsiveness to "soft" versus "loud" sounds, reaction to environmental sounds, sound localization, "tuning out" behavior, responsiveness to nonauditory stimuli, and listening in noise. Before the behavioral assessment, the responses from the questionnaire can be reviewed and concerns about the child's auditory behavior explored.

The overall goal of behavioral audiometry is to obtain a complete frequency- and ear-specific audiogram. Because toddlers and young children have limited attention spans, the audiologist should plan the session and prioritize tests and stimuli accordingly. At any point in the session the child may stop participating. If a child readily tolerates otoscopy, insert earphones should be used from the outset. If there is concern that the child will not tolerate insert earphones or train to the behavioral task, initial testing can be done in the sound field. When there is concern for severe or profound hearing loss, initiate testing with vibrotactile stimuli. Some children, in spite of having the cognitive ability for the task, are unable to respond to conventional behavioral testing because of motor deficits. However, they may be testable when modifications commensurate with their motor capabilities are employed. For example, a child with limited use of his hands and arms may be conditioned to blink his eyes, nod, or give a spoken response (see Chapter 22).

It is reasonable and efficient to initiate VRA testing with frequency-specific stimuli (Widen et al., 2000) rather than speech stimuli. The rationale for this is to minimize the number of responses required of the child prior to habituation while obtaining as much fre-

Table 32–1. Case History Form

Presence of:	***Yes***	***No***	***Details***
Hearing concerns			
Speech/language concerns			
Developmental concerns			
Family history of hearing loss			
Pregnancy/birth complications			
Neonatal intensive care unit (NICU) stay			
Newborn hearing screening			
Hospitalizations			
Medications			
Ear infection/surgery			
Early intervention/educational/therapeutic services			

Risk indicators for permanent congenital, delayed-onset, or progressive hearing loss in childhood (JCIH, 2007)

1. Caregiver concerns for hearing, speech/language, or development.
2. Family history of childhood-onset permanent hearing loss.
3. Stay in the NICU of more than 5 days.
4. In utero infections (e.g., CMV, herpes, rubella, syphilis, toxoplasmosis).
5. Craniofacial anomalies.
6. Physical findings associated with a syndrome known to include hearing loss.
7. Syndromes associated with hearing loss or progressive or late-onset hearing loss (e.g., neurofibromatosis, osteopetrosis, Usher's).
8. Neurodegenerative disorders (e.g., Hunter, sensory motor neuropathies).
9. Culture-positive postnatal infections associated with permanent hearing loss.
10. Head trauma.
11. Chemotherapy.

quency-specific information as possible. If the child does not respond readily to tones, speech or music stimuli can be used. Music stimuli likely cannot be calibrated, but can provide a novel and interesting stimulus for training purposes. The same approach could be applied to CPA testing.

If the child tolerates earphones, alternate testing between the right and left ears. For example, obtain one or two frequency-specific thresholds in the right ear and then do the same for the left ear. Because children with hearing loss present with a wide array of audiometric configurations (Pittman & Stelmachowicz, 2003), the frequency chosen to start testing may not be ideal in every case. It is often efficient to initiate testing at 2000 Hz and then proceed to another test frequency, depending on case history information and previously obtained results. If the child is responding reliably, continue testing additional frequencies until habituation occurs. Speech or music stimuli can be used at any point in the test session for interest and as a cross-check of pure/warble tone thresholds.

Habituation occurs when the child quits responding because of lack of interest or waning attention. Scheduling an optimal evaluation time for behavioral testing, not during the child's typical naptime, is an important consideration in controlling for habituation. Based on parent reports and informal observations, the audiologist can often judge the child's attending skills and ability to stay on task. While listening skills vary, clinical experience suggests that behavioral testing for toddlers and preschoolers should seldom exceed 20 to 30 minutes. When children start to habituate, they can often be brought back to task by increasing signal intensity (e.g., +30 dB from previous level), switching type of test stimuli (e.g., from tones to speech), changing visual reinforcement or play activities, and/or giving short rest periods.

If hearing loss is present, bone conduction testing should be completed, with masking if necessary and as tolerated by the child. Some children are initially confused by the introduction of masking noise. Perhaps just a few frequencies will be obtained reliably at each test session.

The motor and cognitive skills to perform VRA should be achieved by a developmental age of 6 months. For VRA, Widen et al. (2000) used probe stimuli prior to conditioning in order to minimize the number of training trials. For example, a 30 dB HL 2000-Hz tone is presented, and the child is given an opportunity to give an unconditioned head turn. The child who turns is reinforced, and a second 30 dB HL 2000 Hz tone is presented. The child who turns again is reinforced and a threshold search is initiated. However, if the child does not provide a spontaneous head turn at 30 dB HL, the level is increased to 50 dB HL. If a spontaneous head turn is not seen at 50 dB HL, conditioning trials are begun. If the child has had an evoked potential test or previous audiogram consistent with hearing loss, the starting levels for the training trials would be altered accordingly. The reader is referred to Widen et al. (2000) for a complete description of this highly efficient VRA protocol. This research emphasizes the importance of control/catch trials to monitor and minimize false-positive responses during testing. See also Chapter 22 in this volume.

Research suggests that VRA is appropriate for children who are at a developmental age of 6 months to about 2 years of age. That extensive literature is not reviewed here. A limiting factor in moving from a VRA to a CPA task is a child's impulsivity. During this transition phase, children may not find the VRA task interesting, yet the CPA task may be beyond their skill set. Appendix 32–A provides practical suggestions for VRA setup and toy choices.

The motor and cognitive skills to perform CPA typically are achieved by a developmental age of 24 months. The stimuli choices for CPA are similar to VRA. Enthusiastic praise for the child goes a long way to ensure a productive test session.

Engage the parent in the process of CPA game selection. Ask them what the child likes to play. Use that information to set the stage for play audiometry. Have a wide range of game choices that vary in interest level for different age groups and level of motor skills. Flexibility and creativity during play audiometry are two characteristics required of pediatric audiologists and test assistants. As a percentage of children with hearing loss will also have vision impairment, have some game choices that are appropriate for children with low vision. Likewise, have choices for children with compromised motor skills.

Appendix 32–B offers CPA setup suggestions. Appendix 32–C contains additional child-friendly testing tips.

Speech Perception Skills

Language abilities and speech production skills to perform speech awareness/reception or word recognition tasks are largely dependent on the child's age and degree of hearing loss. The continuum of speech audiometry tasks ranges from speech awareness to word-repetition. Informal speech audiometry can be completed as soon as the child can wave "bye-bye" or respond to other simple verbal commands. The child's vocabulary level must be considered during test selection and analysis.

When the child is able to perform object/picture-pointing or word-repetition tasks, it is informative to complete unamplified and amplified tests. Comparisons can be made to demonstrate improvements with amplification in place. These tests also can be done in noise as with the Bench, Kowal, and Bamford (BKB-SIN) 1979 test, but not until 5 years of age.

Physiologic Assessment

Physiologic assessments for audiologic testing include: auditory evoked potentials (AEP), typically ABR; OAEs; and acoustic immittance testing (tympanometry and stapedial reflexes). For children unable to perform VRA or CPA tasks, hearing threshold monitoring will be done using AEP. Toddler and preschool-age children cannot sit quietly enough for conventional AEP tests. Thus, sleep deprivation or sedation may be required to ensure sufficient quiet to obtain high quality recordings and the best estimates of thresholds. Options for

AEPs that do not require sleep or complete stillness are under development.

JCIH (2007) recommends that a child have at least one ABR test if diagnosed with permanent hearing loss before age three years. The purposes of the ABR test are to: (1) obtain frequency- and ear-specific thresholds and (2) assess the integrity of the auditory brainstem pathways. The use of tone-evoked ABR testing to obtain estimates of behavioral hearing thresholds is well established (Gorga et al., 2006; Stapells, 2000). Auditory steady-state responses (ASSR) also have been proposed for this purpose (see Chapter 20 for a complete discussion of electrophysiologic measures).

OAEs generally are used in two ways: (1) as an assessment of preneural auditory function (Gorga et al., 1993; Prieve et al., 1993) for those without middle ear effusion, and (2) as a cross-check of behavioral responses.

For toddlers and preschoolers, tympanograms are completed using a low-frequency probe tone. Acoustic stapedial reflexes are done as a cross-check of diagnostic findings and as a first-tier test for auditory neuropathy/dys-synchrony (AN/D). Berlin et al. (2005) recommended that acoustic stapedial reflexes be tested, at least for the ipsilateral condition, at 1000 Hz and 2000 Hz for infants who have hearing screening consisting of OAEs only. If the reflexes are elevated or absent despite present OAEs and normal tympanograms, an ABR test is indicated to assess for AN/D. In a similar vein, if a child presents with an audiologic profile of normal hearing sensitivity, present OAEs, normal tympanograms, and reportedly atypical auditory behaviors and/or speech/language delays, acoustic stapedial reflex testing is indicated as a "screening" for AN/D.

Due to the relatively high incidence of otitis media (OM) in this age group, tympanometry at every audiology session is justified. OM-related audiologic management issues are discussed later in this chapter (also see Chapter 9).

Developmental Screening and Functional Auditory Assessment

Developmental screening and functional auditory assessments are available for the audiologist to use with the family and/or early intervention specialist. Working in concert with the child's family and early intervention team, the audiologist can assist in determining if any of the concerns for the child's performance: (1) relate to the hearing loss or its effects; (2) are indicative of a need for further referrals; and/or (3) potentially could be ameliorated by changes in the amplification configuration or listening environments.

Corroborating Test Results

Meaningful observations of auditory behavior in toddlers and preschoolers can be made in conjunction with behavioral audiologic evaluations (VRA, CPA) without significantly increasing testing time. Information from these observations can be useful in assessing hearing status, corroborating behavioral or electrophysiologic test results, relating auditory behavior to neurodevelopmental adequacy, suggesting risk for sensory processing disorders (SPD), predicting effectiveness of amplification, and managing hearing impairments.

When behavioral and electrophysiologic tests are completed, the audiologist judges whether or not the child's auditory behaviors corroborate results. In some instances, intertest discrepancies may be noted. For example, while a child might at times give responses consistent with normal hearing, he also might have episodes of being unresponsive to sound regardless of intensity level. These inconsistencies can be documented during behavioral audiometry by recording whether or not a response has occurred to each stimulus presented. If the child has normal AEP test results but the audiogram is suggestive of hearing loss, other conditions should be considered. For example, the child might be at risk for auditory attention or processing challenges. Similarly, a parent may strongly suspect hearing loss despite normal audiologic test findings. In consultation with the family, primary physician and early intervention team, these children should be referred for further evaluations. Depending on the specific concerns, developmental, educational, speech/language, neurologic, or ophthalmologic evaluations might be indicated.

Amplification Issues

When significant hearing loss is confirmed and it is determined that hearing instruments are indicated, ear impressions can be taken and amplification initiated. Medical clearance for use of amplification must be obtained. The JCIH (2007) recommendation is that amplification be initiated within one month of the hearing-loss confirmation. Most toddlers and preschoolers with significant hearing loss already will have been fitted with amplification as infants. The exceptions are those with later identified or later onset hearing loss. Also, some of the children, as they become mobile, will add an FM system to their amplification configuration. Toddlers with severe and profound hearing loss might acquire their first and/or second cochlear implant.

A toddler's ability to walk or run away from his parents has a large impact on distance listening. The greater the hearing loss, the more difficult distance listening becomes. This needs to be considered and discussed with the family as part of the amplification assessment. It is well established that an FM system can provide a clearer signal when distance, noise, and reverberation are present; however, in practice, some families adapt to home-use of an FM system whereas others do not. Cost can be a roadblock to home-use of an FM system for some families.

Children's listening environments become more demanding as they move into larger groups in their daycare or preschool during transition from infancy to toddlerhood. Larger groups mean more noise and greater hearing challenges. Audiologists can provide ideas for decreasing noise at home, at daycare and in the classroom, and advocate for FM use in these situations.

Amplification Guidelines

The American Academy of Audiology (AAA) provides a comprehensive discussion of pediatric fitting considerations in their *Pediatric Amplification Protocol* (2003). It is helpful for both new and experienced pediatric audiologists to be familiar with this document and its anticipated revisions. The importance of verification of amplified audibility with probe microphone measures and validation with functional assessment tools, such as parent or teacher questionnaires, is covered in other chapters (see Chapters 25 and 29). The following discussion focuses on practical implementation of pediatric fitting practices.

The Earmold

Taking earmold impressions can be a challenge with toddlers and preschoolers. Having interesting distracters handy will help keep the child's hands occupied so he does not pull out the otoblock/dam or impression material. Mark the otolight or the otoblock string at an appropriate depth for the child's ear, to help gauge how deeply the dam is inserted. Vented dams provide pressure release and may increase comfort; however, the vent may take up space on impressions for small ear canals. Slim dams may turn in the canal with the force of impression material, and the impression material can move past it, deeper into the ear canal. Impression material with lower viscosity (as found in self-mixing cartridges) takes longer to harden, moves past dams more easily, and may remain in the ear canal if a child pulls out the dam before the impression is ready. If any of these situations are anticipated, the firmer impression materials that are mixed by hand may be more appropriate. The disadvantage of the firmer material is that it can stretch and distort small canals, potentially resulting in an uncomfortable earmold.

When ordering earmolds for atypical ears, ask the technical support staff at the earmold lab for advice. They have a wealth of information and experience, and can provide information about earmold options. When choosing earmold material, consider vinyl for narrow ear canals, as it is less likely to "stretch the canal" as compared to silicone. Because tubing tends to pull out of vinyl material more easily, some labs use special bonding techniques to make the tubing extra secure. If ordering silicone material, consider tubing that has a retention ring so that the tubing stays in place in the earmold. Gluing tubing in silicone molds can be difficult. Tubes with retention rings are easy to change and sometimes parents can learn to change tubing themselves. With a very small ear canal, audiologists must take care that the retention ring does not distort the ear canal portion of the earmold.

The canal length of the earmold may need to be adjusted based on acoustic needs. Venting is important to use for some audiometric configurations and when a child has tympanostomy tubes or tympanic membrane perforations. Parallel vents may be impossible on some small ears, so diagonal vents may be required, with the possible tradeoff of high-frequency acoustic response loss. Use caution when re-tubing earmolds with diagonal vents to avoid covering the vent with the internal tubing. As the child grows, a parallel vent can be added.

Let the child or parents pick out the color for the earmolds. Keep in mind that vibrant colors may be more visible if the child removes the instrument. If the ear has an atypical shape, note that on the order form so the lab can take it into consideration, especially if retention will be an issue. In extreme cases, a photograph of the child's ear can be informative for the lab. Be sure to obtain a photographic release.

Hearing Instrument Retention and Tamper Resistance

Parental involvement is critical to successful amplification use. Persistence is the key to hearing instrument retention, despite the commonly encountered frustrations. There can be many reasons for retention problems, the most common being resistance of the child to wear anything near the head. For some children a barrier is used, such as a thin fabric bonnet, to prevent them from removing the hearing instruments. If this approach is used, the audiologist should ensure that the fabric is acoustically transparent. This can be done by completing output curves in a test box, comparing the microphone output with and without the bonnet fabric over the microphone of the hearing instrument. It is important that the bonnet fits snuggly or fabric noise may affect the signal when the child moves his head.

Inevitably, children manage to put hearing instruments in their mouths, so battery door locks are essential for safety purposes. Also, moisture control options, like desiccant jars or hearing instrument dryers, may minimize repairs. Some children require wearing a helmet for skull-shaping purposes, and for these children it is helpful to work with the helmet designer so that the hearing instrument will work with the helmet. Some simply have no room behind their ears for their hearing instruments and/or their glasses. Double-sided tape or wig/toupee tape can help deter "flopping" of hearing instruments. The tape is placed on the hearing instrument, on the side that will touch the mastoid area. This is especially useful when there is little room behind the pinna or when the pinna is small or absent. However, tape can easily stick to hair and cause discomfort or distress for the child. A wire retention system built into the earmold can be useful to keep the earmold and hearing instrument in place without toupee tape as shown in Figure 32–1.

Retention cords with clips link the hearing instrument to the child's shirt. The clothing clip is affixed to the back of the child's shirt. These work best when they attach to the hearing instruments versus to the earmold tubing because earmolds (and some tone hooks) easily detach from the hearing instruments when the retention cord is pulled. There are retention devices with either a stretchy silicone ring that fits over the behind-the-ear (BTE) case or a "sock" made out of acoustically transparent material that slides over the BTE. Finally, the tubing angle and tone hook size and orientation should be checked to ensure best fit. An optimal fit greatly improves hearing instrument retention and acceptance.

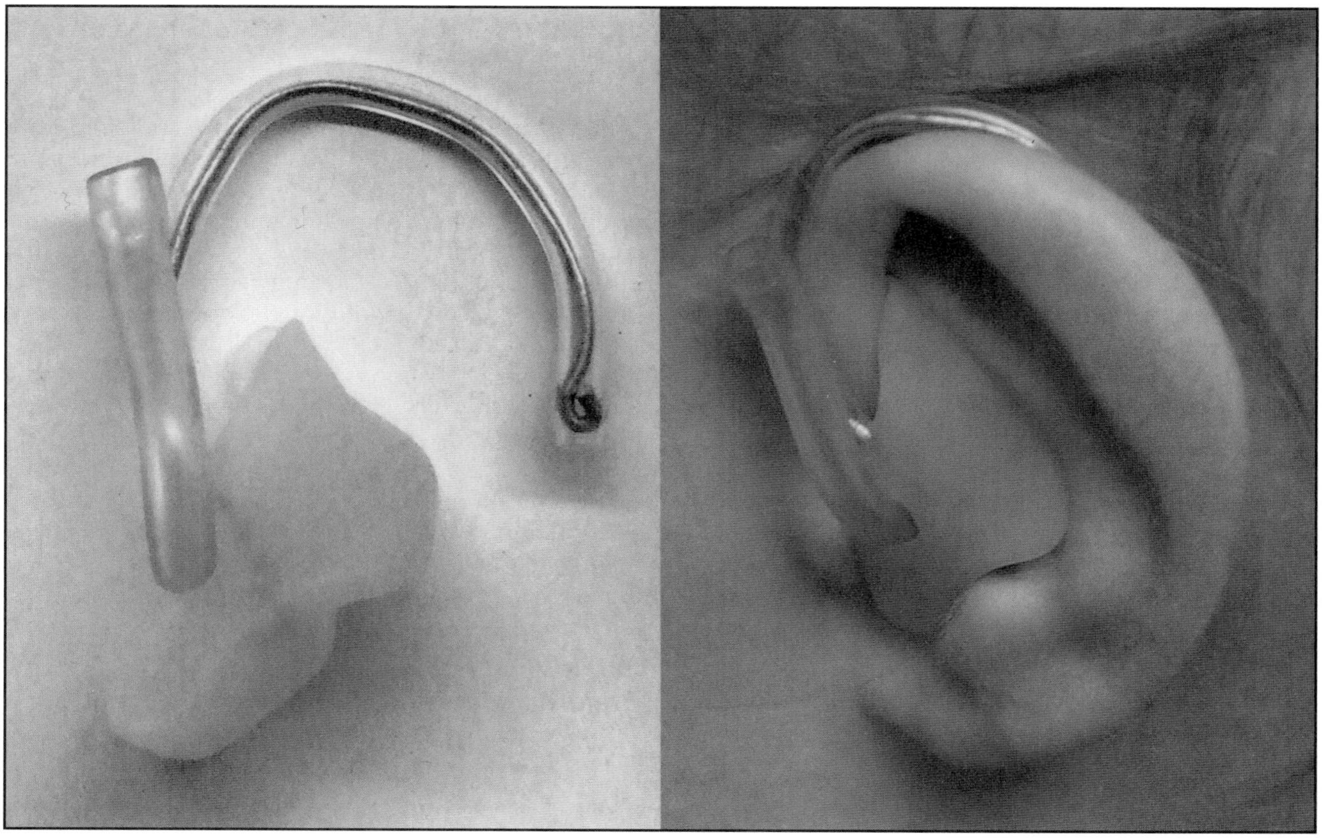

FIGURE 32–1. Earmold with built-in wire retention system (*left*), placed in child's ear (*right*).

For children who *strongly* object to wearing hearing instruments, obvious reasons for their objections should be addressed. For example, do the earmold and hearing instrument fit appropriately? Is the hearing instrument working? Are there other tactile concerns? Does the child object to certain sounds in the environment? Are sounds too loud? When objections have been minimized, a schedule of gradually increasing use over a specified period of time is recommended, growing to full-time use as soon as possible.

Hearing Instruments: Safety Concerns

The dangers of accidental battery ingestion should be stressed to every parent and caregiver. As mentioned above, tamper-resistant battery doors are helpful. Hearing instruments and earmolds, because of their size, are choke hazards. Parents and caregivers must be made aware of these issues so that they can implement precautions.

Selection of Hearing Instrument Characteristics

Most children will wear the same devices for several years. For this reason, the audiologist must think ahead and anticipate the child's hearing instrument needs over about a 5-year time period. If a child is expected to use an FM system at home or at school, the hearing instrument should be FM-compatible. Programs should be set up to be FM compatible in a way that parents can easily use.

Directional microphones may not be appropriate for younger children because: (1) they may need to hear sounds that originate from behind them, and (2) the directional microphone orientation may not be correct when seated on their small ears. However, as the child grows and listening situations change, directional microphones may become appropriate. Therefore, the audiologist may choose a hearing instrument with directional microphones, deactivating this feature initially, and activating it as dictated by the listening needs of the child.

Slim tube and receiver-in-the-ear BTE hearing instrument fittings also may be considered, depending on the size of the child's ear canal; however, both options would require custom earmolds for retention purposes. Slim tubes with custom earmolds should be used with caution with this population as they can create a reverse-horn effect, which decreases the high frequency response (AAA, 2003). Real-ear verification is essential.

At the time of this publication, noise reduction strategies are still being evaluated for use with young children. As with this or any emerging technology, the audiologist should inform parents of currently-understood pros and cons, and monitor the child for potential detrimental effects.

Assessment of Amplification Performance/Verification Measures

Verification measures should be completed using probe-microphone measures at regular intervals, and at least when there are hearing, hearing instrument or earmold changes. Prior to the appointment when hearing instruments are first fitted, it is time efficient to preset the instruments in the test box using age-related real-ear to coupler differences (RECDs). Then, when the child arrives, the hearing instruments are fine-tuned using their custom earmolds and probe-microphone measures. Calibrated inputs, ideally speech, at a variety of levels are recommended, with the real-ear saturation response (RESR) run with a swept pure tone (AAA, 2003).

Impact of Otitis Media on Assessment and Management

Children who have otitis media (OM) and significant hearing loss require additional assessment and management considerations. How often should hearing testing be completed? How aggressive will an ear, nose, and throat (ENT) physician be regarding ventilation tubes in a child with coexisting sensorineural hearing loss (SNHL)? How should the hearing instruments be set if there is a fluctuating conductive component? What are amplification options if there are chronically draining ears? What about children with purely conductive hearing loss whose ears are too small for ventilation tubes? The answers to these questions vary greatly depending on individual characteristics, case history, and the opinions of members of the medical management team. Below are a few considerations to keep in mind when grappling with these decisions.

Scheduling Follow-Up for Children with OM

The AAA protocol (2003) recommends that children have their hearing tested every 3 months during the first 2 years of amplification, and every 4 to 6 months thereafter. Children with OM may require hearing evaluations to be scheduled more often, in conjunction with ENT visits or following medical management.

With chronic OM, children may have fluctuations in hearing levels that may not be detected between visits. Parents may notice when their child is having increased hearing difficulties or an older child may be able to report when they are having a "bad hearing day." Parents should be counseled to make appointments as soon as changes are suspected. One option is to activate the volume control on the hearing instruments so that the parent can adjust the volume until able to come in for an appointment. Multiple memories also can be used for this purpose (AAA, 2003).

Use of Bone-Conduction Devices with OM

In addition to their use for permanent conductive hearing loss, bone-conduction hearing instruments can be a temporary option for children with OM as long as they have normal or near normal bone-conduction thresholds. This is especially useful for those who have chronically draining ears or tiny ears that cannot accommodate ventilation tube insertion or earmolds. Bone-conduction hearing instruments would not need to be adjusted based on the fluctuation of air conduction thresholds.

Hearing Instrument: Ventilation and Aeration of the Ear Canal and Hygiene

Alvord, Doxey, and Smith (1989) found that adequate earmold ventilation and periods of rest (when the instruments are out) tended to result in the least amount of middle and external ear infections. Naptimes or bedtime serve as natural periods when the instruments will be out of the ears, providing air exchange in the ear canals.

When placing an earmold in an ear with a tympanic membrane (TM) perforation or a ventilation tube, special considerations must be made. Occluding earmolds will compromise the air exchange that ventilation tubes are supposed to provide. Even pressure vents or vents smaller than 1 mm may provide little or no ventilation and may tend to get plugged easily (Alvord et al., 1989).

Parents must be educated about the purpose of earmold vents and how to keep them clean with the help of an earmold blower and a cleaning tool. Effective earmold hygiene requires regular cleaning, and in addition to using soap and water, there are ultraviolet light sanitizers available in some hearing instrument drying units.

Hearing Instrument Acoustics: Venting and OM

Ear canal acoustics and hearing thresholds can change with tubes or TM perforations, and providing earmold venting creates additional acoustic changes, primarily loss of low-frequency energy. Earmold venting is also used for patients with normal low-frequency hearing sensitivity. Small ear canals will not always accommodate parallel venting, so a diagonal vent may be needed. Diagonal vents, however, can cause a drop in high-frequency acoustic energy compared with parallel vents (Cox, 1979). The RECDs of ears with TM perforations or tubes commonly show negative values in the low frequencies even with a well-sealed, unvented earmold (Martin, Munro, & Langer, 1997). Additionally, children with tubes may have poorer low-frequency hearing thresholds than those without tubes.

Verification of amplified audibility can be complicated when there are vents in the earmold, ventilation tubes, or TM perforations. Audiologists must know how their verification equipment applies correction factors like RECDs to thresholds. There is some question about how accurately a threshold converted to real-ear SPL using a RECD measured with a TM perforation or tube accurately reflects threshold.

Vented earmolds cause a low frequency acoustic loss in the RECD; however, the RECD does not measure acoustic energy *leaking in* through the vent or *around the earmold*. It is most accurate to obtain conventional probe-microphone measures instead of relying solely on RECD with electroacoustic measures; conventional probe-microphone measures take into account the acoustic contributions of vent leaks, tubes, or TM perforations.

Acoustic energy enters the ear canal unattenuated at 250 and 500 Hz, even with a fully occluding earmold (Hoover, Stelmachowicz, & Lewis, 2000). Therefore, if there is no hearing loss or minimal hearing loss in the low frequencies, low-frequency energy might remain audible to the child even if there is an apparent low-frequency acoustic loss in the RECD. Conventional probe-microphone measures would be more likely to measure these effects and should be used whenever possible.

Both conventional probe-microphone measures and RECD with electroacoustic measures have variability, especially in active toddlers or preschoolers. Depending on the probe-depth and its relationship to the TM, standing waves may be present that further influence results (Dirks & Kincaid, 1987; Gilman & Dirks, 1986). Nonetheless, these measures are an essential part of hearing-instrument verification process, and are *far* more accurate than depending on the computer simulations of hearing-instrument performance.

Summary: Serving a Population in Transition

Families with children between 12 and 60 months are constantly in transition, both in terms of changes in audiologic test techniques, hearing/listening demands, and early intervention strategies. Families go from home-based services with a parent-infant specialist, to enrolling their child in preschool, to enrolling in kindergarten. Children vary in their progress along the typical continuum of educational services. They and their families will not necessarily meet benchmarks and goals set by the audiologist. Clinicians must vary test techniques and management strategies in accordance with the needs, desires, and capabilities of the child and family. Families are more apt to progress toward goals set in collaboration.

Audiologists must respond to the emotional needs of families with appropriate counseling throughout the many stages and transitions of young childhood. They also must recognize when the families' needs for emotional support are beyond what audiologists can provide, necessitating referrals to mental health professionals or family counselors (ASHA, 2008). Matching families with other families facing similar issues is an invaluable resource. Even after families become empowered and able to advocate for themselves, they may have recurring needs for emotional support in times of transition, or if their child's hearing loss progresses.

Assessment and management guidelines and protocols are frameworks for service delivery. They are fluid in that new data and new technologies shape them. Updates and revisions occur over time. Audiologists must remain current with the literature and assume responsibility as a key player in the process of communication skill development in children.

Acknowledgments. The authors thank Brenda Hoover and Elizabeth Runnion for their careful review of this manuscript and for their insightful suggestions.

References

Alvord, L. S., Doxey, G. P., & Smith, D. M. (1989). Hearing aids worn with tympanic membrane perforation: Complications and solutions. *American Journal of Otology, 10*(4), 277–280.

American Academy of Audiology (AAA). (2003). *Pediatric amplification protocol*. Retrieved July 10, 2008, from http://www.audiology.org/NR/rdonlyres/53D26792-E321-41AF-850F-CC253310F9DB/0/pedamp.pdf

American Speech-Language-Hearing Association (ASHA). (2004). *Guidelines for the audiologic assessment of children birth to 5 years of age*. Retrieved August 27, 2008, from http://www.asha.org/NR/rdonlyres/0BB7C840-27D2-4DC6-861B-1709ADD78BAF/0/v2GLAudAssessChild.pdf

American Speech-Language-Hearing Association (ASHA). (2006). *Roles, knowledge, and skills: Audiologists providing clinical services to infants and young children birth to 5 years of age*. Retrieved August 17, 2008, from http://www.asha.org/docs/html/KS2006-00259.html

American Speech-Language-Hearing Association (ASHA). (2008). *Guidelines for audiologists providing informational and adjustment counseling to families of infants and young children with hearing loss birth to 5 years of age*. Retrieved July 10, 2008, from http://www.asha.org/docs/pdf/GL2008-00289.pdf

Bench, J., Kowal, A., & Bamford, J. (1979). The BKB (Bamford-Kowal-Bench) sentence lists for partially-hearing children. *British Journal of Audiology, 13*, 108–112.

Berlin, C. I., Hood, L. J., Morlet, T., Wilensky, D., John, P., Montgomery, E., & Thibodaux, M. (2005). Absent or elevated middle ear muscle reflexes in the presence of normal otoacoustic emissions: A universal finding in 136 cases of auditory neuropathy/dys-synchrony. *Journal of the American Academy of Audiology, 16*, 546–553.

Cox, R. M. (1979). Acoustic aspects of hearing aid-ear canal coupling systems. *Monographs in Contemporary Audiology, 1*(3), 1–4.

Dalzell, L., Orlando, M., MacDonald, M., Berg, A., Bradley, M., Cacace, A., & Prieve, B. (2000). The New York State universal newborn hearing screening demonstration project: Ages of hearing loss identification, hearing aid fitting, and enrollment in early intervention. *Ear and Hearing, 21*(2), 118–130.

Dirks, D. D., & Kincaid, G. E. (1987). Basic acoustic considerations of ear canal probe measurements. *Ear and Hearing, 8*(5 Suppl), 60S–67S.

Gilman, S., & Dirks, D. D. (1986). Acoustics of ear canal measurement of eardrum SPL in simulators. *Journal of the Acoustical Society of America, 80*, 783–793.

Gorga, M. P., Johnson, T. A., Kaminski, J. R., Beauchaine, K. L., Garner, C. A., & Neely, S. T. (2006). Using a combination of click- and tone burst-evoked auditory brain stem response measurements to estimate pure-tone thresholds. *Ear and Hearing, 27*, 60–74.

Gorga, M. P., Neely, S. T., Bergman, B., Beauchaine, K. L., Kaminski, J. R., Peters, J., & Jesteadt, W. (1993). Otoacoustic emissions from normal-hearing and hearing-impaired subjects: Distortion product responses. *Journal of the Acoustical Society of America, 93*, 2050–2060.

Hoover, B. M., Stelmachowicz, P. G., & Lewis, D. E. (2000). Effect of earmold fit on predicted real ear SPL using a real ear to coupler difference procedure. *Ear and Hearing, 21*(4), 310–317.

Joint Committee on Infant Hearing (JCIH). (2007). Year 2007 position statement: Principles and guidelines for early hearing detection and intervention programs. *Pediatrics, 120*, 898–921.

Kile, J., Schaffmeyer, M. J., & Kuba, J. (1994). Assessment and management of unusual auditory behavior in infants and toddlers. *Infant Toddler Intervention, 4*(4), 299–318.

Martin, H. C., Munro, K. J., & Langer, D. H. (1997). Real-ear to coupler differences in children with grommets. *British Journal of Audiology, 31*(1), 63–69.

Pittman, A. L., & Stelmachowicz, P. G. (2003). Hearing loss in children and adults: Audiometric configuration, asymmetry and progression. *Ear and Hearing, 24*(3), 198–205.

Prieve, B. A., Gorga, M. P., Schmidt, A., Neely, S., Peters, J. Schulte, L., & Jesteadt, W. (1993). Analysis of transient-evoked otoacoustic emissions in normal-hearing and hearing-impaired ears. *Journal of the Acoustical Society of America, 93*, 3308–3319.

Schmida, M. J., Peterson, H. J., & Tharpe, A. M. (2003). Visual reinforcement audiometry using digital video disc and conventional reinforcers. *American Journal of Audiology, 12*, 35–40.

Stapells, D. R. (2000). Threshold estimation by the tone-evoked ABR: A literature meta-analysis. *Journal of Speech-Language Pathology and Audiology, 24*, 74–83.

Widen, J. E., Folsom, R. C., Cone-Wesson, B., Carty, L., Dunnell, J. J., Koebsell, K., & Norton, S. J. (2000). Identification of neonatal hearing impairment: Hearing status at 8–12 months corrected age using a visual reinforcement audiometry protocol. *Ear and Hearing, 21*(5), 471–487.

APPENDIX 32–A

An Efficient Setup for VRA

- Test assistant or "play partner" in the test booth to keep the child motivated and at midline
- Infrared or FM system to talk to test assistant
- Sound field system
- A range of distraction toys for the audiologist or assistant to manipulate, from simple to complex to suit different interest levels of children. The toys should not make noise. Consider:
  - Plastic linking or stacking toys
  - Large plastic toy cars
  - Stuffed animals or puppets (to be used by only by test assistant, avoid contact with children as they cannot be sanitized appropriately)
  - Unbreakable mirror
  - Soft, washable colorful books
  - Spring toys
  - Soft balls
  - Flashlight, if needed to distract a child with visual impairment
- An assortment of visual reinforcement toys. More is better.
  - Shadow boxes with toys that light up and move. If space allows, choose larger boxes that are well lit with large animated toys.
  - Computer monitors that play slides showing animated objects or video clips. (Schmida, Peterson, & Tharpe, 2003). Connect the monitors to a main control computer on the tester's side, use a switch box to turn monitors on and off.
  - Make-your-own computerized reinforcement: Add pictures or video to a computerized slide presentation. Add animation features. Place completely black slides in-between each animated slide. Run the "slide show," advancing to animated toy slides for reinforcement, and advancing to black slides between stimuli.
- Speech stimuli for monitored live-voice presentation:
  - "Bye-bye baby"
  - "Okay, okay big girl/boy"
  - "Hey-hey (child's name)"
- Music stimuli: choose common and popular children's music

APPENDIX 32–B

An Efficient Setup for Conditioned Play Audiometry (CPA)

- Test assistant in booth to train the child to the task and to keep the child motivated
- Infrared or FM system to talk to test assistant
- A range of toys for different ages and levels of dexterity. The toys must be easy to clean and have minimal choke precautions
  - Stacking rings or cups
  - Blocks and a bucket
  - Pegs and a pegboard
  - Checkers that stack vertically
  - Plastic cookies and jar
  - Button or switch that makes enough sound when pressed to be picked up over the talk-back microphone
  - Game for older children—"Magic Button": The child is trained to press a button or switch as the response, and the clinician activates a visual reinforcement (shadow boxes or computer monitors) or a computerized slide presentation on an in-booth computer monitor.

APPENDIX 32–C

Child-Friendly Tips and Techniques for Audiologic Assessment

- Examine your manner and how the child and family are reacting to you. Put yourself at the child's eye level. Keep yourself calm with gentle movements when approaching the child. If you are anxious, the child is likely to be anxious. Smile!
- Give the child something to hold in both hands while doing otoscopy, tympanometry, OAE testing, while taking earmold impressions, or during probe microphone measures.
- Keep cords behind the child and out of reach when possible.
- Engage the child in the activity; make it a game.
  - If buttons need to be pressed on tympanometry, OAE or probe-microphone equipment, guide the child's hands to press them.
- Make procedures sound and look less frightening.
  - Cover the tympanometry probe until the soft tip is in place. Tell the child that it is an "ear camera." Show them the "pictures" when the test is complete. Some preschoolers like to have their own printout of the test.
  - Let older children play with excess ear-impression material while it hardens. Use care that they do not put in their mouth.
- Bubbles! Engage parents or test assistant in blowing bubbles when the child needs to sit for OAEs, tympanometry, earmolds, or probe-microphone measures.
- A player to show movies can distract the child during OAEs, tympanometry, earmolds, or probe-microphone measures.
- A supply of stickers for distraction and for reward.
- Speech and language milestones for a variety of ages to give to parents.

33

School-Aged Children

Carolyne Edwards

Introduction

When children reach school age, the focus of our audiologic attention changes in response to the different players involved. Assessment and management of school aged children demands a comprehensive view of their educational setting and the people who now enter their school life. On the professional side, those people include the classroom teacher, special education teacher, principal, teacher of the deaf and hard of hearing, educational audiologist, speech-language pathologist, and other support personnel as needed. On the personal side, children now must interact with a large group of other children, who may or may not have hearing loss depending on the school setting. Family members are the one constant throughout and therefore carry the history of where their child began and the direction for the future.

The audiologist must now focus on how to create the most optimal integration of children with hearing loss into the elementary school setting. Although educational audiologists are best known for their direct mandate in children's auditory needs in the school system, it behooves all audiologists to see themselves as vital contributors to children's educational progress and to ensure that the necessary steps are taken to provide for the learning needs of all children with hearing loss.

Creating Optimal Integration for Children With Hearing Loss

The audiologist contributes to the children's successful integration into the school setting in the following ways:

- assessment of children under a variety of listening conditions to provide:
  - an ongoing picture of the growth in children's listening abilities;
  - the communication strategies necessary for optimal understanding of speech in the classroom;
- description of children's auditory functioning in layperson terms so that all personnel who work with hearing-impaired children develop appropriate expectations of their auditory capabilities;
- description of the social-emotional impact of hearing loss so that personnel working with children with hearing loss can incorporate that knowledge into their strategies;
- evaluation of amplification needs on an ongoing basis in order to respond to the changing auditory demands of the classroom;
- communication with the team of key support personnel at the school level to ascertain concerns and issues that need to be addressed by the audiologist;
- addressing the counseling needs of children and their families as the school demands change.

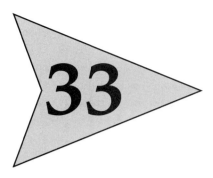

Assessment of Listening Skills

Audiologic assessment has moved well beyond diagnosis and monitoring of hearing levels in the last 25 years. In the early years, the only audiologic information requested at school case conferences was the pure-tone audiogram and the degree of hearing loss. In recent years, educational and clinical audiologists alike have forwarded information to school personnel to describe:

- the type and degree of hearing loss,
- the child's auditory potential based on degree of hearing loss,
- the child's current auditory capacity to understand speech,
- predictors of the child's listening difficulty,
- the effects of middle ear function on the child's hearing levels and everyday functioning,
- the effects of the child's hearing loss on functioning within current school setting,
- the relationship of the child's hearing loss to overall functioning.

Although traditional testing protocols consisted of the pure-tone audiogram, middle ear measurement, speech awareness or reception thresholds and a word discrimination score, there is a wide variety of speech tests now available to measure understanding of speech under varying conditions. The audiologist is able to provide a comprehensive description of a child's listening skills and then measure changes over time. This information is critical to the school staff's understanding of the child's current and future needs in the classroom.

Degree of Hearing Loss

Degree of hearing loss is the most well-reported and understood characteristic of audiologic testing. Anderson's *Relationship of Hearing Loss to Listening and Learning Needs* (2007) continues to provide valuable descriptors of auditory functioning in layperson language for hearing levels ranging from unilateral hearing loss to bilateral minimal to profound sensorineural hearing loss (Appendix 33–A). Audiologists would be wise to include these descriptors in their reports to schools.

Type of Hearing Loss

Often the type of hearing loss is no longer prominent in audiologic reporting as the child enters the school years. However, it is useful to differentiate at the time of school entry the functional differences between the child with conductive hearing loss and the child with sensorineural hearing loss so that educators know what to expect with regard to speech perception and speech intelligibility.

Middle Ear Function

The presence of abnormal middle ear function is significant to educators for one or more reasons and can be reported as such:

- the pure-tone thresholds obtained on the audiogram do not reflect the child's optimal hearing levels;
- the child may perform more poorly than usual and need a higher volume setting or a different program on the hearing aid;
- the child may need more support and communication strategies in the classroom;
- if hearing levels are significantly poorer than typical levels, then the child may be more fatigued than usual.
- Normal middle ear function indicates that the pure tone thresholds reflect optimum potential for understanding of speech.

Speech Perception Ability

The original purpose of speech testing was to obtain a validation of pure tone thresholds and a measure of understanding of speech using speech perception tests. Unlike the adult population where the results are given directly to the individual with hearing loss, results of testing for children are sent to school settings so that educators can better understand the impact of hearing loss. Although speech perception testing continues to be commonly used in clinics, it does not necessarily give a direct representation of the child's ability to function in the classroom under the variety of listening conditions encountered in the school. Therefore, additional tests are useful and round out the audiologic results in order to increase relevance of speech testing to the educational environment.

Testing Different Modalities

The impact of hearing loss is well known to audiologists but those who work with children in the schools often have little background knowledge in the area of audition. Therefore, when the audiologist can present speech perception scores that demonstrate the child's capacity to understand speech by listening only and by listening and speechreading, teachers have a better idea of the impact of various listening conditions.

SAMPLE SPEECH PERCEPTION SCORES

Child #1	
By listening only:	92%
Child #2	
By listening only:	48%
By listening and speechreading:	92%
Child #3	
By listening only:	16%
By listening and speechreading:	76%
By speechreading only:	48%
Child #4	
By listening only:	0%
By listening and speechreading:	56%
By speechreading only:	60%

Although speechreading cues enhance comprehension of speech, child #1 will not be affected by the loss of speechreading cues to the same degree as the other three children in the above examples. When the teacher looks away or turns to the blackboard to write, child #2, #3, and #4 will lose critical information. Notice the difference between child #3 and child #4. Child #4 has little use for auditory information and is functioning primarily through visual information only. In contrast, child #3 improves speech perception with the combination of auditory and visual clues together.

Testing Different Intensity Levels and Speech-to-Noise Ratios

Classroom listening conditions vary considerably depending on the grade level, the classroom activity, the number of students in the class, the location of the student in the classroom and proximity to the teacher and the acoustical conditions of the classroom. Testing at speech-to-noise ratios of +5 dB or 0 dB will best replicate challenging acoustic conditions in most classrooms without the use of classroom amplification systems (Crandell & Smaldino, 2002; Hetu, Truchon-Gagnon, & Bilodeau, 1990).

SAMPLE SCENARIOS

Child #1	
Word recognition at normal conversational speech:	92%
Word recognition at quiet conversational speech:	56%
Word recognition at normal conversational speech in background noise (S/N = + 5 dB):	68%
Child #2	
Word recognition at normal conversational speech:	56%
Word recognition at quiet conversational speech:	12%
Word recognition at normal conversational speech in background noise (S/N = + 5 dB):	16%

Notice that child #2 will have considerably more difficulty than child #1 when the teacher is at a distance (quiet conversational speech levels) or in the presence of background noise when the teacher is within close proximity.

Test results such as the above scenarios can highlight for the audiologist the importance of recommending other technologies such as an FM system, a boom microphone versus a lapel microphone, and strategies such as preferred seating locations in the classroom. The quantitative data offered by speech perception scores are useful in describing the child's auditory difficulties in the classroom, potential problems and recommended solutions to educators.

Testing Different Speech Materials

One of the easiest modifications for word recognition testing is to record the child's responses and then score the number of phonemes correct in addition to the number of words correct.

WORD VERSUS PHONEME SCORING

Child #1	
Word recognition at 50 dB HL	32%
Phoneme recognition at 50 dB HL	66%
Child #2	
Word recognition at 50 dB HL	32%
Phoneme recognition at 50 dB HL	36%

Although the word recognition scores for both children is the same, the phoneme scores are significantly different, suggesting far more auditory perceptual errors for the second child. These difficulties will be apparent on spelling tasks and often will be reflected in the child's speech intelligibility.

For children with high-frequency hearing loss, Gardner's high frequency monosyllabic word list (Berger, 1977) continues to be useful to demonstrate to the child, teacher or parents the listening challenges that are not clearly seen with administration of a conventional word list that has no special emphasis on high-frequency phonemes.

Although word recognition testing is a more reliable and valid indicator of auditory perception, it does not represent the nature of the speech that a child faces in the classroom. The child is faced with sentence material, and often a series of sentences presented without pause in the classroom. It is difficult to standardize norms for children's performance on phrase or sentence material since it is highly language dependent. Therefore, testing that goes beyond word recognition is not used as a precise comparative measure of performance from year to year, but rather as an indication of the degree of enhancement in understanding speech when moving from word to sentence material using materials such as BKB sentences (Bamford, Koval, & Bench, 1979), or the Speech-in-Noise test (SPIN; Kalikow, Stevens, & Elliott, 1977).

In some cases such as precipitous hearing loss, the difference between word recognition and sentence recognition is great, often showing very low scores on word recognition of 30% or less and high scores on sentence materials ranging from 76 to 100% with the addition of the acoustic and contextual clues provided by connected speech. The child's functioning in the classroom can be better described by including both measures than either measure alone.

There are a variety of other speech materials using phrase or sentence recognition or comprehension tasks that can be used to gain a broader understanding of the child's auditory abilities (DeConde Johnson, Benson, & Seaton, 1997a; Edwards 1991, 1999). The reader is referred to these references for further elaboration of pediatric speech test batteries for school-aged children.

Description of Auditory Functioning

Many educators have little familiarity with the nature of audiologic testing. Therefore audiologic assessment and reporting that can translate clinical findings into meaningful descriptions of classroom functioning is essential to produce changes in educators' understanding of the auditory needs of the child.

The audiologist needs to describe the nature of the hearing loss in terms of implications for the classroom, specifically the challenges that the child will have in the classroom. The questions below can be used as a guide to the type of information valuable to educators.

- What is the child's capacity to understand speech?
  - by listening only?
  - by listening and watching the teacher's face?

  How much does the child rely on hearing alone? Will the child be able to understand the teacher when they are not facing each other? Is the child reliant on watching the teacher's face to understand speech?
- Which speech sounds are difficult to hear?
  Does the child have difficulty hearing high frequency speech sounds such as s, f, voiceless "th" or "ch" or t? The /s/ sound is a grammatically loaded sound in the English language that signifies plurals, possessives, and change in verb tense. If a child is unable to hear the /s/, it is useful for the teacher to know so the child can be provided with other grammatical clues instead.
- How will distance affect the child's understanding of speech?
  - without amplification?
  - with hearing aid(s)?
  - with classroom hearing technology?

  School situations such as classroom discussion, listening in the gymnasium during sports activities, gatherings of the whole school for assemblies, the playground and class trips involve distance listening. The degree of difficulty children experience for softer degrees of speech will affect their ability to respond in these situations. Identifying the child's degree of difficulty in these situations will be helpful to the child's teachers. Furthermore, educators will need to know how much change to expect when a child uses a classroom hearing technology.

- How will noise affect their understanding of speech?
  - without amplification?
  - with hearing aid/s?
  - with classroom hearing technology?

  School situations such as small group work, seminar groups, and listening in the gymnasium during sports activities involve listening in noise. The degree of difficulty children experience in noise will affect their ability to respond in these situations. Again, educators need to know how much improvement will occur when classroom hearing technology is used.

- What modifications will assist the child in hearing better?
  - proximity to the teacher
  - use of FM system
  - repetition and buddy systems
  - visual supports—speechreading and written supplements

  For children not using an FM system who have difficulty listening at a distance, sitting close to the teacher during circle time for primary levels or row seating near the teacher for higher grades will be beneficial.

Most children with hearing loss will benefit from the use of classroom hearing technology of some kind IF there are large group teaching situations in which they are involved. Evaluation of candidacy for an FM system is best done at the school level where the educational audiologist and the teacher of the deaf and hard of hearing, and occasionally the speech-language pathologist, are in direct contact with the classroom teacher and can assess the nature of the classroom structure and its suitability for the use of such systems. The clinical audiologist can raise the issue of FM use for consideration with the parents and child as soon as the child enters school. Furthermore, the audiologist needs to ensure that hearing aid settings are compatible with FM use. See Chapter 26 for detailed discussion of FM system use.

Where the child has difficulty in quiet listening situations by listening only, it is wise to ensure that there are other strategies put into place to support comprehension, such as repetition of instructions by the teacher, or a buddy system where a classmate is selected to provide repetition of instructions as required by the child.

When a child is dependent on speechreading for accurate listening, the importance of speechreading needs to be underlined. Educators need to be aware that when they turn their backs to write on the blackboard or to address another child, the understanding by the child with hearing loss will be compromised. Writing key words or instructions on the blackboard, the overhead projector or on interactive white boards will assist the child by supplementing the loss of speechreading information.

In summary, audiologists must ensure that that the implications of audiologic testing are translated into concrete actions for those working with children in the classroom setting.

Social-Emotional Impact of Hearing Loss

Children's sense of difference from their family and friends starts to develop between ages 7 and 9 years (Rall, 2007). Even with the best technology available, we cannot change the fact that children with hearing loss will have more difficulty hearing under degraded listening conditions (such as noise and distance) than their hearing peers. However, what we can change is children's attitudes toward their differences.

Accurate perspective comes from acceptance of both the similarities AND the differences from others. Some children will imagine their difference as greater than it appears to others, and some children may imagine their differences as less than they appear to others. Without adequate input and feedback from others in their environment, either viewpoint can lead to inappropriate use of communication strategies due to an inaccurate perspective of auditory needs.

Children with hearing loss often identify their own listening difficulties, but do not know that normal-hearing peers also have difficulty listening in noise, with the resulting feeling that others will never understand their experience. That feeling of separation from others must be bridged in order to bring a greater sense of self worth.

The audiologist can encourage the classroom teacher to support sharing of listening difficulties by all students in the class so that children with hearing loss begin to understand that everyone, normal hearing or hearing impaired, has difficulty hearing in noise to varying degrees. When children with hearing loss understand that they are not alone in their experience of auditory challenges, it gives them more confidence to ask for help and implement strategies to enhance communication. If the teacher can make all children in the class part of the solution, communication strategies become inclusive rather than isolating (Edwards, 1996, 2005).

Simulation of hearing loss using earplugs (Appendix 33–B) is an effective way to educate individuals about hearing loss (Edwards, 2005). Whether we give earplugs to a child's classmates, teachers, or to the child's parents for a personal experience of mild loss, the experience of simulated hearing loss is powerful and memorable for most people and can elicit a surprising empathy for the person with hearing loss.

Children need an opportunity to share their thoughts and feelings about hearing loss for acknowledgement and validation of their experiences. Sharing can reveal what is working and what is not working in the classroom, what strategies to continue, what strategies need to be discarded and what new strategies need to be implemented. Audiologists can use such tools such as the Listening Inventory for Education (LIFE; Anderson & Smaldino, 1998), Child Home Inventory for Home Listening Difficulties (CHILD; Anderson & Smaldino, 2000) or scales such as the Children's Peer Relationship Scale (English, 2002) to elicit comments on the ease or lack of ease of listening for the child. Alternately, audiologists can use open-ended questions and discussion such as:

- How do you feel about your FM system?
- What do your classmates understand about your hearing loss?
- What is difficult to explain to your classmates?
- What is frustrating about school right now?
- What is working in the classroom and what is not?

Such information can then lead to discussion of strategies that might assist students in the classroom and with their peers.

Audiologists can support the development of children's self-advocacy skills in the clinical setting and the educational setting. Children need to understand their own audiogram, and be knowledgeable about the cause of their hearing loss, the implications of their hearing loss, and any progression of hearing loss through the years. They must have an increasing understanding of their hearing technology and how best to use it, and the types of hearing concerns that they should report to their audiologist: Audiologists can be effective teachers in these subject areas.

The educational audiologist in the school system can engage the child in decisions about the type of education to be provided to their classmates and teacher about hearing loss and the degree of involvement of the child in such programming. Often the student knows more about their hearing devices than their classroom teachers; it is important to encourage the classroom teacher to draw on the student's expertise when possible.

Having children teach others about their hearing loss builds confidence and empowers students to learn how to manage their hearing impairment. The ways in which we support children will change with their age. For younger children, they can show their classmates how their hearing aid works with support personnel such as the educational audiologist or the teacher of the deaf and hard of hearing present as support. Older students can teach others about their hearing loss through science projects, class presentations, lessons on sound, or being part of a hearing awareness day in the school where various booths are created to teach others about hearing loss and hearing aids. Giving children experiences in managing their own hearing needs teaches them what works and what does not, increases their awareness of options, improves their decision-making ability and their ability to negotiate solutions.

Audiologists also need to be aware of a child's educational placement in order to intuit the challenges that may be confronted. Children in the mainstream can feel the pressure to be the same as their peers and therefore may minimize any interventions that demonstrate their differences from others. Children in self-contained classes in the mainstream often feel more secure in their class with other hearing impaired peers, but may need more support for their visits to the general education classes. Children in schools for the deaf often are secure in their school setting with their deaf peers but face their greatest challenges in their social community at home, either as day students who by the time they arrive home on the bus have little energy to interact with people other than their family, or as residential students whose weekend visits with their families leave only brief opportunities to interact with the hearing world.

Ongoing Evaluation of Hearing Technology Needs

Most children with hearing loss are candidates for some form of classroom amplification. As described in detail in Chapter 26 of this volume, there are a myriad of FM system configuration options now available for children with varying degrees of hearing loss as well as for children with normal hearing. Table 33–1 shows many of the possible choices facing the audiologist in

Table 33–1. Selection of Amplification System

Type of Classroom Amplification System	
Personal FM System	***Sound Field System***
FM Receiver Options	*Nature of Signal Transmission*
∞ Ear level hearing aid with FM receiver attached to audio shoe	∞ FM system
∞ universal FM receiver and separate audio shoe	∞ conventional frequency
∞ integrated FM receiver and audio shoe	∞ ultrahigh frequency
∞ Ear level hearing aid and neckloop FM receiver	∞ Infrared system
∞ Ear level hearing aid and body worn FM receiver	*Type of Loudspeaker*
∞ Combined hearing aid—FM in ear level casing	∞ Totable
∞ FM receiver only in ear level casing	∞ Portable
∞ FM body-worn receiver	∞ Stationary
∞ with ear level hearing aid and audio shoe	∞ Single Speaker
∞ with earphones	∞ Multiple speakers
∞ Cochlear implant	• Wall mounted • Ceiling mounted
∞ FM receiver with ear level processor	*Type of Transmitter Options*
∞ FM receiver with body-worn processor	∞ Single-channel transmitter
∞ neckloop FM receiver	∞ Dual-channel transmitter
FM Transmitter Options	∞ Pass around microphone
∞ Single channel transmitter	*Type of Ear Coupling for Transmitter*
∞ Dual channel transmitter	∞ Over-the-ear microphones
∞ Multichannel transmitter	∞ Collar microphone
∞ Pass around microphone	∞ Lapel microphone
∞ Coupling Options for Transmitter	
∞ Lapel microphone	
∞ Boom microphone	
∞ Collar microphone	

order to make a recommendation for an FM system for a school child.

As the reader can see, audiologists must gather information on the child's hearing aids, the type of classroom setting, the structure and scheduling of the classroom setting, the type of instruction, the teacher's use of the system, and the child's willingness to accept a device, to select the optimal FM system for a child. Then these choices must be reviewed annually to ensure the equipment can be modified to include any additional amplification needs arising from changing classroom structure or demands.

The important questions that audiologists must ask to ascertain the need for change are:

■ *What has changed, if anything, in the classroom structure?*

If there is team teaching in the classroom, the FM system will have to provide multiple transmitters working within the same classroom without interference. Different manufacturers have different ways of addressing this. If the child has an educational assistant who does the primary work with the child, one must consider a second transmitter on a different frequency and determine who will wear the "master" transmitter. If there is small group work in the classroom, a pass-around microphone may be necessary. The child may prefer a different type of microphone (boom versus lapel) depending on the vocal characteristics of the teacher's voice.

- *Has the child changed from a single classroom to rotary classes?*

For children with sound field systems, a totable or portable system rather than stationary loudspeaker system, or change to a personal FM system, should be considered.

- *Are there any interference problems reported this year?*

Transmission frequency may need to be changed if the student reports interference. With a change in classrooms, the frequency that the child was previously using may no longer be suitable. Interference may occur in one area of the school and not in another area.

And, of course, any time that the child's hearing aids change, the FM system must be evaluated with the new amplification to ensure compatibility and transparency. The other outstanding issue that occurs with the use of FM systems is the monitoring and maintenance of such systems.

With sound field systems, it is immediately obvious to everyone when the system is not working. However, with personal FM systems, we are dependent on the child reporting a problem or one of the school staff checking the system to ensure adequate functioning. The historical data on adequate functioning of hearing aids are quite discouraging, so it is critical to ensure that a staff member has been trained to check the personal FM system in combination with the hearing aid(s) and does so on a routine basis.

Despite the enhanced speech-to-noise ratio when the FM transmitter is in use by the teacher, children with hearing loss are still acoustically challenged during small group work. Overhearing is an important part of language development for normal hearing children and children with hearing loss (Moeller, 2008), and yet children with hearing loss do not have many technological or acoustic options to assist with overhearing. The FM system is not a viable option for the rapid communication that occurs in small groups and so enhancement of classroom acoustical conditions is the only option available. Unfortunately, there has been less emphasis on improving classroom acoustics in recent years.

Carpeting the classroom is still the most effective way to reduce the noise of classroom chairs scraping on the floor and provide some absorption of children's voices, particularly if carpet underpadding is added (Crandell & Smaldino, 2005). Tennis balls placed on the bottom of chair legs will reduce the noise of chairs scraping against the hard floor surfaces but will not provide any absorption of the overall classroom noise. Precut tennis balls are commercially available through several companies in Canada and the United States. For acoustic design modifications to classrooms, readers are referred to Melancon, Truchon-Gagnon, and Hodgson (1990) for a comprehensive guide.

Working With Other Professionals

The audiologist's mandate within the educational setting is to ensure that every aspect of audition is addressed for the child with hearing loss. Depending on the extent of involvement, the audiologist can be seen on a continuum from a peripheral consultant to an integral part of the team of professionals working with the child with hearing loss.

What is unique about the audiologist's role in providing information regarding auditory perception? The audiologist can:

- Provide the school staff with a clear sense of expectations for the child's understanding of speech in the classroom;
- Identify the communication challenges that the child will have in the classroom;
- Determine the contribution of hearing loss to the child's reported academic, social or behavioral difficulties, especially for children with multiple learning challenges;
- Provide the information necessary for working with the child's hearing aids;
- Provide recommendations for classroom hearing technology;
- Educate the class regarding hearing loss and amplification devices;
- Meet with the child as needed regarding any hearing related concerns;
- Meet with parents regarding any hearing-related concerns;
- Support interactions between the child with hearing loss and other classmates;
- Meet with hearing resource staff regarding auditory programming.

It is important that the audiologist anticipate the areas of difficulty that might arise with school personnel to manage proactively. For example, for children with subtle hearing loss, school personnel often do not notice any obvious hearing difficulties with the child. It is useful to ask the staff if there are *any* areas that they have concern with first, prior to sharing information. That will allow the audiologist to build on staff information and align with them rather than creating resistance at the beginning by assuming that others have also seen the problem.

When other personnel report other speech, language, emotional and learning concerns for the child, the audiologist must be prepared to state which of those issues are likely affected by hearing loss and which are unaffected by hearing loss. This is particularly helpful for teachers, parents, and other staff when too much or too little attention is focused on the effects of the hearing loss.

Counseling Needs of Children and Families

It is essential that children and parents have an opportunity to express their feelings related to the hearing loss as feelings arise. What feelings can emerge? Isolation can occur when the child feels different from his peers. Frustration and anger can occur when the child cannot change the environment, and the differences from his peers become evident. Denial of hearing loss or increased dependency can emerge as default strategies to cope with hearing loss. The child can feel lost or want to give up when there is not enough support available in the environment to cope.

Parents can experience similar feelings when they are unable to change their child's reality and make it better for their child and when they do not have other parents with whom to share. Luterman and Kurtzer-White (1999) found that when parents of preschool hearing-impaired children were asked what the most important factor was in their adjustment to the diagnosis of their child's hearing loss, they indicated that it was meeting other parents, specifically other parents of children with hearing loss.

Often, parents are not aware of the many areas of support that are available to them. The Family Needs Survey (DeConde Johnson, Benson, & Seaton, 1997b) can empower parents to ask for the support they need. By having the family fill out the survey before meeting with the audiologist, parents learn more about the questions they can ask relating to general information, specific information about hearing and hearing loss, communication, services and educational resources, family and social support, child care, and community services and financial support. By the time they see the audiologist, they are better informed as to the support services that could be useful to them at that time and are equipped to ask questions about those services.

Acceptance of the child's hearing loss is often presented as a one-time experience, but in reality, each time there is a new demand in the child's environment that is constrained by hearing loss, parents are faced with a new demand for acceptance of the hearing loss. Parents hold the balance and perspective between the child's current reality and the dream of who their child can be. Audiologists must be sensitive to these demands and be able to acknowledge and discuss both the reality of the current situation and the child's auditory potential in the context of the child's school performance.

Although much attention is given to the tutoring and academic support that parents provide, we must not forget their role in modeling an attitude and approach to hearing loss that will support the child through the school years. Through counseling at different stages of the child's development, audiologists can help parents to model principles essential for acceptance and growth of the child's individuality.

Perspective is key in facilitating a child's understanding of oneself both as a person and as a child with hearing loss. Parents can model perspective by acknowledging and naming difficult communicative situations for the child. When the child recognizes those situations, parents can then teach the child *choice* by discussing and modeling a variety of communication strategies to explore under acoustically challenging situations. When parents reinforce the child's use of strategies to improve listening, they support the development of the child's *decision-making* skills. The child learns that decision-making is an ongoing process in response to the communicative situation, and that there are no mistakes, but rather simply more opportunities to learn. Finally, parents can stand behind the child when the child begins to advocate for their own communicative needs—providing *independence with support*. That is a critical step prior to the child having to advocate independently. The audiologist can show the parents how to model each of these steps for their child in order to co-empower both the child and the family.

Summary

The audiologic management of the child with hearing loss through the school years is broad-ranging and multifaceted, and is directed by the child's clinical and educational audiologists. Audiologists must work with the child, the family, the educators, and other school personnel in order to ensure that the audiologic information is meaningful and relevant to the child's progress. The information from the school staff is essential to shape the audiologic recommendations for further assessment, changes in amplification, implications of hearing loss, and directions for counseling for the child and family. Ease of communication among all of the personnel involved with the child can ensure that all the child's auditory needs are being addressed.

When we reach the stage where young adults with hearing loss who are graduating from high school no longer depend on their parents, clinical or educational audiologists, or the classroom teachers for the management of their communication needs, then we will have done our job well.

References

Anderson, K. (2007). *Relationship of hearing loss to listening and learning needs*. Retrieved from Karen Anderson Audiology Consulting Web site: http://www.kandersonaudconsulting.com/

Anderson, K., & Smaldino, J. (1998). *Listening Inventory for Education (LIFE)*. Westminster, CO: Educational Audiology Association.

Anderson, K. L., & Smaldino, J. J. (2000). Children's Home Inventory for Listening Difficulties (CHILD). *Educational Audiology Review, 17*(3 Suppl).

Bamford, J., Koval, A., & Bench, J. (1979). *Speech hearing tests and the spoken language of partially hearing children*. New York, NY: Academic Press.

Berger, K. (1977). Gardner High Frequency List. In *Speech audiometry materials*. Kent, OH: Herald.

Bess, F. (1982). Children with unilateral hearing loss. *Journal of Rehabilitative Audiology, 15,* 131–144.

Bess, F., Dodd-Murphy, J., & Parker, R. (1998). Children with minimal sensorineural hearing loss: Prevalence, educational performance and functional status. *Ear and Hearing, 19*(5), 339–355.

Crandell, C., & Smaldino, J. (2002). *Classroom acoustics*. Paper presented at the American Academy of Audiology National Convention, Philadelphia, PA.

Crandell, C., & Smaldino, J. (2005). Acoustical modifications in classrooms. In C. Crandell, J. Smaldino, & C. Flexer (Eds.), *Sound field FM amplification: Applications to speech perception and classroom acoustics* (2nd ed.). New York, NY: Thomson Delmar Learning.

DeConde Johnson, C., Benson, P., & Seaton, J. (1997a). Assessment practices. In *Educational audiology handbook* (pp. 478–488). San Diego, CA: Singular.

DeConde Johnson, C., Benson, P., & Seaton, J. (1997b), Family needs survey—Appendix 10-B. In *Educational audiology handbook* (pp. 443–444). San Diego, CA: Singular.

Edwards, C. (1991). Assessment and management of listening skills in school aged children. *Seminars in Hearing 12*(4), 389–401.

Edwards, C. (1996). Auditory intervention for children with mild auditory deficits. In F. Bess, J. Gravel, & A. M. Tharpe (Eds.), *Amplification for children with auditory deficits*. Nashville, TN: Bill Wilkerson Center Press.

Edwards, C. (1999). Current directions in educational audiology. In J. Katz & L. Medwetsky (Eds.), *Handbook of clinical audiology* (4th ed.). Baltimore, MD: Williams & Wilkins.

Edwards, C. (2005). From system selection to enhancement of listening skills: Considerations for the classroom. In C. Crandell, J. Smaldino, & C. Flexer (Eds.), *Sound field FM amplification: Applications to speech perception and classroom acoustics* (2nd ed., pp. 166–191). New York, NY: Thomson Delmar Learning.

English, K. (2002). *Counseling children with hearing impairment and their families*. Boston, MA: Allyn and Bacon.

English, K., & Church, G. (1999). Unilateral hearing loss in children: An update for the 1990s. *Language, Speech and Hearing Services in the Schools, 30*, 26–31.

Hetu, R., Truchon-Gagnon, C., & Bilodeau, S. (1990). Problems of noise in school settings: A review of the literature and the results of an exploratory study. *Journal of Speech Language Pathology and Audiology/Revue d´Orthophonie et d´Audiologie, 14*(3), 31–39.

Kalikow, D., Stevens, K., & Elliott, L. (1977). Development of a test of speech intelligibility in noise using sentence materials with controlled word predictability. *Journal of the Acoustical Society of America, 61,* 1337–1351.

Kenworthy, O. T., Klee, T., & Tharpe, A. M. (1990). Speech recognition ability of children with unilateral sensorineural hearing loss as a function of amplification, speech stimuli, and listening condition. *Ear and Hearing, 11,* 264–270.

Lieu, J. E. (2004). Speech-language and educational consequences of unilateral hearing loss in children. *Archives of Otolaryngology-Head and Neck Surgery, 130*, 524–530.

Luterman, D., & Kurtzer-White, E. (1999). Identifying hearing loss: Parents' needs. *American Journal of Audiology, 8*(1), 13–18.

Melancon, L., Truchon-Gagnon, C., & Hodgson, M. (1990). *Architectural strategies to avoid noise problems in child care centres*. Montreal, Canada: Groupe d'acoustique de l'Universite de Montreal.

Moeller, M. P. (2008). Building sound foundations: What's in a word? In R. Seewald, & J. Bamford (Eds.), *A sound foundation through early amplification 2007: Proceedings of the fourth international conference.* Stäfa, Switzerland: Phonak AG.

Oyler, R., Oyler, A. & Matkin, N. (1988). Unilateral hearing loss: Demographics and educational impact. *Language, Speech and Hearing Services in Schools, 19*, 201–210.

Rall, E. (2007). *Supporting psychosocial development of children with hearing loss*. Poster Session Presentation at the Sound Foundation through Early Amplification. Fourth International Conference, Chicago, IL.

Tharpe, A. M. (2008). Minimal hearing loss in children: The facts and the fiction. In R. Seewald & J. Bamford (Eds.), *A sound foundation through early amplification 2007: Proceedings of the fourth international conference* (pp. 213–219). Stäfa, Switzerland: Phonak AG.

APPENDIX 33–A

Relationship of Hearing Loss to Listening and Learning Needs

16-25 dB HEARING LOSS		
Possible Impact on the Understanding of Language and Speech	**Possible Social Impact**	**Potential Educational Accommodations and Services**
Impact of a hearing loss that is approximately 20 dB can be compared to ability to hear when index fingers are placed in your ears. Child may have difficulty hearing faint or distant speech. At 16 dB student can miss up to 10% of speech signal when teacher is at a distance greater than 3 feet. A 20 dB or greater hearing loss in the better ear can result in absent, inconsistent or distorted parts of speech, especially word endings (s, ed) and unemphasized sounds. Percent of speech signal missed will be greater whenever there is background noise in the classroom, especially in the elementary grades when instruction is primarily verbal and younger children have greater difficulty listening in noise. Young children have the tendency to watch and copy the movements of other students rather than attending to auditorily fragmented teacher directions.	May be unaware of subtle conversational cues that could cause child to be viewed as inappropriate or awkward. May miss portions of fast-paced peer interactions that could begin to have an impact on socialization and self concept. Behavior may be confused for immaturity or inattention. May be more fatigued due to extra effort needed for understanding speech.	Noise in typical classroom environments impede child from having full access to teacher instruction. Will benefit from improved acoustic treatment of classroom and sound-field amplification. Favorable seating necessary. May often have difficulty with sound/letter associations and subtle auditory discrimination skills necessary for reading. May need attention to vocabulary or speech, especially when there has been a long history of middle ear fluid. Depending on loss configuration, may benefit from low power hearing aid with personal FM system. Appropriate medical management necessary for conductive losses. Inservice on impact of "minimal" 15 – 25 dB hearing loss on language development, listening in noise and learning, required for teacher.

26-40 dB HEARING LOSS		
Possible Impact on the Understanding of Language and Speech	**Possible Social Impact**	**Potential Educational Accommodations and Services**
Effect of a hearing loss of approximately 20 dB can be compared to ability to hear when index fingers are placed in ears therefore a 26 – 40 dB hearing loss causes greater listening difficulties than a "plugged ear" loss. Child can "hear" but misses fragments of speech leading to misunderstanding. Degree of difficulty experienced in school will depend upon noise level in the classroom, distance from the teacher, and configuration of the hearing loss, even with hearing aids. At 30 dB can miss 25-40% of the speech signal; at 40 dB may miss 50% of class discussions, especially when voices are faint or speaker is not in line of vision. Will miss unemphasized words and consonants, especially when a high frequency hearing loss is present. Often experiences difficulty learning early reading skills such as letter/sound associations. Child's ability to understand and succeed in the classroom will be substantially diminished by speaker distance and background noise, especially in the elementary grades.	Barriers begin to build with negative impact on self-esteem as child is accused of "hearing when he/she wants to," "daydreaming," or "not paying attention." May believe he/she is less capable due to difficulties understanding in class. Child begins to lose ability for selective listening, and has increasing difficulty suppressing background noise causing the learning environment to be more stressful. Child is more fatigued due to effort needed to listen.	Noise in typical class will impede child from full access to teacher instruction. Will benefit from hearing aid(s) and use of a desk top or ear level FM system in the classroom. Needs favorable acoustics, seating and lighting. May need attention to auditory skills, speech, language development, speechreading and/or support in reading and self-esteem. Amount of attention needed typically related to the degree of success of intervention prior to 6 months of age to prevent language and early learning delays. Teacher inservice on impact of so called "mild" hearing loss on listening and learning to convey that it is often greater than expected.

Please Consider Indicated Items in the Child's Educational Program:

_____Teacher inservice and seating close to teacher
_____Hearing monitoring at school every ____mos.
_____Amplification monitoring
_____Contact your school district's audiologist
_____Protect ears from noise to prevent more loss
_____Educational support services/evaluation
_____Screening/evaluation of speech and language
_____Note-taking, closed captioned films, visuals
_____FM system trial period
_____Educational consultation/ program supervision by specialist(s) in hearing loss
_____Regular contact with other children who are deaf or hard of hearing
_____Periodic educational monitoring such as October and April teacher/student completion of SIFTER, LIFE

NOTE: All children require full access to teacher instruction and educationally relevant peer communication to receive an appropriate education. Distance, noise in classroom and fragmentation caused by hearing loss prevent full access to spoken instruction. Appropriate acoustics, use of visuals, FM amplification, sign language, notetakers, communication partners, etc. increase access to instruction. Needs periodic hearing evaluation, rigorous amplification checks, and regular monitoring of access to instruction and classroom function (monitoring tools at www.hear2learn.com or www.SIFTERanderson.com).

Relationship of Hearing Loss to Listening and Learning Needs

41-55 dB HEARING LOSS		
Possible Impact on the Understanding of Language and Speech	**Possible Social Impact**	**Potential Educational Accommodations and Services**
Consistent use of amplification and language intervention prior to age 6 months increases the probability that the child's speech, language and learning will develop at a normal rate. Without amplification, understands conversation at a distance of 3-5 feet, if sentence structure and vocabulary are known. The amount of speech signal missed can be 50% or more with 40 dB loss and 80% or more with 50 dB loss. Without early amplification the child is likely to have delayed or disordered syntax, limited vocabulary, imperfect speech production and flat voice quality. Addition of a visual communication system to supplement audition may be indicated, especially if language delays and/or additional disabilities are present. Even with hearing aids, child can "hear" but may miss much of what is said if classroom is noisy or reverberant. With personal hearing aids alone, ability to perceive speech and learn effectively in the classroom is at high risk. A personal FM system to overcome classroom noise and distance is typically necessary.	Barriers build with negative impact on self esteem as child is accused of "hearing when he/she wants to," "daydreaming," or "not paying attention." Communication will be significantly compromised with this degree of hearing loss if hearing aids nor worn. Socialization with peers can be difficult, especially in noisy settings such as cooperative learning situations, lunch or recess. May be more fatigued than classmates due to effort needed to listen.	Consistent use of amplification (hearing aids + FM) is essential. Needs favorable classroom acoustics, seating and lighting. Consultation/program supervision by a specialist in childhood hearing impairment to coordinate services is important. Depending on intervention success in preventing language delays, special academic support necessary if language and academic delays are present. Attention to growth of oral communication, reading, written language skills, auditory skill development, speech therapy, self esteem likely. Teacher inservice required with attention to communication access and peer acceptance.

56-70 dB HEARING LOSS		
Possible Impact on the Understanding of Language and Speech	**Possible Social Impact**	**Potential Educational Accommodations and Services**
Even with hearing aids, child will typically be aware of people talking around him/her, but will miss parts of words said resulting in difficulty in situations requiring verbal communication (both one-to-one and in groups). Without amplification, conversation must be very loud to be understood; a 55 dB loss can cause a child to miss up to 100% of speech information without functioning amplification. If hearing loss is not identified before age one year and appropriately managed, delayed spoken language, syntax, reduced speech intelligibility and flat voice quality is likely. Age when first amplified, consistency of hearing aid use and success of early language intervention strongly tied to speech, language and learning development. Addition of visual communication system often indicated if language delays and/or additional disabilities are present. Use of a personal FM system will reduce the effects of noise and distance and allow increased auditory access to verbal instruction. With hearing aids alone, ability to understand in the classroom is greatly reduced by distance and noise.	If hearing loss was late-identified and language delay was not prevented, communication interaction with peers will be significantly affected. Children will have greater difficulty socializing, especially in noisy settings such as lunch cooperative learning situations, or recess. Tendency for poorer self-concept and social immaturity may contribute to a sense of rejection; peer inservice helpful.	Full time, consistent use of amplification (hearing aids + FM system) essential. May benefit from frequency transposition (frequency compression) hearing aids depending upon loss configuration. May require intense support in development of auditory, language, speech, reading and writing skills. Consultation/supervision by a specialist in childhood hearing impairment to coordinate services is important. Use of sign language or a visual communication system by children with substantial language delays or additional learning needs, may be useful to access linguistically complex instruction. Note-taking, captioned films, etc. accommodations often needed. Requires teacher inservice.

Please Consider Indicated Items in the Child's Educational Program:

_____Teacher inservice and seating close to teacher _____Hearing monitoring at school every ____mos. _____Amplification monitoring

_____Contact your school district's audiologist _____Protect ears from noise to prevent more loss _____Educational support services/evaluation

_____Screening/evaluation of speech and language _____Note-taking, closed captioned films, visuals _____FM system trial period

_____Educational consultation/ program supervision by specialist(s) in hearing loss _____Regular contact with other children who are deaf or hard of hearing

_____Periodic educational monitoring such as October and April teacher/student completion of SIFTER, LIFE

NOTE: All children require full access to teacher instruction and educationally relevant peer communication to receive an appropriate education. Distance, noise in classroom and fragmentation caused by hearing loss prevent full access to spoken instruction. Appropriate acoustics, use of visuals, FM amplification, sign language, notetakers, communication partners, etc. increase access to instruction. Needs periodic hearing evaluation, rigorous amplification checks, and regular monitoring of access to instruction and classroom function (monitoring tools at www.hear2learn.com or www.SIFTERanderson.com).

Relationship of Hearing Loss to Listening and Learning Needs

71-90 dB & 91+ dB		
Possible Impact on the Understanding of Language and Speech	**Possible Social Impact**	**Potential Educational Accommodations and Services**
The earlier the child wears amplification consistently with concentrated efforts by parents and caregivers to provide rich language opportunities throughout everyday activities and/or provision of intensive language intervention (sign or verbal), the greater the probability that speech, language and learning will develop at a relatively normal rate. Without amplification, children with 71-90 dB hearing loss may only hear loud noises about one foot from ear. When amplified optimally, children with hearing ability of 90 dB or better should detect many sounds of speech if presented from close distance or via FM. Individual ability and intensive intervention prior to 6 months of age will determine the degree that sounds detected will be discriminated and understood by the brain into meaningful input. Even with hearing aids children with 71-90 dB loss are typically unable to perceive all high pitch speech sounds sufficiently to discriminate them or benefit from incidental listening, especially without the use of FM. The child with hearing loss greater than 70 dB may be a candidate for cochlear implant(s) and the child with hearing loss greater than 90 dB will not be able to perceive most speech sounds with traditional hearing aids. For full access to language to be available visually through sign language or cued speech, family members must be involved in child's communication mode from a very young age.	Depending on success of intervention in infancy to address language development, the child's communication may be minimally or significantly affected. Socialization with hearing peers may be difficult. Children in general education classrooms may develop greater dependence on adults due to difficulty perceiving or comprehending oral communication. Children may be more comfortable interacting with peers who are deaf or hard of hearing due to ease of communication. Relationships with peers and adults who have hearing loss can make positive contributions toward the development of a healthy self-concept and a sense of cultural identity.	There is no one communication system that is right for all hard of hearing or deaf children and their families. Whether a visual communication approach or auditory/oral approach is used, extensive language intervention, full-time consistent amplification use and constant integration of the communication practices into the family by 6 months of age will highly increase the probability that the child will become a successful learner. Children with late-identified hearing loss (i.e., after 6 months of age) will have delayed language. This language gap is difficult to overcome and the educational program of a child with hearing loss, especially those with language and learning delays secondary to hearing loss, requires the involvement of a consultant or teacher with expertise in teaching children with hearing loss. Depending on the configuration of the hearing loss and individual speech perception ability, frequency transposition (frequency compression) aids or cochlear implantation may be options for better access to speech. If an auditory/oral approach is used, early training is needed on auditory skills, spoken language, concept development and speech. If culturally deaf emphasis is selected, frequent exposure to Deaf, ASL users is important. Educational placement with other signing deaf or hard of hearing students (special school or classes) may be a more appropriate option to access a language-rich environment and free-flowing communication. Support services and continual appraisal of access to communication and verbal instruction is required. Note-taking, captioning, captioned films and other visual enhancement strategies necessary. Training in pragmatic language use and communication repair strategies helpful. Inservice of general education teachers is essential.

Please Consider Indicated Items in the Child's Educational Program:

_____Teacher inservice and seating close to teacher _____Hearing monitoring at school every ____mos. _____Amplification monitoring
_____Contact your school district's audiologist _____Protect ears from noise to prevent more loss _____Educational support services/evaluation
_____Screening/evaluation of speech and language _____Note-taking, closed captioned films, visuals _____FM system trial period
_____Educational consultation/ program supervision by specialist(s) in hearing loss _____Regular contact with other children who are deaf or hard of hearing
_____Periodic educational monitoring such as October and April teacher/student completion of SIFTER, LIFE

NOTE: All children require full access to teacher instruction and educationally relevant peer communication to receive an appropriate education. Distance, noise in classroom and fragmentation caused by hearing loss prevent full access to spoken instruction. Appropriate acoustics, use of visuals, FM amplification, sign language, notetakers, communication partners, etc. increase access to instruction. Needs periodic hearing evaluation, rigorous amplification checks, and regular monitoring of access to instruction and classroom function (monitoring tools at www.hear2learn.com or www.SIFTERanderson.com).

Relationship of Hearing Loss to Listening and Learning Needs

UNILATERAL HEARING LOSS		
Possible Impact on the Understanding of Language and Speech	**Possible Social Impact**	**Potential Educational Accommodations and Services**
Child can "hear" but can have difficulty understanding in certain situations, such as hearing faint or distant speech, especially if poor ear is aimed toward the person speaking. Will typically have difficulty localizing sounds and voices using hearing alone. The unilateral listener will have greater difficulty understanding speech when environment is noisy and/or reverberant, especially when normal ear towards the overhead projector or other competing sound source and poor hearing ear towards the teacher. Exhibits difficulty detecting or understanding soft speech from the side of the poor hearing ear, especially in a group discussion.	Child may be accused of selective hearing due to discrepancies in speech understanding in quiet versus noise. Social problems may arise as child experiences difficulty understanding in noisy cooperative learning, or recess situations. May misconstrue peer conversations and feel rejected or ridiculed. Child may be more fatigued in classroom due to greater effort needed to listen, if class is noisy or has poor acoustics. May appear inattentive, distractible or frustrated, with behavior or social problems sometimes evident.	Allow child to change seat locations to direct the normal hearing ear toward the primary speaker. Student is at 10 times the risk for educational difficulties as children with 2 normal hearing ears and 1/3 to 1/2 of students with unilateral hearing loss experience significant learning problems. Children often have difficulty learning sound/letter associations in typically noisy kindergarten and grade 1 settings. Educational and audiological monitoring is warranted. Teacher inservice is beneficial. Typically will benefit from a personal FM system with low gain/power or a sound-field FM system in the classroom, especially in the lower grades. Depending on the hearing loss, may benefit from a hearing aid in the impaired ear.

MID-FREQUENCY HEARING LOSS or REVERSE SLOPE HEARING LOSS MID-FREQUENCY HEARING LOSS or REVERSE SLOPE		
Possible Impact on the Understanding of Language and Speech	**Possible Social Impact**	**Potential Educational Accommodations and Services**
Child can "hear" whenever speech is present but will have difficulty understanding in certain situations. May have difficulty understanding faint or distant speech, such as a student with a quiet voice speaking from across the classroom. The "cookie bite" or reverse slope listener will have greater difficulty understanding speech when environment is noisy and/or reverberant, such as a typical classroom setting. A 25 – 40 dB degree of loss in the low to mid-frequency range may cause the child to miss approximately 30% of speech information, if unamplified; some consonant and vowel sounds may be heard inconsistently, especially when background noise is present. Speech production of these sounds may be affected.	Child may be accused of selective hearing or "hearing when he wants to" due to discrepancies in speech understanding in quiet versus noise. Social problems may arise as child experiences difficulty understanding in noisy cooperative learning situations, lunch or recess. May misconstrue peer conversations, believing that other children are talking about him or her. Child may be more fatigued in classroom setting due to greater effort needed to listen. May appear inattentive, distractible or frustrated.	Personal hearing aids important but must be precisely fit to hearing loss. Child likely to benefit from a sound-field FM system, a personal FM system or assistive listening device in the classroom. Student is at risk for educational difficulties. Can experience some difficulty learning sound/letter associations in kindergarten and 1st grade classes. Depending upon degree and configuration of loss, child may experience delayed language development and articulation problems. Educational monitoring and teacher inservice warranted. Annual hearing evaluation to monitor for hearing loss progression is important.

Please Consider Indicated Items in the Child's Educational Program:

_____Teacher inservice and seating close to teacher _____Hearing monitoring at school every ____mos. _____Amplification monitoring

_____Contact your school district's audiologist _____Protect ears from noise to prevent more loss _____Educational support services/evaluation

_____Screening/evaluation of speech and language _____Note-taking, closed captioned films, visuals _____FM system trial period

_____Educational consultation/ program supervision by specialist(s) in hearing loss _____Regular contact with other children who are deaf or hard of hearing

_____Periodic educational monitoring such as October and April teacher/student completion of SIFTER, LIFE

NOTE: All children require full access to teacher instruction and educationally relevant peer communication to receive an appropriate education. Distance, noise in classroom and fragmentation caused by hearing loss prevent full access to spoken instruction. Appropriate acoustics, use of visuals, FM amplification, sign language, notetakers, communication partners, etc. increase access to instruction. Needs periodic hearing evaluation, rigorous amplification checks, and regular monitoring of access to instruction and classroom function (monitoring tools at www.hear2learn.com or www.SIFTERanderson.com).

Relationship of Hearing Loss to Listening and Learning Needs

HIGH FREQUENCY HEARING LOSS		
Possible Impact on the Understanding of Language and Speech	**Possible Social Impact**	**Potential Educational Accommodations and Services**
Child can "hear" but can miss important fragments of speech. Even a 25-40 dB loss in high frequency hearing may cause the child to miss 20%-30% of vital speech information if unamplified. Consonant sounds t, s, f, th, k, sh, ch likely heard inconsistently, especially in noise. May have difficulty understanding faint or distant speech, such as a student with a quiet voice speaking from across the classroom and will have much greater difficulty understanding speech when in low background noise and/or reverberation is present. Many of the critical sounds for understanding speech are high pitched, quiet sounds, making them difficult to perceive; the words: cat, cap, calf, cast could be perceived as "ca," word endings, possessives, plurals and unstressed brief words are difficult to perceive and understand. Speech production may be affected. Use of amplification often indicated to learn language at a typical rate and ease learning.	May be accused of selective hearing due to discrepancies in speech understanding in quiet versus noise. Social problems may arise as child experiences difficulty understanding in noisy cooperative learning situations, lunch or recess. May misinterpret peer conver-sations. Child may be fatigued in classroom due to greater listening effort. May appear inattentive, distractible or frustrated. Could affect self concept.	Student is at risk for educational difficulties. Depending upon onset, degree and configuration of loss, child may experience delayed language and syntax development and articulation problems. Possible difficulty learning some sound/letter associations in kindergarten and 1st grade classes. Early evaluation of speech and language skills is suggested. Educational monitoring and teacher inservice is warranted. Will typically benefit from personal hearing aids and use of a sound-field or a personal FM system in the classroom. Use of ear protection in noisy situations is imperative to prevent damage to inner ear structures and resulting progression of the hearing loss.

FLUCTUATING HEARING LOSS		
Possible Impact on the Understanding of Language and Speech	**Possible Social Impact**	**Potential Educational Accommodations and Services**
Of greatest concern are children who have experienced hearing fluctuations over many months in early childhood (multiple episodes with fluid lasting three months or longer). Listening with a hearing loss that is approximately 20 dB can be compared to hearing when index fingers are placed in ears. This loss or worse is typical of listening with fluid or infection behind the eardrums. Child can "hear" but misses fragments of what is said. Degree of difficulty experienced in school will depend upon the classroom noise level, the distance from the teacher and the current degree of hearing loss. At 30 dB can miss 25-40% of the speech signal; child with a 40 dB loss associated with "glue ear" may miss 50% of class discussions, especially when voices are faint or speaker is not in line of vision. Will frequently miss unstressed words, consonants and word endings.	Barriers begin to build with negative impact on self esteem as the child is accused of "hearing when he/she wants to," "daydreaming," or "not paying attention." Child may believe he/she is less capable due to understanding difficulties in class. Typically poor at identifying changes in own hearing ability. With inconsistent hearing, the child learns to "tune out" the speech signal. Children are judged to have greater attention problems, insecurity, distractibility and lack self esteem. Tend to be non-participative and distract themselves from classroom tasks; often socially immature.	Impact is primarily on acquisition of early reading skills and attention in class. Screening for language delays is suggested from a young age. Ongoing monitoring for hearing loss in school, communication between parent and teacher about listening difficulties and aggressive medical management is needed. Will benefit from sound-field FM or an assistive listening device in class. May need attention to development of speech, reading, self esteem, or listening skills. Teacher inservice is beneficial.

Please Consider Indicated Items in the Child's Educational Program:

_____Teacher inservice and seating close to teacher _____Hearing monitoring at school every ____mos. _____Amplification monitoring
_____Contact your school district's audiologist _____Protect ears from noise to prevent more loss _____Educational support services/evaluation
_____Screening/evaluation of speech and language _____Note-taking, closed captioned films, visuals _____FM system trial period
_____Educational consultation/ program supervision by specialist(s) in hearing loss _____Regular contact with other children who are deaf or hard of hearing
_____Periodic educational monitoring such as October and April teacher/student completion of SIFTER, LIFE

NOTE: All children require full access to teacher instruction and educationally relevant peer communication to receive an appropriate education. Distance, noise in classroom and fragmentation caused by hearing loss prevent full access to spoken instruction. Appropriate acoustics, use of visuals, FM amplification, sign language, notetakers, communication partners, etc. increase access to instruction. Needs periodic hearing evaluation, rigorous amplification checks, and regular monitoring of access to instruction and classroom function (monitoring tools at www.hear2learn.com or www.SIFTERanderson.com).

APPENDIX 33–B

Simulation of Hearing Loss Handout (Edwards, 2005)

Simulation of Hearing Loss: An In-Service Training Tool

Mirect experience often produces optimum learning. Most teachers who are faced with the prospect of a child with hearing loss in their classroom for the first time, express concern about their ability to address the child's needs in their class. By giving the teacher some direct experience with hearing loss, you can provide them with

- an empathetic understanding of the communication demands on the child with hearing loss in the classroom.
- an understanding of the teaching strategies that are detrimental to communication in the classroom.
- an understanding of the teaching strategies that are beneficial to the child with hearing loss in the classroom.

Use of foam earplugs can simulate a mild conductive hearing loss of approximately 25 to 35 dB. The following points are important to emphasize to school staff.

- The simulation only creates a mild hearing loss, and so students with moderate, severe, or profound hearing loss will experience greater difficulty than that experienced with the earplugs.
- The simulation reflects what children with mild hearing loss may hear without a hearing aid, or what children with moderate or moderately severe hearing loss may hear with the hearing aid on.
- Use of the earplugs simulates a conductive rather than a sensorineural hearing loss, as the earplugs are simply impeding the passage of sound through the external ear. This is an important distinction, as the staff must realize that the distortion of speech sounds and the susceptibility to noise seen with children with sensorineural hearing loss cannot be simulated through the use of earplugs alone.
- The simulation produces an accurate perception of the hearing loss often seen with children with recurrent otitis media. Although many teachers may not have experiences with children with sensorineural hearing loss, all primary teachers will have a number of children in their classes each year with histories of recurrent otitis media (Otitis media is the single most common reason for a child to visit the family physician, and the most common cause of hearing loss in children).

Suggested Procedure

After explaining the purpose of the exercise, hand out a pair of foam earplugs to each group member. Ask the participants to hold the plugs by the rounded edge and roll them between their fingers to compress them to approximately 1/3 to 1/4 of their original size. Then have everyone insert the compressed plugs into their ear canals so that the canals are completely occluded. If the participants do not hear a clear difference in the loudness of the sound after inserting the plugs, the plugs have not been inserted correctly. Have the individuals remove and reinsert the earplugs. Then ask the participants to get out a sheet of paper and pencil to write down what you say. There are a number of concepts that you want to demonstrate during the simulation.

- The farther away the speaker is from the listener, the more difficult the listening task.
- Restricting speechreading cues makes the listening task more difficult.
- Presence of background noise increases the difficulty of the listening task.
- The type of material presented will vary the difficulty of the task. Single words are much more difficult to identify than is sentence material, where contextual clues can provide a great deal of information.
- The intensity of vowels is greater than that of consonants, thus increasing the ease of vowel recognition.
- High frequency consononants such as /s/, /f/, /ch /, /k/, /t/, and the voiceless /th/ are usually the most difficult sounds to hear, particularly the /f/ and voiceless /th/, since they are the softest of all of the consonants.
- Listening under difficult conditions is fatiguing, resulting in a tendency to tune out or daydream.
- Listening can be very frustrating when speakers are far away, or are covering their mouth, or when background noise is present. The listener may experience anger or frustration towards the speaker or towards the sources of background noise.
- Additional visual supplements such as writing on the blackboard or the overhead projector can be of great assistance in following the conversation, and reduce the strain of listening.

Ask participants to write numbers 1 to 15 on the side of the page. In order to demonstrate the above concepts, present words and sentences in the following way.

Write the word . . .

1.	please	BY HEARING ALONE
2.	great	(MOUTH COVERED);
3.	sled	QUIET CONVERSATIONAL LEVEL;
4.	pants	MOVE AROUND WHILE YOU ARE
5.	rat	TALKING

Write the word. . .

6.	bad	BY HEARING ALONE
7.	pinch	(MOUTH COVERED);
8.	such	CREATE BACKGROUND NOISE
9.	bus	(PAPERS RUSTLING, KEYS JINGLING,
10.	need	BOOK DROPPING ON FLOOR.);
		QUIET CONVERSATIONAL LEVEL;
		MOVE AROUND WHILE YOU ARE TALKING

Write the word . . .

11. ways BY HEARING AND SPEECHREADING
12. five (MOUTH UNCOVERED);
13. mouth QUIET CONVERSATIONAL LEVEL;
14. rag BACKGROUND NOISE SPORADIC
15. put

Now ask the participants to number their page from 1 to 10 and tell them that you will now say some sentences.

1. Walking is my favorite exercise.
2. Here's a nice quiet place to rest.
3. Somebody cleans the floors every night.
4. It would be much easier if everyone would help.
5. Open your window before you go to bed.

BY HEARING ALONE
(MOUTH COVERED);
BACKGROUND NOISE SPORADIC

6. Do you think that she should stay out so late?
7. How do you feel about beginning work at a different time every day?
8. Move out of the way.
9. The water is too cold for swimming.
10. Why should I get up so early in the morning?

BY HEARING AND SPEECHREADING
(MOUTH UNCOVERED);
BACKGROUND NOISE SPORADIC

- It is important to use a quiet conversational voice level rather than a normal conversational level for maximum effect.
- Because sentences are considerably easier to identify than are single words, they are presented through hearing alone in noise, rather than in quiet.
- The background noise can be sporadic or continuous; the listeners will experience the frustration in either situation.
- When moving around, ensure that you rotate around the entire room so that everyone can experience both optimal and least desirable listening conditions.

Then have the participants take up their answers WITH THE EARPLUGS STILL INSERTED. When a person gives his or her answer, ensure that the rest of the group has heard it. If not, ask the person to change the way that he or she has presented the answer so that others will understand better (such as repeating the response, saying the word or sentence louder, facing the group, spelling the word, or adding an accompanying gesture). Write down the various answers on a chartboard or overhead to provide a visual supplement. Underline the correct answer from all of the choices provided by the participants.

Once all of the words and sentences have been reviewed, HAVE THE GROUP TAKE OUT THE EARPLUGS. Initiate a group discussion of the following issues:

- their emotional reactions to the overall experience.
- the causes of specific frustrations experienced.
- insights about the experiences of children with hearing loss in the classroom.
- ways in which they could change their teaching strategies to address the needs of children with hearing loss.

The discussion deepens the experience of the simulation of hearing loss and allows participants themselves to determine the necessary changes in teaching strategies.

34

Audiologic Management of Unilateral and Minimal to Mild Bilateral Hearing Loss in Children

Anne Marie Tharpe and William W. Dickinson

Background

In Chapters 10 and 11, we discussed the psychoeducational outcomes of children with permanent unilateral (UHL), and permanent minimal to mild bilateral hearing loss (MBHL). Most audiologists agree that the audiologic management of these children must be made on a case-by-case basis. Although approximately 30 to 40% of children with UHL and MBHL appear to be at high risk for academic difficulty, it is unclear exactly which of these children will fall into that risk category and require some form of intervention and which children will not. Therefore, at this point in time, all children with permanent UHL or MBHL must be considered at risk for psychoeducational difficulties and monitored accordingly. This chapter addresses the components of a comprehensive monitoring plan for these children, including:

- counseling and education
- etiologic evaluation
- daycare and school environments
- hearing aids and assistive technologies
- audiologic monitoring
- functional assessments

Counseling and Education

Before any management can be initiated, family members of children with UHL and MBHL and the professionals who work with them must all be aware of the value of normal hearing and the risks associated with these losses. If not convinced that a risk of developmental or academic problems exists, it is likely that efforts to provide services will be declined.

Keep in mind that depending on the environmental listening conditions, children with UHL or MBHL can often hear much of a speech signal. Therefore, family members and others who observe these children will note that they respond to being called, can hear television, listen to the radio, and so forth. It might be difficult for observers to understand that multiple factors can affect how children with UHL and MBHL hear. That is, if the child is in a noisy and/or reverberant environment, or if speech is presented on the side of the poorer ear, the signal-to-noise ratio (SNR) will be adversely affected and listening will be difficult. One way to educate individuals about the hearing difficulties associated with UHL and MBHL is through the use of hearing loss simulations. Different configurations of UHL and MBHL have been simulated and can be found on the internet, and recorded versions can be obtained from professional audiology organizations. For simulating UHL, one can simply provide a single earplug for a family member or school personnel to wear during a counseling session or meeting, which can provide an effective demonstration of what a child experiences.

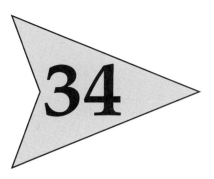

Even if a child receives hearing technology for listening assistance, families should be aware of techniques for improving the acoustic conditions in their home. For example, infants with UHL can be held such that their normal hearing ear is positioned outward, away from their parent's chest. Background noise in the home, such as televisions and stereos, can be turned off during times when the family is conversing (e.g., during meal times) or reading aloud.

It is also important to remind parents and health care professionals of the limitations of newborn hearing screening in identifying minimal degrees of childhood hearing loss. As discussed in Chapter 11, newborn hearing screening programs are not designed to target minimal and mild degrees of hearing loss. Furthermore, the number of children estimated to have MBHL or UHL at birth is 0.36 to .55:1000 (Johnson et al., 2005; Watkin & Baldwin, 1999) and at school age is 5.4:100 (Bess, Dodd-Murphy, & Parker, 1998). It is reasonable to assume that this increase in numbers of children with UHL or MBHL is the result, at least in part, of acquired, late-onset, or progressive hearing loss, in addition to limited screening sensitivity at birth. Thus, just because a child passed a newborn hearing screening does not mean that the child does not need to be tested at a later time, especially in the pre-school years, and especially if risk factors are present.

Etiologic Evaluation

Since the 1960s, reports of UHL have emphasized a lack of information about causative factors. In fact, those early reports as well as more recent ones indicated that between 35% and 65% of children with UHL had unknown etiologies. The most frequently reported known causative factors include viral complications (approximately 25%), meningitis (approximately 15%), head trauma (approximately 8–12%), prenatal or perinatal disorders (approximately 12%), and genetic disorders.

Similarly, little is known about the etiologies of MBHL. The delay in identifying causative factors with this group of children might be related to the later age of identification of the hearing loss. Recall that MBHLs are not targeted by our newborn hearing screening programs and are often not identified until school age. This delay in identification naturally results in a delay of finding a causative factor; a delay that might result in an inability to determine etiology at all. For example, we know that cytomegalovirus (CMV) is the primary cause of nongenetic, sensory hearing loss and the leading cause of unilateral prelinguistic hearing loss in children (Nance, 2007). However, to determine the presence of congenital CMV in children, testing must be conducted in the first week of life, prior to natural exposure to the virus from family members, especially young children. Because we know that congenital, not acquired, CMV is associated with hearing loss, a positive test obtained after the newborn period does not assist us in determining etiology. In addition, delays in identification of hearing loss might affect parental memory of possible maternal illnesses, like signs of CMV, that could account for the loss. Therefore, most of what we know about causation of hearing loss in children is associated with moderate or greater degrees of hearing loss, rather than minimal to mild degrees, because they are identified earlier. It is reasonable to assume that some of the same factors that result in more severe degrees of hearing loss can also cause lesser degrees of loss but, at the time of this writing, we are lacking the data to confirm that.

In addition to the late identification of some of these minimal and mild losses that might be contributing to our inability to define the causative factors, there is reason to believe that the medical community is not as aggressive in searching for etiology of these losses as it is for more severe degrees of hearing loss. Etiologic evaluations of *all* degrees of hearing loss should include a careful history and physical exam, and selective use of genetic, radiographic imaging, and laboratory assessment. Determining hearing loss etiology helps to individualize our parent counseling and inform our management decisions. For a comprehensive review of etiology of UHL and MBHL, see Tharpe and Sladen, 2008.

Daycare and School Environments

As noted in Chapter 11, high levels of noise and/or reverberation can have adverse effects on speech perception of children with UHL and MBHL. The American Speech-Hearing-Language Association and the American National Standard Institute have recommended standards for classroom acoustics (ANSI, 2002; ASHA, 2005). Several steps should be taken to ensure adherence to these guidelines:

- measure background noise levels in dBA
- measure or estimate reverberation time
- measure or estimate signal-to-noise ratio.

Following measurement or estimation of these acoustic conditions, a comparison must be made to acceptable standards. ASHA (2005) recommends the following acoustic conditions in educational settings:

- unoccupied classroom noise levels must not exceed 35 dBA
- unoccupied classroom reverberation times must not surpass 0.6 seconds in smaller classrooms

(<10,000 ft^3) or 0.7 seconds in larger rooms (>10,000 ft^3 and <20,000 ft^3)
- SNR should be at least +15 dB at the child's ears.

In addition, ANSI S12.60-2002 provides acoustic guidelines for learning spaces greater than 20,000 ft^3. There is some evidence to suggest that today's classrooms are not meeting these guidelines for background noise. Reported background noise measurements for typical classrooms range from about 40 to 66 dBA (Crandell & Smaldino, 1995; Knecht, Nelson, & Whitelaw, 2002).

Of course, there is no guarantee that adequate acoustics will overcome the effects of degraded speech across distance for children with hearing loss. Regardless of the degree of hearing loss or whether the child is using hearing technology, the primary signal should be presented in close proximity of the student, when possible. Hearing technology, especially frequency-modulated (FM) systems, can overcome many of these adverse acoustic effects. However, many children with UHL and MBHL do not use hearing technology either because it is assumed that such losses are inconsequential, or school systems do not provide the technology except for more severe degrees of hearing loss. Therefore, in the absence of technologic listening enhancements, or in addition to such equipment, low-tech interventions can be employed. Although many acoustic modifications to the listening environment will require the expertise of acoustical engineers, architects, and audiologists, some modifications can be accomplished via simple steps including:

- strategic placement of carpet remnants throughout the classroom
- placement of sound-absorbing materials on the walls to reduce reverberation times (e.g., cork boards, window curtains)
- sound-reducing pads on feet of chairs (e.g., tennis balls, foot covers)
- acoustic ceiling tiles.

Such modifications to the physical structure of a room improve the SNR, decrease reverberation time, and decrease the overall ambient noise levels.

Hearing Aids and Assistive Technologies

Although audiologists are well aware of the potential psychoeducational and psychosocial difficulties that some children with UHL and MBHL can experience, they remain concerned about the appropriate application of hearing technologies for these children and might question their effectiveness. Specifically, questions abound regarding which technologies should be used, when they should be used, who should use them, and how they should be fitted on children.

Candidacy

National organizations in the United States have agreed that hearing technology recommendations for children with UHL or MBHL should be considered on a child-by-child basis (American Academy of Audiology, 2003; Centers for Disease Control and Prevention, 2005). The reason for this approach is that although children with minimal hearing loss are at risk for academic difficulty, it is unclear exactly which children will require some form of intervention and which children will not. Furthermore, at this point in time, there is no evidence to suggest that the fitting of hearing technology will ameliorate the negative impact of UHL or MBHL on academic performance, although certainly listening in adverse acoustic environments such as classrooms can be improved. Therefore, each child's hearing, speech-language, psychosocial, and educational development should be monitored closely. It also is likely that children with UHL or MBHL will not be considered as candidates for hearing technology in infancy. This is the result of several factors including late identification of MBHL and UHL, audiologic uncertainty, and parental hesitation (see Chapter 11 for a discussion of these topics). Some audiologists also believe that children do not need technology until they enter school where they are faced with difficult listening environments while trying to learn. However, most audiologists would agree that once the degree, configuration, and type of hearing loss has been determined, children with UHL or MBHL should be considered candidates for some type of hearing technology.

Types of Hearing Technology

Much like children with other degrees of hearing loss, there is a variety of technology options for children with UHL or MBHL. The type of technology is selected based on the individual needs and activities of each child. For example, there might be a need for a personal FM system for use outside of the school environment if a child participates in activities that impose a distance from a speaker of interest when good communication is critical (e.g., bike riding, horseback riding).

Therefore, it is important for audiologists to collect information about a child's activities and interests both inside and outside the home when determining the types of technology that might be valuable. Although some types of hearing technologies can be considered by both those with UHL and those with MBHL, some technologies (e.g., CROS hearing aids) are considered only for those with UHL.

Conventional Hearing Aids

As noted previously, one of the reasons that children with mild UHL or MBHL are fitted with hearing technology later than children with more severe degrees of hearing loss relates to audiologic uncertainty. This uncertainty can be the result of concern about an accurate determination of the degree of hearing loss, which drives the concern about the possibility of overamplification. However, as with all amplification fittings, the use of real-ear measurements for verification purposes is of particular importance for the safety and efficacy of hearing aid use in children. Verification is particularly important for children with minimal and mild degrees of hearing loss because of their near-normal hearing and the potential for overamplification or tolerance problems.

Prescriptive methods have been developed for use with infants and young children and incorporate the real-ear-to-coupler difference (RECD) to determine gain and output values for safe and audible sound levels (e.g., Desired Sensation Level Approach [DSL]; Seewald & Scollie, 2003). However, the prescribed targets serve as a starting place, not a final goal, for gain and output settings, and adjustments in fittings should be individualized. See Chapter 25 for more detailed discussion of prescriptive hearing aid fitting for infants and children.

When infants and young children are fitted with conventional hearing aids, the size of their external ear canals will alter their RECD, which in turn will influence how much hearing aid gain is prescribed. Given the expected large RECDs in infants and young children, it is possible that the prescribed gain at each frequency for those with minimal degrees of loss will be only a few decibels. In such circumstances, one should consider whether the expenditures of cost and effort warrant the purchase of a hearing aid or if, alternatively, the goals of improved SNR and audibility could be immediately accomplished by instructing families to use effective communication strategies. For example, families can be counseled to obtain the child's attention prior to initiating communication, maintain close proximity to their infant when speaking, or speak to the better hearing side for those with UHL. These strategies can improve the SNR and lead to improved speech perception. In addition, parents can maintain an acoustically-friendly environment in the home by reducing extraneous background noise such as televisions and stereos, or managing the play activities of siblings. A benefit of this approach is that an acoustically friendly environment is already in place when and if the infant transfers into using hearing aid technology. As an infant moves into childhood and gains mobility and independence, the decision about the need for hearing aids can be revisited. It should be noted that it will be important to monitor a child's RECD over time as growth of an ear canal can reduce the sound pressure level at the tympanic membrane and, thus, change the recommendation for amplification. This concept will be an important one to explain carefully to parents to avoid the fear that the hearing loss is progressing.

When fitting hearing aids on children with MBHL, consideration should be given to specific hearing aid characteristics. Linear processing with compression limiting or low-threshold compression might provide comfortable listening and minimize loudness tolerance problems. Feedback cancellation circuitry might not be necessary because the low amount of recommended gain is unlikely to produce feedback unless coupled to an open earmold. Open-ear fittings might be appropriate to avoid occluding the ear from natural, audible signals in the environment. However, in infants, open-ear fittings might not be possible because of the small size of the ear canal. For those with high frequency hearing loss, the perception of the phonemes /s/ and /z/ are critical for the development of language and speech production. After all, these high-frequency phonemes indicate plurality (e.g., shoe vs. shoes), possession (e.g., the girl's sweater), contractions (e.g., that's right), and third-person present tense (e.g., she sits). For perception of these critical phonemes, audibility is required at least through 8000 Hz (Stelmachowicz, Pittman, Hoover, & Lewis, 2002). However, as already noted, small ears might not accommodate the large sound bores required to enhance these high frequency sounds. Some promising work has been reported on the use of frequency-lowering technology (nonlinear frequency compression) to enhance audibility of high frequency phonemes in children with mild to moderate losses (Glista et al., 2009; Wolfe, Caraway, John, Schafer, & Nyffeler, 2009).

Another consideration when fitting low-gain instruments is that the noise floor inherent in hearing aids typically is not heard by those with greater degrees of hearing loss but might interfere with speech perception in those with minimal and mild degrees of hearing loss. For those with minimal degrees of hearing loss, the amount of benefit from amplification might be negated by the amount of low-level noise that is emitted by the hearing aid.

When considering hearing aids for those with UHL, an oft-repeated concern by audiologists has been how to define the loss as "aidable" or "unaidable." The decision to provide a hearing aid to a child with UHL will depend on the severity of the loss, the age of the child, and other factors such as a child's and family's motivation for using the device. Valente (2007) defined "unaidable" UHL as that which is profound, has very poor word recognition ability, no functional benefit with amplification, and/or marked intolerance for amplified sound. Although the benefits of conventional hearing aid fittings on children with UHL have not been thoroughly documented, it is reasonable to expect that these children would experience some of the advantages of binaural hearing. These advantages include improved speech understanding in noise, binaural summation, and improved localization skills. However, the provision of bilateral hearing does not ensure that a listener will enjoy the binaural benefits that are available from two normal hearing ears. That is, it is possible that by aiding one ear, a reduction in speech perception relative to unaided performance can occur. This phenomenon of decreased bilateral performance when an individual receives asymmetric auditory input is referred to as "binaural interference" (Jerger, Silman, Lew, & Chmiel, 1993). In a study of child and adult listeners, Rothpletz, Tharpe, and Grantham (2004) found evidence of bilateral interference in adults but not children, when listening to asymmetrically degraded speech. However, neither children nor adults demonstrated a binaural advantage under the same listening conditions.

Another consideration in fitting amplification to a child with UHL is that of when to fit the amplification relative to possible auditory deprivation effects. As previously noted, UHL is typically not considered of great importance and, thus, hearing technology is often not considered until school age or later, if at all. However, researchers have speculated that binaural hearing is a skill learned early in childhood and cannot be recovered later in life (Litovsky, Johnstone, & Godar, 2006). It is possible that leaving an impaired ear unaided during infancy and early childhood might limit the benefits (i.e., binaural hearing abilities) a child might receive as compared to being fit earlier in life.

Contralateral-Routing-of-Signal (CROS) Hearing Aids

The traditional option for individuals with UHL whose hearing is considered to be "unaidable" with a conventional hearing aid is a contralateral-routing-of-signal (CROS) hearing aid system (often referred to as a *conventional* CROS). The premise of a CROS system is that signals coming to the poorer ear are routed, via a wired or wireless connection, to a receiver coupled to an open earmold on the normal-hearing ear, thus, eliminating head-shadow effects (i.e., diffraction effects of the head) and allowing better perception of sounds originating on the side of the impaired ear. Figure 34–1 illustrates a wireless CROS aid with an FM transmitter and receiver attachment.

Although a CROS aid can provide an effective option for children with UHL, one must also consider the possible limitations. For example, in classroom settings, it often is difficult to control the dynamic nature of sound throughout the room. A child might be seated such that the desired signal (usually speech) is routed to the normal-hearing ear one minute, but then background noise might be routed to the normal-hearing ear the next. If a CROS aid is under consideration, one must note whether the child possesses the maturity to monitor the environment and adjust his or her location accordingly. Therefore, young children typically are not considered candidates for CROS devices.

Transcranial CROS. Reported limitations of CROS amplification (i.e., having to wear a device on each ear, poor sound quality) led to the application of transcranial hearing technology. The principle behind the transcranial CROS fitting is that by fitting a high-power in-the-ear, completely-in-the-canal, or behind-the-ear hearing aid deep into the osseos portion of the ear canal of the impaired side, enough output will be produced to stimulate the contralateral cochlea via bone conduction. However, evidence supporting the use of transcranial fittings in children with UHL has been lacking and their use with adults has been received with mixed results.

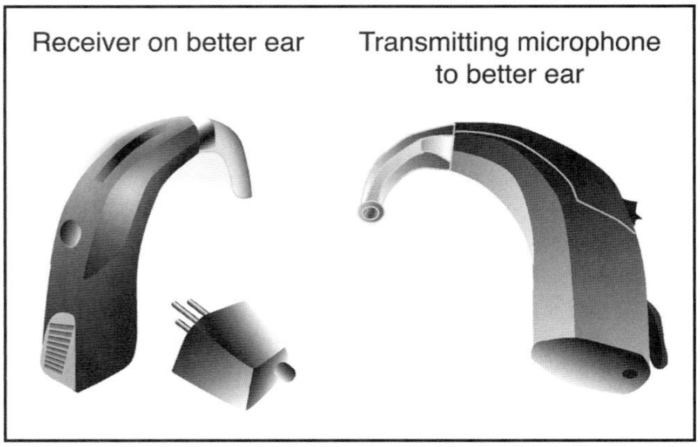

FIGURE 34–1. Example of a CROS hearing aid with FM transmitter.

Bone-Anchored Hearing Aids (Baha). Although originally intended for use by individuals with conductive or mixed hearing loss, the Baha is gaining popularity for individuals who have unaidable UHL. At the time of this writing, the Baha has been approved by the Food and Drug Administration for implanting children over 5 years of age. The Baha provides transcranial delivery of the signal via bone conduction from the impaired side to the normal cochlea (Figure 34–2). Specifically, a Baha utilizes direct percutaneous coupling of the vibrating transducer to a titanium implant anchored in the temporal bone and is now a CROS option for those with UHL (see Chapter 28 for a detailed discussion of Baha devices).

Most of the efficacy research on this device has been with adults, not children. For children younger than the age of 5 years, conventional transcutaneous coupling of bone conduction sound is required. This can be achieved by either a traditional bone conduction hearing aid worn with a rigid headband or the application of the Baha external sound processor coupled to a soft band worn around the child's head. Proper placement, retention, comfort, and overall ergonomics of use have been reported to be superior with the soft band Baha compared to the traditional rigid band bone conduction devices. As the Baha and the transcranial CROS provide transcranial delivery of the signal in individuals with profound UHL, one could speculate that in adverse listening situations, the introduction of noise to the impaired ear, which is sent to the normal hearing ear, would have similar negative listening effects as those associated with a conventional CROS aid.

Frequency Modulation Systems

Three factors that work together to degrade speech perception in listening environments are high levels of background noise, long reverberation times, and long speaker-listener distances. These factors are commonly present in classroom settings and have a more deleterious effect on children with hearing loss than those with normal hearing. In adverse listening environments, the effectiveness of hearing technology such as traditional hearing aids, CROS systems, and bone-anchored instruments is limited relative to their performance in quiet environments. As such, the hearing technology of choice for use in poor acoustic environments or to hear far-field signals is an FM system, if the primary goal is to maximize speech intelligibility, compared to secondary goals of sound awareness, lateralization/localization of signal or issues related to alerting and personal safety.

FM systems have many useful applications for children with MHL or UHL because they incorporate a microphone in close proximity to a talker's mouth, or directly connected to the sound source, and the sound is transferred via FM radio waves to the listener. This arrangement maintains a listening advantage above the level of background noise without reverberation and other effects that degrade the primary signal of interest. FM systems use a low-power radio transmitter to send FM radio signals to a miniature receiver. The FM transmitter and microphone are worn by the primary talker (i.e., teacher or parent) or can be directly coupled to other sound sources of interest such as a

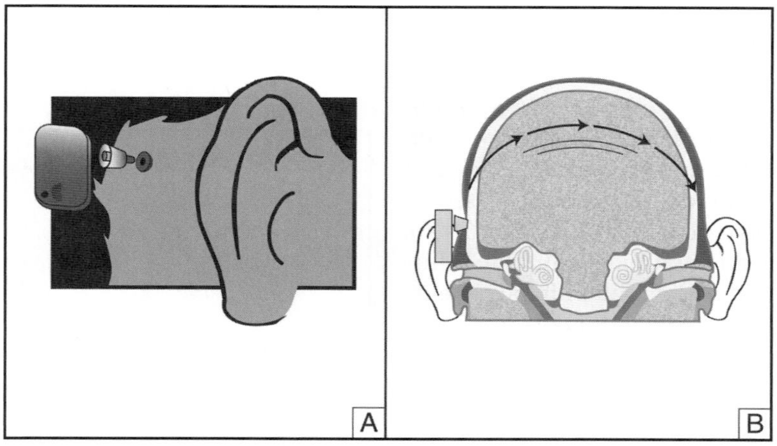

FIGURE 34–2. Example of a Baha device with the percutaneous coupling of the vibrating transducer to a titanium implant anchored in the temporal bone **(A)** and the transduction of sound via the skull to the normal hearing cochlea **(B)**.

television, radio, or computer. A range of transmitter/microphone options is available from boom-style or lavaliere-style microphones to others that are hand-held and incorporate beam-forming technology that highly focuses on the target sounds of interest. The most current transmitters include several digital signal processing advantages such as noise-reduction technology, directional microphone options and other wireless signal delivery formats such as Bluetooth (see Chapter 26 for a more in-depth discussion of FM system technology).

The choice of user-selected directionality allows flexibility in using the FM transmitter/microphone in a variety of settings outside traditional classrooms. Some examples include switching the transmitter to act as a conference microphone to hear several speakers in a restaurant or working around a table. Using a narrow directional microphone setting, the transmitter can be used as a hand-held "pointer" microphone at a family gathering or party setting, where the main talker is frequently changing.

If a child is not wearing personal hearing aids, FM options include use of a low-gain ear-level FM-only device on a normal or near-normal hearing ear; a classroom sound-field FM (or infrared system) with speakers installed in the ceiling or around the periphery of a room; or a desktop style of FM with a speaker placed directly in front of the student. Limited research is available to determine the most preferred configuration, but both ear-level FM systems and desktop FM systems outperform classroom sound-field systems, in terms of improving the SNR, for students with hearing loss. Classroom sound-field systems improve the overall audibility of the teacher's voice for all students in the class and are relatively cost effective. However, in terms of size, portability, and audibility, ear-level FM systems have obvious advantages over larger speaker choices but usually have an increased cost. Moreover, ear-level FM systems are easily worn in settings outside of the classroom; for example, in the car when parents want to converse with their child in the back seat, when a caregiver wants to talk with a child being pushed in a stroller, or on field trips when considerable distances are expected between the primary speaker and listener. For children who already use ear level amplification, another FM option becomes available, that of coupling an FM receiver directly to hearing aids or Bahas. For children with UHL, the decision to route an FM signal to an ear with hearing loss, rather than to the normal hearing ear, will depend on the ability of that ear to process and understand speech. The use of an FM system might not provide any benefit and might even be a detriment if the ear to which the FM signal is routed cannot process the talker's voice adequately.

Recently, Tharpe, Ricketts, and Sladen (2004) examined various fitting configurations (monaural or bilateral with open or skeleton earmolds) of an ear-level FM system on children with minimal to mild degrees of hearing loss (including some children with UHL). Outcome measures included speech perception ability and configuration preference as reported by the children. The children enrolled in the study demonstrated significantly better speech perception ability in noise (originating from a variety of sources around the child's head) when wearing any of the FM configurations as opposed to the unaided condition. This FM benefit was significantly enhanced when using bilateral FM placement relative to monaural placement in only two of the sound source locations. All but one of the children enrolled in this study reported that they liked wearing the ear-level FM device, and their families chose to purchase the system at the end of the study. Furthermore, all of the children who wanted to keep the FM systems wanted a monaural configuration. It was speculated that monaural usage allowed the students to use their opposite ear for communicating with classmates.

Because of the varied amplification and FM coupling options available, FM candidacy should be considered carefully. FM options should be considered for all children with MBHL or UHL in the classroom setting. Current FM options make it possible to choose an FM system for a child to be used as the primary amplification intervention or as an adjunct to the child's primary hearing aid. This makes FM systems a viable option for many individuals with MBHL or UHL.

Audiologic Monitoring

Because UHL and MBHL have less obvious impact on speech and language development than more severe bilateral hearing losses, there might be a tendency for less aggressive audiologic follow up. However, recent data from at least one statewide newborn screening program in the United States suggest that close monitoring is warranted. More than one-third of babies who did not pass a newborn screening in one ear were later found to have bilateral hearing loss upon diagnostic evaluation (Neault, 2005). There are numerous possible reasons for this change in identification of a unilateral to a bilateral loss including progression of a hearing loss caused by CMV, enlarged vestibular aqueduct, and other unknown causes, or a "miss" of the bilateral loss at the initial screen. These data support the need for an additional systematic hearing screening after the newborn period and before the start of school.

An additional concern with permanent, minimal degrees of hearing loss is the possible confounding factor of otitis media with effusion, which could result in a conductive overlay in addition to the permanent loss. Given that many children with UHL or MBHL do not use hearing technology, this conductive overlay could seriously compromise their listening ability and, thus, their speech, language, or academic development. Therefore, air-conduction and bone-conduction testing as well as immittance audiometry are necessary components of audiologic monitoring.

As with all children with hearing loss, it is recommended that infants and young children with UHL or MBHL receive hearing testing at least every six months until the child is able to report if a change in hearing has occurred. If there is reason to believe that a child has a progressive hearing loss or is prone to otitis media with effusion, more frequent monitoring might be justified.

Functional Assessments

Another way to monitor a child's progress is through the use of functional auditory assessments. Functional auditory assessments are designed to assess real-world listening behaviors outside of the clinical setting. These real-world behaviors can be those observed in homes, in schools or other areas where children play and learn. These assessments typically come in the form of checklists and questionnaires and can be completed by parents, teachers, speech-language pathologists, or, when appropriate, the child. Together, these individuals can contribute to the decision of what type of intervention a child might need and help determine the effectiveness of the intervention. As discussed previously, these interventions include acoustic modifications to the child's environment, preferential seating, the use of FM systems, hearing aids, or other hearing technologies. Functional assessment measures designed specifically for evaluating children with UHL and MBHL are discussed in more detail in Chapter 11.

Conclusions

Despite the converging data supporting the conclusion that 30 to 40% of children with permanent UHL or MBHL will have psychoeducational difficulties during their school years, exactly which children will have difficulty and which will not remains a mystery. Therefore, it is necessary to individualize the management of these children and determine through a process of regular monitoring, which interventions are appropriate for each child. Furthermore, there is preliminary evidence to suggest that this monitoring needs to begin early in the preschool years of children with UHL and MBHL. Management and intervention will continue to be informed by our increasing knowledge about causation, demographics, and challenges experienced by these children.

Acknowledgment. The authors appreciate the graphic services of the Vanderbilt Kennedy Center for Research on Human Development, supported in part by NICHD Grant P30 HD15052.

References

American Academy of Audiology (AAA). (2003). Pediatric amplification protocol. *Journal of the American Academy of Audiology, 11*(10), 561–569.

American National Standard Institute (ANSI). (2002). *American National Standard ANSI S12.60-2002*. Acoustical performance criteria, design requirements, and guidelines for schools. Available from http://www.asastore.aip.org/

American Speech-Language-Hearing Association. (2005). *Guidelines for addressing acoustics in educational settings* [Guidelines]. Available from http://www.asha.org/policy

Bess, F. H., Dodd-Murphy, J., & Parker, R. A. (1998). Children with minimal sensorineural hearing loss: Prevalence, educational performance, and functional status. *Ear and Hearing, 19*, 339–354.

Centers for Disease Control and Prevention (CDC). (July 2005). *Early hearing detection and intervention*. National Workshop on Mild and Unilateral Hearing Loss: Workshop Proceedings. Breckenridge, CO. Retrieved February 3, 2010, from http://www.cdc.gov/ncbddd/ehdi/

Crandell, C. C., & Smaldino, J. J. (1995). Classroom acoustics. In: R. J. Roeser & M. P. Downs (Eds.), *Auditory disorders in school children: The law, identification, remediation* (3rd ed., pp. 219–234). New York, NY: Thieme Medical.

Glista, D., Scollie, S., Bagatto, M., Seewald, R., Parsa, V., & Johnson, A. (2009). Evaluation of nonlinear frequency compression: Clinical outcomes. *International Journal of Audiology, 48*(1), 632–644.

Jerger, J., Silman, S., Lew, H., L., & Chmiel, R. (1993). Case studies in binaural interference: Converging evidence from behavioral and electrophysiologic measures. *Journal of the American Academy of Audiology, 4*, 122–131.

Johnson, J. L., White, K. R., Widen, J. E., Gravel, J. S., James, M., Kennalley, T., . . . Holstrum, J. (2005). A multicenter evaluation of how many infants with permanent hearing loss pass a two-stage otoacoustic emissions/automated auditory brainstem response newborn hearing screening protocol. *Pediatrics, 116*, 663–672.

Knecht, H. A., Nelson, P. B., & Whitelaw, G. M. (2002). Background noise levels and reverberation times in unoccupied classrooms: Predictions and measurements. *American Journal of Audiology, 11*, 65–71.

Litovsky, R. Y., Johnstone, P. M., & Godar, S. P. (2006). Benefits of bilateral cochlear implants and/or hearing aids in children. *International Journal of Audiology, 45*(Suppl.): S78–S91.

Nance, W. (2007). *Marion Downs lecture: How can newborn hearing screening be improved?* Presented at Audiology Now conference, Denver, CO.

Neault, M. (2005). Progression from unilateral to bilateral loss. *National Workshop on Mild and Unilateral Hearing Loss: Workshop Proceedings.* Breckenridge, CO. Retrieved January 3, 2010, from htpp://www.cdc.gov/ncbddd/ehdi/

Rothpletz, A. M., Tharpe, A. M., & Grantham, D. W. (2004). The effect of asymmetrical signal degradation on binaural speech recognition in children and adults. *Journal of Speech, Language and Hearing Research, 47*, 269–280.

Seewald, R. C., & Scollie, S. D. (2003). An approach for ensuring accuracy in pediatric hearing instrument fitting. *Trends in Amplification, 7*, 29–40.

Stelmachowicz, P., Pittman, A., Hoover, B., & Lewis, A. (2002). Aided perception of /s/ and /z/ by hearing-impaired children. *Ear and Hearing, 23*, 316–324.

Tharpe, A. M., Ricketts, T., & Sladen, D. P. (2004). FM systems for children with minimal to mild hearing loss. In D. Fabry & C. D. Johnson (Eds.), *ACCESS: Achieving Clear Communication Employing Sound Solutions—2003. Proceedings from the First International FM conference* (pp. 191–197). Stäfa, Switzerland: Phonak AG.

Tharpe, A. M., & Sladen, D. P. (2008). Causation of permanent unilateral and mild bilateral hearing loss in children. *Trends in Amplification, 12*, 17–25.

Valente, M. (2007). Fitting options for adults with unilateral hearing loss. *Hearing Journal, 60*(8), 10–18.

Watkin, P. M., & Baldwin, M. (1999). Confirmation of deafness in infancy. *Archives of Disease in Childhood, 81*, 380–389.

Wolfe, J., Caraway, T., John, A., Schafer, E. C., & Nyffeler, M. (2009). Study suggest that non-linear frequency compression helps children with moderate loss. *Hearing Journal, 62*(9), 32–37.

35

Care of Children Who Use Cochlear Implants

Marilyn Neault

Introduction

In the early 1990s, a child from halfway around the globe appeared in the otolaryngology clinic at Children's Hospital Boston. "My son is deaf," said the father through an interpreter. "He had an operation last year in my country for his hearing, but he can't hear any better than before." Baffled, the resident sent the child to Audiology. The audiologist felt for a slightly raised area on one side of the child's head, behind his ear. "When he had the operation, were you given a box?" she asked. "Yes, it's in our hotel room," replied the father. "Nobody told us what to do with it, so we never opened it."

Absurd but true, this story is the antithesis of the preparation, teamwork, and follow-up steps that characterize most cochlear implant procedures at major pediatric implant centers today. A review of these steps, and the reasons for them, helps to clarify the factors that support a good outcome.

Overview of the Cochlear Implant

The cochlear implant is humankind's first artificial sense organ. It stimulates sensory neurons to fire in a pattern that mirrors aspects of the external environment. A thorough explanation of the function of a cochlear implant, both electrically and electrophysiologically, can be found in Chapter 27. An externally worn processor (Figure 35–1) transforms sounds picked up by a microphone into a complex series of pulses that are transmitted across the skin by radio waves to the implant (Figure 35–2). The processor's transmitting coil attaches to the receiver/stimulator portion of the implant by means of two magnets, one outside and one under the skin. If the child has been implanted with a magnetless internal device because of a projected need for future magnetic resonance imaging (MRI) tests, an adhesive retainer disk, changed weekly and containing a small magnet, can be worn on the scalp to hold the transmitting coil in place. The antenna of the receiver/stimulator under the scalp picks up the signal that has been sent across the skin and sends it to an array of electrodes in the cochlea.

Although the electrode arrays of current models may have 16 to 24 electrodes arranged into 12 to 22 channels, some electrodes may be deactivated in a particular user's program because they are not working (short circuit or open circuit), because they are not fully inserted in the cochlea, or because they elicit facial or vestibular stimulation. With present-day technology, the number of channels available for frequency encoding is limited by current spread and channel interactions. For some implants, additional virtual channels are made possible by current steering to achieve intermediate pitch percepts (Koch, Downing, Osberger, & Litvak, 2007), or by adding temporal encoding to the low frequency channels (Wilson et al., 2005). Although some users can rank more acoustically presented pitches than the number of channels of stimulation, other users may not be able to perceive pitch differences between all the channels employed, because of current spread, depleted neural survival, or learning effects.

The processor analyzes the incoming sound into the same number and boundaries of filtered frequency bands as there are channels included in the user's "map" or program.

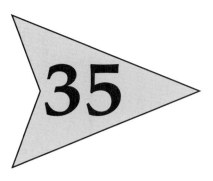

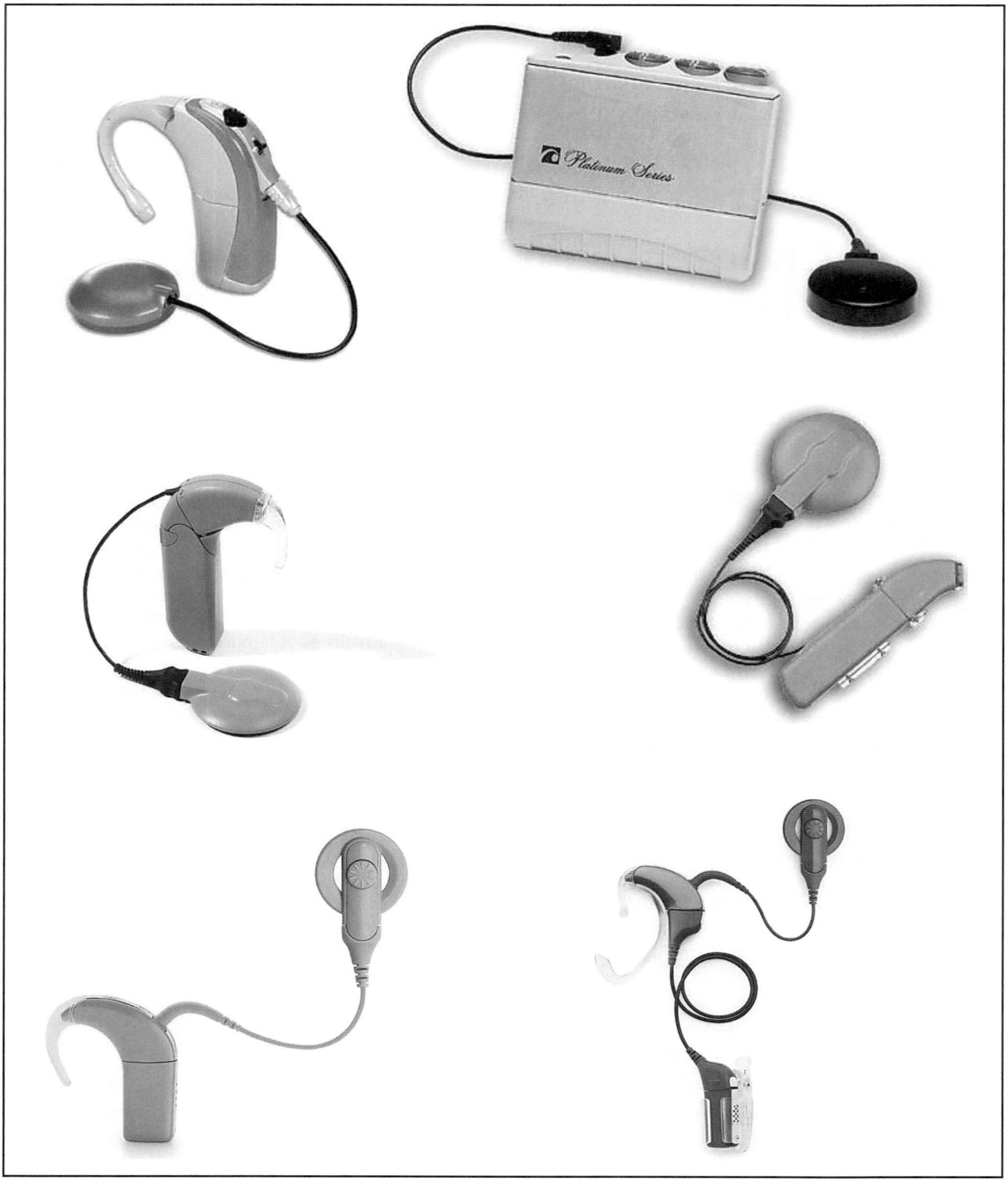

FIGURE 35–1. Examples of sound processors (photos are not depicted to scale). Configurations worn by older children are on the left, and configurations designed for toddlers are on the right. *Top row*: Advanced Bionics Harmony® processor and Platinum Series® Processor (Provided courtesy of Advanced Bionics). *Middle row*: MED-EL OPUS 2 processor (Provided courtesy of MED-EL). *Bottom row*: Nucleus® 5 (CP810) processor (Provided courtesy of Cochlear™ Americas, © 2009 Cochlear Americas).

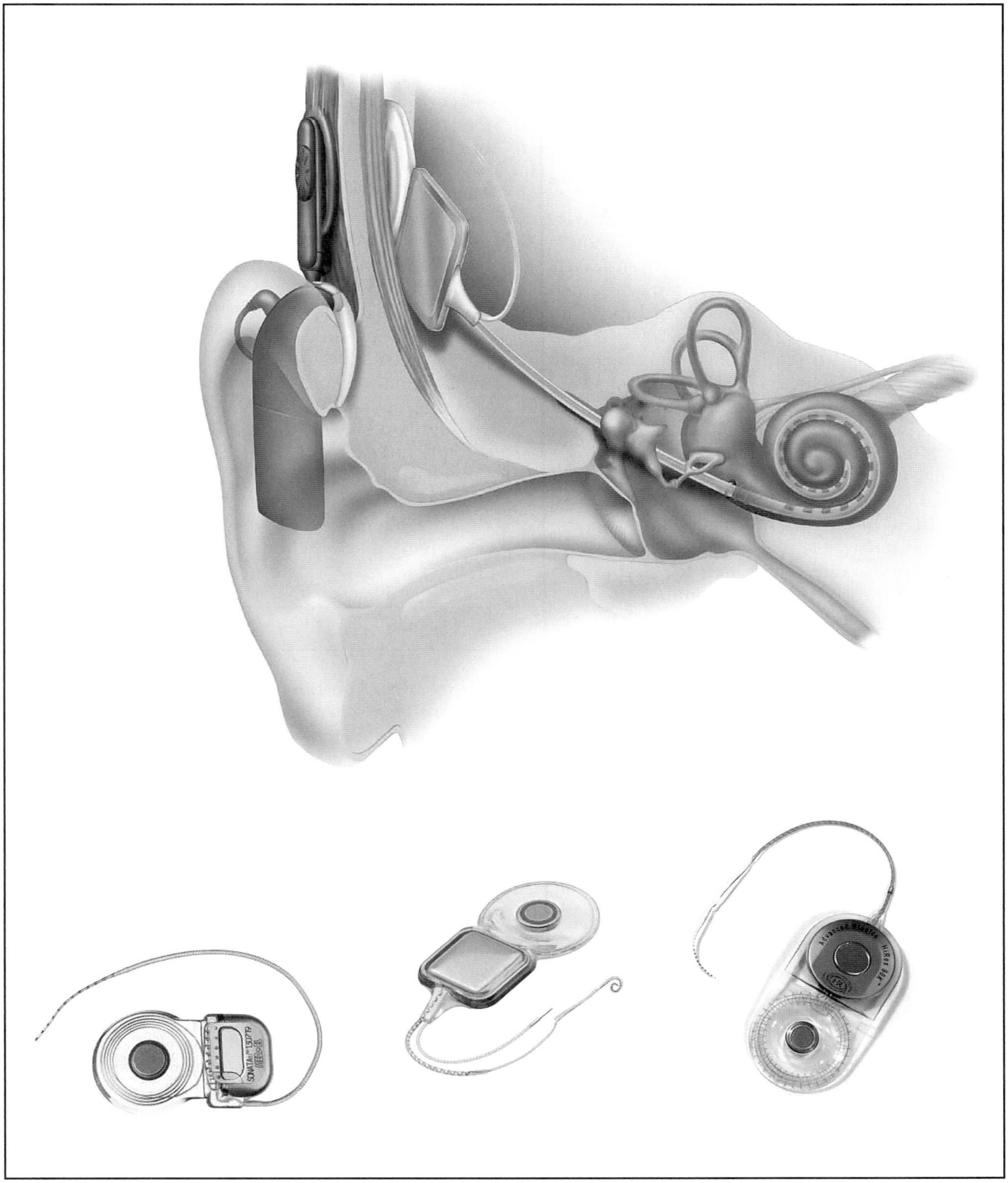

FIGURE 35–2. Examples of cochlear implants (photos are not depicted to scale). *Top*: Nucleus® 5 implant and processor in place (Provided courtesy of Cochlear™ Americas, © 2009 Cochlear Americas). *Bottom left*: MED-EL SONATA$_{TI}^{100}$ implant (Provided courtesy of MED-EL). *Bottom middle*: Nucleus® 5 (CP512) implant (Provided courtesy of Cochlear™ Americas, © 2009 Cochlear Americas). *Bottom right*: Advanced Bionics HiRes 90K® implant (Provided courtesy of Advanced Bionics).

Frequency bands are assigned to channels in tonotopic order from low frequency at the apical tip to high frequency at the basal end of the array. A cogent explanation of the differences in engineering among current implant models may be found in Zeng, Rebscher, Harrison, Sun, and Feng (2008). In the basic paradigm, biphasic pulses are delivered to the electrodes at an assigned stimulation rate. Depending on the implant's design and programmer's decisions, each electrode may function as an independent circuit, or may be grounded to another electrode inside the cochlea (bipolar mode) or outside the cochlea (monopolar mode). The pulses may be delivered to the channels simultaneously or sequentially, depending on the implant design and the coding strategy chosen by the programming audiologist. The pulses are amplitude-modulated according to the intensity of incoming sound in the assigned frequency band. These pulses replace the function of the inner hair cells and stimulate neural elements in the modiolus of the cochlea, causing the generation of compound action potentials in the auditory nerve. The input dynamic range, which used to be set to 30 dB in the 1980s and early 1990s to accommodate the 30 dB range from the weakest to the strongest phoneme, typically is now set to 40 to 60 dB or even larger to accommodate intensity variations in speech, environmental sounds and music. In the amount of current delivered, the pulses are bound at the weaker limit by electrical threshold values (T levels) that are either measured behaviorally or determined by a formula used in the programming software. At the maximal limit, "comfort levels" (M or C levels) are determined based on psychophysical measures or estimated by measurement of the current required to elicit an electrically evoked compound action potential of the auditory nerve or an electrically evoked stapedial reflex. While individuals with normal hearing experience changes in loudness over a 120 dB range, and the processor's input dynamic range typically is set to 40 to 60 dB, the dynamic range for nerve fiber discharge rates is only 4 dB (Kiang & Moxon, 1972). To code intensity changes adequately, therefore, very small increments in electrical current must be used to code greater changes in the intensity of the incoming sound. This amplitude compression is performed by the processor (Rubinstein & Miller, 1999).

Given the cochlear implant's limited number of channels for pitch percepts and its compressed dynamic range for intensity, one would think that its paltry display of auditory "pixels" would yield a grainy, incomplete picture of an incoming sound at best. Why, then, have cochlear implants become the standard of care for children with severe to profound bilateral sensorineural hearing loss whose parents have aspirations for them to speak? Why are legions of children who are congenitally deaf succeeding in transitioning to mainstream education using spoken language with the help of cochlear implants? The fact that cochlear implants work better than their electronics seemingly would allow is a testament to the power of neural plasticity in the young child's brain, with the support of the family and a team of professionals.

In the United States, the Food and Drug Administration (FDA) approved cochlear implantation starting at 24 months in 1990, at 18 months in 1998, and at 12 months for children with profound bilateral loss (24 months for severe loss) in 2002. Even younger infants are implanted when medically indicated. With each drop in age, cochlear implant clinicians strive to employ best practices based on available data. Until recently, however, studies of cochlear implant outcomes were limited to descriptions of small patient cohorts. Now that a substantial number of early-implanted children are in high school and college, a body of literature is evolving that is helping to guide clinical decisions.

The Process of Getting an Implant

For the typical postlinguistically deaf adult, a cochlear implant team often consists only of the surgeon and audiologist, often with a single consultation with a social worker or mental health professional during the evaluation process. For a child, however, the team usually consists of the surgeon, audiologist, speech-language pathologist, psychologist, and deaf education specialist. All team members must be well-versed in working with children who are deaf and their families. If the child depends on sign language to communicate, then sign language should be accessible to the child during clinical encounters. The speech-language pathologist and psychologist in particular should be fluent in order to evaluate the child's language in sign. This same team, aided by an administrative coordinator, provides both evaluation and long-term care. A geneticist, ophthalmologist, radiologist, and neurologist also may see the child during evaluation of the potential benefit of an implant, because the implant evaluation may overlap with the etiologic workup for the hearing loss. For a child with motor disabilities, an occupational therapist may help to optimize seating to participate in listening activities and headrest modifications so that the transmitting coil stays on the head. In addition to a sign language interpreter for a parent or child who primarily signs, an interpreter for a spoken language other than English must be provided when needed. A social worker may participate to assess family dynamics that may interfere with the outcome and to guide the family to resources that will help them to make appointments and support the child.

Although the order of events varies among teams, the evaluation begins with an intake questionnaire and a review of existing audiologic data to determine whether the hearing loss is severe enough for implant candidacy. The hearing aid fitting is optimized and further audiologic evaluation is performed. If the child fits the general guidelines of the implant center for acceptance to the evaluation process, an informational consultation (audiologist with parents or guardians and with the child if older) is often the next step. At this session, parents relay what brings them to learn about the option of an implant, explain what they know about it thus far, share their aspirations for their child, and ask questions about the implant option. The audiologist in turn explains what an implant is and how it works, how the model is chosen, the process of evaluation and follow-up, the need for a concrete plan for expert auditory habilitation therapy postimplant, expectations for outcome in general and for their child. Internal device reliability and reimplantation are discussed. Printed and video materials are given to the family to keep. The parents' knowledge coming into the consultation varies from not knowing surgery is required to asking how different speech processing strategies are implemented on two models. The audiologist's vocabulary level and rate of delivery during this important session should not exceed that of the parents, or the information will not be grasped.

Most parents who seek consultation see the implant appropriately as an opportunity to open the auditory window for their child. Although hesitant parents never should be coerced into implants, those who wish to defer their decision should be familiarized with the better spoken language outcomes of children implanted at younger as compared to older ages. Common causes for parental hesitation to implant a good candidate are as follows: wishing to save the ears for future technology; misinformation from someone who opposes pediatric implantation or from someone who knows a child whose implant did not help; guilt that implanting the child would mean not accepting him as he is; viewing the implant as a failure of the hard-fought battle to make hearing aids work; reluctance to destroy residual hearing; lack of understanding how little the child hears now and how far behind his spoken language may become without auditory access; fear of the surgery; or a variety of cultural beliefs. It may be true that an ear with an implant will not benefit from some future technologies, but nor would an ear with a long-unused auditory pathway. Accurate information must be presented about progress in spoken language development following implantation being supported by expert auditory habilitation, constant exposure to spoken language, and high auditory expectations. The audiologist should not decisively recommend implantation prior to team evaluation, as the other professionals may discover reasons why an implant would not be a beneficial intervention. Particularly when the hearing loss is profound and the computerized tomography (CT) scan and magnetic resonating image (MRI) have not yet been performed, one must keep in mind that the child may prove to have no cochlea or no auditory nerve, rendering a cochlear implant impossible. Parents often ask the audiologist questions about information best presented by the surgeon, such as how the risk of facial nerve damage is avoided and other details of the procedure. The audiologist may outline the topics that the surgeon will discuss, without giving details best left to the surgeon.

Candidacy for Benefit From Cochlear Implantation

Minimum Age for Surgery

The U.S. Food and Drug Administration (FDA, 2010) issues approvals for cochlear implants that are device-specific. The audiologic criteria and minimum age may be determined by the population of subjects and tests used in the clinical trial. Health insurance companies pay attention to these criteria and may question or deny authorization for surgery when the criteria are not met, unless medical necessity can be demonstrated. Current FDA criteria for minimum age are 12 months and up for bilateral profound sensorineural hearing loss and, for Nucleus® devices, 24 months and up for severe (bilateral or better-ear) loss. Some surgeons implant infants well under 12 months, while others wait until 12 months, citing challenges including accuracy of audiologic diagnosis, increased anesthesia risks (lessened in the hands of a pediatric anesthesiologist), limited anatomical access during surgery, increased vulnerability of the facial nerve, blood loss and temporal bone marrow development. However, when careful surgical techniques for infants are employed, extra risks are minimized (Birman, 2009; Vlastarakos, Candiloros, et al., 2010; Waltzman & Roland, 2005). Ossification following meningitis is one factor that many surgeons would agree constitutes medical necessity for implantation under 12 months, if the parents so desire. Although there is convincing evidence that implantation under age 18 months is associated with steeper learning curves for receptive and expressive spoken language than implantation at a later age (Niparko et al., 2010), there are not yet outcome data reported on enough infants to support a widespread policy change regarding implantation under age 12 months (Vlastarakos, Proikas, et al., 2010). Some parents may not be ready for their child to undergo surgery under 12 months. In no case should an implant team recommend that the surgery be scheduled to take place before the parents have an understanding of their child's hearing loss, habilitative therapy services are in place, and there is assurance that the implant offers the child an opportunity worthy of long term commitment. The implant team should support the family in achieving readiness for surgery at an early age, if the family chooses implantation.

Candidacy and Preparation

Most children whose parents are inquiring about cochlear implants fall into certain categories that become familiar to the implant team. The most straightforward is the very young child with congenital severe to profound bilateral hearing loss and no other known developmental challenges. A second large category is that of older children who have acquired spoken language using hearing aids, but have either experienced worsening of hearing in one or both ears, or have not found that hearing aids provide adequate access to speech at conversational intensity. A third category is that of children with auditory neuropathy spectrum disorder (ANSD), whose pure-tone audiogram may not be severe enough for typical guidelines but who benefit from the increased synchrony of neuronal firing provided by the implant. A fourth category is the child with developmental disabilities for whom lack of hearing may not be the greatest challenge. A fifth group is that of older children who are deaf, do not use hearing aids, and use American Sign Language (ASL) to communicate.

The young child who presents under 4 years of age without significant medical or developmental issues other than hearing loss still poses major tasks for the implant team: determining whether the audiologic diagnosis is accurate; performing developmental and language assessments to foresee any previously unsuspected learning or behavioral concerns that should be addressed; and planning appropriate therapy services postactivation if the child is not already receiving expert auditory habilitation. The implant team typically performs an auditory brainstem response (ABR) test, otoacoustic emissions (OAE) and verification of the hearing aid fitting even if these have been performed elsewhere because of the diagnostic responsibility required for a surgical decision. It is helpful for the audiologist who is going to be activating and programming the implant to be the one who performs the last behavioral audiologic evaluation prior to surgery, so that the child's response style can be observed and familiarity and trust can be built.

By FDA guidelines, children who have not developed word recognition ability can meet audiologic criteria by showing lack of progress or developmental lag on a scale such as the IT-MAIS (Infant-Toddler Meaningful Auditory Integration Scale; Zimmerman-Phillips, 2000) or MAIS (Meaningful Auditory Integration Scale; Robbins, Renshaw, & Berry, 1991). A 3- to 6-month period of hearing aid use and therapy is advised to determine adequacy of hearing aid use to support auditory development, but the waiting period is not advised in the case of profound hearing loss following meningitis because ossification may develop in the cochlea within weeks after the illness. With early diagnosis of hearing loss after newborn screening referral, most children have had a period of hearing aid use before the implant evaluation. Hearing aid use should not cause a delay in implantation if there is reason to believe that hearing aids will not provide benefit. The three models of implant most recently approved by the FDA (Cochlear Corporation's Nucleus® System 5, Advanced Bionics Harmony® HiResolution® Bionic Ear System, and MED-EL Sonata TI_{100}) have three different sets of approved indications, which are derived from the subjects and tests used in the clinical trials for each device. The FDA audiologic criteria for a young child include best aided word recognition ability no greater than 20% for the Advanced Bionics and MED-EL devices and no greater than 30% for the Cochlear Corporation device using the Multisyllabic Lexical Neighborhood Test (MLNT) or Lexical Neighborhood Test (LNT; Kirk, Pisoni, Sommers, Young, & Evanson, 1995), whichever is developmentally appropriate. However, the implant team audiologist must judge whether the child is likely to receive more access to sound using an implant than a hearing aid in the ear being considered. Even if the child's word recognition skills are better than FDA guidelines for implantation, the audiologist should compare the child's performance with that of similar children from published data and should consider the presentation level required to achieve best aided performance, when deciding whether to support implantation.

In addition to the speech-language evaluation and the developmental evaluation by a psychologist, the parents meet with a psychologist or social worker to help prepare themselves for the surgery and follow-up, and learn how they can help to prepare their child as well. Even a toddler benefits from playing with surgical masks and stethoscopes, as it can be unnerving to see people with their mouths covered in the operating room area. Learning a few words or signs for the surgery (hospital, bandage, doctor, nurse, etc.) can help give the child confidence. Playing out the surgical experience with a doll or stuffed animal by placing a hospital identification bracelet, having it "breathe" in the anesthetic, go to sleep, and wake up with a head bandage can prepare the child for the experience (Figure 35–3). Parents (if there are two with whom the child feels equally comforted) can decide which parent goes into the operating room for a parent-present anesthesia induction based on which parent is less anxious, as the anxiety can be conveyed to the child.

The child over 4 years of age who has acquired spoken language using hearing aids, whether or not sign language also has been used, can receive great benefit from cochlear implantation to provide greater access to sound. Often these children present with an ear difference in hearing and the poorer ear is implanted first, because the better ear can continue to benefit from acoustic amplification. After the hearing aid fitting is optimized, aided word and sentence recognition tests should be given at 60 dB SPL and, if feasible, 50 dB SPL even if the aided performance would be better at a higher presentation level, because an implant affords perception of speech even at soft conversational intensities (Davidson, 2006). If the child does not have clear enough articulation to administer an open-set monosyllabic word test and does not yet write, closed-set word recognition tests may be given, with the caveat that closed-set tests are "easy" and the open-set test score on which candidacy is judged would be lower. In the case of progressive hearing loss, the poorer ear often is implanted while the better ear does not yet meet rigid candidacy criteria, rather than waiting until audition is a struggle for the child. Older children who can repeat sentences competently sometimes are judged by the implant audiologist using adult criteria (no more than 60% best aided word score on a sentence recognition test such as the Hearing in Noise Test (HINT; Gelnett, Sumida, Nilsson, & Soli, 1995) given in quiet, or 50% in the ear to be implanted). Scores obtained with the test given at 60 dB SPL (average conversational level) or even 50 dB SPL (soft speech) with the hearing aids, rather than 70 dB SPL, often reflect the hearing aid user's struggles to hear speech at an average intensity, which may be improved with an implant. It is likely that the future holds increasing numbers of carefully considered implants for candidates with residual hearing, and eventually expanded FDA criteria for cochlear implantation, based on studies such as Dowell, Hollow, and Winton (2004) that showed that adults having up to 70% sentence recognition scores had greater than 75% chance of improvement with a cochlear implant.

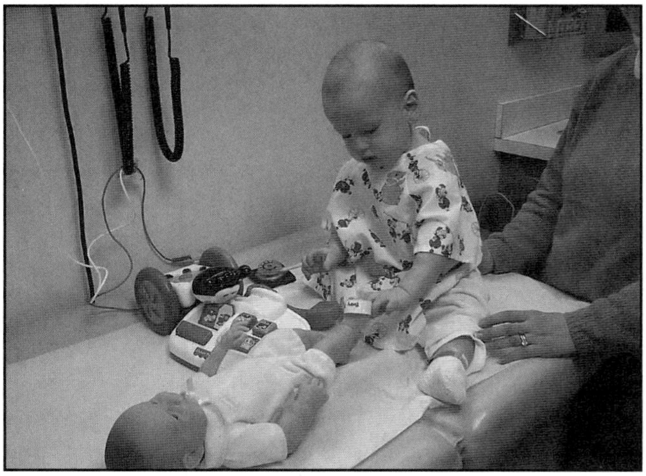

FIGURE 35–3. A 12-month-old boy, well prepared for cochlear implant surgery, places a hospital ID bracelet on his doll's ankle in the preop holding area. Reprinted with permission by George Borhegyi.

Preparing the child over 4 years of age for surgery and activation includes the use of comic/coloring books about the implant, playing with a toy operating room set, and meeting other children who have implants and can explain their experience. The latter recommendation is particularly needed by adolescents, who may have helpful e-mail relationships with peers who use implants. The implant team must assist the parents in determining whether the child's school environment is conducive to learning to use the implant. If not, the team recommends changes in educational programming to foster the use of audition while nurturing language development. For most students, the appropriate environment uses spoken language as the mode of instruction, though some need sign support as well. Classroom acoustics should at least meet the background noise and reverberation requirements of ANSI/ASA S12.60-2002 (R2009), the American National Standard Acoustical Performance Criteria, Design Requirements, and Guidelines for Schools (Acoustical Society of America, 2009). There should be at least one member of the student's educational team, typically a speech-language pathologist or consulting teacher of the deaf, who is expert in language learning and classroom accommodations for children who use cochlear implants. The student should receive individual speech and language therapy specifically geared to auditory skill development. If the school speech and language clinician has little background in auditory development of children who use implants, mentoring by an experienced clinician is an option. Although in the United States the school is not obligated to pay for cochlear implant programming (mapping), the school is responsible for checking that the processor is functioning, providing assistive technology such as an educational amplification system, and providing needed support services (U.S. Department of Education, 2006).

Children with auditory neuropathy spectrum disorder (ANSD) may have pure tone thresholds far better than typical implant candidacy requirements, yet may benefit from cochlear implantation (Roush, 2008). Children with ANSD undergoing cochlear implant candidacy evaluation should undergo MRI to determine the presence of normally sized cochlear nerves (Buchman et al., 2006). Accuracy of audiological diagnosis is critically important, as is determining whether hearing aids help and allowing an adequate time to determine whether neuronal synchrony and functional audition are developing. When the child's audition is holding back his communication development rather than helping it to move forward in a timely fashion, implantation should be considered. Filming a child's communication behavior in a spoken language interchange and watching it with the parents helps in making the implant decision. Functional auditory assessment scales are useful to catalog the child's everyday auditory skills (Can the child hear from front to back seat in the car? Understand words on the phone? Understand speech outdoors? etc.). Cortical evoked potentials may prove to be useful as a correlate to functional speech perception ability (Rance, Cone-Wesson, Wunderlich, & Dowell, 2002). As yet there are inadequate data to know whether children with any particular genetic basis for ANSD, such as certain recessive mutations in the otoferlin (OTOF) gene, are immune from auditory recovery so that they can be implanted very young (Rodriguez-Ballesteros et al., 2003). Although Rance and Barker (2008) found that speech perception outcomes were lower in implanted children with ANSD than in implanted children with typical sensorineural hearing loss, Shallop (2008) reported no such difference between the two groups. However, because roughly half of children with ANSD have spent time in a neonatal intensive care unit (Bolajoko et al., 2008), many have medical and developmental problems apart from hearing loss that may slow their progress with an implant.

Ethical considerations become paramount when evaluating the child with developmental disabilities for cochlear implantation. Although the burning question of 1990 was, "How can you do this surgery **to** this child?" the question now is, "How can we **not** do this surgery **for** this child?" The child first must be healthy enough to undergo an elective surgery safely. The implant team must project what the child might do with some audition if he or she had access to it, and whether the child would be more participatory in family and peer interactions with access to sound. Children with physical but not cognitive disabilities make good progress in auditory skill development, whereas children with cognitive impairment make slower progress, may plateau in their spoken language development at the level of words and rote phrases without mastering grammar, and are more likely to use total communication (Edwards, Waltzman, & Scalchunes, 2007; Holt & Kirk, 2005; Waltzman, Scalchunes & Cohen, 2000; Wiley, Meinzen-Derr,& Choo, 2008). Children with autism spectrum disorder typically make only modest gains in communication function with the implant (Donaldson, Heavner, & Zwolan, 2004) and sometimes do not benefit from the implant, unless they already had spoken language development before becoming deaf.

Older children who use ASL to communicate, do not use hearing aids, interact primarily with signing Deaf peers and teachers, and have not developed awareness of the sounds of speech are at risk for becoming nonusers of their processors if they are implanted. Although the occasional older Deaf recipient enjoys having environmental sound awareness and basic speech pattern detection to support lipreading, most should be counseled that a cochlear implant would not change their communication modality nor enable them to use a voice phone. If the older child who uses ASL to communicate has Usher syndrome or other risk for vision loss, cochlear implantation should be strongly considered, with careful counseling.

The use of a preimplant rating scale helps the implant team remember to weigh the input of all disciplines, to be objective in predicting benefit and to counsel the family regarding expectations. The original Children's Implant Profile (ChIP) developed by Hellman and colleagues (1991) has been adapted by different implant centers to suit their needs (e.g., Dava et al., 1999; Edwards, Thomas, & Raiput, 2009; Lazaridis, Therres, & Marsh, 2010). However, the sum of the ratings (no concern, some concern, great concern) for each category does not always predict the team's recommendation. For example, Lazaridis et al. (2010) found that the ratings predicted 75% of the team's recommendations to implant and 75% of their recommendations not to implant, in a group of 107 children for whom the ratings were completed. However, the rating scale does help to guide expectations and counseling. The rating scale currently in use at Children's Hospital Boston (O'Brien et al., 2007) is shown in Figure 35–4.

Children's Hospital Boston
at Waltham

Cochlear Implant Program
9 Hope Avenue
Waltham, Massachusetts 02453
781-216-2250
www.childrenshospital.org

NAME:
CH#:
DOB:

I. Team Impressions of the Factors Important to Cochlear Implant Use and Success:	No Concern	Some Concern	Great Concern	Not Applicable	Comments
1. Chronological Age [Age:]					
2. Etiology [Cause:]					
3. Duration of Deafness [Age of onset:]					
4. Otolaryngology					
Medical					
Radiology					
5. Other Disabilities:					
6. Audiology					
Test Reliability					
Hearing Aid Use/Use of Residual Hearing (use of available auditory cues)					
Hearing Aid Fitting Optimized/Used					
7. Speech-Language Pathology					
Auditory Training—Past/Present					
Communication Ability—Parental Assessment					
Communication Ability—Clinician Assessment					
Formal Language Use/Comprehension					
Primary Language of the Family [Lang:]					
Primary Language of the Child [Lang:]					
Use of Voice to Communicate					
Speechreading (i.e. Lipreading) Skills					
Communicative Intent					
Parent-Child Language Interactions					
Vocabulary Measure [Score:]					
8. Psychology					
Cognitive Level [Score:]					
Developmental Level [Score:]					
Family Support					
Family System					
Behavioral Traits					
Behavioral Issues					
Behavioral Concerns—Parental					
Expectations (Parents)					
Expectations (Child)					
Adequate Information (Parents)					
Adequate Information (Child)					

FIGURE 35–4. Modification of the Children's Implant Profile used at Children's Hospital Boston to guide discussion, counseling, and expectations for the potential benefit of a cochlear implant (O'Brien et al., 2007). Reprinted with permission.

continues

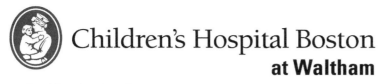

9. Education					
Current Educational Placement					
Future Educational Placement (Transition)					
Access to Auditory-Oral Services					
Educational Staff CI Training					
Ability of Parent to Participate in Educational Process					
Overall impression of team					

II. **PREDICTORS OF HOW ________________ WILL BE COMMUNICATING IN THREE YEARS**
Based on communication continuum (Robbins, 2001). (Circle one of each):

Expressive Communication Continuum

Fully Sign Communicator	Mostly Sign Communicator		Mostly Oral Communicator	Fully Oral Communicator
S	$\mathbf{S_O}$	**SO**	$\mathbf{O_S}$	**O**

Receptive Communication Continuum

Fully Visual Communicator	Mostly Visual Communicator		Mostly Auditory Communicator	Fully Auditory Communicator
V	$\mathbf{V_A}$	**VA**	$\mathbf{A_V}$	**A**

III. **EXPLANATORY NOTES:**

IV. **SIGNATURES:**

Team Members

____

____

____

____

Family Members

____

____

Date ____________________

Page 2

FIGURE 35–4. *continued*

Table 35–1 shows the definitions of the categories that the team audiologists needed to determine in order to use the form the same way. For example, hearing status may be of concern because there is too much residual hearing or conversely, because there has been too little auditory experience for the candidate's age. A second rating scale, developed to guide expectations for outcome of sequential bilateral implantation (Neault et al., 2007) is shown in Figure 35–5. Such rating scales need periodic evidence-based revision as new data continue to emerge regarding factors that contribute to various outcomes.

Intraoperative Testing of the Cochlear Implant

Although some implant centers do not perform intraoperative tests of the function of the implant, many surgeons do elect for the audiologist to test the device following insertion while the surgical field remains sterile. A laptop computer loaded with the programming software, the patient interface box, programming cable, and sound processor are required. The processor and programming cable are inserted into a sterile plastic sleeve such as a camera drape. The surgeon places the transmitting coil over the receiver/stimulator. If the skin flap is not yet closed, either the unsutured flap, a spacer or gauze pads are required to simulate the thickness of the flap, rather than placing the coil directly on the exposed receiver/stimulator.

The audiologist typically performs two tests: impedance telemetry to check for short circuits or open circuits, and measurement of the action potential of the cochlear nerve upon stimulation of individual electrodes. High impedances on one or two electrodes sometimes improve postoperatively, whereas short circuits indicate electrodes that should not be included in the patient's map. The surgeon is advised of any malfunctioning electrodes so that a decision can be made about replacing the device. Following the impedance telemetry, the audiologist typically performs neural response measurements using the manufacturer's software. A good tutorial on neural response testing is found in Hughes (2006a, 2006b). If no interpretable response is seen in the automated version of the test, a more advanced version can be used with user-defined parameters and higher pulse widths available. The neural response should be measured on at least one apical, one medial, and one basal electrode. Lack of typical responses should be followed by an x-ray to check the placement of the electrode array. The impedance telemetry and neural response test can be accomplished while the surgeon is stitching the final layer of the flap, so that no time is added to the anesthesia. It is important for the surgeon to inform the audiologist whether the entire array was inserted into the cochlea, so that no extracochlear electrodes are activated postoperatively.

When a sufficient number of electrodes are tested for neural responses in the operating room, the results yield a contour that helps to predict the contour of the comfort levels of the map at activation of the device (Mason, Cope, Garnham, O'Donoghue, & Gibbin, 2001). Because the current levels required to measure the neural response are perceptually loud for a new user, these intraoperative measures are particularly valuable to have when activating a young child's implant.

Table 35-1. Definitions of No Concern, Some Concern, Great Concern, and Not Applicable for Audiologic Categories of the Form Depicted in Figure 35-4.

AUDIOLOGY	*NO CONCERN*	*SOME CONCERN*	*GREAT CONCERN*	*NOT APPLICABLE*
Test Reliability	Good	Fair	Poor	No behavioral data
Hearing Aid Use/ Use of Residual Hearing	Developed some spoken language or detection/awareness of environmental sounds with limited auditory cues	Inconsistent responses, not clear; or may have too much useful hearing in other ear to appreciate sound of implant	Good amount of residual hearing with no auditory behaviors	Hearing loss too significant to derive any benefit
Hearing Aid Fitting Optimized/Used	Used consistently	Used inconsistently (e.g., couple of hours each day)	Never or infrequently used	

Children's Hospital Boston

NAME:
CHB #
DOB:

BILATERAL CHILDREN'S HEARING IMPLANT PROFILE (BiCHIP)

Predictors for Use and Outcome of 2nd (Sequential Bilateral) Cochlear Implant

#	FACTOR	4	3	2	1	SCORE/DATE	SCORE/DATE
1	AGE AT 2ND CI	0-35 MONTHS	3-4 YEARS	5-8 YEARS	9+ YEARS		
2	GAP BETWEEN 1ST & 2ND CI	0-11 MONTHS	12-35 MONTHS	3-5 YEARS	6+ YEARS		
3	ANATOMY OF 2ND COCHLEA / AUDITORY NERVE	NO CONCERN	MILD CONCERN	MODERATE CONCERN	GREAT CONCERN		
4	COMMUNICATION MODE	AUDITORY/ORAL	AUD W/ VISUAL ASSIST	VISUAL W/ AUD ASSIST	VISUAL		
5	SPOKEN LANGUAGE DEVEL.	AGE APPROPRIATE	MILD DELAY/DISORDER	MODERATE DELAY/DISORDER	SEVERE DELAY/DISORDER		
6	WORD RECOGNITION AT 60 dBSPL WITH 1ST CI (PBK AT 5+ YEARS; NU-CHIPS <5 YEARS)	EXCELLENT 80-100%	GOOD 68-78%	FAIR 50-66%	LIMITED < 50%)		
7	SENTENCE RECOGNITION AT 60 dBSPL WITH 1ST CI (HINT-C IN QUIET AT 5+ YEARS; COMMON PHRASES TEST <5 YEARS)	EXCELLENT 91-100%	GOOD 80-90%	FAIR 50-78%	LIMITED <50%		
8	AUDIBILITY WITH HEARING AID IN 2ND EAR *	>30% OPEN-SET WORD RECOGNITION AT 60 dBSPL WITH HEARING AID	WORD RECOGNITION IN CLOSED SET OR AT HIGH INTENSITY WITH HEARING AID	ONLY SLIGHT BENEFIT FROM HEARING AID	HEARING AID GIVES NO USEFUL AUDIBILITY		
9	PREVIOUS AUDITORY EXPERIENCE OF 2ND EAR **	<100 dBHL WITH HX OF AIDED SPEECH RECOGNITION	<100 dBHL OR CONSISTENT HEARING AID USE	>105dBHL WITH SOME HEARING AID USE	NONE, OR >105 dBHL WITH LITTLE OR NO HEARING AID USE		
10	EQUIPMENT MANAGEMENT	NO CONCERN	MINIMAL CONCERN	MODERATE CONCERN	GREAT CONCERN		
11	EXPECTATIONS (PARENT)	NO CONCERN	MINIMAL CONCERN	MODERATE CONCERN	GREAT CONCERN		
12	READINESS (CHILD)	NO CONCERN	MINIMAL CONCERN	MODERATE CONCERN	GREAT CONCERN		
13	BEHAVIORAL TRAITS (CHILD)	NO CONCERN	MINIMAL CONCERN	MODERATE CONCERN	GREAT CONCERN		
14	COGNITIVE LEVEL	NO CONCERN	MINIMAL CONCERN	MODERATE CONCERN	GREAT CONCERN		
15	ACCESS TO EXPERT THERAPY	NO CONCERN	MINIMAL CONCERN	MODERATE CONCERN	GREAT CONCERN		
16	SUPPORTIVE EDUCATIONAL PROGRAM	NO CONCERN	MINIMAL CONCERN	MODERATE CONCERN	GREAT CONCERN		

* ALTHOUGH HEARING AID BENEFIT MAY PREDICT GOOD CI BENEFIT, CANDIDATES NEED GUIDANCE RE: CHOOSING TO LOSE RESIDUAL UNAIDED HEARING AND HEARING AID BENEFIT

** <100 dBHL MEANS 3-FREQ. PURE TONE AVERAGE BETTER THAN 100 dBHL IN 2ND EAR TO BE IMPLANTED

SCORES LOWER THAN 39 WITH CONCERN ON FACTORS 1, 2, 3, AND 9 WARRANT EXTRA CAUTION.

TOTAL SCORE

(HIGHER SCORE SUPPORTS BETTER CANDIDACY FOR INITIAL ADJUSTMENT, WEARING TIME, AND WORD RECOGNITION WITH 2ND CI)

COMMENTS:

DATE____________________ RATERS____

FIGURE 35–5. Bilateral Children's Hearing Implant Profile (BiChIP) used at Children's Hospital Boston to guide discussion, counseling, and expectations for sequential bilateral implant candidacy (Neault et al., 2007). Reprinted with permission.

If a simultaneous bilateral implantation is performed, the audiologist may be making two trips to the operating room, one to test each device before the patient is turned. When the audiology clinic is located far from the operating suite, remote testing is possible by means of a secure remote computer access program, provided that someone in the operating room can attach the processor to the laptop and place it over the implant.

Activation and Programming of the Cochlear Implant

One to four weeks after surgery, depending on the healing process and the philosophy and schedule of the implant team, the sound processor is programmed so that the child can begin to use it. Between surgery and activation, the child may have been playing with a stuffed animal or doll with a toy processor, reading a coloring book about implants, or getting together with another child who has an implant. For a young child, the appointments should not be scheduled at naptime. Parents of a 1-year-old may wish to purchase a thin cotton "pilot cap" to bring to the activation, to help keep the processor on the ear and to keep little hands away from it while the child becomes accustomed to it. It is very helpful if the parents and older child have watched a video regarding how the processor works before the initial activation, even though the information will be reviewed in detail.

The initial activation and programming typically takes two visits, often scheduled in the same week. Simultaneous bilateral implants may be activated the same day or sequentially. The next visit is no more than a month later, with phone or email contact in the interim, even if reliable measures are obtained in order to create a set of progressively louder maps (programs) to use as the child becomes accustomed to the new sound. Magnet strength should be adjusted and monitored carefully at each visit to avoid skin breakdown. The method used to determine the electrical threshold (T) levels and electrical comfort (C) levels varies with the characteristics of the device, as well as the child's ability to respond. It is in the activation and programming that it becomes clear once more, as it did in the preimplant counseling, that good pediatric audiology skills and a focus on the family spell success.

For a mapping strategy that does not require psychophysical thresholds on each channel, a default set of programming parameters sometimes is used and the processor, connected to the programming computer, is simply turned on at the minimum stimulation level and turned up very slowly while the child's behavior is observed. The contour of the comfort levels (the maximum levels set for each channel) can be determined by the contour of the neural response test results from the operating room, by behavioral observation, or by loudness scaling pictures (Figure 35–6) if the child is about 4 years or older. When the microphone of the processor is turned on, the room is kept quiet until the child begins to make sounds, whereupon a drum, little keyboard, and other musical toys are provided to explore (Figure 35–7). Parents are advised that the initial stage of learning to listen with an implant is to show awareness of sounds that the child is creating. In this phase, if the child is squeezing play-dough and the parent calls from behind, the child may think the sound has been created by the squeezing. When the parent does begin to speak during the session, it is wise to show the child the source of the sound.

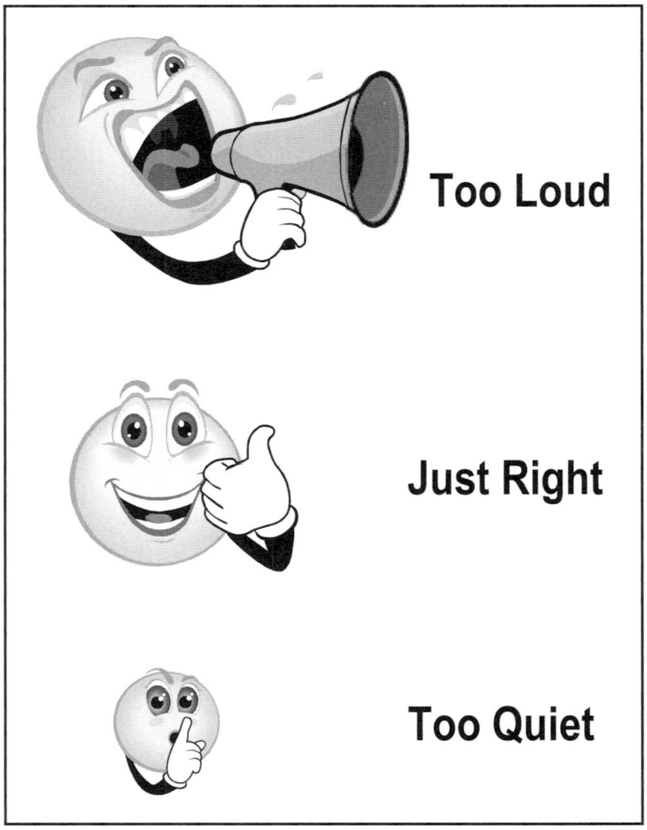

FIGURE 35–6. Example of loudness scaling pictures used by children to help in setting electrical comfort (C) levels when programming a cochlear implant processor.

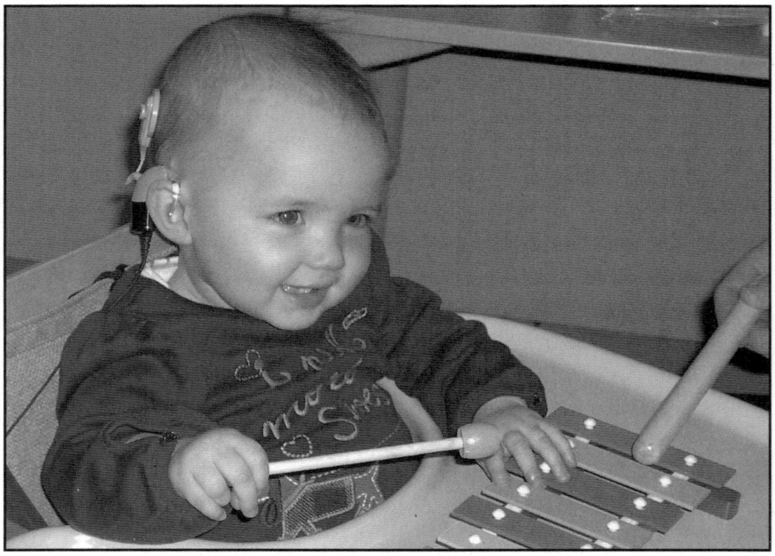

FIGURE 35–7. A 13-month-old girl whose implant was just activated at Children's Hospital Boston enjoys the sound of a xylophone. Her processor is attached to the mapping computer by a programming cable, and the processor microphone is activated following creation of the map. Reprinted with permission.

For a map that will incorporate psychophysical thresholds on individual channels, the audiologist uses developmentally appropriate pediatric test measures. The young child may be on a parent's lap, or preferably in a chair with a tray and properly adjusted footrest. Electrical "beeps" are presented on individual channels to measure thresholds using visual reinforcement audiometry (VRA, Figure 35–8) or conditioned play audiometry (Figure 35–9). The older child or teenager may simply say "yes" or push a response button on hearing a beep. If VRA is used, initial responses may be closer to C levels than to T levels, so the overall levels are adjusted accordingly before activating the microphone. Interpolation of values on intervening electrodes is possible for some types of maps, if not all channels are measured individually. The overall levels should be reduced at least 30 current units below measured T levels, and a small range (no more than 20–30 units) set between T and C levels, before the microphone is activated to avoid an adverse response. Three or four progressively stronger maps are created and stored. The processor is detached from the computer and the family is given instruction in the operation, care, and use of the device.

The parameters that constitute a map include the coding strategy, stimulation rate, pulse width, frequency allocation table, which electrodes are used, grounding (mode), and T and C levels. Preprocessing at the input stage, such as Adaptive Dynamic Range Optimization (ADRO), autosensitivity, and adjustments to the low end of the input dynamic range are part of the map. Output limits determined by voltage compliance may be displayed on the mapping screen. If the processor has an internal telecoil, the ratio of telecoil to microphone input is specified, as is the ratio of accessory input (FM receiver, audio cable, etc.) to microphone input.

It takes most cochlear implant users approximately three months to work up to the C levels they will use for the long term, with periodic fine tuning. It is a goal to achieve equal loudness across frequency bands. However, rate of loudness growth from T to C on the various channels may not be equally steep, so simply balancing the C levels for loudness may not always be enough. Occasionally there are channels with "T-tails" on which loudness begins to grow only partway up the range from T to C, in which case the T level should be reset to the level just below where loudness begins to grow. Likewise, if loudness stops growing below the C level, usually because of voltage compliance limitations, then the C level should be set where loudness stops growing as current units are increased. As speech sound perception develops, the map can be adjusted to optimize awareness and discrimination of individual phonemes. However, one must keep in mind that

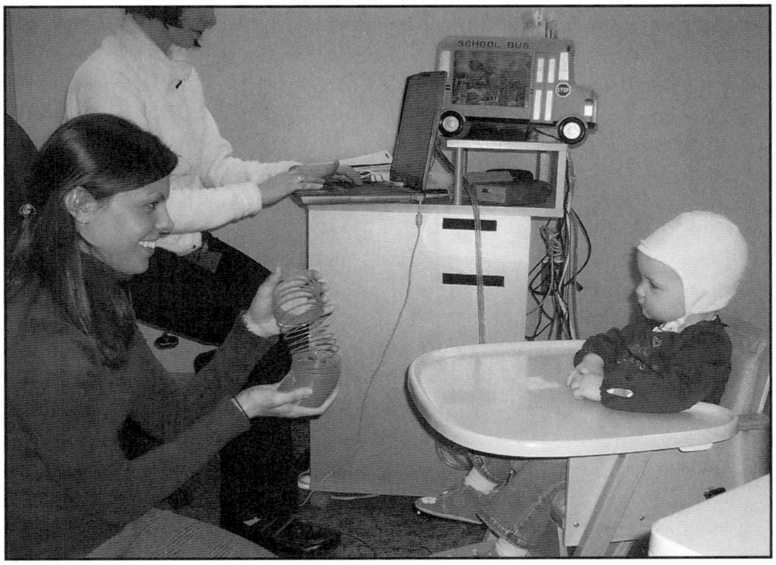

A

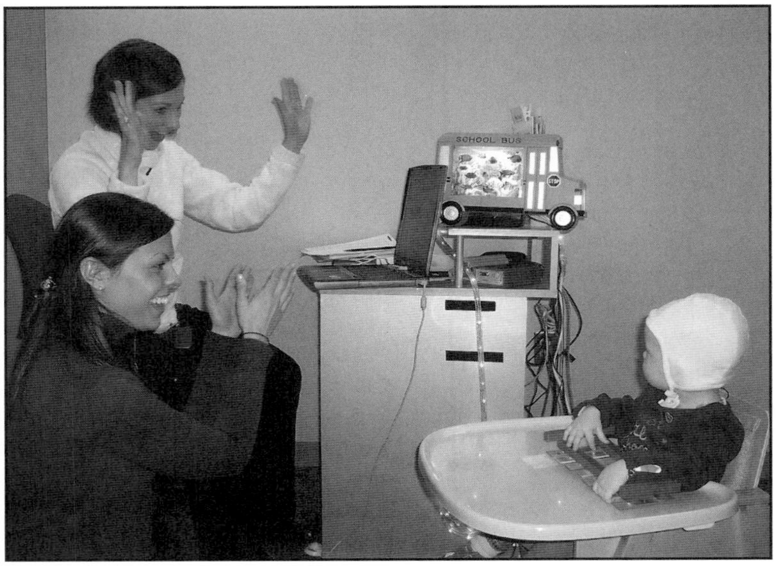

B

FIGURE 35–8. A. A graduate student enchants a 13-month-old girl, while the programming audiologist prepares to measure T levels using Visual Reinforcement Audiometry. The pilot cap worn by the child helps to keep the processor on her head. **B.** The child, whose implant is on the right ear, turns right toward the visual reinforcer in response to a sound. The programming audiologist operates the visual reinforcer with a foot switch. Reprinted with permission.

the child may not yet have developed the auditory skill necessary to recognize certain distinctions, even though the auditory information is accessible to him. Having achieved a phonemic distinction and then losing it may signal the need for a new map, if the processor microphone has not merely become muffled and

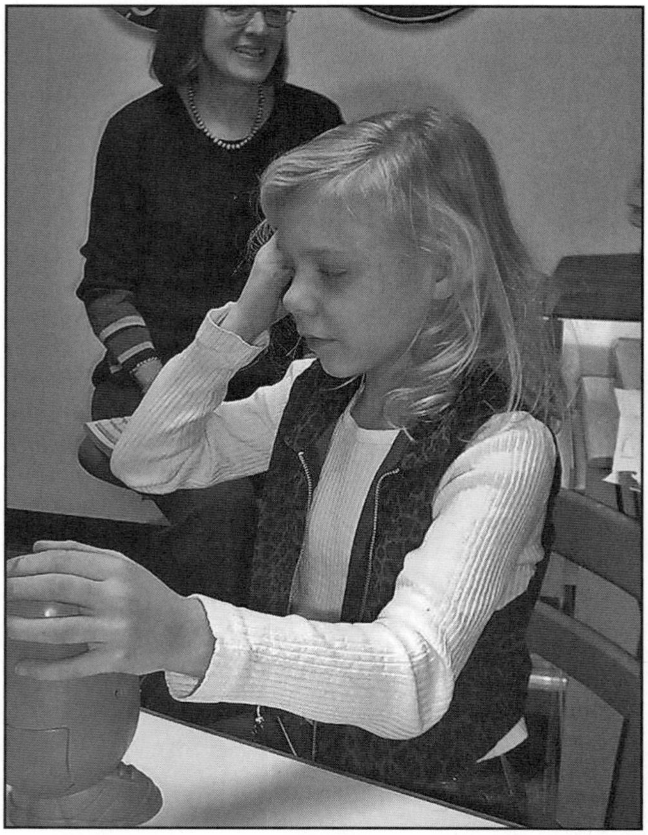

FIGURE 35–9. A child waits for a "beep" before she can place the toy piece, using conditioned play audiometry to measure T levels. Her cochlear implant processor is out of view on her right ear, attached to the computer by a programming cable and interface box. During this portion of the mapping, the processor microphone is not activated, and she cannot hear sounds in the room. Reprinted with permission.

distorted by moisture. Having mastered the production of a phoneme and then losing it also may signal the need for a new map, unless of course the phoneme is /s/ and the front teeth are missing in a 6-year-old!

Communication among the audiologist, speech-language pathologist, and parent (and the child if old enough) before and after a new map helps in determining needs and expectations. After the first three months, mapping typically takes place at 3-month intervals until the map seems fairly stable, then at 6-month intervals. After optimal loudness is achieved, maps are created and stored for different listening situations, such as quiet and noise environments, telephone, and music. Even for experienced users, regular visits are critical for monitoring progress, discussing educational, social, and therapeutic needs and informing the family about technology updates in processors or accessories. Children in an educational setting benefit from FM amplification when participating in group listening activities. Educational audiology support for the use of the processors and FM receivers is important for their benefit. Annual speech and language evaluation and psychological reevaluation at least every 3 years at the implant center maintains good monitoring of progress and adequacy of support services.

The Other Ear

For almost two decades of cochlear implantation, nearly all recipients used only one ear. They were, in fact, encouraged to remove the hearing aid from the other ear to promote adjustment to the implant. Now, however, the two ears are viewed as having both independent and interdependent needs. If the ear contralateral to the implant can benefit from traditional amplification without causing binaural interference, hearing aid use is encouraged. Ample evidence exists to support bimodal speech perception benefit for children who have residual hearing in the unimplanted ear (Ching et al., 2005; Holt et al., 2005; Mok, Galvin, Dowell, & McKay, 2010). Particularly in the early stages of implant adjustment for a long-term hearing aid user, the child may rely on the hearing aid for intonational cues. In the words of a 10-year-old boy who received one implant at age 9 years, "With my cochlear implant, I hear the words; with my hearing aid, I hear the emotion." Unless the child can use the hearing aid independently to understand speech and use the aid on the phone, one may consider rolling off the high frequency gain of the hearing aid, as the implant will provide better access to high frequency sounds. In this way a more comfortable earmold can be used, without feedback. A volume control is useful on the hearing aid in the initial stages of adjustment to bimodal input. When programming the hearing aid, the potential for FM system use should be considered, so that an FM plus environment setting can be accessed by the child. Although the child is more likely to use the cochlear implant than the hearing aid on the telephone, a telecoil setting should be included on the aid if the child might be using a neck loop FM receiver (needing an MT setting), or listening to music through inductive stereo ear hooks.

If the contralateral ear does not have aided thresholds at a level that allows lateralization of sounds and does not have the potential for word recognition, a second implant should be considered to achieve bilateral implant use, which is discussed in depth in Chapter 27. Bilateral cochlear implant use improves speech perception in noise, eliminates the head shadow experienced by unilateral implant users, improves perception of soft speech by binaural summation, and allows some localization ability to develop over time (Johnston et al., 2009). Although the processor on the originally implanted side is removed for some listening therapy sessions and for an hour or so per day at home so that the new ear can "practice," the ultimate goal is for the brain to integrate the input from the two sides. Using an FM receiver on the poorer performing side only, to "train" it, results in poorer hearing in background noise (Schafer & Thibodeau, 2006) and is not recommended.

Programming the two implants may be done at the same or separate visits. Even with slightly different insertion depths, having the frequency allocation tables start at the same frequency allows similar loudness of the user's own voice between the two sides. At the present time, there is no commercially available software that assists in programming the two sides to sound alike. It is hardly expected that they will sound identical and, in fact, the contribution of different bits of information from each side may add more "pixels" to improve the resolution of the grainy overall auditory picture. Each side is programmed as a separate entity, though both may be activated at once if two interface boxes and programming cables can be connected to the computer at the same time, so that adjustments can be made. If only one processor is connected to the programming computer at a time, then after the psychophysical measurements are completed, that processor's map can be adjusted "live" while the other processor is worn on its own battery power. The future may hold correlation of the two maps so as to allow the user to appreciate fine timing differences between sound arrivals at the two ears, which currently is a weakness of bilateral implant use, and to match pitch percepts on the two sides.

Monitoring Progress and Problems

Audiologic evaluation in the audiometric sound suite should occur at least at the 6-month interval and annually. For young children, these evaluations should take place at a separate appointment, not after a long bilateral mapping session. An unaided audiogram should be obtained annually for each ear, to assess any remaining residual hearing and to document the degree of loss in order to support the need for educational accommodations. Sound field thresholds of detection for pulsed or pulsed warbled tones are measured at 250, 500, 1000, 2000, 4000, and 6000 Hz using each processor. Values poorer than 35 dB HL or uneven across the frequency range by more than 10 dB require an explanation. Thresholds typically average 20 to 30 dB HL (slightly better for narrow band noise stimuli than for pulsed tones) and are influenced by the sensitivity control setting, input processing, input dynamic range, and characteristics of the microphone. Unexplained poor thresholds warrant checking the processor function and reprogramming.

If the child is too young or not ready to point to pictures when they are named, early progress can be assessed using a scale such as the IT-MAIS (Zimmerman-Phillips, 2000), Auditory Skills Checklist (Meinzen-Derr, Wiley, Creighton, & Choo, 2007), MED-EL Corporation's LittlEars Auditory Questionnaire (Küehn-Inacker, Weichbold, Tsiakpini, Coninx, & D'Haese, 2003), or other functional auditory scales. Speech recognition testing is accomplished by developmentally appropriate measures, recorded rather than live voice when possible, starting with closed-set picture pointing tests graduating to open-set word recognition tests or another developmentally appropriate recorded sentence test in quiet and noise, given with optimized maps for each ear separately and together. If a hearing aid is used contralateral to the implant, the hearing aid should be checked and the fitting verified prior to speech recognition testing. A presentation level of 60 dB SPL is appropriate for speech recognition testing with a cochlear implant, with at least one test given at 50 dB SPL (soft speech level) if performance at 60 dB SPL is good, for comparison and counseling purposes. Careful sound field calibration and placement of the head in the sound field are important. Decrements in performance should be taken seriously as they may signal a lapse in therapy or a device problem. Any suspicion of internal device malfunction triggers an alert to the surgeon and an integrity test, typically administered at the implant center by a manufacturer's clinical specialist.

Tympanometry should be performed at the first postoperative audiologic evaluation and then annually or as needed in otologic monitoring. The static admittance of the implanted ear typically is lower postoperatively than preoperatively and may remain lower than the unimplanted ear (Neault, O'Brien, Rimmer, Licameli, & Kenna, 2005), so a baseline measure with the implant in place when the ears are clear is helpful in the event of future need for the use of tympanometry to assess middle ear dysfunction. If vestibular evoked myogenic potentials (VEMPs) were recorded and found to be present prior to surgery, the test may be repeated at the first postoperative audiologic evaluation. The VEMP threshold may be elevated and the amplitude reduced postoperatively (Licameli, Zhou, & Kenna, 2009). The use of cortical evoked potentials to assess auditory response development is reviewed in Chapter 27.

Fostering Independence

Just as teenagers with hearing loss need to learn to wake themselves up in the morning with a vibrating or flashing alarm clock, they also need to begin to become independent users of their hearing technology. They may have been implanted when they were too young to understand the process or device and need progressive education about their hearing loss, how they access sound, and how their hearing differs from typical hearing. College preparation group meetings for students with hearing loss and other support groups, in person or on line, foster independence. They can be independent in asking for captions to be turned on. They can begin to handle processor breakdowns independently before they graduate from high school. College preparation requires students with hearing loss to develop organizational skills and knowledge of accommodations including FM systems and real-time text support to access the curriculum at the same time as their classmates, not later by reading notes after class. Young adults who were implanted at age 2 years at the time of FDA approval of implantation for children are in college now, leading the way for a generation of children who have access to the world of sound using cochlear implants. Pediatric implant teams can anticipate the reward of watching them choose and become successful in their vocations.

References

Acoustical Society of America. (2009). ANSI/ASA S12.60-2002 (R2009). *American National Standard acoustical performance criteria, design requirements, and guidelines for schools* (reaffirmation of ANSI S12.60-2002). http://asastore.aip.org

Birman, C. (2009). Cochlear implant surgical issues in the very young child. *Cochlear Implants International, 10*(1), 19–22.

Bolajoko, O., Olusanya, A. B., Shiela, L., Wirz, C., Linda, M., & Luxon, A. (2008). Factors associated with auditory neuropathy/dys-synchrony in a developing country. *Audiological Medicine, 6*(2), 120–128.

Buchman, C. A., Roush, P. A., Teagle, H. F. B., Brown, C. J., Zdanski, C. J. & Grose, J. H. (2006). Auditory neuropathy characteristics in children with cochlear nerve deficiency. *Ear and Hearing, 27*(4), 399–408.

Ching, T. Y., Hill, M., Brew, J., Incerti, P., Priolo, S., Rushbrook, E., & Forsythe, L. (2005). The effect of auditory experience on speech perception, localization, and functional performance of children who use a cochlear implant and a hearing aid in opposite ears. *International Journal of Audiology, 44*(12), 677–690.

Dava, H., Figueirido, J. C., Gordon, K. A., Twitchell, K., Gysin, C., & Papsin, B. C. (1999). The role of a graded profile analysis in determining candidacy and outcome for cochlear implantation in children. *International Journal of Pediatric Otorhinolaryngology, 49*(2), 136–142.

Davidson, L. S. (2006). Effects of stimulus level on the speech perception abilities of children using cochlear implants or digital hearing aids. *Ear and Hearing, 27*(5), 493–507.

Donaldson, A. I., Heavner, K. S., & Zwolan, T. A. (2004). Measuring progress in children with autism spectrum disorder who have cochlear implants. *Archives of Otolaryngology-Head and Neck Surgery, 130*(5), 666–671.

Dowell, R., Hollow, R., & Winton, E. (2004). Outcomes for cochlear implant users with significant residual hearing. *Archives of Otolaryngology-Head and Neck Surgery, 130*, 575–581.

Edwards, L., Thomas, F., & Rajput, K. (2009). Use of a revised children's implant profile (GOSHChIP) in candidacy for paediatric cochlear implantation and in predicting outcome. *International Journal of Audiology, 48*(8), 554–560.

Edwards, L. C., Waltzman, S. B., & Scalchunes, V. (2007). Children with cochlear implants and complex needs: A review of outcome research and psychological practice. *Journal of Deaf Studies and Deaf Education, 12*(3), 258–268.

Gelnett, D., Sumida, A., Nilsson, M., & Soli, S. D. (1995). *Development of the hearing in noise test for children (HINT-C).* Annual Meeting of American Academy of Audiology, Dallas, TX.

Hellman, S. A., Chute, P. M., Kretschmer, R. E., Nevins, M. E., Parisier, S. C., & Thurston, L. C. (1991). The development of a Children's Implant Profile. *American Annals of the Deaf, 136*, 77–81.

Holt, R. F., & Kirk, K. I. (2005). Speech and language development in cognitively delayed children with cochlear implants. *Ear and Hearing, 26*(2), 132–148.

Holt, R. F., Kirk K. I., Eisenberg, L. S., Martinez, A. S., & Campbell, W. (2005). Spoken word recognition development in children with residual hearing using cochlear implants and hearing aids in opposite ears. *Ear and Hearing, 26*(4 Suppl.), 82S–91S.

Hughes, M. L. (2006a). Fundamentals of clinical ECAP measures in cochlear implants. Part 1: Use of the ECAP in speech processor programming. *Audiology Online*, April 10, 2006, Article 1569. Retrieved April 10, 2006, from http://www.audiologyonline.com/articles/article_detail.asp?article_id=1569

Hughes, M. L. (2006b). Fundamentals of clinical ECAP measures in cochlear implants, Fundamentals of clinical ECAP measures in cochlear implants Part 2: Measurement techniques and tips. *Audiology Online*, November 6, 2006,

Article 1717. Retrieved November 6, 2006, from http://www.audiologyonline.com/articles/pf_article_detail.asp?article_id=1717

Johnston, J. C., Durieux-Smith, A., Angus, D., O'Connor, A., & Fitzpatrick, E. (2009). Bilateral pediatric cochlear implants: A critical review. *International Journal of Audiology, 48*(9), 601–617.

Kiang, N. Y., & Moxon, E. C. (1972). Physiological considerations in artificial stimulation of the inner ear. *Annals of Otology, Rhinology and Laryngology, 81*(5), 714–730.

Kirk, K. I., Pisoni, D. B., Sommers, M. S., Young, M., & Evanson, C. (1995). New directions for assessing speech perception in persons with sensory aids. *Annals of Otology, Rhinology, and Laryngology, 104*(Suppl. 106), 300–303.

Koch, D. B., Downing, M., Osberger, M. J., & Litvak, L. (2007). Using current steering to increase spectral resolution in CII and HiRes 90K users. *Ear and Hearing, 28*(2 Suppl.), 38S–41S.

Küehn-Inacker, H., Weichbold, V., Tsiakpini, L., Coninx, S., & D'Haese, P. (2003). *LittlEARS Auditory questionnaire: Parents questionnaire to assess auditory behavior*. Retrieved February 8, 2010, from http://www.medel.com/english/img/PDF/reha/MKT1070E_r20.pdf

Lazaridis, E., Therres, M., & Marsh, R. R. (2010). How is the children's implant profile used in the cochlear implant candidacy process? *International Journal of Pediatric Otorhinolaryngology, 74*(4), 412–415.

Licameli, G., Zhou, G., & Kenna, M. A. (2009). Disturbance of vestibular function attributable to cochlear implantation in children. *Laryngoscope, 119*(4), 740–745.

Mason, S. M., Cope, Y., Garnham, J., O'Donoghue, G. M., & Gibbin, K. P. (2001). Intra-operative recordings of electrically evoked auditory nerve action potentials in young children by use of neural response telemetry with the nucleus C124M cochlear implant. *British Journal of Audiology, 35*(4), 225–235.

Meinzen-Derr, J., Wiley, S., Creighton, J., & Choo, D. (2007). Auditory Skills Checklist: Clinical tool for monitoring functional auditory skill development in young children with cochlear implants. *Annals of Otology, Rhinology, and Laryngology, 116*(11), 812–818.

Mok, M., Galvin, K. L., Dowell, R. C., & McKay, C. M. (2010). Speech perception benefit for children with a cochlear implant and a hearing aid in opposite ears and children with bilateral cochlear implants. *Audiology and Neurotology, 15*(1), 44–56.

Neault, M., Kammerer, B., Clark, T., O'Brien, L., Kenna, M., & Licameli, G. (2007). *Pre-implant rating scale for prediction of outcome with sequential bilateral cochlear implantation in children*. Poster presentation at the 11th International Conference on Cochlear Implants in Children. Charlotte, North Carolina, April 12, 2007.

Neault, M., O'Brien, L., Rimmer, D., Licameli, G., & Kenna, M. (2005). *Effect of cochlear implantation on static admittance of the middle ear*. Paper presented at the10th International Conference on Cochlear Implants in Children Dallas, TX, March 17.

Niparko, J. K., Tobey, E. A., Thal, D. J., Eisenberg, L. S., Wang, N.-Y, Quittner, A. L., & Fink, N. E. (2010). Spoken language development in children following cochlear implantation. *Journal of the American Medical Association, 303*(15), 1498–1506.

O'Brien, L., Kenna, M., Poe, D., Neault, M., Kammerer, B., Clark, T., . . . Licameli, G. (2007). *Validation of a modified cochlear implant profile (mChIP) tool for use in pediatric cochlear implant candidacy evaluation*. Poster presentation at the11th International Conference on Cochlear Implants in Children. Charlotte, North Carolina, April 12.

Rance, G., & Barker, E. J. (2008). Speech perception in children with auditory neuropathy/dyssynchrony managed with either hearing aids or cochlear implants. *Otology and Neurotology, 29*(2), 179–182.

Rance, G., Cone-Wesson, B., Wunderlich, J., & Dowell, R. (2002). Speech perception and cortical event related potentials in children with auditory neuropathy. *Ear and Hearing, 23*(3), 239–253.

Robbins, A. M. (2001). A sign of the times: Cochlear implants and total communication. *Loud & Clear, A Cochlear Implant Rehabilitation Newsletter, 4*(2), 1–4. Advanced Bionics Corporation.

Robbins, A. M., Renshaw, J. J., & Berry, S. W. (1991). Evaluating meaningful integration in profoundly hearing impaired children. *American Journal of Otolaryngology, 12*(Suppl.): 144–150.

Rodríguez-Ballesteros, M., del Castillo, F. J., Martín, Y., Moreno-Pelayo, M. A., Morera, C., Prieto, F., . . . del Castillo, I. (2003). Auditory neuropathy in patients carrying mutations in the otoferlin gene (OTOF). *Human Mutation, 22*(6), 451–456.

Roush, P. (2008). Auditory neuropathy spectrum disorder: Evaluation and management. *Hearing Journal, 61*(11), 36, 38–41.

Rubinstein, J. T., & Miller, C. A. (1999). How do cochlear prostheses work? *Current Opinion in Neurobiology, 9*, 399–404.

Schafer, E. C., & Thibodeau, L. M. (2006). Speech recognition in noise in children with cochlear implants while listening in bilateral, bimodal, and FM-system arrangements. *American Journal of Audiology, 15*, 114–126.

Shallop, J. (2008). *Management of children with Auditory Neuropathy Spectrum Disorder: Cochlear implants. Guidelines for identification and management of infants and young children with auditory neuropathy spectrum disorder*. Guidelines Development Conference at NHS 2008, Como, Italy.

U.S. Department of Education. (2006). *Final regulations to implement the Individuals with Disabilities Education Improvement Act of 2004 (IDEA)*. Federal Register, 71(56, August 14, 2006).

U.S. Food and Drug Administration (FDA). (2010). *Medical Device Premarket Approval (PMA) Database: Cochlear implants*. Rockville, MD: FDA. Accessed on April 30, 2010, at http://www.fda.gov/MedicalDevices/ProductsandMedicalProcedures/ImplantsandProsthetics/CochlearImplants/default.htm

Vlastarakos, P. V., Candiloros, D., Papacharalampous, G., Tavoulari, E., Kampessis, G., Mochloulis, G., & Nikolopoulos, T. P. (2010). Diagnostic challenges and safety considerations in cochlear implantation under the age of 12 months. *International Journal of Pediatric Otorhinolaryngology, 74*(2), 127–132.

Vlastarakos, P. V., Proikas, K., Papacharalampous, G., Exadaktylou, I., Mochloulis, G., & Nikolopoulos, T. P. (2010). Cochlear implantation under the first year of age —the outcomes. A critical systematic review and meta-analysis. *International Journal of Pediatric Otorhinolaryngology, 74*(2),119–126.

Waltzman S. B., & Roland, J. T., Jr. (2005). Cochlear implantation in children younger than 12 months. *Pediatrics, 116*(4), e487–e493 (doi:10.1542/peds.2005-0282).

Waltzman, S. B., Scalchunes, B., & Cohen, N. L. (2000). Performance of multiply handicapped children using cochlear implants. *American Journal of Otology, 21*(3), 329–335.

Wiley, S., Meinzen-Derr, J., & Choo, D. (2008). Auditory skills development among children with developmental delays and cochlear implants. *Annals of Otology, Rhinology and Laryngology, 117*(10), 711–718.

Wilson, B. S., Schatzer, R., Lopez-Poveda, E. A., Sun, X., Lawson, D. T., & Wolford, R. D. (2005). Two new directions in speech processor design for cochlear implants. *Ear and Hearing, 26*(4 Suppl.), 73S–81S.

Zeng, F. G., Rebscher, S., Harrison, W., Sun, X., & Feng, H. (2008). Cochlear implants: System design, integration and evaluation. *IEEE Reviews in Biomedical Engineering, 1*, 115–142.

Zimmerman-Phillips, S., Osberger, M. F., & Robbins, A. M. (1997). *Infant-toddler: Meaningful Auditory Integration Scale (IT-MAIS)*. Sylmar, CA: Advanced Bionics Corp.

36

Audiologic Considerations for Children With Multiple Modality Involvement

Allan O. Diefendorf, Rachel K. Allen, Monica L. Burch, Kathleen R. Corbin, Christine E. Griffiths, Baljit K. Rehal, and Amanda S. Weinzierl

Introduction

The etiology of congenital hearing loss can be derived from four major etiologic classifications including chromosomal origin, genetic origin, environmental teratogens, and low birth weight. Table 36–1 provides "common" selected examples within each classification. Usually, the most frequent examples would be those conditions that themselves are common, with hearing loss being a variably occurring component of the condition. However, for this table, the authors have chosen to define "common" as those patients seen at their home institution (James Whitcomb Riley Hospital for Children) who carry the diagnosis of hearing loss, and who also have another chromosomal feature, genetic feature, or associated congenital clinical condition.

Historically, the past 25 years of demographic data (Gallaudet College Center for Assessment and Demographic Studies, 1983; Gallaudet Research Institute, 2005; Fortnum & Davis, 1997; Mace, Wallace, Whan, & Stelmachowicz, 1991) consistently have reported that 30 to 40% of children with hearing loss have one or more *additional* disabilities. Table 36–2 lists physical and cognitive/intellectual conditions that are most frequently reported to accompany hearing loss. Thus, Table 36–1 and Table 36–2 are complementary; that is, Table 36–1 identifies "cause" and Table 36–2 identifies "effects" that may occur in a high percentage of children with hearing loss. Additionally, the manner in which multiple modality conditions *coexist* and the manner in which multiple modality conditions are *expressed* (by degree of involvement) contribute to each child's unique developmental profile. Therefore, *every child* brings a unique combination of characteristics (hearing loss alone, hearing loss with multiple modality involvement) to their personal developmental profile.

The fact that hearing impairment in children can be accompanied by additional challenging conditions emphasizes the importance of considering each child's developmental profile when implementing an audiologic assessment plan for infants and young children suspected of hearing loss. Additionally, with the goal of audiologic diagnosis by 3 months of age in early hearing loss detection and intervention (EHDI) programs today (Joint Committee on Infant Hearing [JCIH], 2007), it is likely that many infants with hearing loss and multiple modality conditions may not have had these conditions identified at the time of the audiologic assessment. Therefore, audiologists face challenges when dealing with the diversity of characteristics that may be found among children suspected of hearing loss.

Clearly, the presence of physical and cognitive/intellectual conditions will add to the complexity of caring for children with multiple special needs. Furthermore, these conditions can influence audiologic test selection, audiologic outcomes, and subsequent recommendations. As such, audiologic test protocols must be, by necessity, flexible to accommodate individual child differences and preferences. As pointed out by Tharpe (2009) audiologists must be mindful of the possibility that unexpected and/or undiagnosed conditions may influence their testing and subsequent audiologic outcomes.

Thus, the purpose of this chapter is to focus on modifications and adaptations in pediatric audiologic assessment when providing services to children with suspected or confirmed multiple modality conditions.

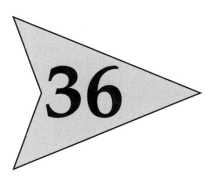

Table 36–1. Etiologic Classification of Congenital Hearing Loss and "Common" Selected Examples Within Each Classification

Etiologic Classification	*"Common" Selected Examples*	
Chromosomal Origin	Trisomy 13 (Patua syndrome)	Fragile X syndrome
	Trisomy 18 (Edward syndrome)	Turner syndrome
	Trisomy 21 (Down syndrome)	
	5P—(Cri-du-chat syndrome)	
	4P—(deletion problem)	
Genetic Origin	Alport syndrome	Mitochondrial disorders
	Branchio-oto-renal syndrome	Neurofibromotosis type II
	CHARGE association	Osteogenesis Imperfecta spectrum
	Chiari malformation	Pendred syndrome
	Crouzon syndrome	Pierre Robin sequence
	de Lange syndrome	Stickler syndrome
	DiGeorge syndrome	Treacher Collins syndrome
	Hemifacial microsomia	Usher syndrome
	Jervell & Lange-Nielsen	Waardenburg syndrome
Teratogens Agents in the environment of the developing embryo and fetus that cause structural or functional abnormalities	Viral disease	Bacterial disease
	Maternal smoking	Thyroid disorders
	Environmental toxins (lead; mercury)	Fetal Alcohol syndrome
	Drugs (substance abuse)	Radiation
Low Birth Weight	Respiratory Distress syndrome	
	Bronchopulmonary dysplasia (BPD)	
	Hyperbilirubinemia	
	Neonatal sepsis	
	Patent ductus arteriosus	
	Peri/Intraventricular hemorrhage	
	Perinatal asphyxia	

Patient History

When assessing infants and young children with suspected or confirmed multiple modality conditions, a thorough patient history is essential. Traditionally, acquiring patient history information has been completed by obtaining answers to a predetermined list of questions. However, this approach may limit audiologists to a "closed-set" of information and prevent a more individualized patient-centered approach to acquiring relevant information about the patient. It is recommended that time for obtaining a patient history be viewed as a valuable opportunity to observe and interact with the child and family, build rapport, and instill confidence and comfort in the child and family, while acquiring patient specific history information. This is especially true when attempting to assess a child with special needs. Furthermore, these initial observations facilitate assessment planning and clinical strategies by determining how much independence, cooperation, communication, and physical ability can be expected.

Table 36–2. Physical and Cognitive/Intellectual Conditions* Frequently Reported to Accompany Hearing Loss in Children

Physical Conditions
Asthma
Brain damage or injury
Cardiovascular defects
Cerebral palsy
Endocrine abnormalities (e.g., hypothyroidism, diabetes, kernicterus)
Epilepsy
Immunologic abnormalities
Kidney defects
Legal blindness
Neurologic abnormalities
Orthopedic abnormalities
Uncorrected or uncorrectable visual problems
Cognitive Intellectual Conditions
Intellectual disability
Specific learning disability which may include: visual/auditory perceptual problems; fine motor coordination problems; attention deficit disorder; developmental delay.
Emotional/behavioral problems which may include: autism spectrum disorder; hyperactivity; passive/withdrawn behavior (social isolation); reduced self-esteem; aggressive/abusive behavior; unfounded physical complaints and symptoms.

*Sixty to 70% of children present with no additional handicapping conditions, whereas 30 to 40% present with one (or more) additional handicapping conditions.

Observation and Interaction

The patient history process begins as early as calling the child's name in the waiting room. Time spent observing the child from the waiting room to the assessment area can provide cues about the child's physical and developmental status. Previous literature has stressed the importance of the "hallway conversation" or the history intake that is completed as the audiologist walks the family from the waiting room to the evaluation area (Renshaw & Diefendorf, 1998). However, in concert with increasingly stringent privacy laws (i.e., Health Insurance Portability and Accountability Act [HIPAA]), strict adherence to protecting confidential patient information in a public area is essential. A HIPAA compliant hallway conversation might be one where instead of asking confidential questions regarding the child's medical history, the brief time is utilized for observation and for casual conversation intended to build rapport with the child and their family.

Observations can be made about behaviors such as, but not limited to:

- Temperament of the child;
- Alertness of the child;
- Clues about the developmental status of the child;
- Clues about the interaction/communication between the child and their family;
- Independence/shyness following introduction; and
- Willingness of the child to engage/participate in conversation.

For example, a child greater than 18 months of age who is not walking independently may signal delays in developmental status. If calling a child's name in the waiting room causes crying, this might suggest fearfulness, a low comfort level or a lack of willingness to engage.

Casual conversation allows the audiologist an initial opportunity to interact with the child for the purposes of building rapport with the child and family. The desired outcome is reducing their anxiety about a new environment, new adults, and entering a room with unfamiliar equipment. Some examples of rapport-building and anxiety-reducing strategies include:

- Introducing yourself to the child and family;
- Complimenting the child on attire or toys;
- Asking about age or grade level;
- Introducing positive reinforcements/rewards that may be used during or at completion of assessment (e.g., showing stickers/toys);
- Providing the child and family with information about the assessment in order to ease anxiety/fears (the benefit of this practice with the child should not be underestimated); and
- Allowing the child to touch equipment (e.g., holding the otoscope; feeling the ear tips; touching the bone oscillator).

The single most important thing that may determine the comfort level of the child is the communication between the family (caregiver) and the audiologist. Positive interactions are more likely to evoke positive feelings in the child about the assessment procedure (Northern & Downs, 2002).

Interview

Audiologists need answers to some very direct and specific questions in order to accurately assess and diagnose hearing loss. One can find examples of various "case history questionnaires" published in audiology literature (ASHA, 2004). Even the most exhaustive of case history questionnaires essentially try to gather information regarding the same basic concepts including family history, birth history, developmental history (including hearing and speech/language development), and medical history. Each concept can be used to generate as many or as few questions as each child's situation may demand to create a meaningful history intake process. Each of these unique concepts should then be viewed collectively to integrate all the information obtained for the purpose of determining appropriate assessment and follow-up (Figure 36–1).

Audiologists must be flexible enough to modify the order in which they ask questions and be intuitive enough to ask appropriate follow-up questions (that might not be on the published questionnaire) based on initial observations and interactions. It also is important to clarify obtained information to ensure accuracy of reporting. Frequently, audiologists may need to ask sensitive questions about things such as visible physical characteristics, performance in school, achieving developmental milestones relative to other siblings, and ability to understand speech and language by relatives, friends, and neighbors. Avoiding direct questions for fear of appearing insensitive may result in failure to learn relevant information about the child.

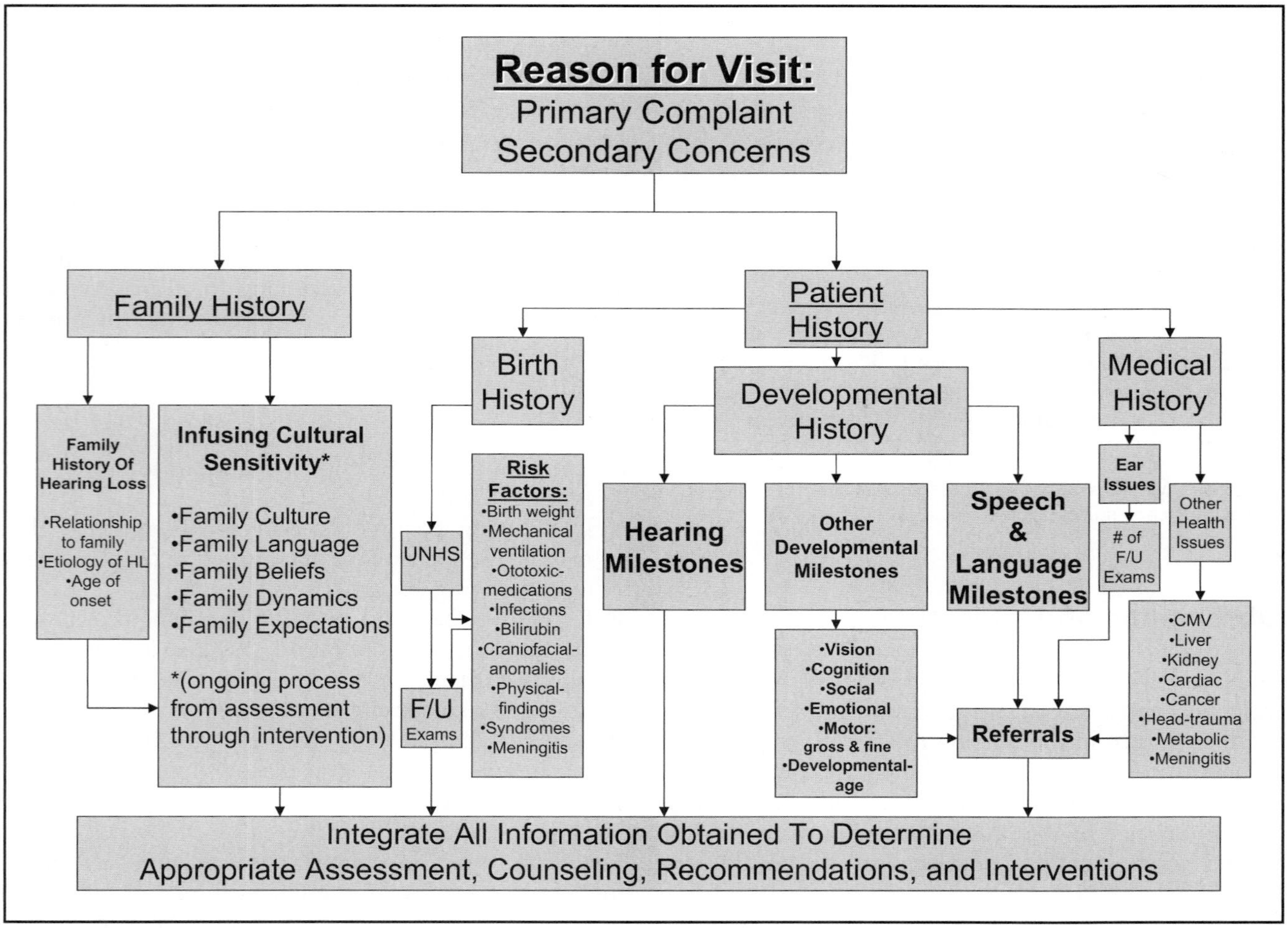

FIGURE 36–1. Flow chart demonstrating information management and integration from family and patient history for achieving optimal audiologic outcomes. F/U = follow-up, UNHS = universal newborn hearing screening, CMV = cytomegalovirus.

Therefore, it is important to pose these questions in an empathetic and professional manner. It also is critical to rely on careful and active listening.

All history intake questions that are asked should never lose track of the main goals of the interview process:

- Child's individuality;
- Family's culture and language;
- Parent/caregiver concern;
- Respect for family coping style;
- Family's expectations from appointment; and
- Support for the development of informed and empowered families.

Interview time also should be viewed as an opportunity to acknowledge the expertise of the caregiver/s in their child's life. Caregiver/s should be viewed as experts about their child because they can provide unique insight about their child's personal preferences, personality, and other characteristics that constitute their individuality. "There are no magical instruments or questionnaires that can substitute for authentic understanding born of lengthy acquaintance, mutual trust, and rapport" (Turnbull, 1991, p. 39).

Multicultural Considerations

The United States population is becoming increasingly diverse as is demonstrated by the U.S. Census data obtained over the last few years. According to data obtained in 2005, one-third of the United States population now belongs to racial and ethnic minority groups and approximately 20% of the population over age 5 speaks a language other than English in the home. These population statistics are expected to increase over time.

The Institute of Medicine (IOM) published a report (2002) that reviewed over 100 studies that assessed the quality of health care for various ethnic and racial minority groups. The report highlighted existing disparities in quality of health care provided to minorities. The IOM committee concluded that very few of these differences in health care quality for minorities/nonminorities can be attributed to patient attitudes and preferences. More significant contributors to these disparities include:

- Ecology of health care systems and environmental factors: these include factors such as cultural or linguistic barriers (e.g., lack of interpretive services) and fragmentation of health care systems (e.g., minorities are less likely to access care at a private physician's office even when insured at the same level; IOM, 2002).
- Discrimination: biases, stereotyping, and uncertainty. The report suggests that these disparities might originate from the provider; that is, prejudice against minorities, clinical uncertainty when interacting with minorities, and stereotypes held about minorities.

This increasing diversity poses unique challenges for health care professionals, including audiologists. Perceptions regarding hearing loss differ across cultures. Some cultures may not attribute much significance to hearing loss and are consequently less likely to seek hearing services. For example, individuals whose values and beliefs are representative of Deaf culture do not view hearing loss as a disability, but as a difference. As such, they may choose to not engage in "treatment and/or interventions" if recommendations are in conflict with personal/cultural views, or their desired short and long-term goals. People from other cultures may recognize hearing loss as a problem but choose to not follow recommended treatment/interventions due to religious or other societal beliefs.

Linguistic barriers and a lack of familiarity with accessing resources may prevent other minority groups from receiving quality care. In the case of a child who speaks any language other than English, testing materials in that language may not be readily available. This potentially could result in less than optimal quality of service delivery and compromise rapport with the family, subsequent recommendations, and future appointments.

Cultural Competence

As health care professionals, audiologists need to be respectful of and responsive to the needs of a diverse patient population by continually increasing their knowledge and skill in cultural competence. Being culturally competent is the ability to ensure that cultural disparities do not influence desired outcomes for patients. "Culturally competent professionals understand the power of culture in shaping family and professional beliefs, attitudes, and practices" (Kaufmann & McGonigel, 1991, p. 55). This skill is especially important during the history intake process. Audiologists should be proficient at the art of "ethnographic interviewing." Westby et al. (2003) define ethnographic interviewing as the means for developing an appreciation of the "child and their family's perception of the communication disability and its effects." General principles for ethnographic interviewing as outlined by Westby et al. include:

- Ask for use instead of meaning;
- Use open-ended questions rather than dichotomous questions;
- Restate what the child/family says in exact words: do not paraphrase or interpret;
- Summarize their statements and give them the opportunity to correct any misinterpretations;
- Avoid multiple questions;
- Avoid leading questions; and
- Avoid using "why" questions because they tend to sound judgmental and assume that the person knows "why."

Interpreter Use

Another useful skill that audiologists must master is the effective use of interpreters when dealing with families that speak other languages. Some techniques to consider for ensuring successful exchange of information include using short concise sentences and pausing frequently between them to allow the interpreter to organize and effectively translate. It also is important to remember to speak directly to the child/family and avoid oversimplification of important explanations. It is necessary to be mindful of nonverbal gestures that may be interpreted differently by different cultures and certain words that may not have the same meaning when translated.

Revising our traditional views of the history intake procedures and implementing progressive strategies that are culturally sensitive and appropriate lays the foundation for providing high quality health care to our diverse patient populations. Additionally, these same principles should be applied throughout the patient care process from assessment to intervention.

Optimizing Audiologic Assessment for Children With Multiple Modality Involvement: Physiologic Measures

Following observations, interactions, and a thorough patient history, the audiologist may decide that the child will not be able to participate in behavioral testing. Therefore, reliance on physiologic measures will be necessary.

Employing optimal test parameters with physiologic measures for children with multiple modality involvement should not be compromised, regardless of the child's disability. However, completing physiologic measures on children with additional disabilities can prove to be a challenge. As such, it is important to have a thorough familiarity with the child's medical history as it may offer insights into test selection, test order, test interpretation, and subsequent recommendations.

Children who are behaviorally, developmentally, and/or cognitively challenged may be lethargic, hyperactive, combative, tactilely defensive, or unable to sit quietly. Additionally, they may be unwilling or unable to comply with instructions and unable to cooperate for a sufficient length of time for test completion. Although evidence-based protocols for administering physiologic measures remain the same with these children, there are several modified strategies that can easily be made to maximize patient compliance.

Customizing your test battery/selection for the child is a skill that comes with experience. By paying careful attention to the subtle details of the child's behavior and demeanor, you may gain some insights regarding their capabilities and level of cooperation. This will save time in the limited window offered by the child. Choosing appropriate audiologic tests and deciding on the appropriate order of test presentation is essential to a successful outcome.

Acoustic Impedance Measures

Acoustic immittance measures are an integral part of the assessment battery when evaluating children with multiple modality involvement. Clinical decisions should be made on a quantitative assessment of the tympanogram, including consideration of equivalent ear canal volume, peak compensated static acoustic admittance, tympanometric width or gradient, and tympnometric peak pressure.

Frequently, a tympanogram is the first test attempted. However, there are times when tympanograms should be deferred until after behavioral testing. The rationale for deferring is that the positive interaction desired in behavioral testing may not be available if the child has found a tympanogram to be a traumatic experience.

In addition to providing confirmation of middle ear status, acoustic reflex measurement is useful in the interpretation of other components in the audiologic test battery. That is, the acoustic reflex may provide supplemental information relevant to the functional status of the middle ear, cochlea, and brainstem pathway. The same distraction techniques used for obtaining tympanograms may be used while measuring acoustic reflexes.

Some suggestions for obtaining impedance measures include:

- Carefully observe the child.
  - Is there readiness to sit quietly or not at all?
  - Is the child calm or afraid?
  - Is the child crying?
- Tailor your approach accordingly.
- Enlist assistance from the parent. This may range from verbal reassurance to gentle restraint of the child. It is well established that involvement of families in the provision of clinical services is crucial for families' acceptance of hearing loss (Luterman, 1999). A family's presence and/or participation allows the audiologist to explain the purpose of each step of the assessment, which in turn improves the family's ability to understand the findings of an otherwise abstract and technical test process.
- Enlist your coworker as a participant (Table 36–3).
- Use a bottle or a pacifier to comfort an infant who is crying.
- Select screening mode when possible rather than the diagnostic mode. This allows the audiologist to physically assist in the maintenance of a proper seal and reduces the overall test time.

Otoacoustic Emissions

Otoacoustic emissions (OAE) expand the pediatric audiology test battery by providing a physiologic means of assessing preneural auditory function. OAE testing provides an efficient method for obtaining hearing screening results for children who may not be able or willing to cooperate for behavioral audiometry.

The presence of OAEs is consistent with normal or near-normal hearing thresholds in a given frequency region. Moreover, measuring OAEs clinically permits the differentiation between sensory and neural components of a sensory-neural hearing loss (Lonsbury-Martin, McCoy, Whitehead, & Martin, 1993). Because of their remarkable stability over time within the same ear, OAEs also are useful for monitoring the status of disease conditions that are progressive, including certain genetic disorders such as Usher syndrome (Meredith, Stephens, Sirimanna, Meyer-Bisch, & Reardon, 1992).

Schemes for trying to determine the degree of hearing loss and/or predicting thresholds using OAEs have been investigated (Boege & Janssen, 2002; Dorn et al., 2001; Gorga, Neely, & Dorn, 2002; Gorga, Stover, & Neely, 1996; Gorga et al., 2003). Although some strategies have met with success, variability is such that threshold predictions should be viewed cautiously. Although OAE testing should not be used to specify hearing thresholds, it can be used to establish an initial impression about hearing. These impressions determine if further assessments need to be completed (Evenhuis, 1996).

Challenges in obtaining OAEs may arise if the child is unable to sit quietly or leave the probe tip in their ear for the duration of the test. Some considerations for obtaining OAE results include:

- Enlist parental support in holding the child on their lap and hold the child's hands as necessary.
- Place younger children in a high chair.
- Allow the child to quietly play with objects of distraction. Examples include: Lego blocks, Mr. Potato Head, pop beads, puzzles, and books.
- Have a small VCR or DVD player available and allow the child to watch a cartoon or children's video without sound. This can help distract and quiet the child for an extended period of time.
- Consider your protocol selection. You may want to use a protocol that assesses a smaller range of frequencies, thus reducing overall test time.

Table 36–3. Distraction Suggestions for Use During Acoustic Immittance Measurements

	Tactile	*Auditory*	*Visual*	*Visual*	*Visual*	*Visual*
Examining Audiologist	Tickle the outer ear	Sing "One, two, three," as you "take a picture"	"Watch the picture that your ear can draw"	—	—	—
Assisting Coworker	—	—	—	Blow bubbles	Play "peek-a-boo"	Use puppets

Auditory Brainstem Response (ABR)

Measurement of auditory evoked potentials, especially the ABR, can provide accurate estimates of threshold sensitivity in children with multiple modality involvement. To maximize reliable electrophysiologic measurements, an adequate signal-to-noise ratio (S/N) must be maintained, and an extended recording window must be used to identify threshold responses. The number of signals averaged may vary depending on the amount of background noise, the response amplitude, and the presence of hearing loss.

Children with multiple modality involvement often present challenges to the interpretation of ABR findings. For example, several studies have reported delayed conduction times in the ABR of children with autism (McCellend, Eyre, Watson, Calvert, & Sherrard, 1992; Rosenthall, Nordin, Brantberg, & Gillberg, 2003; Wong & Wong, 1991). Moreover, children with hydrocephalus may have elevated or absent ABR thresholds (Kraus, Ozdamar, Stein, & Reed, 1984). In children presenting with neurofibromatosis type I or II (NFI or NFII), involvement of the auditory system is indicated by abnormal middle ear muscle reflexes and abnormal ABRs (Pikus, 1995). Additionally, the ABR in children with Down syndrome reveals wave V latency and amplitude differences at reduced intensity levels when compared to normal developing controls. However, at greater stimulus levels (e.g., 60 dB nHL) latency of the ABR is shorter than matched control subjects. Thus, the slope of the intensity-latency function is steeper for children with Down syndrome than for normally developing controls (Folsom, Widen, & Wilson, 1983). Dille (2003) concluded that ABR testing should be interpreted with caution because it is likely that those with Down syndrome demonstrate a neural developmental time course that is uniquely different than the developmental time course of typically developing individuals. As such, it is important to note that ABR results should not be interpreted in isolation.

Additionally, children with auditory neuropathy/auditory dys-synchrony (AN/AD) present with absent and/or distorted ABRs, suggesting abnormal auditory pathway function beginning with the eighth nerve. The diagnosis of AN/AD requires ABR tests *and* tests of cochlear function, such as otoacoustic emissions, cochlear microphonics, and acoustic stapedial reflexes. The JCIH (2007) has included neural hearing loss (e.g., AN/AD) in infants admitted to the neonatal intensive care unit (NICU) in their targeted definition of hearing loss. As such, the audiologic community must be vigilant concerning this disorder because intervention and management is different from those with sensory-neural hearing loss.

It is important to have a thorough acquaintance with the child's medical history, as it may influence clinical decision making prior to testing. Once testing is initiated, further observations may require adapting to unforeseen circumstances during testing. Finally, for children who are neurologically, cognitively, and/or behaviorally involved, interpretation of waveform data must proceed with caution. The ABR findings should be considered as part of a test battery including behavioral audiometry, patient history, and other physiologic measures before developing a definitive diagnosis of the child's hearing status (Kaga, Ohuchi, Kaga, & Tanaka, 1984; Pijl, Stewart, & Laskowski, 1988; Siegenthaler, 1987).

To facilitate electrophysiologic recordings, a relaxed patient state is essential to improve response morphology and subsequent interpretation accuracy. In children with multiple modality involvement, this may be achieved during natural sleep or with the addition of sedation. Although the following suggestions work best for unsedated patients, they also may apply when sedation is administered:

- Request that the child arrive sleepy. This may require that parents awaken the child early. Prevent the child from taking a nap, and emphasize the importance of keeping the child awake while traveling to the appointment.
- Request that the bottle-fed or nursing child arrive hungry. Having the parent feed them immediately prior to the test often facilitates sleep.
- Reduce stimulation in the room. This might include dimming the lights or reducing the number of people present in the room.
- Make the setting more comfortable. Provide a recliner or rocking chair and allow the parent to hold the child during the test. Have a pillow or a blanket available and adjust the room temperature as needed.
- Allow the parent to bring any items that comfort the child. This could include a pacifier, bottle, blanket, stuffed animal, or special toy.

To gain the cooperation of some infants and young children during physiologic assessments of auditory function, sedation may be required. However, sedation of pediatric patients, with or without multiple modality involvement, may be contraindicated due to factors such as airway obstruction, apnea, cardiopulmonary impairment, and hypoventilation. As such, moderate sedation should only be administered by, or in the presence of, individuals skilled in airway management and cardiopulmonary resuscitation. Additionally, the oversight by a sedation team and the availability of age- and size-appropriate equipment, medications, and continuous monitoring are essential during procedures and for resuscitating the child should an adverse sedation event occur.

Optimizing Audiologic Assessment for Children With Multiple Modality Involvement: Behavioral Measures

The literature over the past 50 years has reinforced the widely held view that when children hear a sound, they will react in a stereotyped way that is consistent with their level of developmental/mental functioning (Barr, 1955; Eisenberg, 1969; Greenberg, Wilson, Moore, & Thompson, 1978; Hoversten & Moncur, 1969; Moore, 1995; Primus, 1992; Suzuki & Ogiba, 1960; Talbott, 1987; Thompson & Weber, 1974; Wilson, Moore, & Thompson, 1976). Scientific evidence coupled with clinical observations substantiate that predictable response behavior is characteristic of *typically developing children*. However, for children with multiple modality involvement (e.g., children with autism and children with Down syndrome), auditory response behavior may not be as predictable, nor can it be stereotyped (Tharpe et al., 2006). That is, children with multiple modality involvement may not orient to sound, may be hypersensitive to sound to the extent that they exhibit painful hearing, may have a preoccupation with or agitation to sound, cannot be conditioned to sound, or may demonstrate very poor test-retest reliability within a test session and between test sessions. Despite these challenges in behavioral assessment with children with multiple modality involvement, Tharpe (2009) advocates that, "we must bear in mind that behavioral tests provide an indication of how an individual uses his or her hearing, a very important factor when considering management needs."

Every effort must be made to ensure the comprehensiveness and accuracy of all audiologic results. For children with multiple modality involvements, audiologic results can be difficult to obtain, although no less important. With flexibility, patience, and determination, behavioral results can be obtained that provide valuable information regarding "hearing" in the child relative to their complex developmental profile.

Chapters 22 and 23 review behavioral assessment techniques for infants and children, however, physical conditions and cognitive/intellectual conditions (see Table 36–2) may have a significant influence on behavioral outcomes in audiologic assessment. That is, these conditions can influence reflexive and orienting responses, as well as "mask" conditioned responses (e.g., cerebral palsy, neurologic abnormalities, blindness, and/or uncorrected visual problems). Additionally, cognitive/intellectual conditions can influence the child's dynamic range (threshold responses to loudness discomfort), operant conditioning, overall response behavior, response latency, and habituation to auditory stimuli. As such, the audiologic approach initiated (usually made on the basis of developmental age) must consider these variables on the specific protocol used (behavioral observation audiometry, visual reinforcement audiometry and conditioned play audiometry).

When physical and cognitive/intellectual conditions are considered for each child's unique developmental profile, and appropriate modifications in behavioral protocols are implemented, confidence in behavioral results is improved. This confidence comes not only from experience, but also from the application of techniques and strategies that incorporate each child's abilities to the fullest potential in audiologic assessment.

Behavioral Observation Audiometry (BOA)

Although not a measure of auditory sensitivity, behavioral observation audiometry (BOA) is useful in conjunction with physiologic measures to provide additional insights into the response behavior of children with multiple modality involvement who may be unwilling or unable (cognitively and/or physically) to perform an audiologic procedure requiring a conditioned response. In fact, BOA is the only method of behavioral evaluation appropriate for individuals under approximately 6 months developmental age (a distinction between chronologic age and developmental age must be made, as chronologic age is often not an indicator of developmental age, especially in children with multiple modality involvement; additionally, subtraction of weeks of prematurity from chronologic age is necessary to compute an estimate of developmental age). Moreover, some children with multiple modality involvement are not good candidates for sedated procedures, and audiologists must rely on BOA as their only behavioral measure of a child's "hearing."

In BOA, a child's nonintentional responses to sound are observed by the audiologist. Diefendorf and Gravel (1996) placed these responses in two categories: (1) reflexive responses such as sucking, eye-blink, and startle; and (2) orienting responses such as eye widening, searching, a decrease in movement, and localization. Because of the nonintentional nature of these responses, and because they are often elicited by a suprathreshold level sound, Matkin (1977) suggested use of the term "minimum response level" to describe these responses rather than "auditory threshold." The difference in terminology implies that BOA responses simply provide information regarding gross auditory function, rather than auditory sensitivity.

Renshaw and Diefendorf (1998) listed three categories into which results of BOA testing may be placed: (1) no observable response to sound, (2) responses only to high-intensity stimuli (70–80 dB HL), and (3) responses to relatively soft and comfortable stimuli (30–50 dB HL). These categories provide some delineation about results obtained from BOA testing. In concert with BOA as a test of auditory responsivity (not sensitivity), the categories promote the use of BOA as a behavioral measure, useful to support physiologic findings, and to verify the presence of a general level of functional hearing.

When attempting BOA with a child with multiple modality involvement, it is important to remain unbiased when judging the presence or absence of a response (Gans, 1987). Often, children with cerebral palsy or other neurologic conditions may elicit frequent involuntary movements or vocalizations, making it difficult to determine valid behavioral response patterns. As such, it often is beneficial to enlist the assistance of a second audiologist, who may be able to assess the child's responses from another perspective. Additionally, in order to reduce habituation, it also is recommended to alternate between several different types of stimuli, including narrowband noise, frequency-modulated tones, and speech. Using pulsed stimuli also seems to help reduce habituation. Enlisting the parent/caregiver's assistance in determining a response from children with multiple modality involvements also can be an invaluable strategy. Parents/caregivers typically know their child better than any other participant in the audiologic evaluation. Their input should be regarded as potentially very useful, although the audiologist must also consider their input as potentially biased. Gravel (1992) suggests the parent/caregiver-participant wear earphones delivering a masking noise while involved in the test procedure to neutralize their potential bias. Conversely, Gravel also points out the benefit of allowing parents/caregivers to hear the intensity level at which the child responds to assist in counseling regarding any existing hearing loss.

Visual Reinforcement Audiometry (VRA)

As stated earlier, employing optimal test parameters with physiologic measures for children with multiple modality involvement *should not be compromised* regardless of the child's disability. Yet, when employing behavioral measures for children with multiple modality involvement, adapting test parameters may be necessary to match the physical and behavioral characteristics of the children under test. However, recognizing the impact that may result from these adaptations is essential.

Evidenced-based practice in pediatric audiology has a long history of defining clinical protocols in VRA. In most published studies however, evidence-based protocols have been based on research data with typically developing infants. Examples include: age appropriateness of VRA (Moore, Wilson, & Thompson, 1977), conditioning protocols (Primus & Thompson, 1985; Thompson & Folsom, 1984), use of reinforcement (Moore et al., 1977), types of reinforcement (Lowry, von Hapsburg, Plyler, & Johnstone, 2009; Moore, Thompson, & Thompson, 1975; Schmida, Peterson, & Tharpe, 2003), reinforcement novelty (Primus, 1987), reinforcement duration (Culpepper & Thompson, 1994), reinforcement schedules (Primus & Thompson, 1985), trial durations (Primus, 1992), use of control trials, and validity of findings from infants (Diefendorf, 1988; Nozza & Wilson, 1984; Primus, 1988). In fewer published studies, low-functioning children (Thompson, Wilson, & Moore, 1979), children with Down syndrome (Greenburg et al., 1978), children with autism spectrum disorders (Tharpe et al., 2006), and at-risk premature infants (Moore, 1995; Moore, Thompson, & Folsom, 1992; Widen, 1990), have been used as study subjects. For the most part, studies of children with hearing loss and multiple modality involvement are missing in the literature. Yet, clinical experience suggests that VRA protocols *must be flexible and adapted* to accommodate children with multiple modality involvement to establish behavioral audiologic profiles for these children. In doing so, the risks and benefits of modifying VRA protocols must be acknowledged.

The age at which VRA is optimally successful for the child with multiple modality involvement must be considered. For example, Thompson, Wilson, and Moore (1979) found the VRA technique to be appropriate for children with Down syndrome beginning at a developmental age of approximately 10 to 12 months. While these data serve as an excellent guideline, attempting behavioral audiologic evaluation on children presenting with any neurologic or developmental condition, including Down syndrome, under the age of 10 months is encouraged. In a clinical setting with a diverse and complex patient population, it is helpful to obtain any behavioral information that leads to more informed decision-making and recommendations.

In a discussion that places its primary focus on assessments of typically developing children, Gravel (1992) lists additional factors necessary for optimization of the clinical VRA procedure: (1) judging true responses from false responses, (2) increasing attention and motivation, and (3) decreasing false alarm rate. These three factors also must be considered when utilizing VRA with children presenting with multiple modality involvement.

Judging Response Behavior

Judging the presence or absence of a head-turn response may be more difficult in children with multiple modality involvement (e.g., cerebral palsy, visual impairments, autism spectrum disorders, hyperactive behavior). These children may exhibit involuntary movements, nonpurposeful movements, and/or random head turning that compromise the validity and reliability of the VRA procedure. For these behaviors, increasing the use of control trials (used to judge false response behavior) must be considered. Additionally, the use of a second audiologist within the test room can be extremely helpful in determining the presence or absence of a response. The second audiologist also can assist in optimizing attention and motivation of the child under test.

It may be necessary to increase the trial duration (usually about 4 seconds) during which a true response is acceptable for children who have poor head control and/or are slow responders. However, by increasing trial duration audiologists also risk an increase in judging false responses as true responses. When added control trials are necessary to verify correct response behavior, it is essential that the control trial duration is equal to the test trial duration so that opportunities to judge false response behavior are not biased.

Increasing Attention and Motivation

Initiating and maintaining the attention and motivation of children with multiple modality involvement is essential for establishing an accurate audiogram with VRA. For example, in the case of a child with autism, the presence of unusual sensory responses including preoccupation with or agitation to sound, abnormalities in auditory processing, and failure to condition are clinical features. These children may exhibit behaviors such as a disregard for speech stimuli, a fixation on one object, and/or an aversion for direct eye contact or physical contact. Additionally, children with attention deficits, cognitive delays, and vision impairment often need additional effort on the part of the examiner to ensure that they remain appropriately attentive and motivated throughout the evaluation, and that the results obtained are comprehensive and representative of the child's hearing abilities.

Different strategies may be employed to increase a patient's attention during the VRA procedure. An obvious way to increase attention is to decrease distraction. When presenting stimuli for VRA, decreasing distraction may involve: (1) darkening the control side of the booth, (2) keeping the child in an alert position (e.g., sitting up instead of leaning back on a parent's lap, sitting in a high chair or sitting in a stroller), (3) keeping additional toys, picture boards, and other items that may cause distraction in the control room of the booth or out of the child's line of sight, (4) allowing only one parent/caregiver to be in the booth with the child, and (5) involving a second examiner to serve not only as a second opinion regarding the presence/absence of a response, but also to provide centering distraction for the child, and to provide occasional verbal or tactile reinforcement to the child. In this role, the audiologist must stabilize behaviors that compromise true responses to the auditory stimulus. This can be achieved, although with some challenge, by maintaining the child's attention at midline and returning the child to this position once a response is made. The audiologist must be creative and proactive in keeping the child alert and in a listening posture without the child becoming too focused on the examiner and/or the activity. If the audiologist and distracting technique are not sufficiently interesting, the likelihood of random behavior will continue.

Audiologists also can influence attention and motivation by being flexible with the use of different auditory stimuli. Often, if a child begins to habituate to a specific stimulus, response behavior can be increased by using a different (novel) stimulus. For example, head-turning to speech stimuli or narrowband noise after habituation to a pure-tone stimulus often results in the opportunity for further frequency-specific testing after the introduction of the novel stimulus, and is an excellent strategy to increase the child's attention to the VRA procedure. This strategy is especially useful when attempting to obtain ear-specific information using VRA.

For some children, a very brief presentation of the reinforcement toy/DVD video provides enough motivation to continue the evaluation until the audiologist has gathered all necessary information. Culpepper and Thompson (1994) studied the response behavior of 2-year-olds and found that habituation was delayed when subjects received very brief exposure to reinforcement (0.5 seconds) compared to those children who received longer exposure to reinforcement (4 seconds). For others, especially those with special needs, a longer presentation of the reinforcement may be necessary, possibly as a result of increased processing time, attention deficits, or visual deficits. Extending the reinforcement duration should only be considered when it is deemed necessary to allow the child with special needs full access to the reinforcement. However, by increasing reinforcement duration, the audiologist also may observe more rapid onset of habituation.

One strategy to counteract the consequence of longer reinforcement durations is to employ the use of multiple reinforcers or DVD/video reinforcement. Additionally, the use of conventional reinforcers permits the ability to illuminate the colorful toys only, and select between animation/no animation for enhancing novelty and facilitating motivation.

Decreasing False Responses

Determining a true response from a false response is often one of the most challenging aspects of performing behavioral audiometry on a child with special needs. Decreasing the number of false responses is essential to have confidence in audiometric outcomes. Reliable audiologic data are achievable when attention is focused on response shaping, versatile midline distraction techniques, lengthening interstimulus intervals, and persistent monitoring of false response behavior with control trials.

Response shaping is critical to the success of VRA. The examiner must be skilled in response training and sensitive to the various stages of response acquisition. Two different approaches that can be attempted in the conditioning phase are: (1) pairing the stimulus with the reinforcer and (2) observing a spontaneous response from the infant followed by reinforcement. For the child with special needs, conditioning may take longer to establish the conditioned behavior. Successful completion of the conditioning stage occurs when the child is making contingent responses and random head turning is at a minimum.

Excessive false responses suggest that the infant is not under stimulus control. As such, audiologists should focus on two factors to rectify clinical outcomes: (1) reinstitute response shaping or (2) increase the entertainment level of the activity to engage the child's interest at a midline position before presenting the auditory stimulus.

Northern and Downs (2002) suggest taking a "time-out" subsequent to false responses to permit the child time to relax and regain composure, as this can be a frustrating situation for many children with special needs. Taking "time-out" is essentially increasing the inter-stimulus-interval (ISI). Increasing the ISI increases stimulus novelty thereby increasing the likelihood of a correct response. Additionally, increasing ISI provides optimal time to bring the child to a midline gaze, thereby increasing the likelihood of judging stimulus-related head turn behavior/responses.

Tharpe et al. (2006) found that children with autism provided elevated and less reliable behavioral audiometric responses than their typically developing peers, with no significant difference in physiologic test results between the two groups. In this study, if the child became bored or distracted, the examiners would implement the following: (1) repeat the trial, (2) switch stimulus, or (3) switch transducer.

Although eliminating false responses altogether is not feasible or clinically desirable, these strategies serve to regain the child's focus when it may have lapsed. The desired outcome is achieved when the child's false response rate during control trials is approximately 25% or less (Moore, 1995).

Conditioned Play Audiometry

Conditioned play audiometry (CPA) follows a model of auditory stimulus → response → reinforcement, in which a play activity (blocks in a bucket, pegs in a board) is the response and social praise is the reinforcement. Through conditioning, children learn to engage a response that is within their motor coordination ability and consistently can be completed.

Conditioned play audiometry is considered the most appropriate technique for obtaining ear- and frequency-specific information in children 3 years developmental age and above. Although this is an extremely useful guideline, the audiologist must always remain open to the behavioral test procedure that provides the most reliable responses coupled with facilitating the longest delay of habituation from the child. That is, a general knowledge of the child's developmental abilities will guide the audiologist to an *age-appropriate* test technique, whereas the child's physical abilities, developmental skills, and personal motivations will guide the audiologist to a *developmentally appropriate* test technique. For example, some 2-year-olds can be conditioned to play audiometry (Thompson, Thompson, &

Vethivelus, 1989). Moreover, when 2-year-olds are conditioned for CPA, they are more likely to provide greater responses before habituation than they would if tested by VRA. For this reason, and for others discussed earlier in this chapter, the time the audiologist spends on history intake and building rapport with the child and the family is important in the determination of a test method with which to begin the evaluation.

When teaching children to perform CPA, it is usually not difficult to select a response behavior that children are capable of performing, as long as the audiologist is intuitive in matching the child's motor skill with an appropriate play activity. The challenge in CPA is teaching the child to wait, listen, and respond when the auditory signal is presented. In addition to teaching the child under test the conditioned response in the CPA task, the examiner also must be skilled in delivering social reinforcement at the appropriate time and interval.

Children with multiple modality involvement present unique challenges during audiometric evaluation using CPA. Response acquisition, identifying positive reinforcements, and response time are several challenges that must be carefully considered. Kile (1996) suggests that children with Down syndrome may require longer response intervals following the stimulus to ensure the child has adequate time to process and respond to the signal. The following suggestions will increase the likelihood of successful audiologic outcomes.

- Many factors should be considered prior to choosing an appropriate toy to be used during CPA. The audiologist must consider the child's gross/fine motor skills, vision, attention, developmental level, personal interests/motivators, and social interaction skills, to name several. If the physical demands of the game are too great, the child will give up prior to obtaining the necessary information. If the task is too simple for the child, they are less motivated and may fatigue earlier than the audiologist hopes (Diefendorf, 2003).
- Teaching the CPA task can be slightly more difficult in the child with multiple modality involvement. Holte et al. (2006) suggest using tactile cues (bone oscillator or simple touch), thereby physically training a child who is deaf-blind to perform the CPA task. The bone oscillator can be removed from the headband and held in the child's hand or rested against the child's arm. A 250-Hz signal is presented at the maximum output for the bone oscillator, and the vibratory stimulus is then paired with appropriate reinforcement following the desired response.
- Practicing the task together several times prior to beginning the formal evaluation is also extremely helpful. Northern and Downs (2002) suggest using animated facial cues and body language along with overtly demonstrating the task. Diefendorf (1981) demonstrated the positive effects of a "preplay period" for facilitating response acquisition during conditioning.
- Response patterns may differ greatly from child to child. Others may look to their parent/caregiver or the audiologist for confirmation that they heard the stimulus at every presentation and wait for reinforcement prior to performing the play task (Renshaw & Diefendorf, 1998). Children with Down syndrome may elicit a sound mimicking the stimulus rather than performing the conventional CPA task. These behaviors (if consistent) should be considered valid and representative of reliable conditioned behavior.
- Often, in a busy clinic setting, using two audiologists to perform CPA (one in the test room playing with the child, one in the control room) is not always an option. Utilizing the parent as an assistant in this case often allows the evaluation to flow more quickly while also feeling more natural for the child.
- Even under headphones, pure tones may not be the stimulus that best holds the child's attention. Narrow-band noise or warbled tones may be found more interesting and novel by the child with special needs.

Conventional Audiometry

Once an audiologist has determined a child with special needs has developed the skills necessary to complete conventional audiometry (i.e., make a distinct and agreed-upon response to auditory stimuli), the audiologist must keep the evaluation upbeat, motivating to the child, and as comprehensive as time allows. Often, the window of opportunity to obtain this information is rather small when evaluating a child with special needs due to stress, tolerance, distractibility, habituation, or fatigue. Keeping the child motivated and attentive with intermittent social reinforcement, coupled with a response behavior that is physically easy for the child are key components for obtaining a valid and thorough audiogram. Air conduction and bone conduction data are desirable, and a tradeoff between fewer air conduction thresholds in favor of several bone conduction thresholds may be important as the child begins to fatigue.

The audiologist can introduce different options as fatigue sets in as an attempt to maintain and/or increase the child's motivation and continued response behavior. For example, the audiologist may need to become a more active participant in the evaluation. For a child with special needs, maintaining/increasing any of the conditioned responses for conventional audiometry can be made easier when the audiologist participates from the control side of the booth. That is, if the response option chosen is for the child to clap hands, the audiologist must be willing to clap hands *with* the child upon presentation of the stimulus. This not only aids in teaching the child the desired response, but also reinforces the child for the correct behavior.

Occasionally, the child with special needs may choose a unique response option as a modification of the task introduced by the audiologist. That is, a child may begin to smile and wave at the audiologist in response to auditory stimuli after being instructed to clap hands. As long as this alternate response is consistent and easily observable, the audiologist should not discourage an appropriate behavioral response.

The following options have all been used successfully with children for whom conventional audiometry is physically/developmentally appropriate:

- Raise hand
- High-five to parent/caregiver
- Clap hands
- Nod head
- Push button
- Say "I hear it"
- Say "beep"
- Blink eyes

Social reinforcement such as nodding, smiling, and clapping on the part of the audiologist is often the only reinforcement necessary to obtain a standard audiogram for this age group. The audiologist evaluating a child with special needs must determine how much and how frequent social reinforcement needs to be provided to the child in order to motivate the child, without being overly praiseful (which may encourage false positive responses from the child). Renshaw and Diefendorf (1998) also suggest using VRA toys as reinforcement in addition to social reinforcement for selected children who find this to be motivating.

Optimizing Audiologic Assessment for Children With Multiple Modality Involvement: Speech Audiometry

The inclusion of speech audiometry in the audiological evaluation of an individual with multiple modality involvement must be viewed as essential for developing a complete profile of auditory function and hearing ability. Because of the limitations of pure tone or narrow-band noise thresholds in predicting functional efficiency for speech, additional clinical tests utilizing speech materials must be employed for a complete audiologic evaluation and follow-up description of auditory abilities. Additionally, although an individual's ability to understand speech is influenced by his audiometric threshold configuration, the former cannot always be predicted accurately from the latter, and it is this fact that makes speech audiometry an indispensable clinical tool.

Speech audiometry provides the audiologist with information that can only be obtained through the use of speech stimuli. Audiologists are acquiring information regarding the softest hearing level where speech can be detected, the hearing level at which speech can be recognized, or a percent score reflecting word, phrase, or sentence recognition when these materials are presented at a comfortable or optimal hearing level. All of these components help frame the diagnosis of an individual's hearing function/dysfunction.

Speech Detection/Awareness Thresholds (SDT/SAT)

The speech detection threshold (SDT) or speech awareness threshold (SAT) may be defined as the hearing level at which a listener may just detect the presence of an ongoing speech signal. A SDT/SAT can be obtained with a variety of stimulus words or phrases to gain the child's attention and cooperation. The audiologist often will call the child's name, present words, present numbers, or repeat syllables (bai-bai-bai; uh-oh) and look for a response from the patient. An acceptable response can be a preconditioned head nod, a hand raise, or a head turn toward the speaker when testing in sound field. Threshold is marked when a consistent response is given during approximately 50% of the test trials.

The signal selected is often delivered in repetition until a response is obtained. However, test trial duration should not exceed 5 seconds due to the risk of taking a false response as a true response. The SDT/SAT often relates most closely to the best single pure tone threshold within the frequency range of 250 to 4000 Hz. Considering this, the child will respond to the portion of this broad band of frequencies at which hearing is most sensitive.

When obtaining SDT/SAT it is important to be versatile and flexible with the presented stimulus. The clinician will notice that some stimuli work better than others, reflecting the individual preferences of the child under test. Therefore, it may be helpful to consider using a familiar voice to present the stimulus. Allowing a parent, sibling, or caregiver to speak into the microphone, while the audiologist is monitoring the VU meter, may facilitate the acquisition of speech awareness responses. It also may be necessary to enlist an interpreter or native language speaker to optimize speech awareness testing in the child's primary language. Regulating the VU meter and documenting strategies, as well as results, is essential.

Speech Reception Threshold (SRT)

Speech reception threshold, spondee recognition threshold, or speech recognition threshold are all appropriate terms referring to the lowest hearing level at which the patient can correctly identify spondaic words that are presented. The SRT is recognized as the intensity at which an individual is able to identify simple speech materials approximately 50% of the time.

The standard presentation involves the use of phonetically balanced spondees where the child repeats back or points to the targeted word. However, the conventional protocol can be modified to meet the needs of any child, and particularly those with multiple modality involvement.

When developing a modified test protocol to use with a child with special needs, it is important to consider the familiarity of the words that are attempted. The child must have a familiarity with the words being considered, and eliminating those words that are not within the child's receptive vocabulary is critical. The audiologist also must consider the child's ability to repeat the word. This includes accounting for possible speech and/or articulation disorders that may interfere with proper articulation and pronunciation.

The audiologist can use pointing tasks, game tasks, and/or classic repetition games. A picture board can be used for pointing tasks. Large, brightly colored, easily recognized images are recommended so there is no confusion with busy pictures. The use of either picture- or object-pointing rather than verbal response will require that the number of test items be limited to 12 or less (Olsen & Matkin, 1979). Otherwise, the visual scanning task as well as the demands placed on memory and attention become contaminating variables.

If a child is unable to view the picture board due to vision deficits, a "show me" game may be an effective alternative. The child may be able to point to body parts or a parent's body parts (e.g., "show me your nose," "eyes," "hair," "fingers," "toes," "shoes").

Some children may be more willing to play a game task. Their motor development must be considered to determine if they would be a successful candidate to participate in the game. A few options to choose between would include a familiar objects game or a "put it in" the bucket game. The familiar objects game would consist of placing known objects on the table and having the child point them out. Objects can be pulled from a parent's or child's belongings (e.g., toys, brush, phone, shoes, rings). When playing the bucket game, the child must have the coordination to place a ball, block, or peg into a bucket during conditioning and testing.

The audiologist can play a simpler repetition game for children with compromised cognitive function. For example, the game may be enhanced by calling it "copycat," "mirror," "Simon says," or "being a parrot." The child mimics or copies the word that is being presented through the transducer.

Speech Perception

There are several challenges that must be considered when attempting to measure speech perception skills in children with multiple modality involvement. The selection of test materials within a child's receptive vocabulary competency, the designation of an appropriate response task, the utilization of reinforcement, and the reduction or alleviation of memory load are important factors that may affect the reliability and validity of speech perception measurement.

Clinicians must exercise caution in administering the phonetically balanced kindergarten (PB-K) word lists unless there is relatively good assurance that the receptive vocabulary age of the child approaches at least that of a normal-hearing kindergartner. Alternatively, the use of Word Intelligibility by Picture Identification (WIPI) test is appropriate for those children with receptive vocabulary ages of 4 years and older. The Northwestern University-Children's Perception of Speech (NU-CHIPS) test (Elliott & Katz, 1980) materials are documented to be in the recognition vocabulary of children with normal hearing as young as age 3 years.

Kirk, Pisoni, and Osberger (1995) examined the effect of lexical characteristics on a group of pediatric cochlear implant users' spoken word recognition, and compared their performance on the LNT and MLNT with their scores on the PB-K. Word recognition was significantly higher on the lexically controlled lists than on the PB-K.

When selecting appropriate speech perception measures for use with children (with or without multiple modality involvement) it is essential to match the developmental level of the child with a speech perception measure that reflects the vocabulary level of the child under test. Additionally, an appropriate response task that considers memory, attention, and physical capabilities also must be considered to ensure valid measures of speech perception that are not compromised by test protocols and/or vocabulary levels.

Conclusion

The standard of care in the United States for early hearing detection and intervention is articulated by the Year 2007 Joint Committee on Infant Hearing Position Statement. The 2007 statement advocates universal hearing screening by 1 month of age, audiologic diagnosis of hearing loss by 3 months of age, and intervention by 6 months of age. Compliance with this timeline is intended for *all* children with hearing loss.

For those children suspected of hearing loss who present with multiple modality involvement, meeting this timeline may be more difficult. Although there are evolving and ever-changing priorities for children with multiple modality involvement, optimal care coordination for these children is facilitated when an early and accurate diagnosis of hearing loss is established. Therefore, an appropriate battery of audiologic tests coupled with appropriate protocols must be utilized to achieve a timely diagnosis of hearing loss in these children. When achieved, the goal of optimizing a child's communication development is positively influenced and significantly enhanced.

References

American Speech, Language, Hearing Association (ASHA). (2004). *Guidelines for the audiologic assessment of children from birth to 5 years of age* [Guidelines]. Available from http://www.asha.org/policy

Barr, B. (1954). Pure tone audiometry for pre-school children [in Swedish]. *Nordisk Medicin. 51*(14), 464–468.

Boege, P., & Janssen, T. (2002). Pure-tone threshold estimation from extrapolated distortion product otoacoustic emission I/O functions in normal and cochlear hearing loss ears. *Journal of the Acoustical Society of America, 111*, 1810–1818.

Culpepper, B., & Thompson, G. (1994). Effects of reinforcer duration on the response behavior of preterm 2 year-olds in visual reinforcement audiometry. *Ear and Hearing, 15*, 161–167.

Diefendorf, A. O. (1981). *The effect of a pre-play period on play audiometry*. Paper presented at the Tennessee Speech-Language-Hearing Association Annual Convention, Memphis, TN.

Diefendorf, A. O. (1988). Behavioral evaluation of hearing-impaired children. In F. H. Bess (Ed.), *Hearing impairment in children*. Parkton, MD: York Press.

Diefendorf, A. O. (2003). Behavioral hearing assessment: Considerations for the young child with developmental disabilities. *Seminars in Hearing, 24*, 189–200.

Diefendorf, A. O., & Gravel, J. S. (1996). Behavioral observation and visual reinforcement audiometry. In S. E. Gerber (Ed.), *The handbook of pediatric audiology*. Washington, DC: Gallaudet University Press.

Dille, M. F. (2003). Perspectives on the audiological evaluation of individuals with Down syndrome. *Seminars in Hearing, 24*, 201–210.

Dorn, P. A., Konrad-Martin, D., Neely, S. T., Keefe, D. H., Cry, E., & Gorga, M. P. (2001). Distortion product otoacoustic emission input/output functions in normal-hearing and hearing-impaired human ears. *Journal of the Acoustical Society of America, 110*, 3119–3131.

Eisenberg, R. B. (1969). Auditory behavior in the human neonate: Functional properties of sound and their ontogenetic implications. *International Journal of Audiology, 8*, 34–45.

Elliott, L. L., & Katz, D. (1980). *Development of a new children's test of speech discrimination* [Technical manual]. St. Louis, MO: Auditec.

Evenhuis, H. M. (1996). Dutch consensus on diagnosis and treatment of hearing impairment in children and adults with intellectual disability. *Journal of Intellectual Disability Research, 40*, 451–456.

Folsom, R. C., Widen, J. E., & Wilson, W. R. (1983). Auditory brainstem responses in Down syndrome infants. *Archives of Otolaryngology, 109*, 607–610.

Fortnum, H., & Davis, A. (1997). Epidemiology of permanent childhood hearing impairment in Trent Region, 1985–1993. *British Journal of Audiology, 31*, 409–466.

Gallaudet College Center for Assessment and Demographic Studies. (1983). *Annual survey of hearing-impaired children and youth, 1981–1982*. Washington, DC: Author.

Gallaudet Research Institute. (2005). *Regional and national summary report of data from the 2004–2005 annual survey of deaf and hard of hearing children and youth*. Washington, DC: Author.

Gans, D. P. (1987). Improving behavior observation audiometry testing and scoring procedures. *Ear and Hearing, 8*, 92–100.

Gorga, M. P., Neely, S. T., Dierking, D. M., Dorn, P. A., Hoover, B. M., & Fitzpatrick, D. (2003). Distortion product otoacoustic emission tuning curves in normal-hearing and hearing-impaired human ears. *Journal of the Acoustical Society of America, 114*, 262–278.

Gorga, M. P., Neely, S. T., & Dorn, P. A. (2002). Distortion product otoacoustic emissions in relation to hearing loss. In M. S. Robinette, T. J. Glattke, (Eds.), *Otoacoustic emissions: Clinical applications* (2nd ed., pp. 243–272). New York, NY: Thieme Medical.

Gorga, M. P., Stover, L. T., & Neely, S. T. (1996). The use of cumulative distributions to determine critical values and levels of confidence for clinical distortion product otoacoustic emission measurements. *Journal of the Acoustical Society of America, 100*, 968–977.

Gravel, J. S. (1992). Audiologic assessment of infants and toddlers. In E. Cherow (Ed.), *Proceedings of the ASHA audiology superconference: ASHA Reports, 21*, 55–62.

Greenburg, D., Wilson, W. R., Moore, J., & Thompson, G. (1978). Visual reinforcement audiometry (VRA) with young Down syndrome children. *Journal of Speech and Hearing Disorders, 43*, 448–458.

Holte, L., Prickett, J. G., Van Dyke, D. C., Olson, R. J., Lubrica, P., Knutson, C. L., . . . Brenna, S. (2006). Issues in the evaluation of infants and young children who are suspected of or who are deaf-blind. *Infants and Young Children, 19*, 213–227.

Hoversten, G., & Moncur, J. (1969). Stimuli and intensity factors in testing infants. *Journal of Speech and Hearing Research, 12*, 687–702.

Institute of Medicine (IOM). (2002). *Unequal Treatment: What health care providers need to know about racial and ethnic disparities in healthcare*. Retrieved December 14, 2009, from http://hospitals.unm.edu/health_literacy/pdfs/unequal treatmenthcprovider.pdf

Joint Committee on Infant Hearing (JCIH). (2007) Year 2007 position statement: Principles and guidelines for early hearing detection and intervention programs. *Pediatrics, 120*, 898–921.

Kaga, M., Ohuchi, M., Kaga, K., & Tanaka, Y. (1984). Normalization of poor auditory brainstem response in infants and children. *Brain Development, 6*, 458–466.

Kaufmann, R. K., & McGonigel, M. J. (1991). Identifying family concerns, priorities, and resources. An overview. In M. J. McGonigel, R. K. Kaufmann, & B. H. Johnson (Eds.), *Guidelines and recommended practices for the individualized family service plan* (2nd ed., p. 55). Bethesda, MD: Association for the Care of Children's Health.

Kile, J. E. (1996) Audiologic assessment of children with Down syndrome. *American Journal of Audiology*, 5, 44–52.

Kirk,K. I., Pisoni D. B., Osberger M. J. (1995). Lexical effects on spoken word recognition by pediatric cochlear implant users. *Ear and Hearing, 16*, 470–481.

Kraus, N., Ozdamar, O., Stein, L., & Reed, N. (1984). Absent auditory brain stem response: Peripheral hearing loss or brain stem dysfunction? *Laryngoscope, 94*, 400–406.

Lonsbury-Martin, B. L., McCoy, M. J., Whitehead, M. L., & Martin, G. K. (1993). Clinical testing of distortion-product otoacoustic emissions. *Ear and Hearing, 14*, 11–22.

Lowery, K. J., von Hapsburg, D., Plyler, E. L., & Johnstone, P. (2009). A comparison of video versus conventional visual reinforcement in 7- to 16-month old infants. *Journal of Speech, Language and Hearing Research, 52*(3), 723–731.

Luterman, D. (1999). *The young deaf child*. Baltimore, MD: York Press.

Mace, A. L., Wallace, K. L., Whan, M. Q., & Stelmachowicz, P. G. (1991). Relevant factors in the identification of hearing loss. *Ear and Hearing, 12*(4), 287–293.

Matkin, N. D. (1977). Hearing sensitivity during preschool years. In F. H. Bess (Ed.), *Childhood deafness: Causation, assessment and management* (Ch. 10, pp. 127–133). New York, NY: Grune & Stratton.

McCellend, R. J., Eyre, D. G., Watson, D., Calvert, G. H., & Sherrard, E. (1992). Central conduction time in childhood autism. *British Journal of Psychiatry, 160*, 659–663.

Meredith, R., Stephens, D., Sirimanna, T., Meyer-Bisch, C., & Reardon, W. (1992). Audiometric detection of carrier of Usher's syndrome type II. *Journal of Audiological Medicine, 1*, 11–19.

Moore, J. (1995). Behavioral assessment procedures based on conditioned head-turn responses for auditory detection and discrimination with low-functioning children. *Scandinavian Audiology Suppl., 41*, 36–42.

Moore, J., Thompson, G., & Folsom, R. (1992). Auditory responsiveness of premature infants utilizing visual reinforcement audiometry (VRA). *Ear and Hearing, 13*, 187–194.

Moore, J. M., Thompson, G., & Thompson, M. (1975). Auditory localization of infants as a function of reinforcement conditions. *Journal of Speech and Hearing Disorders, 40*, 29–34.

Moore, J. M., Wilson, W. R., & Thompson, G. (1977). Visual reinforcement of head-turn responses in infants under 12 months of age. *Journal of Speech and Hearing Disorders, 42*, 328–334.

Northern, J. L., & Downs, M. P. (2002). *Hearing in children* (5th ed.). Baltimore, MD: Lippincott Williams & Wilkins.

Nozza, R. J., & Wilson, W. R. (1984). Masked and unmasked pure-tone thresholds of infants and adults: Development of auditory frequency selectivity and sensitivity. *Journal of Speech and Hearing Research, 27*, 613–622.

Olsen, W. O., & Matkin, N. D. (1979). Speech audiometry. In W. F. Rintelmann (Ed.), *Hearing assessment* (pp. 133–206). Baltimore, MD: University Park Press.

Pijl, S., Stewart, I. F., & Laskowski, W. (1988). Limitations of ABR as a hearing test as exemplified in multiply handicapped adults. *Journal of Otolaryngology, 17*, 362–367.

Pikus, A. T. (1995). Pediatric audiologic profiles in type 1 and type 2 neurofibromatosis. *Journal of the American Academy of Audiology, 6*, 54–62.

Primus, M. A. (1987). Response and reinforcement in operant audiometry. *Journal of Speech and Hearing Disorders, 52*, 294–299.

Primus, M. A. (1988). Infant thresholds with enhanced attention to the signal in visual reinforcement audiometry. *Journal of Speech and Hearing Research, 31*, 480–484.

Primus, M. A. (1992). Operant response in infants as a function of time interval following signal onset. *Journal of Speech and Hearing Research, 35*, 1422–1425.

Primus, M. A., & Thompson, G. (1985). Response strength of young children in operant audiometry. *Journal of Speech and Hearing Research, 28*, 539–547.

Renshaw, J. J., & Diefendorf, A. O. (1998). Adapting the test battery for the child with special needs. In F. H. Bess (Ed.), *Children with hearing impairment: Contemporary trends* (Chap. 7, pp. 83–104). Nashville, TN: Vanderbilt Bill Wilkerson Center Press.

Rosenthall, U., Nordin, V., Brantberg, K., & Gillberg, C. (2003). Autism and auditory brainstem responses. *Ear and Hearing, 24*, 206–214.

Ross, M., & Lerman, J. (1970). A picture identification test for hearing-impaired children. *Journal of Speech and Hearing Research, 13*, 44–53.

Schmida, M., Peterson, H., & Tharpe, A. M. (2003). Visual reinforcement audiometry using digital video disc and conventional reinforcers. *American Journal of Audiology, 12*, 35–40.

Siegenthaler, B. M. (1987). Auditory problems. In E. T. McDonald (Ed.), *Treating cerebral palsy: For clinicians by clinicians* (pp. 85–103). Austin, TX: Pro-Ed..

Suzuki, T., & Ogiba, Y. (1960). A technique for pure-tone audiometry for children under three years of age: Conditioned orientation reflex (COR) audiometry. *Revue de laryngologie–otology–rhinologie (BORD), 81*, 33–45.

Talbott, C. B. (1987). A longitudinal study comparing responses of hearing impaired infants to pure tones using visual reinforcement and play audiometry. *Ear and Hearing*, 8, 175–179.

Tharpe, A. M. (2009). Individuals with multiple disabilities. In J. Katz, L. Medwetsky, R. Burkard, & L. Hood (Eds.), *Handbook of clinical audiology* (6th ed., pp. 666–677). Philadelphia, PA: Lippincott, Williams & Wilkins.

Tharpe, A. M., Bess, F. H., Sladen, D. P., Schissel, H., Couch, S., & Schery, T. (2006) Auditory characteristics of children with autism. *Ear and Hearing, 27*(4), 430–441.

Thompson, G., & Folsom, R. C. (1984). A comparison of two conditioning procedures in the use of visual reinforcement audiometry (VRA). *Journal of Speech and Hearing Disorders, 49*, 241–245.

Thompson, G., & Weber, B. (1974). Responses of infants and young children to behavioral observation audiometry (BOA). *Journal of Speech and Hearing Disorders, 39*, 140–147.

Thompson, G., Wilson, W. R., & Moore, J. M. (1979). Application of visual reinforcement audiometry (VRA) to low-functioning children. *Journal of Speech and Hearing Disorders, 44*, 80–90.

Thompson, M. D., Thompson, G., & Vethivelu, S. (1989). A comparison of audiometric test thresholds for 2-year-old children. *Journal of Speech and Hearing Disorders, 54*, 174–179.

Turnbull, A. (1991). Identifying children's strengths and needs. In M. J. McGonigel, R. K. Kaufmann, & B. H. Johnson (Eds.), *Guidelines and recommended practices for the individualized family service plan* (2nd ed., pp. 39–46). Bethesda, MD: Association for the Care of Children's Health.

Westby, C., Burda, A., & Mehta, Z. (2003, April 29). *Asking the right questions in the right ways: Strategies for ethnographic interviewing*. The ASHA leader online feature.

Widen, J. (1990). Behavioral screening of high-risk infants using visual reinforcement audiometry. *Seminars in Hearing, 11*, 342–356.

Wilson, W. R., Moore, J., & Thompson, G. (1976). *Sound-field audiometry thresholds of infants utilizing visual reinforcement audiometry (VRA)*. Paper presented at the American Speech and Hearing Association Annual Convention, November 20–23, Houston, TX.

Wong, V., & Wong, S. N. (1991). Brainstem auditory evoked potential study in children with autistic disorder. *Journal of Autism and Developmental Disorders, 21*, 329–340.

37

Children With Auditory Neuropathy Spectrum Disorder (ANSD)

Patricia A. Roush

Introduction

In 1991, Arnold Starr and colleagues described an 11-year-old child with the paradoxic findings of absent auditory brainstem responses in the presence of normal cochlear microphonics (CMs) and otoacoustic emissions (OAEs). The child demonstrated severely impaired speech understanding despite a mild loss of hearing sensitivity. Further evaluation showed impaired temporal processing as exhibited by abnormal findings on a battery of psychophysical tests that included gap detection and binaural masking level differences. In 1996, Starr and colleagues reported on a group of 10 children and adults with similar findings (Starr, Picton, Sininger, Hood, & Berlin, 1996). Although the patients presented with no apparent neurologic involvement when their hearing impairments were first identified, eight of the ten showed later evidence of other peripheral neuropathies. Starr and colleagues coined the term "auditory neuropathy" (AN) to describe patients whose hearing impairment was attributed to "neuropathy of the auditory nerve."

Since the initial report by Starr and colleagues it has become clear that individuals diagnosed with AN are a heterogeneous group even though they may exhibit common audiologic findings. Some individuals who exhibit the AN pattern may have a congenital form of the disorder resulting from a genetic mutation or pre/perinatal causes, whereas others may have a later onset form of the disorder associated with other peripheral neuropathies. Speculation regarding the underlying mechanisms of AN includes selective inner hair cell loss, a synaptic or myelinization disorder, or an auditory nerve disorder with other peripheral neuropathies (Starr, Sininger, & Pratt, 2000). Over the past decade, as universal newborn hearing screening has expanded and as audiologists have become more familiar with AN and its diagnosis, a growing number of infants and young children have been identified with this disorder. Characteristics of AN have been reported in children with histories of low birth weight, prematurity, neonatal insult, hyperbilirubinemia, perinatal asphyxia, artificial ventilation, and various infectious processes (Dowley et al., 2009; Mason, De Michele, Stevens, Ruth, & Hashisaki, 2003; Xoinis, Weirather, Mavoori, Shaha, & Iwamoto, 2007). Genetic abnormalities have also been identified, including those associated with the genes OTOF, PMP22, MPZ, and NDRG1 (Kovach et al., 1999; Starr et al., 2003; Varga et al., 2006; Yasunaga et al., 1999). In 2006, Buchman and colleagues described a group of children who presented with physiologic test results typical of AN who subsequently were diagnosed by magnetic resonance imaging (MRI) as having cochlear nerve deficiency (CND); that is, absent or small cochlear nerves (Buchman et al., 2006).

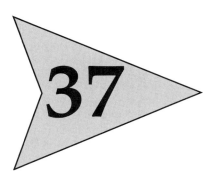

Auditory neuropathy was initially thought to be quite rare; however, current estimates of prevalence range from 7 to 10% of children with permanent hearing loss (Madden, Rutter, Hilbert, Greinwald, & Choo, 2002; Rance, 2005). Considerable controversy exists regarding almost every aspect of the disorder including its etiology, site of lesion, treatment, and even the terminology used to describe it. In an effort to provide recommendations to clinicians working with these children a panel was convened in June, 2008, at an international conference in Como, Italy (Guidelines Development Conference on the Identification and Management of Infants with Auditory Neuropathy, 2008). The panel was charged with developing guidelines for identification and management of infants with AN. After extensive review and discussion, the term "auditory neuropathy spectrum disorder" (ANSD) was adopted as a way of describing the heterogeneous and multifaceted nature of the disorder.[1] Even so, current terminology remains inadequate since the level of dysfunction for many of the children with this condition may be central to the auditory nerve (Rapin & Gravel, 2003, 2006).

Further examination of this disorder, including information about etiology, possible mechanisms, and clinical characteristics is provided in Chapter 13 in this volume. The present chapter addresses clinical management guidelines for pediatric audiologists and other professionals who work with these children.

Audiologic Evaluation

The Joint Committee on Infant Hearing (JCIH; American Academy of Pediatrics, JCIH, 2007) recommends that a comprehensive audiological evaluation be performed for all infants referred from newborn screening by audiologists experienced in pediatric assessment. The recommended test battery includes physiologic measures and, when developmentally appropriate, behavioral measures. The goal of the diagnostic assessment is to determine the type of hearing loss and to estimate hearing sensitivity across a range of frequencies for each ear. The same comprehensive approach is needed to identify ANSD, and care must be taken to select and apply an appropriate electrophysiological test protocol. The initial battery should include: otoscopic examination, immittance measures, auditory brainstem response (ABR) testing, and assessment of otoacoustic emissions (OAEs). When developmentally feasible, behavioral audiometry and speech perception measures should be included.

Diagnostic Criteria

In ANSD there is evidence of hair cell function while afferent neural conduction in the auditory pathway is disordered. Typical audiologic findings include absent or markedly abnormal auditory brainstem response (ABR) in combination with present cochlear microphonics (CM) and/or otoacoustic emissions (Figure 37–1).

Some earlier definitions of auditory neuropathy included present OAEs as a requirement for diagnosis; however, it is now recognized that OAEs may be present initially and disappear over time (Deltenre et al., 1999; Rance et al., 1999; Starr et al., 2001) and many infants with the disorder have present CM with absent emissions at the time of diagnosis, even when middle ear status is normal. Furthermore, both OAEs and CM provide evidence of hair cell function, albeit by different mechanisms. Thus, more recent definitions of ANSD include either present OAEs or a present CM in combination with markedly abnormal or absent ABR.

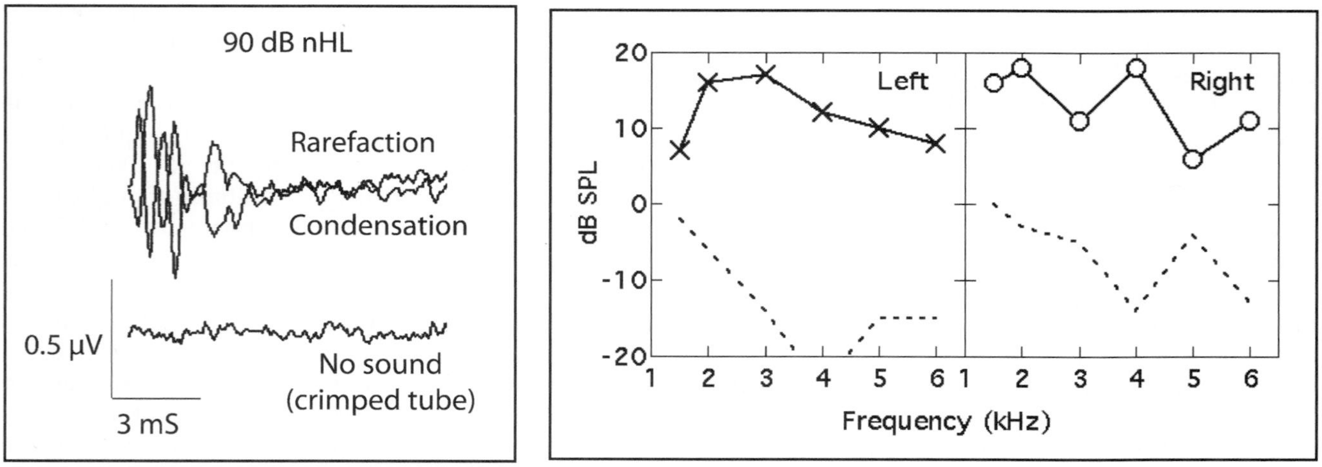

A **B**

FIGURE 37–1. ABR **(A)** and OAE **(B)** test results for a child with ANSD.

[1]The term "auditory neuropathy spectrum disorder" was suggested by Judy Gravel who noted the varied etiologies, presentations, and outcomes for children with similar electrophysiologic test findings.

Physiologic Measures

When diagnostic ABR testing using either click or tone burst stimuli shows no evidence of a neural response at high levels of stimulation, the clinician must determine if a CM is present. To accomplish this, ABR testing should be performed with insert earphones and high-intensity click stimuli (80–90 dB nHL) with separate response averages obtained for both *rarefaction* and *condensation* click polarities (Berlin et al., 1998; Starr et al., 2001). The CM occurs in the first few milliseconds of the response and, unlike neural responses, will show a reversal of the waveform when the stimulus polarity is inverted. If testing is limited to the evaluation of click stimuli with *alternating* polarity, the CM will not be evident because of cancellation and this may result in an incorrect diagnosis of profound sensory hearing loss in a child who actually has ANSD. To eliminate the possibility of incorrectly identifying stimulus artifact as the CM, a "no sound/control run" should be completed by clamping or disconnecting the sound tube from the transducer without altering the spatial relationship between the transducer and the electrodes/leads (Rance et al., 1999). Insert earphones are required instead of standard headphones because inserts introduce a delay between the electrical signal at the transducer and the acoustic signal in the ear canal, further eliminating the possibility of electromagnetic stimulus artifact being incorrectly identified as the CM. Figure 37–2 shows an example of stimulus artifact *incorrectly* identified as CM.

As in all diagnostic ABR procedures, it is important to optimize recording conditions and to complete the testing with the infant sleeping quietly in either natural or sedated sleep. If an infant tested in natural sleep is too active for accurate, artifact-free assessment, it is better to reschedule the procedure and complete a sedated test than to risk an incorrect diagnosis due to poor recording conditions.

Both the amplitude and the latency of the CM vary in ANSD, so clinicians need to be familiar with the full range of possible test results (Starr et al., 2001). The characteristic pattern associated with the diagnosis of ANSD includes a "flat" ABR with no evidence of a neural response but with a present CM (see Figure 37–1). However, it is also possible to have a present CM in combination with markedly abnormal ABR morphology, as shown in Figure 37–3. In this case, early waveforms are absent, but a wave V is present and can be tracked down to lower intensity levels.

With abnormal patterns like these, caution must be exercised in using the ABR to estimate behavioral thresholds since the minimal response levels obtained from the ABR may not correlate with the child's behavioral thresholds. Once the ANSD pattern has been identified, it is no longer possible to use the ABR to estimate the infant's behavioral thresholds, even when there is evidence of distal waveforms. At the time of this writing, controversy exists regarding whether these patients should be diagnosed as having ANSD. However, this electrophysiologic pattern is clearly abnormal, and these children should be closely monitored until behavioral audiograms are obtained and functional abilities can be determined.

Caution is also needed when interpreting abnormal ABR findings obtained in infants prior to 34 to 36 weeks gestation as maturation of the auditory pathway may be incomplete. Furthermore, because cases of transient ANSD have been reported when the initial ABR was obtained in the first few months of life, the ABR should be repeated at a later point in time to confirm the diagnosis (Madden et al., 2002; Psarommatis et al., 2006;

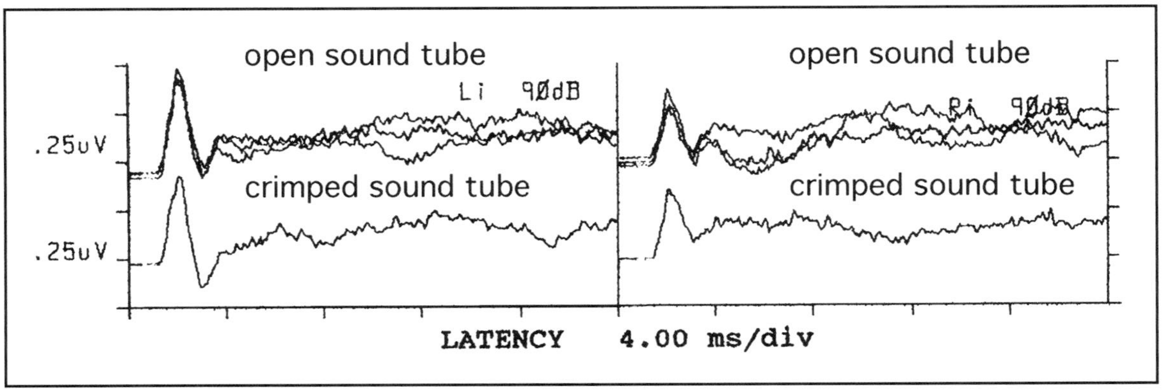

FIGURE 37–2. Example of stimulus artifact that may be misinterpreted as CM.

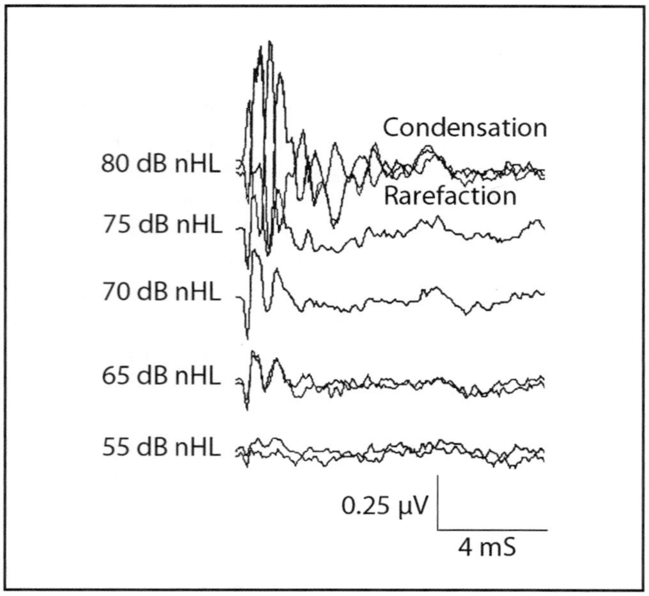

FIGURE 37–3. Abnormal ABR showing CM with presence of distal waveforms.

Raveh, Buller, Badrana, & Attias, 2007). This is especially important if there is a history of prematurity or hyperbilirubinemia (Xoinis et al., 2007).

In some clinics, auditory steady-state responses (ASSR) are used as the primary electrophysiologic measure in the evaluation of hearing loss. Although auditory steady state responses may be measured in patients with ANSD, they do not correlate with behavioral thresholds and, therefore, should not be used to estimate behavioral thresholds (Rance et al., 1999, 2005). In cases where the ASSR is absent or when an infant is at risk for ANSD, ABR testing should be completed using single polarity click stimuli at a high intensity level to determine if a cochlear microphonic is present; otherwise, an infant with ANSD may be incorrectly diagnosed as having a profound sensory hearing loss.

Other electrophysiologic measures such as cortical evoked potentials and electrocochleography have also been explored in children with auditory neuropathy in an effort to determine the site of lesion (Rea & Gibson, 2003; Santarelli, Starr, Michalewski, & Arslan, 2008), to predict outcomes following treatment with amplification or cochlear implantation (Narne & Vanaja, 2008; Rance, Cone-Wesson, Wunderlich, & Dowell, 2002) and to evaluate children with AN who are young or difficult to test (Pearce, Golding, & Dillon, 2007). These procedures, although still under investigation, hold promise for the future and warrant continued research.

Acoustic immittance measures (tympanometry and acoustic reflex testing) are also included in the comprehensive evaluation of ANSD. Middle ear muscle reflexes (MEMR; both ipsilateral and contralateral) are usually absent or elevated in cases of ANSD (Berlin et al., 2005). For infants under 6 months of age it is important to include a high-frequency (e.g., 1000 Hz) probe tone frequency (Margolis, Bass-Ringdahl, Hanks, Holte, & Zapala, 2003).

Behavioral Audiometry

Physiologic measures such as ABR and ASSR are not true tests of hearing in the perceptual sense, yet for many years these tests have enabled pediatric audiologists to make predictions regarding behavioral hearing thresholds. It is important to emphasize that in children with ANSD, thresholds cannot be predicted using ABR or ASSR. Thus, accurate behavioral audiometric procedures must be completed as soon as the child is developmentally capable of providing reliable responses. Behavioral audiometry using a conditioned response procedure such as visual reinforcement audiometry (VRA) can be initiated at a developmental level of 6 to 7 months. Using insert earphones attached to either foam tips or the infant's custom earmolds, it is often possible to obtain ear and frequency-specific measures by 7 to 9 months of age for typically developing infants (Widen et al., 2000). However, many infants identified with ANSD are born prematurely or have complex medical conditions putting them at risk for delayed motor and/or cognitive development (Teagle et al., 2010). These children are less likely to perform conditioned response procedures at the same age as healthy, typically developing infants, and testing at multiple intervals over a period of weeks or months may be required to obtain a complete audiogram. Furthermore, some infants with complex medical conditions or developmental delays may never be able to perform behavioral audiometry well enough to provide reliable estimates of hearing thresholds. In these cases behavioral observation audiometry (BOA) may be used; however, it is important to recognize the inter- and intra-subject variability inherent in this procedure (Widen, 1993) and the limitations of BOA for purposes of hearing aid fitting. In cases where it is unlikely the infant will perform VRA reliably in a reasonable timeframe for decisions regarding intervention, cortical evoked potentials may be a useful supplement to BOA for determining the child's auditory capacity (Pearce et al., 2007; Wunderlich & Cone-Wesson, 2006).

Medical Assessment

A comprehensive examination by an otolaryngologist is recommended for all children suspected of having ANSD. The otolaryngologist will obtain a medical history, perform a head and neck examination, and order laboratory studies needed to determine the etiology of the hearing loss or to identify coexisting conditions. Radiologic assessment using MRI is essential in ANSD since the auditory neuropathy phenotype is often present in children who have cochlear nerve deficiency (small or absent VIII nerves; Buchman et al., 2006). Furthermore, children with ANSD also have a higher incidence of other abnormal MRI findings. In a group of 118 children with ANSD who had available imaging studies at the University of North Carolina, nearly 65% had at least one abnormal finding on MRI (Roche et al., 2010). The abnormalities identified in addition to cochlear nerve deficiency included: prominent temporal horns; abnormalities of the brainstem, cerebellum, midbrain or cerebrum; cerebrospinal fluid (CSF) and ventricular abnormalities; white matter changes; Dandy Walker malformation; and Arnold Chiari Type I malformation. In contrast, only approximately 30% of children with non-ANSD hearing loss have been reported to have abnormal MRI findings (Mafong, Shin, & Lalwani, 2002; Simons, Mandell, & Arjmand, 2006).

Other medical consultations include evaluation by an ophthalmologist to assess visual acuity and to rule out concomitant visual disorders, and referral for medical genetics to determine if there is a genetic basis for the disorder. Although not routinely recommended for children with sensory hearing loss, referral to a pediatric neurologist is recommended for children diagnosed with ANSD as some may have neurologic disease or other conditions requiring medical treatment. It is important to inform the child's primary care physician of the ANSD diagnosis and related findings, and to provide information regarding the disorder and how it will be treated.

Evidence to Guide Management Decisions

Studies of children with ANSD show considerable variability in auditory capacity. Among the clinical characteristics reported are pure tone thresholds that range from normal to profound; disproportionately poor speech recognition abilities for the degree of hearing loss; difficulty hearing in noise; and impaired temporal processing (Rance et al., 2002; Rance, McKay, & Grayden, 2004; Starr et al., 1996; Zeng & Liu, 2006; Zeng, Oba, Garde, Sininger, & Starr, 1999). It is important to recognize that the characteristics of ANSD vary, and not every individual diagnosed with the condition will present with the same symptoms or level of severity. Some children with ANSD have disproportionately poor speech recognition ability for their degree of hearing loss, whereas others perform at a level similar to peers with non-ANSD hearing loss. For example, Rance and colleagues in Australia compared unaided and aided speech perception abilities for a group of 15 children with ANSD to a group with typical sensory hearing loss matched for age and hearing level (Rance et al., 2002). Their results showed that approximately 50% of the children with ANSD had speech recognition scores that were similar to the children with sensory hearing loss; the other 50% showed essentially no open-set speech perception ability. Interestingly, the children showing no open-set speech perception had absent cortical evoked potentials, whereas the children who had measureable speech recognition scores had present cortical evoked potentials.

Similarly, although it has been reported that children with ANSD have particular difficulty hearing in the presence of background noise (Gravel & Stapells, 1993; Kraus et al., 2000), a recent study by Rance and colleagues showed that children with typical sensorineural hearing loss and those with ANSD had more difficulty in noise than children with normal hearing. However, the effects were not consistent across subjects and some children with ANSD showed relatively good speech perception abilities even at low signal to noise ratios (Rance et al., 2007).

Following the initial report by Starr and colleagues (1991) describing patients with what appeared to be a "neural" hearing loss, several journal articles and book chapters have included recommendations for clinical management. Recommendations include: low gain hearing aids or FM systems; low gain hearing aids in one ear only; or the avoidance of hearing aid use altogether (Berlin, 1996, 1999; Berlin, Morlet, & Hood, 2003). Furthermore, because early reports described what appeared to be pathology of the auditory nerve, it was initially thought that cochlear implantation would not be beneficial (Cone-Wesson, Rance, & Sininger, 2001; Miyamoto, Kirk, Renshaw, & Hussain, 1999). Over time, as more young children diagnosed with ANSD have been evaluated, investigators have shown that both hearing aid use and cochlear implantation can be of benefit to some children with ANSD

(Buss et al., 2002; Rance et al., 1999; Rance et al., 2002; Rance & Barker, 2008; Rance, Barker, Sarant, & Ching, 2007). The clinician's challenge is to determine, as soon as possible, the hearing technology that will provide the most benefit for a particular child. Further research is needed to guide the clinician in predicting, at an early age, the technology and communication strategies that will be most beneficial for each child.

Hearing Aids and FM Systems

Currently available clinical tests provide limited information regarding site of lesion and, in many cases, it is difficult to predict whether a given child will benefit from amplification. In cases where there is residual hearing, and once reliable threshold estimates have been obtained, a trial period with amplification using an evidence-based hearing aid fitting protocol should be completed (American Academy of Audiology Pediatric Amplification Guidelines 2003; Bagatto, Scollie, Hyde, & Seewald, 2010). This recommendation was also endorsed by the panel convened for the Guidelines Development Conference on the Identification and Management of Infants with Auditory Neuropathy (2008) in Como, Italy.

Established protocols for children include real ear measures or simulated real ear measures based on real-ear-to-coupler differences (RECD) and use of a prescriptive hearing aid fitting method (e.g., Desired Sensation Level or National Acoustics Laboratory Approaches), to ensure that speech at conversational levels is audible and comfortable. When managing amplification in these children the clinician must keep in mind that ANSD is thought to cause a disruption in temporal rather than spectral processing (Rance et al., 2004; Zeng et al., 1999). As such, improving the audibility of the signal may not be sufficient to allow a child to make adequate progress with spoken language. Studies also have shown that in children with ANSD it is possible to have varying degrees of temporal disruption (Rance et al., 2004). Thus, one might expect better performance with acoustic amplification in individuals who have milder forms of the disorder, although at the present time there is limited peer-reviewed literature regarding the benefits of amplification in children with ANSD.

Finally, considering the likelihood of difficulty hearing in the presence of background noise, use of a personal FM system by parents and other caregivers may be beneficial. As with children who have non-ANSD hearing loss, the use of an FM system in the classroom is especially important to reduce problems related to distance, reverberation, and background noise.

Evaluating Outcomes

Once hearing aids have been provided it is important to evaluate the child's speech perception ability. Although evaluation of speech perception abilities in young children is challenging, a battery of age-appropriate tests such as those used by cochlear implant teams allow the pediatric audiologist to evaluate a child's unaided and aided performance. Parent questionnaires such as the Infant-Toddler Meaningful Auditory Integration Scale (IT-MAIS; Zimmerman-Phillips, Robbins, & Osberger, 1997), informal tests such as identification of body parts, as well as closed set speech perception tests such as the Early Speech Perception test (ESP; Moog & Geers, 2003) may be useful in assessing progress when children are too young for open-set testing. Once the child is able to perform open-set speech recognition testing, measures such as the Multisyllabic Lexical Neighborhood Test (MLNT) and the Lexical Neighborhood Test (LNT; Kirk, Pisoni, Sommers, Young, & Evanson, 1995) may be used. These tests use vocabulary in the lexicon of children under 5 years of age. For a review of speech recognition testing in children less than 3 years of age, see Eisenberg, Johnson, and Martinez (2005).

When children reach 5 years of age, the phonetically balanced kindergarten words (PBKs; Haskins, 1949) may be used. It is important to use recorded speech materials whenever possible. In addition to evaluation of speech perception abilities, the child's speech and language development must carefully be evaluated to monitor communication milestones. As with young children who have sensory hearing loss, the pediatric audiologist is advised to partner with speech-language pathologists and early intervention specialists. Experienced clinicians who know what to expect from children with varying degrees of sensory loss are essential to the process of monitoring communication development. Changes to the intervention strategy may be needed based on the child's progress and the preferences of the family.

Considerations for Cochlear Implantation

Children diagnosed with ANSD who exhibit severe to profound detection levels with stable thresholds over a period of several months, and whose families desire a spoken language approach, often are good candidates for cochlear implantation. For children without additional disabilities, decisions regarding cochlear implantation usually are uncomplicated once MRI has confirmed auditory nerve sufficiency (Buchman et al., 2006).

Because of reports describing spontaneous improvement in auditory function in a subset of children with the ANSD phenotype, the guidelines developed at the Lake Como Conference recommend postponement of cochlear implantation until auditory test results (ABR and behavioral audiometry) are stable and demonstrate unequivocal evidence of permanent ANSD.

Decisions regarding the advisability of cochlear implantation for children with lesser degrees of hearing sensitivity loss are more challenging, due to the range of functional abilities seen in this population and the difficulty determining the degree of impairment in very young children with ANSD. Because the behavioral pure-tone audiogram is of limited prognostic value in the prediction of aided benefit in children with ANSD, cochlear implantation should be considered even if audiometric thresholds are better than what typically would be considered when progress with conventional amplification is inadequate. For children with ANSD who have substantial residual hearing, an adequate trial with amplification, appropriate early intervention services, and comprehensive evaluation by a team of professionals experienced in the evaluation and management of young children with hearing loss, are all prerequisites to cochlear implantation. For any child with a hearing disorder a variety of factors may influence developmental outcomes. These include age at diagnosis and hearing aid fitting, consistency of hearing aid use, quality and intensity of early intervention, degree of parental involvement, and presence of additional developmental and/or medical conditions. The amount of time needed to determine benefit from hearing aid use will vary depending on each of these factors. Rather than identify an arbitrary time period for determining whether the child is receiving sufficient benefit from amplification, it is the role of the pediatric audiologist, in partnership with the family and other team members, to identify the possible influence of each factor and its impact on developmental outcomes. Optimal management requires careful observation and a comprehensive team approach.

In the United States, candidacy for cochlear implantation is based on criteria developed by the Food and Drug Administration (FDA) using information obtained during clinical trials; the criteria specified on the device labeling varies by manufacturer. At the time of this writing, children between 12 and 18 to 24 months may be considered for cochlear implantation if they have a profound bilateral sensorineural hearing loss. Children older than 18 months with severe to profound hearing loss may be considered for cochlear implantation if there is a "failure to meet auditory milestones" or if performance in the best aided condition is less than 20 to 30% for MLNT or LNT at 70 dB SPL. The criteria for one manufacturer states that in children older than age 4 years, cochlear implantation may be considered if the score is less than 12% on PBK words or 30% on open-set sentences presented at 70 dB SPL. Although no specific FDA guidelines for cochlear implant candidacy currently exist for children with ANSD, professionals attempting to determine CI candidacy for children with ANSD who have less than a profound hearing loss should consider these general guidelines.

Counseling Families

Professionals who work with families of infants and young children with newly diagnosed hearing loss understand the critical role of counseling in helping a family understand the nature of the child's hearing loss and the implications of the diagnosis. Families need assistance with the emotional aspects of the new diagnosis and information they will need to make the best decisions for their child. This is a challenging process for the family and for the clinician. Families receiving a diagnosis of ANSD face additional challenges due to the uncertainties inherent at the time of the diagnosis and the complexities associated with management decisions for their child. When delivering a diagnosis of ANSD it is important to share information based on the best available scientific evidence while providing the family with hope. For the young infant diagnosed with ANSD through electrophysiologic testing, the audiologist knows little more at the time of diagnosis than that the infant has an electrophysiologic pattern that is abnormal. Considering the heterogeneous nature of the disorder and range of functional outcomes, it makes little sense to make definitive predictions to the family regarding "expected" auditory behaviors until additional diagnostic information has been obtained.

For an infant only a few weeks of age, it may be appropriate to simply advise the family that the results of the ABR are not normal and that testing should be repeated in a few weeks. If the infant returns for a repeat study that yields similar results, additional information regarding ANSD should be provided to the family. For some families this may include showing them the ABR waveforms and contrasting them with expected results for children with non-ANSD hearing loss, as well as for a child with normal hearing sensitivity. Other families will prefer a more basic explanation. It is important for families to understand that an MRI will be needed to rule out cochlear nerve deficiency. Once cochlear nerve status has been determined, families will benefit from knowing the heterogeneous nature of ANSD and the variable outcomes associated with the disorder. It is important for families to understand that, unlike with non-ANSD hearing loss, the ABR does not assist in predicting the degree of hearing loss or in establishing thresholds for purposes of hearing aid fitting.

It is helpful for families to have a timeline for management during the first year including the need for medical evaluations, enrollment in intervention and for behavioral audiometry to establish thresholds beginning at 6 to 7 months of age. They will need to understand that decisions regarding amplification may need to be deferred until behavioral audiometric thresholds can be established.

If the child is determined to be a good candidate for amplification, the family must understand the importance of full time hearing aid use and the need to monitor communication milestones. Cochlear implantation may be discussed as one of several interventions that might be considered, but it should be explained that decisions regarding implantation need to be deferred until behavioral thresholds are established and benefit from hearing aid use has been determined. As discussed earlier, decisions regarding continuation of hearing aid use versus cochlear implantation must be made on an individual basis and determined by the needs of the child and the preferences of the family. Further research is needed to understand ANSD, its diagnosis, and its optimal management, but families should leave the clinic knowing that much can be done to facilitate their child's acquisition of functional communication ability.

Case Studies

As discussed above, the electrophysiologic test results that are characteristic of ANSD show a wide range of functional outcomes. The following case illustrations will demonstrate the variable results obtained from children who exhibit the audiologic profile of ANSD. Key points are made to highlight the different habilitative recommendations made and/or outcomes obtained for each case.

Case 1

This child was born at 25 weeks gestation, with a history of hyperbilirubinemia that required an exchange transfusion. He was ventilated for six weeks and was on oxygen for 3 months. He did not pass his newborn hearing screen with automated ABR and was referred for diagnostic ABR testing. Following the ABR testing with tone bursts and clicks, the parents were told that the infant had a profound hearing loss, and he was fitted with high gain hearing aids. The father had a job transfer and the family moved into our state. They were told that another ABR would be needed prior to acceptance into our program. On the day of the sedated ABR evaluation, the family reported that in spite of the diagnosis of profound hearing loss, they observed the baby respond to a variety of sounds at home and had even observed him startle to a loud sound.

Subsequent ABR testing showed an absent ABR with only a large CM present consistent with a diagnosis of ANSD. Otoacoustic emissions were absent bilaterally (Figure 37–4).

The diagnosis was explained to the family, and it was recommended that they discontinue use of the high gain hearing aids until behavioral audiometry could be completed. The child was enrolled in an early intervention program, and the family was informed of various communication options. They chose spoken language as their initial communication approach and were assigned an auditory verbal therapist who provided weekly visits to the family's home. The child was seen by an otolaryngologist who recommended an MRI. The MRI showed normal inner ear anatomy with present auditory nerves bilaterally. Subsequent behavioral audiometric testing at 10 months of age (7 months adjusted age) using VRA showed a moderate bilateral sensorineural hearing loss (Figure 37–5).

Once behavioral thresholds were obtained the family decided to move forward with amplification, and the child was fitted with hearing aids appropriate for a moderate hearing loss. In addition to hearing aids, the family used a personal FM system at home once the child began to walk, and there was increasing distance between the child and the speaker. Aided speech perception measures showed aided benefit, and subsequent speech and language evaluations showed the child was making excellent progress in meeting communication milestones. At 3½ years of age, the child had recurrent middle ear problems and was scheduled for placement of tympanostomy tubes. ABR testing was repeated and again showed no neural responses to click stimuli at high intensity levels with only a CM present. The child is now 5½ years old and has successfully completed kindergarten in a mainstream classroom. At the time of his most recent audiologic evaluation his speech reception thresholds were 60 dB

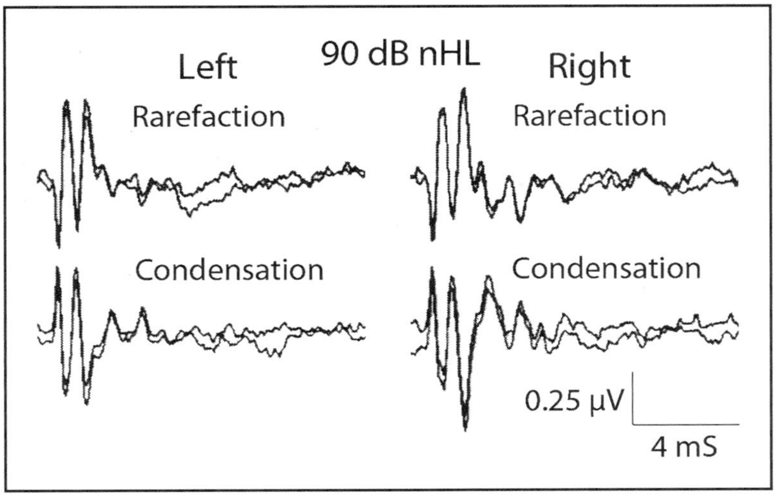

A

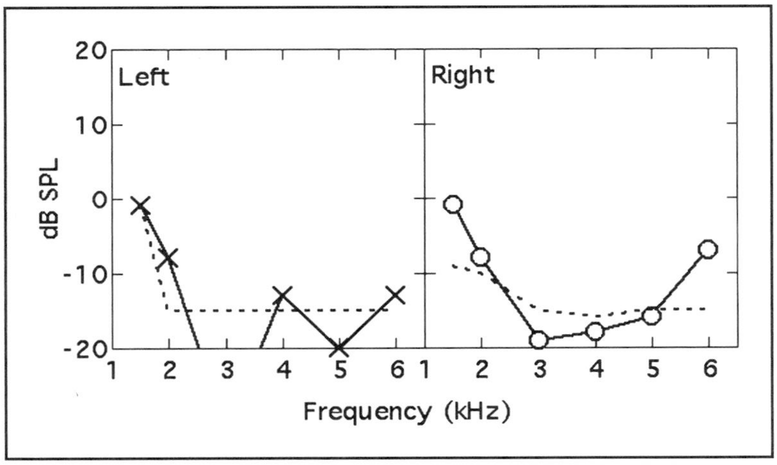

B

FIGURE 37–4. A. ABR for child in Case 1. Note large CM with reversal of waveform when stimulus polarity is inverted and lack of neural response. **B.** OAEs for Case 1.

HL unaided and 35 dB HL aided and he scored 0% on a monosyllabic word test (LNT) at 55 dB HL unaided and 100% aided. His most recent speech and language evaluation showed age-appropriate language skills with some mild speech production problems. He continues to receive support from a teacher of the deaf and a speech and language pathologist and uses FM in the classroom.

Key points: In this case, the first ABR was done at a clinic that used alternating polarity rather than single polarity clicks. This resulted in an incorrect diagnosis of profound bilateral sensory hearing loss. Fortunately, the family's move to another state resulted in the child having a repeat ABR study. The case illustrates the importance of asking the family about their observations of the child's auditory behaviors. Although the child was initially diagnosed with profound hearing loss, it was obvious to the family that their baby was responding to moderately loud sounds at home even without amplification, an unexpected finding with profound bilateral hearing loss. It also illustrates the importance of accurate initial diagnosis, as habilitative recommendations are often based on the initial diagnostic ABR evaluation. Finally, this is an example

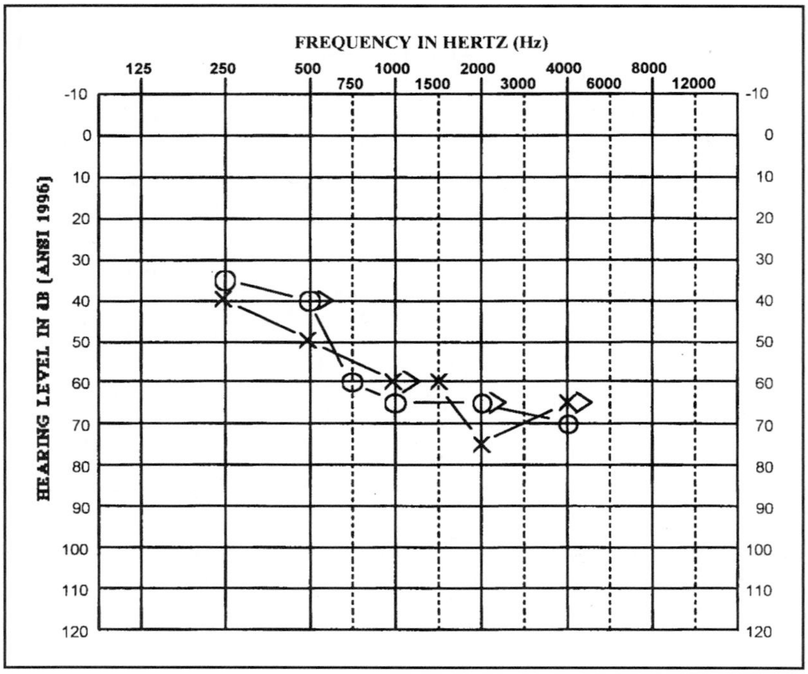

FIGURE 37–5. Audiogram for child in Case 1.

of a child who shows electrophysiologic findings that are characteristic of auditory neuropathy, yet receives significant benefit from acoustic amplification.

Case 2

The second case is a child who was born at full term in a hospital that used only otoacoustic emissions for their infant hearing screening program. The child passed his newborn OAE screen bilaterally. At age 3½ years, he subsequently developed recurrent middle ear problems and was scheduled for myringotomy and tube placement. His postoperative hearing evaluation showed normal hearing sensitivity for the right ear and a profound bilateral sensorineural hearing loss for the left ear (Figure 37–6A). Unexpectedly with a profound hearing loss in one ear, otoacoustic emissions were present bilaterally (Figure 37–6B).

The child was referred to our center for further evaluation. Diagnostic ABR testing showed, in the right ear, normal waveform morphology with responses consistent with normal hearing sensitivity; in the left ear, the ABR indicated absent neural responses with only a prolonged CM present at high intensity levels (Figure 37–7). MRI testing was completed and revealed a normal study for the right ear and an absent auditory nerve for the left ear.

Key points: As previously noted in this chapter, individuals who have cochlear nerve deficiency (small or absent VIII nerves) often present with the phenotype of ANSD (absent ABR, present CM and present OAEs; Buchman et al., 2006). MRI is useful in identifying the site of lesion in these cases and will assist the audiologist and intervention specialist in making appropriate management recommendations. Use of radiologic imaging is particularly important when determining cochlear implant candidacy in cases of profound bilateral hearing loss when there is no evidence of residual hearing. In this child's case, availability of MRI findings allowed the pediatric audiologist to make recommendations for management that were the same as those recommended for a child with profound, unilateral, sensory hearing loss.

Another key point is that it is possible to pass OAE-based newborn hearing screening and yet have a profound hearing loss in one or both ears. Professionals must be aware that passing newborn hearing screening does not ensure normal hearing and further diagnostic study is warranted when there is concern about hearing status even when an individual has passed a newborn hearing screen.

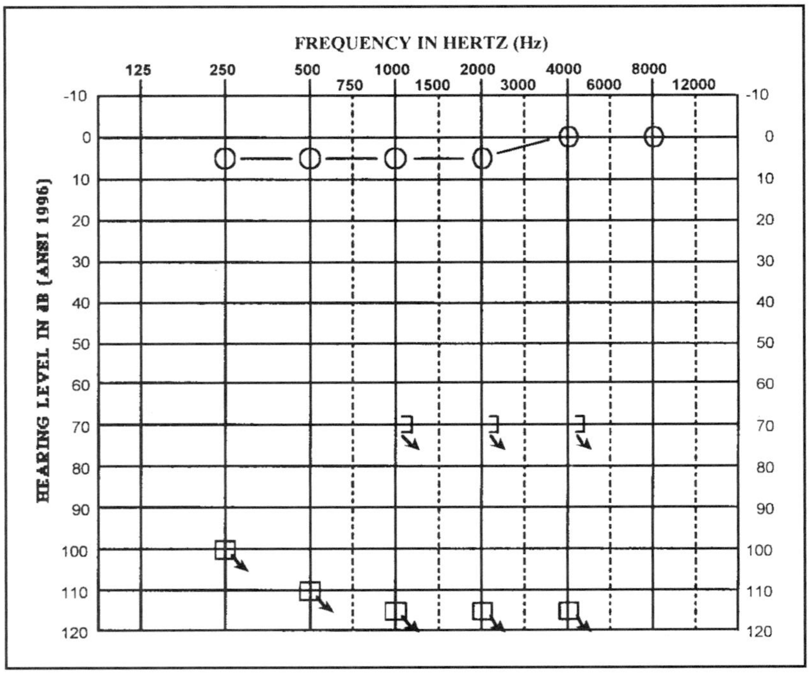

A

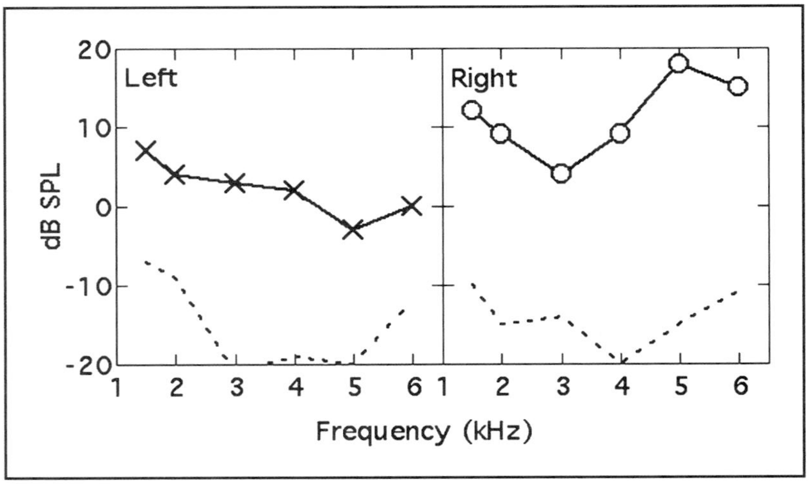

B

FIGURE 37–6. A. Audiogram for child in Case 2. **B.** OAEs for Case 2.

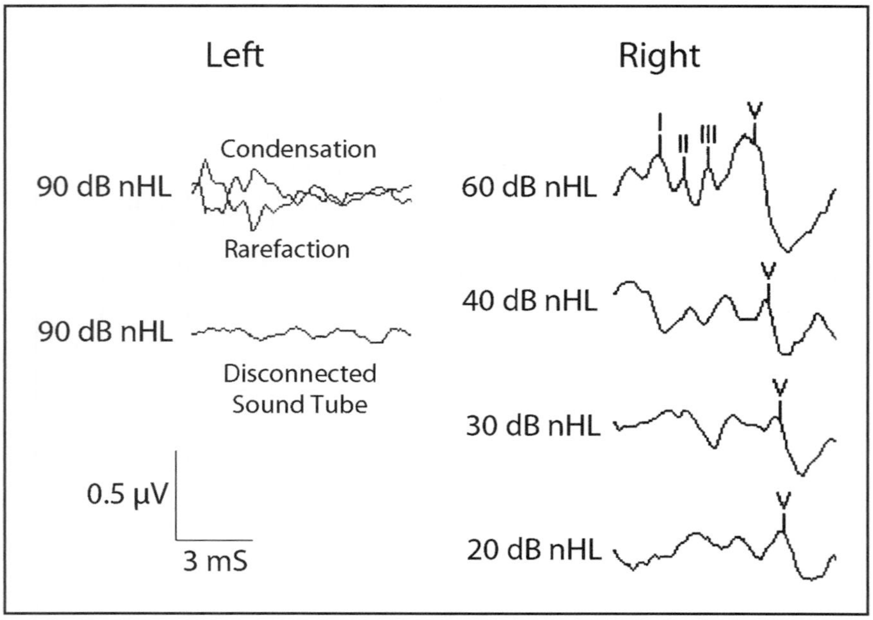

FIGURE 37–7. ABR for Case 2 showing normal ABR for right ear; left ear shows absent neural responses with only a CM present.

Case 3

This is a child who was born prematurely at 24 weeks gestation. He was hospitalized in the newborn intensive care nursery (NICU) where he received ventilation. He did not pass his initial newborn hearing screen or a repeat screen using automated ABR. Subsequent diagnostic ABR testing at 4 months of age showed absent neural responses with only a CM present for single polarity clicks at a high intensity level (Figure 37–8A). Otoacoustic emissions were present bilaterally (Figure 37–8B).

Behavioral audiometry was attempted at regular intervals beginning at 7 months adjusted age. At 12 months of age (8 months adjusted age), a sound-field audiogram showed normal hearing sensitivity for 250 to 4000 Hz. At 13 months of age (9 months adjusted age), individual ear measures were completed with insert earphones and confirmed normal hearing sensitivity for each ear (Figure 37–9).

The results were discussed with the family and the importance of monitoring the child's communication status in view of the abnormal ABR pattern was discussed. The child was enrolled in an early intervention program, and a teacher visited the home on a monthly basis. Because of reports of "recovery" in cases of ANSD, ABR testing was repeated at 17 months of age and test results again showed an abnormal ABR with no neural responses at maximum intensity levels for click stimuli with only a CM present.

It was recommended that the child return for audiologic evaluation every six months to monitor the stability of his thresholds and to obtain speech perception measures once he was developmentally able to perform this testing. At age 3, the child scored 100% on a closed-set monosyllabic word test (Early Speech Perception Test; ESP). The child developed spoken language and at 3½ years of age he was able to comprehend speech and use multiple word sentences expressively. He was also able to repeat monosyllabic words in quiet without difficulty in an auditory only condition.

Key points: In this case, although the child's ABR was grossly abnormal showing absent neural responses, the child's audiogram demonstrates normal hearing sensitivity. While the child is not currently exhibiting any functional difficulty and is developing speech and language appropriately, it will be important to monitor performance at regular intervals and continue early intervention services. It also will be important to monitor the child's ability to hear in the presence of background noise and consider use of FM in the classroom if the child experiences difficulty hearing in noise.

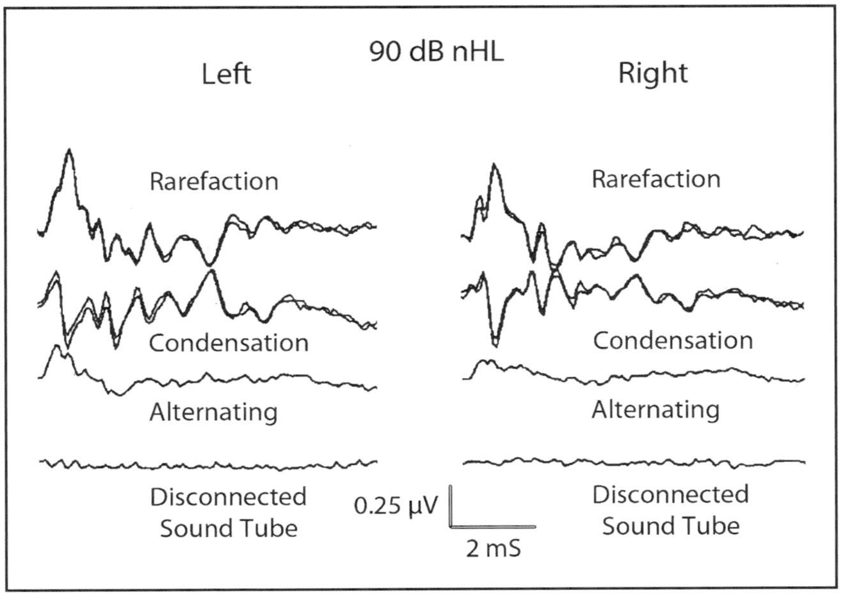

A

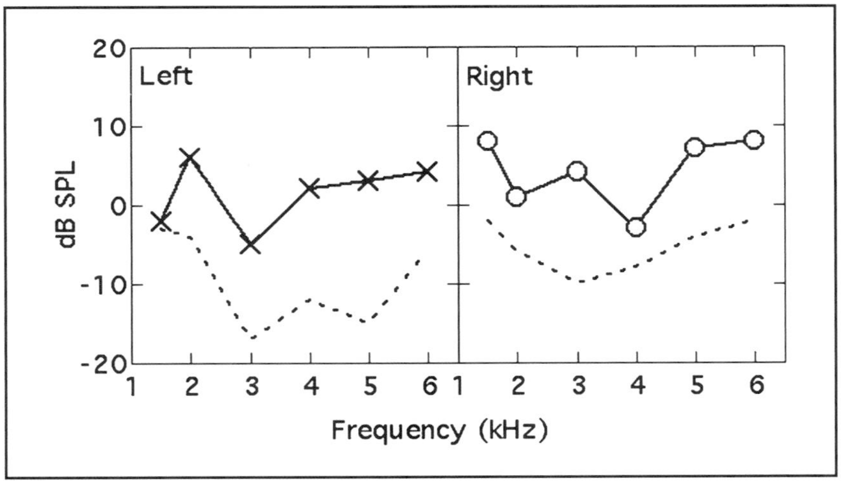

B

FIGURE 37–8. A. ABR showing no neural response with only a CM for child in Case 3. **B.** OAEs for child in Case 3.

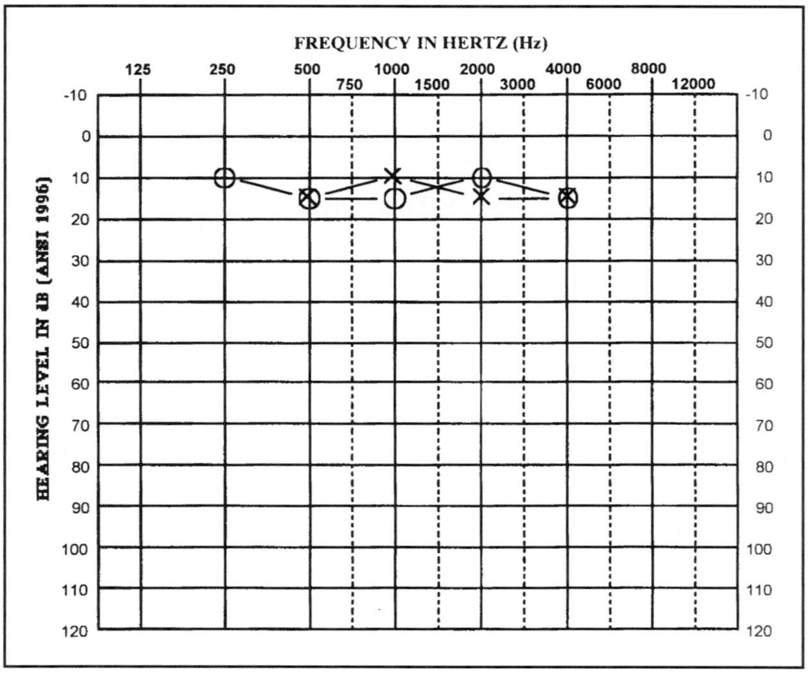

FIGURE 37–9. Audiogram for child in Case 3.

Case 4

This child was born at full term without any significant complications. There was no family history of hearing loss. This child did not pass an automated ABR hearing screen at birth but passed a re-screen with otoacoustic emissions at an outside ENT office, and her parents were told she had normal hearing. At 8 months of age, her parents became suspicious that she was not hearing and brought her to our university hospital clinic for a diagnostic ABR. The results of the diagnostic ABR evaluation showed absent neural responses to clicks with only a CM present at high intensity levels (Figure 37–10A). Otoacoustic emissions were present bilaterally (Figure 37–10B).

MRI evaluation was normal and indicated the presence of auditory nerves bilaterally. Behavioral audiometry at 9 months of age using VRA was consistent with a profound bilateral sensorineural hearing loss (Figure 37–11).

She was fitted with high gain hearing aids; however, her parents did not observe any improvement in her responses to sound with amplification, and she was subsequently referred to the cochlear implant team for evaluation. She received a right cochlear implant at 21 months of age.

Key points: In this case, the child's profound hearing loss would have been identified earlier if the outside clinic had recognized the importance of not re-screening with otoacoustic emissions when the child failed the ABR screen. Fortunately, the family obtained a second opinion in sufficient time for her to receive appropriate management. If a child does not pass a hearing screen with ABR, the child either should have a second level screen with ABR or a diagnostic ABR as a follow up. In many clinics ABR has replaced OAE screening in the intensive care nursery due to the high prevalence of ANSD in this population; however, screening with OAEs is still common in many well baby nurseries. Although the majority of cases of ANSD will be found in the NICU, it is possible to have a full term birth without complications yet present with ANSD. Clinicians must be mindful of the possibility of ANSD when there is suspicion of hearing loss in a full-term infant who has passed a newborn hearing screen with OAEs. In some of these cases, a genetic basis for the ANSD may be the etiology of the disorder

Case 5

This is a child who had normal development for the first two years of life and then developed peripheral neuropathies including optic neuropathy. She was hospitalized at 3 years of age and underwent several diagnostic studies including electromyography and mus-

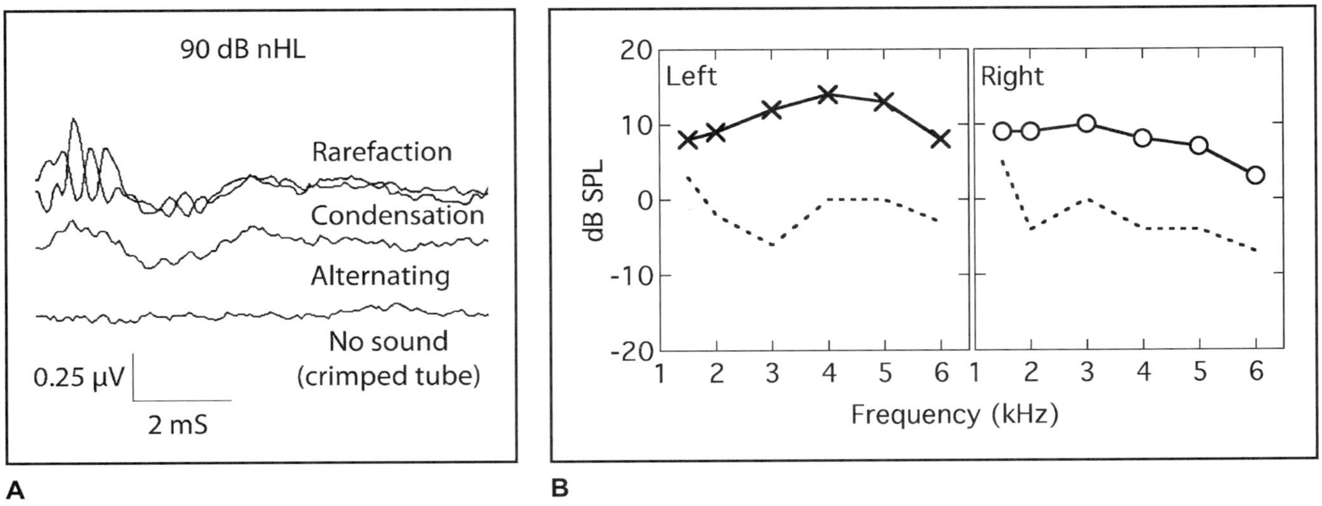

FIGURE 37–10. A. Abnormal ABR for Case 4 showing no neural response with only a CM. **B.** Present OAEs for child in Case 4 with profound hearing loss.

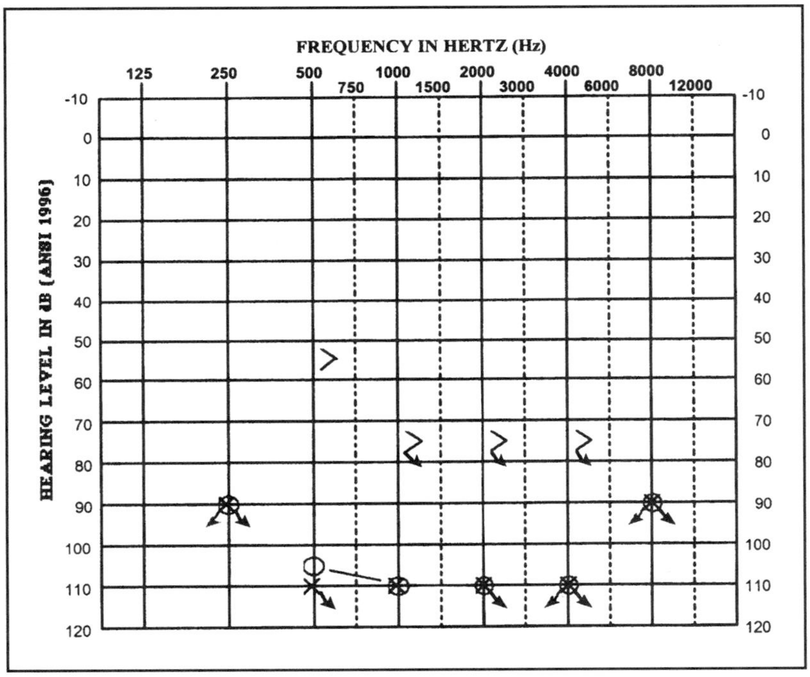

FIGURE 37–11. Audiogram for child in Case 4 showing profound hearing loss.

cle biopsies. She has had numerous specialty medical consultations including: otolaryngology, genetics, neurology, ophthalmology, and infectious disease. The etiology for her medical problems was never determined; Guillain-Barré, Charcot-Marie-Tooth and mitochondrial disease were all ruled out. An audiogram obtained at age 6 years showed a bilateral low-frequency hearing loss with unaided speech recognition scores of 100% for the right ear and 84% for the left (Figure 37–12).

An audiogram at age 10 years showed a bilateral rising audiogram; mild on the right and moderate on the left with speech recognition scores using monosyllabic words of 40% for the right at 65 dB HL and 24% for the left at 95 dB HL (Figure 37–13).

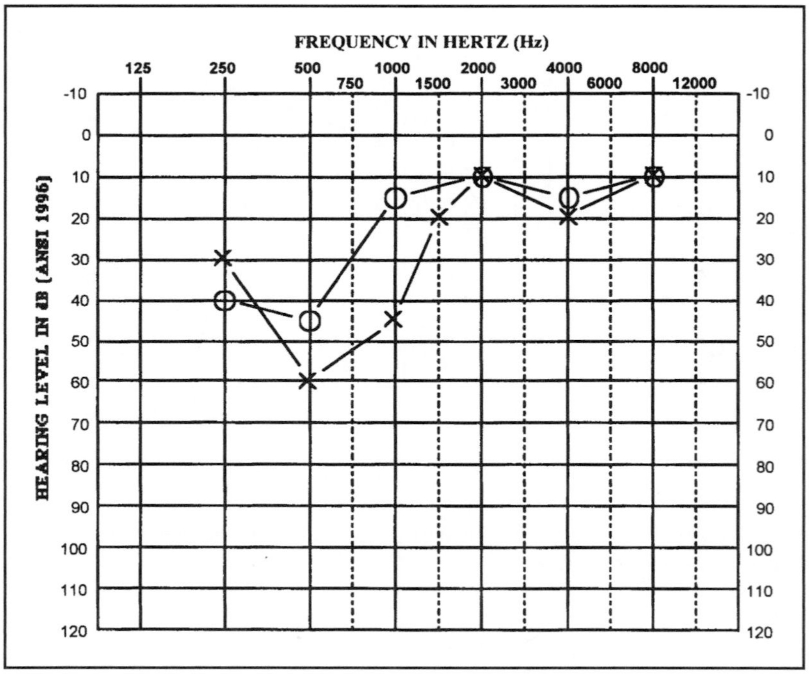

FIGURE 37–12. Audiogram showing rising low frequency hearing loss for child in Case 5 (age 6 years).

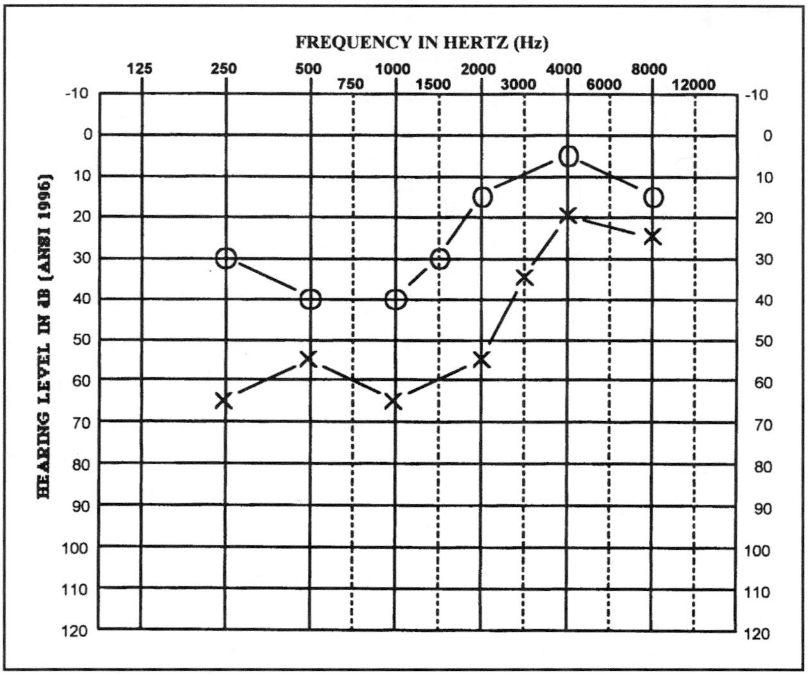

FIGURE 37–13. Audiogram showing left ear worse than right for child in Case 5 (age 10 years).

Subsequent hearing evaluations showed fluctuating speech recognition scores and a subsequent diagnostic ABR evaluation showed a pattern consistent with ANSD. Hearing aids were tried; however, the child and family reported they were of minimal benefit. By age 11 years, despite an audiogram showing significant residual hearing (Figure 37–14A), the child was unable to repeat any monosyllabic words on a speech recognition test and successful communication could only be accomplished at close range with lip reading. Robust otoacoustic emissions were present bilaterally (Figure 37–14B).

The family was counseled extensively regarding potential benefits and limitations of cochlear implantation, particularly in view of her history of multiple peripheral neuropathies. After careful consideration, the

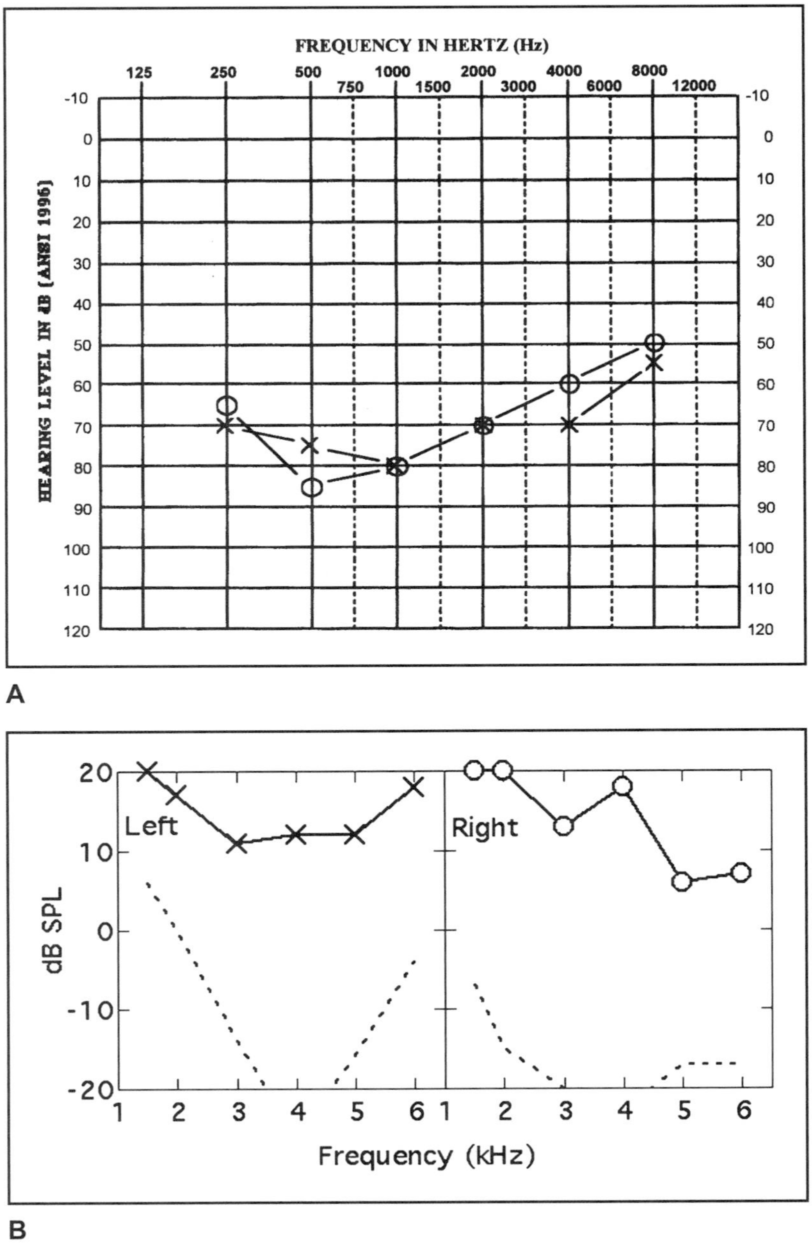

FIGURE 37–14. A. Audiogram showing severe hearing loss for child in Case 5 (age 11 years). **B.** Present OAEs for child in Case 5.

family decided to proceed with a left cochlear implant. After one year of device use, the child's monosyllabic word score with her cochlear implant was 32% on words and 66% on phonemes. Her parents reported that while she continued to have significant communication difficulty, they felt that the need for repetitions was reduced with the device on. After four years of device use, her speech recognition score while wearing her CI was only 20% and she continued to have deterioration in her motor abilities. The parents reported that she had significant difficulty understanding anyone other than her family members with her implant. Since the child still had significant residual hearing in her right ear, a decision was made to attempt hearing aid use again in the right ear. At the age of 17 and after six years of implant use and with a hearing aid in the contralateral ear, this child only achieves a score of 20% for monosyllabic words.

Key points: This child's case is complex and is similar to cases described by Dr. Arnold Starr and his colleagues in 1996. It likely represents a true case of "auditory neuropathy." Despite the use of hearing aids, a cochlear implant, supplemental visual input, and the best effort of her parents and the professionals who work with her, this child continued to have significant communication difficulty.

Conclusion

The disorder described as AN is more complicated than originally thought and the patient population is more heterogeneous. Early recommendations were often based on findings in adults with other peripheral neuropathies. Hearing aids, cochlear implants and other management strategies were both promoted and discouraged based on minimal evidence. There is now a considerable body of clinical evidence that indicates some children with ANSD are good candidates for amplification while others obtain greater benefit from cochlear implantation. With either technology a child's performance may differ from that expected in children with cochlear hearing loss, and in some cases neither strategy provides sufficient benefit. There is a growing body of literature, but the available evidence to guide clinical management of ANSD remains limited and more research is needed, especially with infants and young children. Considering the likelihood of varied etiologies, sites of lesion, age of identification, and risks of cognitive/developmental delays, it is unlikely that a single management strategy will apply to all infants and young children who present with this profile of audiologic findings. As with other sensorineural hearing loss, a continuum of multidisciplinary care is needed to provide optimal management of infants and children with ANSD.

References

American Academy of Audiology Pediatric Amplification Guidelines. (2003). http://www.audiology.org/resources/documentlibrary/Documents/pedamp.pdf

American Academy of Pediatrics, Joint Committee on Infant Hearing (JCIH). (2007). Year 2007 position statement: Principles and guidelines for early hearing detection and intervention programs. *Pediatrics, 120*(4), 898–921. doi:10.1542/peds.2007-2333

Bagatto, M., Scollie, S. D., Hyde, M., & Seewald, R. (2010). Protocol for the provision of amplification within the Ontario infant hearing program. *International Journal of Audiology, 49*(Suppl.), S70–S79.

Berlin, C. I. (1996). Hearing aids: Only for hearing impaired patients with abnormal otoacoustic emissions. In C. I. Berlin (Ed.), *Hair cells and hearing aids*. San Diego, CA: Singular.

Berlin, C. I. (1999). Auditory neuropathy: Using OAEs and ABRs from screening to management. *Seminars in Hearing, 20*, 307–315.

Berlin, C. I., Bordelon, J., St John, P., Wilensky, D., Hurley, A., Kluka, E., & Hood, L. J. (1998). Reversing click polarity may uncover auditory neuropathy in infants. *Ear and Hearing, 19*(1), 37–47.

Berlin, C. I., Hood, L. J., Morlet, T., Wilensky, D., St John, P., Montgomery, E., & Thibodaux, M. (2005). Absent or elevated middle ear muscle reflexes in the presence of normal otoacoustic emissions: A universal finding in 136 cases of auditory neuropathy/dys-synchrony. *Journal of the American Academy of Audiology, 16*(8), 546–553.

Berlin, C. I., Morlet, T., & Hood, L. J. (2003). Auditory neuropathy/dyssynchrony: Its diagnosis and management. *Pediatric Clinics of North America, 50*(2), 331–340, vii–viii.

Buchman, C. A., Roush, P. A., Teagle, H. F., Brown, C. J., Zdanski, C. J., & Grose, J. H. (2006). Auditory neuropathy characteristics in children with cochlear nerve deficiency. *Ear and Hearing, 27*(4), 399–408. doi:10.1097/01.aud.0000224100.30525.ab

Buss, E., Labadie, R. F., Brown, C. J., Gross, A. J., Grose, J. H., & Pillsbury, H. C. (2002). Outcome of cochlear implantation in pediatric auditory neuropathy. *Otology and Neurotology: Official Publication of the American Otological Society, American Neurotology Society [and] European Academy of Otology and Neurotology, 23*(3), 328–332.

Cone-Wesson, B., Rance, G., & Sininger, Y. (2001). Amplification and rehabilitation strategies for patients with auditory neuropathy. In Y. Sininger & A. Starr (Eds.), *Auditory neuropathy: A new perspective on hearing disorders* (pp. 233–249). San Diego, CA: Singular Thompson Learning.

Deltenre, P., Mansbach, A. L., Bozet, C., Christiaens, F., Barthelemy, P., Paulissen, D., & Renglet, T. (1999). Auditory neuropathy with preserved cochlear microphonics and secondary loss of otoacoustic emissions. *Audiology: Official Organ of the International Society of Audiology, 38*(4), 187–195.

Dowley, A. C., Whitehouse, W. P., Mason, S. M., Cope, Y., Grant, J., & Gibbin, K. P. (2009). Auditory neuropathy: Unexpectedly common in a screened newborn population. *Developmental Medicine and Child Neurology, 51*(8), 642–646. doi:10.1111/j.1469-8749.2009.03298.x

Eisenberg, L. S., Johnson, K. C., & Martinez, A. S. (2005). *Clinical assessment of speech perception for infants and toddlers.* Audiology Online, 2005. Retrieved from http://www.audiologyonline.com/articles/pf_article_detail.asp?article_id=1443

Guidelines Development Conference on the Identification and Management of Infants with Auditory Neuropathy. (2008). International Newborn Hearing Screening Conference. June 19–21. Como, Italy. Retrieved from http://www.thechildrenshospital.org/conditions/speech/danielscenter/ANSD-Guidelines.aspx

Gravel, J. S., & Stapells, D. R. (1993). Behavioral, electrophysiologic, and otoacoustic measures from a child with auditory processing dysfunction: Case report. *Journal of the American Academy of Audiology, 4*(6), 412–419.

Haskins, H. (1949). *A phonetically balanced test of speech discrimination for children.* Unpublished master's thesis. Evanston, IL.

Kirk, K. I., Pisoni, D. B., Sommers, M. S., Young, M., & Evanson, C. (1995). New directions for assessing speech perception in persons with sensory aids. *Annals of Otology, Rhinology & Laryngology (Suppl.), 166*, 300–303.

Kovach, M. J., Lin, J. P., Boyadjiev, S., Campbell, K., Mazzeo, L., Herman, K., . . . Kimonis, V. E. (1999). A unique point mutation in the PMP22 gene is associated with charcot-marie-tooth disease and deafness. *American Journal of Human Genetics, 64*(6), 1580–1593.

Kraus, N., Bradlow, A. R., Cheatham, M. A., Cunningham, J., King, C. D., Koch, D. B., . . . Wright, B. A. (2000). Consequences of neural asynchrony: A case of auditory neuropathy. *Journal of the Association for Research in Otolaryngology: JARO, 1*(1), 33–45.

Madden, C., Rutter, M., Hilbert, L., Greinwald, J. H., Jr., & Choo, D. I. (2002). Clinical and audiological features in auditory neuropathy. *Archives of Otolaryngology-Head & Neck Surgery, 128*(9), 1026–1030.

Mafong, D. D., Shin, E. J., & Lalwani, A. K. (2002). Use of laboratory evaluation and radiologic imaging in the diagnostic evaluation of children with sensorineural hearing loss. *Laryngoscope, 112*(1), 1–7. doi:10.1097/00005537-200201000-00001

Margolis, R. H., Bass-Ringdahl, S., Hanks, W. D., Holte, L., & Zapala, D. A. (2003). Tympanometry in newborn infants—1 kHz norms. *Journal of the American Academy of Audiology, 14*(7), 383–392.

Mason, J. C., De Michele, A., Stevens, C., Ruth, R. A., & Hashisaki, G. T. (2003). Cochlear implantation in patients with auditory neuropathy of varied etiologies. *Laryngoscope, 113*(1), 45–49. doi:10.1097/00005537–200301000-00009.

Miyamoto, R. T., Kirk, K. I., Renshaw, J., & Hussain, D. (1999). Cochlear implantation in auditory neuropathy. *Laryngoscope, 109*(2 Pt. 1), 181–185.

Moog, J. S., & Geers, A. E. (2003). Epilogue: Major findings, conclusions and implications for deaf education. *Ear and Hearing, 24*(1 Suppl.) 121S–125S. doi:10.1097/01.AUD.0000052759.62354.9F

Narne, V. K., & Vanaja, C. S. (2008). Speech identification and cortical potentials in individuals with auditory neuropathy. *Behavioral and Brain Functions, 4*(15) 1–8.

Pearce, W., Golding, M., & Dillon, H. (2007). Cortical auditory evoked potentials in the assessment of auditory neuropathy: Two case studies. *Journal of the American Academy of Audiology, 18*(5), 380–390.

Psarommatis, I., Riga, M., Douros, K., Koltsidopoulos, P., Douniadakis, D., Kapetanakis, I., & Apostolopoulos, N. (2006). Transient infantile auditory neuropathy and its clinical implications. *International Journal of Pediatric Otorhinolaryngology, 70*(9), 1629–1637. doi:10.1016/j.ijporl.2006.05.005

Rance, G. (2005). Auditory neuropathy/dys-synchrony and its perceptual consequences. *Trends in Amplification, 9*(1), 1–43.

Rance, G., & Barker, E. J. (2008). Speech perception in children with auditory neuropathy/dyssynchrony managed with either hearing AIDS or cochlear implants. *Otology & Neurotology: Official Publication of the American Otological Society, American Neurotology Society [and] European Academy of Otology and Neurotology, 29*(2), 179–182. doi:10.1097/mao.0b013e31815e92fd

Rance, G., Barker, E., Mok, M., Dowell, R., Rincon, A., & Garratt, R. (2007). Speech perception in noise for children with auditory neuropathy/dys-synchrony type hearing loss. *Ear and Hearing, 28*(3), 351–360. doi:10.1097/AUD.0b013e3180479404

Rance, G., Barker, E. J., Sarant, J. Z., & Ching, T. Y. (2007). Receptive language and speech production in children with auditory neuropathy/dyssynchrony type hearing loss. *Ear and Hearing, 28*(5), 694–702. doi:10.1097/AUD.0b013e31812f71de

Rance, G., Beer, D. E., Cone-Wesson, B., Shepherd, R. K., Dowell, R. C., King, A. M., . . . Clark, G. M. (1999). Clinical findings for a group of infants and young children with auditory neuropathy. *Ear and Hearing, 20*(3), 238–252.

Rance, G., Cone-Wesson, B., Wunderlich, J., & Dowell, R. (2002). Speech perception and cortical event related potentials in children with auditory neuropathy. *Ear and Hearing, 23*(3), 239–253.

Rance, G., McKay, C., & Grayden, D. (2004). Perceptual characterization of children with auditory neuropathy. *Ear and Hearing, 25*(1), 34–46. doi:10.1097/01.AUD.0000111259.59690.B8

Rance, G., Roper, R., Symons, L., Moody, L. J., Poulis, C., Dourlay, M., & Kelly, T. (2005). Hearing threshold estimation in infants using auditory steady-state responses. *Journal of the American Academy of Audiology, 16*(5), 291–300.

Rapin, I., & Gravel, J. (2003). "Auditory neuropathy": Physiologic and pathologic evidence calls for more diagnostic specificity. *International Journal of Pediatric Otorhinolaryngology, 67*(7), 707–728.

Rapin, I., & Gravel, J. S. (2006). Auditory neuropathy: A biologically inappropriate label unless acoustic nerve involvement is documented. *Journal of the American Academy of Audiology, 17*(2), 147–150.

Raveh, E., Buller, N., Badrana, O., & Attias, J. (2007). Auditory neuropathy: Clinical characteristics and therapeutic approach. *American Journal of Otolaryngology, 28*(5), 302–308. doi:10.1016/j.amjoto.2006.09.006

Rea, P. A., & Gibson, W. P. (2003). Evidence for surviving outer hair cell function in congenitally deaf ears. *Laryngoscope, 113*(11), 2030–2034.

Roche, J., Huang, B., Castillo, M., Bassim, M., Adunka.,O., & Buchman, C. (2010). Imaging characteristics in children with auditory neuropathy spectrum disorder. *Otology & Neurotology, 31*(5), 780–788.

Santarelli, R., Starr, A., Michalewski, H. J., & Arslan, E. (2008). Neural and receptor cochlear potentials obtained by transtympanic electrocochleography in auditory neuropathy. *Clinical Neurophysiology: Official Journal of the International Federation of Clinical Neurophysiology, 119*(5), 1028–1041. doi:10.1016/j.clinph.2008.01.018

Simons, J. P., Mandell, D. L., & Arjmand, E. M. (2006). Computed tomography and magnetic resonance imaging in pediatric unilateral and asymmetric sensorineural hearing loss. *Archives of Otolaryngology-Head & Neck Surgery, 132*(2), 186–192. doi:10.1001/archotol.132.2.186

Starr, A., McPherson, D., Patterson, J., Don, M., Luxford, W., Shannon, R., . . . Waring, M. (1991). Absence of both auditory evoked potentials and auditory percepts dependent on timing cues. *Brain: A Journal of Neurology, 114*(Pt. 3), 1157–1180.

Starr, A., Michalewski, H. J., Zeng, F. G., Fujikawa-Brooks, S., Linthicum, F., Kim, C. S., . . . Keats, B. (2003). Pathology and physiology of auditory neuropathy with a novel mutation in the MPZ gene (Tyr145→Ser). *Brain: A Journal of Neurology, 126*(Pt. 7), 1604–1619. doi:10.1093/brain/awg156

Starr, A., Picton, T. W., Sininger, Y., Hood, L. J., & Berlin, C. I. (1996). Auditory neuropathy. *Brain: A Journal of Neurology, 119*(Pt. 3), 741–753.

Starr, A., Sininger, Y., Nguyen, T., Michalewski, H. J., Oba, S., & Abdala, C. (2001). Cochlear receptor (microphonic and summating potentials, otoacoustic emissions) and auditory pathway (auditory brain stem potentials) activity in auditory neuropathy. *Ear and Hearing, 22*(2), 91–99.

Starr, A., Sininger, Y. S., & Pratt, H. (2000). The varieties of auditory neuropathy. *Journal of Basic and Clinical Physiology and Pharmacology, 11*(3), 215–230.

Teagle, H., Roush, P., Hatch, D., Woodard, J., Zdanski, C., . . . Buchman, C. (2010). Cochlear implantation in children with auditory neuropathy spectrum disorder. *Ear and Hearing, 31*(3), 1–11.

Varga, R., Avenarius, M. R., Kelley, P. M., Keats, B. J., Berlin, C. I., Hood, L. J., . . . Kimberling, W. J. (2006). OTOF mutations revealed by genetic analysis of hearing loss families including a potential temperature sensitive auditory neuropathy allele. *Journal of Medical Genetics, 43*(7), 576–581. doi:10.1136/jmg.2005.038612

Widen, J. E. (1993). Adding objectivity to infant behavioral audiometry. *Ear and Hearing, 14*(1), 49–57.

Widen, J. E., Folsom, R. C., Cone-Wesson, B., Carty, L., Dunnell, J. J., Koebsell, K., . . . Norton, S. J. (2000). Identification of neonatal hearing impairment: Hearing status at 8 to 12 months corrected age using a visual reinforcement audiometry protocol. *Ear and Hearing, 21*(5), 471–487.

Wunderlich, J. L., & Cone-Wesson, B. K. (2006). Maturation of CAEP in infants and children: A review. *Hearing Research, 212*(1–2), 212–223. doi:10.1016/j.heares.2005.11.008

Xoinis, K., Weirather, Y., Mavoori, H., Shaha, S. H., & Iwamoto, L. M. (2007). Extremely low birth weight infants are at high risk for auditory neuropathy. *Journal of Perinatology: Official Journal of the California Perinatal Association, 27*(11), 718–723. doi:10.1038/sj.jp.7211803

Yasunaga, S., Grati, M., Cohen-Salmon, M., El-Amraoui, A., Mustapha, M., Salem, N., . . . Petit, C. (1999). A mutation in OTOF, encoding otoferlin, a FER-1-like protein, causes DFNB9, a nonsyndromic form of deafness. *Nature Genetics, 21*(4), 363–369. doi:10.1038/7693

Zeng, F. G., & Liu, S. (2006). Speech perception in individuals with auditory neuropathy. *Journal of Speech, Language, and Hearing Research, 49*(2), 367–380. doi:10.1044/1092-4388(2006/029)

Zeng, F. G., Oba, S., Garde, S., Sininger, Y., & Starr, A. (1999). Temporal and speech processing deficits in auditory neuropathy. *NeuroReport, 10*(16), 3429–3435.

Zimmerman-Phillips, S., Osberger, M. F., & Robbins, A. M. (1997). *Infant-Toddler: Meaningful Auditory Integration Scale (IT-MAIS)*. Sylmar, CA: Advanced Bionics Corp.

VIII

Family and Educational Considerations

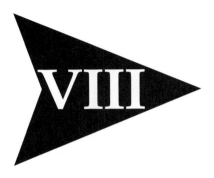

38

Family-Centered Approaches

Aneesha Pretto and Melody Harrison

Introduction

Today, in the United States, early hearing detection and intervention (EHDI) programs have been successful in the identification of most children with moderate to profound losses within the first three months of life. The success of the transition to newborn hearing screening and early identification is underscored by research on age of identification. In 1996, Harrison and Roush reported that approximately one-half of children with severe to profound hearing loss did not receive diagnosis until after the age of 12.5 months. Other retrospective studies found that the average age of identification in deaf school-age children occurred later, around 14.5 months (Meadow-Orlans, Mertens, Sass-Lehrer, & Scott-Olson, 1997). In most instances, a diagnosis of hearing loss was motivated by parental concerns about speech, language, or auditory development. Although it was often a traumatic experience, the diagnosis frequently confirmed suspicions that families had developed over a period of months. This shift in age of identification has meaningfully altered the canvas of emotions experienced by families who generally have not had time or reason to anticipate that their infant might have a hearing loss.

The family of a child with a significant hearing loss very quickly confronts a variety of daunting decisions. Although the journey from their child's birth to the diagnosis of hearing loss may occur over the course of only a few weeks, within that period of time parents will be asked to determine: "How will my child interact with the world for years to come, and for potentially the rest of his (or her) life?" Their response to this question will influence caregiver decisions to pursue assistive technology (e.g., hearing aid fitting, cochlear implantation); learn about and select a communication approach (e.g., manual, oral, or combination); change employment (e.g., work inside or outside the home; seek positions offering benefits); or relocate (e.g., moving closer to desired services or programs). Given the potentially life-altering decisions families are asked to make, early intervention programs must be responsive to the priorities, concerns, and resources specific to each family.

The potential complexity of the family adjustment process requires a framework of services that encourages empowerment of the caregivers of children with hearing loss. The litmus test of any such family-centered approach is its ability to guide the routine decisions confronted by families and professionals in both audiologic management and early service provision. As such, a true family-centered framework is dynamic and must therefore incorporate an ongoing conversation among *all* stakeholders (e.g., caregivers, audiologists, early interventionists, policy makers, etc.) who are invested in promoting the child's development.

Goals of the Chapter

The following discussion offers, to the existing dialogue, additional considerations about how professionals as help-givers may best empower the families of children with hearing loss. Specifically, the authors seek to:

1. Describe the essential components of family-centered practice in the management of children with hearing loss;
2. Illustrate through a case study how early interventionists can encourage family-centered practice within their existing system of care.

Family-Centered Practice in Early Hearing Detection and Intervention

Family-centered early intervention describes a broad agenda that values family strengths instead of deficits, advancement of family choices, control of desired resources, and collaboration between caregivers and professionals (Dunst, Trivette, & Deal, 1994). In this way, family-centered programs strive to empower families to access and use the services they desire for their child with hearing loss. Within this view, caregivers are recognized as *already competent* or possessing the facility to achieve the competencies necessary to make informed decisions. They have only failed to find a health care system that allows them to demonstrate or learn the skills necessary to promote their advancement. In this manner, professionals are not called to "intervene" in the family's functioning but rather to help caregivers as they acquire new competencies and mobilize the resources that will satisfy their needs and aspirations for their child. To the extent that families recognize their own efficacy in fulfilling these goals, they are empowered.

Evidence regarding the efficacy of the empowering practices that support families of children with hearing loss can be found in clinical research (DesJardin, 2005, 2006; Jackson & Turnbull, 2004; Zaidman-Zait, 2007). For example, caregivers with a greater sense of self-efficacy often express confidence in their ability to manage their child's audiologic and habilitation needs. DesJardin (2006) demonstrated that maternal beliefs of self-efficacy about hearing aid management were positively associated with specific strategies that mothers used to facilitate communication with their child. Moreover, the mothers who employed these facilitative language techniques typically had children with more advanced receptive and expressive language skills; and this trend was consistent irrespective of the child's degree of hearing loss or length of hearing aid use. Although preliminary, this evidence underscores the potential for family-centered care to meaningfully influence the linguistic development of children with hearing loss.

The scope of family-centered care, however, can and should extend beyond the goal of improving child-focused outcomes. To embrace family-centered practices requires a commitment to enhance the quality of life for all members as it relates to the child with hearing loss. Family "quality of life" describes the extent to which each member has his or her needs fulfilled, enjoys time with other members and can pursue goals that he or she values (Jackson & Turnbull, 2004). Rearing a child with a hearing loss affects multiple dimensions of family life including, family interaction, material and emotional resources, parenting approaches, and the family support system. A holistic approach toward family-centered care will seek not only to promote the development of the children to whom services are provided but also to address and ease the challenges that families confront in nurturing a child with hearing loss.

What are the activities that cultivate empowered caregivers, particularly those who are adjusting to a recent diagnosis? The following discussion offers additional considerations about how pediatric audiologists can promote empowerment of families to maintain or improve their quality of life. Specifically, it will address how family-centered thinking can inform choices caregivers make regarding audiologic assessment and management. Because family empowerment best addresses each family's specific concerns and priorities as they exist in their immediate context, a vignette will be used to illustrate opportunities for engaging in a family-centered approach.

The vignette presented in this chapter is based on an actual family and the timeline and findings from their child's assessments are real. Family-centered care requires that families receive the services they desire at the time they need them. As their child ages, the needs and interests of the parents will change as a function of the child's strengths and challenges, the support systems available to the family, their decisions regarding amplification and device use, as well as access to professional services. A brief discussion following each segment of the vignette will explore how the family's system of care provided by audiologists and other professionals can be most responsive to their developing concerns.

> Following an uneventful pregnancy, Jamie Anderson was born at a university medical center on September 13, 2007. Her in-hospital screening revealed a possible unilateral hearing loss in the left ear. The family was scheduled to return to the hospital with Jamie for a follow-up screen 2 weeks later. Jamie lives with her biological mother, father, and older brother and sister.

As a result of the successful implementation of newborn hearing screening, many families, like the Andersons, first receive the news of a potential hearing loss shortly after their child's birth. Because a family may have had little or no information about hearing screening prior to their child's birth, it is important that the early detection process provide sufficient information and support to assist parents in their efforts to confirm the status of their child's hearing. At a minimum, this support should include information written at a level the parents can understand and access to follow-up appointments. If the parents are illiterate or do not speak the national language(s), information should be made available in a format and/or language they can understand. In the United States, the challenge of providing information to families who lack basic literacy or who are non-English speaking is growing. The U.S. Department of Education estimates that 32 million adults lack basic literacy skills. In the 2000 census, the U.S. Census Bureau reported that 47 million people (18% of the population) over the age of five years indicated they spoke a language other than English at home. While this does not necessarily mean that these individuals are non-English speakers, it is an indicator of a demographic shift and highlights a potential barrier to adequate communication to promote screening follow-through by the family.

Building Ties Between Early Screening and Follow-Up

Universal newborn hearing screening (UNHS), now available in all 50 American states, provides the initial contact in the early identification of children with hearing loss. Barriers to accessing desired services following screening often present an acute strain for families of children who are deaf or hard of hearing. Earlier access, particularly for children with significant congenital hearing loss, increases the likelihood that age-appropriate language skills are achieved within the first five years of life (Yoshinago-Itano, 2003). Despite these documented advantages, the time saved in early detection through universal screening can be easily compromised by ineffectual follow-up care after referral.

In order to preserve the benefits of early detection, pediatric audiologists can establish strong collaborative relationships with the newborn hearing screening programs in their communities. Creating links with birthing facilities that do not provide follow-up services to families referred from an initial screening is particularly valuable in providing continuity of care from initial screening to diagnosis and management of an identified hearing loss.

Rescreening is a critical juncture in the process of identification at which families are frequently lost to follow-up. In 2007, approximately 44% of children referred from their most recent hearing screening (e.g., the in-hospital initial screen or the outpatient rescreen) had no subsequent documentation confirming a hearing loss or providing evidence of normal hearing (CDC, 2009). It is unclear whether these children were in fact lost to follow-up, or if they were seen for diagnostic evaluation and the results were unreported. To lessen this trend, EHDI professionals have advocated that re-screening serve as the initial point of audiologic service provision (Gravel & McCaughey, 2004). Some proponents favor reserving a scheduled block of time for appointments at the referral facility (Roush, 2000), although flexibility in rescreening may suit families with challenging work schedules or travel concerns. A combination of rescreening time blocks with flexibility for scheduling outside of those blocks may capture more of the children who do not pass the initial screen.

In 2008, the National Initiative for Childhood Healthcare Quality established a learning collaborative among state newborn hearing screening programs to improve the system of care for children with hearing loss. Each member state within the collaborative developed a plan to facilitate transition from the initial screening to referral, diagnosis, and receipt of intervention services. The initiative emphasized increased support for families within the medical home, as well as enhanced communication between the medical home and professionals involved in specialty care. The strategies identified as most helpful in supporting families after early detection appear in Table 38–1. Some of these strategies are the responsibility of the screening program while others relate more specifically to service providers in audiology or other disciplines.

Providing Information to Families About the Screening and Referral Process

Informed decision making is a vital component of family-centered practice. Availability of a pediatric audiologist early in the referral process can enhance family follow-through by assisting the family in understanding the scope and goals of the screening and referral processes, providing them with information about what will occur at appointments and why, and helping families understand the consequences of childhood hearing loss. Tattersall and Young (2006) interviewed caregivers about their personal family experiences subsequent to newborn hearing screening. Families reported that, "what counted as a diagnostic process was hugely variably perceived" (p. 39). Some reported confirmation of hearing loss after one follow-up appointment,

Table 38–1. National Initiative for Childhood Healthcare Quality (NICHQ) Strategies to Improve the System of Care in Newborn Hearing Screening Programs

1. Verify the results of the initial screening with the parent and primary care provider before family leaves.
2. Schedule the follow-up appointment at the time of the initial referral.
3. Collect a second point of contact and additional information for the family.
4. Create a letter template to fax results of the screening to primary care provider.
5. Use a fax-back form at the time of the diagnostic evaluation to alert the primary care provider of the results and the need for prompt follow-up.
6. Make reminder calls before the diagnostic audiology appointment to reinforce the importance of the visit and to verify appointment time and place.
7. Obtain consent for release of information at first contact with early intervention services so as to facilitate information-sharing.

while others reported as many as five appointments were required. Although there were parents who viewed the multiple audiologic visits as an information-seeking process, others interpreted it more negatively as a series of "one-off" appointments. The interviews conducted by Tattersall and Young revealed that the rationale and purpose of each session were often unclear. One possible consequence is that families who do not understand that hearing screening is a process involving multiple steps and that each of the steps provides information to facilitate decision making regarding next steps may be less inclined to complete it.

To circumvent the problems created when parents are uninformed about referral and possible diagnosis of hearing loss, Gravel and McCaughey (2004) encourage audiologists to provide families with informational handouts about the scope and potential length of the diagnostic process. One of the most comprehensive sources of information regarding newborn hearing screening, the diagnostic process, and early services in the United States is available at National Center for Hearing Assessment and Management (http://www.infanthearing.org). This website provides information for both families and professionals.

Audiologists who conduct screenings are encouraged to contact those families with an infant who is referred from an initial screen to answer any questions about the results or what should happen next. As shown in the vignettes, an informed approach is no less important for families of children with suspected unilateral hearing loss, especially as loss to follow-up rates may be higher for children with mild or unilateral hearing loss.

AGE: 2 months

The results of Jamie's second screening replicated those of the newborn screen. The family was referred for an audiologic assessment in mid-November with a pediatric audiologist in the ear, nose, and throat (ENT) clinic at the hospital. At that visit, auditory brainstem response testing (ABR) using tone-burst stimuli was conducted under natural sleep conditions. Air and bone conduction thresholds were used to identify the type of hearing loss. Otoacoustic emissions (OAEs) were absent in the left ear. Jamie received a diagnosis of moderate sensorineural hearing loss (SNHL) in her left ear.

Following the evaluation, the possibility of a hearing aid fitting for Jamie's left ear was discussed with her parents; however, they were reluctant to pursue the use of a hearing aid for her at that time. Jamie was scheduled for an MRI with an ENT consult and an appointment for comprehensive behavioral assessment 5 months later at 7 months of age. The family also received a referral to a statewide parent advocacy program for families of children with hearing loss.

Parental Needs at the Time of Confirmation of Hearing Loss

At the time of confirmation of hearing loss, the likelihood of a significant condition with the potential to affect their child's development is verified. At the point of confirmation, the need for both informational and emotional adjustment counseling becomes most acute. Parents' need for information at the time hearing loss is diagnosed has been a topic of research and discussion for years. Almost three decades ago, Williams and Darbyshire (1982) queried parents regarding their experiences surrounding the diagnosis of their child's hearing loss. The need for factual information about the hearing loss and its effects upon their child's development was reported by 88% of the families. When, however, they were asked to describe their understanding of the hearing loss and potential consequences, 40% were unable to do so and another 24% responded inaccurately. It is not possible to determine whether the information was ever provided to them, or if parents were unable to retain the information. Additionally, it was unclear whether the audiologists included in the study had a pediatric focus in their practice or saw children only occasionally and were thus less aware of parental need for information and support. Regardless, the finding demonstrates the need for information to be provided in a variety of formats, including print, and at multiple times during the management of the child's hearing loss. More recently, Roush and Harrison (2002) reported that parents' number one priority for information, regardless of the degree of their child's hearing loss, was to understand the cause of the hearing loss. With today's array of diagnostic imaging resources, such as MRI, as well as genetic consultation, audiologists and early intervention professionals can support the family in fully investigating the etiology of the diagnosis, not only because this is typically the family's most immediate concern, but also because, as will be shown, etiology may contribute to informed decision making when planning hearing loss management options.

Coping with the emotional aspects of the diagnosis was also listed as a high priority by families. Thus, pediatric audiologists are asked to be a source of both information and emotional support, as well as to be aware when factual information is a higher parental priority than emotional support and vice versa. Simply asking parents, "What information or assistance do you need to leave here with today?" demonstrates responsiveness to their needs and concerns, and allows the audiologist to support the family in moving forward with the information or support they require. It may be that members of a family have differing informational or emotional needs. In such a situation, meeting the competing needs of various family members can be truly challenging. Developing a network with other professionals such as speech-language pathologists, teachers, and early intervention specialists, who work with and can be resources for families of children with hearing loss is especially important when serving those who have multiple and often competing needs. It sometimes may be the case that the family's needs are beyond the scope of the pediatric audiologist's role in providing emotional support. In these instances, referral to appropriate services is always advised.

In this same study of parent priorities, Roush and Harrison (2002) asked pediatric audiologists to identify what *they* believed parents' priorities were at the time of diagnosis. *Coping with the emotional aspects of hearing loss* was most frequently selected as the top priority by the audiologists, and *explaining the cause of hearing loss* was a close second. Clearly, many pediatric audiologists who provide services to children and their families understand parents' needs for both information and support in coping with the emotional aspects of a diagnosis of hearing loss for their child (Table 38–2).

Fostering Informed Decision Making

Notwithstanding the value of informational and emotional support, Dunst and his colleagues (1994) have asserted that, "effective help-giving encourages and promotes movement from *concerns* to *needs and actions* as rapidly as possible" (*emphasis added*, p. 11). From a family-centered empowerment approach, caregivers are assumed to be competent decision-makers who can

Table 38–2. Parent Priorities at the Time of Diagnosis

Parent Priorities for Children with Mild-to-Moderate Hearing Loss	*Parent Priorities for Children with Severe-to-Profound Hearing Loss*
1. Learning about the causes of hearing loss	1. Learning about the causes of hearing loss
2. Understanding the audiogram	2. Coping with the emotional aspects of hearing loss
3. Realistic timelines for learning speech and language	3. Learning to listen and speak
4. Coping with the emotional aspects of hearing loss	4. Understanding the ear and hearing

Roush & Harrison, (2002).

identify the options that best serve their interests and those of their child once information regarding options is made available. However, families may find it difficult to make informed decisions, or to make decisions professionals feel they can support, when little or no empirically driven information is available. Faced with multiple treatment options, families often select a course of management with the highest potential to fulfill their expectations for their child's development.

For families of children with unilateral hearing loss (UHL), limited information is available on the efficacy of amplification. Children with UHL have been reported to wear amplification less often than children with mild bilateral hearing loss (Davis, Reeve, Hind, & Bamford, 2002). However, hearing aid use for children with UHL and hearing thresholds at or below moderately severe range has met with some success in comparison to those with severe or profound losses (Kiese-Himmel, 2002). These findings suggest that unilateral amplification can help achieve a more balanced sense of hearing between the ears with a lesser degree of hearing loss, but not when the loss is severe or profound.

In cases such as these, the audiologist may encourage parents to rely upon their own judgment which is influenced by cultural, familial, and socioeconomic experience. Families may actively participate by investigating their intervention options. Two popular avenues to determine the most suitable management include consulting other parents of children with a similar hearing loss, or engaging in a trial period of treatment with amplification where possible. These activities promote caregiver confidence in their ability to address their child's needs as well as continued progress in their child's development.

Bolstering Family Support

After diagnosis, the family system is invariably altered as members of the family begin to recognize and accommodate the diagnosed child's unique needs. One of the best known supports to the adjustment process is the creation of an informal social support network (e.g., child care programs, extended family) to bolster the intervention process. Social support research has revealed that informal help-giving bears a stronger relationship to parental well-being, child rearing practices, and child outcomes (Dunst, 2000) than formal services. The desire for these social supports among parents of children with hearing loss has also been firmly documented in the literature (ASHA, 2008). In a 1996 national survey of 404 parents deaf and hard of hearing children, informal supports (e.g., spouse, relatives, other parents, deaf adults, friends) dominated the top 10 ranks of most helpful resources (Meadow-Orlans et al., 1997). Only two professional roles (i.e., the teacher and therapist) figured prominently in the list; and these findings indicate that although key formal services are highly influential, informal help within the social environment can exert a consistent influence on daily family functioning.

Through informal parent interviews, the audiologist can gauge the degree to which informal social supports are available and accessible to each family and can play an important role in developing available sources of support by coaching the family to identify the specific individuals among their family and friends to whom they are most likely to turn. Specific questions might be: "With whom will it be easiest (or most important) for you to share the information about Jamie's hearing loss?," "Is there anyone who can come to Jamie's next appointment with you?," "Is there anyone who can take care of Jamie's older brother when you come for your next appointment?" These types of questions not only assist the family in identifying those who can help them manage the logistical challenges of caring for a young child with a hearing loss, they also affirm the need to reach out to invaluable sources of emotional support.

Meeting families of other children with hearing loss who have successfully dealt with the challenges of diagnosis and management can be a particularly helpful form of support to many families. With permission, the pediatric audiologist can facilitate contact among families from nearby communities who may share many similar experiences. In some instances, parents have created well-organized support groups, welcoming families of children with all degrees of hearing loss and inclusive of any form of communication. For example, HITCH-UP (Hearing Impaired Children Have Unlimited Potential) was founded on the premise that parents, given accurate information about hearing loss, could make sound decisions for their child. These decisions involve placement, communication methodology, and related service needs. Members of HITCH-UP are committed to sharing information in a family-centered atmosphere to facilitate active involvement of parents in their child's social, emotional, and educational growth.

Mutual reflection with other parents has also been reported to alleviate stress, especially in mothers (Calderon & Greenberg, 1999). In this regard, parent support groups serve this purpose as well. Establishing connections through such formal groups enables parents to discuss their firsthand experiences, view the progress of children similar to their child, and collectively discover unique solutions to daily parenting challenges. Thus, the installment of a robust social support system after identification can help insulate families from the demands and stress of parenting a child who is deaf.

The decision to engage peer support varies from family to family. Caregivers of children with mild and/or unilateral hearing loss may be less likely to identify with the needs of families with deaf or hard of hearing children. However, most parents of children with severe to profound hearing loss are known to benefit from peer support. After in-depth interview of 15 families, Zaidman-Zait (2007) also found that over 90% of parents viewed shared experiences with other parents of children who are deaf as critical to their coping in parenting a child with a cochlear implant.

Immediate referral to family support agencies is another strategy that can extend the family's support network while also helping to prevent loss to follow-up. In the vignette, preliminary counseling was initiated by the audiologist who then referred the family to a parent advocacy program that could provide individualized counseling and information on local resources. Although family support agencies vary from state to state, organizations like Hands and Voices (http://www.handsandvoice.org) have established 19 chapters in the United States and Canada. It is a nonprofit, parent-driven national organization dedicated to supporting families of children with hearing loss without bias. Hand and Voices also offers resources for parents and professional, parent-to-parent mentoring, and support in educational advocacy. Whatever the resource, it is essential that professionals identify programs that deliver *impartial* and comprehensive information on communication and educational options to families in need.

> ***AGE: 4 months***
>
> Two months later, Jamie's family met with the ENT physician who had reviewed her MRI. The physician explained the presence of bilateral enlarged vestibular aqueducts seen in the MRI. The vestibular aqueduct connects the inner ear (vestibule) to the cranial cavity. It is commonly, but not always, associated with sensorineural hearing loss. At this visit, Jamie's family was referred for genetic testing.

Equal Access to Comprehensive Services

Referral of Jamie's family for genetic testing aligns with the 2007 EHDI guidelines endorsed by the Joint Committee on Infant Hearing (JCIH) to provide genetic counseling to children with *any* degree of hearing loss. Despite the JCIH recommendation, some families choose not to pursue a genetic consultation. This is often the case when hearing loss is the only presenting concern or family planning is no longer an issue. In other instances, referral for genetic testing is not recommended, particularly when it is known that the family will incur additional financial expense and anxiety about the risk of recurrence in future children is low. The inclination to advocate for only those services that fit the family's array of resources can prevent professionals from encouraging the maximal level of care among all families. One of the many roles of the pediatric audiologist is to dispel misconceptions about the value of genetic counseling for all families. Among other things, genetic counseling can identify and alert the family to the presence of an underlying condition. Knowledge of the condition can guide immediate as well as future decisions regarding intervention options.

The tendency to make recommendations to families based on their economic status can be seen at a variety of decision points in audiologic management. For example, Sass-Lehrer (2004) remarked that "audiologists often balance cost and effectiveness in their recommendations for hearing aids," suggesting that available family resources may deter professionals from advocating for the same level of care among all families. Steinberg and colleagues (Steinberg, Bain, Li, & Ruperto, 2003) reported that non-English speaking families or low income households are less likely to receive encouragement to pursue cochlear implants for their child. Although these decisions relate to device use and technology, perception may guide audiologic recommendations for families to engage other professional services for their child, such as genetic counseling.

It is critical to remain attuned to changes in each family's circumstance. Early on in the diagnostic process, parents empower each professional with their confidence that he or she will recommend the services best suited for their child's needs. If informed decision-making is to be the cornerstone of family-centered practice, then professionals must foster empowered parenting by providing families with access to the services and tools necessary to understand their child's hearing loss. They ultimately may make a decision not to pursue genetic counseling or opt for hearing aids that are adequate rather than optimal; however, the decision, based on the full array of options, should be theirs.

It will be demonstrated as Jamie's case develops that her family's ability to make planned and informed decisions was strongly influenced by information provided by the MRI and genetic testing.

> *AGE: 7 to 8 months old*
>
> Jamie returned with her mother for behavioral assessment with visual reinforcement audiometry (VRA). After multiple attempts, "thresholds" were identified at three frequencies (1, 2, 4 kHz; Figure 38–1A). One month later, the two returned for behavioral testing; Jamie provided reliable responses to VRA stimuli in the right ear across a range of frequencies (Figure 38–1B). Following the visit, the family received results from a genetic counselor that confirmed a diagnosis of Pendred syndrome. The syndrome presents with multiple conditions including, an enlarged thyroid during puberty, progressive hearing loss, and sometimes vestibular dysfunction. Jamie's older brother was also diagnosed with Pendred syndrome, although he did not have a hearing loss.

Jamie's first exposure to behavioral testing was marginally successful. She and her mother became acquainted with the audiologic testing booth, the visual reinforcement test paradigm, the testing assistant and better acquainted with the pediatric audiologist. With encouragement and information from the audiologist, Jamie's mother began to assume a larger role in the assessment and ongoing monitoring of her daughter's hearing status. Her contributions will enrich their mutual understanding of how Jamie responds to sound both inside and outside of the test booth.

Providing Opportunities for Parent Participation

Best-practice in pediatric audiology has recently moved towards a wider involvement of the family in the clinical setting (ASHA, 2008). Audiologists can involve parents in the report and monitoring of their child's auditory development through multiple means. For example, parents can validate the child's performance during behavioral testing and participate in demonstration of their child's auditory or other skills during the session (ASHA, 2008). Caregivers may also occupy active roles as informal reporters of their child's auditory behaviors. Some audiologists may promote the

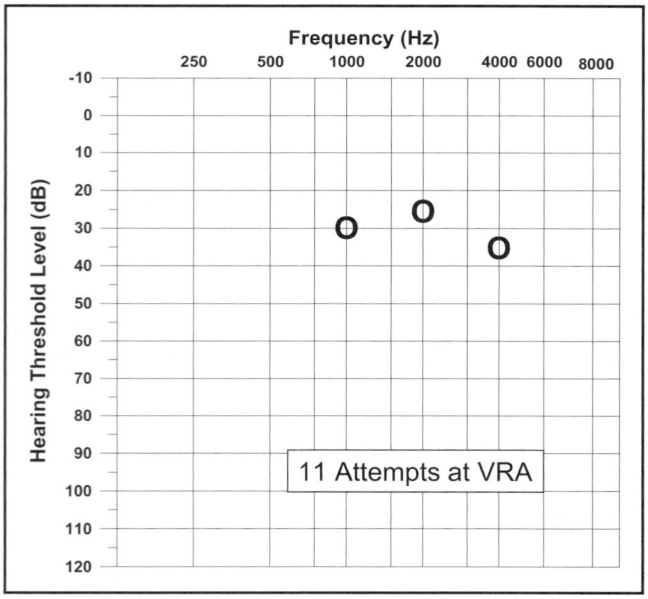

A

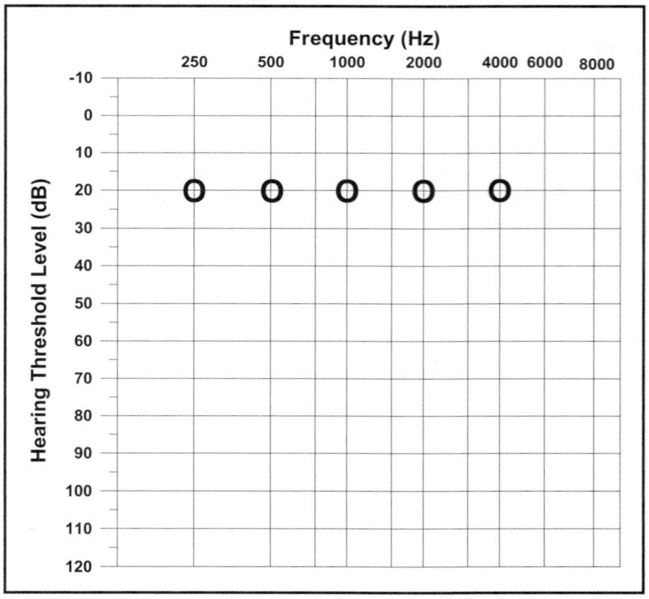

B

FIGURE 38–1. A. Early visual reinforcement audiometry (VRA) test results, right ear. **B.** Right ear VRA results one month later.

regular use of diaries to track the child's response to auditory stimuli that can promote the caregiver's ongoing awareness of auditory development over time. Others may favor use of formal parent report tools to gauge performance in diverse environmental contexts. Parent report instruments such as the ELF (Early Listening Function) test can be used by parents to obtain an estimate of their child's functional use of hearing as it relates to distance and noise. The ELF (http://www.phonak.com/professional/pediatrics/diagnostic.htm) describes twelve contrived listening activities that can easily be performed at home. Parents are guided to determine if their child exhibits a behavioral response at specified distances, in quiet and "typically noisy" conditions. As the parents become more aware of their child's range of listening in a variety of noise environments and at varying distances, they become much more knowledgeable about the interaction between the environment and their child's specific auditory ability. In addition to the information they can provide about their child's auditory functioning, asking families to participate in formal and informal assessments can result in other benefits. Rather than assuming the role of "bystanders" families are more likely to see themselves as contributors to the hearing aid fitting process. This may result in a sense of partnering with their audiologist in optimally maintaining the hearing aids and assuring that they are consistently used.

The benefits of these participatory practices have been confirmed in the larger research of children with special needs. In a meta-analytic synthesis of family-centered help-giving research, Dunst and his colleagues (Dunst, Trivette, & Hamby, 2007) found that family involvement in achieving their desired goals and outcomes enhanced the caregiver's satisfaction with program delivery and feelings of self-efficacy. Use of participatory practices also exhibited a stronger association to these outcomes than relational practices (e.g., active listening, empathy, respect) provided during adjustment counseling. Many early intervention program models have acknowledged the role of the family in their child's development. Yet, the degree to which these programs involve families in a manner that allows them to strengthen their existing skills or develop new ones varies dramatically (Dunst, Boyd, Trivette, & Hamby, 2002).

AGE: 18 months old

Approximately 16 months after the diagnosis, Jamie's mother has become more directly involved with her daughter's audiology services and most frequently accompanies Jamie to the appointments. At the most recent session, air conduction thresholds indicated that thresholds in the better (right) ear have worsened. The family was scheduled to return for behavioral assessment on a monthly basis to monitor the status of Jamie's hearing. Her subsequent visit confirmed increased thresholds in the right ear via bone conduction (Figure 38–2). A second ABR was requested to confirm the shift in thresholds. At that time, the audiologist recommended the daily use of bilateral amplification. Ms. Anderson agreed that amplification was needed and earmold impressions were taken that day. It was also recommended that a speech and language assessment be completed to ascertain whether or not her hearing loss had affected Jamie's communication development.

The Benefits of Early Counseling

In the vignette, the MRI and genetic evaluation that were completed in the first year of Jamie's life laid the foundation for the present discussion. Children with

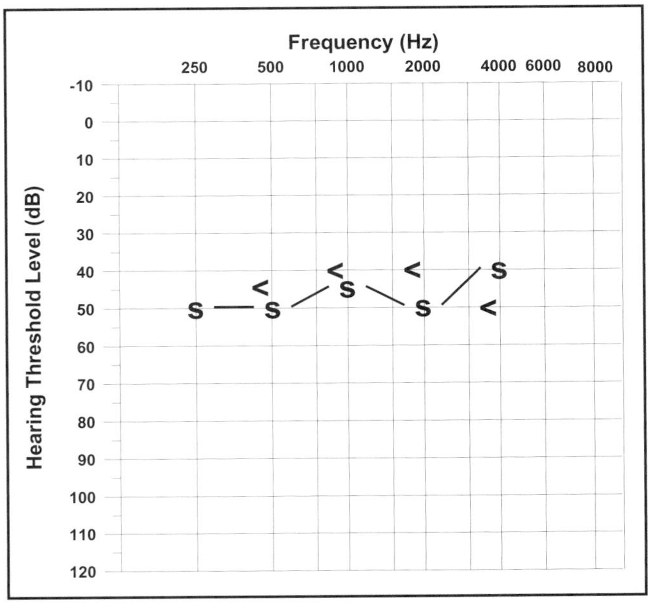

FIGURE 38–2. Auditory thresholds at 18 months of age.

enlarged vestibular aqueducts, and Pendred syndrome in particular, often experience a progression in their hearing loss. The change in hearing may be sudden, and can negatively affect the family's adjustment to their child's hearing loss. Some families, at the onset of change in hearing status, may reenter an early phase of the grieving process and respond with feelings of denial, anger, or withdrawal. As a result, their ability to make decisions to implement changes in both audiologic and early service intervention can be diminished. For the Anderson family, early counseling regarding both the presence of enlarged vestibular aqueducts and Pendred syndrome facilitated discussion about a newly detected hearing loss in their daughter's previously unaffected ear. Similarly, because she was aware that Jamie's hearing loss could progress and might affect her other ear, Jamie's mother was better equipped to revisit the decision to pursue the use of hearing aids. Given the increasing severity of their toddler's condition, the family opted to obtain conventional amplification for their child. Prior to involvement of her right ear, audiologic management for the family had focused exclusively on monitoring Jamie's hearing levels and auditory development. However, development of a bilateral hearing loss led to the addition of another critical level of services to the family's current needs and the decision to have Jamie fitted for hearing aids.

Hearing Aid Counseling

Hearing aids and other assistive listening devices (i.e., FM/infrared, cochlear implant) introduce a new component of follow-up care. Here again an opportunity to facilitate family empowerment and address major areas of concern has arisen. The primary concern for most parents at hearing aid fitting relates to proper maintenance of the device (Table 38–3). These concerns can supersede anxieties about the appearance and the potential benefit of the hearing aids for their child (Sjoblad, Harrison, Roush, & McWilliam, 2001). Later, Desjardin (2005) published findings that also underscored the need for *routine* informational counseling on device use and maintenance beyond the initial hearing aid fitting. In her study, mothers of children with hearing aids perceived themselves as less knowledgeable and competent than mothers of children with cochlear implants in checking and adjusting child's sensory device. This trend was more prevalent among mothers of children who received amplification later or delayed enrollment in early intervention. Accordingly, it seems that families with later access to services are less likely to develop comfort and skill in their use and maintenance of hearing aids over time. Routine counseling on how to optimize device performance is a much needed support, particularly when a change in technology or the child's hearing status has occurred.

For most families, optimal device functioning will necessitate additional appointments to remake earmolds or receive repairs particularly in the first three years of a child's life. Educating families on the proper use and maintenance of hearing aids can reduce the need to provide services in a clinical setting. In the early years, clinical contact is vital to insure the maximal use of the device. A frequent need to remake and fit earmolds, particularly in the early years, is a recognized component of device care but often a source of frustration to families. Providing clinical services in a flexible manner can alleviate this strain by allowing families to access services at the times and locations that are convenient to their schedule. Flexibility in service delivery can occur in a variety forms. If a family has a long commute to the clinic, local providers, even those audiology practices with a predominantly adult clientele, can provide routine services for earmolds. Over time, caregivers of children who are long-

Table 38–3. Parental Concerns About Hearing Aid Fitting

Parents Reported Anxiety About:	*Parents Desired:*
changing batteries	careful explanation & demonstration
cleaning earmolds	providing clear simply written instructions
insertion of earmolds	providing instructional videos
hearing aid retention	scheduling a follow-up appointment within 2 weeks

Sjoblad, Harrison, Roush, & McWilliam, (2001)

term hearing aid users may be trained to cut tubing and attach new molds to their child's hearing aids. When molds are delivered directly to the family, the number of clinic appointments and demands upon the pediatric audiologist's time can be reduced. Earmolds have a limited shelf life and maximizing their use by even 1 to 2 weeks is worthwhile. In the United Kingdom, teachers of the deaf who provide regular home visits to families have been trained and accredited by health services staff to take earmold impressions (Early Support, 2009, Jun 9). If the early service system and its providers are mobilized to deliver services across a variety of settings, the demands of effective follow-up care are reduced for caregivers and this factor can directly impact the overall quality of life for families. Although reducing the number of audiologic visits may be beneficial to family resources, it is important to recognize that the earmold is a permanent part of the hearing aid system and effectively accounting for its' influence on device output is most accurately done by reassessing hearing thresholds through new earmolds and obtaining real-ear to coupler difference (RECD) measures. When the audiologist is available to do this, the best estimate of the sound pressure level (SPL) at threshold in the child's ear is obtained (see Chapter 25 of this volume for greater detail). Thus, this strategy should be employed in moderation with visits to the audiologist for at least every other set of earmolds.

AGE: 18 to 36 months old

Over the course of the next 18 months, Jamie's thresholds continued to worsen. She continued to receive audiologic assessment to monitor her status on nearly a monthly basis. At 22 months of age, Jamie was fitted with an FM system to enhance her digital hearing aids in conditions of noise and distance; however, concerns of poor word recognition motivated the discussion regarding her potential candidacy for a cochlear implant. At 30 months of age, Jamie was evaluated by a speech-language pathologist from the local cochlear implant team to assess her current receptive and expressive language skills. Based upon the results of a comprehensive cochlear implant evaluation, implantation was recommended. Surgery was scheduled to occur at 32 months but had to be rescheduled because of a family emergency. Jamie received a cochlear implant at 34 months of age (Figure 38–3).

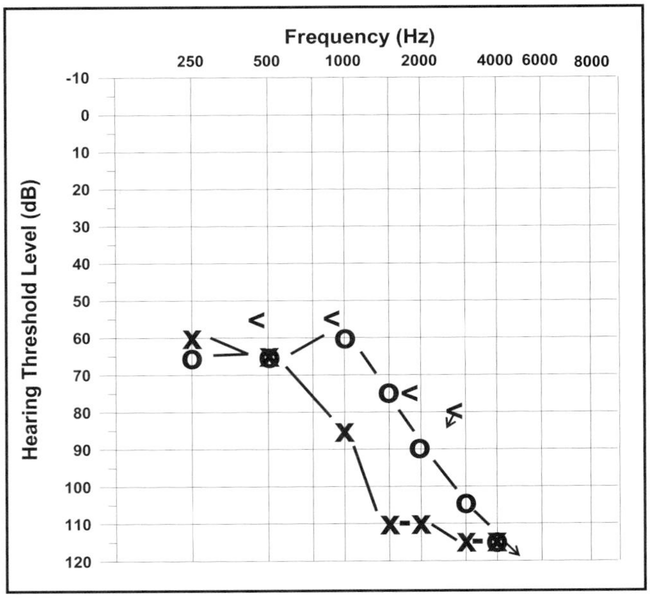

FIGURE 38–3. Results of audiometric testing at 30 months of age.

Professional Collaboration

Over the first 2½ years of Jamie's life, her hearing loss progressed from a moderate, unilateral loss to bilateral and severe-profound. The Andersons experienced multiple revisions to the decisions they made about managing their daughter's hearing loss and their expectations for how it would affect her life as well as theirs. They dealt with the increasing demands on their time and resources for audiology and medical appointments, and they absorbed information related to anatomy, genetics, hearing aid management, measures of audibility, and many other related topics. They are now being asked to make decisions regarding cochlear implantation that will require interacting with a different team of audiologists.

Fortunately for the Andersons, at this site, the pediatric audiologists and the cochlear implant team have developed a formal collaborative network. They meet as a group once a week to discuss any children whose diagnosis and hearing status potentially could result in a move from hearing aids to cochlear implants. Thus, the implant team is fully aware of Jamie's medical and audiologic history. They are knowledgeable about the family's commitment to Jamie's consistent use of amplification and their understanding of the environmental factors that affect their daughter's ability to hear. The C.I. team's speech-language pathologist evaluated Jamie's speech and language when she was 18 months old and is familiar with her and her mother. In fact, when the speech and language evaluation was conducted, it occurred at the cochlear implant center. Thus, the Andersons have already visited the site and are familiar with some of the staff. In addition, the possibility of the eventual need for cochlear implantation was discussed with the Andersons when enlarged vestibular aqueducts and Pendred's syndrome were diagnosed. The recommendation for implantation is therefore not a surprise and the family, who has observed deterioration in Jamie's ability to hear, especially in noise or at a distance is emotionally prepared.

Collaboration between Jamie's audiologist, her parents, and the audiologists and speech language pathologists on the implant team should not only reduce duplication of assessment measures, but also help to build a sense of trust and confidence in the Andersons as they approach the next phase of their journey in managing their child's hearing loss.

Conclusion

The discussion presented here adds to the current understanding of family-centered practice a context-based illustration relevant to the some of the decisions confronted by families after the early detection of hearing loss followed by diagnosis and management. In this view, professionals who operate from an approach that supports and empowers families will:

1. Collaborate with EHDI programs to facilitate family's journey from screening to diagnosis in a timely, effective manner;
2. Regard the newborn hearing screening and identification as an educational process that seeks to facilitate informed-decision making among parents of children with hearing loss;
3. Address the family's concerns at the time of diagnosis and beyond;
4. Advocate for the optimal level of services and supports across all families;
5. Encourage opportunities for parent participation in assessment of hearing and device performance;
6. Adapt the service delivery model to accommodate the family's resources and strengths as they evolve over time; and
7. Communicate consistently and effectively with the medical and/or habilitation providers who routinely serve the family in other settings.

An empowerment philosophy for families of children with hearing loss emphasizes the capacity of caregivers to recognize, procure, and manage the supports that contribute to their own priorities and needs. To the measure that families regard clinicians as supportive agents in their own process of change, they are empowered. Undoubtedly, systemic factors such as lack of institutional support or technical resources may limit the service options that the practitioner can offer. Nonetheless, empowered family-centered practice constitutes a collaborative and evolving *relationship* between parents and professionals. Although external stressors may affect the kind of decisions made in this relationship, the audiologist and family will collectively determine its nature and quality.

References

American Speech-Language-Hearing Association (ASHA). (2008). *Guidelines for audiologists providing informational and adjustment counseling to families of infants and young children with hearing loss birth to 5 years of age* [Guidelines]. Available from http://www.asha.org/policy

Calderon, R., & Greenberg, M. (1999). Stress and coping in hearing mothers of children with hearing loss: Factors affecting mother and child adjustment. *American Annals of the Deaf, 144*(1), 7–18.

Centers for Disease Control (CDC). (2009, May 29). *Annual EHDI Data 2006*. Retrieved June 3, 2008, from http://www.cdc.gov/ncbddd/ehdi/data.htm

Davis, A., Reeve, K., Hind, S., & Bamford, J. (2002). Children with mild and unilateral impairment. In R. C. Seewald & J. S. Gravel (Eds.), *A sound foundation through early amplification 2001* (pp. 179–186). Proceedings of the Second International Conference, Great Britain: St. Edmundsbury Press.

DesJardin, J. (2005). Maternal perceptions of self-efficacy and involvement in the auditory development of young children with prelingual deafness. *Journal of early intervention, 27,* 193–209.

DesJardin, J. (2006). Family empowerment: Supporting language development in young children who are deaf or hard of hearing. *Volta Review, 106*(3) (Monograph), 275–298.

Dunst, C. (2000). Revisiting "Rethinking early intervention." *Topics in Early Childhood Special Education, 20,* 95–104.

Dunst, C., Boyd, K., Trivette, C., & Hamby, D. (2002). Family-oriented program models and professional helpgiving practices. *Family Relations, 51,* 221–229.

Dunst, C., Trivette, C., & Deal, A. (1994). Enabling and empowering families. In C. J. Dunst, C.M., Trivette, M., & A.G. Deal (Eds.), *Supporting and strengthening families. Vol. 1. Methods, strategies and practices* (pp. 171–186). Cambridge, MA: Brookline Books.

Dunst, C., Trivette, C., Hamby, D. (2007). Meta-analysis of family-centered helpgiving practices research. *Mental Retardation and Developmental Disabilities, 13*, 370–378.

Early Support. (2009, Jun 9). *Informed choice, families and deaf children: Professional handbook.* Retrieved June 9, 2009, from http://www.earlysupport.org.uk/decMaterialZone/modResourcesLibrary/HtmlRenderer/Informed%20choice.html

Gravel, J., & McCaughey, C. (2004). Family-centered audiologic assessment for infants and young children with hearing loss. *Seminars in Hearing, 25*, 309–317.

Harrison, M., & Roush, J. (1996). Age of suspicion, identification, and early intervention in infants with hearing loss: A national study. *Ear and Hearing, 17*, 55–62.

Jackson, C., & Turnbull, A. (2004). Impact of deafness on family life: A review of the literature. *Topics in Early Childhood Special Education, 24*(1), 15–29.

Joint Committee on Infant Hearing (JCIH). (2007). Year 2007 Position statement: Principles and guidelines for early hearing detection and intervention programs. *Pediatrics, 120*, 898–921.

Kiese-Himmel, C. (2002). Unilateral sensorineural hearing impairment in childhood: Analysis of 31 consecutive cases. *International Journal of Audiology, 41*, 57–63.

Meadow-Orlans, K., Mertens, D., Sass-Lehrer, M., & Scott-Olson, K. (1997). Support services for parents and their children who are deaf or hard of hearing: A national survey. *American Annals of the Deaf, 142*, 278–288.

Roush, J. (2000). What happens after screening? *Hearing Journal, 53*, 56–60.

Roush, J., & Harrison, M. (2002). What parents want to know at diagnosis and during the first year. *Hearing Journal, 55*, 52–54.

Sass-Lehrer, M. (2004). Early detection of hearing loss: Maintaining a family-centered perspective. *Seminars in Hearing, 25*, 295–307.

Sjoblad, S., Harrison, M., Roush, J., & McWilliam, R. (2001). Parents' reactions and recommendations after diagnosis and hearing aid fitting. *American Journal of Audiology, 11*(1), 24–31.

Steinberg, A., Bain, L., Li, Y., & Ruperto, V. (2003). Decisions Hispanic families make after the identification of deafness. *Journal of Deaf Studies and Deaf Education, 8*, 291–314.

Tattersall, H., & Young, A. (2006). Deaf children identified through newborn hearing screening: Parents' experiences of the diagnostic process. *Child: Care, Health and Development, 32*, 33–45.

Williams, D., & Darbyshire, J. (1982). Diagnosis of deafness: A study of family responses and needs. *Volta Review, 84*, 24–30.

Yoshinago-Itano, C. (2003). Early intervention after universal neonatal hearing screening: Impact on outcomes. *Mental Retardation and Developmental Disabilities, 9*, 252–266.

Zaidman-Zait, A. (2007). Parenting a child with a cochlear implant: A critical incident study. *Journal of Deaf Studies and Deaf Education, 12*(2), 221–241.

39

Family Informational and Support Counseling

Kris English

You don't really understand human nature unless you know why a child on a merry-go-round will wave at his parents every time around—and why his parents will always wave back.

William D. Tammeu

Merry-go-rounds and waving . . . a charming image, but what does it have to do with family counseling? Please keep this question in the back of your mind. It will be posed again at the end of the chapter, and at that point, you will have at least one answer.

Introduction

Pediatric audiologists engage in counseling in virtually every family interaction. But what *kind* of counseling is occurring? It is important to remember that we have two kinds of counseling options available to us. One option is *informational counseling*, which is a formal name for our efforts to educate families about their child's hearing loss. While in "informational counseling mode," we explain to families what their child can and cannot hear, why amplification is needed, the nature of early intervention, and so on. In fact, the content of this textbook represents the body of information the pediatric audiologist will likely want to convey to families at the appropriate time.

However, conveying information is only one aspect of counseling. While adjusting to the diagnosis of their child's hearing loss, families experience a range of psychological and emotional reactions. Those reactions are not easily resolved, nor are they filed away as "finished business" at some point. Rather, these reactions recur in some fashion throughout their child's development, and can disrupt the overall adjustment process. Because audiologists are the primary service provider for children's hearing loss, their families are right to expect us to provide ongoing *support counseling* for these adjustment challenges.

Informational and support counseling are two sides of the same coin, the coin being "family care." Therefore, counseling should be perceived as a dual-consciousness activity. That is, while information is being conveyed, the audiologist also should watch for reactions to the information. And when support counseling is being provided, the audiologist also must determine if including information will help or hinder the support process.

This chapter describes basic strategies for effective informational and support counseling, including the skill needed to determine which type of counseling to provide.

Informational Counseling

Conveying information is *teaching*. We teach when we explain and demonstrate new information to family members, an activity that could occur at every appointment. However, audiologists are not always familiar with the science of *teaching effectively*. The fact that something was explained does not ensure that the learner understood it. In fact, research shows that explaining alone usually does not result in real understanding.

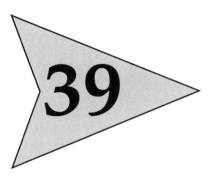

So, how do professionals convey information effectively? That is, how do audiologists help families not only understand, but also remember and apply the information we convey? This section summarizes current research on how adults learn, and how best to facilitate that learning.

How People Learn

Learning is a specialty area in the fields of neurology, cognitive psychology, and patient education. Learning involves an organized and permanent change in brain function; synaptic connections become more efficient, allowing the learner to create new connections to previously learned information, making it easier to retrieve and use at a later point. These changes most likely will occur when the brain is fully engaged. Here is how Zull (2002) describes a fully engaged brain while in learning mode:

- the sensory cortex takes in new auditory and visual input;
- the back integrative cortex engages in memory formation;
- the frontal integrative cortex engages in problem-solving; and
- the motor cortex carries out plans originating from the frontal integrative cortex.

Effective learning occurs when all of these activities take place. When we only explain, we only engage the sensory cortex, minimizing the likelihood of complete understanding.

Following are two "timeless principles of learning" (Suter & Suter, 2008) with applications for pediatric ("fully-engaging-the-brain") informational counseling.

Knowledge Is Enhanced by Activity: Learners Remember What They Do

It is quite reasonable for parents to doubt the diagnosis of a hearing loss when their own observations do not support that diagnosis. Indeed, children with mild and moderate loss will still startle to loud sounds and notice voices, so parents become understandably skeptical. They have been told there is a hearing loss, but their observations indicate no hearing problems.

To help parents work their way through this dilemma, in 2002 Anderson created the Early Listening Function (ELF; http://www.phonak.com/com_elf_questionnaire_gb.pdf). The ELF is a "discovery tool" to help parents actively test their child's age-expected auditory responses to sounds that are loud or soft, near or far, low or high pitched (male versus female voices). As they hold their child, present sounds and watch reactions, parents begin to understand and remember because they are "doing"—they are cross-checking their own observations to expected behaviors, and they are also learning a concept called the "listening bubble." The listening bubble is the space around the child where hearing is optimal; beyond that bubble, hearing will be a challenge. The size of the bubble will be different for every child, and it will change when using amplification. The ELF helps parents "learn by doing" and is an invaluable exercise to help parents move forward.

Learning Is Enhanced by Social Interaction: Learners Need Social Engagement in Learning

When asked what they need most, parents often will place "contact with other parents" at the top of their list. This request is consistent with the need for social engagement.

Parent support groups should be run by parents, and pediatric audiologists can help by providing a meeting place, childcare arrangements, and other logistical support. Support via the internet is also available, especially through special interest groups or communities of practice (Shirky, 2008). Social engagement helps parents ask other parents "How do you do this?"—for instance, how do you handle discipline, hearing aid problems, questions from strangers, sibling issues, pressure from grandparents? How do you navigate the special education system? How do you help your child develop and maintain friendships?

Whether in person or online, only "seasoned parents" can answer these kinds of parenting questions with credibility. Pediatric audiologists can establish relationships with these groups and keep families apprised about events and membership. See "Resources" at the end of this chapter for the names of some parent support groups.

Beyond Audiology 101: Looking Ahead to Literacy

In addition to providing information about *hearing*, pediatric audiologists also need to help families understand the concept of *listening* as part of their child's cognitive development. We know (but parents may not yet realize) that a direct relationship exists from hearing to academic success. Specifically:

- hearing leads to listening;
- listening leads to understanding language;

- understanding language leads to using language;
- using language leads to phonemic awareness and other preliteracy skills; and
- preliteracy skills must be mastered before first grade (reading readiness).

All parents want their child to read! We know (but parents may not yet realize) that if hearing is not optimal, the subsequent steps will be delayed, perhaps irreparably (Cole & Flexer, 2007).

"Learning language" is an abstract concept, and early interventionists and speech-language pathologists face the challenge of explaining that concept to parents. However, all parents know what learning to read means (Bus, van Ijzendoorn, & Pellegrini, 1995; Yarosz & Barnett, 2001). Yet, they typically are not aware that *years of consistent auditory input* are a prerequisite to learning to read. For example, children need to clearly hear a phoneme (for example, /b/) literally thousands of time before they are *cognitively ready* to associate the sound of that phoneme ("buh") with its written symbol. This skill is called "sound-symbol association." Children who do not use amplification consistently will not receive the necessary early exposure to speech sounds, and thus will not be ready to make the cognitive connection between sound and symbol when they enter the first grade.

Audiologists should be sufficiently conversant in literacy development to help parents understand the linked relationships from hearing to listening, to phonemic awareness and preliteracy skills (Figure 39–1). Audiologists can and should also provide direction to parents regarding their state's first grade learning standards, most of which rely on age-level listening skills.

Caveat: This topic must be approached differently when families actively identify with Deaf culture. New strategies such as Visual Phonics (Tresek & Malmgren, 2005) are being used to improve reading skills for children who are not accessing the world of sound. Even though 95% of children with hearing loss have at least one hearing parent (Mitchell & Karchmer, 2004), the audiologist cannot predict a family's cultural identification.

How can we help the family focus on helping the child achieve "reading readiness" when entering first grade? The pediatric audiologist should consider this topic as routine as any other issue discussed during appointments. In the United States, every state's Department of Education has a Web site with materials written for parents, describing specific benchmarks for each grade. A section on language arts, for example, will indicate, "what is expected in Grade 1" (from http://www.OhioAcademicStandards.com):

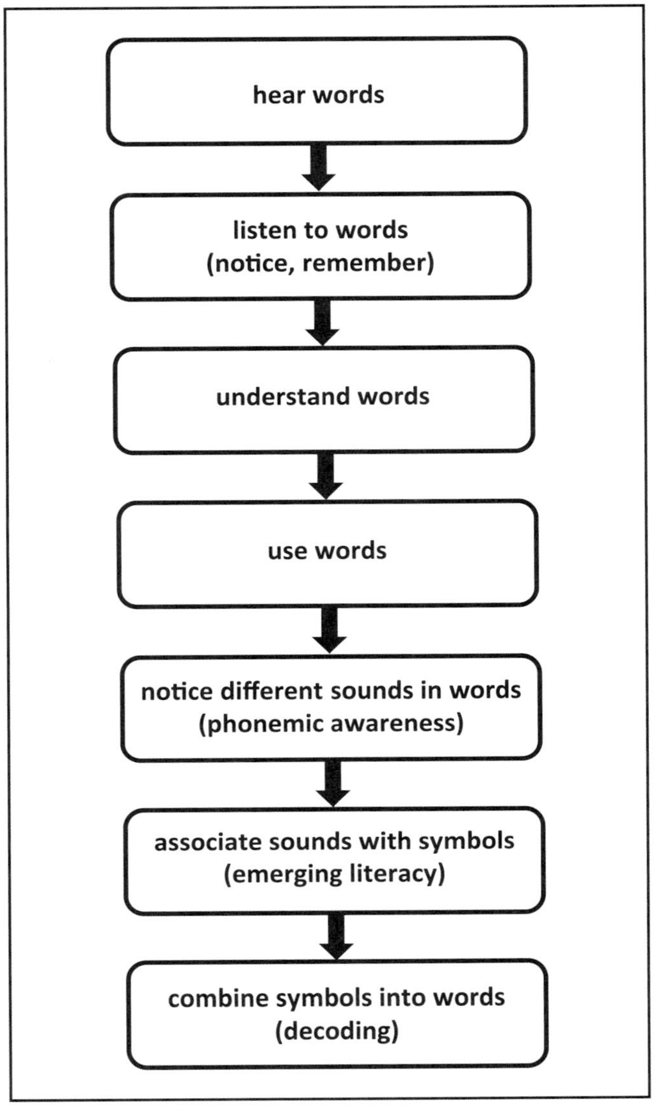

FIGURE 39–1. Sequence of skills leading to literacy.

- being able to read well by sounding out words;
- being able to recognize clues in writing, ask questions, listen, and converse with adults and peers;
- know the meaning of compound words (raindrop, daydream) using what is already known about the individual words; and
- using the steps of pre-writing, drafting, revising, and editing to produce different types of writing.

All of these skills are predicated on age-appropriate listening skills. Families are well served when they are aware of these standards, and also given information on how to support their child's development toward reaching these standards. Following are some examples, with "enhanced listening components" for children with impaired hearing:

- Gather pictures, alphabet letters, or other objects. Let your child tell you which objects are alike, which are different, and why. *Enhanced listening component:* pronounce two sounds (ay/ee or sh/sh) while covering your mouth (without muffling your speech), and ask your child, Are these two sounds the same or different?
- Say a word or show your child a picture. Let your child write or say the beginning and final sounds. *Enhanced listening component:* pronounce two words (dog, dad) and ask, are the first two sounds the same? Are the last two sounds the same?
- Write four to five words that would make a complete sentence. Make sure the beginning of the sentence begins with a capital letter and the last word ends with a period. Next, have the child put the words in an order than makes sense. *Enhanced listening component*: Say the words in any order and ask the child to organize the words in the order given.

An important note: the suggested "enhanced listening components" are not part of these educational materials. The audiologist will need to add them. We can help families develop their child's listening skills by building on predeveloped parent materials.

The Child Connected to These Ears

One mother reports:

> When our son was diagnosed with profound hearing loss, we immediately committed ourselves to his success. We kept every appointment, religiously put his hearing aids on every day; we hired specialists to improve his speech. His early years consisted of appointments, therapy, and homework.
>
> We were so focused on helping him with his hearing loss, we forgot to attend to his social development—his development as a person. We arranged no play dates, were oblivious to the other children in the neighborhood, drove right past the park and the local preschool.
>
> Now he is 8 years old. We've changed schools to give him a fresh start because his friendship skills were nonexistent, but that didn't help. He doesn't know how to approach other children, share or talk to them, or just be nice to them. The other children actively avoid him.
>
> If even one professional had asked us about his social development, we would have pulled our heads out of the treatment "sand" and realized we were overlooking something. And at this stage in his life, it's become the most important thing!

Do pediatric audiologists ask about children's social development? Do we ask parents if their child has a friend to play with, or other social opportunities? We may be the "one professional" who reminds parents that their child needs practice communicating with their peers and support in learning how to make and keep friends.

In addition to adding this topic to our repertoire, we can also suggest reading materials on overall child development, or provide brochures that summarize this topic. For instance, pediatrician Greenspan and colleagues (Greenspan & Greenspan, 1985; Greenspan & Lewis, 1999) write about parents' roles in supporting their child's social and emotional growth, and summarizes key points in a functional developmental growth chart. Children with hearing loss may experience some initial delays while finalizing the diagnosis and waiting for amplification; however, if parents are consistent in hearing aid use, they should be able to expect their child to catch up.

Stage 1: Regulation and Attention

By 3 months of age, infants should be showing an interest in things in the environment. They should be able to focus while remaining calm and regulated. Even with a hearing loss, infants should be visually attentive. Ask families about those behaviors.

Stage 2: Engaging in Relationships

By 5 months of age, infants should seem happy or pleased when they see favorite people by looking and smiling, making sounds or moving arms and legs that indicate delight. In this stage, infants "fall in love" with their caregivers, and one of the inputs that affect this development is the human voice. When infants cannot hear "the love in one's voice" because of hearing loss, there is all the more reason to stress the value of amplification to parents. Focusing on the development of the parent-child relationship and bonding is very meaningful to parents, probably more so than the development of speech and language.

Stage 3: Interacting in a Purposeful Manner and Becoming a Two-Way Communicator

By 9 months, children should be able to show what they want by pointing at something, reaching out to be picked up, and making purposeful noises. Children using amplification should also be developing as communicators, so at this stage we should be asking not only for parents' reports on auditory responses, but also on two-way communication.

Stage 4: Organizing Chains of Interaction for Simple and Complex Problem-Solving and Forming a Sense of Self

By age 14 to 18 months, toddlers are able to show parents what they want by using actions, such as leading them by the hand to the refrigerator, tugging on the handle, and pointing to juice or milk. Toddlers also use imitation to interact, with sounds, words, or gestures.

Stage 5: Using Ideas (Words/Symbols) to Convey Intentions or Feelings

By age 24 to 30 months of age, toddlers imitate familiar pretend actions ("driving" or "cooking"). The toddler's world expands to include peers, and to engage in parallel play with another child. This kind of play is not heavily dependent on verbal communication. This is the time to ask the family about peer play opportunities.

Stage 6: Creating Logical Bridges between Ideas

By 36 months of age, children engage in pretend play and are occasionally able to use feelings to explain behaviors or desires ("Because I'm mad/happy"). Understanding one's emotions and being able to name them is a cornerstone skill to social development; children are not able to understand their peers' feelings until they understand their own feelings.

Summary

Pediatric audiologists should be able to converse with parents about their child's overall development. While not being expected to have a high level of expertise in child development, we should have enough background to ask parents informed questions about their child's overall development, provide relevant materials, and make referrals when necessary.

The Merry-Go-Round

We started this chapter with the image of a child on a merry-go-round. Has the first part of this chapter helped you understand why child and parent wave? Does the audiologist as an effective *information counselor* help parent and child enjoy this moment? Keep thinking about this dynamic and what it means to families.

Support Counseling

Staying in Step with Families

During each moment that family members process information, they also experience a range of emotional reactions. The reactions cannot be predicted, but they may include shock, fear, confusion, vulnerability, doubt, guilt, and grief (Luterman, 2008).

PET scan studies confirm that we think and feel simultaneously. Typically, one process (for example, thinking) takes precedence over the other (feeling) depending on the circumstance, but the second process is never completely out of the picture.

Goleman (2006) describes "emotional intelligence" as the ability to perceive whether someone is communicating with a "thinking mind" or a "feeling mind." Communicating with the "thinking mind" includes discussing data, specific details, and other types of information. Communicating with a "feeling mind" includes recognizing and discussing psychological and emotional states. The pediatric audiologist's challenge is not only to recognize which "mind" a family member is using at a given moment, but also how to respond accordingly. That is, a "thinking mind" comment or question should be given a "thinking mind" response (information). On the other hand, a "feeling mind" comment or question should be given a "feeling mind" response (acknowledging the emotions or psychological reactions that were expressed).

If we are not paying attention, we are likely to "mismatch" our response (English, Rojeski, & Branham, 2000). This mismatch most often occurs when families describe *how they feel*, whereas our response indicates *what we think*. This mismatch is often a result of training, wherein we are prompted to give information to demonstrate to our supervisor that we indeed know specific information. However, family members are not our supervisors; a different audience needs a different approach. Here is an example of a typical exchange:

Dialogue #1

Parent: My in-laws claim that our little boy Aaron was born deaf because I worked until the last week of pregnancy.

Audiologist: Our research indicates otherwise; there is no reason to worry about that.

In this exchange, listen to the parent's subtext: she is indirectly reporting *how she feels* (guilt, stress, fear). Regrettably, the audiologist did not notice, and instead indicated *what she thinks* (by citing data and research). A "matched" response would have actively addressed the "feeling mind," such as, "That sounds like a difficult situation." Audiologists can learn to avoid communication mismatches by "raising their antenna" to listen at a deeper level to the subtext, and then respond with reflective comments that invite more conversation (Clark & English, 2004; English et al., 2000). This skill is an important one to develop. Mismatching our responses frustrates the family and interferes with the development of a supportive relationship.

How do we prevent mismatches? When in doubt, address both possibilities. After providing content or data, step back and ask the patient about the emotional components of the comment, or inquire if they are not explicitly stated, as we see demonstrated in this exchange:

Dialogue #2

Audiologist: Your suspicions were correct, Ms. Watson, your son does have hearing loss in both ears.

Parent: I should have done something about this much sooner.

Audiologist: The main thing is, we can do something now. (Stops, recognizes the mismatch). But . . . much sooner? Are you thinking about an earlier time?

Parent: Yes, back on his first birthday, some loud sound happened and I wondered about it then. But he is pretty hard to read in a lot of ways, you know?

Audiologist: Sure. You had no real information to work with.

Parent: That's it exactly. I couldn't be sure of what I saw, and I didn't know what to do when I did see it. But (ready to move forward), here we are, what do we do next?

The "sidebar" conversation took an extra 20 seconds, and yet it made an important and positive difference in relationship-building. The audiologist perceived a clear call for help, and was aware that unacknowledged feelings do not disappear; they fester (Pipher, 2006), so she took the time to ask for an elaboration. When it was provided, she accepted it as a gift, as it were, without judgment. The parent is learning that the audiologist is listening carefully, and will accept whatever the parent has to say. The audiologist has indicated that she trusts the parent, and the parent is starting to decide she can trust the audiologist.

The desired outcome for both kinds of counseling (informational and support) is to establish a therapeutic relationship with the patient. Research shows that relationships are a vital component to health care, as explained in the next section.

Relationship-Centered Care

Present-day medical care is based on the principle of patient autonomy. That is, patients are recognized to have the "final say" regarding health care recommendations. This reality is a challenge for audiologists. We often see families who, even in the face of strong evidence and their own experiences, still decide against our recommendations. Why?

When a recommendation is rejected, the decisions are often related to fear and distrust. On the other hand, when families adhere to recommendations, they are quite likely to report experiencing a supportive relationship with their health care provider. Studies have examined the variables that affect patients' decisions to adhere to recommendations for diabetes management, smoking cessation, weight control, and other health concerns. Patients who reported a sense of trust and partnership with their health care provider were far more likely to adhere to their provider's recommendations. The supportive relationship between patient and provider makes the difference. As Taylor (2002) puts it, "Social support is good medicine" (p. 81).

Relationship-centered care (Tresolini, 2000) is especially applicable to audiologic counseling. Families may wish they could disregard the diagnosis and live the life they had expected to live. Our recommendations ask families to modify their expectations, make decisions, and take on unfamiliar responsibilities. It is human nature to pull back rather than move toward change. However, it is also human nature to "choose growth" (Rogers, 1979) when we perceive we are in an environment of support and genuine care. Hence, families are far more likely to move forward when they perceive a supportive relationship with their audiologist.

The foundation for any relationship is trust. It is difficult to explain how to earn and foster trust, but one example might help us start to understand this process. Imagine an audiologist conveying to a parent (unaccompanied by other family members) that her 1-month-old child has a hearing loss in both ears. The mother becomes distraught and starts to cry. The audiologist politely slides a box of tissues toward her and says, "I'll return when you feel better," and then leaves the room.

What message is the mother left with? "This situation is too personal for me." "Your lack of emotional control embarrasses me." "I am only able to communicate with you when you maintain your composure." Will the mother ever again trust the audiologist with her emotional reactions? Not likely; instead, she will work with the distance that the audiologist has created. The relationship will be stilted and superficial, and the family will be challenged to follow recommendations from a professional who does not seem to care.

Imagine now an alternative response. The audiologist slides over the box of tissues, moves her chair closer and puts her hand on the mother's arm, and waits. The parent may feel embarrassed about crying but knows the audiologist is not embarrassed. The parent may feel forlorn but will not feel abandoned. This time the message is, "We are in this together." The mother feels support, not distance. If she feels she can trust the audiologist in this difficult moment, she will more likely be able to trust her for the course of their partnership.

The audiologist has the ability to set the tone for the relationship, and, if the relationship is deteriorating, the audiologist can at least attempt to repair it. A consultative meeting might be needed, with this type of preamble: "We seem to be at odds lately, would you agree? If so, I'd like to start afresh, if you are willing. Where should we begin?" For example, imagine receiving this phone call:

Dialogue #3

Colleague:	I am working with a parent who is especially frustrating. She calls me at least twice a week with the same questions she's asked me before, and I can't figure out why she isn't listening to me. Our exchanges are getting more and more tense. I may need to refer her to you.
You:	Before you make that referral—how would you describe your relationship with this parent?
Colleague:	Not adversarial, but close to it. I'd say it's confusing, stressed, and disconnected.
You:	Trusting?
Colleague:	(Pauses) No . . . I would say I trust her ability to handle things and make decisions, but she keeps challenging me, so I guess she doesn't trust me. I don't know how that happened.
You:	Any possibility of making a fresh start?
Colleague:	Sure, anything is possible. How would I do that?
You:	Maybe visualize it—what would work best for your setting?
Colleague:	I could set aside some time so that we could just talk. I would need to control my tendency to dive in with all those answers. When she peppers me with all those questions, I immediately answer them—using my "thinking mind," as they say. But I actually don't know WHY she is asking the questions.
You:	That's why the relationship is a little confusing?
Colleague:	I think it's part of the problem. I've been implying I'm the "go-to" expert, while also saying she is the "captain" of this team. Mixed messages!

Occasionally, a family member may not know how, or is unwilling, to sustain a trusting relationship, but at least the audiologist can make the attempt. Usually, families will appreciate the genuine effort and will adjust to the new start. Those kinds of conversations would draw heavily on the counseling/listening strategies discussed in the following section.

Counseling Strategies

Counseling involves a complex skill set, supported by a deep theoretical base and scientific evidence. Three basic skills will be described here: differentiation, reflective listening, and—something *not* to do—refrain from answering every question. For additional information on counseling strategies, see Clark and English (2004) and English (2002).

Differentiation

In an earlier section, we discussed the concept of communicating with a "thinking mind" versus a "feeling mind." The pediatric audiologist needs to determine which "mind" the family is using at any given time, in order to avoid a communication mismatch. The skill used to perceive the difference is called *differentiation* (Cormier & Hackney, 2008). Differentiation is the cognitive act of listening carefully and asking oneself, "Is this a request for information or support?" It takes perhaps one second to ask oneself this question, so it would seem that differentiation is an easy skill to acquire. In fact, it is easy to learn but hard to maintain: almost anyone can demonstrate its use when asked to, but applying it on a regular basis throughout a busy workday, as an internal dialogue, is an ongoing challenge. See "Suggested Learning Activities" #4 and #5 for structured practice.

Reflective Listening

If our differentiation leads us to conclude that the comment or question was from the "feeling mind," our challenge is to match our response with a "feeling mind" comment. This skill is more formally called reflective listening (Rogers, 1979). Some principles of reflective listening include these three subskills:

- More listening than talking;
- Responding to what is personal rather than to what is impersonal or abstract;
- Restating and clarifying what the other has said, not telling what the listener feels or thinks.

The first subskill (more listening than talking) is much harder than it sounds. We may feel obligated to fill the "talk time" with our professional direction and advice, because is not that why the family is here? We will need to use mature professional judgment to determine if in fact that assumption is true; at any given point, the family may actually want us to listen, and share the talk time more than we expect.

The second subskill (responding to what is personal) again is a challenge in settings that value science, research, facts, and test results. Audiologists seem to need to be routinely reminded that the "ears belong to a person," and that the person is struggling with quality of life issues. Families seek help expecting an improvement in the quality of life, not a 50% improvement in recognition of single-syllable words per se. Responding to what is personal requires us to develop a comfort level with families' emotional states, and a willingness to discuss them.

The third subskill was "restating and clarifying what the other has said, not telling what the listener feels or thinks." An example of this strategy can be found in Dialogue #3, when the audiologist says, "You had no real information to work with." Restating the parent's point tells the parent: (1) "I am following you (and please correct me if I am not following you)," and (2) "I am waiting for the next thing you want to tell me." The parent can continue her train of thought, and is not obligated to answer distracting questions.

Reflective listening has been described as a figurative sounding board (Clark & English, 2004). If you have played the piano or violin, you already know that a sounding board is a piece of wood that is especially porous. It is built into those instruments in order to enhance the quality of the music being produced. It makes all the difference—and yet it does not actually create the music itself. It only resonates to the music.

Do Not Answer Every Question

You might have noticed in Dialogue #2 that when the colleague asked, "How would I do that?" a direct answer was not offered. Instead, another question was submitted: "What would work best for your setting?" And with that prompt, the caller answered his own question. His friend trusted his colleague's ability to manage the situation. In most counseling situations, the person with the problem does have his or her own answer—but at the moment when the question is asked, the person lacks clarity. The challenges are not well understood, and possible solutions are elusive. However, given an opportunity to verbally organize one's thoughts, explore options, weigh consequences, and sort out good and bad ideas, the speaker gains clarity and begins to understand the problem and hence the solution. For over 100 years, this process has been called "talk therapy," and recent neurologic evidence indicates that talking out one's problems helps the brain shift from chaotic random activity to focused and specialized activity (Friedman, 2002; Vaughn, 1997). When we say, "Now I understand!" our brains have literally changed its patterns and have found a way to operate more efficiently.

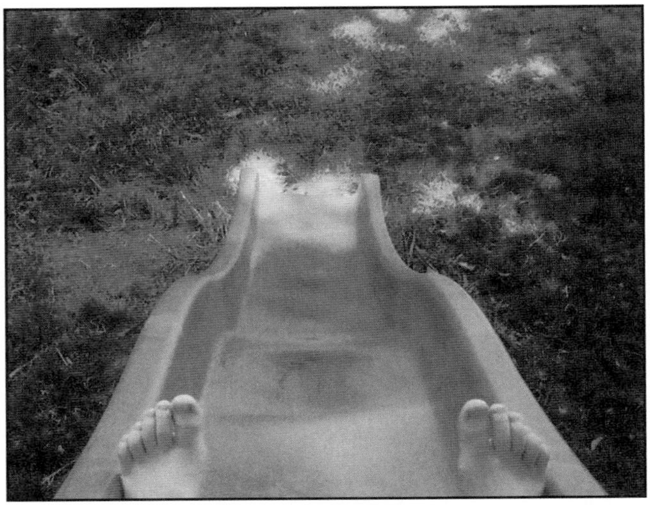

FIGURE 39–2. Child on the playground. Photo credit: Michael Donovan, age 7.

Summary

The second part of this chapter presented the concept of support counseling and its philosophical underpinnings as well as a few practical applications. Developing these skills requires practice and feedback. Evaluation tools designed to provide practice and feedback are listed in a subsequent section ("Evaluations for Counseling Skill Development").

Conclusion

We began this chapter with a quote about children and parents and waving (Figure 39–2). Visualize the situation and ask yourself: How does the child feel about his parent as he circles around and around? And how does the parent feel as he keeps his eye on the child and watches for that wave? If the child had a hearing loss, does that change how child and parent feel? Is the essential parent-child bond at risk? If so, what can pediatric audiologists do to support its development?

Suggested Learning Activities

1. Choose a typical topic of family informational counseling and design a teaching strategy that gives the learner something to do, or includes social interaction, or both.
2. Develop a sample parent brochure describing the "hearing-listening-reading" connection, including information drawn from your state's Department of Education on expected preliteracy skills for first grade.
3. Prepare a short presentation on general child development principles and describe how a pediatric audiologist can incorporate this perspective into family care.
4. Over the course of a semester, complete three or four "Listen For It" exercises. Open your ears, increase your attention to notice and write down comments heard from patients or family members that reflect adjustment concerns (e.g., "Are my daughter's processing problems caused by the year I home-schooled her?"). In addition to writing down the comment, describe possible emotions underlying the comment.
5. Perform the "Watch for It" exercise (similar to #4 above, developed by John Greer Clark, Ph.D., University of Cincinnati). Over the course of a semester, watch for and write down examples of effective communication "matching." When a patient or parent makes a "feeling mind" comment (e.g., "The kids at school make fun of me when I wear this FM thing"), make note of the audiologist's "feeling mind" response.
6. Download Tresolini's (2000) monograph on relationship-centered care (http://www.futurehealth.ucsf.edu/pdf_files/RelationshipCentered.pdf) and read pages 1–37. Write a paper on the apparent applications of relationship-centered care to the practice of pediatric audiology. Discuss with peers and instructors.

Resources

Alexander Graham Bell Association for the Deaf and Hard of Hearing, Parent Section: http://www.agbell.org

Boys Town: http://www.boystown.org

Early Listening Function (ELF): http://www.phonak.com/com_elf_questionnaire_gb.pdf

Hands and Voices: http://www.handsandvoices.org

John Tracy Clinic: http://www.jtclinic.org

Karen Anderson, Pediatric Consultant: http://www.kandersonaudconsulting.com

Evaluations for Counseling Skill Development

Audiologic Counseling Evaluation (ACE)
Described in English, K., Naeve-Velguth, S., Rall, E., Uyehara-Isono, J., & Pittman, A. (2007). Development of an instrument to evaluate audiologic counseling skills. *Journal of the American Academy of Audiology, 18*(8), 675–687. Available at http://gozips.uakron.edu/~ke3/ACE.pdf

Audiology Counseling Growth Checklist (ACGS)
Described in Clark, J. G. (2006). The Audiologic Counseling Growth Checklist for student supervision. *Seminars in Hearing, 27*(2), 116–126.

The 4 Habits Counseling Skills Rubric
Described in: English, K. (2008). Counseling issues in the delivery of aural rehabilitation services. *Contemporary Issues in Communication Sciences and Disorders, 35*, 93–101.

References

Bus, A.G., van Ijzendoorn, M., & Pellegrini, A. D. (1995). Joint book reading makes for success in learning to read: A meta-analysis on intergenerational transmission of literacy. *Review of Educational Research, 65*(1), 1–21.

Clark, J. G., & English, K. (2004). *Counseling in audiological practice: Helping patients and families adjust to hearing loss.* Boston, MA: Allyn & Bacon.

Cole, E., & Flexer, C. (2007). *Children with hearing loss: Developing listening and talking birth to six.* San Diego, CA: Plural.

Cormier, S., & Hackney, H. (2008). *Counseling strategies and interventions* (7th ed.). Boston, MA: Allyn & Bacon.

English, K. (2002). *Counseling children with hearing impairments and their families.* Boston, MA: Allyn & Bacon.

English, K., Rojeski, T., & Branham, K. (2000). Acquiring counseling skills in mid-career: Outcomes of a distance education course for practicing audiologists. *Journal of American Academy of Audiology, 11*, 84–90.

Friedman, R. A. (2002, August 27). Like drugs, talk therapy can change brain chemistry. *New York Times*. Retrieved June 30, 2008, from http://query.nytimes.com/gst/fullpage.html?res=9C06E1DF113CF934A1575BC0A9649C8B63&sec=&spon=&pagewanted=1

Goleman, D. (2006). *Emotional intelligence: Why it might matter more than IQ.* New York, NY: Bantam Books.

Greenspan, S., & Greenspan, N. (1985). *First feelings: Milestones in the emotional development of your baby and child.* New York, NY: Penguin Books.

Greenspan, S. & Lewis, N.B. (1999). *Building healthy minds: The six experiences that create intelligence and emotional growth in babies and young children.* New York, NY: Da Capo Press.

Luterman D. L. (2008). *Counseling persons with communication disorders and their families* (5th ed.). Austin, TX: Pro-Ed.

Mitchell, R., & Karchmer, M. (2004). Chasing the mythical ten percent: Parental hearing status of deaf and hard of hearing students in the United States. *Sign Language Studies, 4*(2), 138–163.

Pipher, M. (2006). *Writing to change the world* (p. 100). New York, NY: Riverhead Books.

Rogers, C. R. (1979). Foundations of the person–centered approach. *Education, 100*(2), 98–107.

Shirky, C. (2008). *Here comes everybody: The power of organizing without organizations* (p. 101). New York, NY: Penguin Press.

Suter. P. M., & Suter, W. N. (2008). Timeless principles of learning: A solid foundation for enhancing chronic disease self-management. *Home Healthcare Nurse, 26*(2), 82–88.

Taylor, S. (2002). *The tending instinct: How nurturing is essential to who we are and how we live.* New York, NY: Henry Holt.

Tresek, B., & Malmgren, K. (2005). The efficacy of utilizing a phonics treatment package with middle school deaf and hard-of-hearing students. *Journal of Deaf Studies and Deaf Education, 10*(3), 256–271.

Tresolini, C. P. (2000). *Health professions education and relationship-centered care.* San Francisco, CA: Pew-Fetzer Professions Commission. http://www.futurehealth.ucsf.edu/pdf_files/RelationshipCentered.pdf

Vaughn, S. (1997). *The talking cure: The science behind psychotherapy.* New York, NY: Putnam.

Yarosz, D. J., & Barnett, W. S. (2001). Who reads to young children? Identifying predictors of family reading activities. *Reading Psychology, 22*, 67–81.

Zull, J. (2002). *The art of changing the brain: Enriching the practice of teaching by exploring the biology of learning.* Sterling, VA: Stylus.

40

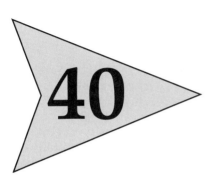

Potential Meets Reality in Early Intervention for Children With Hearing Loss

Amy McConkey Robbins

Introduction

This chapter explores issues related to the gaps that currently exist between the technology available to identify babies with hearing loss (HL) at very early ages and the reality of serving those babies and their families in a timely and comprehensive way. I explore these gaps recognizing the monumental progress that has been made in this arena over the last 15 years. It has taken the perseverance, creative use of resources, devoted energies and the best minds in our field to make Universal Newborn Hearing Screening (UNHS) possible in the United States and in many other countries. That UNHS is so widely used is a dream come true for many, including this author. The screening of all infants, though a necessary and momentous first step, was never intended to be the end goal, but rather the beginning of a long-term process to ensure communicative competence and ultimately, improve the quality of life of these children (Bamford, 1998). This is reflected in the term early hearing detection and intervention (EHDI), which is becoming more commonly used in place of UNHS and which implies a more comprehensive continuum of care.

The challenges clinicians face in serving babies and families after HL has been diagnosed in infancy are formidable. As with any health care movement that involves rapid changes in technology, legislative policies that impact multiple agencies, and urgency for widespread professional education, challenges are inevitable. It is incumbent on those of us working in EHDI to recognize the many ways in which we have succeeded, to acknowledge where we are falling short in our service to deaf and hard of hearing (D/HH) babies and their families, and to explore what might be done to manage children and families effectively, even within this gap between the vast potential of early detection of HL and the reality—the gap between "what could be" and "what is."

The Value of Early Screening and Diagnosis of Hearing Loss

The undeniable value of early screening and diagnosis of HL is covered at length elsewhere in this volume and is not repeated here, as this chapter deals primarily with communication intervention after HL is diagnosed. From the standpoint of a speech-language pathologist, I reinforce the importance of EHDI by noting that babies who are identified in the first six months of life and who shortly thereafter receive appropriate early intervention demonstrate substantially better communication outcomes than do later-identified children (See Joint Commission on Infant Hearing [JCIH] Year 2007 Position Statement for extensive references). Conversely, if HL is not identified and treated early, the consequences to spoken language are detrimental and often irreparable.

The issues in this chapter relate to families who have made an informed choice to value auditory development, who want their children to wear amplification, and who place importance on the development of spoken language, whether through methods of auditory-oral, auditory-verbal, cued speech, or spoken language augmented by manual signs. Issues of families who choose a strictly manual communication approach for their child, and/or where amplification is not a priority are beyond the scope of this chapter.

Advances in Serving This Population

Considering the tremendous changes over the last decade, we must acknowledge that many improvements have occurred in how D/HH babies and their families are served. Such improvements include the fact that hearing screening of newborns is now commonplace, thereby dramatically lowering the average age at which HL is diagnosed:

- Many techniques have been designed specifically to assess hearing and fit hearing aids and cochlear implants on infants and toddlers;
- Curricula have been published to help early-interventionists guide families in developing the baby's communication potential;
- Research on brain plasticity provides evidence to families and clinicians of the benefits of early auditory stimulation and the critical time-sensitive windows for auditory cortical development;
- Some universities have recognized the need to include early identification (EI) topics in their students' curricula and practicum;
- Preservice and in-service programs are becoming available so that clinicians who previously served only older children may learn the principles and practices of EI; and
- IDEA, the United States federally mandated Individuals with Disabilities Education Act legislation, stipulates that parents be informed of and offered choices about communication methods, and that they have a voice as full members of the team that writes the Individualized Family Service Plan (IFSP).

All of these actions represent improvement in our efforts to serve very young children with HL and their families.

The Potential of Early Intervention for D/HH Babies and Families

There is general agreement that the purpose of identifying HL through UNHS is not just to "know early" but to "act early." Extracting key points from the Joint Committee on Infant Hearing (JCIH) Year 2007 Position Statement, we could define "acting early" as diagnosing the hearing loss accurately before age three months, fitting appropriate amplification within one month of initial confirmation of HL, and providing family-centered early intervention by a clinician knowledgeable and experienced with this population before age 6 months. For purposes of this chapter, the term "early intervention" (EI) is used to mean parent-baby services directed at improving communication skills (i.e., auditory, speech, language, and pragmatics). The term "audiologic management" is used to mean the diagnosis and monitoring of the HL, and the fitting and maintaining of appropriate hearing instruments, recognizing that there may be considerable overlap between the two.

There has been overwhelming success in screening nearly all newborns in the United States, yet the steps that follow this screening in the widely used 1-3-6 month time frame of infant hearing management have a much lower rate of success. This represents one of the first gaps between potential and reality: the technology exists to successfully screen almost all newborns, but approximately half of those who fail the screening do not undergo further evaluation for HL by the recommended 3-month benchmark. In a technical paper (American Speech and Hearing Association [ASHA], 2008b) written by an ASHA working group and commissioned by the Centers for Disease Control and Prevention (CDC), it was noted that various EHDI jurisdictions designate infants and their families who miss the three-month benchmark for confirmation of HL as "lost to follow up" or "lost to documentation," without agreement about the definition of those terms. More recently, it has been suggested that these two designations might be combined under the broader heading of "lost to system" (LTS). State EHDI programs are working diligently to reduce the number of LTS infants. Indeed, progress toward this end is being made, with some EHDI jurisdictions reporting impressively low numbers of children who are LTS. Solutions to reducing overall LTS rates are ongoing and described elsewhere in this volume, but it is important to mention the issue here because high LTS rates early in the process create another gap between the potential and the reality of EI, largely due to a cascade effect. Based on national data, at least one-third of the children eventually referred for therapy services are behind the recommended schedule (i.e., older than age six months) when starting early intervention, in many cases because they did not meet the previous benchmark on time (i.e., confirmation of HL before 3 months; CDC, 2008).

Early Intervention Begins with the Audiologist

In 1998, as UNHS was just becoming a reality, Bamford (1998) cautioned that:

> It is important for us to reestablish in pediatric audiology a wider perspective; there is always a danger that pediatric audiology may be implemented as a narrow health-based discipline in which the outcome measures of importance stop at age of identification and age of HA fitting. (p. 353)

Taking Bamford's broader view of success, not just as the fitting of amplification, the long-term goals of early identification of HL are the child's achievement of communicative competence and enhanced quality of life. Achieving these goals becomes more realistic if pediatric audiologists recognize the important role they play in fostering a baby's communication development during the weeks and months of early confirmation of HL and fitting of amplification. A traditional model of the management of infants with HL would assign this role to early interventionists: speech-language pathologists or deaf educators. However, the foundation that is established by the audiologist during the earliest weeks and months with a family whose baby has a HL often sets the stage for either informed, involved families who have high expectations, or for passive families who struggle with managing their D/HH child and with achieving full-time use of amplification in a timely way. If audiologists begin the discussion of communication progress with families, EI can be thought of as overlapping with the fitting of amplification in infants. This is a role some audiologists are willing but unprepared to play, largely because they do not have tools readily available to: (a) guide families who are struggling with full-time HA use; and (b) connect such use directly to the development of auditory and spoken language proficiency. Throughout this chapter, suggestions are provided to help audiologists discuss with parents the direct connection between full-time use of amplification and spoken language development.

Features of Early Intervention for Infants With Hearing Loss and Their Families

We have acknowledged that an initial gap exists between the technology available to screen babies at birth and the success rate of confirming HL before age 3 months, and that this creates an additional gap by delaying the age at which a substantial number of D/HH infants begin receiving EI. Another gap between potential and reality is covered in detail in the next section: the gap between what have been identified as appropriate EI practices and the actual services many D/HH babies and families receive through federally-mandated IDEA Part C programs (In the United States, Part C of IDEA governs early intervention services for infants and toddlers with disabilities under age 3 years). Several official documents outline the characteristics of appropriate EI. For example, a position paper from an ASHA Ad Hoc Committee (ASHA, 2008a) addresses recommended practices for speech-language pathologists who conduct EI with infants or toddlers who have disabilities. This document outlines four guiding principles of EI:

1. Services are family centered and culturally and linguistically responsive;
2. Services are developmentally supportive and promote children's participation in their natural environments;
3. Services are comprehensive, coordinated, and team based;
4. Services are based on the highest quality evidence that is available.

As we shall discover, the EI services many D/HH children receive fall short of adhering to one or more of these principles. For some families, there are considerable barriers to receiving EI that approximates the four principles above. Barriers to meeting these four guiding principles are multilayered and differ widely across EHDI jurisdictions. The next section reviews the four principles and provides examples illustrating the barriers some families and clinicians encounter.

Principle 1: Services Are Family Centered and Culturally and Linguistically Responsive

"Family-centered" service has been the term of choice in EI for at least a decade, yet it remains an unattained goal in some cases. An often reported obstacle to family-centered services is that many clinicians were trained in a traditional therapy model and are accustomed to conducting intervention as a "teacher-student" dyad. In a traditional therapy model, interactions are primarily controlled by the clinician, while the parent quietly observes, or in some cases, is not even present in the room. This is in conflict with a family-centered philosophy of EI in which the clinician does not "teach" the baby, but rather models effective communication techniques, coaches and encourages parents who gradually assume a greater leadership role during sessions. The goal of a family-centered model is that parents naturally incorporate techniques learned in EI to foster good language, speech, auditory and pragmatic skills with their baby during everyday activities. This shift in philosophy may be difficult for some seasoned clinicians to embrace.

A fundamental feature of "family-centered" EI is that it honors the choice of communication methodology and the goals families have expressed and written in the IFSP. This is also directly related to services being "culturally and linguistically responsive," as culture and language are deeply entwined in the fabric of families. Parents have reported facing multiple barriers to securing EI that is consistent with their communication choice and language. Five common barriers are reviewed in the following section. First, there may be no clinician in the geographic area who is trained to conduct EI in the communication method chosen by the parents. Second, the family may speak a language other than English, and there are neither clinicians nor interpreters in the geographic area who speak the language, or interpreters are available but the Part C program will not authorize their services. Third, there may be clinicians in the geographic area trained in the chosen communication method but their caseloads are full and families must wait until a therapy spot becomes available, which may be a matter of 6 months or more. Fourth, highly trained and experienced EI clinicians are available but may not approved as Part C providers because they conduct primarily center-based EI rather than home-based EI. This will be discussed further as it relates to "natural environment" policies. These four barriers result from the paucity of EI clinicians who are knowledgeable about HL, or fluent in another language, or authorized as Part C providers, relative to the number of babies being diagnosed and referred for EI services.

Communication Bias

The fifth barrier to "family-centered and culturally/linguistically responsive" EI is of a different nature. It relates to the bias toward a particular communication method that may exist among members of the eligibility determination (ED) team that confirms a child's eligibility and authorizes EI services (such teams and their titles vary across states; ED team is used here as a generic term). Professional bias at this level may be overt, with families being told outright that one communication method is superior to others, or it may be insidious, where team members make subtle remarks in verbal or written form that families worry about, find offensive, or begin to internalize. For example, the parents of one deaf toddler receiving Part C services attended her annual IFSP review with their ED team. The parents reported that she had recently received a cochlear implant and was making excellent progress learning to listen with it. An audiologist on the team asked the parents, "Do you realize you have just tethered your child to a fragile technology for the rest of her life?" The mother later reported:

> Clearly this was not a legitimate question but a statement of concern or even opposition about the irreversible choice we had made for our child. My husband and I were not dissuaded by this insensitive and hurtful "question" because we were well-informed when we decided on the cochlear implant, and our decision was reinforced by the amazing changes in our daughter's listening and speech since her initial stimulation. But we were angered to think what effect this insidious question might have had on the confidence level of less secure families attempting to do what they believed was in the best interest of their child.

Communication bias may manifest itself as a failure by professionals to describe the range of options available to families, including support groups or parent advocacy groups consistent with the family's choice. Parents sometimes report that only in hindsight, as they look back at their early experiences with the ED Team and the IFSP, do they realize what they were NOT told. One parent remarked,

> I knew there was a program in the city that taught deaf children using an oral method, but it was never mentioned as an option when the ED team described EI choices to us. Only one option was mentioned and given all-around accolades by the team, so knowing absolutely nothing about deafness, we assumed every D/HH child and their parents were taught American Sign Language (ASL) during EI. We enrolled her in ASL EI and followed their recommendation to join an ASL parent-child playgroup at our state school for the deaf. [Author note: In this particu-

lar case, most members of the ED team were dually employed as Part C providers and by the state school for the deaf.] The ED team eventually authorized speech therapy services as well, but recommended a speech-language pathologist with no experience or knowledge of HL. Only later, as our daughter was approaching age three and we explored preschool options, did we realize that through Part C, she had been eligible to receive EI from oral therapists experienced and knowledgeable about HL, either instead of or in addition to our ASL involvement.

A Therapeutic Alliance on Behalf of the Child

Central to the integrity of a professional who evaluates, authorizes and/or conducts EI should be the conviction that parents have a right to know of all the communication options available to D/HH children, to make choices for their child, and know that these choices will be honored and supported, even if they are not the same choices the professional would make. For example, a clinician with a strong bias toward oral education was deeply puzzled by a family's choice to teach sign to their baby and used pressure to dissuade the family from this option, stating erroneously that, "no child who uses sign will ever learn to talk." Such actions clearly violate the spirit of respect for family choice. The ethical, professional code demands that in all of these cases, parent choice must be honored after the family has been informed of all communication options in an unbiased way. A negative and often long-lasting consequence occurs when professionals do not honor parent choice in that the clinician and the family fail to form what has been termed a "therapeutic alliance on behalf of the child" (ASHA, 2008a; Dinnebeil, Hale, & Rule, 1996). Such an alliance is required if a child is to benefit from the collaboration between professionals and parents who demonstrate mutual respect and are united in their efforts on behalf of the child.

"Proving" a Child With Hearing Loss Requires Intervention

Another family's experience involved their 2-month-old infant with a moderate-to-severe loss diagnosed after UNHS. During the IFSP process, they expressed their goal that he develop auditory skills, learn to talk and be mainstreamed in regular school by age five years. The EI service offered to the family through Part C was to send a deaf, signing, and nonspeaking adult into their home to conduct EI, accompanied by a reverse oral interpreter. When the family protested that this was not consistent with their communication choice, they were told that although it is known that D/HH babies have "language" delays from birth, a "speech" delay cannot be documented until 12 months of age, and therefore the team could not authorize an oral therapist until the child was one year old. The team explained that at age 12 months, the baby's speech could be tested and a speech delay possibly "proven." They mentioned that even at that time, there would be a long wait for a provider if the baby did show a speech delay. The family's response was to borrow money from relatives to pay for oral EI for their baby, outside of the Part C program. Although rules for eligibility differ across states, the state in which this family lived considers children immediately eligible for EI services, "if they have a diagnosed medical condition [permanent hearing loss being one of them] that has a high probability of resulting in a delay." The regulations state that children with these medical conditions are eligible for EI even if they are not exhibiting delays at the time of diagnosis. Therefore, a specific "speech" delay should not need to be documented for a child with permanent HL to be eligible for services; the presence of the HL already puts the baby at risk for language, auditory and speech delays, much in the same way that clinicians following babies with Down syndrome do not have to "prove" the child will be delayed; the presence of Down syndrome automatically qualifies the child for services.

The JCIH Year 2007 Statement lists as one of the obstacles to successful EHDI implementation the fact that "Children may not qualify for services before demonstrating language delays (a prevention model versus deficit model)" (p. 23). This document also asserts that, "All families of infants with any degree of bilateral or unilateral permanent hearing loss should be considered eligible for early intervention services" (p. 3). The wait-and-see, failure-based model of intervention has been shown to be ineffective and a disservice to families, going back many decades in the literature. It also is more costly over time, because children who do not begin intervention until a later age make slower progress than those who begin intervention early (Moeller, 2000), take longer to "catch up," require such intervention for a longer period of time, and are more likely to require special education placement rather than typical classroom placement when they begin school.

Principle 2: Services Are Developmentally Supportive and Promote Children's Participation in Their Natural Environments

The first part of this principle, that services be developmentally supportive, faces several obstacles. We have already noted that there is a severe shortage of clinicians who are experienced and knowledgeable about working with D/HH babies and their families. The legislation and policies mandating services from birth onward to children with HL were set in place years before an adequate number of clinicians received training and practice in working within an EI context. Because of this severe shortage, some EI services currently are being provided by those with no experience or knowledge of HL, and/or no experience with children younger than age 3 years. Professionals are hired, despite their lack of experience, because of the mandate to provide EI under Part C. However, doing therapy with a 4- or 5-year-old is very different from working with a 7-month-old and his parent(s), regardless of whether the baby has a HL or not. As noted earlier, a shift in intervention philosophy is needed when working with babies. One of the characteristics effective EI clinicians tend to possess is flexibility, given that infants and toddlers have less reliable behavior than older children, will often fluctuate in their compliance, or may spend the entire session sleeping. The creative clinician adequately trained and experienced in EI, recognizes these behaviors as an expected part of working with such young children. A productive session still is entirely possible by abandoning a lesson plan to do something that grabs the baby's attention, or in the case of a sleeping infant, focusing more on parent discussion and information-sharing. Robbins (2003) outlines four essential differences between parent-infant EI and traditional therapy and provides suggestions for clinicians who must make adjustments in the way they approach intervention with infants and toddlers with HL.

Natural Environment Policies

The second part of this principle, that services *promote children's participation in their natural environments* is a well-intentioned goal, given that the purpose of any intervention is to develop skills that carry over into real life. Nonetheless, misguided implementation of the natural environments policy has had negative consequences for many D/HH children and families. Increasingly rigid interpretation of "natural environments" has meant that in some EHDI jurisdictions, the location in which EI occurs (i.e., intervention always must take place in the child's home) takes precedence over any other considerations, including a clinician's knowledge and experience, efficient use of the expertise of a limited number of specialists in HL, the conditions within the home environment, and family choice. Some families strongly prefer that EI take place in their home, citing the reduction in stress at having a clinician come to their residence, or the elimination of the hardship of locating transportation to appointments, or the desire to see communication techniques demonstrated in their own home, among others. For these families, no one would argue that home-based EI be available to them (JCIH, 2007). Other families express a preference for center-based services, noting that, as parents, they can give their full attention to their baby and the therapy session when they are not distracted by the frequent interruptions that occur in their home. Some families live in homes that are not conducive to conducting EI for children with HL, such as the case of a multigenerational extended family where the D/HH baby and her mother lived with many relatives, including two uncles who worked night shifts and slept during the day, requiring complete silence in the home. A reason cited by some families who prefer center-based EI is the frequent contact available there with other parents who are also raising a child with HL, alleviating a sense of isolation. Some families report that center-based services allow them to observe other children with HL, to see the range of performance and individuality of each child, and to feel optimism at seeing older children who are making good progress. Such contact is also possible for families who received home-based EI, but this involves organizing additional meetings or groups, rather than spontaneous interactions.

No One Solution Fits All Families

Given that there is no research evidence that demonstrates that early intervention with D/HH children is more effective if it is conducted in the home rather than in a clinic or other setting (Yoshinaga-Itano, Stredler Brown, & Beams, 2004), it seems logical that different families require different settings for EI, and many families may benefit from a combination of home sessions and clinic sessions. Ultimately, "natural environment" is a *family-centered philosophy* of dealing with parents and their infants, not a definition of the physical space in which intervention takes place. Some have commented that, for an infant in particular, the "natural environment" is wherever the mother [or other caregiver] is.

Another issue that must be considered in relation to "natural environment" policies with D/HH children is how we can make the most effective use of the available clinical time of the relatively few trained EI professionals. We have noted repeatedly that there is a severe shortage of EI specialists trained to work with D/HH babies. As written in a summary document (Marge & Marge, 2005) from the 2004 Consensus Conference, *Effective Interventions for Infants and Young Children with Hearing Loss*, "In some instances [of early intervention delivery] . . . when the service provider must travel long distances, home visitation may not be practical or financially feasible" (p. 16).

Auditory Conditions in the Child's Home

Experts agree that controlling the auditory environment is critical when a baby is first learning to listen with hearing aids (HAs) or cochlear implant (CIs), but achieving this control may be impossible if a family lives in an apartment complex next to neighbors who play loud rock music during EI sessions, or for a family with four other children who disrupt sessions, and pull the parent's attention away from the task at hand. The deleterious effects on auditory development of a baby living in a chaotic, noisy environment with constant background auditory "clutter" cannot be overstated. This is an example of a case where a home visit by the EI provider would be critical, to see the characteristics of this family's daily life. By noting the excessive background noise, the clinician could make recommendations about reducing this noise, including educating the family about the negative effects of loud background noise on the baby's communication development, moving the television or video games to another location in the home, engaging one of the other children during EI activities and rotating between sessions so that everyone feels included, or finding quiet, motivating activities for the other children to do on their own during the EI sessions. For long-term productive intervention, this may well be a family that is best served by conducting most sessions at a center where the auditory environment can be controlled and the child's listening skills developed. Just as each family has individual characteristics, so EI solutions should be individualized to meet current best practices and be consistent with parent choice.

It is widely accepted that the goal of intervention is to enable children to participate in their natural environments; that is, in the venues and activities in which nondisabled children participate. However, to say we wish to *promote* learning that will be transferred to the natural environment is very different from saying that intervention must always be *conducted* in the natural environment. An increasing number of formal documents have expressed concern about the overly-restrictive interpretation of "natural environment" and have recommended that multiple options be offered to families. For example, under the "Early Intervention section," the JCIH Year 2007 document states that, "the committee recommends that both home-based and center-based intervention options should be offered" (p. 3). In a Fact Sheet approved by the Joint Committee of ASHA and the Council on Education of the Deaf (CED), "Natural Environments for Infants and Toddlers who are Deaf or Hard of Hearing and their Families" (ASHA, 2004), the committee noted that the individual needs of a child should be given considerable weight in the IFSP team's decision about location of services. The document states:

> While the IFSP team is required to justify why services may need to be provided in settings other than a natural environment, ASHA-CED believes the team should not feel compelled to provide an undue burden of justification, *as this would violate the spirit of the requirement that the IFSP be based on the individual needs of the child.* (Sec. 303.340)

Principle 3: Services Are Comprehensive, Coordinated, and Team-Based

Providing coordinated rather than fragmented services is often a challenge when children are receiving services from more than one professional or agency, but the problem is compounded in the case of EI with D/HH babies. Reasons for this include the ways different states in the United States transition children from the hearing detection program to Part C services, restrictions on agencies sharing information due to the U.S. Family Education Rights and Privacy Act (FERPA) regulations, policies limiting reimbursement for clinical hours spent in team meetings or team conference calls, and the sheer number of D/HH children who receive a variety of therapies from different clinicians. The latter reflects the fact that approximately 40% of children with hearing loss also have at least one other disability (Parrish & Roush, 2004; Yoshinaga-Itano, Sedey, Coulter, & Mehl, 1998) meaning that almost half of D/HH children will require EI services from two or more clinicians. Many clinicians do not have training or experience in working with D/HH children with multiple disabilities and must rely on a team of experts from different disciplines for guidance.

Cotreatment of Children with Multiple Disabilities

Published literature and clinical experience suggest that an excellent way to provide coordinated, team-based services, particularly to children with multiple disabilities, is to cotreat a child. Using this model, two clinicians work together for a few sessions to share with each other techniques and expertise in their respective areas. This author has had the experience of working with a child with both HL and vision impairment (VI), and learned valuable information over a period of three joint sessions from the VI therapist. Her input changed how I positioned the child in therapy and taught me to utilize the limited vision he had to its fullest potential. Conversely, the VI therapist was unaware of the value of full-time HA use or the amount of residual, aidable hearing the child had. In three sessions together, she was amazed at the power of audition to connect this child to his environment, to give him the security of knowing his parents were near by the sound of their voices, and to provide access to musical experiences. As a result of teaming for just three sessions, she became an advocate for this child's full-time use of HAs and incorporated many listening techniques into her EI with him.

Principle 4: Services Based on the Highest Quality Evidence That Is Available

A glaring barrier to meeting this principle within EI is the shortage of clinicians qualified, experienced, and knowledgeable about working with D/HH babies and their families. As previously noted, some therapists providing EI do not have even basic training working with D/HH children, nor familiarity with current literature that would guide evidence-based practices. Because Part C programs cannot locate a sufficient number of clinicians trained to provide EI to D/HH babies and families, many of the clinicians serving this population have no experience with issues of communication choice, the impact of hearing loss on language development, how hearing aids or cochlear implants work, or techniques to achieve full-time device use in the home. This is a cause of great concern, considering that the JCIH (2007) statement asserts that, "The key component of providing quality EI service is the expertise of the provider specific to HL" (p. 17). This assertion is borne out by published research studies (Moeller, 2000; Yoshinaga-Itano et al., 1998).

Early Intervention and Qualified Providers

The reality of the shortage of qualified providers became apparent to a family whose D/HH baby was authorized to receive speech-language EI services. After an exhaustive search, the family discovered that all the trained Part C EI clinicians in their geographic area had caseloads with a six- to nine-month waiting list. As an alternative, the Part C program authorized a developmental therapist to visit the home on a weekly basis, in spite of the fact that the child had no disabilities except HL (developmental therapist is a generic term, varying across jurisdictions, which refers to persons providing "general" EI. Persons labeled as developmental therapists span the continuum from clinicians highly knowledgeable about children with developmental disabilities to former second-grade teachers who have experience with neither special needs children nor family-centered EI. Developmental therapists with no EI experience are required to work under the "direct supervision" of a credentialed developmental therapists for 12 months, although in many cases the supervisor has no expertise or experience with D/HH children, hearing aids or other issues relevant to this population.) The family, fully self-educated about the importance of acting early, decided to pay privately for EI from a speech-language pathologist specialized in HL and to receive Part C services from the developmental therapist.

The baby's mother noted that the developmental therapist was kind and nurturing, but could offer no guidance on issues specific to HL. The developmental therapist was amazed that the baby wore his HAs full-time within a few weeks after fitting, as a result of sessions with the private SLP. The developmental therapist asked the mother to give her tips on how she might help her other families with D/HH babies achieve this. The mother was distressed to learn: (a) that this developmental therapist was the primary EI provider for families of D/HH babies, given that she admitted having no training or knowledge of this area; and (b) that the D/HH babies the developmental therapist was following were all inconsistent users of amplification even after extended periods of time, largely because the developmental therapist was not familiar with the techniques to achieve this goal. Given that this was not her area of expertise, the developmental therapist was unfamiliar with the research literature regarding the powerful influence of early auditory experiences that HAs and CIs provide, how brain development is changed when babies receive consistent auditory input at early ages, and how young an age was meant by "early." All these factors combined to unintentionally deny the D/HH babies in this therapist's practice access to services that met even basic standards of care, much less were evidence-based.

Families as the Source of Some Barriers

The sources of some of the barriers found in EI service provision are created by the families of D/HH children themselves. Even in a perfectly planned program, clinicians report family-related challenges that are daunting and discouraging. A few illustrations of such challenges are given, not as a comprehensive list, but as examples of a much broader set of challenges and include the following:

- Families do not show up for scheduled appointments or are not home when clinicians have traveled long distances to conduct EI at a child's residence;
- Personal family conflicts interfere with the delivery of EI, such as when divorced parents cannot agree upon services for their child or when a baby is at the father's home when the clinician arrives at the mother's home for the scheduled EI session;
- Parents fail to follow through with suggestions provided by the EI clinician, causing the child's communication progress to plateau;
- Parents experience prolonged periods of anger or resentment after the diagnosis, treating the EI clinician with hostility in a "blame the messenger" scenario, or become depressed to the point of requiring mental health care;
- Families do not have a predictable schedule for the D/HH child, with regular routines for meals, bathing, and bedtime. Without these routines, which are essential for babies to feel secure in their world, there are often concomitant problems with behavior and compliance; and
- Families question the presence of a HL in their baby and/or doubt the benefit provided by the HAs.

Under these conditions, the chances of success in achieving full-time HA use are severely compromised. The clinician will need to reevaluate various supports and information that may be important for the family to have.

Summary of Barriers Within EI Service Provision

In the sections above, some of the barriers that contribute to the gap between "what could be" and "what actually is" in the provision of EI services for D/HH babies and their families were reviewed. Though these barriers differ across jurisdictions and individual families, some common themes re-appear. These are:

- Inadequate number of early interventionists with D/HH expertise, relative to the number of babies being identified and referred for EI services;
- Regulations within Part C that create roadblocks or prevent clinicians from providing state-of-the-art EI;
- Interpretation of certain regulations, particularly those related to "natural environments" that constrain the EI services available, create disincentives for experienced clinicians to become Part C providers and limit parent choice;
- Failure of some ED teams or other EI professionals to provide families unbiased information about the range of communication options available to babies with HL; and
- Barriers that originate within the child's home or family that limit the child's auditory or language progress. Chief among the latter is the lack of full-time HA use by some babies with HL.

Full-Time Device Use— A Disconnect?

Let us consider the last point mentioned above, that of failure to achieve full-time HA use, even among some early-identified infants. Because early interventionists vary so greatly in their knowledge of HAs and their ability to advise families about a baby's acceptance of amplification, audiologists become fundamental partners in this critical aspect of EI: achieving full-time HA use. The reasons for lack of full-time HA use result from a number of different factors that we have already mentioned, and certainly differ widely. However, for some families, there may be a disconnect between our explanation of highly technical, computer-generated test results (i.e., auditory brainstem response [ABR], auditory steady-state response [ASSR], otoacoustic emissions [OAEs], and speech-mapping) and the parent's understanding of hearing loss and importance of full-time use of HAs, thereby undermining the potential of EHDI to mitigate the detrimental effects of HL on communication development.

Traditionally, many audiologists included parents as part of the audiologic assessment. Rather than presenting technically complex graphic results obtained with limited parent input, the child was often tested in a sound booth when seated on a parent's lap. During testing the audiologist would periodically query, "Mrs. Jones, do you think Johnny heard that last sound?" The parents became a part of the assessment team and developed ownership and belief in the test results. With newborn infant hearing assessment, a natural shift occurred to a reliance on technology (i.e., ABR, OAE), with the unfortunate consequence of a dramatic reduction in parent involvement in the assessment process. Similarly, digital hearing aid verification procedures, such as real-ear speech-mapping and simulated real ear measurements utilizing real-ear-to-coupler differences (RECD) and prescriptive targets, are wonderful tools that are technologically superior for predicting speech audibility than traditional pure tone aided audiograms obtained in the sound booth. These new measurements represent "good science." Unfortunately, these technologies that more accurately assess the appropriateness of the hearing aid's programming *do not automatically improve parents' understanding of hearing aid benefit*. On the contrary, it is not uncommon in this author's experience for parents to come away from real-ear verification appointments with several sheets of printouts and no understanding of what the testing showed or what the printouts mean. From the standpoint of being user-friendly, a traditional audiogram with aided and unaided results made sense to parents; they could clearly see the difference between what their child heard with and without HAs. In addition, most parents sat in the sound booth while their child was tested and actually experienced the intensity levels of the presentation stimuli. This involvement in the testing made their child's hearing loss real to them.

One Parent's Story

A mother of a 4-year-old child with bilateral severe sensorineural hearing loss explained her experience this way:

> Billy's dad and I certainly believed the ABR results that confirmed he had a significant HL at three months of age and intellectually understood the importance of aiding him right away. But the reality of HL and the value of his HAs didn't truly sink in for us until a few months later. That's when he sat on my lap in the sound booth, and I watched his responses to sound without his HAs, and then while wearing them. The difference was so dramatic that I re-committed myself to ensuring Billy always had access to sound via his HAs. Over time, I became familiar with audiograms and could explain Billy's HL to others by showing them the difference between his aided and unaided results. This was especially important because early on, his grandparents didn't seem to believe he had a HL; they kept saying he looked so "normal." They certainly didn't grasp the importance of the HAs and didn't insist he keep them in during his frequent visits with them. It was only after I showed and explained the audiogram to them that they became "believers" in the importance of HAs and were firm about the rule that he always wear them. After a few predictable but unsuccessful attempts to test limits about this rule, Billy complied with full-time HA use at his grandparents' home. It has never been an issue since then.

This mother continues,

> Recently, Billy completed real-ear verification testing and in contrast to booth testing, I felt completely removed from the process of whatever they were assessing, which actually was unclear to me. Upon completion, I was given a paper with squiggly lines accompanied by techno-jargon with which I was unfamiliar. As the audiologist pointed to various marks on the graph and pronounced the aids appropriate for Billy, I began to feel the knowledge I thought I had about Billy's hearing sucked right out of me. I sensed I knew less now than I had before! I pondered a question in my mind for a long time after the real-ear speech mapping was performed, "How do I gain access to what those test results really mean for Billy and his listening skills with hearing aids?"

This is a poignant question for a parent to pose and one that deserves a frank answer. Although no one would advocate returning to an inferior technology, such as relying exclusively on aided audiograms, we might wonder how a better balance could be achieved between the use of newer, more accurate assessment technologies and ensuring that parents understand those assessment results as well as they understood aided audiograms. Is there a user-friendly protocol for graphically displaying the results of such tests as real-ear verification that clearly communicates the findings to parents or nonaudiology colleagues? Clearly, no professional intentionally sacrifices a parent's comprehension of test results, yet if parents come away from testing confused and unsure about the value of HAs, we may be setting into motion a chain of events that leads to an under-valuing of HAs by the parents, and more difficulty achieving full-time amplification in early-identified babies. This possibility is supported by data from Moeller (2007) showing that some parents of early-identified babies struggle to achieve full-time HA use, even over an extended period of time. In fact, when the children in the Moeller study were 24 to 28 months of age, only five of 14 early-identified children had achieved use of HAs during all waking hours. Although the causes of part-time use in these infants are likely multifaceted, we could hypothesize that the type of assessment used and the way results were shared with families might be contributing factors.

The Two Owners of Test Results

Is it possible that, with the advent of newer and more accurate technologies, our profession has thrown the baby out with the bath water? Have we abandoned aided testing in the sound booth completely? Perhaps a combination of assessments is the most pragmatic approach, given that hearing test results have two "owners." The first owner is the audiologist, who interprets the test information to make the most accurate diagnosis and provide the best care on the baby's behalf. This first owner finds real-ear verification measures to be the superior technique. But, there is a second "owner" of test results—the parents—and it may be appropriate to utilize aided audiograms focusing on speech stimuli in the booth, not in place of real-ear measures but in addition to them, to be certain that parents understand the results and the enormous benefits of full-time amplification to their baby's development.

To summarize, the development of more accurate technology to confirm hearing loss does not automatically transfer to better ability to convey the results to parents or to nonaudiology colleagues, such as early interventionists. This represents an additional gap between potential and reality: the difficulty clinicians encounter in translating highly-technical test results so that parents can understand and believe the results. If doubt remains in a parent's mind about whether their baby really needs to wear HAs full-time, the "therapeutic alliance on behalf of the child" may take a long time to develop, or may never be an alliance that has mutual trust and confidence at its core.

The Amplification-Communication Connection: A Three-Phase Program for Audiologists

Audiologists who treat a baby with newly diagnosed HL typically focus on the critical jobs of verifying the degree of HL and fitting HAs as early as possible. The pediatric audiologist is often the professional with whom the parents have the most contact in the early period following diagnosis of HL. In that capacity, audiologists have the potential to establish with parents a foundation that fosters communication development in their child with HL. If this foundation is established convincingly, progress during the subsequent stages of EI and educational placement may be highly effective. Conversely, if parents do not understand the direct connection between the consistent, full-time use of HAs and the role they, the parents, play in nurturing communication development, the speech and language achievement of even early-identified babies may be adversely affected. For more information about the program outlined below, see Robbins (2002, 2007). The Three-Phase program described here encompasses the period immediately following diagnosis of HL in babies. The timeframe for this period may be only a few weeks or may last up to six months, a point when all babies and their parents should be enrolled in an ongoing EI program with an experienced and knowledgeable therapist. As we have noted, unfortunately, this is one of the goals of EHDI that is not yet a reality for every family. Even after an EI program is established, the audiologist often has more knowledge and experience with HL than the EI provider. Thus, the audiologist remains an integral part of the child and family's support team.

Three Phases and Their Goals

The three phases within the program are as follows: Phase I starts at diagnosis and lasts until the first fitting of HAs (often loaners); Phase II encompasses the early weeks after the initial fitting of amplification; Phase III begins after HA adjustment and tapers, but does not end when the baby and family are enrolled in an EI communication program. The audiologist's role in giving input related to communication development differs at each of the three phases, largely because the emotional status, needs, and processing capabilities of parents change over time. Families respond to the news of deafness in a variety of unique ways, yet there are some common reports parents have given. These reports often tell of a sense of helplessness or despair families felt as they waited for upcoming appointments, after receiving the diagnosis of HL. These parents have reported their desire to DO something, to take action that would help their child rather than simply waiting for the next audiology appointment. In these cases, it is important to give parents some tasks on which to focus so they feel empowered to have a positive effect on their child's communication. Receiving this news from the audiologist is essential. Some parents later lament that the audiologist handled issues of hearing and the HAs but deferred questions of communication to the speech-language pathologist or other early interventionist whom the parents did not meet until weeks or months later. Importantly, if the audiologist treats the HAs as a domain separate from communication, families may not make the connection that the full-time use of amplification is the foundation of auditory and spoken language progress.

Because parents of newly identified D/HH babies are likely to best retain information if it is presented in both oral and written forms, audiologists are advised to accompany their verbal discussion of the communication goals with a printed sheet that reviews this information. A handout version of the goals at each of the three stages was created by Martilla (2007) and entitled *Journey with Hearing Loss*. Reprints of Martilla's parent handouts for Stages I, II, and III appear in the following figures. Hearing health care professionals may assume it is self-evident that HAs and communication development are inextricably linked, though data and clinical experience suggest that parents of D/HH babies may not recognize that link unless it is explicitly and repeatedly explained.

Phase I

At Phase I (Figure 40–1), caution is advised in supplying too much technical information, as many parents experience disbelief, grief, and a sense of being overwhelmed at the time of diagnosis. This is a period when parents require time to absorb the news and react emotionally. If professionals are uncomfortable responding to parents' emotional reactions in Phase I, they may inadvertently utilize the counter-productive "technical jargon" or "hit and run" approaches (Hersch & Amon, 1973) with families. Feedback from parents suggests that these approaches often leave families feeling lost and powerless to effect change in their child with HL. At Phase I, audiologists will, of course, review the hearing test results and respond to the many questions parents ask at this stage. A sense of optimism may be conveyed to families if the audiologist also reviews the communication goals on the Phase I, *Journey with Hearing Loss*, handout (see Figure 40–1).

Phase II

When families come for the initial HA fitting at Phase II, our first communication advice is an equipment issue, where the audiologist gives the family multiple opportunities to become familiar with the HAs themselves. Giving the parents Handout II at this time (Figure 40–2) will serve as a reminder to cover these points, knowing that the audiologist has much to accomplish in the limited appointment time. But, at this appointment both parents, not just one, should repeatedly practice opening the battery door, inserting the battery, and manipulating other parts of the HA. The majority of parents have never held a HA in their hands, much less tried to insert a tiny earmold in the ear of a 6-week-old baby. Demonstrating putting the aid in, then letting both parents practice at least twice can make the difference at this stage. The author has had initial EI sessions with babies who have already had several audiology appointments, including HA fitting, but whose families do not know how to change the battery, struggle to the point of frustration to insert the earmold, or have one parent who feels incapable and always defers to the other parent to handle the HAs. This point is mentioned, not as a criticism of audiologists, but as a reminder that practice makes perfect. To save time during audiology appointments, families can practice inserting the HAs and changing batteries while the audiologist is engaged in other tasks.

Professional standards dictate that we approach each family about the importance of full-time HA use with sensitivity to their unique situation and coping skills. If the data from Moeller (2007) are representative of the larger group of children with HL, this is a discouraging trend. However, it remains unknown whether audiologists are explicitly making the connection for families early and often, as in, "Your baby needs full-time HA use if her brain's auditory centers are to develop fully." Some families may be given this information repeatedly, provided with appropriate

MISSISSIPPI
BEND AREA
EDUCATION
AGENCY

The Journey with Hearing Loss – Phase I

Lifetime Goals

Be confident! You can and will master what you need to know about raising a child with hearing loss.

Have high expectations! Your child can and will achieve much if you expect that he or she can do much.

Develop autonomy and responsibility! Your child can and will grow up to be an independent and responsible person.

Here are three things you can do right now to reach these lifetime goals:

1. **Continue to talk to your child.** Speak close to your child's face and use plenty of facial expression.
2. **Write down your thoughts and feelings in your journal.** You can also write down any questions you might have for the audiologist or teacher so you can remember to ask them.
3. **Sign up for the home instruction class through the John Tracy Clinic.** (800-522-4582 or www.johntracyclinic.org)

FIGURE 40–1. Handout to use during Phase I with families of newly-diagnosed babies. Used with permission from Robbins, A. M. (2002). Empowering parents to help their newly diagnosed child gain communication skills, *Hearing Journal*, *55*(11), 55–59. Created by Mississippi Bend Area Education Agency/Dr. Joan Marttila, Bettendorf, IA. http://www.aea9.k12.ia.us/documents/filelibrary/pdf/Hearing_Loss_1.pdf

support and techniques and still elect not to insist on full-time HA use. But if families have never been told, gently but bluntly, that listening development depends on the baby having consistent and dependable auditory input all day long, how do we expect them to figure this out?

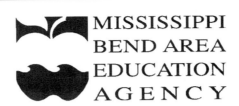

MISSISSIPPI
BEND AREA
EDUCATION
AGENCY

The Journey with Hearing Loss - Phase II

<u>Lifetime Goals</u>

Be confident! You can and will master what you need to know about raising a child with hearing loss.

Have high expectations! Your child can and will achieve much if you expect that he or she can do much.

Develop autonomy and responsibility! Your child can and will grow up to be an independent and responsible person.

Here are four things you can do right now to reach these lifetime goals:

1. **Use the hearing aid calendar to record when your child is wearing the hearing aids.** You can record your child's responses to sound, any equipment problems or questions you have for the teacher or audiologist.

2. **Use your child's name with a purpose.** It's important for your child to know his name. Make sure you are calling your child's name for a reason, not just to see her response to her name.

3. **Help your child become aware of important sounds in your home.** Use a hand-to-ear response at home when sounds occur. When you hear something your child should attend to, say "I hear that!" and put your hand to your ear.

4. **Pay attention to the sounds your child is making.** As your child learns how to use sound, she will become more aware of how to use her voice to get your attention. Your child will also continue to learn to correctly identify sounds in your home. Use your journal to record changes in your child's responses. Writing them down will be helpful for you, your audiologist and your teacher.

FIGURE 40–2. Handout to use during Phase II with families of newly-diagnosed babies. Used with permission from Robbins, A. M. (2002). Empowering parents to help their newly diagnosed child gain communication skills, *Hearing Journal*, *55*(11), 55–59. Created by Mississippi Bend Area Education Agency/Dr. Joan Marttila, Bettendorf, IA. http://www.aea9.k12.ia.us/documents/filelibrary/pdf/Hearing_Loss_2.pdf

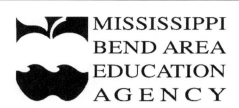

Providing parents with real-life examples creates a mental snapshot that may be worth a stack of pamphlets or research articles. I have shared with parents the importance of consistent auditory input for their baby by relaying stories such as,

> I worked with a 4-year-old boy whose parents did not insist on full-time HA use when he was first fitted as an infant, because he went through phases of pulling them out or whining when they were inserted. When he behaved this way, his family allowed him to leave the HAs out, not recognizing that all babies will pull the aids out and require re-insertion, and most babies will whine at HA insertion until the parents get very adept and swift with the process. The parents hoped the baby's full-time use would happen naturally as he got older. On the contrary, as the baby became a toddler, the harder it was to change the "rule" that had been established. That rule, unintentionally reinforced, was that the child, not his family, was in control of the HAs. A child who fails to achieve full-time device use within three months of initial fitting is at high risk for ongoing power struggles over the HAs for years to come, as was this four-year-old boy.

The clinician should express optimism to parents that, with the team's support, their child's full-time HA use is achievable.

Phase III

At Phase III (Figure 40–3), the audiologist should gently but thoroughly query the parents about HA adjustment and hours of daily use. It is particularly important at this interval to remind the family that the earlier a baby accepts HAs and wears them full-time, the sooner the benefit and the more consistent the auditory input to the baby's brain. Toward that end, the audiologist can provide assistance only if the family feels secure enough to honestly report HA adjustment problems. If asked, "Katy is wearing her HAs full-time, isn't she?" parents may feel a sense of failure at admitting that Kathy is not wearing the HAs full-time. Techniques for probing families about full-time use must be sensitive to the family's desire to please the professionals or the family's embarrassment at not achieving full-time use. Horton (personal communication, 2008) suggests some nonthreatening ways to gain an accurate picture of a child's HA use. These suggestions include asking parents:

- "When was the last time you changed the battery in Sally's HA?"
- "How comfortable is Dad (or the child care provider or other significant person) with inserting the HAs?"
- "Tell me about situations when Sophie doesn't wear her HAs," as this gives parents "permission" to provide an honest report;
- "When do you get the most resistance from Sophie about wearing her HAs?" as this implies that all babies show some resistance; and
- "What problem with Sophie's HA use could I help you most with today?"

Resources for Families Struggling With Full-Time Hearing Aid Use

If the parents report challenges or frustrations with their baby's acceptance of HAs, an array of resources are available to support families in working toward the goals of full-time use of amplification. Such resources include the following:

- Printed or video materials discussing HA adjustment issues unique to infants and toddlers. Parent-friendly suggestions are found in the first several lessons of the "Listen Around the Clock" section of Rossi's (2003) parent-infant program. Rossi gives many practical examples of how a baby benefits from full-time device use and emphasizes that a baby's listening development is jeopardized if full-time use is not established;
- Samples of products designed specifically to keep a baby's HAs in place, such as special clips and some styles of bonnets of caps (www.listen-up.org is a Web site with a wealth of practical tips from experienced parents of children with HL);
- A dedicated weekly HA calendar on which parents record the number of hours of HA use each day, as well as pertinent information about equipment problems, baby's resistance to putting HAs on, or problems pulling them out. Parents may also note whenever their child responds to sounds, and the nature of the response, such as a startle, cessation of activity, or eye widening. Some families find it useful to fax the audiologist the HA use calendar at the end of each week to ensure they complete it. Families should bring the calendar to audiologic appointments to discuss HA use and problems;

MISSISSIPPI
BEND AREA
EDUCATION
AGENCY

The Journey with Hearing Loss - Phase III

Lifetime Goals

Be confident! You can and will master what you need to know about raising a child with hearing loss.

Have high expectations! Your child can and will achieve much if you expect that he or she can do much.

Develop autonomy and responsibility! Your child can and will grow up to be an independent and responsible person.

Here are three things you can do right now to reach these lifetime goals:

1. **Imitate the sounds your child makes.** Babies and young children enjoy playing with sounds and they love to use them to communicate to you.
2. **Help your child put meaning to sound.** For example, if you've been playing "How Big is (your child's name)? SOOO Big!" with your child face-to-face, try to get the same response from your child standing behind him.
3. **Choose a few sounds in your home that will help your child learn.** Many children love to hear the telephone ring, the dog bark, or someone knocking at the door. When you hear one of those sounds, make a big deal about it.

FIGURE 40–3. Handout to use during Phase III with families of newly-diagnosed babies. Used with permission from Robbins, A. M. (2002). Empowering parents to help their newly diagnosed child gain communication skills, *Hearing Journal*, *55*(11), 55–59. Created by Mississippi Bend Area Education Agency/Dr. Joan Marttila, Bettendorf, IA. http://www.aea9.k12.ia.us/documents/filelibrary/pdf/Hearing_Loss_3.pdf

- A discussion of baby seats that are conducive to HA use and fully port an infant's trunk and upper body without any padding across the back of the head. This contrasts to most infant seats or high chairs where the baby's head rests back on a surface, often causing the HAs to move out of position or to be pulled out by the baby;
- Some HAs have a data logging device that allows families and clinicians to keep track of actual use time;
- An invaluable source of support is advice from other families, as they are able to share real-life tips about things that have worked with their babies.

To complete the visit at Stage III, the *Journey with Hearing Loss* handout may be reviewed and given to parents, focusing on the child's developing communication skills through listening. Families should be advised that another fundamental reason to establish full-time HA use quickly is to ascertain whether HAs provide adequate access to spoken language. If they do, we expect to see certain positive changes in the baby's speech and listening behaviors. If not, the family should know there are other options, including educational ones, such as visual communication (sign language or cued speech) and medical ones (cochlear implantation).

The Power of Parental Influence

Parents continue to have powerful influence over their child's communication development, long after Stage III when they are enrolled in an ongoing intervention program. Moeller et al. (2007) cite statistics from Dunst (2001) that indicate that 2 hours per week in therapy make up only 2% of a normal-hearing toddler's waking hours, whereas everyday activities such as diapering and feeding occur at least 2,000 times before the first birthday. This statistic is a convincing statement about the power of families to influence, positively or negatively, their child's communication after HA fitting. Parents who take advantage of only 10 interactions each waking hour of a child's day will have provided more than 36,000 teachable moments between ages 1 and 2 years (Moeller et al., 2007). Consider the lost opportunity if the child is not wearing amplification during these interactions. If this is case, are audiologists and other hearing health care professionals emphasizing this fact to parents repeatedly? If families are struggling with HA compliance months after initial fitting, Horton (personal communication, 2008) suggests providing additional stories that demonstrate the detrimental effect of inconsistent HA use. She has shared with families in her EI practice this example of a 4-year-old boy with moderate-severe hearing loss who said, "My parents smarter than me. When we makin' microwave popcorn, it ready every time them open the door! But when I open it, popcorn sometimes ready and sometimes not. Them is lucky!" This story makes the point that first, this 4-year-old has delayed syntactic development as a result of inconsistent auditory input via HAs, particularly because grammatical morphemes in English are often at the ends of words and are acoustically subtle. For example, without HAs, the child did not hear the difference between "it ready" and "it's ready." The second point is that children must hear a grammatical form hundreds of times before they begin to use it. Suppose half of this child's exposure to those forms occurred when he was not wearing HAs; his mastery would be slower than that of a child with similar loss who wore HAs full-time, or might never occur. Finally, the story shows parents that, without full-time HA use, the child did not hear the microwave buzzer often enough to associate it with food being ready. He never made the connection that his parents knew the popcorn was ready because they heard a buzzer go off, erroneously interpreting this as luck.

Parents' Most Important Decisions

Audiologists may offer a realistic optimism to families that has a lasting effect on the attitude and coping skills of parents. Moeller and Condon (1998) have noted that most of the decisions parents are required to make after diagnosis relate to communication mode, amplification and educational choices. But, they suggest that professionals reinforce that the most important decision parents will make are not these technical ones but rather: (1) the decision to have high expectations for their child; (2) the decision to give the child autonomy and responsibility; and (3) the decision to be confident in their ability to parent a child with a hearing loss. These decisions are so fundamental that they are included at the top of each of the handouts in Figures 40–1 through 40–3 to remind families they are capable of handling the difficult but rewarding task of raising their baby who is D/HH.

Cochlear Implants Provide Another Viable Intervention Option

The now common option of providing cochlear implants to profoundly deaf babies has far-reaching implications for EI services and the qualifications of

EI providers. Although the topic of early cochlear implantation is too extensive to cover here, the reader is referred to Chapters 27 and 35 in this volume. In almost every instance in which "hearing aids" have been used in this chapter, the words "cochlear implants" could be substituted. That is, issues of full-time device use, knowledge, and experience of the clinician, valuing of family choice, parent understanding of test results, and the need for urgency in treatment to take advantage of sensitive periods of development, are as applicable to babies who receive cochlear implants as to those who wear HAs. Due to the vast body of published literature demonstrating the effectiveness of early cochlear implantation, families should be made aware of this treatment option during discussions of communication and educational choices.

A Review of the Gaps Between Potential and Reality

This chapter has described some of the gaps that currently exist between the potential and the reality of EI services for infants with HL and their families. Readers will recognize that none of these gaps exist in isolation; rather they are interrelated, forming a web of challenges facing our profession:

- Almost all newborns are screened for HL with the primary goals of early diagnosis and HA fitting, EI services and subsequent competence in communication; yet half of newborns needing further audiologic evaluation before age 3 months are lost to the system (LTS).
- Children who are LTS experience a chain reaction of delays: their HL is not confirmed through diagnostic evaluation by age 3 months, causing them to miss the next goal of enrollment in Part C EI before age 6 months.
- A substantial number of infants with confirmed hearing loss are not fitted with HAs within one month of diagnosis, as recommended by JCIH (2007).
- Once babies are fitted with HAs and families are enrolled in Part C intervention, the services they receive may not meet professional standards of care.
- Clinicians providing EI encounter system roadblocks and family circumstances that limit the effectiveness of their intervention.
- The technologies used to more accurately assess hearing and to confirm HA benefit in children may not yield results that are easily interpreted by some parents and therapists.
- Though babies are identified at young ages, a substantial number may not wear HAs on a full-time basis. This undermines one of the primary goals of infant hearing screening: providing access to sound to ensure communicative competence.

Finding Solutions and Closing the Gaps

Acknowledging the gaps that exist between what is and what could be brings us to the ongoing work of closing these gaps. Early in this chapter we cited some positive advances toward improving our services to D/HH babies and families. Some of these are mentioned again as they directly relate to improving the quality of EI that professionals provide:

1. An urgent need exists to rapidly increase the number of specialists trained to provide EI to D/HH babies and their families. Current action to address this need includes:
   - University training programs in Audiology, speech language pathology and deaf education have begun to include EI coursework or practicum in their curriculum so that students graduate with some basic knowledge in this area. Some programs provide the option of obtaining an "emphasis" in EI.
   - For clinicians who have already completed college degrees, a range of continuing education options are available to learn about (a) EI practices and (b) children with HL. Beginning with those that involve short-term commitments, there are one-hour on-line courses or multiple hour "virtual conferences" offered through such agencies as ASHA, hearing aid companies, and cochlear implant manufacturers.
2. Clinicians conducting EI require materials specifically designed for D/HH babies and their parents. A key ingredient to successful EI with D/HH children is the use of developmentally-appropriate materials. Fortunately, excellent resources are available for this population.
   - Rossi's "Learn to Talk Around the Clock Toolbox" (2003) has step-by-step lessons that are

user-friendly, even for early interventionists who lack extensive experience with HL. An accompanying videotape demonstrates the Signature Behaviors that parents learn to use with their D/HH child to enhance listening and spoken language.

- A second program by Rossi (2007) is written specifically for child care providers. "Learn to Talk Around the Clock at Childcare" addresses a need that has existed for a long time because a considerable number of D/HH babies spend most of their waking hours with a childcare provider, not with their parents. Though parent education remains our primary focus, materials written for childcare providers require a different level of complexity and a realistic approach to the amount of time the provider can give any one child. Rossi's child care lesson kits come with colored bracelets, each of which is a reminder to childcare providers of a skill they should target that day.
- The John Tracy Correspondence Course free home lessons (http://www.johntracyclinic.org) can be accessed anywhere in the world and give parents a sense of empowerment as they observe their baby's progress.
- The Cottage Acquisition Scales for Listening, Language & Speech (CASLLS) help clinicians monitor progress in D/HH children and select communication goals that are developmentally appropriate (http://www.sunshinecottage.org). Other materials from this Web site incorporate Learning-to-Listen sounds and the concept of Listening Age.

3. Support from other parents is needed by families of newly-identified D/HH babies.
   - A marvelous parent-to-parent link is the Listen-Up Web site (http://www.listen-up.org). This website has a vast array of information, resources, Web site links for parents, with particular emphasis on families helping families by sharing tips, products, and services they have found useful with their D/HH child.
   - State chapters in the United States of the Guide-by-Your-Side program (http://www.handsandvoices.com) of Hands and Voices helps families make connections with other families of D/HH children and encourages mentoring of families with newly identified babies by experienced parents.
4. Professionals working with D/HH infants require training about presenting unbiased options to families. Daylong workshops and other materials from such groups such as Hands and Voices (http://www.handsandvoices.org) address issues of discussing communication options with parents of D/HH children in an unbiased and family-centered manner.
5. Government agencies need feedback from clinicians and parents whose lives are directly affected by EHDI and Part C Policies.
   - Grass-roots and organizational pressures are needed to influence the ways in which Part C policies are interpreted, particularly those related to natural environments and the qualifications of those who provide EI services for infants with HL.
   - NCHAM, the National Center for Hearing Assessment and Management, Utah State University, has resources and data available on their extensive Web site (http://www.infanthearing.org) that cover all aspects of EHDI, including legislative mandates and public policies.
6. The development of user-friendly ways to translate highly technical hearing test results for parents should be a priority. The best technology is only as good as the parents' belief in its validity and their subsequent commitment to full-time HA use. Newer, more precise measurements of hearing are questionable leaps forward if families understand less about their child's HL and cannot easily recognize the benefit provided by HAs. Audiologists report a desire for training in how to counsel families, including how to explain test results to parents (Harrison & Roush, 2002), yet most university programs in audiology offer limited coursework on the principles and techniques of counseling. "Counseling" within the context of managing infants and families should not be viewed as a separate service, but as an approach to conveying information, providing support, and listening to families that is infused into ongoing clinical services. An excellent resource about the audiologist's roles in counseling is the Guidelines for Counseling document (ASHA, 2008c).
7. Continued funding for research is imperative to further explore such topics as brain plasticity, sensitive windows for cortical development, and evidence-based clinical practices. Results from research studies should inform clinical procedures so that professionals provide intervention consistent with best practices. Conversely, clinical reports and dilemmas help frame the questions that lead investigators in new research directions.

Conclusion

There is a maxim in quantum physics, "When you change the way you look at things, the things you look at change." Change for the better is within our profession's grasp, but is not guaranteed. The same level of energy and commitment of resources that brought UNHS into existence against many odds must be mustered if we are to improve EI services as dramatically as UNHS changed early identification of HL. This becomes a requirement that we "change the way we look at things" by taking a different perspective, both individually and collectively, altering the way we look at what we do. This requirement is a call, not just to examine the relatively small realm of our own specialized role in serving D/HH babies and their families but to view the entire EHDI system broadly, and to re-commit ourselves to moving "what is" ever closer to "what could be."

Acknowledgment. The author wishes to thank Naomi Horton and Julia Renshaw for reviewing drafts of this chapter and providing input to the author.

References

American Speech Language Hearing Association (ASHA). (2008a). *Ad hoc committee. Roles and Responsibilities of speech-language pathologists in early intervention: Technical report.* Retrieved August 16, 2010, from http://www.asha.org/policy

American Speech Language Hearing Association (ASHA). (2008b). *Working group. Loss to follow-up in early hearing detection and intervention programs: Technical report.* Retrieved August 16, 2010, from http://www.asha.org/policy

American Speech Language Hearing Association (ASHA). (2008c). *Guidelines for audiologists providing informational and adjustment counseling to families of infants and young children with hearing loss birth to 5 years of age.* Retrieved August 16, 2010, from http://www.asha.org/policy

American Speech Language Hearing Association (ASHA). (2004). *Fact sheet. Natural environments for infants and toddlers who are deaf or hard of hearing and their families. Joint committee of ASHA and CED.* Retrieved August 16, 2010, from http://www.asha.org/policy

Bamford, J. (1998). Early identification . . . what then? In F. Bess (Ed.), *Children with hearing impairments: Contemporary trends* (p. 353). Nashville, TN: Vanderbilt Bill Wilkerson Press.

Centers for Disease Control and Prevention (CDC). (2008). *Summary of 2006 national EHDI data.* Retrieved July 21, 2008, from http://www.cdc.gov/ncbddd/ehdi/data.htm

Consensus Conference. (2004). *Effective interventions for infants and young children with hearing loss.* September 10–12. Washington, DC.

Dinnebeil, L. A., Hale, L. M., & Rule, S. (1996). A qualitative analysis of parents' and service coordinators' descriptions of variables that influence collaborative relationships. *Topics in Early Childhood Special Education, 16,* 322–347.

Dunst, C. J. (2001). *Parent and community assets as sources of young children's learning opportunities.* Asheville, NC: Winterberry Press.

Harrison, M., & Roush, J. (2002). Information for families with young deaf and hard of hearing children: Reports from parents and pediatric audiologists. In R. C. Seewald, & J. S. Gravel (Eds.), *A sound foundation through early amplification: Proceedings of the second international conference* (pp. 233–249). Stäfa, Switzerland: Phonak AG.

Hersch, B., & Amon, C. (1973). An approach to reporting the diagnosis of hearing loss to parents of a hearing-impaired child. In J. Northern & M. Downs (Eds.), *Hearing in children* (pp. 167–170). Baltimore, MD: Williams & Wilkins.

Joint Committee on Infant Hearing (JCIH). (2007). Position statement: Principles and guidelines for early hearing detection and intervention programs. *Pediatrics, 120,* 898–921.

Marge, D., & Marge, M. (Eds.). (2005). *Report and recommendations for the 2004 national consensus conference on effective educational and health care interventions for infants and young children with hearing loss.* Syracuse, NY: SUNY Upstate Medical University.

Martilla, J. (2007). *The journey with hearing loss.* Online handouts available at: http://www.aea9.k12.ia.us/documents/file library/pdf/Hearing_Loss_3.pdf

Moeller, M. P. (2000). Early intervention and language development in children who are deaf and hard of hearing. *Pediatrics, 106*(3):e43. Retrieved August 16, 2010, from http://www.pediatrics.org/cgi/cntent/full/106/3/e43

Moeller, M. P. (2007). Building sound foundations: What's in a word? In R. Seewald & J. Bamford (Eds.), *A sound foundation through early amplification 2007. Proceedings of the fourth international conference* (pp. 19–31). Stäfa, Switzerland: Phonak AG.

Moeller, M. P., & Condon, M. (1998). Family matters: Making sense of complex choices. In F. Bess (Ed.), *Children with hearing impairment, contemporary trends.* Nashville, TN: Vanderbilt Bill Wilkerson Press.

Moeller, M. P., Hoover, B., Putman, C., Arbataitis, K., Bohnenkamp, G., Peterson, B., . . . Stelmachowicz, P.G. (2007). Vocalizations of infants with hearing loss compared to infants with normal hearing—Part I: Phonetic development. *Ear and Hearing, 28*(5), 605–627.

Parrish, R., & Rousch, J. (2004). When hearing loss occurs with other disabilities. *Volta Voices 11,* 20–21.

Robbins, A. M. (2002). Empowering parents to help their newly diagnosed child gain communication skills. *Hearing Journal, 55*(11), 55–59.

Robbins, A. M. (2003). Communication intervention for infants and toddlers with cochlear implants. *Topics in Language Disorders, 23,* 16–33.

Robbins, A. M. (2007). Monitoring communication progress in early intervention. In R. Seewald & J. Bamford (Eds.), *A sound foundation through early amplification 2007: Proceedings of the fourth international conference* (pp. 95–105). Stäfa, Switzerland: Phonak AG.

Rossi, K. (2003). *Learn to talk around the clock*. Washington, DC: A. G. Bell Publications.

Rossi, K. (2007). *Learn to talk around the clock at childcare*. Omaha, NE: Learn to Talk Around the Clock Products.

Yoshinaga-Itano, C., Sedey, A. L., Coulter, D., & Mehl, A. (1998). Language of early- and later-identified children with hearing loss. *Pediatrics*, *102*, 1161–1171.

Yoshinaga-Itano, C., Stredler Brown, A., & Beams, D. (2004). *Evidence-based programming for infants and young children with hearing loss*. Paper commissioned for Consensus Conference: Effective interventions for infants and young children with hearing loss, September 10–12. Washington, DC.

41

Providing Services in Educational Contexts: Defining the Role of the Pediatric Audiologist

Patricia M. Chute and Mary Ellen Nevins

Introduction

Deafness is global. Physiologically, deafness and all levels of hearing loss affect the poor living in small villages in underdeveloped countries in the same manner as the wealthy who live in metropolitan areas of affluent societies. Its population is age-encompassing from the tiniest newborn to the oldest citizen. It can be present at birth, develop slowly over time, or occur suddenly. Communication through sound and spoken language is affected immediately, thus breaking the bond between mother and child and changing family dynamics with those members who are hearing. In all cases, the auditory system is limited in function or rendered nonfunctional. For all its similarities around the world, however, cultures respond to hearing loss in different ways. Despite the fact that it is the manifestation of damage to the auditory system, how it is treated varies depending on finances, location, medical care, socioeconomic status, and philosophical approach.

In an attempt to gather data on variation across societies, the International Directory of Communication Disorders (IDCD), a free internet resource (www.comdisinternational.com), was developed through a consortium of diverse professionals (Bleile, Ireland, & Kiel, 2006). Kotby (2006) and McLeod and Bleile (2007) report that a key indicator of the degree of attention that a country gives to speech and hearing problems is found in its "history, cultural views of language and disability, economics and availability of services" (p. 2). Economically, countries with limited health and education resources will fair more poorly than those with an infrastructure that supports the education of *all* children regardless of disability. Worldwide, 100 million primary-aged school children (60% of whom are girls) are not in school, thereby contributing to poverty and higher childhood mortality (World Bank Group, 2005). The Millennium Project of the World Bank Group has identified training more professionals, in the areas of health and education, as a necessary step toward fighting childhood mortality.

In order for training to take place, there must be sufficient funding and educational opportunities. The IDCD notes that professionals around the world in the fields of speech pathology and audiology may have different titles, responsibilities, and education levels. Degrees awarded for these "titles" may vary markedly with little equivalency from one country to the next. In some cases, education may be a single course rather than a broad-based curriculum as it is in the United States and other first world nations. Consequently, services delivered by under-prepared speech and hearing professionals are affected as well. Limited education for pediatric audiologists and speech-language pathologists in countries where the fields are new or nonexistent results in service provision that is often relegated to family members, volunteers or those from a different discipline (Ndigirwa, 2006; Topbas & Ozdemir, 2001). The effect this has on the overall (re)habilitation of children with disabilities can be devastating.

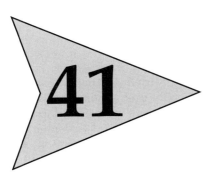

Treatment of hearing loss in some of the more underdeveloped regions of the world becomes a low priority when governments and agencies must deal with diseases such as malaria, HIV, and malnutrition. In addition, the multiplicity of languages and dialects within a household, community, or school frequently exacerbates communication difficulties. In many cases, school systems do not have an infrastructure to support children with disabilities. The social stigma attached to children with handicaps often results in their being sent out of the household at young ages to live on the streets. For children who are unable to communicate, the problems may be insurmountable. Most recently, Shafer (2008) reported an initiative undertaken by the University of Texas Callier Center to provide hearing aids and audiologic services to citizens of Mozambique. Prior to this well-intentioned program, individuals living in this country had never been fitted with hearing aids. Providing sensory devices, however, was only part of the solution to the larger problem of educating children with hearing loss. In a rather misguided step to duplicate systems in more developed countries, Mozambique decided to mainstream its deaf children without the necessary support or understanding of the language deficits from the hearing loss. Needless to say, the overall result of these efforts has been disastrous.

Central to the education of children with hearing loss is the selection of a communication approach. Two extremes of the continuum include the use of residual hearing with sensory devices to assist in developing spoken language skills at one end, and sign language with no verbal output at the other. A mixture of these and other variations of communication choices fall between the two; controversy abounds regarding which method provides the deaf/hard-of-hearing child with the greatest potential for a better quality of life. As with most circumstances, there is no one answer and no one treatment. However, technologic advances have changed the face of hearing loss around the world as more sophisticated hearing aids are developed and surgical interventions such as the cochlear implant have become treatment alternatives. In addition, governmental mandates also have contributed to identifying hearing loss in children at earlier ages.

In the United States, Canada and many countries throughout Europe, governments have begun to authorize the screening of newborns for detection of hearing loss at birth. Universal newborn hearing screening (UNHS) has provided the impetus for treating auditory deficits in the first months of life in an effort to intervene during the period when learning language is physiologically and developmentally more efficient. Initiatives to identify and provide intervention to infants and toddlers have been a direct result of studies on cost/benefit ratio analyses that look at the lifetime costs of educating children with hearing loss (Cheng et al., 2000; Easterbrooks, O'Rourke, & Todd, 2000; Francis, Koch, Wyatt, & Niparko, 1999; Mohr et al., 2000) The majority of recent studies have investigated the savings afforded by mainstreaming children, especially those with cochlear implants.

Thus, changes in both the technologic and political climate of the 21st century have set the stage for early identification and treatment of hearing loss for greater numbers of children around the globe. It is against this backdrop that educational considerations for children with any degree of hearing loss must be viewed with the expectation for improved outcomes that reflect contemporary and future possibilities. Today, it is by parental choice or limited programming options that a child, whose sole challenge is peripheral hearing loss, uses manual communication through sign language. Auditory access provided by any one of a number of sensory devices unleashes the potential for spoken language learning through the natural auditory channel. The pendulum of communication methodology is once again swinging toward auditory and oral education, today, more commonly referred to as a listening and spoken language option. In many cases, it is the pediatric audiologist who serves as a portal through which children identified with hearing loss access the intervention system. This professional requires knowledge of the law, evidenced-based practices and communication choices. The influence of the pediatric audiologist cannot be overstated as the need for positive exchanges with the child's parents at the time of diagnosis is crucial for timely follow up. The pediatric audiologist is the professional with the most knowledge regarding the level of hearing loss and the sensory device best suited to achieve communication goals set by the parents. As the degree of hearing loss increases, the complexity of the decision-making process for communication choice and educational options increases commensurately. Offering cautious optimism for the potential of spoken language outcomes through utilization of available technology gives hearing parents a sense of hope at an extraordinarily difficult time. Surprisingly, residual effects from the Deaf President Now movement in 1988, and a long-standing association of deafness and sign language in the media may lead parents to believe that there is only one option for communication. Colleges and universities associated with residential schools for deaf children who prepare teachers have supported the proliferation of early intervention and preschool programs that promote visual communication systems over listening and spoken language.

It is unfortunate to note that there appears to be a correlation between socioeconomic status (SES) and communication competence; children from homes (and countries) with a higher SES tend to have greater access to listening and spoken language educational options than do their less affluent peers (Geers & Brenner, 2003; Hoff & Tian, 2005; Hyde & Power, 2006; Sorkin & Zwolan, 2008). As indicated previously, economic well-being of a country will affect the manner in which children with hearing loss are treated. Distressingly, Swanepoel (2008) reported that almost 90% of infants born with hearing loss live in developing countries where early identification or intervention is virtually nonexistent. The high prevalence of childhood hearing loss in tandem with both the lack of early indicators of impairment and a low priority for non-life-threatening conditions has created what he has called a "silent epidemic." The enviable position of advocating for one communication option over another pales in light of a global look at hearing loss. Nevertheless, much research in industrialized countries cites parental involvement as a critical component of language outcomes for children with hearing loss (Calderon, 2000; Moeller, 2000; Spencer, 2004). One might conclude that access to professionals knowledgable and skilled in developing listening and spoken language has been reserved for the economically advantaged. The correlate of this observation is that children from poorer backgrounds have limited options. Auditory access should be a basic right of every child with hearing loss. It is only with technology and education provided by expert professionals that the effects of childhood hearing loss can be ameliorated and allow a child the opportunity to develop spoken communication skills that contribute to a productive adult life. The pediatric audiologist is often the gatekeeper to this process.

Whether counseling parents of newly diagnosed infants or toddlers or working with school-aged children, the pediatric audiologist is considered the foremost professional charged with assessing and monitoring the auditory abilities of a child with hearing loss. This individual is the most knowledgable concerning issues of amplification and classroom acoustics and is a major source of information for the collaborative teams of which they will be a part. It also is critical for the educational audiologist to be articulate about the educational options that are available to children with hearing from which parents can choose.

Educational Placement Options for Children With Hearing Loss

Each placement option has certain features that might make it more or less attractive and suitable for any individual child. Unfortunately, population density and geographic locale may preclude the possibility that parents will have access to a continuum of options from which to select. Furthermore, family goals for the child with hearing loss, as well as whole family priorities, create a filter that may constrain the field of appropriate options. Although not all placements fit neatly into one of the following categories, the basic descriptions may provide a starting point from which to consider the child-program match that is best for any family. It is not unlikely that a child will attend a number of different program types throughout an educational career as the child's instructional needs change over time.

General Education/Mainstream Placement

The largest number of children with hearing loss will be educated in the general education environment. Degree of hearing loss seems to be the key aspect of the profile of a child with hearing loss in general educational settings. Simply stated, the lesser the degree of hearing loss, the more likely it is that a child will fare well in general education programs. As the degree of educationally significant hearing loss increases, so does the importance of the placement decision. Children with the cognitive, academic, and linguistic capacity to learn alongside their typically developing peers can attend school in their local neighborhoods. In its truest sense, mainstream education should be reserved for children with sufficient skills to directly learn in this environment through the instruction of a classroom teacher. In-class accommodations, such as FM systems, CART (Communication Access Realtime Translation) or C-Print (speech-to-text system developed at the National Technical Institute for the Deaf), may be required to assure access, but once access is provided, the child in the mainstream is expected to "keep pace." Supported as needed, by an audiologic manager, a speech-language pathologist and oftentimes a teacher of deaf children, mainstreamed children are academically and socially integrated in a public or private general education school. In many circumstances, children in the mainstream are "singletons" and may represent the first child with educationally significant hearing loss enrolled in a particular school program.

General Education/Inclusion

The term inclusion is often used synonymously with mainstream education; however, here it represents a different classroom configuration and a different staffing model from that of the mainstream. For the most part, children in included classrooms have good linguistic and academic potential, but benefit from instruction that is co-delivered by a general education teacher and a certified teacher of children who are deaf/hard of hearing. Oftentimes, inclusion is manifested by a small group of children with hearing loss clustered within a general education classroom (that is reduced in class size overall to provide accommodations for instructional needs of the children with hearing loss). The unique staffing of two teachers in a single classroom allows children with hearing loss the best of both worlds: grade-level academic content with the instructional vigilance of the teacher of children with hearing loss. When well executed, inclusion models create instructional teams that have equal status in the classroom, while at the same time assigning equal status to all students regardless of hearing acuity. There are a number of co-teaching models that have been used successfully in inclusion classrooms; administrative support and teams that are well suited for collaboration are essential. Often, this model can be found in densely populated urban areas where there is a critical mass of children with hearing loss such that this is one option on the continuum of service delivery models. Alarmingly, the term inclusion is often overextended and is used when a child with hearing loss is placed, regardless of educational ability, in a class of typically developing children.

Regional Cooperatives/Urban Programs

Metropolitan areas with a large number of children with hearing loss can often support a "program" for children that may have many classrooms, different communication tracks, and instruction across the age span. Similarly, suburban counties or intermediate unit/districts form cooperatives to pool resources to better serve children with all special needs, including hearing loss. Small instruction or self-contained classrooms may be more numerous at the younger ages as children with hearing loss receive the language foundation that may allow them to move on to other instructional environments with their typically-developing peers. Often, regional/urban programs provide opportunities for social mainstreaming. Although content instruction takes place in classrooms with other children with hearing loss, activities such as physical education, art, and music, as well as lunch and recess are scheduled so that all children participate. Partial academic mainstreaming may be offered, subject by subject, as a child's individual achievement may warrant. It generally is the case that programs within this designation have the critical mass (and the administrative vision) to provide a full continuum of placement options.

Private (OPTION) Schools for Children With Hearing Loss

There is a long-standing history of private schools as a placement choice for students with hearing loss that offer listening and spoken language instruction (previously referred to as auditory/oral). Ever increasing auditory access has created recent demand for more of this instructional emphasis, and in a number of major cities, new private school programs have been developed to meet this need. Often considered model programs, many OPTION schools (http://www.auditoryschools.org) specialize in meeting the needs of the preschool to primary aged student with hearing loss and often employ "reverse mainstreaming" in which children with typical hearing are invited to enroll and participate in their language-rich instruction. Early intervention services may also be part of the comprehensive services that these programs offer.

State Schools for Deaf Children

Although not every state in the United States has a school designated as a state school for the deaf (and a few have more than one state school), these campuses and the staff and community that surround them have become centers for the majority of individuals who identify with Deaf Culture. These schools' longstanding presence in the state bureaucracy has made them a natural place to turn for the management of early intervention in many states. However, strong ties to the community of deaf individuals may make it difficult, if not impossible, for professionals to offer parents a realistic world view that reflects a hearing culture. Respect for and a desire to provide auditory access through hearing aids and cochlear implants may not be a priority at some state schools for the deaf. At other state schools, however, sweeping legal and technological changes in the last 30 plus years have created the dissonance that has resulted in a more egalitarian approach to the audiologic management of hearing loss in young children of both deaf and hearing parents.

Regardless of the particular educational environment in which an educational audiologist might function, there are clear roles for this professional, which include aspects of *assessment*, *(re)habilitation*, and *advocacy*. *Counseling* is an integral part of each of these and is infused within the pediatric audiologist's responsibilities. The relative weight of each of these components will change over time as the child moves through early intervention and the educational system.

Early Intervention

In order for children to reach their fullest potential, early detection and intervention are key. In the United States, a federal program (Individuals with Disabilities Education Act [IDEA]) stipulates that parents be informed of and offered choices about communication methods, and that they have a voice as full members of the team that writes the Individualized Family Service Plan (IFSP). Part C of IDEA governs early intervention services for infants and toddlers with disabilitiesunder the age of age 3 years. It is an unfortunate reality that the path of a deaf or hard-of-hearing child's entry into the Part C, birth-to-3, educational system, is often controlled by the least specialized and underprepared professional in the chain of referral: the service coordinator. In order to assist the service coordinator, the pediatric audiologist should be knowledgable of the vast store of information that exists for early hearing detection and intervention services. The most comprehensive resource is the National Center for Hearing Assessment and Management NCHAM (http://www.infanthearing.org). Although developed as an unbiased organization, the NCHAM Web site provides links to agencies and materials that support aggressive auditory management of young children with hearing loss. Keeping in mind that parental choice drives service delivery, recommending resources that are user-friendly to parents who have chosen a listening and spoken language option may assist them in securing the necessary services to launch communication competence. Since the pediatric audiologist is the lead professional that parents encounter when the hearing loss is confirmed, it is critical for this professional to have knowledge of the resources available to assist parents in making subsequent decisions.

If parents are relying on audiologic input to make decisions about communication choices (i.e., should sign language be introduced, should a cochlear implant be considered, should the hearing aid be changed?), then hearing data cannot exist in a vacuum that only measures performance under carefully controlled conditions. It is vital that the pediatric audiologist collaborate with other key professionals to provide the context in which services are linked to the parents' desired outcome for their child. Collaboration encompasses communication, coordination, and cooperation and is more than any one of these entities.

Communication is not synonymous with report dissemination. This relegates communication to a product-oriented outcome. True communication requires interaction between and among the parties of interest. When parents become the messengers and are demoted to the role of distributing reports among agencies, the result is often a disjointed collection of information with no substantive integration. For communication to be truly effective, there must be coordination that facilitates the communicative *exchange* in response to agency reports.

Coordinating appointments, activities, and outcomes is a role that is assigned to the various health and education professionals providing services to the child with hearing loss. Although every professional has an individual role, coordination requires that *one* individual bear the responsibility of managing the information that is being generated across disciplines. The coordination of this effort requires cooperation among professionals to ensure that all relevant data are considered, thus encouraging the best possible outcome.

The nature of a collaborative relationship is dependent upon a cooperative spirit among professionals. It must be respectful and have as its goal a genuine concern for the child without bias or prejudice for one particular outcome; it allows for individual expertise to be considered fully within the context of mutual esteem. Thus, communication, coordination, and cooperation represent the foundation of a true collaborative effort.

Collaboration can be interdisciplinary and intradisciplinary in nature. Interdisciplinary collaboration occurs between and among professionals who may *not share* a common professional education, value system, identity, or experience. Conversely, intradisciplinary collaboration occurs among colleagues who *do share* common experiences (Streeter, 1999). When previous experiences with collaboration have been positive, it is more likely that there will be expectations for a positive outcome; unfortunately, the reverse is often true. Negative experiences with collaborative groups may color the outcomes of future efforts. Furthermore, if collaboration is imposed by administration and not viewed as a best practice approach to service delivery, the quality of the interactions may be compromised. In order to be a productive member of a collaborative group, one must project a sincere belief in the value of the professional expertise of the other members of the group. There should be no sense of competition among service providers; the needs of the child transcend each individual's area of expertise. It is the collective construction of a comprehensive plan to meet the child's needs that becomes the desired outcome of this effort. Clear and unambiguous communication about the implications of hearing loss and its effect on the development of spoken language is imperative to this process that starts at the pediatric audiologist's point of intersection with other professionals: the initial evaluation.

Assessment

Pediatric audiologists evaluate children for many purposes: initial diagnosis, sensory device fitting, or monitoring progress with auditory skill development. The initial identification of hearing loss may occur as a result of the referral process of universal newborn hearing screening, physician recommendation or parental concern. The diagnosis is often a culmination of data gathered over multiple visits. A comprehensive battery of tests provides a cohesive picture of the status of the auditory system. It is at this point that the pediatric audiologist as counselor is most critical. As parents learn the news of their child's hearing loss, there is often a tendency for them to pass through the various stages of grief that have been documented in the psychological literature. These stages take into account denial, anger, bargaining, depression, and acceptance (Kubler-Ross, 1969). Professionals must respect parents' actions during this challenging time. Although there is an urgency to begin habilitation through the dispensing of a sensory aid, some parents may disengage from the process as a mechanism for coping and appear to be noncompliant.

For pediatric audiologists, there is a need to offer both information and support at this time. Most pediatric audiologists are trained to provide informational counseling concerning the degree, type, and severity of hearing loss along with the sensory aid recommendation for ameliorating the loss. However, parents are often in the early stages of grief when a large amount of this information is being imparted. For this reason, a great deal of the subject matter is poorly received and often misunderstood. Research indicates that patients forget 40 to 80% of the information provided at any medical appointment (Kessels, 2003). Half of the information that is remembered is incorrect. Furthermore, pediatric audiologists who address only the informational aspects of hearing loss and not the emotional effects of that information will not engender the important relationship necessary to move parents past the initial stage of grief. As parents enter subsequent stages they may "shop around" to identify another professional who will provide a diagnosis they find more acceptable or one who will be more sensitive to the family's needs. Seeking second and third opinions often causes delays in the ultimate fitting of amplification and in accessing early intervention services. Professionals walk a fine line in providing necessary support as parents adjust to the diagnosis, yet encouraging intervention in a timely manner. Families who have been given the news that they have a child with a disability must first learn to make room in their life for the disability but not make the disability their life. This concept is not one that can be grasped in a single session, and as assessment progresses it requires continual attention.

The assessment process that begins in early intervention persists throughout childhood to monitor changes that may occur in functional auditory capacity. The introduction of new technologies may be required to remediate hearing loss that changes over time. Assessment should be viewed as an activity that is dynamic and is constructed to ensure the best outcome for the child. Parents who embrace this concept will contribute to their child's progress; parents who withdraw will increase the likelihood that additional roadblocks might impede positive growth. Assessment is seen as a shared responsibility of the pediatric audiologist, the family, and the early intervention system. Once habilitation is initiated, the early intervention period creates a productive intermingling of evaluation, response, and reevaluation.

Habilitation

If assessment answers the question "What is the level of hearing loss?" then habilitation must answer the question, "How can the hearing loss be treated in the most effective manner?" The habilitation process begins with the selection of the proper sensory device/s (see Chapters 25–29) coupled with appropriate intervention. Monitoring performance with hearing aids or cochlear implants is necessary to ensure development of age-appropriate auditory, speech and language skills. It is incumbent on the pediatric audiologist to stay current with technology that can affect the outcomes of the early intervention plan.

A primary factor in determining the appropriateness of a prescribed sensory aid is to benchmark performance against other children with hearing loss of the same magnitude. The pediatric audiologist cannot merely check the sensory device for proper function but must evaluate it relative to the child's outcomes in the areas of spoken language, auditory perception, and educational progress. The view from the sound-treated audiometric test suite should not be simply one of measuring functional gain or even word recognition scores but rather an all encompassing measurement of child performance in light of the age at identification, duration of sensory aid use, and philosophical approach to communication. In order to make a truly informed decision about the successful use of the selected sensory device, mode of communication, or educational environment, the pediatric audiologist should gather information from a variety of sources to consider the role audition is playing in the child's overall development. Anything less would be ineffective.

It is never more critical to be part of a transdisciplinary collaborative team than in evaluating the effectiveness of the sensory device and the habilitation plan during the EI period. There has been long-standing association between pediatric audiologists, and speech-language pathologists. Communication with teachers of deaf children is customary, but the early intervention system has created an even wider circle of professional colleagues with whom the pediatric audiologist must interact. With a mandate for considering all the child's needs during the period of greatest development, the pediatric audiologist is challenged to make the implications of hearing loss clear to nonspeech and hearing professionals as they deliver services within their scope of practice.

Thus the role of the pediatric audiologist does not begin and end with the fitting of a sensory device. The overall benefits of amplification and its contribution to the development of spoken language skills must be monitored. In addition, this professional should, in fact, provide oversight of the use of amplification, the amount and type of services and the venue in which these services are available.

The hallmark of the EI period is the provision of family-centered services in the natural environment. To date, this generally has been interpreted as home-based interventions in which parents are counseled and guided in learning to facilitate their child's language development. Currently, studies are underway to investigate the efficacy of non-home-based or center-based services for young children with hearing loss (Tharpe, 2008). Evidence-based research that informs the pediatric audiologist regarding service delivery models and their outcomes allows for better advocacy during the EI process.

Advocacy

Advocacy can take many forms. It can include negotiating for services, ensuring device function or educating others about the implications of hearing loss in daily living. There are components of advocacy that are legal while others are personal. Those that are legal require parents to be knowledgable about rights and privileges within their local education communities. As most parents have no legal background or knowledge of special education law, becoming an advocate may seem overwhelming. This task is compounded by the fact that parents may still be struggling with the diagnosis of hearing loss. There are multiple resources that parents can access both locally and nationally, through advocacy organizations, to assist them in the process.

Personal advocacy issues focus on the day-to-day usage of the sensory device in conjunction with the development of an identity as an individual with hearing loss. Self-awareness of auditory access should be targeted as an early intervention goal. Even young children can learn personal advocacy skills by informing teachers or interventionists when there are problems with their sensory aids. By developing responsibility at a young age, the early intervention professional is supporting the acquisition of the more complex advocacy skills that will be required in the future.

The pediatric audiologist may assume the role of chief advocate for the child and family during the birth-to-three period. For computer savvy and Internet secure families, this may not be necessary as the Internet can provide a wealth of information and resources to assist in the development of advocacy skills. For families with less computer access or those who live in remote areas, learning about hearing loss and its implications for education may require more time. Modeling the types of questions that should be addressed during the Individual Family Service Plan (IFSP) process may be one method of assisting parents in the development of advocacy skills. Part of the pediatric audiologist's role is to transition the parent to become the key individual advocating for the child. Regardless of who performs advocacy activities during the early intervention period, plans should be initiated for transferring this role to the child over time.

Preschool and School-Aged Children

While hearing loss is identified early for many children, there remain a number of youngsters for whom identification is delayed until academic pressures raise questions about hearing acuity. In addition, there are other children who are born with normal hearing, which later diminishes over time. Regardless of when diagnosis occurs, audiologic management within the educational system is required to ensure that a child has every advantage to access curriculum. Generally, a pediatric audiologist who works solely within a school district is known as an educational audiologist. Educational audiologists are certified and licensed individuals who identify their primary place of employment as a local school or educational agency. The Educational Audiology Association is an international organization of pediatric audiologists and related professionals who deliver hearing services to children in educational settings. Their Web site (http://www.edaud.org) has numerous publications and position statements to assist professionals working in schools.

Emphasis on audiologic services for children with confirmed hearing loss does not negate the need for additional programs that focus on identification of auditory processing problems and the promotion of hearing conservation education. The responsibilities of an education audiologist also can be captured in assessment, (re)habilitation and advocacy.

Assessment

The primary role of the educational audiologist is to monitor those children within the school district who have already been identified with hearing loss so that changes in performance are documented over time. The educational audiologist will also screen typically developing children based on local mandates or referrals by teachers. Children with normal hearing acuity but poor auditory perception may be evaluated for auditory processing disorders by the educational audiologist to determine whether additional referral or technology is required.

In addition to assessing individual children, it is also the responsibility of the educational audiologist to assess the acoustic environment of learning spaces within the school. Evaluation of classroom ambient noise and reverberation and identification of strategies to reduce noise are within the purview of the educational audiologist. Measuring the functionality of any sensory device and/or personal or classroom FM system should also be part of the educational audiologist's scope of practice. (For more detailed information on Classroom Acoustics and FM systems, see Chapter 26 in this volume). The educational audiologist can assess a child's listening capabilities within any learning space through a number of questionnaires as rated by the classroom teacher or other professionals. These instruments include the Functional Listening Evaluation (FLE; Johnson & VonAlmen, 1997), Screening Identification for Targeting Educational Risk (SIFTER; Anderson, 2004), Listening Inventories for Education (LIFE; Anderson & Smaldino, 1999), Early Listening Function (ELF; Anderson, 2002), and Children's Home Inventory for Listening Difficulty (CHILD; Anderson & Smaldino, 2000).

(Re)habilitation

Stated job responsibilities or personal preference may determine whether or not the EA takes an active role in providing (re)habilitation services to children with hearing loss. This is well within recognized scope of practice but often is dependent on the needs of an individual school district. The educational audiologist's primary (re)habilitative responsibility is to participate in a collaborative team to ensure that the child is receiving the most appropriate services.

The educational audiologist collaborates with a teacher of deaf children and/or speech-language pathologist in a partnership to emphasize the interrelationships of hearing acuity, auditory skill development, spoken language acquisition, and academic success. Within this collaborative team, the educational audiologist communicates the potential and limitations of a child's sensory device while the teacher and speech-language pathologist share information regarding the child's language and academic development. The complex relationship between listening and language is explored through the dialogue that occurs during these professional exchanges. As audiology is the platform on which subsequent skills are developed, no discussion of a child's performance can take place without an audiologist to contextualize it as a function of access to sound. When access is the issue, the pediatric audiologist assumes responsibility to explore the appropriate options so that learning can commence. When access issues have been ruled out, attention should be placed on provision of services. Specifically, professionals providing services and the quality of those services should be examined. Finally, once access and service provision have been verified, the team can turn its attention to the possibility that learning challenges are limiting performance.

Even when children in the mainstream are operating at their "personal best" in listening, spoken language and academics, there continue to be linguistic issues that may not be obvious to a general education teacher. The acquisition of Tier Two vocabulary (Beck, McKeown, & Kucan, 2002), which is a challenge that many children face, is even more pronounced in children with hearing loss as acoustic access is not precise. With deficits in vocabulary, reading comprehension at increasingly more complex levels is at risk. The educational audiologist must be knowledgable of the potential hurdles that obstruct a child's continued success by raising awareness of vocabulary development issues with the classroom teacher. Similarly, difficulty in understanding colloquial or figurative language may preclude a child from being able to understand narratives written with a rich use of idiomatic language. These linguistic "hazards" are not always associated with children who have hearing loss and may be equally problematic for the child with auditory processing problems.

Children with learning issues related to auditory processing require the attention of the educational audiologist to make available and monitor technology that enhances signal reception. It is not enough to simply provide technology; the educational audiologist must educate school personnel in its proper use and maintenance. Finally, the educational audiologist is also responsible for hearing conservation education. With the growing number of young children using MP3 players, there is increasing concern regarding the potential for noise-induced hearing loss at earlier ages (Vogel, Brug, Hosli, van der Ploeq, & Raat, 2008).

Advocacy

During the school-aged period, the child requiring audiologic services should begin to assume the responsibilities for self-advocacy. Clearly, younger children will be limited in this task by their cognitive and linguistic abilities. It should not be presumed, however, that children are unable to have their auditory needs and wants met. As they grow physically, linguistically, and emotionally, children may be ready to assume more responsibility for management of both their sensory aids and acoustic environment. It is likely that these skills will not develop without coaching. Conscious and intentional instruction in self advocacy should be a part of children's Individualized Educational Programs (IEPs).

A self-advocacy curriculum often includes components of identity, self image, technology, legal rights and community resources for children with hearing loss. These should be guided by professionals with expertise in each of these areas and engage parents and children in the process. Discussions regarding identity and self-image might emphasize how hearing loss affects relationships. Strategies that teach children how to negotiate communication outside the academic setting likely will assist them into their teenage years.

Adolescents and Young Adults

Generally speaking, the child who enters high school will often emerge as a very different young adult. Each child's journey is individual and will be influenced by personality, learning style, talents, and motivation. Fitting in with peers is sometimes a function of the use of colloquial expressions, slang and, in some cases, even sarcasm. Children with hearing loss may have more challenges in this area as the subtleties of the language get "lost." The use of technologies that provide the child with auditory access may be the very reason that the child feels disconnected. Strategic counseling by the educational audiologist may help the child to accept the tradeoff between auditory access and peer pressure to conform.

Assessment

Adolescents often will bring years of sensory device use and therapy experience with them to the high school. The role of the educational audiologist is to ensure that technology is the most advanced and appropriate for the student. In addition, the educational audiologist should guide the selection of other electronics that interface with listening devices to ensure proper use. Like the majority of their peers, teens with hearing loss wish to utilize wireless telephones that are internet accessible and also act as a source of entertainment. The educational audiologist can guide students to the best technology that will yield the greatest advantage given the constraints of any particular hearing loss.

The various assistive technologies that are available for independent living should be reviewed at this juncture. As teenagers begin to consider life outside the cocoon of the home environment, it is important for them to be able to respond to the myriad sounds that are used for signaling or alerting. Exploring the wide range of devices that are available to support independence is an important part of the role of the EA in the high school years.

(Re)habilitation

It is not unexpected that during the adolescent years, students will reject previously prescribed technology that sets them apart from their age-mates. Research indicates that the largest number of nonusers of hearing aids, cochlear implants and FM systems is in the adolescent population (Tyler et al., 1997). In order to circumvent limited use, a good relationship with the educational audiologist and other educational team members is necessary. Contrasting performance outcomes with and without sensory aids is often a mechanism for demonstrating benefit for this age group. In addition, the use of contracts to shape behavior has been successfully implemented by professionals who work with the adolescent population.

Traditional one-on-one therapy paradigms should not be the only service offered to this age group. Self-study that is accessible at any hour of the day may better fit the adolescents' learning and life style. With more information available through the Internet, students with hearing loss can now access listening exercises that are online and available 24 hours per day. Many sites designed for English as Second Language (ESL) users provide excellent resources that can be accessed for guided practice at home. Music videos can also serve as "therapy material" that engages the adolescent in a manner that can enhance listening and speaking. Pragmatics and functional communication in group settings with peers may be emphasized at this age rather than specific listening targets or speech production.

Functional communication takes place in listening environments that are often degraded by competing noise. For the student with hearing loss, strategies to reduce the effects of background noise rely heavily on speech-reading. The use of Continuous Discourse Tracking (CDT; DeFilippo & Scott, 1978) encourages the development of speechreading skills and diminishes the deleterious effects of communicating in less than optimal listening conditions.

(Re)habilitation strategies for the adolescent include functional practice and continued counseling. A broader view of the lifelong implications of hearing loss and acceptance of the strengths and limitations that it brings to the student is required. This creates a seamless transition from rehabilitation to self-awareness and self-advocacy.

Advocacy

The current information-driven society has made advocacy more important than ever before. New technology has made communication easier; new technology has made it more difficult. The adolescent or young adult with hearing loss can now exchange information more easily with the advent of text messaging on a local or global scale. Texting has removed the isolation of the individual with hearing loss but has simultaneously placed communication skills on display to a larger audience. Social networking through sites such as Facebook, Twitter, and My Space provide opportunities for individuals to exchange information in a forum that is not face-to-face. However, such forums can create a false sense of communicative competence. In the virtual world, communication is only limited by the ability to create comprehensible text messages. In the nonvirtual world, communication challenges are real: background noise, insufficient lighting, and poor acoustics. Once individuals with hearing loss step into the real world, they must advocate for support systems to allow equal access. These might include closed-captioning, infrared technology in theatres, and accommodations in travel and public buildings. At no time is this more important than for the student with hearing loss entering college.

The technology of the cochlear implant has enabled children to attend regular district schools and progress through the educational system to enter colleges alongside their hearing age-mates. In the past, most students with severe hearing loss attended colleges specifically designed for deaf students. Services were provided without question; there was no need for the student to practice advocacy skills. Today, public and private institutions of higher education are now among the choices available to students with hearing loss with sufficient skills to compete for admission. It is imperative that students know their legal rights and the systems that must be in place to accommodate their needs. Once in college, student success will be dependent on a variety of factors one of which is student engagement.

Data from the U.S. National Survey of Student Engagement indicate that students who are engaged in curricular and/or extracurricular activities are more likely to be successful and graduate within four years of entertaining college (Wasley, 2006). When a student is fully integrated both in and out of class, there is a greater need for self advocacy skills that transcend the academic environment. Some students find the advocacy role more challenging due to limited opportunities in their youth. Parents who diligently assumed the role of advocate without training their children for a future as independent students were unwittingly shortsighted. Although the "helicopter parent" is a familiar sociological phenomenon for many millennial children, the overall effect often is counterproductive for the student who is striving for independence. An autonomous student is one who presents with the typical skills of registering for classes, paying bills, and managing a class schedule. In addition, the student with hearing loss also must secure services that will support learning. The audiologist may be part of the transition team that provides information to the student and parent to help prepare for the postsecondary culture.

Similarly, students who enter directly into the workforce should ensure that the work environment is conducive to communicative success. As transition plans are developed within the educational setting, consideration of the acoustics of the workplace and the assistive technology that can aid the individual in the proper performance of work responsibilities may be offered by the educational audiologist. Whether in the workplace or the college setting, the greatest obstacle to success occurs when the individual fails to self identify. Recognizing hearing loss as part of the fabric that makes each individual unique, removes its stigma and strengthens the personal adjustment that opens the door to lifelong success.

Summary

Never has it been a more exciting time to be a pediatric audiologist than today. The role of this professional spans the educational lifetime of children with hearing loss. From assessment to advocacy, the educational audiologist can play a vital role in ameliorating the effects of hearing loss be it unilateral, minimal, or profound. Efforts in industrialized countries to train and produce the best audiologists may have far-reaching effects to countries that are less fortunate. The ultimate goal, whether it is in a small village in Mozambique or a large metropolitan center in New York is to create circumstances that will allow children with hearing loss to reach their personal best, whatever that may be. The children of today are the leaders of tomorrow; it should not matter whether they present with or without a hearing loss. The world awaits them.

References

Anderson, K. (2002). Early Listening Function (ELF). Parent involvement: The magic ingredient in successful child outcomes: Improving parent participation using the ELF and the CHILD. *Hearing Review*, *9*(11), 24–27, 56.

Anderson, K. (2004). *Secondary Screening Instrument for Targeting Educational Risk (SIFTER)*. Retrieved November 24, 2009, from http://www.hear2learn.com

Anderson, K., & Smaldino, J. (1999) Listening inventories for education: A classroom measurement tool. *Hearing Journal*, *52*(10), 74–76.

Anderson, K., & Smaldino, J. (2000). Children's Home Inventory of Listening Difficulties (CHILD). *Educational Audiology Review*, *17*, 3.

Beck, I. L., McKeown, M. G., & Kucan, L. (2002). *Bringing words to life*. New York, NY: Guilford Press.

Bliele, K. M., Ireland, L., & Kiel, T. (2006). The professions around the world: New Web-based directory goes global. *Asha Leader*, *11*(17), 8–9, 26–27.

Calderon, R. (2000). Parental involvement in deaf children's education programs as a predictor of child's language, early reading, and social-emotional development. *Journal of Deaf Studies and Deaf Education*, *5*(2), 140–155.

Cheng, A. K., Rubin, H. R., Powe, N. R., Mellon, N. K., Francis, H. W., & Niparko, J. K. (2000). Cost-utility analysis of the cochlear implant in children. *Journal of the American Medical Association*, *284*(7), 850–856.

DeFilipo, C., & Scott, B. (1978). A method for training and evaluating the reception on ongoing speech. *Journal of the Acoustical Society of America*, *63*, 1186–1192.

Easterbrooks, S. R., O'Rourke, C. M., & Todd, N. W. (2000). Child and family factors associated with deaf children's success in auditory-verbal therapy. *Otology and Neurotology*, *21*(3), 341–344.

Francis, H. W., Koch, M. E., Wyatt, J. R., & Niparko, J. K. (1999). Trends in educational placement and cost-benefit considerations in children with cochlear implants. *Archives of Otolaryngology-Head & Neck Surgery*, *125*(5), 499–505.

Geers, A., & Brenner, C. (2003). Background and educational characteristics of prelingually deaf children implanted by five years of age. *Ear and Hearing*, *24*(1 Suppl.), 2S–14S.

Hoff, E., & Tian, C. (2005). Socioeconomic status and cultural influences on language. *Journal of Communication Disorders*, *38*(4), 271–278.

Hyde, M., & Power, D. (2006). Some ethical dimensions of cochlear implantation for deaf children and their families. *Journal of Deaf Studies and Deaf Education*, *11*(1), 102–111.

Johnson, C. D., & Von Almen, P. (1997). The functional listening evaluation. In C. D. Johnson, P. V. Benson, & J. B. Seaton (1997), *Educational audiology handbook* (pp. 336–339). San Diego, CA: Singular.

Kessels, R. (2003). Patient's memory for medical information. *Journal of the Royal Society of Medicine*, *96*(5), 219–222.

Kotby, M. N. (2006). Egypt: Four decades of voice research. *Asha Leader*, *11*(7), 30–32.

Kubler-Ross, E. (1969). *On death and dying*. New York, NY: MacMillan.

McLeod, S., & Bleile, K. (2007). Speech acquisition: A framework. In S. McLeod (Ed.), *The international perspective on speech acquisition*. New York, NY: Thomson Delmar.

Moeller, M. P. (2000). Early intervention and language development in children who are deaf and hard of hearing. *Pediatrics*, *106*, 43.

Mohr, P. E., Feldman, J. J., Dunbar, J. L., McConkey-Robbins, A., Niparko, J. K., Rittenhouse, R. K., & Skinner, M. W. (2000). The societal costs of severe to profound hearing loss in the United States. *International Journal of Technology Assessment in Health Care*, *16*, 1120–1135.

Ndigirwa, P. (2006). A view from Tanzania. *International Directory of Communication Disorders.* Retrieved November, 24, 2009, from http://www.comdisinternational.com/world_views.html

Shafer, D. N. (2008). Audiology in Mozambique. *ASHA Leader, 13*(10), 28–29.

Sorkin, D. L., & Zwolan, T. A. (2008). Parental perspectives regarding early intervention and its role in cochlear implantation in children. *Otology and Neurotology, 29*(2), 137–141.

Spencer, P. E. (2004, Fall). Individual differences in language performance after cochlear implantation at one to three years of age: Child, family, and linguistic factors. *Journal of Deaf Studies and Deaf Education, 9*(4), 395–412.

Streeter, C. J. (1999). *Strategic partnership through collaborative leadership* (Class Notes SW 393T19). Retrieved July 20, 2007, from: http://citeseerx.ist.psu.edu/viewdoc/download?doi=10.1.1.109.3066&rep=rep1&type=pdf

Swanepoel, D. (2008). Infant hearing loss in developing countries: A silent priority. *Audiology Today, 20*(3), 16–24.

Tharpe, A. M. (2008). *A comparison of home- and center-based intervention settings for infants and toddlers with hearing loss.* Paper presented at the Early Hearing Detection & Intervention Conference. New Orleans, LA.

Topbas, S., & Özdemir, S. (2001, July). An emerging profession in Turkey: Speech and language therapy. *Abstract Proceedings of International Special Education Congress.* Antalya, Turkey.

Tyler, R. S., Fryauf-Bertschy, H., Kelsay, D. M., Gantz, B. J., Woodworth, G. P., & Parkinson, A. (1997). *Archives of Otolaryngology-Head and Neck Surgery, 117*(3 Pt. 1), 180–187.

Vogel, I., Burg, J., Hosli, E. J., van der Ploeq, C. P., & Raat, H. (2008). MP3 players and hearing loss: Adolescents' perceptions of loud music and hearing conservation. *Journal of Pediatrics, 152*(3) 400–404.

Wasley, P. (2006). Underrepresented students benefit most from 'engagement'. *Chronicle of Higher Education, 53*(13), A39–A40. Retrieved November 30, 2009, from Education Module (Document ID: 1191531481).

World Bank Group. (2005). *Global monitoring report—Millennium development goals: From consensus to momentum (English).* Retrieved November 24, 2009, from http://go.worldbank.org/EKZ6C0NN60.

Index

A

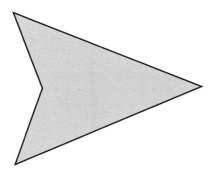

B

C

D

E

G

H

I

J

K

L

M

N

O

P

Q

R

S

T

U

V